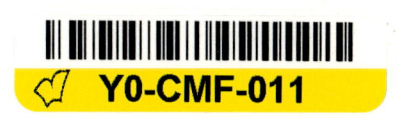

Dedicated to the memory of
Richard Nickel

Richard Nickel (1905–1964), Dr. med. vet. habil., Dipl.-Landwirt,
Professor of Veterinary Anatomy, Histology and Embryology at Hanover 1948–1964

MSU LIBRARIES
JUL 1 1 2018

RETURNING MATERIALS:
Place in book drop to remove this checkout from your record. FINES will be charged if book is returned after the date stamped below.

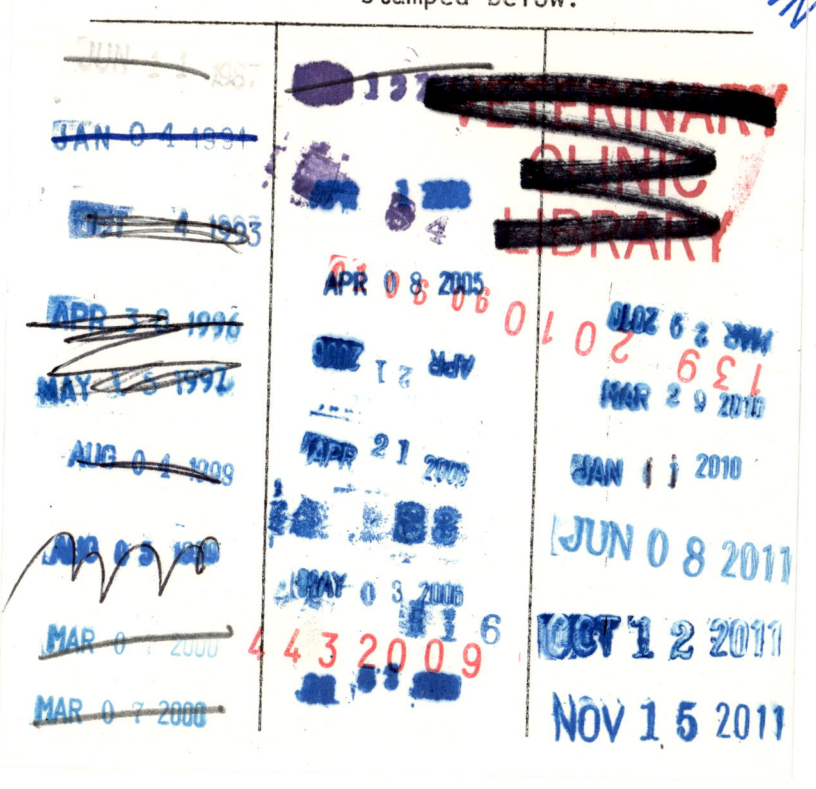

MICHIGAN STATE UNIVERSITY LIBRARY
JUL 24 2025
WITHDRAWN

R. Nickel, A. Schummer, E. Seiferle
The Anatomy of the Domestic Animals
Volume 3

The Circulatory System, the Skin,
and the Cutaneous Organs
of the Domestic Mammals

The Anatomy of the Domestic Animals

founded by Richard Nickel, August Schummer, and Eugen Seiferle

Volume 1: The Locomotor System of the Domestic Mammals
by Richard Nickel, August Schummer, Eugen Seiferle, Josef Frewein, and Karl-H. Wille (prob. published 1983)

Volume 2: The Viscera of the Domestic Mammals
by August Schummer, Richard Nickel, and Wolfgang Otto Sack, 2nd revised Ed. 1979

Volume 3: The Circulatory System, the Skin, and the Cutaneous Organs of the Domestic Mammals
by August Schummer, Helmut Wilkens, Bernd Vollmerhaus, and Karl-H. Habermehl. Translation by Walter G. Siller and Peter A. L. Wight 1981

Volume 4: The Nervous System, the Endocrine Glands, and the Sensory Organs of the Domestic Mammals
by Eugen Seiferle (prob. published 1984)

Volume 5: Anatomy of the Domestic Birds
by August Schummer. Translation by Walter G. Siller and Peter A. L. Wight 1977

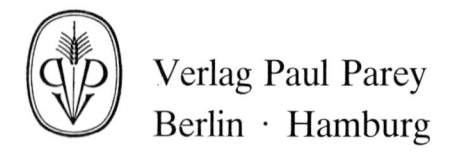

Verlag Paul Parey
Berlin · Hamburg

The Circulatory System, the Skin, and the Cutaneous Organs of the Domestic Mammals

by August Schummer, Helmut Wilkens,
Bernd Vollmerhaus, and Karl-Heinz Habermehl

Translation
by Walter G. Siller and Peter A. L. Wight

With 439 illustrations, 173 in colour

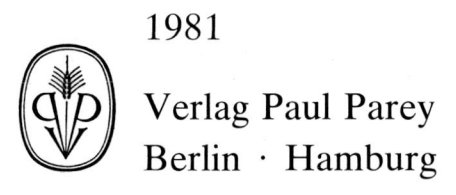

1981

Verlag Paul Parey
Berlin · Hamburg

This volume is an authorized translation of R. Nickel, A. Schummer, E. Seiferle (Ed.), *Lehrbuch der Anatomie der Haustiere (The Anatomy of the Domestic Animals)*, Volume 3: *Kreislaufsystem, Haut und Hautorgane (The Circulatory System, the Skin, and the Cutaneous Organs of the Domestic Mammals)* by A. Schummer, H. Wilkens, B. Vollmerhaus, and K.-H. Habermehl, © 1976. Verlag Paul Parey, Berlin and Hamburg, Germany.

Richard Nickel †, Dr. med. vet., Professor and Head of the Department of Anatomy, Tierärztliche Hochschule Hanover, D-3000 Hanover, Germany

August Schummer †, Dr. med. vet., Professor and Head of the Department of Veterinary Anatomy, Justus-Liebig-Universitaet Giessen, D-6300 Giessen, Germany

Eugen Seiferle, Dr. med. vet., Dr. med. vet. h. c., Professor and Head of the Department of Veterinary Anatomy, Universitaet Zurich, CH-8057 Zurich, Switzerland

Helmut Wilkens, Dr. med. vet., Professor and Head of the Department of Anatomy, Tierärztliche Hochschule Hanover, D-3000 Hanover, Germany

Bernd Vollmerhaus, Dr. med. vet., Professor and Head of the Department of Veterinary Anatomy, Ludwig-Maximilians-Universitaet Munich, D-8000 Munich, Germany

Karl-Heinz Habermehl, Dr. med. vet., Professor and Head of the Department of Veterinary Anatomy, Justus-Liebig-Universitaet Giessen, D-6300 Giessen, Germany

Walter G. Siller, Dr. med. vet., Ph. D., M.R.C.V.S., F.R.C. Path., F.R.S.E., University of Edinburgh

Peter A. L. Wight, F.R.C.V.S., Ph. D., D.V.S.M., F.R.C. Path., F.R.S.E., University of Edinburgh

Synopsis of the English edition: *The Anatomy of the Domestic Animals*
Volume 1: *Locomotor System of the Domestic Mammals.* By R. Nickel, A. Schummer, E. Seiferle, J. Frewein, and K.-H. Wille. Translation from the German. Approx. 560 pages, with about 517 illustrations in the text and on 11 colour plates. In preparation
Volume 2: *The Viscera of the Domestic Mammals.* By A. Schummer, R. Nickel, and W. O. Sack. 2nd revised edition. Translated and revised from the 4th German edition. 1979. 446 pages, with a total of 559 illustrations in the text and on 13 colour plates
Volume 3: *The Circulatory System, the Skin, and the Cutaneous Organs of the Domestic Mammals.* By A. Schummer, H. Wilkens, B. Vollmerhaus, and K.-H. Habermehl. Translated from the German by W. G. Siller and P. A. L. Wight. 1981. 630 pages, with a total of 439 illustrations, 173 in colour
Volume 4: *Nervous System, Sensory Organs, Endocrine Glands of the Domestic Mammals.* By E. Seiferle. Translation from the German. Approx. 442 pages, with a total of about 250 illustrations, about 95 in colour, in the text and on 10 colour plates. In preparation
Volume 5: *Anatomy of the Domestic Birds.* By A. Schummer. Translated from the German by W. G. Siller and P. A. L. Wight. 1977. 214 pages, with 141 illustrations in the text and on 7 colour plates

Synopsis of the German edition: *Lehrbuch der Anatomie der Haustiere*
Volume I: *Bewegungsapparat.* By R. Nickel, A. Schummer, E. Seiferle, J. Frewein, and K.-H. Wille. 4th revised edition. 1977. 560 pages, with a total of 517 illustrations in the text and on 11 colour plates
Volume II: *Eingeweide.* By A. Schummer and R. Nickel. 4th edition. 1979. 446 pages, with a total of 559 illustrations in the text and on 13 colour plates
Volume III: *Kreislaufsystem, Haut und Hautorgane.* By A. Schummer, H. Wilkens. B. Vollmerhaus, and K.-H. Habermehl. 1976. 662 pages, with a total of 439 illustrations, 172 in colour
Volume IV: *Nervensystem, Sinnesorgane, Endokrine Drüsen.* By E. Seiferle. 1975. 442 pages, with a total of 250 illustrations, 95 in colour in the text and on 10 colour plates
Volume V: *Anatomie der Hausvögel.* By A. Schummer. 1973. 215 pages, with a total of 141 illustrations in the text and on 7 colour plates

---

CIP-Kurztitelaufnahme der Deutschen Bibliothek

Nickel, Richard:
The anatomy of the domestic animals / founded by Richard Nickel, August Schummer, and Eugen Seiferle. – Berlin ; Hamburg : Parey
  Dt. Ausg. u.d.T.: Nickel, Richard: Lehrbuch der Anatomie der Haustiere. – Vol. 2 u. 5 erschienen nicht als Teil d. Gesamtwerks

NE: Schummer, August: ; Seiferle, Eugen:

Vol. 3. → The circulatory system, the skin and the cutaneous organs of the domestic mammals

The circulatory system, the skin and the cutaneous organs of the domestic mammals / by August Schummer . . . Transl. by Walter George Siller and Peter Albert Laing Wight. – Berlin ; Hamburg : Parey, 1981.
  (The anatomy of the domestic animals / founded by Richard Nickel, August Schummer, and Eugen Seiferle ; Vol. 3)
  ISBN 3-489-55618-6

NE: Schummer, August [Mitverf.]

Cover design: Christian Honig, D-5450 Neuwied/Rhein, Germany

This work is subject to copyright. All rights are reserved, whether the whole or part of the material is concerned, specifically those rights of translation, reprinting, re-use of illustrations, recitation, broadcasting, reproduction by photocopying machine or similar means, and storage in data banks. Under § 54,1 of the German Copyright Law where single copies are made for other than private use, a fee is payable to the publisher according to § 54,2 of the German Copyright Law. The amount of the fee is to be determined by agreement with the publisher.

© 1981 by Verlag Paul Parey, Berlin and Hamburg, D-1000 Berlin 61, Germany

Printed in Germany by Felgentreff & Goebel Buch- und Offsetdruckerei GmbH & Co. KG, D-1000 Berlin 61, Germany

Binding by Lüderitz & Bauer, D-1000 Berlin 61, Germany

ISBN 3-489-55618-6 Verlag Paul Parey, Berlin and Hamburg
ISBN 0-387-91193-6 Springer-Verlag, New York. Published simultaneously by Springer-Verlag New York for distribution in the United States and its possessions, Canada and Mexico.

Translators' preface

The publication of this translated volume provides English versions of three of the five books which comprise the "Lehrbuch der Anatomie der Haustiere". Some revision was necessary in the English edition of the second volume largely to adapt the nomenclature, but this was not required in the present book in which terms listed in the Nomina Anatomica Veterinaria were used in the original German text. This is, therefore, an unrevised, unabridged translation which follows faithfully the German text. As in the English version of Volume V, translated by ourselves, the Latin terminology is used the first time a name occurs but subsequently the Englisch equivalent is generally substituted.

It should be pointed out that some of the breeds of farm animals mentioned may not be well known outside their native Central Europe, but descriptions of many of them can be found in Mason, I. L. (1951) "A world dictionary of breeds, types and varieties of livestock," Commonwealth Agricultural Bureau, England.

In the chapter on the lymphatic organs, many references will be found to meat inspection and the German legal requirements for the examination of lymph nodes in the abatoir. We were in some doubt whether these should be omitted from the English edition because obviously legislation is not identical in all countries. However, it was decided to retain them because they may be found useful as a general guide but it must be remembered that they are based on the German regulations.

It is our pleasant duty to acknowledge the invaluable advice on the integument given by Dr. W. M. Stokoe of the Department of Anatomy, Faculty of Veterinary Medicine, University of Edinburgh, and Dr. M. L. Ryder of the Agricultural Research Council's Animal Breeding Research Organisation, Edinburgh. We would also like to thank Mrs. Kathleen Wight for the accurate preparation of the typescript. Finally, we must thank Dr. F. Georgi and his staff at the publishing house Paul Parey, Berlin, for their patience and friendly consideration.

Edinburgh, March, 1981.   W. G. Siller and P. A. L. Wight.

Preface to the German Edition

The publication of volume III completes the five-volume Textbook of Anatomy of Domestic Animals.

The authors of the chapter on the blood vascular system are Professor A. Schummer of Giessen (blood vessels – general considerations, blood and heart) and Professor H. Wilkens of Hanover (blood vessels – arterial and venous systems). The section on the lymphatic system was compiled by Professor B. Vollmerhaus of Munich and that on the skin and cutaneous organs was written by Professor K.-H. Habermehl of Giessen. Dr. W. Münster of Hanover also contributed to the section on arteries and veins.

This summarizes the general content of volume III in which the individual species of animals are treated according to the same basic principle as in the previous volumes.

The introductory chapter discusses the cardiovascular system in a general way because the clinical diagnosis of pathological conditions depends on a thorough knowledge of the entire system. The formation, composition, function and destruction of the blood are dealt with and this is followed by a discourse on the structure and function of the blood vessels, including their nervous and hormonal control. The description of the heart follows the same scheme, the first part dealing with fundamental cardiac anatomy applicable to all mammals while subsequently consideration is given to species peculiarities and the comparative characteristics of the organ.

In describing the origin, course and topography of the blood vessels it was important to include all pertinent detail and yet avoid too lengthy a text. This could only be achieved by a comparative presentation of the vessels of all species, region by region. This chosen method also served to emphasize the fact that in each region the organization and distribution of the blood vessels is basically similar in all species, thus allowing rules of nomenclature to be established for individual blood vessels. Once this fundamental concept is understood, it is possible to extract all the desired information about any one species from the descriptive text and illustrations. The principle is used throughout except in the blood vessels of the foot where, because of the obvious differences in the structure of the extremities, it is necessary to give a detailed description for each species of animal.

The discussion on the function of the lymphatic system is appropriate to the importance of this subject, because much current research on it is of great medical interest. For this reason it seemed advisable to record the present (1975) state of our knowledge in this field, although we are well aware that theories are more quickly outdated in this area than in other medical disciplines. In accord with the general principal of the book, the systematic description of the lymphatic organs in the various species has been compiled so as to provide both basic knowledge and information of value in veterinary practice.

The fundamental descriptions of Baum and his students and the more recent investigations of other authors proved of great service in compiling this chapter. Numerous valuable illustrations from older monographs, long out of print, were reproduced by kind permission of Springer Verlag.

As befits the importance of the carnivores, pig and ruminants, these species are dealt with more liberally in the chapter on skin and the cutaneous organs than has been the custom in previous textbooks of anatomy. Particular stress is placed on the account of special skin glands which are of great importance as scent, marker and signal glands in conspecific communication.

We had numerous collaborators in the Institutes of Veterinary Anatomy in the Universities of Giessen and Munich and of the Veterinary School of Hanover and we thank them all for their valuable assistance.

Our thanks go to Mrs. V. Gube of Giessen for illustrating the chapters on the heart and skin and cutaneous organs, which she accomplished with the artistic skill, understanding and insight for which she is well known. We also thank Mrs. S. Pletscher of Zurich for some illustrations in the section on the hoof. Dr. K.-H. Wille of Giessen provided expert criticism and correction of these chapters and, last but not least, we are grateful to the secretary of the Institute at Giessen, Miss H. Seip, for the careful preparation of the typescript.

We thank Mrs. R. Rochner, Mr. W. Heinemann and Mr. G. Kapitzke of Hanover for the careful graphic work and exemplary artistic illustrations to the chapters on the blood vascular system and the skin and cutaneous organs. We thank M.-L. Meinecke for the conscientious typing and Mrs. G. Voigt and many other members of the institute for their help. We are grateful to Professor Dr. Wissdorf for his valuable and stimulating cooperation.

We are indebted in Munich to Mrs. L. Körner for the drawings, to Dr. H. Roos, Dr. B. Hossenfeldner, Dr. H. Waibl and Dr. H. E. König for their valuable help in preparing the list of contents and the index and for proof-reading. Our thanks also go to Mrs. A. Speiser and Miss Ch. Drechsler for typing the manuscript.

It is largely due to the constant and personal interest of Dr. Friedrich Georgi, a proprietor of the publishing house, that this third volume, and, indeed, the whole project, was so satisfactorily completed. He had great patience and understood the problems which confronted the authors. Our special thanks are likewise extended to Mr. E. Topschowsky, manager of the publishing house, whose vast experience spanning many decades, contributed considerably to the outstandingly high standard of the book.

We hope that this third volume will be as well received as those which preceded it.

Giessen, Hanover, Munich Summer 1976	August Schummer, Karl-Heinz Habermehl, Helmut Wilkens, Bernd Vollmerhaus

Contents

	Page
Organs of the circulation	1
Bloodvascular system	1
Blood (A. Schummer, Giessen)	1
Blood plasma	2
Blood cells	2
Erythrocytes	2
Leucocytes	4
Granulocytes	4
Monocytes	5
Lymphocytes	5
Thrombocytes	5
Organs of the haematopoiesis	6
Development of blood cells	6
Blood vessels, structure and function	7
Arteries	8
Veins	10
Capillaries	11
Arteriovenous anastomoses	12
Nutrition of the vessel wall	13
Innervation of the blood vessels	14
Hormones acting on the blood vessels	14
Heart	15
Pericardium	15
Conformation of the heart	16
Position of the heart	17
Tissue components of the heart	19
The skeleton of the heart	20
Architecture of the heart musculature	21
The chambers of the heart and their internal structure	23
The atria of the heart	23
Right atrium	25
Left atrium	26
The ventricles of the heart	27
Right ventricle	27
Left ventricle	32
Excitation and conducting system of the heart	34
Innervation of the heart	37

Contents

Blood vessels of the heart	38
Arteries	38
Veins	40
Structure and special organization of the blood vessels of the heart	40
Lymph vessels of the heart	41
Species characteristic of the heart, general considerations	41
Size, weight and measurements of the heart, general consideration	41
The heart of the dog and the cat	42
Interior of the ventricles	42
Size and weight of the dog's heart	43
Position of the heart in the dog	44
Heart of the cat, size and weight	45
Blood vessels of the heart of the dog and cat	46
Arteries	46
Veins	48
Heart of the pig	49
Internal structure of the ventricles	49
Size and weight	49
Position of the heart	51
Blood vessels of the heart	52
Arteries	52
Veins	53
Heart of the ox	54
Internal structure of the ventricles	56
Size and weight of the heart	57
Heart of the sheep and goat	58
Internal structure of the ventricles (sheep)	58
Size, weight and position	58
Blood vessels of the hearts of ruminants	58
Arteries of the heart of the ox	58
Veins of the heart of the ox	62
Heart of the horse	62
Internal structure of the ventricles	62
Size and weight of the heart	63
Position of the heart	63
Blood vessels	64
Arteries	64
Veins	65
Species-diagnostic features of the hearts of domestic mammals	68
Dog	68
Pig	69
Sheep and goat	69
Ox	70
Horse	70
Arteries (arteriae) (H. Wilkens in collaboration with W. Münster, Hanover)	71
Truncus pulmonalis	71
Aorta	71

Arcus aortae and truncus brachiocephalicus	72
Arteries of the pectoral limb	77
Comparative topography and nomenclature of the blood vessels of the autopodium	92
Deep vessels of the metapodium	92
Superficial vessels of the metapodium	93
Vessels of the acropodium	93
Arteries of the forefoot of carnivores	94
Arteries of the forefoot of the pig	95
Arteries of the forefoot of ruminants	98
Arteries of the forefoot of the horse	99
Arteries of the head and neck	99
Aorta thoracica	120
Visceral arteries of the thoracic aorta	123
Aorta abdominalis	126
Arteries of the pelvic limb	137
Arteries of the hindfoot of carnivores	148
Arteries of the hindfoot of the pig	150
Arteries of the hindfoot of ruminants	151
Arteries of the hindfoot of the horse	154
Arteries of the pelvic and tail regions	155
Visceral arteries of the abdominal aorta	159
Visceral arteries of the internal iliac and internal pudendal interna	176
Veins (venae)	184
Venae pulmonales	184
Vena cava cranialis	184
Vena azygos	185
Veins of the pectoral limb	197
Veins of the forefoot of carnivores	209
Veins of the forefoot of the pig	211
Veins of the forefoot of ruminants	214
Veins of the forefoot of the horse	214
Veins of the head and neck	215
Vena cava caudalis	233
Veins of the pelvic limb	240
Veins of the hindfoot of carnivores	251
Veins of the hindfoot of the pig	254
Veins of the hindfoot of ruminants	255
Veins of the hindfoot of the horse	256
Veins of the pelvic and tail regions	256
Visceral veins of the caudal vena cava	260
Visceral veins of the internal iliac and internal pudendal veins	266
Lymphatic system (B. Vollmerhaus, Munich)	269
Introduction	269
Lymphatic organs	269
Phylogenesis of lymphatic organs	269
Immune system	270

Structure and function of lymphatic organs	272
Fixed cells of the lymphatic organs	272
Free cells of the lymphatic organs	273
Classification of organs of the immune system	275
Peripheral lymphatic organs	275
Lymphatic tissue	275
Tonsils	277
Lymph nodes	278
Haemolymph nodes	280
Spleen	281
Thymus	283
Ontogenesis	283
Microscopic structure and function	283
Macroscopic description of the thymus	285
Thymus of carnivores	286
Thymus of the pig	287
Thymus of ruminants	288
Thymus of the horse	292
Lymphatic vessel system	**292**
General considerations	292
Phylogenesis of lymphatic vessels	293
Ontogenesis of lymph vessels and nodes	293
Structure and function of lymphatic vessels	294
Lymph capillaries	295
Extravascular circulation	296
Lymph formation	298
Lymph vessels	301
Special arrangement of lymph capillaries and lymph vessels in various organs	303
Lymph collecting vessels and lymphovenous anastomoses	305
Systematic and topography of lymph vessels and lymph nodes	307
General considerations	307
Comparative description of the lymph vessel system	308
Lymph vessel system of the head	308
Outflow of lymph from the head	310
Lymph vessel system of the neck	312
Lymph vessel system of the forelimb	314
Outflow of lymph from the forelimb	317
Lymph vessel system of the chest wall and thoracic organs	317
Ductus thoracicus	322
Lymph vessel system of the dorsal abdominal wall and the abdominal viscera	323
Cisterna chyli	330
Lymph vessel system of the lateral and ventral abdominal wall, the pelvis, the pelvic viscera and the pelvic limb	331
Outflow of lymph from the pelvis and pelvic limb	335
Concluding remarks on comparative aspects	337
Lymph nodes of the dog	337
Lymph collecting ducts	352

Lymph nodes of the cat	354
Lymph collecting ducts	364
Lymph nodes of the pig	364
Lymph collecting ducts	382
Lymph nodes of the ox	383
Lymph collecting ducts	403
Lymph nodes of the goat and sheep	404
Lymph collecting ducts	419
Lymph nodes of the horse	419
Lymph collecting ducts	438

Skin and cutaneous organs (K.-H. Habermehl, Giessen) 441

Common integument, integumentum commune 441

General and comparative considerations 441

Phylogenesis of skin	443
Ontogenesis of the skin and its appendages	443
Subcutis, tela subcutanea	445
Corium	446
Epidermis	448
Hairs, pili	450
Outer hair (Capilli)	452
Wool hair (Underwool, pili lanei)	452
Long or horse hairs	454
Bristles (setae)	454
Tactile hairs (pili tactiles)	454
Arrangement of the hair	454
Hair colour	456
Hair replacement	457
Skin glands	458
Sebaceous glands (glandulae sebaceae)	458
Sweet glands (glandulae sudoriferae)	458
Blood supply to the skin	459
Nerve supply to the skin	460

Specialized structures of the skin 461

General skin modification 461

Localized special glandular apparatus (cutaneous scent glands) 461

Perioral glands, glandulae circumorale	463
Infraorbital organ, sinus infraorbitalis	463
Horn gland, glandula cornualis	463
Ceruminous glands, glandulae ceruminosae	464
Mental organ, organum mentale	464
Carpal organ, organum carpale	464
Metatarsal glandular organs, organa metatarsalia	465
Interdigital sinus, sinus interdigitalis	465
Tail gland, organum caudae	466
Subcaudal gland, glandula subcaudalis	467
Anal sac, sinus paranalis	467
Circumanal glands, glandulae circumanales	468

Inguinal sinuses, sinus inguinalis	468
Preputial glands, glandulae praeputiales	468
Preputial diverticulum, diverticulum praeputiale	468

Mammary gland, mamma ... 469
   Ontogenesis of the mammary gland ... 469
   General and comparative considerations ... 470
   Mammogenesis and lactopoiesis ... 474

Specific hairless skin organs ... 476
   Ontogenesis of the specific hairless skin organs ... 476
   General and comparative considerations ... 476
      Pads ... 477
   Digital organ, organum digitale ... 478
      Hoof ... 479
      Claw ... 481
      Nail ... 482
   The horn of ruminants, cornu ... 483

The skin and its appendages of carnivores ... 487
   Skin of the dog ... 487
   Skin of the cat ... 489
   Mammary gland of the dog ... 491
   Mammary gland of the cat ... 493
   Digital organ of carnivores ... 493

Skin and cutaneous organs of the pig ... 496
   Skin of the pig ... 496
   Mammary gland of the pig ... 498
   Digital organ of the pig ... 500
   Blood vessels of the digital organ of the pig ... 502
      Arteries ... 502
      Veins ... 502

Skin and cutaneous organs of ruminants ... 503
   Skin of the ox ... 503
   Skin of the goat ... 505
   Skin of the sheep ... 505
   Mammary gland of the cow ... 506
   Blood vessels of the udder of the cow ... 514
      Arteries ... 514
      Veins ... 517
      Lymph vessels ... 519
      Nerves ... 519
   Mammary gland of the sheep ... 521
   Blood vessels of the udder of small ruminants ... 522
      Arteries ... 522
      Veins ... 523
   Digital organ of the ox ... 524
      General considerations ... 524
      Subcutis of the claw ... 525
      Corium of the claw ... 525

Epidermis of the claw	527
Digital organ of the small ruminants	532
Blood vessels of the digital organ of ruminants	533
Arteries	533
Veins	534
Skin and cutaneous organs of the horse	537
Skin of the horse	537
Mammary gland of the horse	538
Blood vessels of the mammary gland of the horse	539
Arteries	539
Veins	540
The digital organ of the horse	541
General considerations	541
Subcutis of the hoof	542
Corium of the hoof	543
Epidermis of the hoof	546
Differences between the hoofs of the fore- and hind-limbs	549
Histological structure of the horn tubules	550
Chestnuts and ergots	550
Blood vessels of the digital organ of the horse	552
Arteries	552
Veins	555
Bibliography	558
Index	598

Source of non-original illustrations

Fig. 1: Scheunert, A., and A. Trautmann, Lehrbuch der Veterinär-Physiologie, 5th ed., Paul Parey, Berlin and Hamburg, 1965.

Fig. 2: Grau, H., and P. Walter, Grundriß der Histologie und vergleichenden mikroskopischen Anatomie der Haussäugetiere, Paul Parey, Berlin and Hamburg, 1967.

Fig. 3: Staubesand, J., in M. Ratschow, Angiologie, ed. by Heberer/Rau/Schoop, 2nd ed., Thieme, Stuttgart, 1974.

Figs 24, 136–139, 140–143: Ackerknecht, E., in Ellenberger/Baum, Handbuch der vergleichenden Anatomie der Haustiere, 18th ed., Springer, Berlin, 1943.

Figs 60, 76, 83, 84, 93, 135, 166, 211, 367, 368, 375, 413, 429: Zietzschmann, O., in Ellenberger/Baum, Handbuch der vergleichenden Anatomie der Haustiere, 18th ed., Springer, Berlin 1943.

Figs 65, 66, 197: Ellenberger, W., and H. Baum, Handbuch der vergleichenden Anatomie der Haustiere, 17th ed., Springer, Berlin, 1932.

Figs 103, 104, 110, 114, 123, 124, 249, 419, 421–423, 428, 433: Martin, P., Lehrbuch der Anatomie der Haustiere, vol. II, 2nd ed., by Schickhardt and Ebner, Stuttgart, 1915.

Fig. 206: Schmaltz, R., Atlas der Amatomie des Pferdes, part 2: Topographische Myelogie, 5th ed., Schoetz, Berlin, 1939.

Fig. 222 A: Grau, H. in Krölling/Grau, Lehrbuch der Histologie und vergleichenden mikroskopischen Anatomie der Haustiere, 10th ed., Paul Parey, Berlin and Hamburg, 1960.

Fig. 232: Töndury, G., and St. Kubik, Zur Ontogenese des lymphatischen Systems. In: Handbuch der allgemeinen Pathologie, vol. 3, part 6, Springer, Berlin, Heidelberg, New York, 1972.

Fig. 234: Leak, L. V. and J. F. Burke, in L. V. Leak, The Fine Structure and Function of the Lymphatic Vascular System. In: Handbuch der allgemeinen Pathologie, vol. 3, part 6, Springer, Berlin, Heidelberg, New York, 1972.

Fig. 235 A: Sushko, A. A., in J. Wentzel, Normale Anatomie des Lymphgefäßsystems. In: Handbuch der allgemeinen Pathologie, vol. 3, part 6, Springer, Berlin, Heidelberg, New York, 1972.

Fig. 235 B: Kampmeier, O. F. in J. Wenzel, Normale Anatomie des Lymphgefäßsystems. In: Handbuch der allgemeinen Pathologie, vol. 3, part 6, Springer, Berlin, Heidelberg, New York, 1972.

Fig. 236: Courtice, F. C., The Chemistry of Lymph. In: Handbuch der allgemeinen Pathologie, vol. 3, part 6, Springer, Berlin, Heidelberg, New York, 1972.

Fig. 238: Casley-Smith, J. R., in: New Trends in Basic Lymphology, ed. by Collette/Jantet/Schofeniels, Birkhauser, Basel, 1967.

Figs 240 A, 253, 256, 282–294: Baum, H., and H. Grau, Das Lymphgefäßsystem des Schweines, Paul Parey, Berlin, 1938.

Figs 244, 248, 262–273: Baum, H., Das Lymphgefäßsystem des Hundes, Hirschwald, Berlin, 1918.

Figs 246, 255, 257, 321–335: Baum, H., Das Lymphgefäßsystem des Pferdes, Springer, Berlin, 1928.

Figs 250, 251, 258, 259, 296–309: Baum, H., Das Lymphgefäßsystem des Rindes, Hirschwald, Berlin, 1912.

Figs 280, 281: Zietzschmann, O., in Schönberg/Zietzschmann, Tierärztliche Fleischuntersuchung, 5th ed., Paul Parey, Berlin and Hamburg, 1958.

Figs 359, 396, 398: Martin, P., and W. Schauder, Lehrbuch der Anatomie der Haustiere, vol. 3, 3rd ed., by Schickhardt and Ebner, Stuttgart, 1938.

Other illustrations have been reproduced from dissertations and journals which are listed in the bibliography at the end of the book.

List of Abbreviations

(In the plural form the last letter of the abbreviation is duplicated)

a.	= arteria	int.	= internus	proc.	= processus
art.	= articulatio	lam.	= lamina	prof.	= profundus
can.	= canalis	lat.	= lateralis	propr.	= proprius
caud.	= caudalis	lc.	= lymphocentrum	prox.	= proximalis
com.	= communis	lig.	= ligamentum	r.	= ramus
cran.	= cranialis	ln.	= lymphonodus	reg.	= regio
dext.	= dexter	lob.	= lobus	rostr.	= rostralis
dist.	= distalis	m.	= musculus	s.	= seu, sive
dors.	= dorsalis	mand.	= mandibularis	sin.	= sinister
duct.	= ductus	max.	= maxillaris	str.	= stratum
ext.	= externus	med.	= medialis	sup.	= superior
fiss.	= fissura	min.	= minor	supf.	= superficialis
for.	= foramen	n.	= nervus	transv.	= transversus
ggl.	= ganglion	nl.	= nodus lymphaticus	trunc.	= truncus
gl(d).	= glandula	palm.	= palmaris	tub.	= tuberculum
inc.	= incisura	plant.	= plantaris	v.	= vena
inf.	= inferior	post.	= posterior	ventr.	= ventralis

Text references to figures

These appear in parenthesis in the text, mostly thus: (36/*a*). The number before the oblique line refers to the illustration; the symbol in italics following the oblique refers to a labeled part in that illustration. Therefore, notation (36/*a*), for instance, refers to structure *a* in figure 36. The notation (36, 37, 38/*b*) refers to structure *b* in all three figures 36, 37 and 38.

When the italicized index applies to several illustrations, then all the preceding figure numbers are separated by commas thus (36, 37, 38/*b*); if, on the other hand the italicized indices apply only to some figures, then the figure numbers are separated by semicolons as, for instance (54; 60, 61/*a*). This refers to figure 54 and structure *a* in figures 60 and 61.

ORGANS OF THE CIRCULATION

The organs of the circulation *(angiologia)* include the bloodvascular system and the lymphatic system.

The **bloodvascular system** *(systema cardiovasculare)* consists of the heart, its central organ, and the blood vessels among which we differentiate the arteries, running centrifugally from the heart, and the veins which are directed towards the heart. The arterial and venous networks are connected by the capillaries. The blood circulating within these vessels, the organs of blood formation (haematopoiesis) and the organs responsible for the breakdown of the blood cells are also part of the bloodvascular system.

The **lymphatic system** *(systema lymphaticum)* is composed of the lymph and the lymph vessels, the latter generally accompanying the veins. Another important component of this system is the lymphoreticular tissue which varies in structure and appearance and is widely distributed throughout the body.

Bloodvascular system

(4)

The functions of the **blood** circulating within the vascular system include supplying the cells and tissues of the body with the nutrients required for their maintenance and function, removing break-down products and conveying them to the organs of excretion and transporting surplus metabolites to the storage organs. Further functions are regulation of water and electrolyte metabolism, involvement in the maintenance of body temperature and assisting the body's defence against foreign substances and pathogenic organisms.

An essential prerequisite for the fulfilment of these duties is the correct functional construction of the system as a whole and its appropriate relationship with the other organs.

Very high demands are made on the efficiency of the circulation, and especially the heart, in warmblooded animals. In the transition to a terrestrial existence numerous changes in life pattern took place as the animals adapted to their new environment and these led to an intensification of metabolism. An increase in the oxygen requirement was mainly involved and this was achieved by a transition to pure pulmonary respiration which necessitated the division of the heart and the circulation into two "halves". Both anatomically and functionally, therefore, the heart of birds and mammals is divided into two (double heart) consisting of an arterial part which carries oxygenated blood and a venous part in which the blood is rich in carbon dioxide. The left (arterial) and the right (venous) halves of the heart each consist of an *atrium* and a *ventricle* and they supply completely separated vascular systems known as the *systemic* or *large circulation* and the *pulmonary* or *small circulation* respectively.

Blood

The **blood** consists of blood plasma, a viscous fluid possessing the ability to coagulate, the blood cells and the blood platelets, the latter being formed elements which are non-cellular in nature.

Blood plasma

The **blood plasma** is an aqueous solution of blood proteins, such as fibrinogen, albumin, various types of globulins and blood sugar. The inorganic substances contained in the blood plasma ensure the maintenance of the chemico-physical properties of the blood and they include, amongst others, sodium, potassium, calcium and magnesium ions. As bicarbonate and phosphate salts they have a buffering effect, taking up, for instance, the carbon dioxide and lactic acid liberated by the tissues and so keeping the reaction of the blood at the requisite slightly alkaline level.

Other components of blood plasma are lipids in fine suspension. The plasma serves as a carrier of nutrients, taken up during digestion, for the supply of the body's cells and tissues. Similarly it carries vitamins, hormones and enzymes. It contains products of intermediary metabolism which are break-down products that have to be eliminated from the body. As part of the defence mechanism, the plasma contains enzymes, such as proteinases or peptidases, and antigens, antibodies and antitoxins for the neutralization of foreign protein and bacterial toxins.

The blood remains fluid while within the circulation but it clots when it leaves the vessels. *Blood coagulation*, a vital protective mechanism, depends on the ability of the fluid fibrinogen contained in the plasma to become transformed by the interaction of thrombin, into a delicate elastic network of fibrin. This complex process, initiated by the breakdown of thombocytes, is, according to modern theories, dependent on the interaction of nearly thirty different factors. In the pathological condition of thrombosis blood coagulation can also take place in the unopened blood vessel, when its inner lining, which in the healthy state prevents coagulation, bears lesions which bring about the formation of thrombi.

Blood collected in a container will clot unless some anticoagulant substance has been added. The coagulation time varies considerably among the different species. In birds it is only 1–2 minutes, the pig 10–15 minutes and the horse 15–20 minutes. When blood coagulates, a clot of fibrin and sedimented blood cells forms at the bottom of the vessel, the supernatent being the clear, yellowish, fibrin-free blood serum which contains antibodies and is thus employed in serum therapy.

Mention should also be made of the *sedimentation rate* of the erythrocytes. If blood which has been prevented from clotting is allowed to stand in a test tube, the blood cells will settle out after some time. The duration of this process is termed the sedimentation rate. In certain diseases this rate may deviate from the values established for the respective species under physiological conditions, the reason for this presumably being the altered composition of the blood plasma.

Blood cells
(1 and table)

The **blood cells** or corpuscular elements of the blood derived from cells are listed according to frequency as follows: 1. the red blood corpuscles (erythrocytes), 2. white blood cells or corpuscles (leucocytes) and 3. platelets (thrombocytes) (1).

Blood films are used in *haematology* to examine the morphology, number, size and reaction to chemical substances such as dyes, of the blood cells. A very thin film of freshly drawn blood is spread onto a slide so that the individual blood cells lie side by side in a single layer to facilitate recognition. The tinctorial differentiation of the different types of cells and their intracellular structures is carried out with a mixture of neutral, acid and basic dyes. Special facilities are required to examine the cells in the living state, for which purpose the blood is greatly diluted with an isotonic fluid. The blood cells are counted with the aid of a haemocytometer.

Erythrocytes

In the domestic mammals the **red blood corpuscles** *(erythrocytes)* of the blood are circular, biconcave and anucleate discs. *Tylopods* (e.g. camels, llamas, etc.) have erythrocytes which are anucleate but oval. The diameters of the erythrocytes differ in the various species of domestic mammals. In the dog, for instance, they are 7.3 μm in diameter but in the goat they measure only 4.1 μm (see table). The thickness of the erythrocytes, measured at the edge of the disc, also varies between 2.1 μm in the horse and 1.5 μm in the goat. The same disparity between species is found in the number of red cells per cubic millimeter of blood and their numbers are influenced further by breed, sex, age, husbandry, nutrition,

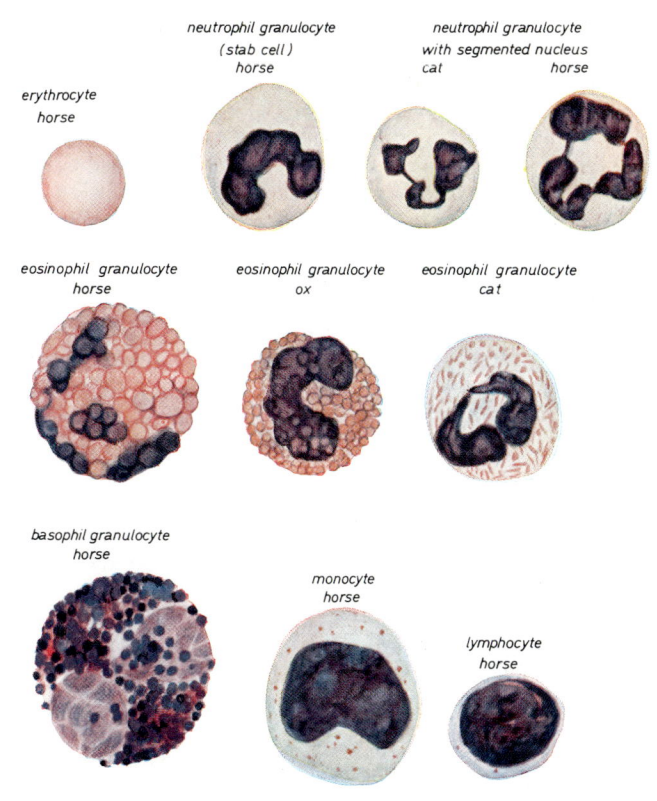

Fig. 1. Various blood cells of the domestic mammals. (Staining by Pappenheim's method; from Schubert, Lehrbuch der Veterinär-physiologie, 5th ed. 1965.)

performance and various other factors. An individual erythrocyte is yellowish-green and only the concentration of large numbers is responsible for the red colour of the blood. The red blood cells are elastic and consequently their shape may be temporarily altered, a property which permits them to pass through capillaries whose lumen is narrower than the diameter of the erythrocytes. In mammals the most striking characteristic of the mature erythrocyte is the absence of a cell nucleus (all other vertebrates have nucleated, oval erythrocytes). Because of the absence of a nucleus their life is relatively short, being about 120 days. It has been shown by electronmicroscopy that they have a semipermeable cell membrane consisting of three layers. They therefore exhibit a characteristic behaviour in media of different molar concentrations. In an isotonic solution, such as physiological saline, they maintain their normal form because the same osmotic tension is present both inside and outside the cell. In hypertonic media, however, the cell loses water and shrivels to the shape of a thorn-apple, while in hypotonic solutions they swell, rupture and release their contents. The latter process is known as (osmotic) *haemolysis*, the fluid medium taking on a red paint-like appearance. After haemolysis the erythrocyte cell membranes can be demonstrated as pale ghosts.

The cytoplasm of the red blood corpuscle consists of various proteins and lipids. A special cytoplasmic structure in the form of a network of delicate granules, the *substantia reticulofilamentosa*, can be demonstrated with specific staining methods only in the incompletely matured cells known as *reticulocytes* or *proerythrocytes*.

Functionally the most important component of the erythrocyte is the red pigment *haemoglobin* which is concerned with oxygen transport. It consists of a protein component, globin, and the iron-containing pigment haem. Haemoglobin has the ability to bind oxygen in a readily dissociable form during its passage through the lung, as a result of which it is converted to bright-red oxyhaemoglobin. Subsequently the oxygen is given off to the tissue cells and, due to this reduction of the oxyhaemoglobin, the colour of the blood becomes dark red. This function of the erythrocytes is directly dependent on their haemoglobin content, which content can be measured by various methods. The removal of carbon dioxide from the cells and tissues and its elimination in the lung is accomplished mainly by binding to alkaline salts of the blood plasma and these also easily dissociate.

In order that the blood may perform its numerous functions it must, in the first place, be present in sufficient amount. Its total volume, which can be assessed by various methods, amounts to 6–8% of the body weight. The percentage of the blood volume occupied by the red blood cells is equally important; this is referred to as the haematocrit value and is dependent on the total number and size of the erythrocytes and on the plasma volume. Determination of the number of blood cells and the relative proportion of the various blood cells to one another is also of great importance (see table).

Red blood corpuscles can show various abnormal features such as different staining affinity; *hyperchromasia* if the haemoglobin content is too great and *hypochromasia* if it is too small. Abnormalities in size are termed *anisocytosis*, in shape *poikilocytosis* and in number *hypererythrocytosis* (normal state in neonates) or *oligoerythrocytosis* (in anaemia). Information regarding these, as well as other morphological, quantitative and qualitative values, provides an important diagnostic aid for the clinician, especially in diseases of the haemopoietic system but also in numerous other illnesses.

Leucocytes

Unlike the red blood corpuscles, the **white blood cells** *(leucocytes)* are colourless, round and nucleated. Certain characteristics, such as differing cell size, nuclear shape, cytoplasmic inclusions and different tinctorial properties make it possible to classify three genetically and functionally seperate types of leucocytes. These are the polymorphonuclear granulocytes, the lymphocytes and the monocytes. The number of white blood corpuscles, between 4,000 and 24,000 per mm^3 of blood, is far less than the number of erythrocytes which are about 500 to 1,500 times as numerous. One of the most striking characteristics of the leucocytes is their amoeboid movement and their consequent ability to leave or enter the capillary by migrating through its wall. In so doing the granulocytes considerably alter the shape of both their cytoplasm and nucleus.

Granulocytes

The **granulocytes** (1) develop, like erythrocytes, in the red bone marrow. They have a diameter of 10–15 μm and thus exceed the red blood cell in size and volume (1:7). During the immature stage their nucleus is unsegmented, rod or "S"-shaped, whereas the nucleus of the mature cells is polymorphic, with a degree of segmentation which depends on the age of the cell. Granulocytes have particularly well-developed amoeboid movement. They leave the capillaries in response to chemotactic stimuli (leucodiapedesis) and collect in areas of vascular damage or loci of bacterial accumulation where they phagocytose and incorporate cell fragments or bacteria and subject them to enzymic digestion. Because of this phagocytic activity, the granulocytes represent a significant part of the complex defense mechanism of the body. Despite their importance they only survive in the circulating blood for 1–1$^1\!/_2$ days.

As already mentioned, we differentiate between granulocytes with rod-shaped and those with segmented nuclei. An increase in the cells with rod-shaped nuclei indicates the appearance of immature forms and these provide the clinician with important indications about the progress of certain diseases. By means of special stains, which consist of a mixture of neutral, acid and basic dyes, it is possible to distinguish three groups of granulocytes. This is because the granules contained in their cytoplasm have a different pH-dependent affinity for these dyes. The delicate granules of one group stain with both the basic (blue) and acid (red) dyes, being thus coloured violet and these cells are termed the *neutrophil granulocytes*. The coarse granules of the second type, the *acidophil* or *eosinophil granulocytes,* stain selectively with the acid, red dye (e.g. eosin). Making up only 2–15% of the total granulocytes, they are far less common than the neutrophils which, depending on the species, amount to 40–75% of the white blood cells. The *basophil granulocytes,* sometimes referred to as *blood mast cells,* comprise only 0.5–1% of the total leucocyte count. As their name indicates, their coarse granules react with the basic component of the stain (e.g. haematoxylin or methylene blue) which colours them dark blue or metachromatically dark violet. The light-blue-stained nucleus of the basophils is more or less completely covered by the granules.

Monocytes

The **monocytes** are large cells 10–15 μm in diameter and they have a round or kidney-shaped nucleus and ample cytoplasm. They, too, display amoeboid movement and their phagocytic activity is well developed. They are therefore termed *macrophages*. Special staining methods will demonstrate delicate granules in their cytoplasm. Their number varies, according to species, from a minimum of 2%–3% to a maximum of 4%–10% of the total leucocytes. There is doubt about their origin but is seems likely that they can develop from the reticulum of the red bone marrow as well as from the reticulum of the lymphatic organs.

Lymphocytes*

The **lymphocytes** (1) constitute the second large group of white blood cells. They differ morphologically, functionally and genetically from the granulocytes. Their number per μl of blood varies considerably between species and also shows considerable individual and age variation but it ranges between a minimum of 20% and a maximum of 70% of the leucocytes. It is possible to differentiate two forms with the light microscope. By far the most common, comprising about 90%, are the small lymphocytes, the remainder being the large lymphocytes. The *small lymphocytes* measure about 6.5 μm and are therefore of similar size to the erythrocytes. They are, however, spherical in structure and possess a relatively large, chromatin-rich nucleus which is surrounded by a narrow border of cytoplasm. They are not able to phagocytose and their amoeboid movement is less than that of the granulocytes. The *large lymphocytes* have a diameter of 10–15 μm. Their nucleus is looser in structure and surrounded by a broader rim of cytoplasm in which isolated granules can be demonstrated with the aid of special stains. The lymphocytes originate in the bone marrow, in the cortex of the thymus and in the germinal centres of peripheral lymphatic organs. Accounts of their differentiation into immune cells may be found in textbooks of histology.

Thrombocytes

The **thrombocytes** (1), also known as **blood platelets,** have a diameter of 2–4 μm and are approximately round or spindle-shaped. Determination of the number of platelets requires special methods because they quickly disintegrate after leaving the circulation; there are said to be 200,000–800,000 per μl of circulating blood.

Blood cell numbers of the most important domestic mammals[1]

Species	Erythrocytes Number mill./μl	Erythrocytes Diameter μm	Leucocytes Number thousand per μl	Neutrophils	Eosinophils	Basophils	Lymphocytes	Monocytes	Thrombocytes Number millions per μl
Dog	5.5– 8	7.3	8–18	55–75	3–10	œ 1	20–25	2– 6	0.2–0.8
Cat	7.2–10	5.7	9–24	55–60	3– 6	œ 1	30–35	2– 5	0.2–0.8
Pig	5 – 8	6.1	8–16	45–55	2– 3	œ 1	40–50	2– 6	0.2–0.8
Ox	5 – 7	5.7	5–10	25–35	5– 6	œ 1	55–65	5–10	0.2–0.8
Sheep	8 –13	5.1	4–12	30–40	5–15	œ 1	45–70	2– 5	0.2–0.8
Goat	13 –17	4.1	8–12	40–45	3– 5	œ 1	50–55	3– 5	0.2–0.8
Horse	6 – 9	5.5	7–11	55–60	2– 4	œ 1	30–40	3– 4	0.2–0.8

[1] After Eder: Das Blut. In: Scheunert/Trautmann, Lehrbuch der Veterinär-Physiologie, 6th Ed. 1976.
* See also chapter "lymphatic system".

These anucleate structures consist of a stainable groundsubstance, the *hyalomer*, and a centrally situated *granulomer* which consists of a number of granules. The thrombocytes are the product of the bone marrow giant cells, the *megakaryocytes*, from which they arise by budding-off of cytoplasmic excrescences. When their cytoplasm has been used-up in this manner the megakaryocytes die. The function of the thrombocytes is to liberate prothrombin, when they break up, from which thrombin then develops. This in turn converts the fibrinogen of the blood plasma into fibrin which stops the flow of blood.

Organs of haematopoiesis

In the embryo both the earliest formation of blood and the primary anlage for blood vessels occur in the *mesoderm of the yolk sac*. At this site the mesenchymal stem cells of the blood give rise first to the **haemocytoblasts**. The latter are capable of perpetual division and from them originate, amongst other cells, the primitive haemoglobin-containing *erythroblasts*.

As blood cell formation (haematopoiesis) ceases in the yolk sac, it is taken over by the mesenchymal component of the *liver anlage*, where not only primitive erythroblasts but also *granulocytes* and *megakaryocytes* develop. Subsequently the *spleen* becomes a site of blood cell formation.

As development of the foetus advances these organs cease to form blood cells and haematopoiesis is taken over by the *red bone marrow (medulla ossium rubra)* which continues to maintain the supply of myeloid cells, that is the erythrocytes, granulocytes, monocytes and thrombocytes, throughout life. This process of continually renewing the blood cells continues in the adult. The bone marrow is situated in the marrow cavity and in the spaces of the spongy substance of the bones. Despite its scattered distribution the bone marrow, which is under humoral and neurovegetative control, is a functional unit. While in the growing individual the bone marrow is responsible for increasing the absolute number of blood cells, its function in the adult is to maintain the normal quality and quantity of the blood cells. For this reason the marrow cavity of young animals consists almost entirely of bloodforming *red marrow*, whereas in the adult the latter is confined to the spongiosa of the short and flat bones and the ends of long bones while about half the marrow organ is converted into *yellow* or *fatty marrow (medulla ossium flava)*.

The **bone marrow** consist of *reticular connective tissue*, the cells of which form a delicate meshwork within the marrow cavity permeated by numerous thin-walled blood vessels which arise from the *vasa nutritia*. The blood passes from the arterial capillaries through funnel-shaped connections into the ramifications of the *venous sinuses* (2/F). The specially constructed, extremely thin endothelial wall of these sinuses allows the easy entrance of young blood cells. Within the intercellular spaces of the reticular tissue one can find all the immature and adult stages of blood cells formed by the active red bone marrow.

The red bone marrow is not only an organ of haematopoiesis but also an important component of that complex defence mechanism of the body which is collectively referred to as the *reticuloendothelial system (RES)*. Both the reticulum cells and the vascular endothelia of the marrow are competent in phagocytosis. They can take up and deal with particles and substances originating from within or outwith the body and they participate in the formation of antibodies. However, macrophages and plasma cells arising from the reticulum cells are capable of similar functions.

Formation of the fat marrow is also a function of the reticulum cell which, by storing lipids, assumes the appearance of a typical adipose cell. The fat marrow is a reserve fat depot which is utilised in prolonged fasting and in the course of serious illness. It then becomes changed into what is termed gelatinous marrow.

Development of blood cells

The **erythrocytes** go through a number of intermediate stages in the course of their development. *Erythropoiesis* commences during embryonic development when reticulum cells are transformed into *haemocytoblasts*. These give rise to the erythrocyte stem cells, the *proerythroblasts*. With the formation of haemoglobin the latter change into *macroblasts (erythroblasts)* which have a nucleus of loose structure. The erythroblasts decrease in size, their nucleus becomes dense and the tinctorial behaviour of the cytoplasm is altered as they change into *normoblasts*. The normoblasts are still able to divide. The transition from the normoblast to the anuclear erythrocyte is completed by the extrusion, or more rarely the break-down, of the nucleus. Nucleated erythrocytes can be observed in the circulation for short periods after, for instance, severe loss of blood or during diseases which are associated with an increased turnover of red blood corpuscles.

The stem cells of the **granulocytes** are also derived from the haemocytoblasts; they are the *myeloblasts* which have spherical nuclei and basophilic cytoplasm. The next intermediate stage is the *promyelocyte* and this is followed by the *myelocyte* which contains granules of specific staining reaction. The cells arising from the myelocytes show striking changes in their nuclei. At first the nucleus is rounded but it then becomes indented and thus characterises these cells as *metamyelocytes* or immature forms. With further transformation of the nucleus the cell enters the circulation as the rod-shaped form of the granulocyte which has been discussed earlier. The final stage in the development of the *polymorphonuclear* granulocyte (1) is attained when the nucleus segments into several connected limbs.

The **thrombocytes** originate, as has already been described, by budding from the megakaryocytes of the bone marrow. The latter, which may measure up to 50 μm in diameter when mature, develop through several intermediate stages from the *megakaryoblast*. Megakaryoblasts originate from the *haemocytoblasts*.

A proportion of **monocytes** develop in the bone marrow by an essentially similar route, since they mature through one intermediate stage from the *monoblasts* which also originate from the haemocytoblasts. The remaining monocytes develop from the reticulum cells of the lymphatic organs.

The **plasma cells** of the bone marrow and of the peripheral lymphoid organs are reactive forms of the reticulum cells. Antigens, such as bacterial break-down products, stimulate the development of these immunoglobulin-producing cells.

The **lymphocytes** belong to the lymphatic series of blood cells. Because of their origin in the mesenchymal connective tissue they possess throughout life a multipotentiality which gives them the power to differentiate as necessity dictates. Proliferation and differentiation to immuno-competent cells takes place in all lymphoid organs.

Blood vessels, structure and function
(2–4)

If one compares the total blood volume of the body to the capacity of the blood vascular system, it is obvious that not all the organs and body regions can be supplied all the time with a constant amount of blood. If we further consider that substantial amounts of blood can be temporarily retained in various organs which act as blood reservoirs, it is evident that the peripheral circulation must possess a mechanism by which the blood flow can be regulated. This mechanism is able, in balanced interrelationship with the central organ, the heart, to supply the various organs with the appropriate amount of blood required to perform their specific functions. This thesis is supported firstly by the morphological demonstration of numerous specialised structures in different regions of the vascular tree and, secondly, by their interpretation on a haemodynamic basis.

From the heart arise the arteries (2/A; 4/black) which spread throughout the body, ever decreasing in size until the very narrow arterioles or precapillary arteries 2/B) terminate in innumerable capillaries (/E) which form an extensive vascular bed. Thence the blood is released into the narrow venules or postcapillary veins (/C). The precapillary arteries, the capillaries and the postcapillary veins form what is sometimes known as the *terminal circulation*; here the exchange takes place between blood and tissues or cells of all those substances which are required for their multifarious functions. The venules, following on from the capillaries, carry the blood into the venous side of the circulation. This consists of the veins which progressively increase in lumen diameter and which eventually carry the blood back to the heart (2/D; 4/long lines).

The walls of the vessels, excluding those of the terminal circulation, consist of three layers: the *tunica interna s. intima* (2/a, b, c), the *tunica media* (/d) and the *tunica externa* (/e, f). It should be noted that the vessels show quantitative, qualitative and structural differences in response to the different mechanical demands made on them and the special functions they have to perform in the different regions of the body. This applies especially to the structure of the tunica media of the arteries and partly also to that of the veins.

Arteries
(2/A; 4)

Two structural types of **arteries** can be recognised even on gross examination. The first type includes the vessels near the heart, the aorta and its cranially-directed branches as well as the pulmonary trunk and its large branches which enter the lungs. The yellow colour of all these vessels and their extreme distensibility are due to the large amounts of elastic fibres and membranes present in the media (2/d). These are, therefore, *elastic arteries*. Towards the periphery these elastic arteries gradually merge into the second type which are reddish or white, thick-walled *muscular arteries*.

The *intima* (/a, b, c) of both types of arteries consists of *endothelium* (/a), a single layer of flat, rhomboid cells which lies upon an elastic membrane known as the *lamina elastica interna* (/c). Between these two layers there is sparse collagenous tissue representing the *lamina subendothelialis* (/b).

The *lamina elastica interna* of the *elastic* arteries gradually merges with the concentrically layered elastic membranes which form the basic ground structure of the *media* (/d). The elastic lamellae are connected to the muscle cells which regulate the tension of the arterial wall. The significance to the circulation as a whole of the structure of the media of these arteries can best be demonstrated using the aorta as an example. Blood which has been pumped into the aorta under systolic pressure puts the media under elastic tension, whereby some of the power produced by the heart is temporarily retained as potential energy. During the diastolic pause this is changed into kinetic energy by the contraction of the vessel wall so that the blood expelled from the heart in rhythmic strokes is transported to the periphery in a much more even stream. The function of the aorta, and the succeeding arteries of elastic type, may thus be compared with that of an expansion chamber.

The arteries of muscular type act as distributing vessels and have the task of carrying the blood to the appropriate organs. As they do so, the pressure of the blood causes their walls to stretch in both longitudinal and circular directions. Depending on the relationship between the arteries and their surrounding tissues there is, especially in the region of the limbs, considerable stretching in the longitudinal direction. The muscular arteries respond to these pressure changes by the organisation of the various tissues in the media and the tunica externa. There is usually a well-developed internal elastic lamina (2/c) followed by a media (/d) largely composed of smooth muscle. The vascular lumen is surrounded by tracts of muscle tissue which contain different amounts of elastic fibres and which are arranged in spiral layers orientated in various directions and variable gradients. The media, being able to respond to this transverse tension, is therefore in a position to adapt to changing demands by constricting or dilating the lumen and so regulating the blood pressure within the arterial system and maintaining it within physiological limits. If, due to degenerative changes or hardening of the arterial wall, this constantly-active regulatory mechanism is lost, then permanent hypertension may follow with a danger of rupture of the brittle arteries. The variable longitudinal tension and distension of the arterial wall are taken up by the *tunica externa* which is made up of a *lamina elastica externa* and *tunica adventitia*. The tunica externa (/e, f) consists of collagenous and elastic fibres which are interwoven and crossed in helical fashion. Furthermore, the tunica externa ensures that the arteries are built into their surroundings in a functionally correct manner.

There are some organs, such as the brain and the kidneys, which have so high and constant a requirement for oxygen that they need a blood supply independent of other circulatory fluctuations. Other organs, like the gastrointestinal tract, lung and skeletal musculature are supplied with a variable amount of blood depending on their changing degrees of activity. In order to prevent excessive demands being made on the heart and to obtain the most economical use of the available volume of blood, the circulatory system is able to provide certain areas with a preferential supply and others with less blood whenever this is necessary.

Although arteries of all sizes can reduce the diameter of their lumina to a certain extent, they cannot completely occlude them, and consequently there are other blood vessels which participate in the regulation of blood flow to the organs. These are the *arterioles* or *precapillaries* which are an important component of the terminal circulation (2/B). Their lumina are often no wider than those of the capillaries following them. Since their media consists of but a single layer of muscle fibres and the elastica interna is broken up into a network of fibres, they can completely close their lumina thus achieving an alternative method of controlling the blood stream.

Blood stream regulating structures of another type occur, their occlusive mechanism being characterised by the presence of swellings or cushions of longitudinal muscles or *epithelioid muscle cells* which bulge the intima into the lumen during contraction and thus bring about their complete closure.* These special structures occur in the skin, lungs, erectile tissue and in certain other organs.

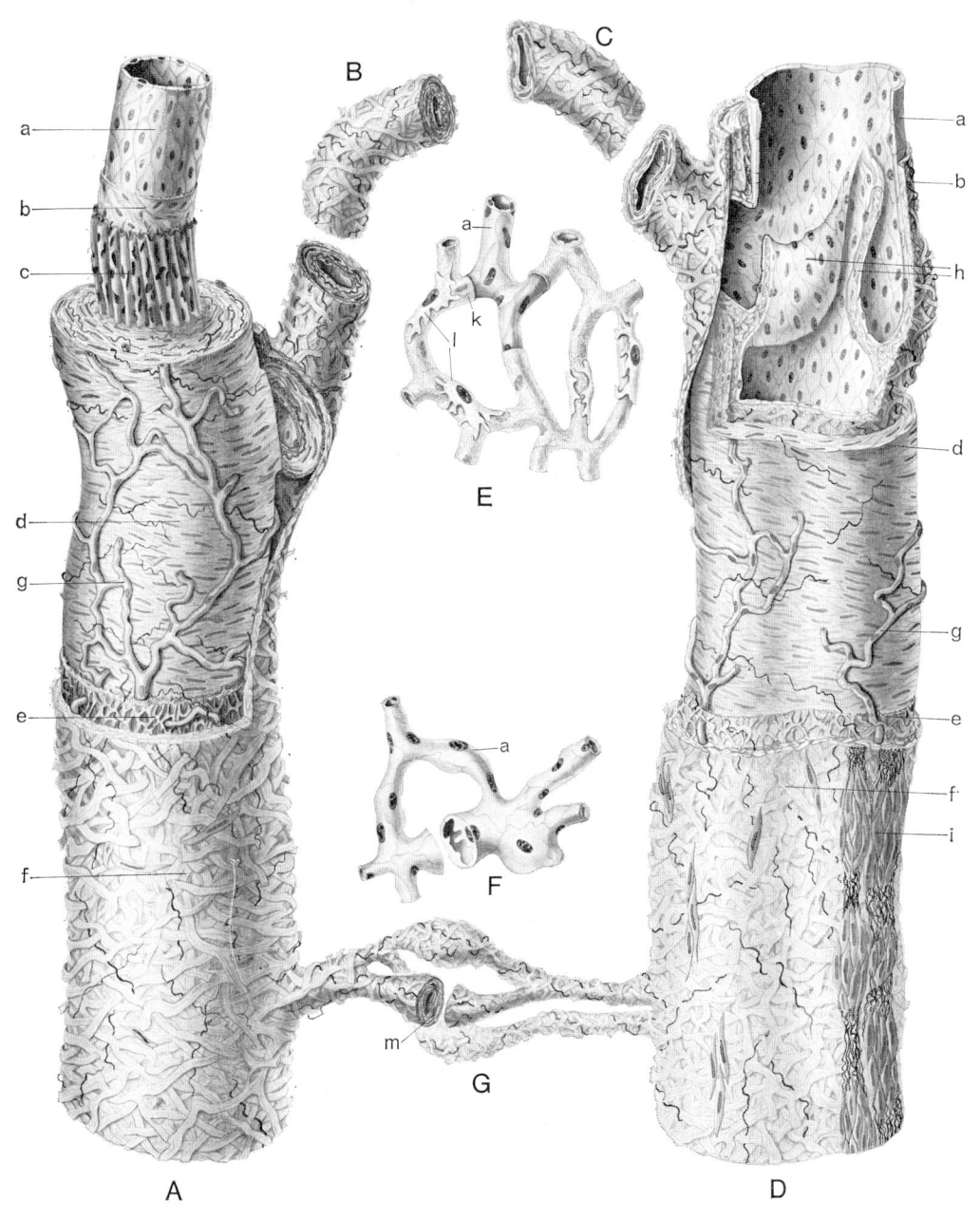

Fig. 2. Structure of the walls of blood vessels.
(After Grau and Walter, 1967.)

A artery; *B* arteriole; *C* venule; *D* vein; *E* capillary, *F* sinus capillary; *G* arterio-venous anastomosis

a, b, c tunica int. s. intima, *a* lamina endothelialis, *b* lamina subendothelialis, *c* lamina elastica int.; *d* media s. tunica muscularis; *e, f* tunica ext., *e* lamina elastica ext., *f* tunica adventitia; *g* vasa vasorum; *h* venous valve; *i* longitudinal musculature of the tunica adventitia; *k* basal membrane; *l* pericytes; *m* intimal cushion

* The German term *Drosselarterien* (throttle arteries) graphically describes their mode of action.

Veins
(2/D; 4)

The **Venous side** of the circulation has the function of returning to the heart a continuous stream of blood which has lost more than 80% of its systolic pressure through the flow-resistance of the arteries, arterioles and capillaries. A completely different haemodynamic function is demanded from the venous system than from the arterial side of the circulation. This is achieved by the general make-up of the veins and their specialized structures and, in particular, by the topography and specialized function of certain parts of the venous system. Firstly it should be pointed out that the number of veins is much greater than the number of arteries because the latter are often accompanied by two, or even more, *collateral veins*. Furthermore, their number is increased, especially in the skin, by veins and collateral vessels with which there is no accompanying artery. Added to this the lumina of the veins are always wider than those of their accompanying arteries and in many sites they form networks so that the potential volume of the venous system is much greater than that of the arterial counterpart.

In this connection one must stress that the spleen, liver, lungs and skin are able to store large amounts of blood and then return it to the circulation when required. The necessity to shunt blood into venous branches, comparable with railway-sidings, explains the presence of haemodynamically active specialized formations and the structural and material differences in the make up of veins from different regions.

The walls of the veins consists of the same three layers that have been described in the arteries, namely the tunica interna, media and externa (2/D) but the boundaries between these are not so clearly distinguished as in the arteries.

The *endothelial sheet* (/a) of the veins lies on a layer of collagenous and elastic fibres of varying thickness (/b). This layer is followed, without sharp definition, by the media (/d) and the tunica externa (/e, f).

The *media* consists of collagen and elastic fibres which are woven into a functional system and which may contain variable amounts of muscular tissue. In different regions one or the other component may predominate and this will determine whether the particular veins are passively distensible tubes or, if there is an excess of musculature, whether they actively participate in the work of the circulation. The former situation occurs mainly in veins near the heart, while the more muscular vessels are at the periphery where they are exposed to greater haemodynamic pressure. This is especially true of the veins of the limbs and of erectile tissue.

The *tunica externa* is the thickest layer in most veins. It consists of a network of collagen and elastic fibres which are situated in the longitudinal musculature. This layer is responsible for providing a correct functional relationship with the surrounding tissues and for protecting the veins from injury and excessive stretching.

A remarkable feature of the veins is the passively mobile **valves** (2/D, h) which project into the lumen. These consist of a double endothelial fold on a connective tissue base. Each valve is made up of two, rarely three or more, *individual cusps*, the free borders of which are half-moon or sickle shaped, while their base is confluent with the vessel wall. The distance between valves varies with the body region and organ system. The valve sinus, delineated by the cusp and the vessel wall, is directed towards the heart. The veins of almost all organs, even those veins with a diameter of but 50 μm, carry valves. They are especially numerous in the veins of the extremities. Their function is to prevent the centrifugal backflow of the blood which is being carried to the heart by hydrostatic pressure and other forces. They are therefore, comparable in action to a non-return valve.

Other flow-regulating structures of the veins correspond to similar occlusive mechanisms in arteries; projecting into the lumina of these small veins are intimal swellings which are formed by muscle tissue or groups of epithelioid cells lying below the intima. In other cases the veins are furnished at intervals with ring muscles or sphincters. These structures can hold the blood for a time in the veins, producing a pearl-string-like appearance. The blood is also held up in the capillaries preceding these throttle veins. Such structures have been demonstrated in the veins of such organs as the adrenal and thyroid glands, the uterus, oviduct, erectile tissue, intestinal mesentery and the corium of the hoof.

There are various forces and factors which cause the blood, flowing under greatly reduced pressure through the capillaries and postcapillary venules into the peripheral veins, to be propelled towards the heart in a continual stream. These include the so-called *vis a tergo*, the driving force which originates from the heart and maintains the blood in motion even through the venous half of the circulation. Then there is *systolic suction* which commences from the heart through the two venae cavae and their larger branches. By this means the negative pressure of the thoracic cavity, which is further increased during inspiration, causes the thin-walled veins to become dilated and be held under tension. Other driving forces exerted on the venous blood arise from the skeletal musculature. The way in which the veins are situated in the intermuscular and interstitial connective tissue causes them to be alternately dilated and compressed during muscular activity and this, coupled with the reflux-preventing action of the valves, drives the blood towards the heart.

In many sites of the locomotor apparatus there are "*arterio-venous linkages*" which represent a special topographical and structural relationship between the arteries and their accompanying veins. In these sites the arteries and their accompanying veins are bound together in a tube of connective tissue, the outer layer of which consists of acutely-angled ring fibres, while the fibres of the inner layer surround the artery and veins in figures of eight. Because of this close binding together it was assumed that the pulse wave running in the complex brought about a rhythmic compression of the collateral veins which, with the help of the valves, propelled the blood towards the heart. However, more recent experimental investigations have shown that there is no such functional interplay.

Capillaries
(2/E; 4)

It is the purpose of the *terminal vascular bed* to facilitate the two way exchange between blood and body cells which is necessary for their survival and function. The actual exchange takes place in the thin-walled capillaries which carry the blood from the *precapillary arterioles* to the cells and tissues. The terminal vascular bed performs another important function in regulating the body temperature of warmblooded animals; it allows the body to loose excessive heat by increasing the blood flow through the skin or, alternatively, it prevents excessive heat loss by displacing a larger proportion of the blood volume into the interior of the body.

The diameter of the capillaries can be altered but ranges between 6 and 30 μm. In rare cases, so-called "*giant capillaries*" may be up to 40 μm in diameter. The length of the capillaries is very difficult to establish but varies between 0.5 and 1.0 mm. Very many wide capillaries are found in the *sinusoids* (2/F) as, for instance, in the liver, the bone marrow and the pituitary. The density of the capillary network depends on the intensity of the metabolic activity of the organs supplied by them. The number is especially great in endocrine organs, in the grey matter of the central nervous system, in kidneys, heart and skeletal musculature as well as in the skin and adipose tissue.

Less well supplied with capillaries are tissues which are mainly "passive" or bradytrophic such as tendons, fasciae, ligaments and bones. The cornea of the eye and hyaline cartilage are entirely devoid of capillaries. It should be noted, however, that the surface area available for metabolic exchange is not dependent only on capillary density. An increase in the function of an organ is always accompanied by a considerable widening of the capillaries and this not only increases the exchange surface but also enhances the blood flow through the terminal vascular bed.

The distribution of the arteries and veins within an organ always follows a characteristic pattern and similarly there is a close correlation between the spatial arrangement of the capillaries and the structure of the tissues. It is thus possible to recognise without difficulty from which organ a corrosion preparation of blood vessels and capillaries was made. In parenchymatous organs the capillaries form three-dimensional networks and in the lungs and glands they surround the alveoli and acini. In the papillary body of the skin and in cutaneous mucous membranes there are capillary loops, in the musculature elongated meshes and in the renal corpuscle capillary skeins known as glomeruli.

The walls of the **capillaries** consist of *endothelium* (2/E, a), *basal membrane* (/k) and pericytes or *adventitial cells* (/l), the latter being closely applied externally.

The endothelium is an extremely thin *simple squamous epithelium*. Its cells are rhomboid and their wavy and notched plasma membranes are in contact except for a space of 100–150 Å which is free of ground substance. Apart from their elongated nucleus which slightly bulges the plasmalemma into the lumen, the endothelial cells contain, like other cells, organelles such as mitochondria, lysosomes, Golgi apparatus, endoplasmic reticulum and ribosomes. The occurrence of these organelles and certain enzymes in the endothelial cells indicate that they can actively participate in the organ-specific, selective metabolic exchange between the blood and the tissue cells (blood-tissue barrier).

The capillary endothelial cells of various organs, such as the kidneys, endocrine glands, the choroid plexus and the synovial villi, carry submicroscopic "windows" closed by *thin membranes (diaphragma)* and also *true pores* which indicate intensive fluid exchange. We must differentiate these structures from the *intercellular spaces* of the hepatic, splenic and bone marrow capillaries, which decrease the barrier effect of the endothelial sheet and permit the passage of corpuscular elements. Increased capillary permeability is seen in the course of inflammatory processes of the tissues.

The exchange of materials can also occur through transcellular transport, a process which is called *cytopempsis* and depends on the *micropinocytotic* ability of the endothelial cell. During this process minute fluid droplets are taken up by little bays in the luminal or basal plasmalemma and then enter the cytoplasm as vesicles. They are finally discharged into the subendothelial region or the capillary lumen. Large-molecular substances, especially plasma proteins, are passed through the capillary wall by this means.

In the endothelium of the capillaries, or more correctly the sinusoids, of the liver, spleen and bone marrow there are cells (known in the liver as *Kupffer cells*) which have an abundance of cytoplasm and cytoplasmic projections which leave gaps between individual cells. They resemble the reticulum cells of the lymphoreticular organs both in appearance and in phagocytic capacity. Their processes project into the capillary lumen and they can become dislodged and carried away in the blood stream. These cells are an important constituent of the reticuloendothelial system (*RES*) and, together with similar cells of the lymphoreticular system, they are involved in the body's defence against foreign substances and pathogenic organisms and in the break-down of red blood cells.

The *basal membrane* of the capillaries (2/E, k) appears homogeneous under the light microscope. With silver stains, however, reticulum fibres can be demonstrated. These give the membrane the property of reversible elasticity and make the capillaries into elastic tubes which can adjust their diameter according to changes in blood pressure.

Electronmicroscopic, polarisation and histochemical examinations have given important insight into the complex ultrastructure of the basal membrane. These methods have shown that the basal membrane has not only a mechanical action but, as the only continuous component separating blood and tissues, it fulfills an important function as a filter.

The *pericytes* or adventitial cells (2/E, l) surround the capillaries with their branched processes and are molded closely to the outside of the basal membrane. The theory that these are contractile elements capable of constricting the capillary lumen is disputed today. Their phagocytic property and their ability to migrate into the surrounding tissues as macrophages, would suggest that they participate in the exchange of materials.

In conclusion, it should be pointed out that the exchange of substances between the blood and the intercellular fluid is a complex and still partly unexplained process and that, as already mentioned, various mechanisms are involved in the penetration of the *blood-tissue barrier* formed by the capillary walls.

Arteriovenous anastomoses

(2/G)

In certain regions of the circulation there are special vascular segments known as *arteriovenous anastomoses*. These precede the capillaries and the diameters of their lumina can be regulated up to complete occlusion. They are a direct link between small arteries and veins and in the dilated condition they shunt the blood, without an intervening metabolic exchange, from the arterial high pressure area directly into the venous low pressure region. However, if the lumina of these by-pass vessels are closed the blood proceeds via its normal course through the capillary bed.

These haemodynamically active arteriovenous anastomoses thus regulate the blood flow. They connect the artery and vein in various ways. The so-called **bridge anastomosis** joins the vessels in a short arch, "S"-shaped vessel or more tortuous link. We can differentiate an active arterial and a passive venous limb. It is interesting to compare the thickness of the wall of the arterial limb with that of the artery of origin. The increase in thickness is due to the addition of circular muscle fibres and longitudinal muscle bundles (2/G, m) in the media. The media is devoid of elastic fibres. Varying numbers of subintimal epithelioid cells are also present.

Such bridge anastomoses occur in many regions. They may be seen in the gastrointestinal wall, salivary glands, nasal mucosa, lungs, endocrine organs, penis, ovary, uterus, placenta and in the skin.

One can draw certain conclusions about the function of the bridge anastomoses from experimental investigations and also from their structure and occurrence in certain vascular regions. Their most important function is haemodynamic. When patent they transfer the blood from the arterial high pressure to the venous low pressure side and thus increase the flow of blood in the veins. At the same time they relieve the distal capillary system in the same manner as an overflow valve. They can thus also play a part in decreasing or increasing the function of those organs which are subject to periodic variation of activity such as the gut, glands and lungs. The thermoregulatory function of these arteriovenous anastomoses depends on the fact that, in the open state, they increase the flow of blood in certain regions of the circulation, particularly those relatively unprotected parts of the body which are exposed to the environmental temperature. These regions include the extremities, the pinna of the ear, the nose, the comb of fowls and other exposed skin appendages.

Glomus anastomoses are morphologically and functionally different from the bridge anastomoses. They consist of vessels having skein-like convolutions. Again, in comparison with the artery from which they originate, they appear as thickened vessels which form a stretched or twisted connection between artery and vein. The wall of their active limb contains bundles of longitudinal muscle fibres and characteristic subintimal cells which surround the narrow lumen in several layers. The tunica elastica interna of the media is absent. The numerous veins, usually narrow and thin-walled, are clustered around the centrally situated connecting pieces and are themselves surrounded by a connective tissue capsule. Another feature of these glomus anastomoses is their rich supply of non-myelinated nerve plexuses originating from the nerves to neighbouring vessels. Because of their complicated structure these types of anastomoses appear as if some organ were interposed in the course of the vessel. These structures are present in the terminal phalanges of both man and animals and in the skin and comb of cockerels. The *glomera caudalia* of animals and the *glomus coccygeum* of man are similar structures.

These *glomus organs* do not have any haemodynamic action on the circulation; their complex clustering of narrow venous convolutions and their inability rapidly to alter the lumen diameter militates this possibility. Because of the remarkably large number of epithelioid cells and their extensive innervation, it was at one time thought that the glomera might have a humoral function. At first experimental evidence seemed to confirm that they could produce a locally-active, vasodilatory, acetylcholine-like substance but electron-microscopical and histochemical examinations have failed to demonstrate the typical features of secretory cells in the epithelioid cells of the glomus organs. Thus the function of these glomus organs remains obscure.

Nutrition of the vessel wall
(2/A, g; 3)

The walls of small blood vessels are nourished by the circulating blood through diffusion and cytopempsis. Such a direct supply is insufficient, however, for thick walled vessels. In the latter only the innermost layers are supplied through the intima while nourishment of the greater part of the media is taken over by the *vasa vasorum*, the "vessels of the vessels". The vasa vasorum do not arise directly from the lumen of the vascular segments they supply. On the contrary, they originate from recurrent branches of collateral arterial plexuses, which then enter the vessel wall and break up into capillaries.

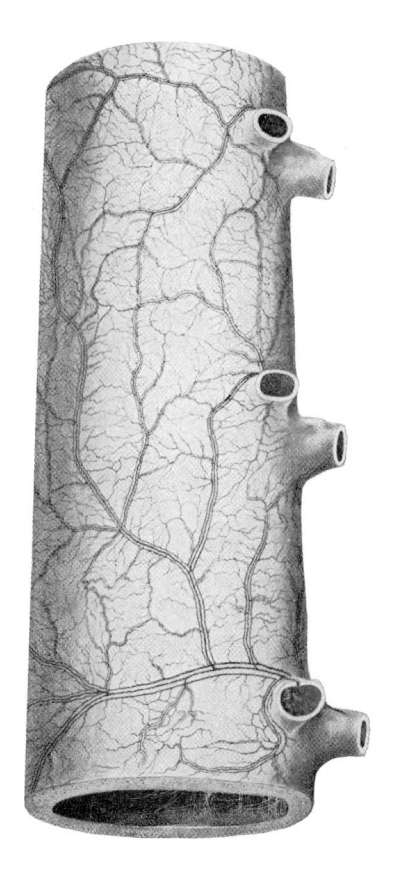

Fig. 3. Part of the thoracic aorta of a horse, showing the dorsal intercostal arteries giving rise to the arterial vasa vasis, accompanied by two veins.
(After Staubesand, 1974.)

Innervation of the blood vessels

As the autonomic, mainly non-myelinated, nerves approach the vessels they form coarse networks in the adventitia and then divide into delicate ramifications which enter the vessel and even extend to the intima. Their main purpose is to supply the vascular musculature and thus they are known as the **vasomotor nerves.** Some fibres may also be concerned with depth sensitivity. Stimulation of the sympathetic fibres generally causes narrowing of the vessels (vasoconstriction) while vasodilatory action is attributed to the parasympathetic fibres.

The sympathetic nerves which innervate the blood vessels of the skin and skeletal musculature are switched in the vertebral ganglia of the sympathetic trunk to the postganglionic fibres and they reach the organs which they ultimately stimulate as part of the mixed cerebrospinal nerves. The *vasoconstrictors* which innervate the vessels of the internal organs originate as the preganglionic fibres of the truncus sympathicus which are switched to their second neurons in the prevertebral ganglia related to the particular organs. Apart from the vasoconstrictor, *adrenergic* sympathetic nerves, there are also *cholinergic* sympathetic *vasodilators,* which widen the blood vessels of the skeletal musculature and, presumably, also the coronary vessels.

It is doubtful whether the vascular nerves originating from the various regions of the parasympathetic system act as vasodilators. A dilatation of the vessels which results in a drop in the blood pressure with lowering of the peripheral resistance, is believed to be due rather to reduction in the impulse frequency of the vasoconstrictors. A dilatation of the vessels is also caused by *bradykinin* which is an enzyme secreted, without parasympathetic participation, by the digestive glands and sweat glands.

Hormones acting on the blood vessels

Another important role in the regulation of the circulation is played by various vasopotent hormones. These include the vasodilating substances *acetylcholine* and *histamine* as well as *vasopressin, hypertensin* and *serotonin* which have a vasoconstrictor action. *Noradrenalin* has a double action in that it constricts most vessels but dilates the coronary vessels. The same is true of *adrenalin* which dilates the vessels of the skeletal musculature while otherwise having a decidedly vasoconstrictor action.

The regulation of an optimal blood supply, adapted to the functional status of the various organs, organ systems and body regions, commences at the terminal vascular bed. An increased requirement for oxygen by the activated organs or an increased accumulation of metabolic products such as carbon dioxide and lactic acid, of acetylcholine and adenosine triphosphoric acid (ATP) and of bradykinin, effect a dilatation of the precapillary arteries.

This local chemical regulation of the circulation leads to a passive dilatation of the capillaries and thus an increased blood flow through the organs, with the result that a larger volume of blood is withdrawn from the total circulation. In view of the disparity which exists between the blood volume and the greater capacity of the circulatory system, such a reaction can cause a sudden drop in blood pressure and an insufficient supply to some vital organs. This risk is counteracted by the **circulatory centre.** This centre regulates the action of the heart and the tonus of the vessels thus maintaining both normal blood pressure and the distribution of the available blood volume according to the requirements of all systems.

The main site of the circulation regulatory centre is in the pons of the metencephalon and the medulla oblongata but blood pressure regulating impulses can also originate from the spinal cord, the sympathetic system, the midbrain and tweenbrain and the cortex. Although the vasomotor centre, which has vasoconstrictor and vasodilator subcentres, is largely autonomous, it is nevertheless under the constant influence of the *baroreceptors,* which control blood pressure, and of the *chemoreceptors* which register the chemical composition of the blood. The baroreceptors are neurovegetative receptor areas located in the adventitia of the aortic arch, in the bifurcation of the common carotid artery (carotid sinus), in the termination of the vv. cavae and in the wall of the atria of the heart. The baroreceptors of the aortic arch are connected with the vasomotor centre by the vagus nerve, those of the carotid sinus by the glossopharyngeal nerve. If they register an excessively high or low tension of the vessel walls then, via the centre, the blood pressure is accordingly decreased or increased. An increase in the pressure of the vv. cavae and the pulmonary veins causes their baroreceptors to elicit an intensification of the heart's action. Other blood pressure receptors are found in the coeliac, mesenteric and renal arteries. However, the reflexes originating from these go via subordinate spinal centres and they are therefore confined to circumscribed vascular regions.

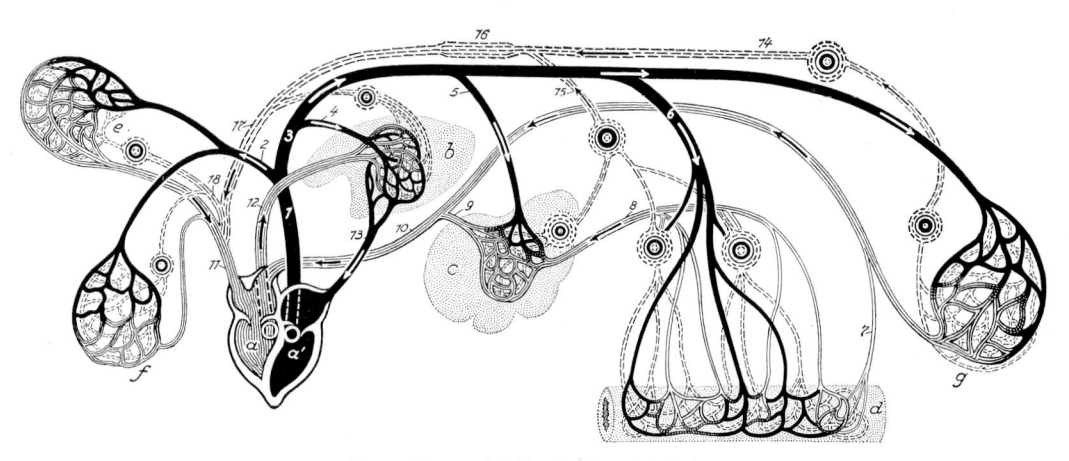

Fig. 4. Diagram of the blood and lymph circulation
(After Nickel, 1939.)(Black: arterial blood; continuous lines: venous blood; interrupted lines: lymph)

a right, *a'* left ventricle; *b* lung; *c* liver; *d* intestine; *e* capillaries in the head and neck region; *f* capillaries of the forelimb; *g* capillaries of the trunk, the pelvic limb, the urogenital apparatus

1 aorta; *2* arteries of the head, neck and forelimb; *3* descending aorta; *4* a. bronchialis; *5* a. hepatica; *6* intestinal arteries; *7* vv. rectales; *8* v. portae; *9* vv. hepaticae; *10* v. cava caud.; *11* v. cava cran.; *12* a. pulmonalis; *13* vv. pulmonales; *14* lymph vessels from the caudal part of the body; *15* visceral lymphatic trunk; *16* lumbar cysterna; *17* ductus thoracicus; *18* lymphatic trunk from the cranial part of the body. The position of the lymph node groups is marked on the course of the lymph vessels.

Chemoreceptors are the *glomus caroticum* and the *glomus aorticum* or *glomus supracardiale* which are located in the carotid sinus and the aortic arch respectively. These are paraganglia which originate from the vagus and glossopharyngeal nerves and are characterised by the production of noradrenalin and the absence of chromaffin cells. A drop in oxygen tension and increase in carbon dioxide tension or a rise in the H^+ concentration cause impulses to travel along the vagus and glossopharyngeal nerves to the vasomotor centre; from this centre the heart rate is then raised, vasoconstriction is stimulated, blood stores are emptied and respiration is intensified. However, the immediate relationship between these paraganglia and the receptor areas of the aorta and carotid sinus might also mean that these areas are sensitive to the hormone produced by these endocrine organs.

Heart (Cor, Cardia)
(5–49)

The **heart** is the muscular central organ of the blood-vascular system which, by its rhythmic contractions, acts like a double suction and pressure pump and thus maintains the motion of the blood through the closed system of tubes, the blood vessels. Although somewhat variable from species to species, its shape resembles that of a more or less pointed and bilaterally flattened cone. It is surrounded by the completely closed pericardium.

Heart and pericardium are located within the thorax in the *spatium mediastini* which is limited by the pleural layers of the *mediastinum medium*. The heart and pericardium are covered dorsally and laterally by the lungs which are moulded accordingly *(impressio cardiaca)*. Lateroventrally a small surface of the pericardium is exposed to the thoracic wall in the region of the *incisura cardiaca dext.* and *sin.* of the lungs, and this exposed surface varies in extent not only between species but also between left and right sides.

Pericardium

The **pericardium** accommodates, within its *cavum pericardii*, the heart and the initial portions of the aorta and truncus pulmonalis and the terminal segments of the vv. caevae and the vv. pulmonales (see vol. 2 Figs 351 and 352). The shape of the pericardium corresponds to the form of the heart and its dimensions correspond to the functionally-determined volume changes of that organ. *Intra vitam* and *post mortem* the pericardium closely encloses the heart, its opposing surfaces being moistened by a thin film of serous fluid, the *liquor pericardii*. The pericardium can only be lifted from the heart after perforation has allowed air to enter the pericardial space.

Including its pleural covering, the pericardium consists of three layers, the *pleura pericardiaca*, the *pericardium fibrosum* and the *lamina parietalis* of the *pericardium serosum*. Loose connective tissue containing variable amounts of fat lightly binds the *pleura pericardiaca* to the *pericardium fibrosum*. The latter is made up of several layers of collagen fibres running in various directions. The movable intertwining of the collagen fibres and supplementary elastic elements of the *pericardium fibrosum*, allow the pericardium to adjust to changes in the volume of the heart and to transmit to the heart the suction effect produced by the lungs during respiration. Dorsally the *pericardium fibrosum* continues onto the *tunica externa* of the blood vessels. It is thus connected, especially above the aorta and its branches to the *fascia endothoracica* which forms the suspension of the heart to the vertebral column.

In carnivores the fibrous layer of the pericardium is joined to the diaphragm near the sternum by means of the *lig. phrenicopericardiacum*. In pigs and ruminants, at the level of the 5th and 6th costal cartilages respectively, there are two tendinous *ligg. sternopericardiaca*. In the horse the pericardium is joined to the sternum by the *lig. sternopericardiacum* which extends from the 4th or 5th costal cartilage to the diaphragm and has a broad insertion into the *fascia endothoracica*.

The third and inner layer of the pericardium, the *lamina parietalis* of the serous pericardium, consists of a richly vascularised and innervated connective tissue layer containing elastic fibres and a single layered mesothelium. This serous membrane is considered to be the source of the small quantity of serous fluid, the *liquor pericardii*, which is present in the *cavum pericardii*. Inflammatory processes (pericarditis), are associated with the excessive production and simultaneous retarded reabsorption of the pericardial fluid; this causes excess fluid, *hydrops pericardii*, which may restrict the heart's action because of the limited elasticity of the pericardial sac. Severe haemorrhage into the cavity of the pericardium can produce a pericardial tamponade and consequent cardiac arrest.

At the base of the heart the serous membrane of the pericardium, the *lamina parietalis*, is reflected onto the heart as the *lamina visceralis* or *epicardium*. This visceral layer also envelops the first part of the large arteries and veins as they leave the heart, forming the *vaginae serosae arteriorum et venarum*. The pericardial space between these great vessels forms recesses of which the *sinus transversus pericardii*, lying between the aorta, pulmonary trunk and atrial wall is particularly prominent. This sinus allows independent movement for the arteries and the atrium during cardiac activity. The *sinus obliquus pericardii* is a pouch between the left and right pulmonary veins and the left atrium.

Conformation of the heart
(5–12, 21–49)

The **heart** can be differentiated into a *right venous* and a *left arterial* part. Each of these two parts consist of an atrium *(atrium cordis dext. et sin.)* (9, 10, 11, 12/a, b; 21–23/a) and a ventricle *(ventriculus cordis dext. et sin.)* (8/E, F; 9/c, d; 10/d, e; 11/s, t; 12/r, s; 21–23).

The two atria rise dome-like above the *basis cordis* and each surrounds the origin of the *aorta* and the *truncus pulmonalis* with a blind diverticulum, the *auricula atrii* (8/A, B; 9/a', b; 21–23/b). The venous blood from the body is carried to the *right atrium* through the *v. cavae cran. et caud.* (10/1, 3) and through the *v. azygos dext.* (/2) or *sin.* (37/17; 39/e). From the cardiac veins the blood returns to the right atrium via the *sinus coronarius* (10/14; 37/16; 39/13). The *left atrium* receives arterial blood from the lungs (8/1, 1; 9/10; 10/7; 11/3) through the *vv. pulmonales*.

The two *ventricles*, of which the left gives rise to the aorta (8/a; 11, 12/1) and the right to the pulmonary trunk (8/k; 9/3; 12/4), are joined together in the form of a cone which is laterally slightly flattened and more or less pointed, according to the species. On this cone we differentiate the *facies auricularis* (8; 9) and the *facies atrialis* (10), the convex *margo ventricularis dext.* (8/C; 9/m) and the straight or slightly concave *margo ventricularis sin.* (/D; /n). The external boundary between the atria and ventricles is formed by the deep coronary groove *(sulcus coronarius)* (8/I; 9/k; 10/p), which is interrupted by the pulmonary trunk. An imaginary plane running through the coronary groove corresponds to the base of the heart *(basis cordis)*. Since the valvular apparatus of the ventricles, the aorta and the pulmonary trunk, are situated on the same plane, we speak of this as the *valvular plane* (13, 27,

30, 34, 37, 43, 46). The left and right ventricles are limited externally by two *longitudinal grooves*, which originate from the *sulcus coronarius* and run towards the point of the heart *(apex cordis)* or the *incisura apicis* (38/K, L). One of these commences caudal to the *conus arteriosus* (8/H; 9/p) of the right ventricle and is therefore known as the *sulcus interventricularis paraconalis (/G; /1)*. The second longitudinal groove starts below the *sinus venarum cavarum* of the right atrium and is therefore termed *sulcus interventricularis subsinuosus* (10/q). The coronary and longitudinal grooves accommodate, within a variable amount of adipose tissue, the subepicardially situated blood vessels of the heart *(arteriae coronariae* and *venae cordis* with their branches) as well as lymph vessels and cardiac nerves.

Position of the heart
(5–7)

The position of the heart of the domestic mammals within the thorax corresponds to their wedge-shaped sternum which, especially in ungulates, is bilaterally flattened. In comparison with the position of the human heart in the more barrel-shaped thorax of man, the heart of these animals appears as if turned to the left through 90° on its long axis. In consequence, the right atrium and ventricle are orientated to the right and craniad (5–7/a, f; 9/d) while the left atrium and ventricles are directed to the left and caudad (5–7/c, h). It follows, then, that the *margo ventricularis dext.* corresponds to the cranial (/g) contour of the heart and the *margo ventricularis sin.* to its *caudal* contour (/i). At the same time the left surface *(facies auricularis)* and the *sulcus interventricularis paraconalis* (5–7/e; 9/1) are turned towards the left thoracic wall, while the *facies atrialis*, with the *sulcus interventricularis subsinuosus* (10/q), together face towards the right wall. Both auricular and atrial surfaces have atrial and ventricular components.

In the dog (5) the long axis of the heart forms an angle of 40°, open anteriorly, with the sternum. In the cat the angle is 25–30° and the apex of the heart points towards the diaphragm. In the pig the heart is aligned somewhat more steeply, its apex pointing towards the sternum. The heart axis is almost vertical in ruminants (6) and especially so in the horse (7) where the apex is tilted slightly to the left, so that it lies 2–3 cm from the sternum. In all domestic mammals the *base* of the heart lies at the level of an imaginary

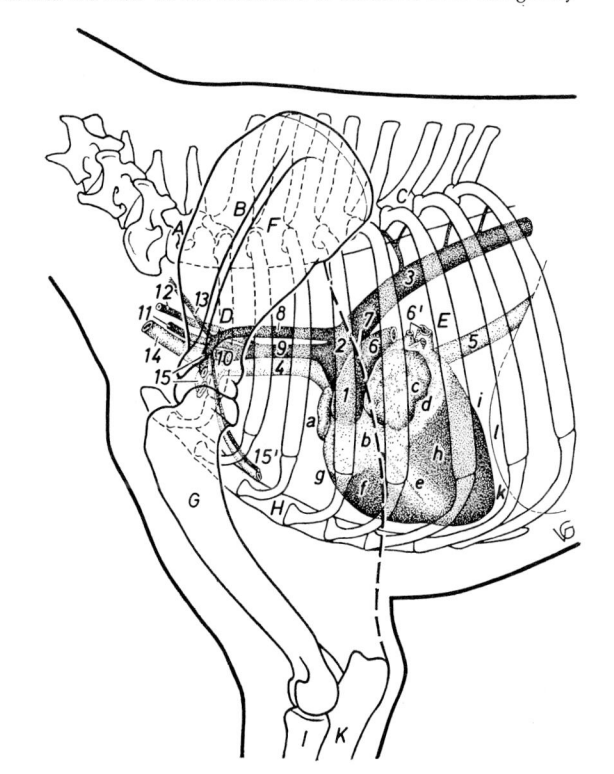

Fig. 5. position of the heart in a formalin-preserved dog in the erect posture.

A 7th vertebra; *B* 1st thoracic vertebra; *C* 6th thoracic vertebra; *D* 1st rib; *E* 6th rib; *F* scapula; *G* humerus; *H* sternum; *I* radius; *K* ulna

a right auricle; *b* conus arteriosus; *c* left atrium with its auricle; *d* sulcus coronarius; *e* sulcus interventricularis paraconalis, *f* right ventricle, *g* its margo ventricularis dext.; *h* left ventricle, *i* its margo ventricularis sin.; *k* apex cordis, *l* contour of the diaphragm

1 truncus pulmonalis; *2* arcus aortae; *3* aorta thoracica with aa. intercostales dorss.; *4* v. cava cran.; *5* v. cava caud.; *6* a. pulmonalis sin., *6'* vv. pulmonales; *7* lig arteriosum (Botalli); *8* a. subclavia sin., *9* a. brachiocephalica; *10* a. subclavia dext., *11* a. carotis comm. dext.; *12* a. carotis comm. sin.; *13* a. vertebralis; *14* v. jugularis ext. sin.; *15* a. and v. axillaris sin.; *15'* a. and v. thoracica int. The interrupted line represents the caudal border of the m. triceps brachii (linea anconaea)

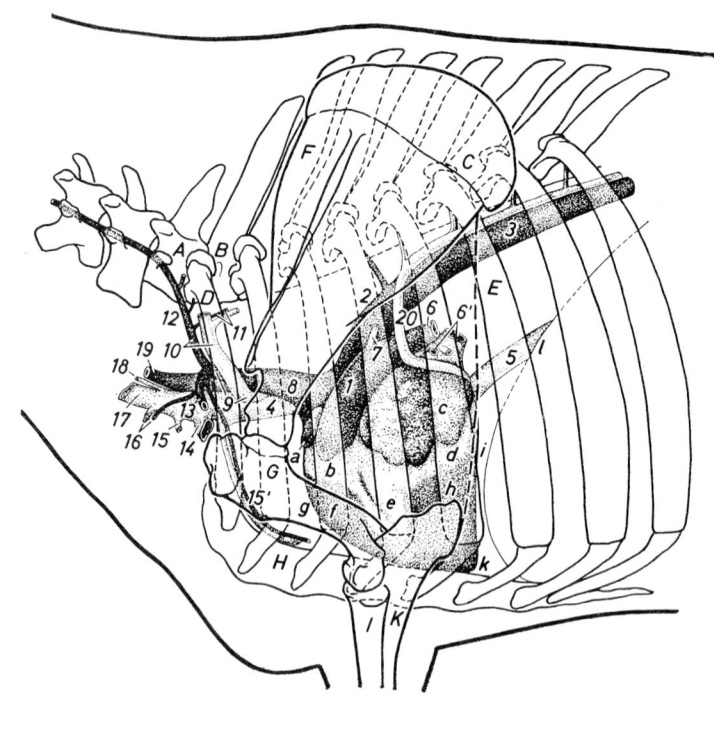

Fig. 6. Position of the heart in a formalin-preserved ox in the erect posture. Left aspect.

A 7th cervical vertebra; *B, C* 1st and 6th thoracic vertebrae; *D, E* 1st and 6th ribs; *F* scapula; *G* humerus, *H* sternum; *I* radius; *K* ulna

a right auricle; *b* conus arteriosus; *c* left atrium with its auricle; *d* sulcus coronarius; *e* sulcus interventricularis paraconalis; *f* ventriculus dext., *g* its margo ventricularis dext.; *h* ventriculus sin., *i* its margo ventricularis sin.; *k* apex cordis; *l* contour of the diaphragm

1 truncus pulmonalis; *2* arcus aortae; *3* aorta thoracica with aa. intercostales dorss.; *4* v. cava cran.; *5* v. cava caud.; *6* a. pulmonalis sin.; *6'* vv. pulmonales; *7* lig. arteriosum; *8* truncus brachiocephalicus; *9* a. and v. subclavia sin.; *10* arterial and venous truncus costocervicalis; *11* a. and v. intercostalis suprema; *12* a. vertebralis; *13* a. axillaris; *14* v. axillaris; *15* v. cephalica; *15'* a. and v. thoracica int.; *16* a. and v. cervicalis superfic.; *17* v. jugularis ext. sin.; *18* v. jugularis int.; *19* a. carotis comm. sin.; *20* v. azygos sin. with vv. intercostales dorss. Interrupted line represents the caudal border of the m. triceps brachii

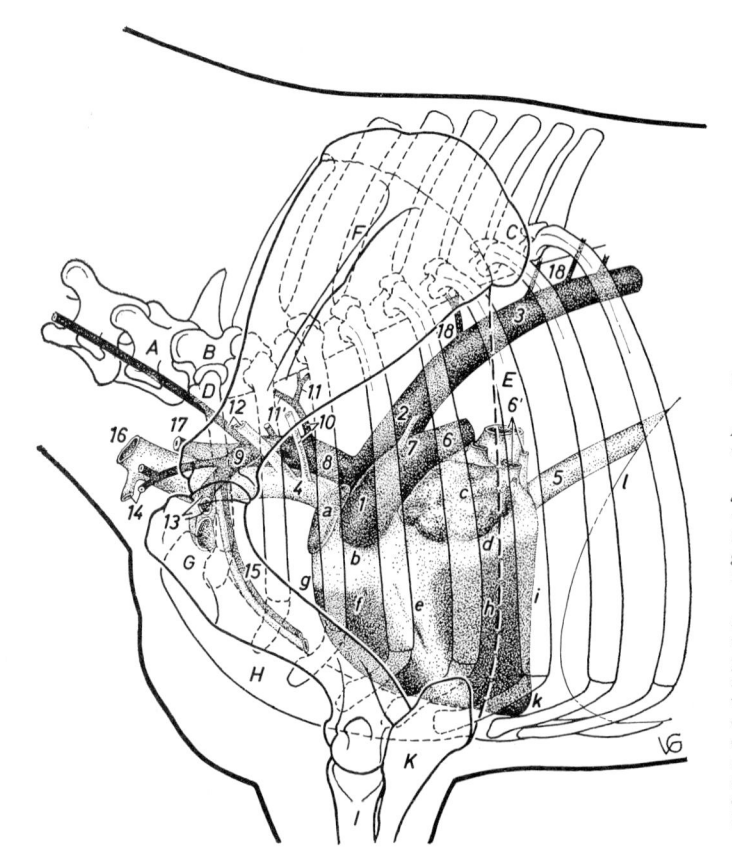

Fig. 7. Position of the heart in a formalin-preserved horse in the erect posture. Left view.

A 7th cervical vertebra; *B, C* 1st and 6th cervical vertebrae; *D, E* 1st and 6th ribs; *F* scapula; *G* humerus; *H* sternum; *I* radius; *K* ulna

a right auricle; *b* conus arteriosus; *c* left atrium with its auricle; *d* sulcus coronarius; *e* sulcus interventricularis paraconalis; *f* ventriculus dext., *g* its margo ventricularis dext.; *h* ventriculus sin., *i* its margo ventricularis sin.; *k* apex cordis; *l* contour of the diaphragm

1 truncus pulmonalis; *2* arcus aortae; *3* aorta thoracica; *4* v. cava cran.; *5* v. cava caud.; *6* a. pulmonalis sin.; *6'* vv. pulmonales; *7* lig. arteriosum; *8* truncus brachiocephalicus; *9* a. subclavia sin.; *10* arterial and venous truncus costocervicalis; *11* a. intercostalis suprema; *11'* a. scapularis dors.; *12* a. and v. vertebralis; *13* a. and v. axillaris; *14* a. and v. cervicalis superficialis; *15* a. and v. thoracica int.; *16* v. jugularis ext. sin.; *17* a. carotis comm. sin.; *18, 18* aa. intercostales dorss. Interrupted line represents the caudal border of the *m. triceps brachii*

horizontal plane, drawn through the centre of the first rib, while the convex *margo ventricularis dext.* follows the internal contour of the sternum (5–7). The craniocaudal extent of the heart is between the 3rd (4th) and 6th (7th) ribs in the dog; in the cat it is from the 4th to the 7th; in the pig from the 3rd to the 6th; in the ox from the 3rd to the 5th (6th); in the sheep and goat from the 2nd to the 5th and in the horse from the 3rd (2nd) to the 6th ribs. Relative to the median plane $^4/_7$ths of the heart of the dog lies in the left half and $^3/_7$ths in the right half of the thorax. In the ox this ratio is $^5/_7$ to $^2/_7$ths and in the horse it is $^3/_5$ to $^2/_5$ths. It follows, therefore, that the *facies auricularis* is nearer to the left wall of the thorax than the *facies atrialis* is to the right thoracic wall, a fact which is of significance in clinical examination of this organ. Unlike the heart of man, which is entirely accessible for clinical exploration by palpation, auscultation and percussion, from the anterior thoracic wall, in domestic mammals this organ does not lend itself to these procedures to the same extent because of the different topography of the chest wall. In these animals the anterior part of the thorax, which accommodates the heart, is covered by the extensive shoulder girdle musculature, which is connected to the shoulder blade and the humerus, and by the massive triceps brachii muscle which fills the angle between these two bones. The thick *margo tricipitalis (linea anconaea)* of the latter muscle extends down to the 4th or 5th intercostal space (5–7).

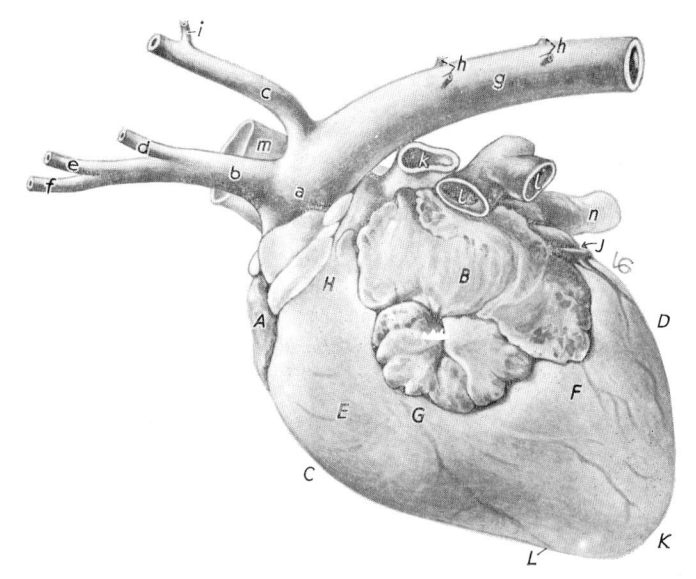

Fig. 8. Auricular surface of a feline heart formalin-preserved in situ (After Habermehl, 1959)

A right auricle; *B* left auricle; *C* margo ventricularis dext.; *D* margo ventricularis sin.; *E* ventriculus dext.; *F* ventriculus sin.; *G* sulcus interventricularis paraconalis; *H* conus arteriosus; *J* sulcus coronarius, pars sin.; *K* apex cordis; *L* incisura apicis

a arcus aortae; *b* a. brachiocephalica; *c* a. subclavia sin.; *d* a. carotis comm. sin.; *e* a. carotis comm dext.; *f* a. subclavia dext.; *g* aorta thoracica; *h, h* aa. intercostales dorss.; *i* a. vertebralis; *k* truncus pulmonalis; *l, l* vv. pulmonales; *m* v. cava cran.; *n* v. cava caud.

Tissue components of the heart

The wall of the heart is made up of three layers, the epicardium, the myocardium and the endocardium.

The **epicardium** is identical with the *lamina visceralis* of the *pericardium serosum* and it forms a smooth, glistening and transparent serosal covering over the surface of the heart. We can distinguish in the epicardium an outer mesothelial layer whose cells are able to alter their shape from squamous to cuboidal in response to the changing tension of the heart wall. These cells lie on a lamina propria, the fibres of which are mainly collagenous and are so orientated that they can follow changes in shape and form undergone by the heart. Below this lamina lies the subepicaridal layer consisting of collagen and elastic fibres continuous with the interstitial framework of the heart musculature. The large blood and lymph vessels and nerves are situated in this layer; it also contains, especially in the coronary and interventricular sinuses, deposits of adipose tissue. The extent of these fat depots is dependent on the species and also on the age and nutritional status of the individual.

The dark red muscular wall, the **myocardium,** consists of muscle cells which have centrally situated nuclei and are enclosed by a membrane, the sarcolemma. The sarcoplasm contains the cross-striated myofibrils, which are concentrated at the periphery and are made up of filaments (elementary fibrils). Because of the great amount of work performed by the heart, the muscle cell contains many mitochondria. Endoplasmic reticulum is located between the myofibrils and, near the nucleus lies the

Golgi apparatus. The myocardial cells are rich in glycogen and contain lipids and brownish-yellow lipofuscin granules. Unlike skeletal muscle fibres, the heart muscle fibres give off branchlets at an acute angle and they thus form a close knit network with neighbouring cells. The muscle cells and their branches are formed into longer fibres by means of intercalated discs, also known as the cement lines. These discs are cell membranes and the myofibril bundles are interlocked by them although they do not transgress this boundary. This gives rise to a formation of muscle fibres which are united into bundles to make a network of long fibres. The spaces between the bundles are filled by delicate connective tissue which, together with the plasmalemma, constitutes the sarcolemma. In certain regions of the heart muscle the fibres of the endomysium continue as collagenous tendons so that in the papillary muscles they form the connection between the muscle cells and the *chordae tendineae* of the membranous valves. Similarly they form the connection between the musculature and the skeleton of the heart.

The rich capillary supply of the heart muscle is consistent with its great output of work. In fact, there are rather more capillaries than there are muscle cells; in the human heart the ratio is 1:1.06 in favour of the capillaries.

The **endocardium** is an elastic connective tissue membrane which lines the interior of the heart chambers and covers the heart valves. It consists of an endothelial layer and a reticulated layer of collagen and elastic fibres intermingled with smooth muscle fibres. Connective tissue fibres join to the perimysium internum and serve to form a movable junction between the endocardium and its underlying tissue. Its tissue components and their organisation permit the endocardium to adjust to changes in tension which occur during heart action.

The skeleton of the heart*

(15)

This term incorporates structures and tissue components which are made up partly of connective tissue and partly of cartilage or bone. They are insinuated between the heart on the one hand and the aorta and pulmonary trunk on the other. They are also found between the atrial and ventricular musculature and they are an important prerequisite for normal heart function. Included in this concept are the *anuli fibrosi* and the *heart skeleton* in the narrow sense.

The *anuli fibrosi arteriosi* are ring-like connective tissue structures which form the transition between the ostia of the ventricles and the aorta and pulmonary trunk (15/8, 9). They are each composed of three arches whose convexity is turned towards the heart and whose neighbouring limbs unite as they project upwards. The course of these three garland-like arches does not follow the line of insertion of the tricuspid valve lying next to it. On the contrary, the valve's crescentic lines of origin cross the fibrous rings, as their heartward pointing concavities go past the boundaries of the vessels and help to link the arterial tube to the ventricular wall. Another similarly stabilising element which contributes to the union between the arterial wall and the myocardium is the *filum tendineum intermedium* which can be demonstrated as a specialized structure within the *anulus fibrosus*. Since the aortic insertion is under greater strain, its anulus fibrosus and filum tendineum are more strongly developed than in the region between the pulmonary trunk and the conus arteriosus. When viewed in three dimensions the anulus fibrosus presents as a conical ring which narrows towards the ventricle; its oblique surfaces are inserted between the vessel wall and the ventricular musculature from above and outside to below and inside.

The immediately-proximate sites of origin of the aorta and pulmonary trunk are joined at their ostia by a figure of eight crossing of the fibres of their anuli fibrosi. These structures have also been referred to as the *chiasma anuli fibrosi*. These are supplemented by areas of fusion or bandlike connections which complete the chiasma and thus help to fuse the base of the two arteries to the muscular ostia.

The *anuli fibrosi atrioventriculares* are similar to the *anuli fibrosi arteriosi* both in shape and structural make up (/10). They surround the atrioventricular orifice and consist of a connective tissue fibre network which continues into the interstitium of the arterial and ventricular musculature without making direct contact with the muscle fibres themselves. This fibrous ring also has a *filum tendineum intermedium* which maintains a close relationship to the membranous valves which are inserted here and to their chordae tendineae. It is important to note that, unlike the two great arteries, the anular rings of

---

* Based on a study by Schmack (1974).

the left and right side of the heart are not linked in any way. Their obliquely descending walls are in the form of conical rings and are interposed between the thickened muscular edge of the ventricle and the atrial muscle which lies inside it.

The anulus fibrosus is broadened distally in the region of the *cuspis septalis* of the right ventricle. This is the site where the connecting fibres of the atrioventricular node pierce the fibrous ring (/11). In the region of the septal cusp the muscular ring surrounding the left atrioventricular orifice is interrupted by the tendinous *septum ventriculoconale aortale* which continues into the non-muscular part of the interventricular septum, the *pars membranacea septi interventricularis*. The latter is present in all domestic mammals with the exception of the ox.

The significance of the *anuli fibrosi atrioventriculares* lies in the fact that it achieves both a morphological and a functional separation of the atrial and ventricular musculature, thus ensuring the unimpeded coordination of atrial and ventricular action.

The *skeleton* of the heart in the strict sense consists of tendinous, cartilaginous and osseous tissue. Situated in the immediate neighbourhood of the aortic orifice and therefore in the centre of the heart valve plane, it is able to prevent detrimental distortions of the ostium during cardiac activity. At the same time it affords a place of origin and insertion for much of the musculature of the ventricle.

In the horse the heart skeleton in the strict sense, consists of two layers of tendinous structure which are completely independent of the anuli fibrosi. These are the *trigonum septale, ventriculare sin. et dext.* Their tendinous elements are supported by two cardic cartilages, the *cartilago cordis septalis sin. et accessoria*. The large septal cartilage lies on the proximal border of the interventricular septum next to the aortic conus. In old animals it measures 2.5–3 cm in length and appears triangular in cross section. It is situated on the base of the interventricular septum with its concave surface hard against the origin of the aorta. The *cartilago cordis sin.*, approximately the size of a cherry-stone, is found in 65–70% of cases embedded in the wall of the aorta. The *cartilago cordis accessoria* is still smaller and is also enclosed in the aortic wall.

In the ox the heart skeleton in the strict sense consists of the large *os cordis dext.*, measuring 5–6 cm in length, and the smaller *os cordis sin.* Both have insignificant cartilaginous and fibrous components. In position and function they correspond to the *trigona fibrosa* of the horse and they are therefore frequently referred to as *trigona ossea*. They are independent structures which belong to the conus region of the left ventricle and they serve to maintain the shape of the aortic ostium by stabilising it in the haemodynamically most favourable position. At the same time they offer a locus for the insertion of muscle fibres of the interventricular septum.

The large cardiac bone of the ox, the *os cordis dext.* (15/A) is a rhomboid. Its four processes (/a, b, c, d) carry cartilaginous caps from which originate connective tissue tracts connected to the interstitium of the ventricular musculature. The *os cordis sin.* is of irregularly triangular shape. It is embedded in the left conal region of the ventricular muscle and with two of its three processes it clasps the left part of the aortic origin.

In the dog, as in the horse and ox, the heart skeleton in the strict sense is a morphologically independent structure. It shows species-specific peculiarities and consists of the *trigonum cartilagineum dext.* and the *cartilago cordis septalis*. The trigonum contains an island of cartilage which is insinuated superficially into the interventricular septum and which, according to its position, corresponds to the right osseous trigonum of the ox. By means of various tendinous tracts it is fixed both to the surrounding tissues and to the origin and insertion of the subsinous part of the septum musculature. Tendinous tracts connect the cartilaginous trigonum to the *cartilago septalis*. The latter corresponds to the large septal cardiac cartilage of the horse although it consists of but a small triangular piece of cartilage which is inserted between the closely apposed origin of the aorta, and the right ventricle.

No detailed studies of the heart skeleton of the pig, sheep and goat are available. We know, however, that these species do possess supporting cartilaginous structures and that they can become ossified in older pigs and sheep.

Architecture of the heart musculature

Although it is exceedingly difficult to demonstrate the overall architecture of the atrial and, especially, the ventricular wall by dissection of the various muscle fibre tracts and their courses, morphological observations have been made which correlate well with our understanding of the heart's action.

The *subepicardial* layer of the remarkably thin muscular wall of the atria contains both long and short muscle fibres. While the former span both atria, the short fibres are confined to one atrium. The more deeply situated tracts originate from the anulus fibrosus and run an arched course or encircle the blind auricles and the termination of the pulmonary veins. Other *subendocardial* fibres form the bases of the *musculi pectinati* which form an anastomosing network and are a prominent feature of the internal relief of the atria.

In the musculature of the ventricular wall and septum we differentiate a subepicardial, a middle and a subendocardial layer, but the fibres run between one layer and another in an intricate interlacement. We

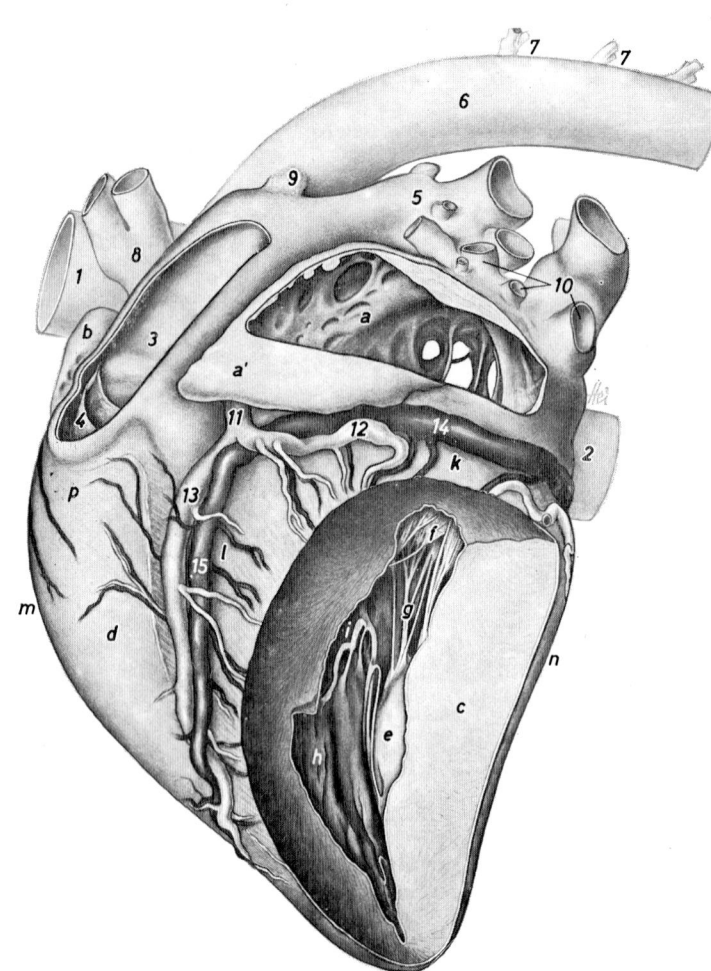

Fig. 9. Auricular surface of a horse's heart. Left atrium and left ventricle have been opened and the pulmonary trunk fenestrated. The subepicardial adipose tissue has been removed.

a atrium sin with mm. pectinati; *a'* auricula sin.; *b* auricula dext., *c* ventriculus sin.; *d* ventriculus dext.; *e* m. papillaris subatrialis; *f* valva atrioventricularis sin.; *g* chordae tendineae; *h* trabeculae carneae; *i* mm. transversi s. trabeculae septomarginales; *k* sulcus coronarius; *l* sulcus interventricularis paraconalis; *m* margo ventricularis dext.; *n* margo ventricularis sin.; *o* apex cordis; *p* conus arteriosus *1* v. cava cran.; *2* v. cava caud.; *3* truncus pulmonalis (fenestrated); *4* valva trunci pulmonalis; *5* a. pulmonalis sin.; *6* aorta thoracica; *7* aa. intercostales dorss.; *8* truncus brachiocephalicus; *9* lig. arteriosum; *10* vv. pulmonales; *11* a. coronaria sin., *12* its r. circumflexus (sin.), *13* its r. interventricularis paraconalis; *14* r. circumflexus of the v. cordis magna, *15* its r. interventricularis paraconalis

are therefore dealing with the same muscle fibres which produce the three layers by merely altering their direction. We thus have a construction that is in accord with the function of any hollow muscular organ.

Both the suction of the blood from the atria into the ventricles and its subsequent expulsion are associated with a lowering of the valvular plane of the heart. This effect takes place because of the arrangement of the musculature of the ventricles. The bundles of the *subepicardial* layer, arising from the heart skeleton, take an oblique course towards the heart's apex and there, at the *vortex*, they descend into the depth of the wall. Continuing in a steep spiral course towards the base, they form the *subendocardial* layer and at the same time form the basis for the *trabeculae carneae* and the *mm. papillares*. The *middle* layer is made up of muscle fibres which leave the subepicardial layer before the apex is reached and enter the substance of the wall. The more superficial of these fibres encircle both ventricles in spirals and the more deeply situated fibres enclose one ventricle each, by entering the septum in the region of the longitudinal grooves. These fibres also subsequently ascend to the heart skeleton. Because of its function, the circular muscle stratum of the middle layer is known as the "powerhouse" of the heart.

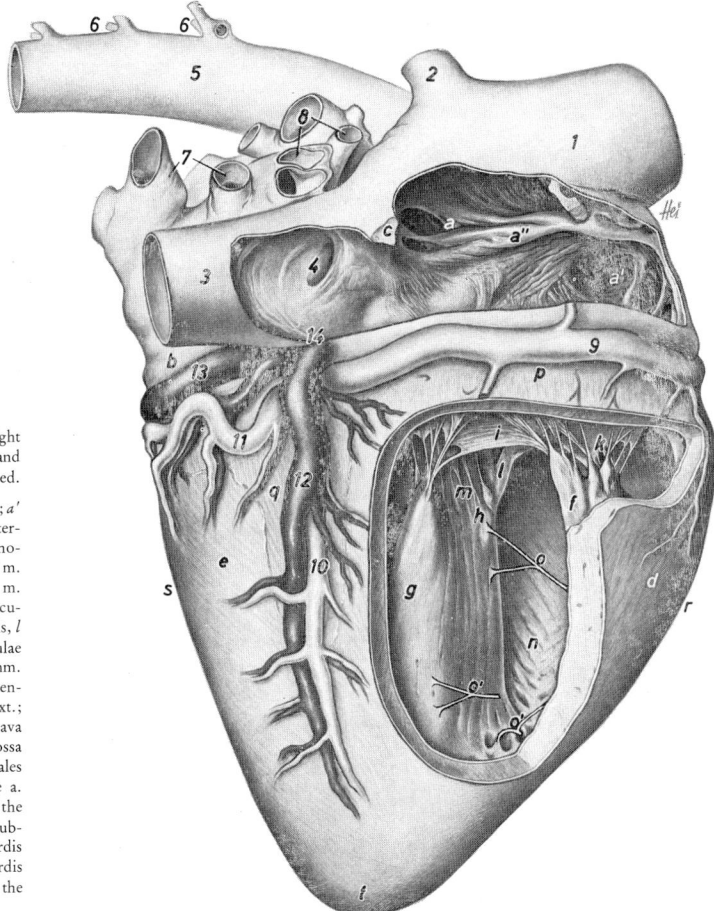

Fig. 10. Atrial surface of a horse's heart. Right atrium and right ventricle have been opened and the subepicardial adipose tissue has been removed.

a atrium dext. with the sinus venarum cavarum; *a'* auricula dext. with mm. pectinati; *a"* crista terminalis; *b* atrium sin.; *c* tuberculum intervenosum; *d* ventriculus dext.; *e* ventriculus sin.; *f* m. papillaris magnus; *g* mm. papillares parvi; *h* m. papillaris subarteriosus; *i, k, l* valva atrioventricularis dext., *i* cuspis parietalis, *k* cuspis angularis, *l* cuspis septalis; *m* chordae tendineae; *n* trabeculae carneae; *o* trabecula septomarginalis; *o'* mm. transversi; *p* sulcus coronarius; *q* sulcus interventricularis subsinuosus; *r* margo ventricularis dext.; *s* margo ventricularis sin.; *t* apex cordis *1* v. cava cran.; *2* v. azygos dext.; *3* v. cava caud.; *4* fossa ovalis; *5* aorta thoracica *6,6* aa. intercostales dorss.; *7* vv. pulmonales; *8* branches of the a. pulmonalis dext.; *9* r. circumflexus (dext.) of the a. coronaria dext., *10* its r. interventricularis subsinuosus, *11* its r. coronarius sin.; *12* v. cordis media s. interventricularis subsinuosa; *13* v. cordis magna; *14* sinus coronarius (obscured by the caudal vena cava).

The chambers of the heart and their internal structure
(4, 9–14, 16–24)

The manner in which the heart is divided into a right venous (4/*a'*) and a left arterial (/*a*) part, each consisting of an atrium and a ventricle has already been described. We shall now discuss the structure and organisation of the four cavities of the heart and describe how they have become adapted to the special function they perform.

The atria of the heart (atria cordis)
(9–12, 14, 15, 21–23)

The **right** and **left atria** (*atrium dext. et sin.*) are separated from each other by the *septum interatriale* (14/*c*; 27/*m*). Of the two atria, the right is the more voluminous but both rise as a flat cupola over the *sulcus coronarius* and communicate with the ventricle of the same side through the *ostium atrioventricu-*

24   Atria of the heart

lare dext. (11, 12/*d* → *d'*; 21/*c*) and *sin.* (11. 12/*e* → *e'*; 23/*c*) respectively. Each of the atria has a blind diverticulum, the *articula cordis* (8/*A, B;* 9/*a', b;* 12/*a, b;* 21, 22, 23/*b*), which are turned towards the *facies auricularis* of the heart and curve around the origin of the aorta and the pulmonary trunk. Thus they occupy, together with subepicardial adipose tissue, the space next to the two great arteries.

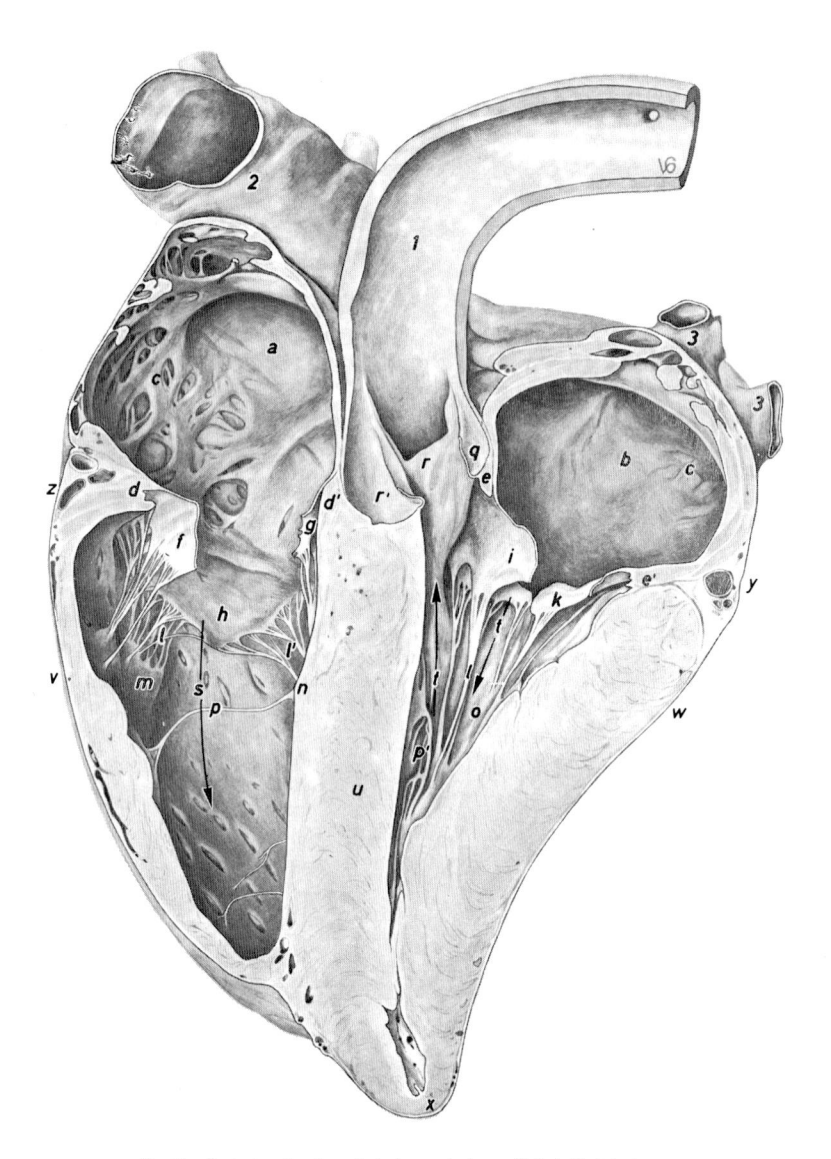

Fig. 11. Sagittal section through the heart of a horse. Right half of the heart.

a atrium dext.; *b* atrium sin.; *c* mm. pectinati; *d, d'* ostium atrioventriculare dext.; *e, e'* ostium atrioventriculare sin.; *f* cuspis parietalis; *g* cuspis septalis; *h* cuspis angularis of the valva atrioventricularis dext. s. tricuspidalis; *i* cuspis septalis, *k* cuspis parietalis of the valva atrioventricularis sin. s. bicuspidalis s. mitralis; *l, l'* chordae tendineae (*l'* going to the mm. papillares parvi); *n* base of the m. papillaris subarteriosus of the right ventricle; *m* m. papillaris magnus; *o* m. papillaris subatrialis of the left ventricle; *p, p'* trabeculae septomarginalis of the right and left ventricles respectively; *q, r, r'* valva aortae in the ostium aortae (between *d'* and *e*), *q* its valvula semilunaris sin., *r* dext. and *r'* septalis; *s* inflow tract of the right ventricle; *t, t* inflow and outflow tracts of the left ventricle; *u* septum interventriculare; *v* margo ventricularis dext.; *w* margo ventricularis sin.; *x* apex cordis; *y* sulcus coronarius, pars sin. with the r. circumflexus of the v. cordis magna and branches of the a. coronaria sin.; *z* sulcus coronarius, pars dext. with the r. circumflexus of the a. coronaria dext. and the accompanying veins

1 arcus aortae; *2* v. cava cran.; *3, 3* vv. pulmonales

Right atrium (atrium dext.)

On the exterior of the **right atrium** (10–12/*a*; 14/*b*; 21, 22/*a*) one can recognize a groove, the *sulcus terminalis*, which is generally shallow and which corresponds internally with the *crista terminalis* (10/*a*"). The sulcus and crista form the border between the embryonic *sinus venarum cavarum* and the true atrium. Through the *ostium venae cavae caud.*, which bears the *valvula v. cavae caud.*, the sinus receives the *caudal vena cava* (8/*n*; 10, 21, 23/3; 24/*b*) and through the *ostium venae caevae cran.* the

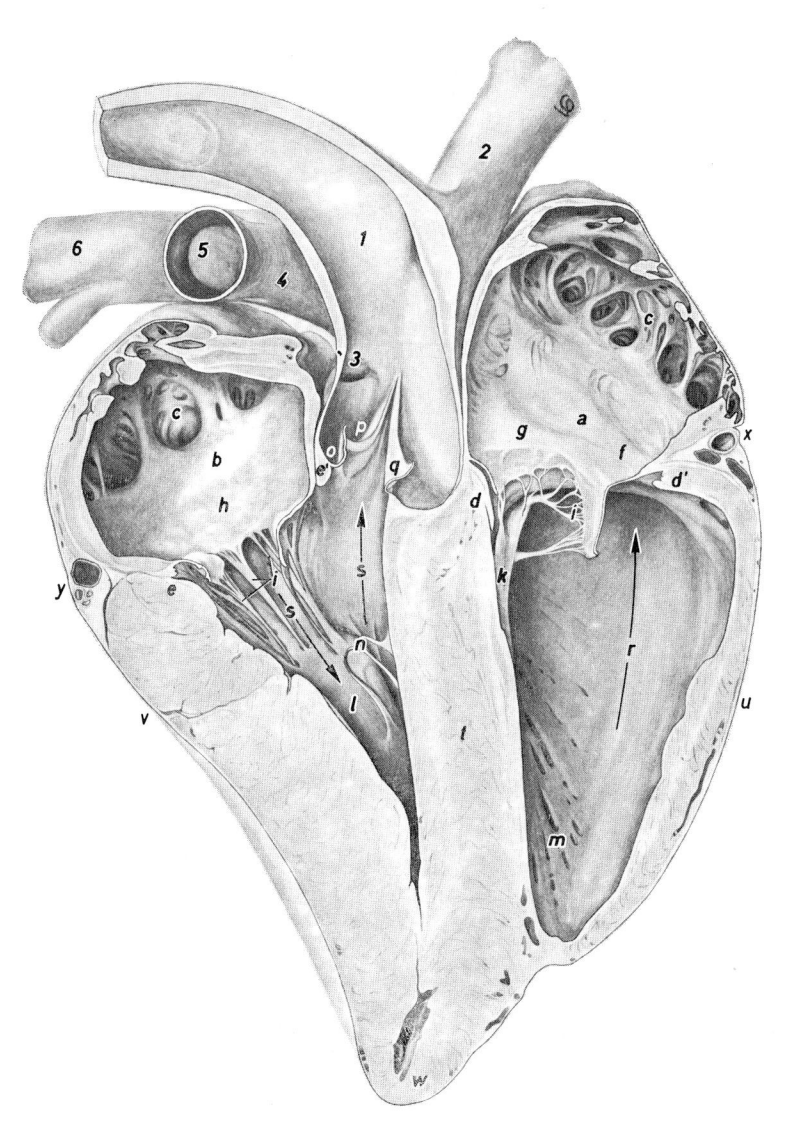

Fig. 12. Sagittal section through the heart of a horse. Left half.

a atrium dext. with view into the right auricle; *b* atrium sin. with view into the left auricle; *c, c* mm. pectinati; *d, d,* ostium atrioventriculare dext.; *e, e'* ostium atrioventriculare sin.; *f* cuspis parietalis; *g* cuspis septalis of the valva atrioventricularis dext. s. tricuspidalis; *h* cuspis parietalis of the valva atrioventricularis sin. s. bicuspidalis s. mitralis; *i, i* chordae tendineae; *k* m. papillaris subarteriosus of the right ventricle; *l* m. papillaris subauricularis of the left ventricle; *m* trabeculae carneae; *n* trabecula septomarginalis; *o, p, q* valva aortae in the ostium aortae (between *e'* and *d*), *o* its valvula semilunaris sin., *p* dext and *q* septalis; *r* outflow tract of the right, *s, s* inflow and outflow tracts of the left ventricle; *t* septum interventriculare; *u* margo ventricularis dext.; *v* margo ventricularis sin.; *w* apex cordis; *x* sulcus coronarius, pars dext. with the r. circumflexus of the a. coronaria dext. and accompanying veins; *y* sulcus coronarius, pars sin. with the r. circumflexus of the v. cordis magna and the r. circumflexus of the a. coronaria sin.

1 arcus aortae; *2* truncus brachiocephalicus; *3* origin of the a.coronaria sin.; *4* truncus pulmonalis; *5, 6* a. pulmonalis dext. and sin. respectively

cranial vena cava (8/*m*; 10, 21, 22/*1*) enters the sinus. There is also the short, tubular *sinus coronarius (10/14; 22/4; 29/11; 37/16)*, whose aperture below the orifice of the caudal vena cava is furnished with an indistinct *valvula sinus coronarii* (Thebesii) (24/*h*). The coronary sinus carries the blood from the cardiac veins and, in pigs and ruminants, also from the *v. azygos sin.* (36/8; 39/*e*) and discharges it into the *sinus venarum cavarum*. The blood from the *vv. cordis minimae* (Thebesii), draining the wall of the right atrium, enters the atrial cavity by way of numerous *foramina venarum minimarum*, In the roof of the sinus venarum cavarum between the ostia of the two caval veins, and projecting into their blood stream, is a muscular protruberance, the *tuberculum intervenosum* (10/*c*; 14/*d*) which diverts the blood, coming in the opposite direction from the caval veins, into the right atrioventricular orifice. More striking still is the function of the intervenous tubercle in the foetal heart which guides the blood from the caudal vena cava into the *foramen ovale* of the interatrial septum. In the left atrium occurs the *valvula foraminis ovalis* of the *septum primum* of the embryonic heart, which prevents the back flow of the blood which has passed from the right into the left atrium. The valve fuses with the *septum secundum* after birth and closes the foramen ovale which then becomes the *fossa ovalis*. The fossa remains surrounded by the more or less insignificant *limbus fossae ovalis;* its floor is derived from the former valve of the oval foramen. The fossa ovalis (10/*4*; 24/*f*) can be recognized as a depression in the interatrial septum between the orifice of the caudal vena cava and the intervenous tubercle.

In addition to the oval foramen, mention should be made of another special structure associated with the foetal circulation. This is the *ductus arteriosus*. Even in the foetus the venous blood from the head, neck, anterior part of the trunk and from the forelimbs passes through the cranial vena cava to gain access to the right atrium and right ventricle and thence to the truncus pulmonalis. But the lung does not function during intrauterine life because the placenta is responsible for the entire exchange process, so the blood from rhe pulmonary trunk is shunted through the wide ductus arteriosus into the neighbouring aorta. From here it is passed to the systemic and placentar circulation together with the blood which enters the left heart through the foramen ovale. Only a small amount of blood, necessary to nourish the organ, passes from the pulmonary trunk through the pulmonary artery into the lung. As the lung unfolds after birth, the route is opened for the blood to enter the pulmonary circulation. At the same time the pressure in the two atria is equalised so that, as well as from the closure of the foramen ovale, there is an obliteration of the vascular bridge between aorta and pulmonary trunk. The vestigial ductus arteriosus remains throughout life as the *ligamentum arteriosum* (Botalli) (9/*9*; 38/*d*) which links the two great arteries. The closure of the foramen ovale (10/*4*) and of the ductus arteriosus takes place during the first weeks of post-natal life. In the case of the oval foramen, however, this process may occupy several months as it does, for instance, in the ox, or it may remain incompletely closed throughout life without causing clinical manifestations of malfunction.

The *tuberculum intervenosum* of the right atrium continues as the muscular swelling known as the *crista terminalis* (10/*a"*). It encircles the orifice of the cranial vena cava (/*1*) and continues on to the ostium of the caudal vena cava (/*3*) or to the mouth of the coronary sinus (/*14*). The *mm. pectinati* arise from the crista terminalis and dominate the interior of the atrium and its auricle. They branch freely and so form, especially in the auricle, a network with meshes of varying size (9/*a*; 10/*a'*; 12/*c, c*; 14). Between these muscles the atrial wall is very thin and in those areas where the musculature is totally absent, the wall of the atrium is made up solely of endocardium and epicardium.

Left atrium (atrium sin.)

The **left atrium** (10–12; 14, 23/*a*) is less spacious than the right. The border of its *auricle* (9/*a*; 12, 23/*b*) is in contact with the pulmonary trunk (9/*3*; 28/*4*) and is notched in similar manner to that of the right atrium of ruminants. The left atrium receives arterial blood from the *vv. pulmonales* (8/*l, l*; 9/*10*; 10/*7*; 11/*3*; 23/*5*) through the *ostia venarum pulmonarum* (14/*f*). The number of these varies between 5 and 8 but usually there are 7, two of which stand out because of their wide lumina. The variable number of pulmonary veins is accounted for by the fact that during the development of the heart two pulmonary veins arise first from the pulmonary trunk and subsequently and indeterminate number of its branches are assimilated into the wall of the enlarging left atrium.

In the *septum interatriale* the scar resulting from the closure of the *foramen ovale* by the *valvula foraminis ovalis* can be recognised. The internal relief of the left atrial wall (14/*a*) resembles that of the right atrium because of the presence and arrangement of the *mm. pectinati*. There is also a similarity in the appearance of the wall between these muscular pillars. As in the case of the sinus venarum cavarum of the right atrium, that part of the wall of the left atrium which receives the pulmonary veins remains free of muscle pillars. The wall of the atrium sin. is also supplied with *vv. cordis minimae*.

The ventricles of the heart (ventriculi cordis)
(8–12, 16–23)

Right ventricle (ventriculus cordis dext.)

The **right ventricle** (*ventriculus dexter*) (8/E; 10/d; 11/s; 12/r; 16–22) receives blood from the right atrium through the *ostium atrioventriculare dext.* (11, 12/d → d'; 21, 22/c) and conveys it, under relatively low pressure, through its *conus arteriosus* (9/p; 22/e) and the truncus pulmonalis (/3; /8) to the lung. The wall of the right ventricle is only about half as thick as that of the left, because its work load is relatively low. The right ventricle forms the *margo ventricularis dext.* (10/r), extends from the *sulcus interventricularis subsinuosus* (/q) to the *sulcus interventricularis paraconalis* (9/l) and does not reach the apex of the heart. The lumen of the right ventricle appears semilunar in cross section because, especially during systole, its outer wall is moulded against its convex inner wall, the *septum interventriculare* (11/u; 22, 25, 26).

The cavity of the right ventricle has two functionally distinct sections. The first, the true ventricular cavity, extends towards the apex from the interventricular orifice, and is termed the *inflow route* (11/s). The second is the *expulsion route* (12/r) which, starting at the apex, includes the conus arteriosus which continues into the truncus pulmonalis. In the region of the inflow route the ventricular wall carries the *trabeculae carnae*, which are particularly well developed in the area near the interventricular grooves. They are not present in the region of the expulsion route and the conus arteriosus.

Apart from the trabeculae carnae there are a variable number of rounded muscular beams which form cross connections between the septum and the outer wall of the ventricle. One of these is especially

Fig. 13. Base of the bovine heart. The ventricles, atria and in part also the aorta and pulmonary trunk have been removed close to their origin. Basal aspect. (After Preuss, 1955.)

a ostium trunci pulmonalis; *b* ostium aortae; *c* a. coronaria dext.; *d* a. coronaria sin.; *e* r. interventricularis paraconalis of the v. cordis magna; *f* v. cordis media s. interventricularis subsinuosa

1, 2, 3 valva trunci pulmonalis, *1* its valvula semilunaris sin., *2* dext. and *3* intermedia; *4, 5, 6* valva aortae, *4* its valvula semilunaris sin., *5* dext and *6* septalis; *7, 8* valva atrioventricularis sin. s. bicuspidalis (mitralis), *7* its cuspis septalis and *8* parietalis; *9, 10, 11* valva atrioventricularis dext. s. tricuspidalis, *9* its cuspis septalis, *10* parietalis and *11* angularis; *12* trabecula septomarginalis; *13* auricula dext.; *14* auricula sin.; *15* m. papillaris subauricularis; *16* m. papillaris subatrialis of the left ventricle; *17* position of the m. papillaris subarteriosus; *18* m. papillaris magnus; *19* mm. papillares parvi of the right ventricle; *20, 20* sinus coronarius; *21* margo ventricularis dext.; *22* margo ventricularis sin.; *23* sulcus interventricularis subsinuosus; *24* sulcus interventricularis paraconalis; *25* conus arteriosus

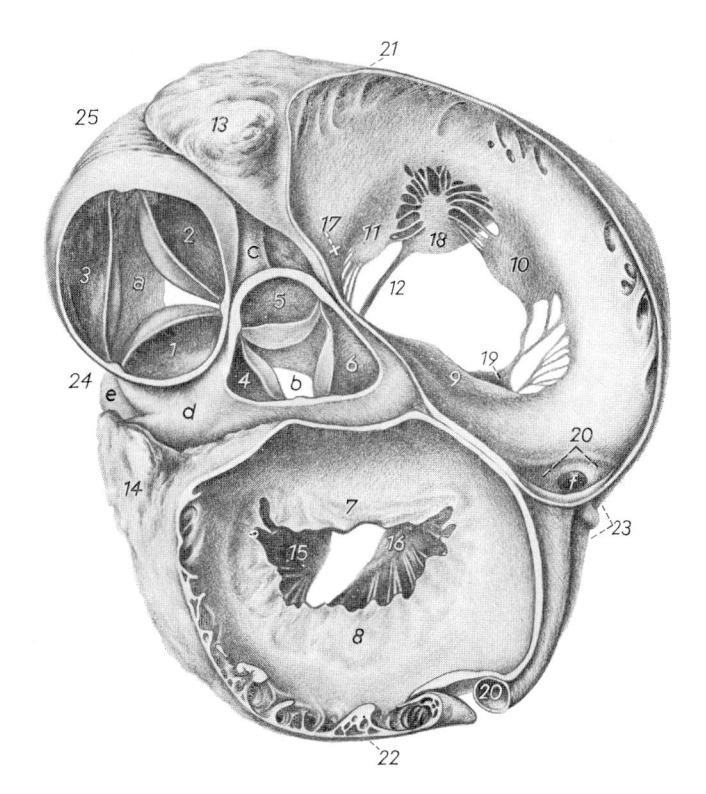

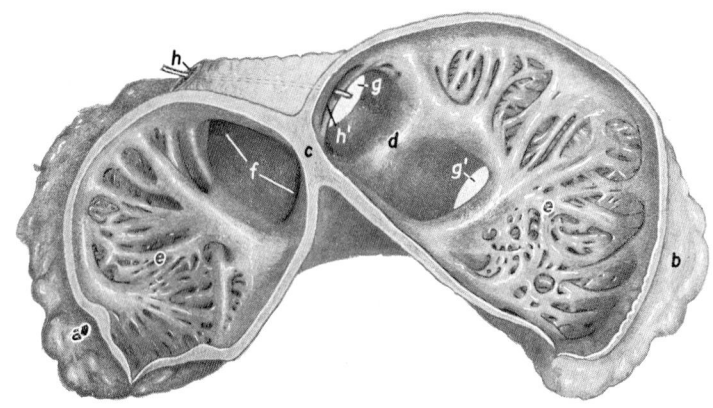

Fig. 14. View into the atria of the heart of a pig which has been transected at the coronary groove. (After Steger, 1927.)

a left, *b* right atrium; *c* septum interatriale; *d* tuberculum intervenosum; *e, e* mm. pectinati; *f* ostia of the vv. pulmonales; *g, g'* ostia of the v. cava cran. and caud.; *h* v. azygos sin. (hemiazygos), *h'* its mouth

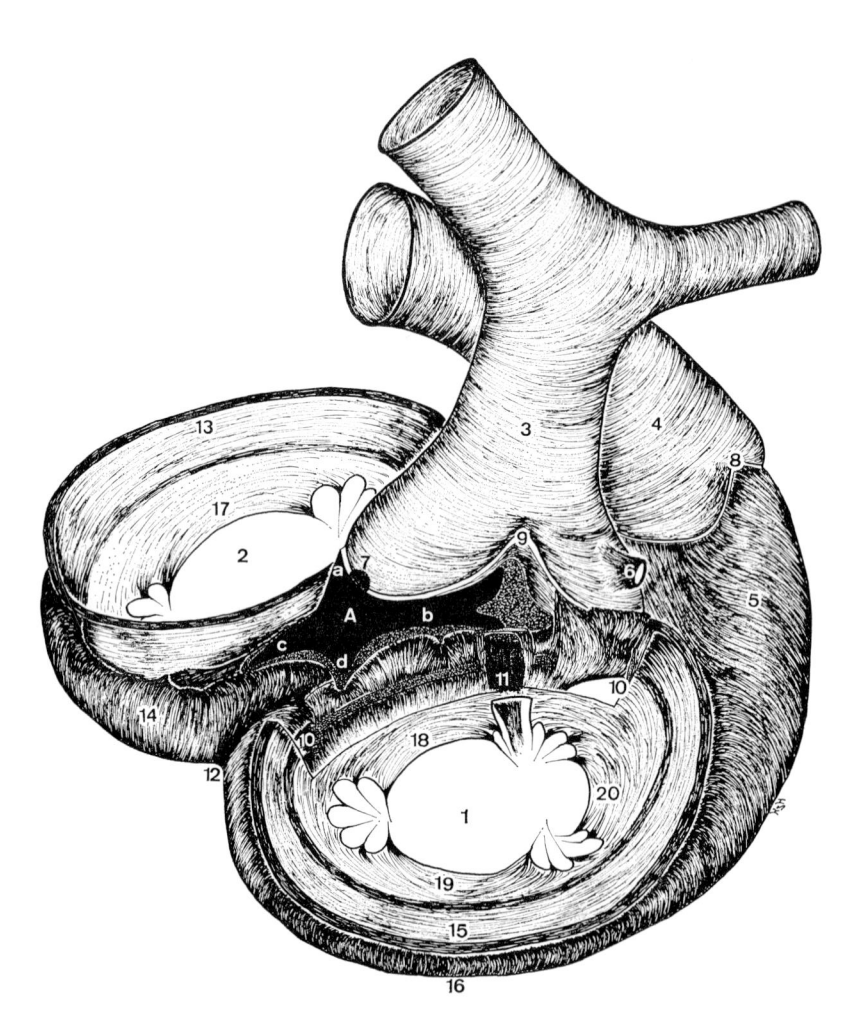

Fig. 15. Heart skeleton of the ox. Right dorsal view. (After Schmack, Diss. med. vet., Giessen, 1974.)

A os cordis dext. with its processes *a, b, c, d*

1 ostium atrioventriculare dext.; *2* ostium atrioventriculare sin.; *3* aorta; *4* truncus pulmonalis; *5* conus arteriosus; *6* a. coronaria dext.; *7* origin of the ligament between the aorta and vena cava caud.; *8* anulus fibrosus trunci pulmonalis; *9* anulus fibrosus aortae; *10* anulus fibrosus atrioventricularis dext.; *11* nodus atrioventricularis; *12* sulcus interventricularis subsinuosus; *13* wall of the atrium sin.; *14* wall of the ventriculus sin.; *15* wall of the atrium dext.; *16* wall of the ventriculus dext.; *17* cuspis parietalis of the valva bicuspidalis; *18* cuspis septalis, *19* cuspis parietalis, *20* cuspis angularis of the valva tricuspidalis

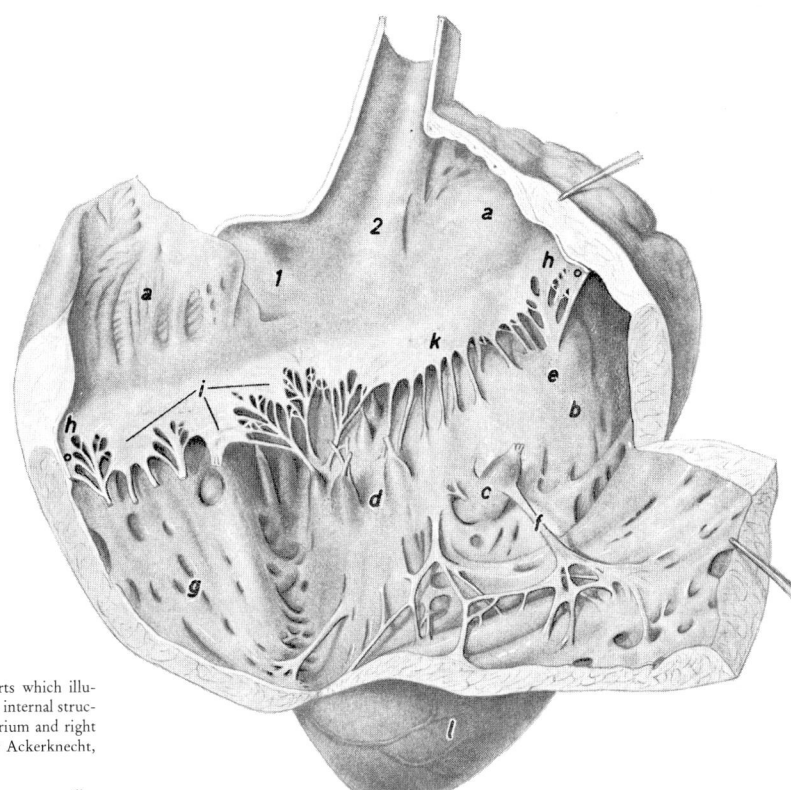

Figs. 16 and 17. Two canine hearts which illustrate the individual variation of the internal structure of the heart. Both the right atrium and right ventricle have been opened. (After Ackerknecht, 1918.)

a, a atrium dext.; *b* ventriculus dext.; *c* m. papillaris magnus; *d, d* mm. papillares parvi; *e* m. papillaris subarteriosus; *f, f* trabecula septomarginalis; *g* trabeculae carneae; *h, i, k* valva atrioventricularis dext., *h, h* cuspis angularis, *i.* cuspis parietalis, *k* cuspis septalis; *l* ventriculus sin.

1 and *2* termination of the v. cava cran. and caud.; *3* (in fig. 17) conus arteriosus

In fig. 16 all the papillary muscles are situated on the septum while in the heart illustrated in fig. 17 not only the m. papillaris magnus but also some of the mm. papillares parvi arise from the outer wall. Note also the attachment of the tendinous chords of the septal cusp to the so-called mm. papillares proprr. septales and the pleomorphism of the mm. transversi in fig. 16

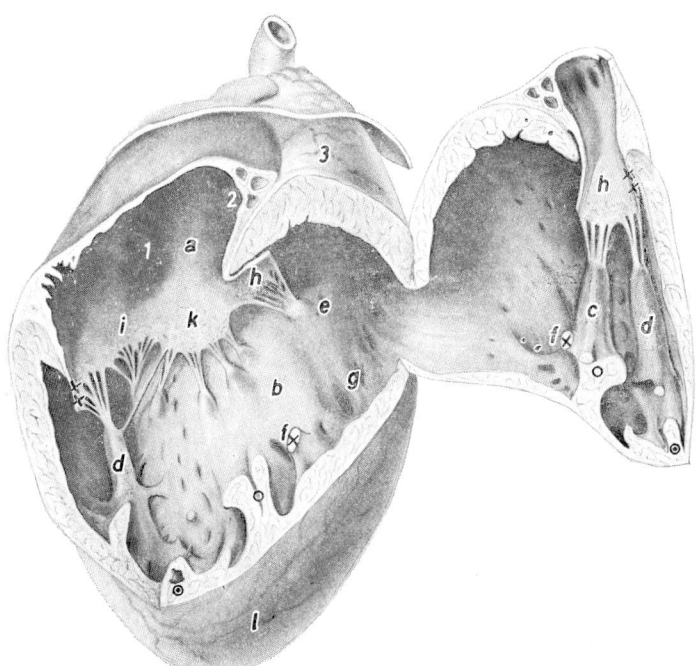

powerful and runs from the septum below the *subarterial m. papillaris* (13/*17*; 19, 20/*e*) to the base of the *m. papillaris magnus* /*18*;/*c*). It represents the *trabecula septomarginalis* (11/*p*; 13/*12*; 19/*f*), an integral part of the conduction system of the heart which will be discussed below. Besides these muscular beams which are always present, there are generally other cross linkages which consist either of active musculature or connective tissue. These structures may contain the specialized cell complexes of the conduction system known as *Purkinje fibres*.

Three papillary muscles (*mm. papillares*) project into the right ventricle. They have a special function and show species and individual variations in shape. One of these papillary muscles of the septum of the right ventricle is termes *m. papillaris subarteriosus* (10/*h*; 12/*k*; 13/*17*; 19, 20/*e*) because of its proximity to the pulmonary trunk. The second comprises a group of muscles, also situated on the septum, which forms a functional unit known collectively as the *mm. papillares parvi* (10/*g*; 11/*l'*; 13/;»; 19, 20/*d*). The third and largest papillary muscle is the *m. papillaris magnus* (/*f*; /*m*; /*18*; /*c*), which is generally located on the outer wall but, especially in carnivores, can extend on to, or even be entirely displaced to, the septum (16/*c*).

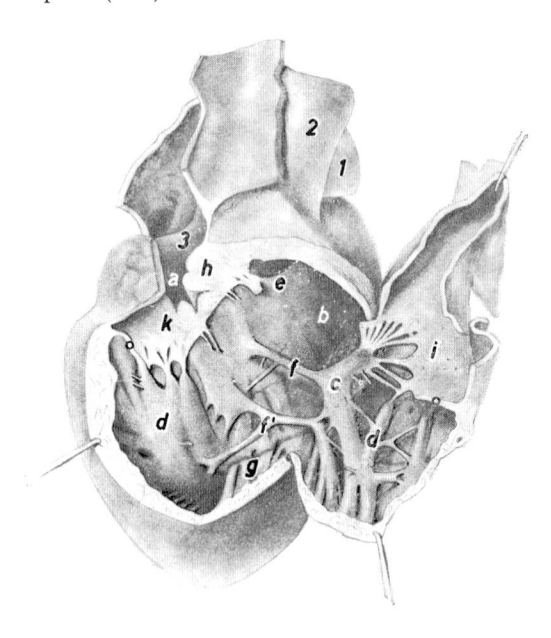

Fig. 18. Heart of a cat. Right atrium and right ventricles have been opened. (After Ackerknecht, 1918.)

a atrium dext.; *b* ventriculus dext.; *c* m. papillaris magnus; *d* mm. papillares parvi; *e* m. papillaris subarteriosus; *f* trabecula septomarginalis; *f'* mm. transversi; *g* trabeculae carneae; *h*, *i*, *k* valva atrioventricularis dext., *h* cuspis angularis, *i* cuspis parietalis, *k* cuspis septalis

1 aorta; *2* truncus pulmonalis; *3* tuberculum intervenosum between the termination of the two caval veins

The papillary muscles give rise to groups of *chordae tendineae* (11/*l*, *l'*) which fan out and radiate into the free borders and onto the luminal surface of the tricuspid valve (*valva atrioventricularis dextra s. tricuspidalis*) (13/*9*, *10*, *11*; 20, 30, 34, 37, 43, 46). The latter originates at the anulus fibrosus (cf. p. 78), surrounds the *ostium atrioventriculare dext.*, and divides into three *cusps* which projects into the lumen of the ventricle and can give rise to secondary cusps. Each of the main cusps is fixed by means of cordae to two papillary muscles. The *valva atrioventriculare dext.* has three cusps, the *cuspis septalis* (13/*9*) which originates from the interventricular septum; the *cuspis parietalis* (/*10*) from the outer wall and the third and smallest the *cuspis angularis* (/*11*) which is situated in the angle between the other two cusps. The framework of these valves is a tendinous membrane, the collagenous fibres of which arise from the anulus fibrosus of the atrioventricular orifice and are linked with the fibres of the tendinous chords. In the basal region of the valves there are also muscle fibres and blood vessels which are confined exclusively to this area. The fibrous middle layer of the valve is covered on both surfaces with endocardium, and this also envelops the chordae tendineae.

The *valva atrioventricularis dext.* acts as a non-return valve. The papillary muscles have the function of maintaining the tendinous chords under tension when the valve plane is displaced during the phases of heart action. During the *diastolic* filling phase the open valve allows the blood to pass freely from the atrium to the ventricle; it is partly sucked in due to the lowering of the valve plane and partly propelled by the atrial musculature. With the commencement of *systole* and onset of the phase of increased pressure the atrioventricular valve closes. This is achieved by contraction of the papillary muscles which, through the tendinous chords, exert a pull on the cusps, which are then unfolded and apposed at their broad rims. The only route for the blood to reach the truncus pulmonalis is through the expulsion route (12/r), which consists mainly of the conus arteriosus.

Thus, during systole, the blood cannot return into the atrium because the atrioventricular valve is closed. Similarly, during diastole, its return into the ventricle is prevented by the tricuspid *valva trunci pulmonalis* (13/1, 2, 3) which is located in the orifice of the pulmonary trunk (/a) and is made up of the three half-moon-shaped *valvulae semilunares*. In accordance with their position they are known respectively as *valvula semilunaris sin.* (/1), *dext.* (/2) and *intermed.* (/3). They consist of a double layer of endothelium supported by an intervening layer of collagen fibres. They are attached to the fibrous ring of the aperture of the pulmonary trunk and their crescentic forms project into the lumen of the vessel, so that their cavities point peripherally (9/4). Their free borders are slightly thickened and in the middle carry a small, hard nodule, the *nodulus valvulae semilunaris,* which is flanked on either side by a crescent transparent part, the *lunulae valvulae*. In the region of the valves the vessel wall is bulged to form the *sinus trunci pulmonales* (22/7, 7).

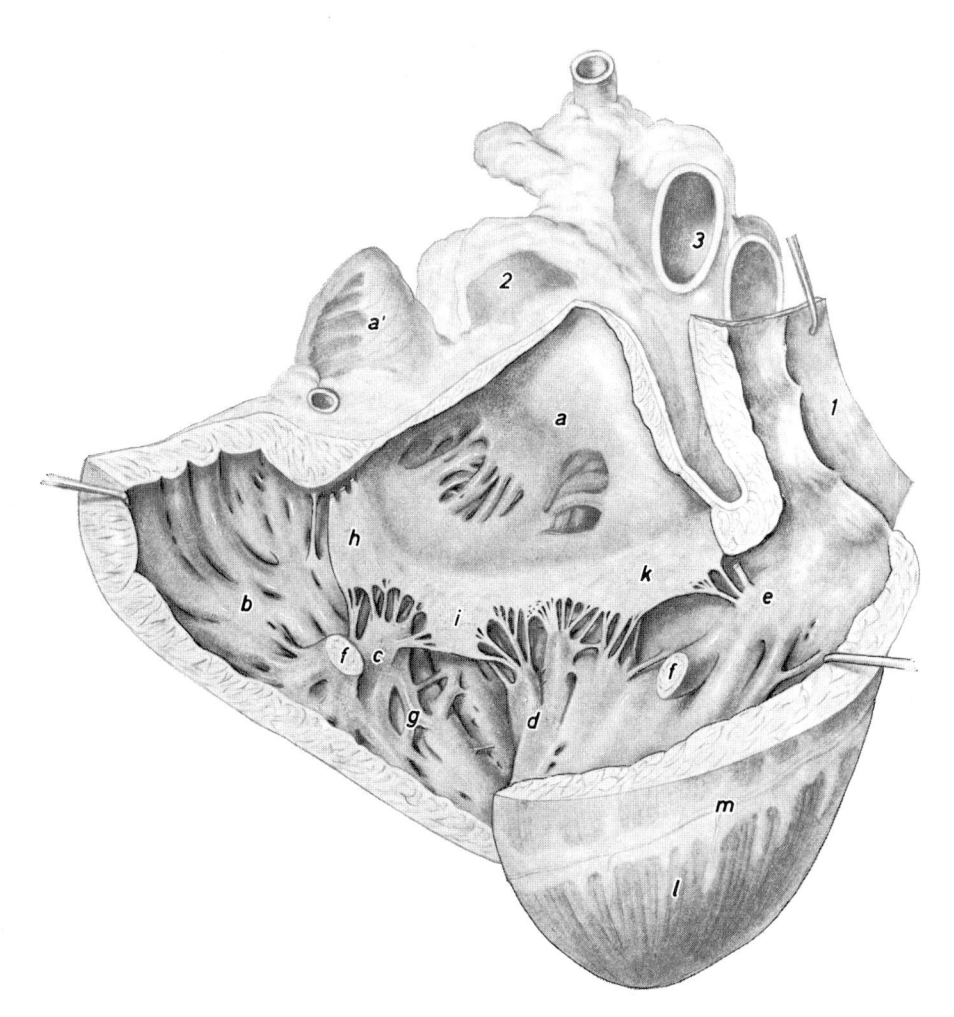

Fig. 19. Heart of a pig. Right atrium and ventricle exposed. (After Huwyler, 1926.)

a atrium dext. with mm. pectinati; *a'* auricula dext.; *b* ventriculus dext.; *c* m. papillaris magnus; *d* mm. papillares parvi; *e* m. papillaris subarteriosus; *f, f* trabecula septomarginalis, transected; *g* trabeculae carneae; *h* cuspis angularis, *i* parietalis and *k* septalis of the valva atrioventricularis dext.; *l* ventriculus sin.; *m* sulcus interventricularis paraconalis

1 truncus pulmonalis, has been opened to provide a better view of its valves; *2* v. cava cran.; *3* aorta

This pulmonary valve, like the atrioventricular, acts as a non-return valve in the orifice of the pulmonary trunk. During the expulsion phase the upstream-directed blood pressure causes the valves to lie against the vessel wall. With the onset of diastole the downstream-directed pressure of the column of blood in the pulmonary trunk causes the valves to fill and so close the orifice. During this process the valvular nodules are said to close the central part of the vessel's lumen.

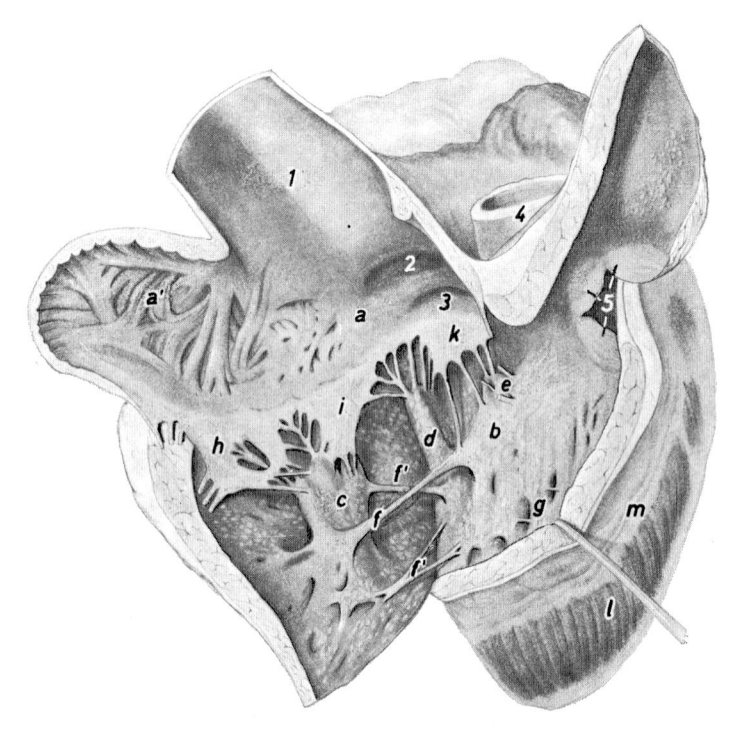

Fig. 20 Heart of a sheep. Right atrium and right ventricle have been opened. (After Angst, 1928.)

a atrium dext.; *a'* auricula dext. with mm. pectinati; *b* ventriculus dext.; *c* m. papillaris magnus; *d* mm. papillares parvi; *e* m. papillaris subarteriosus; *f* trabeculae septomarginalis; *f'*, *f'* mm. transversi; *g* trabeculae carneae; *h* cuspis angularis, *i* parietalis and *k* septalis of the valva atrioventricularis dext.; *l* ventriculus sin.; *m* sulcus interventricularis paraconalis

1 v. cava cran., exposed; *2* termination in the atrium of the v. cava caud. and *3* of the sinus coronarius into the atrium; *4* truncus pulmonalis; *5* ostium and valva trunci pulmonalis. Note the patchy distribution of the subendocardial adipose tissue

Left ventricle (ventriculus cordis sin.)

The **ventriculus sinister** (9/c; 11/t; 12/s; 23) receives its blood from the left atrium through the *ostium atrioventriculare sin.* (11, 12/e–e') and it pumps it with great force through the aorta into the systemic circulation. To accomplish this its muscular wall is very thick being, indeed, two to three times thicker than the outer wall of the right ventricle. The same is true of the *septum interventriculare* (11/u) which forms a functional unit with the outer wall of the left ventricle, and, in fact, the contour of the outer wall is continued by the septum, so that it bulges into the lumen of the right ventricle (25, 26). The capacity of the left ventricle is less than that of the right although its cavity reaches down to the apex where the muscular wall is only a few millimeters thick. In the left, as in the right ventricle, we can differentiate an *inflow* and an *expulsion route* (11/t, t; 12/s, s). The former is situated under the atrioventricular orifice and extends to the apex of the heart. The expulsion route extends from the apex as a groove-like channel passing into the *bulbus aortae* and is limited on the one hand by the interventricular septum and on the other by the septal cusp of the left atrioventricular valve (11/i). The *trabeculae carneae* are less numerous than in the right ventricle but are concentrated in the apical region and shallow recesses are formed between them.

A thick, bifurcated cross-beam, the *trabecula septomarginalis* (moderator band) which is part of the conducting system, runs from the intervertebral septum to the base of the two papillary muscles (9/*i*; 12/*n*). In addition to this cross-beam one may find smaller bands, especially in the apical region. The two papillary muscles of the left ventricle are situated on the outer wall and are termed, according to their location, *m. papillaris subauricularis* (12/*l*; 13/*15*) and *subatrialis* (9/*e*; 11/*o*; 13/*16*). Their *chordae tendinaea* go to the bicuspid *valva atrioventricularis sin. s. valva bucuspidalis s. valva mitralis*. The valve originates at the fibrous ring which surrounds the left atrioventricular orifice (9, 11, 12, 13, 27, 30). Because of their location the two cusps are termed *cuspis septalis* (11/*i*; 13/*7*) and *cuspis parietalis* (11/*k*; 12/*h*; 13/*8*) respectively. The septal cusp is very large and divides the *ostium aortae* from the *ostium atrioventriculare* and also therefore, separates the inflow from the expulsion route (11, 12). The tissue components are similar in the bicuspid and the tricuspid valves of the left and right ventricles respectively.

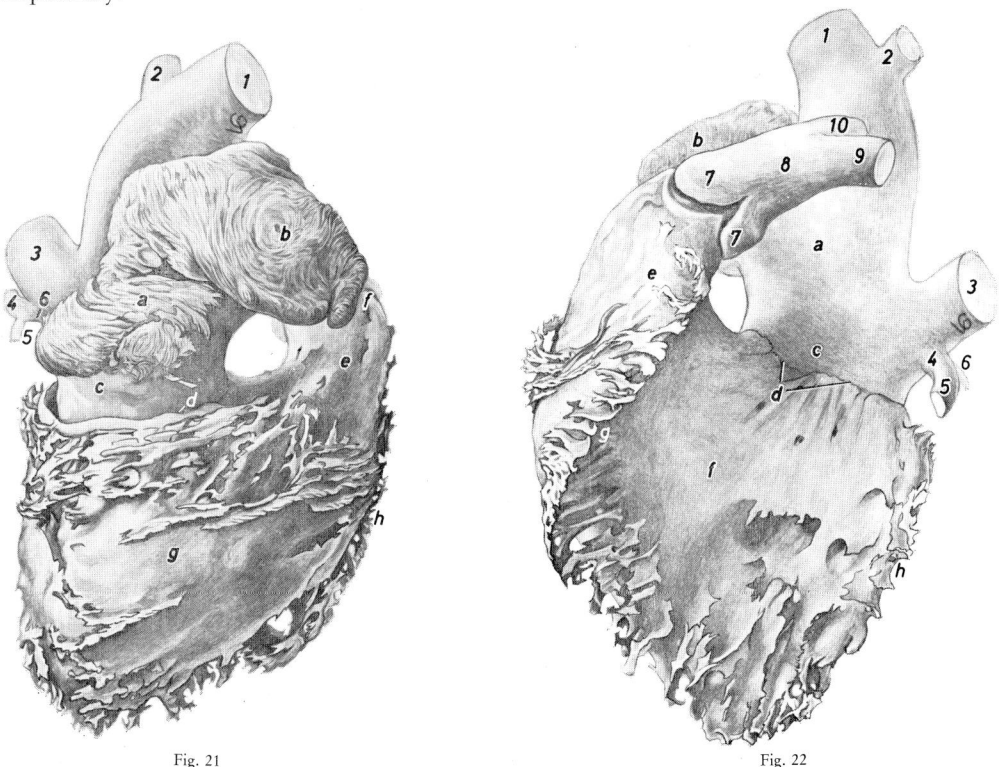

Fig. 21   Fig. 22

Fig. 21 Plastoid cast of the right half of a dog's heart. Right-cranial view. It shows the internal irregularities of the atrial and ventricular walls which are due to the mm. pectinati and the trabeculae carneae.

a atrium dext.; *b* auricula dext.; *c* ostium atrioventriculare dext.; *d* sulcus coronarius; *e* conus arteriosus; *f* truncus pulmonalis; *g* ventriculus dext., *h* its border lying nearest the sulcus interventricularis paraconalis

1 v. cava cran.; *2* v. azygos dext.; *3* v. cava caud.; *4* v. cordis magna; *5* v. cordis media; *6* sinus coronarius

Fig. 22. Plastoid cast of the right half of a dog's heart. Viewed as from the septum. It shows the internal irregularities of the atrium and ventricle caused by the mm. pectinati, the trabeculae carneae and the mm. papillares.

a atrium dext.; *b* auricula dext.; *c* ostium atrioventriculare dext.; *d* insertion point of the valva atrioventricularis dext.; *e* conus arteriosus; *f* ventriculus dext., *g* its border neighbouring on the sulcus interventricularis paraconalis; and *h* on the sulcus interventricularis subsinuosus

1 v. cava cran.; *2* v. azygos dext; *3* v. cava caud.; *4* sinus coronarius; *5* v. cordis magna; *6* v. cordis media; *7, 7* sinus of the valva trunci pulmonalis; *8* truncus pulmonalis; *9* and *10* a. pulmonalis sin. and dext. respectively

The *valva aorta* (11, 12, 13), located in the *ostium aortae*, consists, like the valve of the pulmonary trunk, of three parts, the *valvula semilunaris septalis* (11/*r'*; 12/*q*; 13/*6*) and the *valvulae semilunares dext.* (/*r*; /*p*; /*5*) *et sin.* (/*q*; /*o*; /*4*). Because of the greater demand made upon it, it is more strongly developed than the corresponding valve of the pulmonary trunk and its noduli valvarum are more prominent than in the former. In the region of the semilunar valves the wall of the aorta is distinctly bulged to form the three *sinus aortae*. It should be mentioned here that the *a. coronaria dext.* arises from the right sinus and the *a. coronaria sin.* (13/c, d) from the left sinus. The atrioventricular and aortic valves of the left heart perform the same function during systole and diastole as the corresponding valves of the right heart.

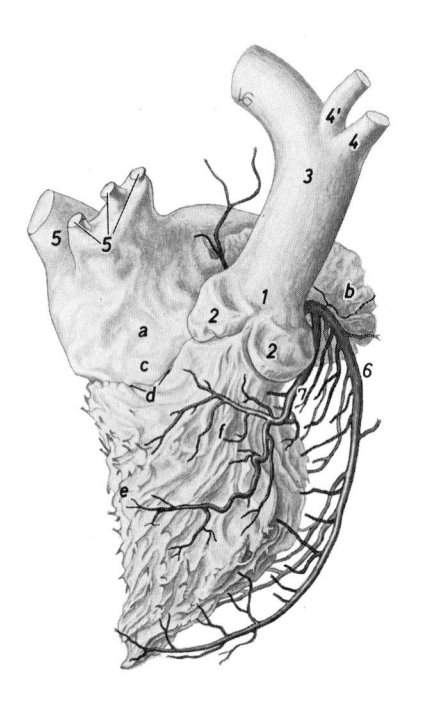

Fig. 23. Plastoid cast of the left half of the heart of a dog. Right cranial view. It shows the internal irregularities of the atrium and ventricle caused by the mm. pectinati and the trabeculae carneae.

a atrium sin.; *b* auricula sin.; *c* ostium atrioventriculare sin.; *d* site of insertion of the valva atrioventricularis sin.; *e* septal surface of the left ventricle showing the numerous stumps of the vv. cordis minimae; *f* right lateral surface of the left ventricle

1 ostium aortae; *2* sinus of the valva aortae; *3* arcus aortae; *4* a. brachiocephalica; *4'* a. subclavia sin.; *5, 5* vv. pulmonales; *6* r. interventricularis paraconalis of the a. coronaria sin.; *7* r. septi interventricularis

Excitation and conducting system of the heart
(24, 24 a)

It has already been pointed out that when birds and mammals became homeothermic they had to undergo numerous adaptations which included intensification of metabolism and a consequent increased demand for oxygen. This, in turn, led to an increase in the requirements made on the circulatory system which, in the course of phylogenetic development, has brought about an anatomical and functional division of the heart into an arterial half and a venous half. It became necessary for the heart, in its most advanced functional form to have independent automatic control over its atrial and ventricular musculature, so that the individual phases of action could be coordinated and the overall rhythm maintained. Warm-blooded animals were phylogenetically the first to have a morphologically recognisable *excitation* and *conducting system* (24, 24 a). In mammals this system consists of two nodes which have been named the *Keith-Flack* and the *Aschoff-Tawara* nodes after their discoverers; they are also known, according to their topography, as the *nodus sinuatrialis* (24/1) and *nodus atrioventricularis* (/2) respectively. The system also contains the bundle of His *(fasciculus atrioventricularis)* consisting of the *truncus fasciculi* (/3) and the *crus dext.* (/4) and *sin.* (/5). These branch and finally terminate in a network of remarkable cell complexes known as the *Purkinje fibres*. Each section of this system, which ensures the autonomy of the heart, has the basic ability to initiate excitation but there is a gradual decrease in grequency from the sinuatrial node to the Purkinje fibres. Under physiological conditions the stimulus commences in the sinuatrial node which is the dominant site of the system and determines the rhythm of the heart; it is therefore called the *"pacemaker."*

The sinuatrial node (24/1) is situated in the region of the *sulcus terminalis* of the right atrium and the opening of the cranial vena cava. It is embedded without sharp demarcation in the musculature which continues from the atrium onto the cranial vena cava. In the heart of large mammals it can be demonstrated by dissection since it is of lighter colour than the atrial musculature. In smaller species it can only be demonstrated microscopically and it is then identified by its specific musculature, its overall structure and by the fact that it contains connective tissue and nerves and has a special type of blood supply.

Compared with the contractile musculature which surrounds it, the sinuatrial node is much looser in structure because of its rich content of connective tissue. The muscle fibres of the node have a circular

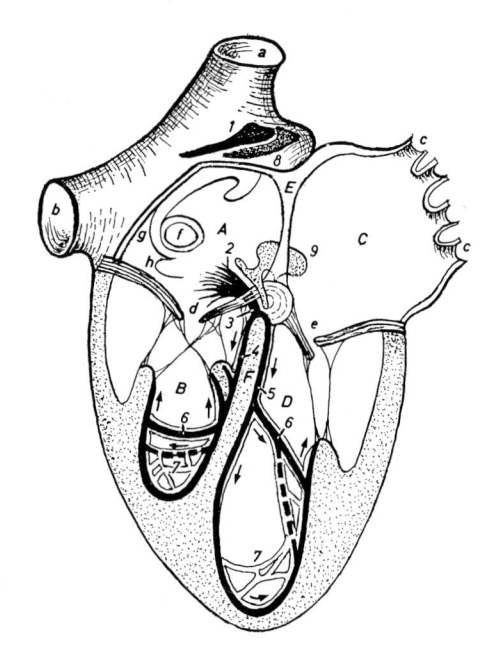

Fig. 24. Diagram of the excitation and conducting system. (After Ackerknecht, 1943.)

A atrium dext.; *B* ventriculus dext.; *C* atrium sin.; *D* ventriculus sin.; *E* septum interatriale; *F* septum interventriculare

a v. cava cran.; *b* v. cava caud.; *c* vv. pulmonales; *d, e* ostium atrioventriculare dext. and sin. with their valves; *f* fossa ovalis; *g* valvula v. cavae caud.; *h* valvula sinus coronarii;

1 nodus sinuatrialis; *2* nodus atrioventricularis; *3, 4, 5* fasciculus atrioventricularis, *3* its truncus, *4, 5* its crus dext. and sin.; *6, 6* trabeculae septomarginales; *7, 7* mm. transversi; *8* ganglion sinuatriale; *9* ganglion atrioventriculare

course in the neighbourhood of blood vessels, whereas they are longitudinally orientated elsewhere. In some animals, such as the sheep, they form muscular plexuses, and in the dog their course is irregular. Adjacent to the node there are also ganglion cells (*ganglion sinuatriale*) (24/8) whose nerve fibres enter the nodes. The connective tissue surrounding the node contains variable quantities of adipose tissue and provides only an indistinct delineation from the surrounding structures. The specialized muscle cells and their processes are connected by intercalated discs to neighbouring cells to form fibres whose diameter and length are distinctly less than those of the atrial musculature. Also, the round nuclei of the nodal cells are distinguishable from the elongated nuclei of the atrial muscle cells. The cross-striated fibrils are mainly located at the periphery of the cells of the node and they thus leave a space in the centre of the cell for the nucleus, the mitochondria, the endoplasmic reticulum and the Golgi apparatus.

Specialized impulse-conducting muscle fibres connecting the sinuatrial and the atrioventricular nodes have not been demonstrated in the atrial musculature. The *excitation wave* starts at the sinuatrial node and spreads throughout the entire contractile musculature of the right atrium and, with a delay of a fraction of a second, to the left atrium, thus causing them both to contract (atrial systole). From there the excitation wave reaches the atrioventricular node and finally, by way of the bundle of His, its two limbs and the Purkinje fibres, it spreads to the papillary muscles and the contractile musculature of the ventricles.

Before proceeding with a description of the topography of the atrioventricular node and the bundle of His, one should again stress that the contractile musculature of the atria is not connected to that of the ventricles, a fact which is of paramount importance to the function of the mammalian heart. The anuli fibrosi of the ostia represent an absolute demarcation between the musculature of the atria and the ventricles. The fibrous rings are bridged only and exclusively by the specialised musculature of the conducting system which carries the excitation from the musculature of the atria to that of the ventricles.

This second part of the excitation and conduction system commences at the elongated oval or club-shaped *nodus atrioventricularis* (24/2). In the dog it measures 3–4 mm long by 1–2 mm broad. In the ox it has a lenght of 0.8–1.3 cm and a breadth of 0.6–0.8 cm and it consists of an upper part lying against the large os cordis, and a lower part which is embedded in the atrial septum. In the horse the node measures 6–10 mm long, 5–7 mm broad and 0.6–2.5 mm thick. The node is embedded in the musculature of the atrial septum in which it fans out without any distinct demarcation or, as in the ox, it is surrounded by a connective tissue capsule. It is located in the floor of the right atrium not far from the mouth of the coronary sinus, above the *chiasma anuli fibrosi arteriosi*, a site at which the two *anuli fibrosi arteriosi* meet in a connective tissue bridge.

The short, circular or flat *bundle of His (truncus fasciculi atrioventricularis)* (/3), resembles a nerve trunk. It arises from the atrioventricular node, perforates the fibrous ring and reaches the apex of the interventricular septum subendocardially at the site of insertion of the *cuspis septalis* of the right ventricle. In the dog this is the site of transition from the *pars membranacea* to the *pars muscularis septi*. It now divides into the *crus dext.* and *sin*. The left limb (/5) crosses the apex of the interventricular septum and continues down its left surface towards the apex of the heart, initially in an intramuscular and later subendocardial position. About half way down the septum the left limb starts to branch; it gives off small ramifications to the septum, others enter the trabeculae carneae and yet others attain the base of the papillary muscles via the *trabeculae septomarginales* (/6, 7). Finally they terminate in the Purkinje fibres.

The right limb of the bundle of His (/4) is initially covered by the septal musculature as it runs behind the *mm. papillares parvi*. It gives off branches to the latter as well as to the *m. papillaris subarteriosus* and the interventricular septum. Subsequently this limb enters the thick *trabecula septomarginalis* (/6) of the right ventricle to reach the base of the *m. papillaris magnus*. Smaller branches go in other trabeculae to the outer wall of the ventricle. Like the ramifications of the left branch, those of the right terminate in Purkinje fibres.

The histological structure of the atrioventricular node is very similar to that of the sinuatrial node. They are both recognised by specific cells which are joined to muscle fibres by intercalated discs. The impulse conducting fibres form a network embedded in connective tissue and having a rich supply of blood vessels, nerve cells and nerve fibres. The overall structure is very loose in the ox and horse but denser in the pig and sheep. No structural differences have been demonstrated between the upper atrial part and the lower ventricular part of the node of the ox.

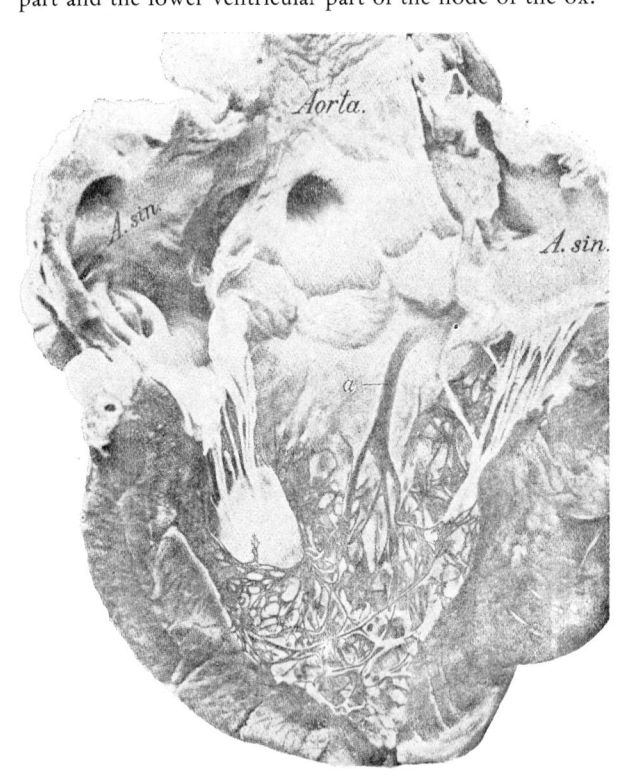

The specific fibres of the atrioventricular node (24/2) are continued in the trunk of the bundle of His (*truncus fasciculi atrioventricularis*) (/4) where they also form a network permeated by connective tissue and supplied by blood vessels and nerves. The fibres run parallel to the direction of the two limbs of the trunk and enter the much thicker Purkinje fibres which in ungulates can arise in close proximity to the limbs. The Purkinje fibres spread subendothelially in a netlike manner and link directly with the contractile musculature. In dogs and cats the specific fibres of the bundle of His are less distinctly differentiated from the fibres of the contractile musculature.

Fig. 24 a. Impulse conducting system in the heart of the ox. (After Aagaard and Hall, 1914.)

The left atrium (atrium sin.) and the left ventricle are opened. The course of the left limb of the bundle of His (a) and its terminal ramifications have been visualised by injection of their connective tissue sheaths

In cattle and horses the typical Purkinje fibres may reach a diameter of 80 to 100 μm and they are thus easily differentiated from the fibres of the contractile musculature which have a diameter of about 10 μm. They are made up of cells with extremely thin plasma membranes. Several neighbouring cells link to become fibres which are surrounded by a structureless basal membrane. The Purkinje cells have abundant cytoplasm which is rich in glycogen but contains few myofibrils. The latter are situated towards the periphery of the cell and connected with the fibril bundles of neighbouring cells by means of intercalated discs.

The fibre bundles of the conducting system are surrounded by a connective tissue capsule which can be demonstrated by the injection of dyes. The injected fluid enters the space between the capsule and the fibres and extends right up to the Purkinje fibres. It is thus possible, especially in ungulates, to visualise the entire system (24 a). These connective tissue capsules are not lymph sheaths since they have no endothelial lining. The fluid within the space facilitates the exchange of metabolites. Furthermore, the capsule allows the fibres of the excitation and conducting system freedom of movement without risk of stretching or tearing during myocardial contraction.

Innervation of the heart

In addition to the automatic control of its action by the impulse generating and conducting system, the heart's function is also controlled by **cardiac nerves.** These ensure that the heart adapts to the requirements of the body, which often change rapidly, by providing an adequate supply of blood and making the most economical use of its reserve power.

The innervation of the heart is by the *autonomic sympatho-parasympathetic nervous system.*

The efferent preganglionic cardiac nerves of the **sympathetic trunk** are derived from the 1st to the 4th or 5th thoracic segment of the spinal cord and reach the *truncus sympathicus* via the *rami communicantes albi.* A proportion of these fibres have already made synaptic connections with the second neurone in the vertebral ganglion of the sympathetic trunk but in the majority of fibres this occurs only in the ganglia of its cervical part, namely the *ggl. cervicale medium* and *caudale,* and to a variable extent also in the *ggll. vertebralia* of the sympathetic trunk and the ganglia of the *plexus cardiacus.*

The 1st, 2nd and often also the 3rd and 4th *ggl. vertebrale* are fused into a large node which is situated at the thoracic entrance in the neighbourhood of the 1st to 3rd ribs. In all domestic mammals with the exception of the dog, the *ganglion cervicale caud.* also participate in this fusion, producing the *ggl. cervicothoracale,* also known, because of its appearance, as the *ggl. stellatum* (for further details see vol. IV). In some animals, such as cats, pigs and ruminants, there is an independent *ggl. cervicale medium* which gives rise to the *nn. cardiaci medii.* The *nn. cardiaci cervicales caudd.* arise from the cervicothoracic ganglion. Finally, the 1st to 6th vertebral ganglia of the sympathetic trunk give rise to the *rami cardiaci thoracales.* Together with the parasympathetic nerves (*infra*), these nerves form a network, the meshes of which are at first wide and then narrow, which contains the *ggll. cardiaca.* The wide-meshed superficial plexus is found mainly on the left side on the concavity of the aortic arch and the branches of the pulmonary trunk. The close-meshed *deep plexus* is situated more to the right, lying between the aortic arch and the bifurcation of the trachea and branches of the pulmonary trunk. Both plexuses are interconnected by numerous branches.

The **parasympathetic innervation** of the heart derives from the *n. vagus* which, after giving rise to the *n. laryngeus recurrens,* carries only parasympathetic fibres to the organs of the thoracic and abdominal cavities. Shortly after entering the thoracic cavity the vagus nerve gives rise to two or three *rami cardiaci crann.* and the recurrent laryngeal nerve gives off the *rami cardiaci caudd.,* all of which enter the *plexus cardiaci* along with the previously mentioned cardiac nerves of the sympathetic system.

Both *plexus cardiaci* give off intracardiac nerves. They supply the cardiac blood vessels, all the layers of the myocardium and the impulse generating and conducting system. They enter the atrial musculature in several groups and are said to maintain a close relationship to the conducting system. Some of the nerve fibres which presumably stem from the vagus are preganglionic and their transference to postganglionic fibres occurs in the numerous *intramural ganglia* of the atrial musculature. A large ganglion, the *ggl. sinuatriale* (24/8), lies next to the sinuatrial node, while another, the *ggl. atrioventriculare* (/9), is situated next to the atrioventricular node. Other stout branches of the plexus form into networks in the coronary groove, whence they follow the coronary arteries and their branches to form a subendocardial ramification which also contains ganglia. Fibres originating from this network enter the myocardium along with the blood vessels, make contact with the muscle fibres by encircling them with delicate offshoots and finally form a subendocardial network.

The function of the sympathetic and parasympathetic nerves extends to both the contractile musculature of the heart and the specific musculature of the impulse generating and conducting system. Stimulation of the *sympathetic* cardiac nerves causes a speeding up of impulse generation in the sinuatrial node and of impulse conduction. Associated with this is a reduction of the impulse transmission time and an increased excitability and contractability of the heart musculature. This leads to an increased heart rate and energy output by the heart with a resultant increase in blood pressure. Because of these effects, the sympathetic nerve of the heart is also spoken of as *n. accelerans*.

The *parasympathetic* or vagus has the opposite action. It retards impulse generation and conduction as well as the transmission time. It lowers the excitability of the musculature. It retards the heart action and therefore preserves the power of the heart and ensures its economic utilisation. Under physiological conditions it reduces the action of the sympathetic to such an extent that the heart maintains a satisfactory basal rate.

The sympathetic-parasympathetic cardiac nerves carry not only efferent but also afferent fibres. These end in delicate branchlets having various types of terminal receptors located in the subepicardial, subendocardial and intramuscular regions. They regulate alterations in the muscle tension of the atria and ventricles and react to chemical or painful stimuli. The impulses originating from them are carried to cardiovascular centres in the brain and spinal cord and elicit a response through various reflexes.

The influence on cardiac action of the baroreceptors and chemoreceptors present in the peripheral circulatory system and of the various hormones which act through the circulation regulating centre, have already been discussed on page 14.

Blood vessels of the heart
(27–49)

Because it has only short diastolic rests, the work output and energy requirements of the heart are very great. Consequently it is outstandingly well supplied with its own blood vessels and, indeed, these carry 10% of the total volume pumped by the organ during systole. Since the structure and function of the heart is essentially the same in all mammals, it is not surprising that the arrangement of its blood supply is also fundamentally similar.

All the blood vessels of the surface of the heart are subepicardial in position although, especially in the pig and to some extent in the carnivores, the vessels may be bridged by thin strips of myocardial tissue. This arrangement is also occasionally encountered in sheep and goats but not in the ox or horse. The subepicardial vessels are embedded in adipose tissue in amounts which vary according to species and nutritional status. The superficially situated arteries give off, usually at right angles, myocardial branches which enter the musculature where they branch extensively forming an exceptionally dense capillary network.

Arteries

The blood necessary to sustain the continuous work of the heart is carried to the organ in two large arteries. These are the first vessels to arise from the aorta and, because of their topographic disposition, they are termed **aa. coronariae**. The distribution pattern and the proportion of the whole organ supplied by the **a. coronaria sin.** and the **a. coronaria dext.** differ in the dog and ruminants from the pig and horse (25, 26).

In the dog and the ruminants the **a. coronaria sin.** arises from the left sinus of the aortic bulbus (28/8; 38/1; 44/1) and divides into the *r. interventricularis paraconalis* and the *r. circumflexus (sin.)*. The former follows the *sulcus interventricularis paraconalis* to the apex of the heart, while the latter follows the left part of the coronary groove and reaches the *facies atrialis* as a stout vessel, to continue thence to the heart apex as the *r. interventricularis subsinuosus* situated in the right longitudinal groove (29/12; 39/2; 45/2).

In the pig and horse the left coronary artery (35/9; 47/1) forks, after a short course, into the *r. interventricularis paraconalis* (/11; /2) which runs towards the *sulcus paraconalis,* and the *r. circumflexus* (/10; /3) which follows the left part of the coronary groove. The latter branch attains the *margo ventricularis sin.* or even the *facies atrialis* (right surface of the heart), where it divides into several branches.

The **a coronaria dext.** (27/9; 37/8; 43/9) of the dog and ruminants is thinner than the left vessel. It originates from the right sinus of the aortic bulbus, initially as the *r. circumflexus (dext.)*, and runs in the right part of the coronary groove towards the atrial surface of the heart where it divides into branches for the right ventricle and atrium (29/16; 39/8; 45/8). It does not extend as far as the subsinuosal interventricular groove.

The **a. coronaria dext.** of the pig and horse arises at the same site as in the previous species and runs in the right part of the coronary groove as the *r. circumflexus (dext.)* (34/8; 46/10). It reaches, without decreasing appreciably in diameter, the right longitudinal groove in which it continues towards the apex of the heart as the *r. interventricularis subsinuosus* (36/15; 48/2).

From this description it is clear that in dogs and ruminants both the paraconal and the subsinuosal interventricular rami arise from the left coronary artery. Thus, in these species, the supply area of the left coronary artery encompasses the whole of the left heart, including the interventricular septum and that part of the right ventricular wall which adjoins the longitudinal groove. The right coronary artery supplies, in these species, only that region of the right ventricular wall near the *margo ventricularis dext.* and the right atrium. This arrangement is known as the left coronary type of supply (25).

Although in the pig and horse the paraconal interventricular ramus also arises from the left coronary artery, the subsinuosal ramus is given off from the right coronary artery and thus is different from the situation in the dog and ruminant. In the pig and horse, therefore, both coronary arteries participate about equally in the supply of the heart musculature including the septum (26). This is known as a bilateral coronary type of supply.

The distribution pattern of the coronary arteries in the cat is variable in that in the majority of cases the left coronary artery behaves as in the dog, giving rise to both interventricular rami. In a few cases, however, the pattern resembles that of the pig and horse in that the paraconal ramus originates from the left and the subsinuosal ramus from the right coronary artery. In rare instances one may even encounter two *aa. interventricularis subsinuosi,* both coronary arteries being involved in their formation. The most

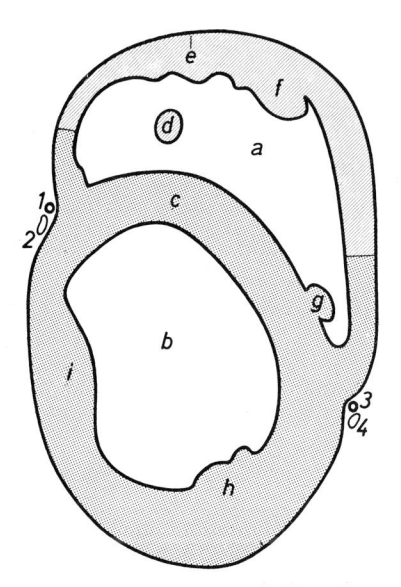

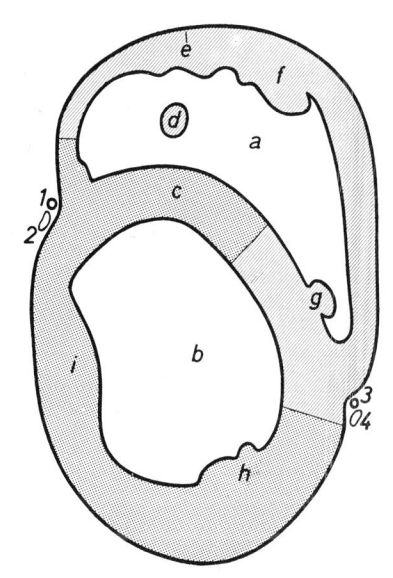

Figs 25, 26. Cross section through the ventricles of the heart. This is a diagramatic representation of the species difference in the supply regions of the coronary arteries. The stippled parts of the wall are supplied by the left coronary artery while the hatched portions are supplied by the right coronary artery.

a ventriculus dext.; *b* ventriculus sin.; *c* septum interventriculare; *d* trabecula septomarginalis; *e* margo ventricularis dext.; *f* m. papillaris magnus; *g* mm. papillares parvi; *h, i* m. papillaris subatrialis or subauricularis;

Fig 25. *1* r. interventricularis paraconalis of the a. coronaria *sin.*; *2* v. interventricularis paraconalis of the v. cordis magna in the sulcus interventricularis paraconalis; *3* r. interventricularis subsinuosus of the a. coronaria *sin.*; *4* v. cordis media in the sulcus interventricularis subsinuosus. *Left-coronary type of supply* in the *dog* and *ruminants.*

Fig. 26. *1* and *2* as in fig. 25; *3* r. interventricularis subsinuosus of the a. coronaria dext.; *4* v. cordis media in the sulcus interventricularis subsinuosus. *Bilateral coronary type of supply* in the *pig* and the *horse.*

common form is thus the left coronary type, the bilateral type is less common and the bilateral coronary variant comprises the remainder.

Veins

The venous blood from the heart empties directly into the right atrium through a variable number of veins or through the coronary sinus. This **sinus coronarius** is a tubular dilatation of the right atrium and it is situated under the *ostium venae cavae caud.* in the coronary groove on the atrial surface of the heart. This sinus measures 2–3 cm in length in the dog (29/*11*), 2–3 cm in the pig (36/*d*), 3.5–5 cm in the ox (39/*13*) and 3–5.5 cm in the horse (48/*15*). In the horse the termination of the sinus in the right atrium is furnished with indistinct *valvula sinus coronarii* (24/*h*).

The coronary sinus continues in the direction of the left, caudal ventricular border as the **v. cordis magna** (great coronary vein). The dividing line between the sinus and vein is indicated in carnivores and horses by the origin of the distinct *v. obliqua atrii sin.* (27/*20*; 46/*24*); in pigs and ruminants it is located at the origin of the *v. azygos* (36/*8*; 39/*e*), a vessel which is characteristic of these species. Some authors look upon the left oblique atrial vein as a rudiment of the left sinus horn of the embryonic heart, while others interpret it as the remnant of the azygos vein which, as implied above, is absent in carnivores and horses. In addition to the great coronary vein, the coronary sinus also gives rise to the **v. cordis media** *s. interventricularis subsinuosa*, which arises directly from the right atrium in the horse.

By their course and drainage area the *v. cordis magna* and *v. cordis media* (middle cardiac vein) correspond in carnivores and ruminants to the branches of the left coronary artery. Its left circumflex and interventricular paraconal rami are accompanied by the *v. circumflexa* (*sin.*) and the *v. interventricularis paraconalis* of the great coronary vein (27, 28/*18, 19*; 37/*19, 20*; 38/*11, 12*). The accompanying vein of the interventricular subsinuosal ramus of the left coronary artery is the middle cardiac vein (29/*12*; 39/*14*). In the pig and the horse (36/*21*; 48/*12*) it also follows the *r. interventricularis subsinuosus* which in this case, however, stems from the right coronary artery.

The **vv. cordis parvae** (*dextrae*) are 4–5 smaller veins which collect the blood from the region near the coronary groove of the right ventricle and empty, either individually or after uniting into a common trunk (34/*20*), into the right atrium (27/*10–13*; 34/*10–12, 21*; 37/*9–12, 22*; 46/*12, 13, 16*; 47/*12, 13*; 48/*3, 4*).

Finally, mention should be made of the **vv. cordis minimae** (*Thebesii*). These are very narrow veins of only a few millimeters length which arise from the capillaries of the myocardial musculature and deliver blood through the *foramina venarum minimarum* directly into the chambers of the heart. Although there are species differences, these foramina are numerous in the atria and less common in the ventricles (23).

Structure and special organization of the blood vessels of the heart

The large and medium sized arteries of the heart are of the elastic-muscular type, while the smaller arteries are of muscular type. Their circular and longitudinal layers vary in thickness and arrangement.

Circulation-regulating structures in the form of cushion or throttle arteries are present and there are also arteries which have epithelioid muscle cells. Because of the great energy-demand of the heart muscle, it has an extremly dense, three-dimensional capillary network the meshes of which are arranged according to the structure of the muscle bundles or the muscle cells.

Anastomoses between branches of the two coronary arteries, referred to as interarterial connections, are relatively rare whereas *intraarterial* connections, that is links between small branches of larger subendocardial arteries, are found frequently. It is important to point out that the supply areas of the individual ventricular branches remain in strictly separated sectors down to their capillary ramifications. Although the capillaries of two bordering regions may interdigitate, there are no connections between them. Thus the branches of the coronary arteries are true end-arteries each of which is responsible for the supply of a distinct and circumscribed area of myocardial tissue of a size which depends on the calibre of the branch vessel. When such an end-artery becomes occluded, the area which it supplies no longer receives blood.

The structure of the media of subepicardial veins is predominantly muscular although in medium-sized and small myocardial vessels only a connective tissue media remains. In all the domestic mammals valves are present in the subepicardial veins, particularly at the origin of branches but also in non-branching parts of the vessels. In pigs such valves are also found in myocardial veins, even in those with a calibre of only 120 μm.

Veno-venous anastomoses are very numerous in the hearts of all domestic mammals. They connect and interconnect the subendocardial and myocardial veins and even form junctions between veins of the right and left ventricles.

It is noteworthy that in the dog, cat and horse the smaller subepicardial arteries are each accompanied by two collateral veins and these veins are connected to each other by *bridge anastomoses*. On the other hand, arteriovenous anastomoses, that is direct connections between precapillary arteries and postcapillary veins, have not been demonstrated in the heart of domestic animals.

Lymph vessels of the heart

In all the domestic mammals the **lymph vessels** of the heart originate from the subendocardial, myocardial and subepicardial networks of *lymph capillaries*. These plexuses unite into larger vessels which follow the courses of the blood vessels in a subepicardial location running towards the coronary groove. This applies both to the lymph vessels of the ventricles and of the atria. The most common lymph vessel collecting site in the heart is at the point where the interventricular paraconal sulcus enters the coronary groove. The larger lymphatics proceed from there to various lymph centres or lymph nodes depending on the species. In the dog they go to the *lymphocentrum bronchale* and the *lnn. mediastinalis crann. et medii;* in the pig to the *lnn. tracheobronchales sinn. et crann.;* in ruminants to the *lymphocentrum bronchale* and the *lnn. tracheobronchales crann. et mediastinales crann.* and in the horse to the *lnn. tracheobronchales sinn. et mediastinales crann.*

In the dog and the horse the lymph vessels from the atrial (right) surface and from the atria may pass directly to their lymph nodes.

Species characteristic of the heart, general considerations

It is difficult to determine the species from which an isolated heart originates by its external appearance and size alone. However, various reliable identifying criteria are available. These include the distribution pattern of the cardiac vessels and the characteristic mode of origin from the heart of the right and left azygos veins, which differ in various species (cf. pg. 40). Another diagnostic feature is the variable amount, colour and consistency of the subepicardial adipose tissue and the presence of subendocardial fat. Fatty tissue occurs in the coronary groove and the interventricular sulci and inside the cavities of the heart. The internal structure of the heart also shows species differences. In this context it should be recalled that in all mammals the trabeculae carneae, the mm. papillares transversi and pectinati, the chordae tendineae and the atrioventricular valves all develop from the embryonic muscular spongy tissue of the ventricles. This complicated developmental process is responsible not only for species differences in the structure of the interior of the heart but also for the fact that, even within one and the same species, no one heart is exactly the same as another.

Size, weight and measurements of the heart, general considerations

The size, the absolute weight and, surprisingly, the relative weight and measurements of the heart are dependent on a number of different factors. These include, above all, the breed and resultant size and body weight of the individual animal. Age and nutritional status are important and the various parameters are considerably influenced by the life style of the animal. The significance of the measurements will also depend on whether, at the time of examination, the heart was in diastole or systole, whether it was full of blood and whether it was, or had been, in rigor.

Consideration must be given to diseases which may influence the circulation. In the dog, for instance, chronic nephritis is very common and may severely influence the size and weight of the heart. If all these factors are taken into consideration, it is not surprising that widely divergent data on the weights and sizes of the hearts of domestic animals are cited in the literature. It is thus important to ascertain in each case what methods were used for the statistical assessment.

The heart of the dog and the cat
(5, 16–18, 21–23, 27–33)

The **heart** of the carnivore is in the form of a blunt, almost spherical cone. The internal structure of its ventricles presents some species-specific characteristics worthy of note.

Interior of the ventricles

The left ventricle of the dog and cat contains numerous bulging, longitudinally directed *trabeculae carneae* which are attached to the ventricular wall to varying extents. Only that part of the interventricular septum which lies below the septal cusp of the mitral valve is entirely smooth. The interior of the right ventricle is of similar structure. In this case the smooth part of the septum will be found in the region of the *conus arteriosus* and the septal cusp of the tricuspid valve.

In the left ventricle there are generally two muscular bands which extend from the septum to the two papillary muscles. The two muscular bands of the right ventricle are less constant. The first, which is always present, is the *m. transversus (trabecula septomarginalis)* (16, 18/*f*) which goes to the *m. papillaris magnus* (/*c*) while the second, which may be absent, takes its course to the *mm. papillares parvi* (18/*f'*, *d*).

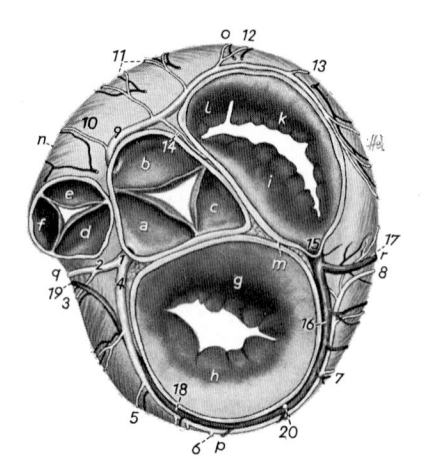

Fig. 27. Base of the canine heart after removal of the atria. The larger arteries and veins are labelled independently, the smaller ones together. (After Lücke, Diss. med. vet., Hanover, 1955.)

a, b, c valva aortae (*a* valvula semilunaris sin., *b* valvula semilunaris dext., *c* valvula semilunaris septalis); *d, e, f* valva trunci pulmonalis (*d* valvula semilunaris sin., *e* valvula semilunaris dext., *f* valvula semilunaris intermed.); *g, h* valva atrioventricularis sin. s. bicuspidalis (*g* cuspis septalis, *h* cuspis parietalis); *i, k, l* valva atrioventricularis dext. s. tricuspidalis (*i* cuspis septalis, *k* cuspis parietalis, *l* cuspis angularis); *m* septum interatriale; *n* conus arteriosus; *o* margo ventricularis dext.; *p* margo ventricularis sin.; *q* sulcus interventricularis paraconalis; *r* sulcus interventricularis subsinuosus

1 a. coronaria sin.; *2* r. interventricularis paraconalis; *3* r. collateralis prox., *4* r. circumflexus (sin.); *5* r. prox. ventriculi sin.; *6* r. marginis ventricularis sin.; *7* r. and v. dist. ventriculi sin.; *8* r. interventricularis subsinuosus; *9* a. coronaria dext., the r. circumflexus (dext.); *10* a. and v. coni vasculosi; *11* r. and v. prox. ventriculi dext.; *12* r. and v. marginis ventricularis dext.; *13* r. and v. dist. ventriculi dext.; *14* r. atrii dext.; *15* ostium of the sinus coronarius; *16* sinus coronarius; *17* v. cordis media; *18* r. circumflexus and *19* r. interventricularis paraconalis of the v. cordis magna; *20* v. obliqua atrii sin.

In the right ventricle the *m. papillaris subarteriosus* (16–18/*e*) is solitary and relatively more substantial in the cat than in the dog, while the *m. papillaris magnus* can consist of two to three components in both the dog and the cat (/*c*). In the dog the great muscle can be situated either on the septum alone (16/*c*) or on the outer wall (17/*c*), although in the latter instance it is intermediate since it still has some relation to the septum. In the cat it is usually intermediate or based entirely on the outer wall (18/*c*). The *mm. papillares parvi* (16–18/*d*) of both species tend to form groups and they are made up of two limbs.

The two papillary muscles on the outer wall of the left ventricle are usually stouter than those of the right ventricle. In the dog the *m. papillaris subatrialis* is usually weaker than in the cat, has a broader base and rises from the outer wall of the ventricle as a single blunt peak from which extend the tendinous cords. The *m. subauricularis* varies in shape. It has a solid base from which several pointed secondary papillae usually project. In addition to these two or three papillary muscles which are inevitably present, there may be a number of additional small papillary muscles in both ventricles of the cat and dog.

Size and weight of the dog's heart

In the following tables 1–4 are given a selection of values for the weight and size of the hearts of dogs which may serve as useful guidelines. The information recorded includes the absolute and relative weights of the hearts of various breeds of dogs, the measurements of the circumference, transverse and

Table 1   Heart weights (in g.) of various breeds of dogs (After Balmer, 1937.)

Breed	Absolute heart weight	Mean	Relative heart weight
Great Dane	130–470	293.1	0.71 %
St. Bernhard	200–500	301.0	0.64 %
Pointer	100–350	233.8	0.78 %
Setter	100–200	158.6	0.73 %
German Shepherd	100–300	199.6	0.75 %
Doberman	90–275	178.0	0.73 %
Airdale	100–300	185.0	0.76 %
Schnauzer	40–150	95.6	0.71 %
Spaniel	30–120	92.8	0.76 %
Spitz	15–100	58.4	0.76 %
Dachshund	40–110	75.2	0.73 %
Pinscher (miniature)	10– 80	48.0	0.70 %
Fox terrier	24–120	67.7	0.73 %
Mongrel	25–320	111.7	0.74 %

Table 2   Transverse and sagittal diameter in cm. (After Kunze, 1952);
Heart circumference in cm. (After Schubert, 1909)

Heart weight in g.	Transverse diameter	Mean	Sagittal diameter	Mean	Circumference of the heart*	Mean
27– 58	3.5–5.5	4.5	4.0– 6.1	5.0	11.3–21.3	16.0
74– 99	3.8–6.5	5.3	5.7– 7.1	6.6	13.7–23.7	18.6
201–237	5.5–7.5	7.0	7.7–11.0	8.5	19.9–33.7	26.8

* Below the coronary groove

Table 3   Height of the margo ventricularis dext. (margo cran.) and of the margo ventricularis sin. (margo caud.) *

Heart weight in g.	Margo ventricularis dext.	Mean	Margo ventricularis sin.	Mean
27– 58	6.9–10.8	8.9	4.5– 8.3	6.4
74– 90	9.0–12.5	12.2	6.5– 8.6	7.5
201–237	13.0–19.0	13.6	10.0–12.0	11.0

* Measured between the sulcus coronarius and the apex cordis; measurements in cm. (After Kunze, 1952)

Table 4   Thickness of the ventricular wall*

Heart weight	Right ventricle	Left ventricle
27– 58	0.3–0.8	0.8–1.3
74– 96	0.4–0.6	1.1–1.5
170–237	0.5–0.9	1.5–2.2

* Measured in cm. above the papillary muscle. (After Kunze, 1952)

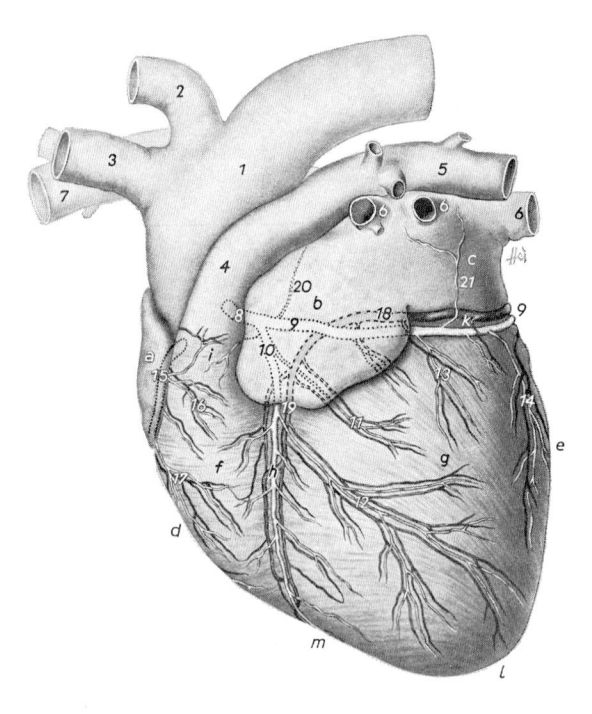

Fig. 28. Auricular surface of a dog's heart. The larger arteries and veins are labelled individually, the smaller ones together. (After Lücke, Diss. med. vet. Hanover, 1955.)

a auricula dext.; *b* auricula sin.; *c* atrium sin.; *d* margo ventricularis dext.; *e* margo ventricularis sin.; *f* ventriculus dext.; *g* ventriculus sin.; *h* sulcus interventricularis paraconalis; *i* conus arteriosus; *k* sulcus coronarius, pars sin.; *l* apex cordis; *m* incisura apicis

1 arcus aortae; *2* a. subclavia sin.; *3* a. brachiocephalica; *4* truncus pulmonalis; *5* a. pulmonalis sin.; *6* vv. pulmonales; *7* v. cava cran.; *8* a. coronaria sin., *9* its r. circumflexus (sin.), *10* its r. interventricularis paraconalis; *11* r. collateralis prox.; *12* r. collateralis dist.; *13* r. prox. ventriculi sin.; *14* r. marginis ventricularis sin.; *15* a. coronaria dext., its r. circumflexus (dext.); *16* a. and v. coni arteriosi; *17* r. and v. prox. ventriculi dext.; *18* v. cordis magna, its r. circumflexus, *19* its r. interventricularis paraconalis; *20* r. prox. atrii sin.; *21* r. intermed. atrii sin.

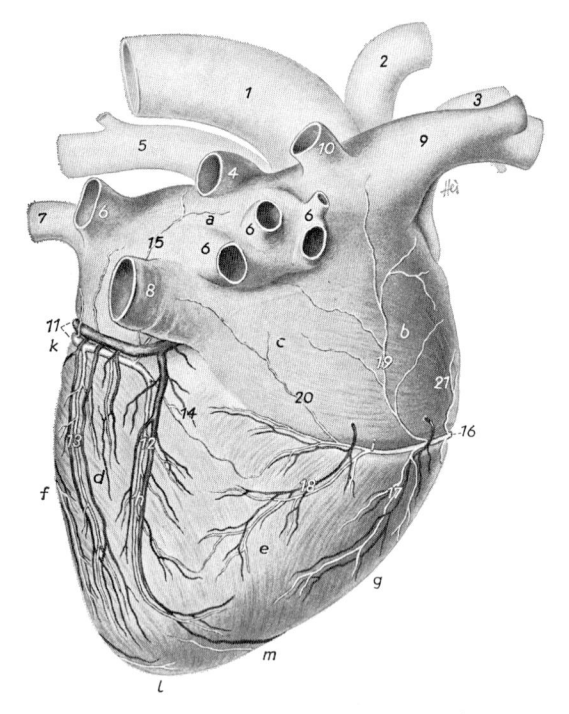

Fig. 29. Atrial surface of a dog's heart. The larger arteries and veins are labelled individually, the smaller ones together. (After Lücke, Diss. med. vet., Hanover, 1955.)

a atrium sin.; *b* atrium dext.; *c* sinus venarum cavarum; *d* ventriculus sin.; *e* ventriculus dext.; *f* margo ventricularis sin.; *g* margo ventricularis dext.; *h* sulcus interventricularis subsinuosus; *i* sulcus coronarius, pars dext.; *k* sulcus coronarius, pars sin.; *l* apex cordis; *m* incisura apicis

1 arcus aortae; *2* a. subclavia sin.; *3* a. brachiocephalica; *4* right, *5* left a. pulmonalis; *6, 6, 6, 6*, right, *7* left vv. pulmonales; *8* v. cava caud.; *9* v. cava cran.; *10* v. azygos dext.; *11* sinus coronarius and r. circumflexus of the a. coronaria sin.; *12* r. interventricularis subsinuosus and v. cordis media; *13* r. and v. dist. ventriculi sin.; *14* v. ventriculi dext.; *15* r. dist. atrii sin.; *16* r. circumflexus (dext.) of the a. coronaria dext.; *17* r. and v. marginis ventricularis dext.; *18* r. and v. dist. ventriculi dext.; *19, 20* r. dist. atrii dext.; *21* r. intermed. atrii dext.

longitudinal diameters at the base of the heart, the height of the ventricles at the right and left ventricular borders and finally the thickness of the ventricular walls.

Position of the heart in the dog[*]

(5)

The long axis of the heart forms with the sternum an angle of about 40° which is open cranially. Its base is craniodorsally directed and lies at about half the height of the thoracic cavity, corresponding to a horizontal level through the centre of the 1st rib or a line connecting the acromion of the shoulder blade with the end of the 13th rib. The *margo ventricularis dext.* follows at some distance the contour of the sternum while the *margo ventricularis sin.* accompanies the cranial border of the 7th rib. Both these borders meet at the apex of the heart which is slightly deflected to the left and reaches the level of the 7th costal cartilage. About $^4/_7$ths of the heart lies on the left side of the midline and $^3/_7$ths on the right and it

---

[*] Data relating to clinical examination are taken from Marek and Mocsy (1956)

occupies the thoracic space between the 3rd and 7th ribs and between the sternum and half the height of the thoracic cavity. Situated mostly at a distance from the thoracic wall, it is imbedded in the cardiac impression of both lungs and only in the region of the *incisura cardiaca*, which is smaller on the right side, does the heart makes contact with the thoracic wall. The topography of the thoracic wall limits the application of clinical examination of the heart by palpation, percussion and auscultation, as well as by radiological means. This is because the thorax is covered in its cranial region by the shoulder blade and part of the humerus and their musculature. The caudal contour of the *m. triceps brachii (linea anconaea)* commences at the third costo-vertebral joint and crosses the lower end of the 5th rib. However, the thoracic wall can be exposed for examination in an area between the 4th and 7th rib, by pulling forward the forelimb. (cf. vol. II. figs 375 and 376).

A knowledge of the topography of the heart permits various diagnostic methods of cardiac examination to be carried out in the living animal. These include palpation of the apex beat which originates from the rhythmic contractions of the myocardium and resultant pounding against the chest wall. In the dog it can be distinctly felt in the lower third of the chest between the 4th and 6th, and especially over the 5th, intercostal spaces. It can also be detected on the right side between the 4th and 5th intercostal spaces but is less distinct.

It is possible to demonstrate by percussion an area of absolute cardiac dullness in that part of the heart which is not covered by the lungs. This will be found on both sides between the 4th and 6th intercostal spaces. The dorsal limit of this area of dullness is formed by the symphyses of the 4th and 5th ribs and medioventrally the areas of dullness from the left and right side meet in the 4th to 6th intercostal spaces.

In the dog auscultation of physiological and pathological heart sounds is carried out in the 5th intercostal space for the left ventricle and for the right ventricle in the 4th intercostal space, the lower third of the chest being examined on both sides. These sites are also suitable for eliciting the normal and adventitious sounds of the heart valves.

Heart of the cat, size and weight
(5, 18)

Some of the peculiarities of the interior of the feline heart have already been described. The following table presents data on the weight and measurements of the heart.

Weight and size of the cat's heart*

Sex	Body weight in g	Heart weight absolute (g)	Heart weight relative %	Diameter (mm) sagittal	Diameter (mm) transverse	Height of the margo ventricularis (mm) dext.	Height of the margo ventricularis (mm) sin.	Circumference of the heart
Male	3360.0	18.4	0.55	33.0	24.3	48.5	39.9	90.3
Female	2480.0	12.7	0.51	26.5	19.3	42.4	31.9	77.6

* Average values (After Sichert, 1935)

The sex dimorphism in favour of the male of this species is significantly reflected in the various parameters of the heart.

The topography of the cat's heart differs from that of the dog as the anteriorly open angle between the axis of the heart and the sternum is only 25–30° and the heart occupies the lower half of the thorax between the 4th and 7th ribs. Since the caudal border of the triceps brachii muscle ends at the 4th rib, the heart of the cat is entirely retroscapular, its left surface being nearest to the thoracic wall between the 4th and 6th ribs and its right surface being closest at the 5th rib. These are also the areas where the *apex beat* is most readily palpated and where the heart sounds can be satisfactorily auscultated.

Blood vessels of the heart of the dog and cat
(27–33)

Arteries

The **a coronaria sin.** (28/8; 31/1) forks into two main branches while still within the coronary groove. One of these, the *r. interventricularis paraconalis*, descends in the groove of the same name to the *incisura apicis* (28/10; 30/2 31/2) while the other, the *r. circumflexus (sin.)* (28/9; 31/3), follows the left part of the coronary groove. In the cat the interventricular paraconal branch gives rise to the *r. angularis* (31/4) and subsequently, both in the cat and the dog, the *rr. collaterales sin. prox. et dist.* (28/11, 12; 31/7, 8) are given off. These last two also go to the *facies auricularis* of the left ventricle. Both branches supply the *m. papillaris subauricularis* of the left ventricle. In the cat the interventricular paraconal branch gives off the *r. coni arteriosi* (31/11) to the wall of the right ventricle and several small branches

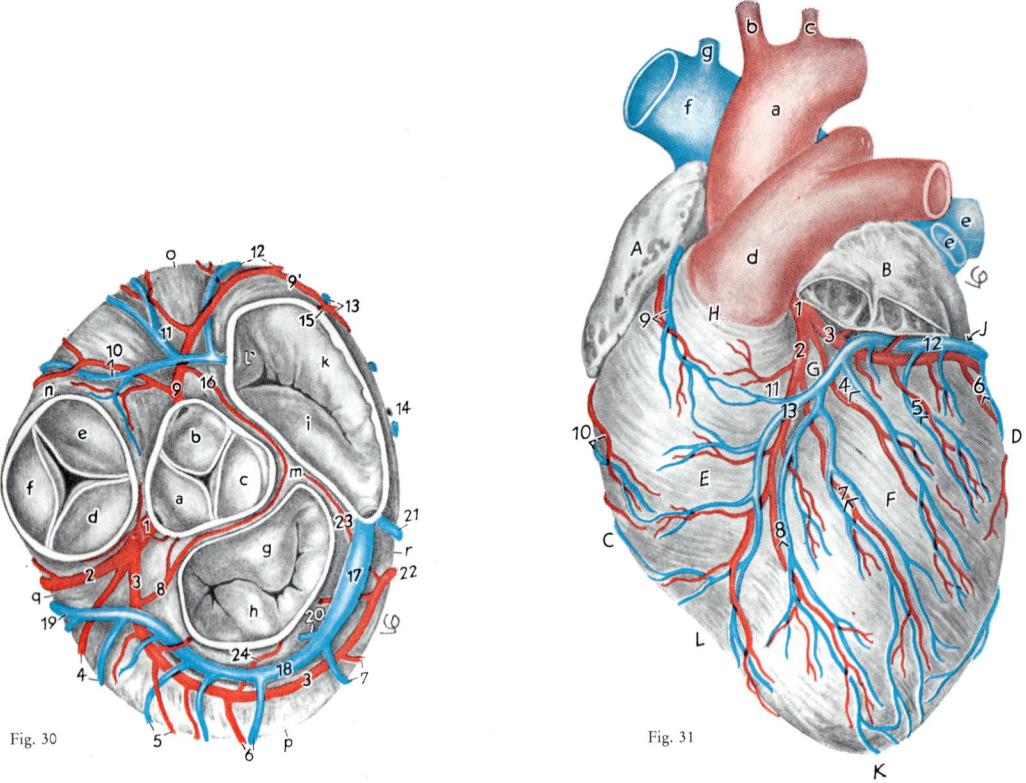

Fig. 30. Base of the heart of a cat, after removal of the atria. (After Habermehl, 1959.)

a, b, c valva aortae (*a* valvula semilunaris sin., *b* valvula semilunaris dext., *c* valvula semilunaris septalis); *d, e, f* valva trunci pulmonalis (*d* valvula semilunaris sin., *e* valvula semilunaris dext., *f* valvula semilunaris intermed.); *g, h* valva atrioventricularis sin. s. bicuspidalis (*g* cuspis septalis, *h* cuspis parietalis); *i, k, l* valva atrioventricularis dext. s. tricuspidalis (*i* cuspis septalis, *k* cuspis parietalis, *l* cuspis angularis); *m* septum interatriale; *n* conus arteriosus; *o* margo ventricularis dext.; *p* margo ventricularis sin.; *q* sulcus interventricularis paraconalis; *r* sulcus interventricularis subsinuosus

1 a. coronaria sin., *2* its ramus interventricularis paraconalis, *3, 3* its r. circumflexus; *4* r. and v. angularis; *5* r. and v. prox. ventriculi sin.; *6* r. and v. marginis ventricularis sin.; *7* r. and v. dist. ventriculi sin.; *8* r. prox. atrii sin.; *9* a. coronaria dext., *9'* its r. circumflexus; *10* a. and v. coni arteriosi; *11* r. and v. prox. ventriculi dext.; *12* r. and v. marginis ventricularis dext.; *13* r. and v. dist.ventriculi dext.;*14* r. dist. atrii dext.; *15* r. intermed. atrii dext.; *16* r. prox. atrii dext.; *17* sinus coronarius; *18* v. cordis magna, pars circumflexa; *19* v. interventricularis paraconalis; *20* v. obliqua atrii sin.; *21* v. cordis media; *22* r. interventricularis subsinuosus of the a. coronaria sin.; *23* r. dist. atrii sin.; *24* r. intermed. atrii sin.

Fig. 31. Arteries and veins of the auricular surface of the cat's heart. (After Habermehl, 1959.)

A auricula dext.; *B* auricula sin., partly removed; *C* margo ventricularis dext.; *D* margo ventricularis sin.; *E* ventriculus dext.; *F* ventriculus sin.; *G* sulcus interventricularis paraconalis; *H* conus arteriosus; *J* sulcus coronarius, pars sin.; *K* apex cordis; *L* incisura apicis

a arcus aortae; *b* a. brachiocephalica; *c* a. subclavia sin.; *d* truncus pulmonalis; *e, e* vv. pulmonales sin.; *f* v. cava cran.; *g* v. azygos dext.

1 a. coronaria sin., *2* its v. interventricularis paraconalis, *3* its r. circumflexus sin.; *4* r. and v. angularis; *5* r. and v. prox. ventriculi sin.; *6* r. and v. marginis ventricularis sin.; *7* r. and v. collateralis sin. prox.; *8* r. and v. collateralis sin. dist.; *9* r. and v. coni arteriosi; *10* r. and v. proximalis ventriculi dext.; *11* r. and v. coni arteriosi; *12* v. cordis magna; *13* v. interventricularis paraconalis

which are distributed to the region of the interventricular septum bordering on the longitudinal groove. However, by far the greatest part of the interventricular septum, as well as the *nodus* and *fasciculus atrioventricularis*, are supplied by its *r. septi interventricularis* (33/4) and this also undertakes the vascularization of the three papillary muscles of the right ventricle.

The *r. circumflexus* (*sin.*) of the left coronary artery (28/9; 29/11; 30/3; 31/3) runs, initially under the cover of the left auricle, in the left part of the coronary groove to the *sulcus subsinuosus* on the atrial surface and finally, as it runs in the longitudinal groove towards the apex of the heart, it becomes the *r. interventricularis subsinuosus* (29/12; 32/2).

In those few cats where the *r. circumflexus* does not reach the subsinuosal groove, the *r. interventricularis subsinuosus* (33/1, 2) is supplied by the **a. coronaria dext.**

During its course the left circumflex branch gives off several small vessels which supply that part of the left ventricular wall which lies next to the coronary groove. Three of its largest branches, the *r. prox. ventriculi sin.* (28/13; 31/5), the *r. marginis ventricularis sin.* 28/14; 31/6) and the *r. dist. ventriculi sin.*

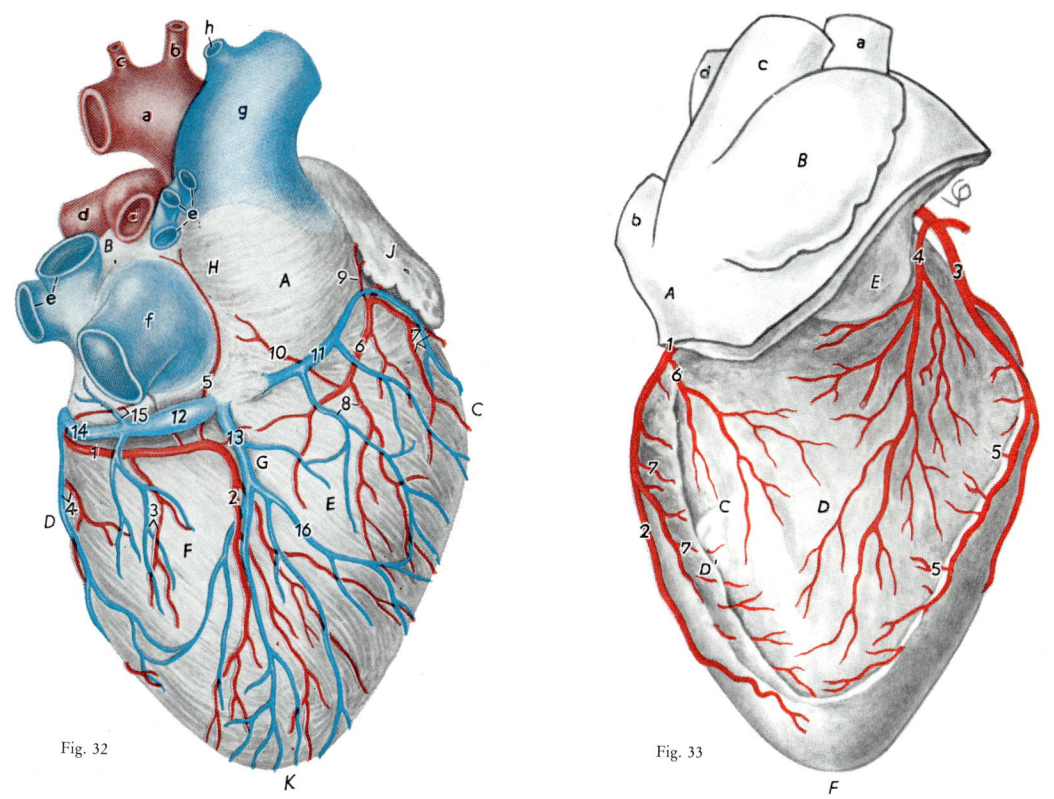

Fig. 32.

Fig. 33.

Fig. 32. Arteries and veins on the atrial surface of the heart of the cat. (After Habermehl, 1959.)

A atrium dext.; *B* atrium sin., *C* margo ventricularis dext.; *D* margo ventricularis sin.; *E* ventriculus dext.; *F* ventriculus sin.; *G* sulcus interventricularis subsinuosus; *H* sinus venarum cavarum; *J* auricula dext.; *K* apex cordis

a arcus aortae; *b* a. brachiocephalica; *c* a subclavia sin.; *d, d* branches of the truncus pulmonalis; *e, e* vv. pulmonales; *f* v. cava caud.; *g* v. cava cran.; *h* v. azygos dext.

1 r. circumflexus of the a. coronaria sin.; *2* its r. interventricularis subsinuosus; *3* r. and v. dist. ventriculi sin.; *4* r. and v. marginis ventricularis sin.; *5* r. dist. atrii sin.; *6* r. circumflexus of the a. coronaria dext.; *7* r. and v. marginis ventricularis dext.; *8* r. and v. dist. ventriculi dext.; *9* r. intermed. atrii dext.; *10* r. dist. atrii dext.; *11* v. semicircumflexa dext.; *12* sinus coronarius; *13* v. cordis media; *14* v. cordis magna; *15* r. intermed. atrii sin. or v. obliqua atrii sin.; *16* v. collateralis dext. prox.

Fig. 33. Arterial supply to the interventricular septum of the heart of a cat. The wall of the right ventricle has been removed. (After Habermehl, 1959.)

A atrium dext.; *B* auricula dext.; *C* mm. papillaris parvi; *D, D'* septum interventriculare and wall of the ventricle; *E* m. papillaris subarteriosus; *F* apex cordis

a arcus aortae; *b* v. cava caud.; *c* v. cava cran.; *d* branch of the truncus pulmonalis

1 r. circumflexus of the a. coronaria dext.; *2* r. interventricularis subsinuosus of the a. coronaria dext.; *3* r. interventricularis paraconalis of the a. coronaria sin.; *4* r. septi interventricularis with its branches to the septum and the mm. papillares subarteriosus and magnus; *5, 6, 7* further septal branches of the r. interventricularis subsinuosus and paraconalis

(29/13; 32/3), also descend the wall of the left ventricle. The last named also vascularizes the *m. papillaris subarterialis* which also receives branchlets from the *r. interventricularis subsinuosus* as described below.

Further offshoots from the *r. cirsumflexus* (*sin.*) supply the wall of the left atrium. These are the *rr. prox. intermed. et dist. atrii sin.* (28/20, 21; 29/15; 30/8, 23, 24; 32/5), which also give off delicate twigs to the interatrial septum.

As already pointed out, in the dog the interventricular subsinuosal branch always represents the continuation of the left circumflex branch. During its course in the subsinuosal groove it sends small branches to the myocardium next to the longitudinal groove. They supply a broad strip of right ventricular tissue and a narrower strip of left ventricle.

In the cat, on the other hand, the interventricular subsinuosal branch arises from the left circumflex ramus of the left coronary artery in only 50% of cases whereas in 30% of cases it springs from the right circumflex branch of the right coronary artery. The former pattern is spoken of as a left coronary type and the latter as a bilateral coronary type. Another possibility (about 12%) is the bilateral coronary variant with two interventricular subsinuosal branches, whereby the two collateral branches supply the neighbouring parts of the wall. Finally, complete absence of this artery is a rare exception.

In the dog the continuation of the **a. coronaria dext.** (27/9; 29/16; 30/9; 32/6) consists solely of its *r. circumflexus* (dext.) which, covered by the right auricle, courses in the right part of the coronary groove and terminates on the atrial surface. This also applies to cats having the left coronary type. In the bilateral coronary type on the other hand, the right circumflex ramus continues in the interventricular subsinuosal groove as the *r. interventricularis subsinuosus* and it passes to the apex of the heart. In both types the right circumflex ramus gives off, as well as some smaller twigs, four large branches to the wall of the right ventricle. These are the *r. coni arteriosi* to the similarly named part of the right ventricle (27/10; 28/16; 30/10; 31/9), the *r. prox. ventriculi dext.* (27/11; 28/17; 30/11; 31/10), the *r. marginis ventricularis dext.* (27/12; 29/17; 30/12; 32/7) and the *r. dist. ventriculi dext.* (27/13; 29/18; 30/13; 32/8). In cats with the bilateral coronary type, the *r. interventricularis subsinuosus* (33/2) is present as already described. Apart from supplying the above mentioned parts of the ventricular wall, it also sends smaller branches and its *r. septi interventricularis* to the interventricular septum (33/6, 7). Other branches of the right circumflex ramus vascularize the wall of the right atrium. These are the *rr. prox. intermed. et dist. atrii dext.* (27, 29 and 30, 32 respectively) which also participate in the supply of the atrial septum. The *r. dist. atrii dext.* of the dog regularly gives off an artery to the sinuatrial node whereas the *r. prox. atrii sin.* only occasionally participates in supplying the sinuatrial node.

Veins

(27/16; 29/11; 30/17; 32/12)

The **sinus coronarius** precedes the right atrium (cf. p. 40) and it is a collecting vessel for the bulk of the venous blood from the heart. From this coronary sinus one of the two great veins of the heart, the **v. cordis media** *s. v. interventricularis subsinuosa* (27/17; 29/12; 30/21; 32/13), arises first. It enters the interventricular subsinuosal groove and by the time it reaches the apex it has divided into several branches which anastomose there with others from the *v. interventricularis paraconalis*. Since the *v. cordis media* has the same course and supply area as the arterial *ramus interventricularis subsinuosus*, it is given the alternative name of *v. interventricularis subsinuosa*. A stout branch springs from it and runs to the wall of the right ventricle; in the cat this is termed the *v. collateralis prox. dext.* (32/16) and in the dog the *v. ventriculi dext.* (29/14). The next vessels arise simultaneously from the coronary sinus and are the *v. obliqua atrii sin.*, the *v. dist. ventriculi sin.* and the largest of the cardiac veins, the **v. cordis magna**, which might be regarded as a continuation of the coronary sinus. The *v. obliqua atrii sin.* (27/20; 30/20; 32/15) forms the division between the coronary sinus and the great cardiac vein. It supplies the wall of the left atrium especially at the site of termination of the pulmonary veins. The *v. dist. ventriculi sin.* (27/7; 30/7) corresponds to the artery of the same name with which it also shares its drainage area.

The **v. cordis magna** (27/18, 19; 30/18; 32/14) runs in the coronary groove and follows the course of the (left) circumflex ramus of the left coronary artery. With its, generally paired, terminal branch it enters the paraconal longitudinal groove as the *v. interventricularis paraconalis* (28/19; 31/13) and accompanies the analogous artery to the apex of the heart. The anastomoses between the terminal branches of this vein and those of the interventricular subsinuosal vein have already been described.

On its way to the interventricular paraconal groove the great cardiac vein gives off the *v. marginis ventricularis sin.* (27/6; 28/14; 30/6; 31/6), the *v. prox. ventriculi sin.* (27/5; 28/13; 30/5; 31/5) and, in the cat, the *v. angularis* (30/4; 31/4) which share a common drainage area with the corresponding arterial branches.

The *v. interventricularis paraconalis* gives rise to the following branches which drain the same area as supplied by their accompanying arteries: the *v. coni arteriosi* (31/11), the *v. collateralis dist. sin.* (28/12; 31/8) and the *v. septi interventricularis*.

A group of small veins, the *vv. cordis parvae*, carries the blood from a part of the atrial surface of the right ventricular wall directly into the right atrium (29, 32). In the cat four of these arise, sometimes in pairs, from the right atrium above the coronary groove and they cross the arterial *ramus circumflexus dext.* as they course towards the apex of the heart to reach their drainage area. These four vessels are the *v. coni arteriosi*, the *v. prox. ventriculi dext.*, the *v. marginis ventricularis dext.* and the *v. dist. ventriculi dext.* In the cat the three last named veins may unite into a common stem which commences below the *sinus venarum cavarum* and is known as the *v. semicircumflexa* (32/11).

Some of the blood draining from the myocardium is carried directly into the interior of the heart by the *vv. cordis minimae* (*Thebesii*). These thin veins, measuring only a few mm. in length, have already been referred to on page 40. They are most numerous in the right atrium and their number decreases progressively in the left atrium, the right ventricle and the left ventricle respectively.

Heart of the pig
(19, 34–36)

The heart of the pig is in the form of a blunt cone and its height only slightly exceeds its greatest craniocaudal diameter.

Internal structure of the ventricles

As in the other domestic mammals the interior of the pig's ventricles exhibits some species peculiarities, especially in its papillary muscles.

Both papillary muscles of the left ventricle arise from the outer wall but the *m. papillaris subatrialis*, which borders on the interventricular septum, is broad and low. Its base is formed by several muscular columns which unite into a single structure. Its cupola, which rises towards the *cuspis septalis*, usually carries two or, less commonly, three projections. The system of muscular bands running from the papillary muscle to the septum consists of a rounded muscle column which divides repeatedly after its origin from the septum. The *m. papillaris subauricularis* can be clearly distinguished against the ventricular wall by its rounded, beam-like shape. Its cupola is either uniformly rounded or bears several small, wart-like processes. Isolated or interwoven muscular bands extend from its plinth to the septum. In addition to these two papillary muscles there are usually several small *accessory papillary muscles* on the outer wall of the left ventricle

Two of the three papillary muscles of the right ventricle are situated on the septum whereas the third is on the outer wall. The *m. papillaris subarteriosus* (19/e) is but a small cupola-like eminence on the septum, while the plinth of the *m. papillaris magnus* is formed by a number of muscular beams which unite into a single complex (/c). The body of the latter extends prominently from the outer wall and carries on its top two to four small excrescences. Always present between the base of the great papillary muscle and the septum is the *trabecula septomarginalis* (/f) which measures between one and nine mm. in diameter. The *mm. papillaris parvi* (/d) form a pleomorphic muscle group consisting of several components. It is not uncommon to find a single muscular eminence arising from the septum, the apex of which carries one or more pointed projections. The right ventricle may also contain *accessory papillary muscles*.

Size and weight

The following tables of the heart weights of pigs are taken from a study by Rühl (1971).

These data are of particular value because of the way in which they were obtained. One hundred and seventy one animals were examined and during their entire life, on the average 205 days, they were kept under exactly the same conditions of management and nutrition. The animals were of five different

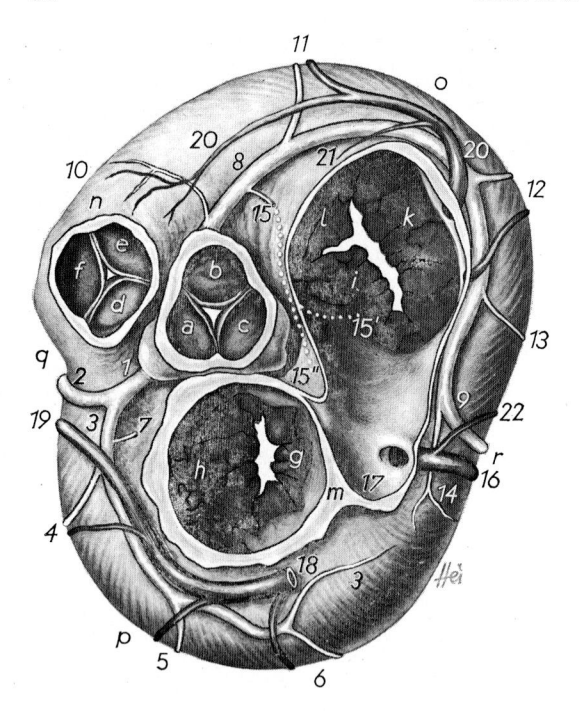

Fig. 34. Base of the pig's heart after removal of the atria. (After Rickert, Diss. med. vet., Hanover, 1955.)

a, b, c valva aortae (*a* valvula semilunaris sin., *b* valvula semilunaris dext., *c* valvula semilunaris septalis); *d, e, f* valva trunci pulmonalis (*d* valvula semilunaris sin., *e* valvula semilunaris dext., *f* valvula semilunaris intermed.); *g, h* valva atrioventricularis sin. s. bicuspidalis (*g* cuspis septalis, *h* cuspis parietalis); *i, k, l* valva atrioventricularis dext. s. tricuspidalis (*i* cuspis septalis, *k* cuspis parietalis, *l* cuspis angularis); *m* septum interatriale; *n* conus arteriosus, *o* margo ventricularis dext.; *p* margo ventricularis sin.; *q* sulcus interventricularis paraconalis; *r* sulcus interventricularis subsinuosus

1 a. coronaria sin.; *2* r. interventricularis paraconalis; *3, 3* r. circumflexus; *4* r. and v. prox. ventriculi sin.; *5* r. and v. marginis ventricularis sin.; *6* r. and v. dist. ventriculi sin.; *7* r. prox. atrii sin.; *8, 9* a. coronaria dext., *8* its ramus circumflexus and *9* its r. interventricularis subsinuosus; *10* a. and v. coni arteriosi; *11* r. and v. prox. ventriculi dext.; *12* r. marginis ventricularis dext. and its accompanying vein; *13* r. dist. ventriculi dext.; *14* r. ventricularis sin.; *15* r. prox. atrii dext., *15'* its terminal branch to the v. cava cran., *15"* its branch to the right atrium; *16* v. cordis media; *17* entry of the sinus coronarius; *18, 19* v. cordis magna, *18* its r. circumflexus, *19* its r. interventricularis paraconalis; *20, 20* v. circumflexa dext.; *21* its r. prox. atrii dext.; *22* r. dist. ventriculi dext. of the v. cordis media

breeds of which the German landrace and the Piétrain pig represented early maturing pork varieties while the German pasture pig and the Mangalitza were examples of late-maturing fattening pigs. Dwarf pigs of a special type were used as controls.

Using the body weight for calculating the relative heart weight may be criticised because it is known that growth of the heart does not keep pace with the increase in body weight in breeds with extensive subcutaneous layers of fat. Calculation of the relative heart weight by comparing, not the body weight, but the weight of the skeletal musculature (theoretical proportion of meat) with that of the heart is a more reliable procedure.

It can be seen from the table that when relative heart weight is calculated on a body weight basis, the pig's heart has a relative weight of 0.3% which is small compared with other domestic mammals. When

Table 1*

Breed (age of animals: 202–205 days)	No. of animals	Body Weight in kg (range)	Absolute heart weight in g — arithmetic mean	Standard deviation	Range	Relative heart weight as % of body weight — arithmetic mean	Standard deviation	Range
German Landrace	33	92–128	335	† 32	258–396	0.32	† 0.03	0.26–0.35
Piétrain	34	71–108	273	† 31	219–352	0.31	† 0.03	0.26–0.39
German Pasture pig	49	98–130	319	† 30	259–374	0.28	† 0.03	0.21–0.37
Mangalitza	21	61–96	213	† 27	172–253	0.27	† 0.03	0.23–0.37
Dwarf pig	37	21–50	122	† 20	91–172	0.33	† 0.05	0.26–0.52

* Modified from Rühl (1971)

the values in table 1 are compared with those of table 2 it will be found that by using the body weight as reference the relative heart weight is greater in the early maturing than in the later maturing breeds. On the other hand, comparison of the absolute heart weight with the whole-body muscle weight indicates that the late maturing breeds have a larger heart and one which is therefore capable of greater performance.

Position of the heart

The craniocaudal limits of the heart extend from the 3rd to the 6th ribs. Its base is craniodorsally directed and lies at about half the height of the thoracic cavity. The right ventricular border follows the contour of the sternum at a little distance from it, while the left ventricular border runs parallel to the cranial border of the sixth rib. The apex of the heart reaches the region of the sixth costal cartilage on the left side. The major part of the heart is embedded in the cardiac impression of both lungs. The *incisura cardiaca* of the left lung leaves a fairly large area of the left surface of the heart uncovered and in

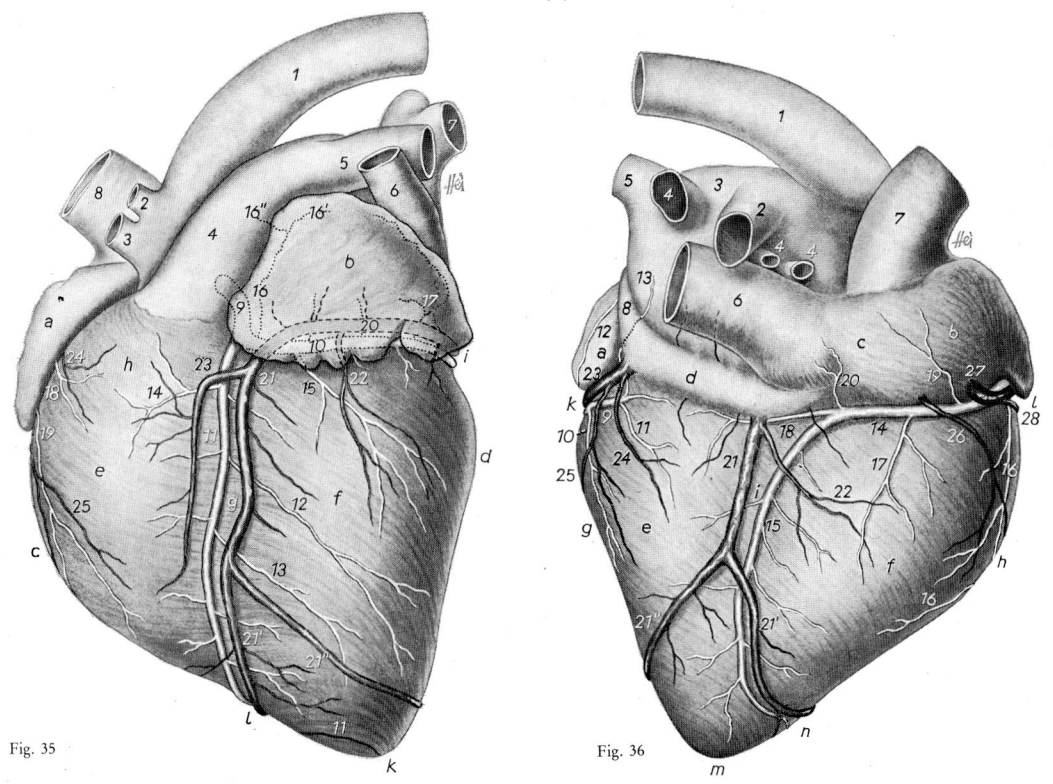

Fig. 35. Facies auricularis of the heart of the pig. (After Rickert, Diss. med. vet., Hanover, 1955.)

a auricula dext.; *b* auricula sin.; *c* margo ventricularis dext.; *d* margo ventricularis sin.; *e* ventriculus dext.; *f* ventriculus sin.; *g* sulcus interventricularis paraconalis; *h* conus arteriosus; *i* sulcus coronarius, pars sin.; *k* apex cordis; *l* incisura apicis

1 arcus aortae; *2* a. subclavia sin.; *3* a. brachiocephalica; *4* truncus pulmonalis; *5* a. pulmonalis sin.; *6* v. azygos sin.; *7* left pulmonary vein; *8* v. cava cran.; *9* a. coronaria sin., *10* its r. circumflexus, *11* its r. interventricularis paraconalis; *12* r. collateralis prox.; *13* r. collateralis dist.; *14* a. coni arteriosi of the a. coronaria sin.; *15* r. prox. ventriculi sin.; *16* r. prox. atrii sin., *16'* its branch to the base of the auricle, *16"* its branch to the wall of the left atrium; *17* r. intermed. atrii sin.; *18* a. coni arteriosi of the a. coronaria dext.; *19* r. prox. ventriculi dext., *20, 21* v. cordis magna, *20* its r. circumflexus, *21* its r. interventricularis paraconalis; *21', 21"* terminal branches of the r. interventricularis paraconalis; *22* v. ventriculi sin.; *23* collateral branch of the v. cordis magna accompanying the r. interventricularis paraconalis; *24* v. coni arteriosi; *25* r. ventricularis dext. of the v. semicircumflexa dext.

Fig. 36. Facies atrialis of the heart of the pig. (After Rickert, Diss. med. vet., Hanover, 1955.)

a atrium sin.; *b* atrium dext.; *c* sinus venarum cavarum; *d* sinus coronarius; *e* ventriculus sin.; *f* ventriculus dext.; *g* margo ventricularis sin.; *h* margo ventricularis dext.; *i* sulcus interventricularis subsinuosus; *k* sulcus coronarius, pars dext.; *l* sulcus coronarius, pars sin.; *m* apex cordis; *n* incisura apicis

1 arcus aortae; *2* right, *3* left pulmonary artery; *4, 4, 4* right pulmonary veins; *5* a left pulmonary vein; *6* v. cava caud.; *7* v. cava cran.; *8* v. azygos sin.; *9* r. circumflexus of the a. coronaria sin.; *10* r. marginis ventricularis sin.; *11* r. ventricularis dist.; *12* r. intermed. atrii sin.; *13* r. dist. atrii sin.; *14, 15* a. coronaria dext., *14* its r. circumflexus, *15* its r. interventricularis subsinuosus; *16, 16* r. marginis ventricularis dext.; *17* r. dist. ventriculi dext.; *18* r. ventriculi sin.; *19* r. intermed. atrii dext.; *20* r. dist. atrii dext.; *21* v. cordis media, *21', 21"* its terminal branches, *22* its r. dist. ventriculi dext.; *23* r. circumflexus of the v. cordis magna, *24* its r. dist. ventriculi sin.; *25* its r. marginis ventricularis sin.; *26* v. marginis ventricularis dext.; *27* v. semicircumflexa dext., *28* its r. prox. ventriculi dext.

Table 2 *

Breed	No. of animals	Proportion of meat in kg arithmetic mean	range	Heart weight relative to meat weight in % arithmetic mean	range
German Landrace	29	18.23	16.06–20.27	1.84	1.5–2.1
Piétrain	32	17.71	15.13–19.62	1.55	1.2–1.8
German pasture pig	48	15.70	12.98–19.14	2.04	1.4–2.5
Mangalitza	21	10.61	8.76–14.73	2.02	1.3–2.8
Dwarf pig	37	5.07	3.34–6.28	2.41	1.8–3.0

* Modified from Rühl (1971)

Weight and dimensions of heart of a pig with a body weight of 73.2 kg are given here as a general example. Absolute heart weight 249.5 g; height of interventricular septum 79.0 mm; height of left ventricle 79.0 mm; height of right ventricle 57.9 mm; thickness of the wall (measured immediately below the atrioventricular orifice) left 20.5 mm, right 10.9 mm; sagittal diameter at the base of the heart 78.4 mm; transverse diameter 62.2 mm.**

apposition to the thoracic wall but the minor incision of the right lung exposes only a small part of the heart surface (cf. Vol II, figs 383 and 384). The *caput longum* of the *m. triceps brachii*, the caudal border of which runs as the *linea anconaea* from the 5th costovertebral joint to the 6th costal cartilage, completely covers the lateral thoracic wall in the region of the heart. However, by pulling the forelimb forward the heart can be made accessible for clinical examination. Examination of the heart in pigs presents considerable difficulties because of the animals excitable reaction to restraint.

Under favourable conditions the apex beat is palpable in the 3rd and 4th intercostal spaces but only faintly so. An indistinct relative cardiac dullness can be elicited by percussion in the left ventral region of the 2nd to 5th intercostal spaces of thin animals.

The left ventricular heart sound can be auscultated in the 4th intercostal space and the right ventricular sound in the 3rd intercostal spaces on the right side (first or muscular sound). The pulmonary sound can be heard on the left side in the 2nd intercostal space and the aortic sound in the 3rd intercostal space (second valvular sound).

Blood vessels of the heart
(34–36)

Arteries

The **a coronaria sin.** (34/1; 35/9) arises from the *sinus bulbi aortae* which belongs to the left semilunar valve. Between the pulmonary trunk and the left auricle it reaches the interventricular paraconal groove in which one of its main branches, the *r. interventricularis paraconalis*, proceeds to the apex of the heart. Its second main branch, the *r. circumflexus (sin.)*, is covered by the left auricle as it follows the *pars sin.* of the coronary groove to reach the *facies subsinuosa* of the heart where it divides into several small ramifications.

The interventricular paraconal branch (34/2; 35/11) gives off numerous innominate branches to the wall of the right ventricle and it also gives off the *a. coni arteriosi* (35/14) to the *conus arteriosus*. The wall of the left ventricle receives, in addition to some smaller vessels, two larger branches the *r. collateralis*

** After Stünze et al. (1959).

prox. (/12) and the *r. collateralis dist.* (/13). Furthermore, there are many small vessels which supply that part of the interventricular septum which lies next to the left longitudinal groove, while the central part of the septum is vascularized by the *r. septi interventricularis.*

The *left circumflex branch* (34/3; 35/10; 36/9), originates from the left coronary artery, and then, as its first off-shoot, gives rise to the *r. prox. ventriculi sin.* (34/4; 35/15) which supplies the left ventricular wall. Next the *r. marginis ventricularis sin.* (36/10) to the caudal border of the heart is given off and this is followed by the *r. dist. ventriculi sin.* (34/6; 36/11) which conveys blood to the wall of the left ventricle between the interventricular subsinuosal groove and the left ventricular border.

The left circumflex branch is also responsible for supplying the wall of the left atrium which it does via the *rr. prox.* (34/7), *intermed.* (35/17) *et dist.* (36/13) *atrii sin.*

The *a. coronaria dext.* (34/8, 9; 36/14, 15) originates from the *sinus bulbi aortae* of the right semilunar valve and its *r. circumflexus (dext.)* (36/14) follows firstly the *pars dext.* of the coronary groove and then, as the subsinuosal interventricular groove (36/15), the *sulcus interventricularis subsinuosus* to the apex of the heart. Thus in the pig we have the so-called bilateral coronary type (26). The first branch of the right circumflex branch to the right ventricular wall is the *r. coni arteriosi* (34/10; 35/18). then follow the *r. prox. ventriculi dext,* (34/11; 35/19), the *r. marginis ventricularis dext.* (34/12; 36/16) and the *r. dist. ventriculi dext.* (34/13; 36/17).

Small branches, including the *rr. prox.* (34/15), *intermed.* (36/19) *et dist.* (/20) *atrii dext.*, supply the wall of the right atrium.

The interventricular subsinuous branch (34/9; 36/15) of the right coronary artery supplies, via numerous smaller branches, the septum and those parts of the right and left ventricular wall which lie near the longitudinal groove. Also participating in the supply of the interventricular septum is the stouter *r. ventriculi sin.* (36/18) which runs below the coronary sinus.

Veins

The tubular **sinus coronarius** (36/*d*) measures about 2–3 cm in length and is the rudiment of the right sinus horn of the embryonic heart. Its orifice in the right atrium carries the *valvula sinus coronarii* and lies below the *ostium venae cavae caud.* The sinus lies on the atrial surface in the coronary groove and continues without any demarcation into the *v. azygos sin.* (36/8) which ascend the left atrium. Its first large branch is the **v. cordis media** *s. v. interventricularis subsinuosa* (34/16; 36/21). In the interventricular subsinuosal groove this vein accompanies the interventricular subsinuosal artery which is a branch of the right coronary artery. In the lower third of the longitudinal groove this medial cardiac vein divides into two vessels of equal calibre (36/21′, 21″). Before reaching the apex of the heart, one of these branches curves round the left ventricular border and the other curves round the right ventricular border, so that they reach the *facies auricularis* where they anastomose with corresponding branches of the great coronary vein. Numerous unnamed branches of the middle cardiac vein drain blood from the neighbouring areas of the ventricular walls and the interventricular septum. A more substantial tributary of this middle cardiac vein is the *v. dist. ventriculi dext.* (36/22).

The *v. cordis magna* (great coronary vein) (34/18; 35/20; 36/23) arises from the coronary sinus at its point of transition to the left azygos vein (36/8). The great coronary vein continues as the *r. circumflexus (sin)*, corvered by the left auricle, in the coronary groove and then enters the interventricular paraconal groove where it is known as the *r. descendens paraconalis* (35/20, 21). In addition to small vessels to the wall of the left ventricle, the left circumflex branch gives off the *r. dist. ventriculi sin.* (36/24), the *r. marginis ventricularis sin.* (/25) and the *r. prox. ventriculi sin.* (35/22) which are the accompanying veins of similarly named arteries that issue from the circumflex branch of the left coronary artery.

The *r. interventricularis paraconalis* of the great coronary vein (35/21) gives off a branch (/23) which runs first at an acute angle and then parallel to it. Within the longitudinal groove the interventricular paraconal ramus gives rise to several smaller branches which supply the right and left ventricular wall and it then divides into two stout limbs (/21′, 21″) which, as already mentioned, anastomose with the terminal branches of the middle cardiac vein.

The *v. marginis ventricularis dext.* (34/12; 36/26) and the stout *v. semicircumflexa dext.* (34/20; 36/27) spring directly from the right atrium. The latter vein acts as a collecting vessel for the *r. prox. ventriculi dext.* (35/25; 36/28), the *v. coni arteriosi* (34/10; 35/24) and the *r. prox. atrii dext.* (34/21).

The *vv. cordis minimae* measure only a few millimeters and they carry blood from the myocardium of the atria and ventricles directly into the interior of the heart. They are most numerous in the wall of the right atrium, less occur in the left atrium and the right ventricle, and finally they are least common in the left ventricle.

Heart of the ox
(6, 37–40)

In the diastolic state the heart of the ox has the form of an even, squat cone but in systole it becomes more pointed with a slightly concave *margo ventricularis sin.* It carries a shallow third longitudinal groove, the *sulcus intermedius* (intermediate or caudal groove), which runs along the left ventricular border but does not reach the apex of the heart. Another striking species characteristic is seen in the auricles; their sharp borders extend far beyond the base of the ventricles and they are so notched and serrated (38/B) that they resemble a cock's comb.

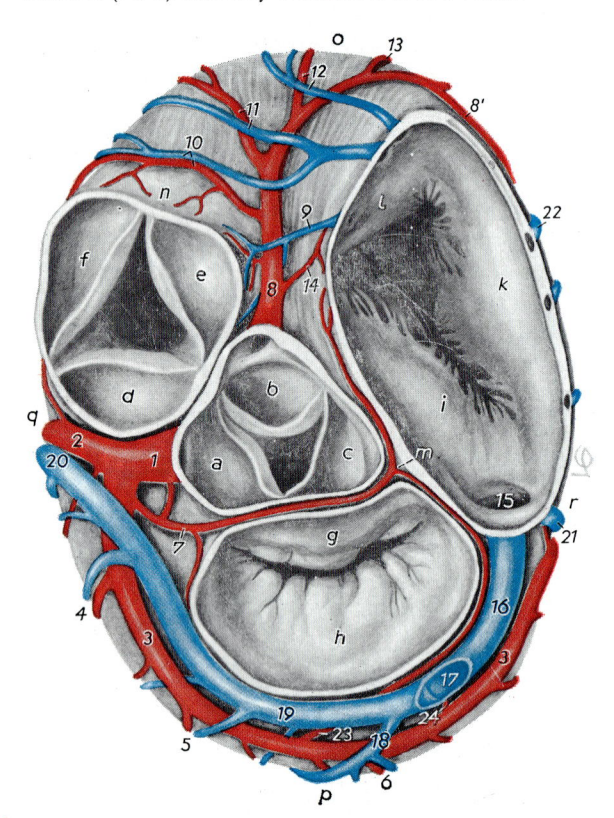

Fig. 37. Base of a bovine heart after removal of the atria. (After Hegazi, Diss. med. vet., Giessen, 1958.)

a, b, c valva aortae (*a* valvula semilunaris sin., *b* valvula semilunaris dext., *c* valvula semilunaris septalis); *d, e, f* valva trunci pulmonalis (*d* valvula semilunaris sin., *e* valvula semilunaris dext., *f* valvula semilunaris intermed.); *g, h* valva atrioventricularis sin. s. bicuspidalis (*g* cuspis septalis, *h* cuspis parietalis); *i, k, l* valva atrioventricularis dext. s. tricuspidalis (*i* cuspis septalis, *k* cuspis parietalis, *l* cuspis angularis); *m* septum interatriale; *n* conus arteriosus; *o* margo ventricularis dext.; *p* margo ventricularis sin.; *q* sulcus interventricularis paraconalis; *r* sulcus interventricularis subsinuosus

1 a. coronaria sin., *2* its r. interventricularis paraconalis, *3, 3* its r. circumflexus (sin.); *4* r. and v. prox. ventriculi sin.; *5* r. and v. marginis ventricularis sin.; *6* r. and v. dist. ventriculi sin.; *7* r. prox. atrii sin.; *8* a. coronaria dext., *8'* its r. circumflexus (dext.); *9* v. coni arteriosi; *10* a. coni arteriosi with its collateral vein; *11* r. and v. prox. ventriculi dext.; *12* r. and v. marginis ventricularis dext.; *13* r. dist. ventriculi dext.; *14* r. prox. atrii dext.; *15* orifice of the sinus coronarius; *16* sinus coronarius; *17* termination of the v. azygos sin. in the sinus coronarius; *18* v. cordis caud.; *19* v. cordis magna; *20* r. interventricularis paraconalis of the v. cordis magna; *21* v. cordis media s. interventricularis subsinuosa; *22* v. dist. ventriculi dext.; *23* r. intermed. atrii sin.; *24* r. dist. atrii sin.

Accumulations of adipose tissue are remarkably abundant in certain parts of the heart and they can amount to up to 24% of the weight of the heart muscle. This adipose tissue is yellowish white and in the cold state of a tallow-like firmness and slightly brittle consistency. It completely fills the entire length and depth of the coronary groove, extending below the auricles so that the conus arteriosus is enclosed in a extensive cushion. An isolated strip-like complex of adipose tissue covers the roof of the right atrium at the insertion of the pericardium. The adipose tissue follows the large blood vessels so that it fills the three longitudinal grooves. Even the smaller blood vessels are accompanied by similar tissue and on other parts of the heart's surface one can also find thin layers of fat tissue. Since this adipose tissue is not removed to any extent even in thin ruminats, it must be considered as comprising what has been referred to as structural fat which is associated with the function of the heart. It fills up all the incongruities of the heart's surface and smooths over the borders between the atria and between their auricles and the base of the ventricles. Another peculiarity of this species is the frequent presence of subendocardial adipose tissue, especially in the region of the papillary muscles and also at other sites on the inner wall of the heart.

Heart of the ox

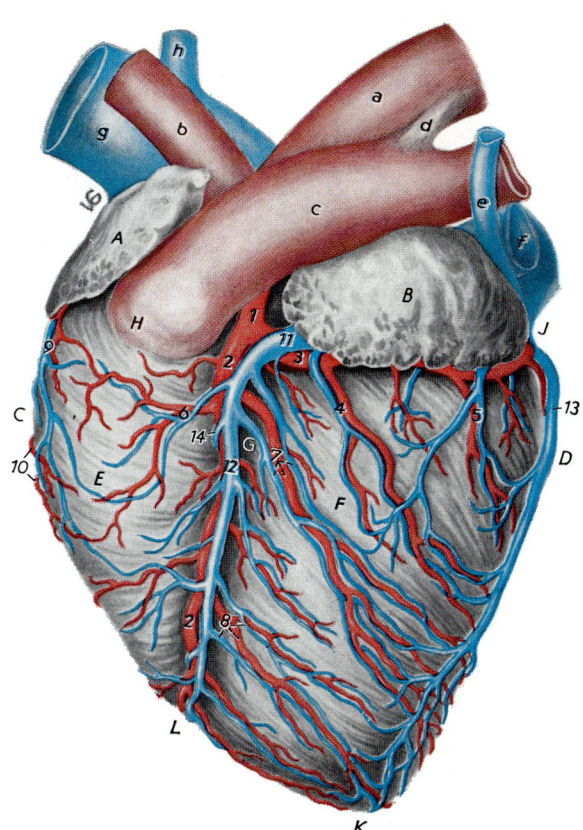

Fig. 38. Arteries and veins on the facies auricularis of an ox heart. (After Hegazi. Diss. med. vet., Giessen, 1958.)

A auricula dext.; *B* auricula sin.; *C* margo ventricularis dext.; *D* margo ventricularis sin.; *E* ventriculus dext.; *F* ventriculus sin.; *G* sulcus interventricularis paraconalis; *H* conus arteriosus; *J* sulcus coronarius, pars sin.; *K* apex cordis; *L* incisura apicis

a arcus aortae; *b* truncus brachiocephalicus communis; *c* truncus pulmonalis; *d* lig. arteriosum (Botalli); *e* v. azygos sin.; *f* left pulmonary vein; *g* v. cava cran.; *h* v. costocervicalis

1 a. coronaria sin., *2*, *2* its r. interventricularis paraconalis with branches to both ventricles, *3* its r. circumflexus (sin.); *4* r. and v. prox. ventriculi sin.; *5* r. and v. marginis ventricularis sin.; *6* a. and v. coni arteriosi; *7* r. and v. collateralis prox.; *8* r. and v. collateralis dist.; *9* a. and v. coni arteriosi; *10* r. and v. prox. ventriculi dext.; *11* v. cordis magna, *12* its r. interventricularis paraconalis with branches to both ventricles; *13* v. cordis caud. with its branches to the left ventricle; *14* r. septi interventricularis of the v. cordis magna

Fig. 39. Arteries and veins of the atrial surface of the ox heart. (After Hegazi, Diss. med. vet., Giessen, 1958.)

A atrium dext., *B*, *B* atrium sin.; *C* margo ventricularis dext.; *D* margo ventricularis sin.; *E* ventriculus dext.; *F* ventriculus sin.; *G* sulcus interventricularis subsinuosus; *H* sinus venarum cavarum; *J* sulcus coronarius dext.; *K* apex cordis; *L* incisura apicis

a arcus aortae; *b* truncus brachiocephalicus communis; *c* branches of the a. pulmonalis; *d* vv. pulmonales; *e* v. azygos sin.; *f* v. cava caud.; *g* v. cava cran.; *h* v. costocervicalis

1 r. circumflexus sin. of the a. coronaria sin., *2* its r. interventricularis subsinuosus with its branches to the right ventricle; *3* terminal branches of the r. interventricularis paraconalis of the a. coronaria sin. and the v. cordis magna; *4* r. dist. ventriculi sin.; *5* r. intermed. atrii sin.; *6* r. dist. atrii sin.; *7* r. ventriculi dext. of the a. coronaria sin.; *8* r. circumflexus of the a. coronaria dext., *9* its r. marginis ventricularis dext., *10* its r. and v. dist. ventriculi dext., *11* its r. intermed. atrii dext., *12* its r. dist. atrii dext.; *13* sinus coronarius; *14* v. cordis media with its branches to the two ventricles, *15* its r. dist. ventriculi sin.; *16* v. cordis magna; *17*, *17* v. cordis caud.; *18*, *18* its r. dist. ventriculi sin.; *19* terminal branches of the v. cordis caud. and the r. collateralis prox. of the a. coronaria sin.

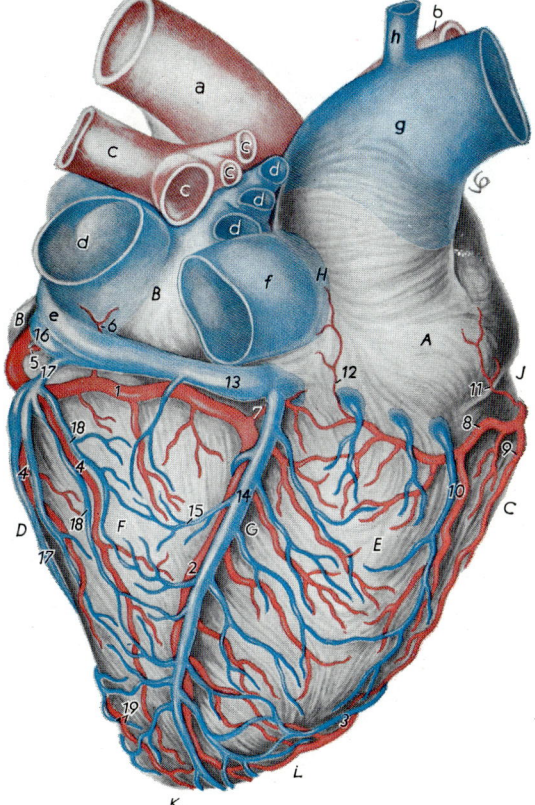

Internal structure of the ventricles

Both ventricles have certain distinctive features but these are only useful in identifying the species to a limited degree.

The outer wall of the right ventricle carries numerous stout trabeculae carneae in the inflow region, that is to say, below the right atrioventricular orifice. In the region of the outflow tract, which extends into the conus arteriosus, the outer wall is smooth. The septum and almost the entire left ventricle are also smooth walled.

The two papillary muscles of the left ventricle are considerably thicker than those of the right ventricle.

The *m. papillaris subauricularis* appears as a column on the outer wall of the left ventricle. The presence of a deep longitudinal groove clearly divides it into two parts each of which terminates at the ostial end in a prominent papilla from which chordae tendineae extend to the membranous valves. The *m. papillaris subatrialis,* which is more distally situated, also presents as a muscular column which is fused to the outer wall and carries several monticules for the insertion of tendinous chords. The thin *mm. transversi* form a wide-meshed network between the septum and the base of the papillary musle. Furthermore there are other, irregularly arranged but also thin, transverse muscles (moderator bands) which connect the septum with the outer wall.

Of the three papillary muscles of the right ventricle, the *m. papillaris magnus* is situated on the outer wall while the *mm. papillares parvi* and the *m. papillaris subarteriosus* arise from the septum.

The base of the great papillary muscle consists of several trabeculae carneae and this muscle also bears several protuberances. It is either broadly fused to the outer wall or rises from it in the form of a multinodular cupola. Its tendinous chords go to the *cuspis parietalis* and *angularis.* The small papillary muscles are situated on the septum where the latter meets the subsinuous part of the outer wall of the right ventricle in an acute angle. They each have a uniform base which carries two or three free-standing wart-like processes and give rise to the chordae tendineae stretching to the septal and parietal cusps. The subarterial papillary muscle arises from the septum as a low swelling and extends to below the *crista supraventricularis* where it gives rise to double rows of tendinous chords running to the septal and angular cusps.

The trabecula septomarginalis (moderator band) of the right ventricle is a thick strand, circular in cross-section and up to one centimeter in diameter. It arises from the base of the subarterial papillary muscle and, pointing towards the apex, crosses the ventricle and is inserted into the outer wall by several branches. There are no other transverse muscles in the right ventricle.

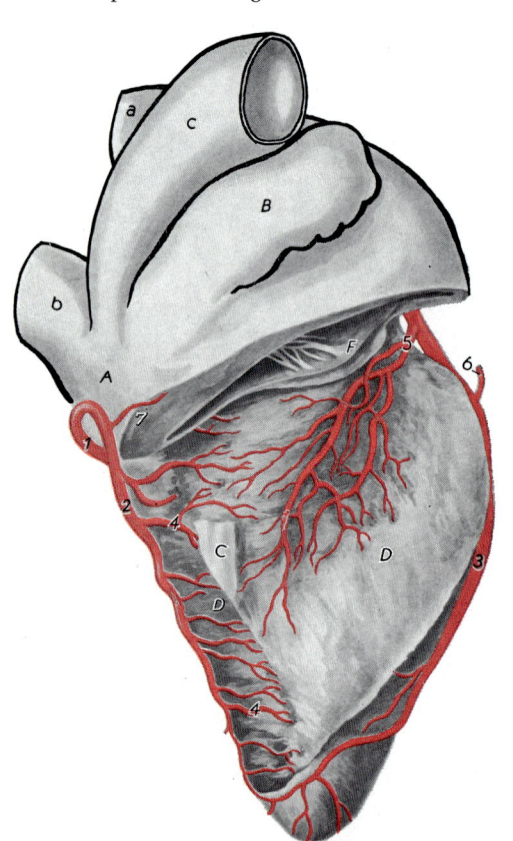

Fig. 40. Arterial supply of the interventricular septum of the ox heart, right side. (After Hegazi, Diss. med. vet., Giessen, 1958.)

A atrium dext.; *B* right auricle; *C* m. papillaris subarteriosus; *D, D* septum interventriculare; *E* apex cordis; *F* mm. papillares parvi

a arcus aortae; *b* v. cava caud.; *c* v. cava cran.

1 r. circumflexus of the a. coronaria sin.; *2* r. interventricularis subsinuosus of the a. coronaria sin.; *3* r. interventricularis paraconalis of the a. coronaria sin.; *4, 4* branches of the r. interventricularis subsinuosus to the septum and papillary muscles; *5* r. septi interventricularis of the r. interventricularis paraconalis with its branches to the septum and papillary muscles; *6* a. coni arteriosi of the a. coronaria sin.; *7* r. ventriculi dext. of the a. coronaria sin.

Size and weight of the heart

As may be seen from the following table, the ox has a small heart, both in absolute and relative weights, when compared with other species but this accords with its style of life.

Size and weight of the heart of the ox *

Sex	Age in years	Body weight in kg	Heart weight in kg absolute	Heart weight in kg relative	Diameter in cm sagittal	Diameter in cm transverse	Length in cm of the margo ventricularis dext.	Length in cm of the margo ventricularis sin.	Circumference of the heart at the coronary groove in cm
female	8	648.6	2.40	0.37 %	17.2	15.0	22.0	20.5	47.4
female	3 1/2	601.5	2.34	0.389 %	15.0	12.0	22.0	18.0	51.0
female	4	480.0	2.40	0.5 %	17.1	14.0	21.2	21.6	50.2
female	7	462.0	2.31	0.5 %	15.4	13.0	21.1	17.2	48.5
female	3	442.5	2.18	0.493 %	17.0	14.0	21.0	21.0	53.0
female	3	419.0	2.2	0.518 %	15.0	13.0	21.0	20.0	44.0
female	6	416.6	2.17	0.48 %	15.0	13.0	18.0	16.2	50.3
female	5	383.3	2.30	0.6 %	15.0	13.0	22.0	19.0	52.0
female	8	330.3	2.16	0.654 %	17.3	12.0	25.0	20.8	49.9
female	7	326.6	1.95	0.597 %	15.2	12.0	21.0	17.0	42.5
female	4	319.0	2.20	0.689 %	13.2	10.7	18.0	15.8	42.2
bull	5	776.6	3.33	0.428 %	17.4	14.0	21.1	21.0	47.4
bull	5	485.4	2.16	0.445 %	13.9	13.0	21.8	19.2	51.8
bullock	5	705.9	3.40	0.441 %	15.3	12.5	19.8	21.0	46.3
bullock	7	575.0	2.30	0.40 %	18.4	12.0	24.0	20.4	47.0
calf	1/12	79.0	0.69	0.87 %	9.0	8.0	12.4	11.3	31.2
calf	2/12	153.3	0.70	0.45 %	9.2	8.7	12.5	11.2	31.7

* After Schubert (1909)

Position of the heart
(6)

In the craniocaudal direction the heart extends from the 3rd to the 5th or 6th ribs. Its long axis is relatively steep. The base of the heart is craniodorsally directed and reaches to about half the height of the thoracic cavity; the apex lies a few centimeters from the sternum in the region of the 5th left costochondral junction. The slightly concave border to the left ventricle lies a short distance from the diaphragm and follows the contour of the cranially arched cupola of this structure. Five sevenths of the heart lies to the left of the median plane and it is in contact with the left thoracic wall between the 4th and 5th intercostal spaces. The lightly curved contour of the ventral border of the double cranial lobe of the left lung leaves a considerable part of the left cardiac surface uncovered whereas the right surface of the heart, which is placed some distance from the thoracic wall, is covered to a greater extent by the cranial and medial lobes of the right lung. In the ox the caudal border of the relatively small long head of the triceps brachii muscle (*linea anconaea*) follows the 5th intercostal space. (cf. vol. II. Figs 207, 208, 351, 352, 398 and 399).

The apex beat in the ox is most distinctly palpable on the left side in the 4th intercostal space. It can also be felt on the right side in the same area but less clearly. In heavy, well nourished animals the apex beat is less distinct.

The area of relative cardiac dullness lies on the left side in the 3rd to 4th intercostal space but its limits are indistinct even in lean animals. The left ventricular and aortic sounds are most clearly audible in the 4th intercostal space, the pulmonary sound being most clearly detected in the 3rd intercostal space. The right ventricular sound is audible in the 3rd intercostal space.

Heart of the sheep and goat
(20, 41–45)

The heart of the sheep is in the form of a blunt cone and resembles in shape that of the ox (41; 42). The goat's heart, on the other hand, has the form of a pointed cone (43; 44). Both species have a less distinct intermediate groove on the left ventricular border, a feature characteristic of the ruminant heart. The edges of both auricles are serrated and the description given above of the colour, consistency and distribution of subepicardial adipose tissue of the ox heart applies equally to the small ruminants.

Internal structure of the ventricles (sheep)

In the sheep both papillary muscles of the outer wall of the left ventricle are stout. The subauricular papillary muscle has a cylindrical shape and two apices. The subarterial papillary muscle is better developed than the preceding and invariably has a double-pointed cupola.

Two of the papillary muscles of the right ventricle are situated on the septum and the third is placed on the outer wall. The latter is the *m. papillaris magnus* (20/c) and usually has a three-pointed apex. The *m. papillaris subarteriosus* (/e) is the smallest and appears as a protrusion the size of a pea on the septum. The *mm. papillares parvi* (/d) vary in shape. They consist of a united group which usually carries two distinctly separated papillae.

The papillary muscles of the goat are similar.

According to Schröder (1922), the absolute heart weight of rams is 241 g, of castrated males 220 g and of ewes 232 g. The corresponding figures for the relative heart weights are 0.51%, 0.46% and 0.49%.

The positions of the heart in the sheep and goat correspond closely to that recorded for the ox (cf. Vol. II, Figs 236, 237) and the topographical data for clinical examination of the heart of the ox are similarly applicable.

Blood vessels of the hearts of ruminants
(37–45)

The cardiac blood vessels of the ox, sheep and goat are similar not only in respect of their origin and course but also in that they supply the same regions of the heart. In all three species the left coronary artery supplies a far greater proportion of the organ than does the right coronary artery and they are thus all of left coronary type (25). In order to avoid repetition when describing the cardiac vascular pattern of the three domestic ruminants, the following account is confined to the ox but, with the aid of the illustrations and corresponding legends, the data presented for the ox can be applied without difficulty to the sheep and goat. Differences in the course of the vessels, especially smaller vessels, in the heart of sheep and goats, which may be of some significance for identification of the species, are shown in the appropriate illustrations.

Arteries of the heart of the ox
(37–40)

The **a. coronaria sin.** (37/1; 38/1) arises from the left sinus of the aortic bulbus. Its short trunk is situated between the truncus pulmonalis and the left auricle and divides into the interventricular paraconal and the left circumflex branches which are of approximately equal diameter.

The *r. interventricularis paraconalis* (37/2; 38/2) runs in the sulcus of the same name to the *incisura apicis* where its branches anastomose with those of the terminal ramifications of the *r. interventricularis subsinuosus*. In addition to small branches to the left and right ventricular musculature in the vicinity of the longitudinal grooves, the interventricular paraconal branch gives off the *r. coni arteriosi* (38/6), to the conus arteriosus of the right ventricle, and the *rr. collaterales prox. et dist.* (38/7, 8) to the auricular face and the border of the left ventricle where it anastomoses with branches of the *r. interventricularis subsinuosus*. The interventricular paraconal branch also provides a stout ramus, the *r. septi interventricularis* (40/5), and numerous smaller vessels for the vascularization of the interventricular septum.

Arteries of the ox's heart

Fig. 41. Arteries and veins of the auricular surface of the sheep heart. (After Hegazi, Diss. med. vet., Giessen, 1958.)

A right auricle; *B* left auricle; *C* margo ventricularis dext.; *D* margo ventricularis sin.; *E* ventriculus dext.; *F* ventriculus sin.; *G* sulcus interventricularis paraconalis; *H* conus arteriosus; *J* sulcus coronarius, pars sin.; *K* apex cordis; *L* incisura apicis

a arcus aortae; *b* truncus brachiocephalicus communis; *c* truncus pulmonalis; *d* lig. arteriosum (Botalli); *e* v. azygos sin.; *f* vv. pulmonales sinn.; *g* v. cava cran.; *h* v. costocervicalis

1 a. coronaria sin., *2* its r. descendens paraconalis with branches to both ventricles, *3* its r. circumflexus (sin.); *4* r. and v. prox. ventriculi sin.; *5* r. marginis ventricularis sin.; *6* a. and v. coni arteriosi; *7* r. and v. collateralis prox.; *8* r. and v. collateralis dist.; *9* a. coni arteriosi; *10* r. and v. prox. ventriculi dext.; *11* v. cordis magna, *12* its r. interventricularis paraconalis with branches to both ventricles; *13* v. cordis caud. with branches to the left ventricle

The *r. circumflexus (sin.)* (37/3; 38/3; 39/1) of the left coronary artery courses in the left part of the coronary groove to reach the interventricular subsinuosal groove. It sends the *r. interventricularis subsinuosus* (39/2) into the latter groove and this extends to the apex of the heart. The circumflex branch also supplies the wall of the left ventricle with several small and three larger arteries, the latter being the *r. prox. ventriculi sin.* (37/4; 38/4), the *r. marginis ventricularis sin.* (37/5; 38/5) and the *r. dist. ventriculi sin.* (37/6; 39/4). From the left circumflex branch the wall of the left atrium receives the *rr. prox.* (37/7), *intermed.* (39/5) and *dist.* (39/6) *atrii sin.*

Fig. 42. Arteries and veins of the atrial surface of the sheep heart. (After Hegazi, Diss. med. vet., Giessen, 1958.)

A atrium dext.; *B, B* atrium sin.; *C* margo ventricularis dext.; *D* margo ventricularis sin.; *E* ventriculus dext.; *F* ventriculus sin.; *G* sulcus interventricularis subsinuosus; *H* sinus venarum cavarum; *J* sulcus coronarius dext.; *K* apex cordis; *L* incisura apicis

a arcus aortae; *b, b, b* truncus brachiocephalicus communis; *c* branches of the a. pulmonalis; *d, d* vv. pulmonales dext.; *e.* v. azygos sin.; *f* v. cava caud.; *g* v. cava cran.; *h* v. costocervicalis

1 r. circumflexus sin. of the a. coronaria sin.; *2* r. interventricularis subsinuosus of the a. coronaria sin. with its branches to the right ventricle; *3* terminal branch of the r. interventricularis paraconalis of the a. coronaria sin.; *4* r. dist. ventriculi sin.; *5* r. dist. atrii sin.; *6* r. ventriculi dext.; *7* r. circumflexus of the a. coronaria dext.; *8* its r. marginis ventricularis dext.; *9* its r. and v. dist. ventriculi dext.; *10* its r. intermed. atrii dext., *11* its r. dist. atrii dext.; *12* sinus coronarius; *13* v. cordis media s. v. interventricularis subsinuosa with its branches to both ventricles, *14* its r. dist. ventriculi sin.; *15* v. cordis magna; *16* v. cordis caud.; *17* vena dist. ventriculi sin.

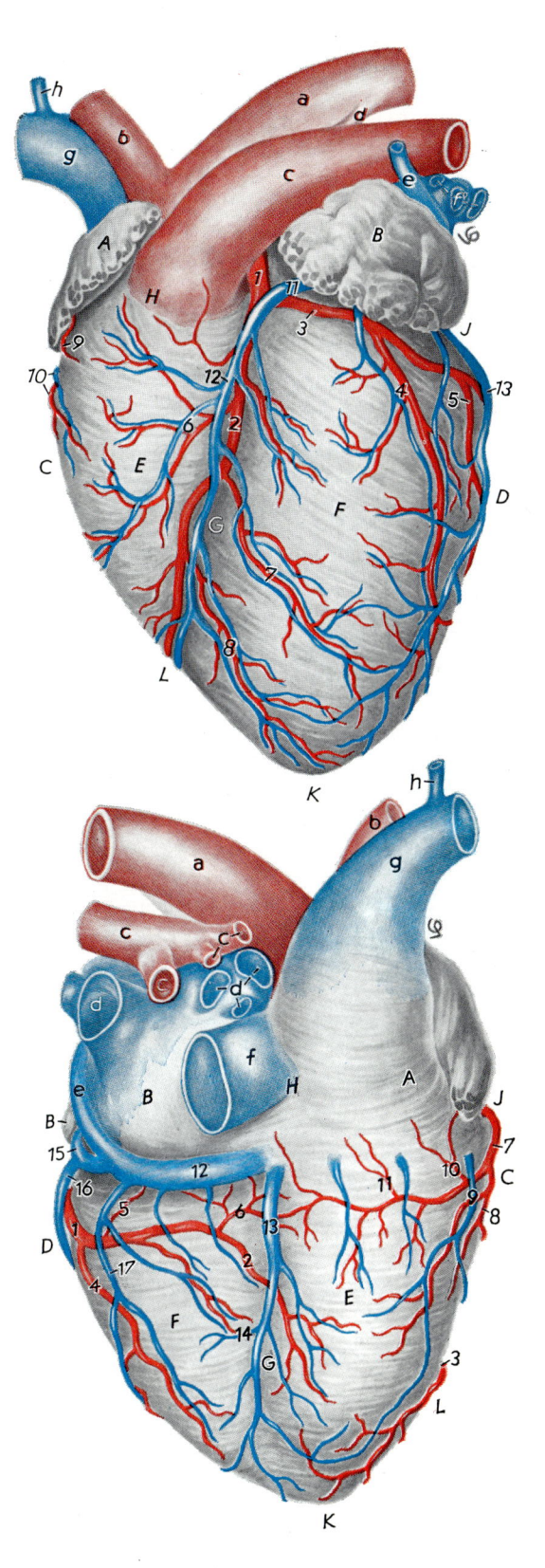

The *r. interventricularis subsinuosus* (39/2) is the immediate continuation of the left circumflex ramus of the left coronary artery and it vascularizes, by means of branches of varying diameter, the interventricular septum (40/4) and those parts of the left and right ventricular wall which are situated next to the longitudinal groove. It also gives off the *r. ventriculi dext.* (39/7) which has subsidiaries supplying the septum of the atria and running to the ventricles. The anastomoses between the terminal branches of the two interventricular arteries in the region of the incisura apicis have already been mentioned.

The **a. coronaria dext.** (37/8; 39/8) is a considerably smaller vessel than its left counterpart. It arises from the sinus of the right semilunar valve of the bulbus aortae and enters the right part of the coronary groove to attain the atrial surface of the right ventricle where its terminal branches anastomose with those of the *r. ventriculi dext.* and the *r. interventricularis subsinuosus* of the left coronary artery. From

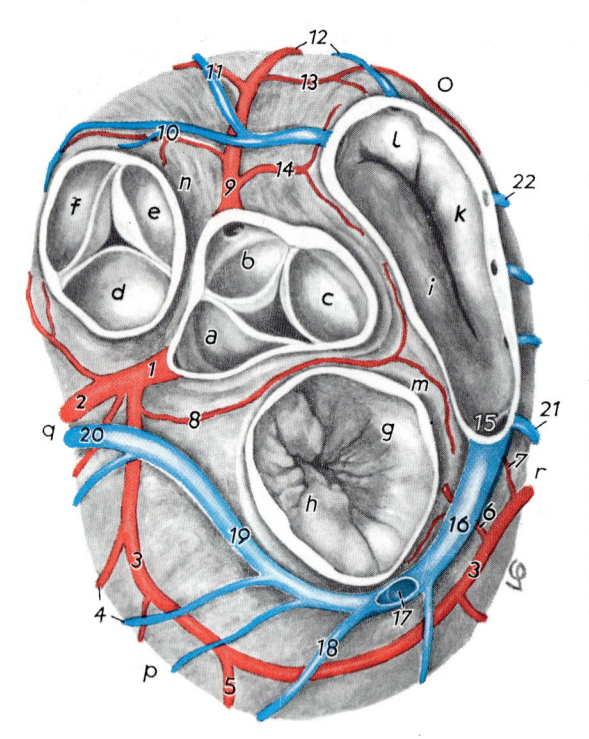

Fig. 43. The base of the goat's heart from which the atria have been removed. (After Hegazi, Diss. med. vet., Giessen, 1958.)

a, b, c valva aortae (*a* valvula semilunaris sin., *b* valvula semilunaris dext., *c* valvula semilunaris septalis); *d, e, f* valva trunci pulmonalis (*d* valvula semilunaris sin., *e* valvula semilunaris dext., *f* valvula semilunaris intermed.); *g, h* valva atrioventricularis sin. s. bicuspidalis (*g* cuspis septalis, *h* cuspis parietalis); *i, k, l* valva atrioventricularis dext. s. tricuspidalis (*i* cuspis septalis, *k* cuspis parietalis, *l* cuspis angularis); *m* septum interatriale; *n* conus arteriosus; *o* margo ventricularis dext.; *p* margo ventricularis sin.; *q* sulcus interventricularis paraconalis; *r* sulcus interventricularis subsinuosus

1 a. coronaria sin., *2* its r. interventricularis paraconalis, *3, 3* its r. circumflexus (sin.); *4* r. and v. prox. ventriculi sin.; *5* common stem of the r. marginis ventricularis sin. and of the r. dist. ventriculi sin.; *6* r. dist. atrii sin.; *7* r. ventriculi dext.; *8* r. prox. atrii sin.; *9* a. coronaria dext.; *10* a. and v. coni arteriosi; *11* r. and v. prox. ventriculi dext.; *12* r. circumflexus of the a. coronaria dext. and the v. marginis ventricularis dext.; *13* r. intermed. atrii dext.; *14* r. prox. atrii dext.; *15* orifice of the sinus coronarius; *16* sinus coronarius; *17* entry of the v. azygos sin. into the sinus coronarius; *18* v. cordis caud.; *19* v. cordis magna, *20* its r. interventricularis paraconalis; *21* v. cordis media s. v. interventricularis subsinuosa; *22* v. dist. ventriculi dext.

it spring small vessels by which it supplies the wall of the right atrium and it also sends larger branches to the right ventricle in the region of the coronary groove. The first of these large branches, the *r. coni arteriosi* (37/10; 38/9), anastomoses in the region of the *conus arteriosus* with branches of a similarly named artery deriving from the left coronary artery. The second offshoot from the right coronary artery, the *v. prox. ventriculi dext.* (37/11; 38/10), attains the atrial surface of the right ventricle, where it forks into two vessels which anastomose with branches of the *r. interventricularis paraconalis* of the left coronary artery. The *r. marginis ventricularis dext* (37/12; 39/9) is given off next and it descends towards the apex on that border of the heart; its branches anastomose with those of the *rr. interventriculares paraconalis et subsinuosus* of the left coronary artery. The fourth of these larger branches of the right coronary artery is the *r. dist. ventriculi dext.* (37/13; 39/10). Together with the last two arteries it participates in the supply of the right ventricular wall. The wall of the right atrium is supplied by the three smaller vessels, the *rr. prox., intermed.* and *dist. atrii dext.* which arise either from the right coronary artery or its circumflex ramus.

The subauricular papillary muscle of the left ventricle receives branches from the *r. collateralis prox.* of the interventricular paraconal ramus and the *rr. proxx. et distt. ventriculi sin.* from the circumflex branch of the left coronary artery. The subatrial papillary muscle is supplied by arteries from the interventricular paraconal and the interventricular subsinuosal branches as well as by vessels from the *r. marginis ventricularis sin.* of the circumflex branch of the left coronary artery.

Arteries of the ox's heart

The large papillary muscle of the right ventricle is supplied by branches of the *r. prox. ventriculi dext.* and the *r. marginis ventricularis dext.* of the *r. circumflexus* (*dext.*) of the right coronary artery. Blood is carried to the small papillary muscles by branches of the *r. septi interventricularis* of the *r. interventricularis paraconalis* (40/5).

Fig. 44. Arteries and veins of the auricular surface of the heart of the goat. (After Hegazi, Diss. med. vet., Giessen, 1958.)

A right auricle; *B* left auricle; *C* margo ventricularis dext.; *D* margo ventricularis sin.; *E* ventriculus dext.; *F* ventriculus sin.; *G* sulcus interventricularis paraconalis; *H* conus arteriosus; *J* sulcus coronarius, pars sin.; *K* apex cordis; *L* incisura apicis

a arcus aortae; *b* truncus brachiocephalicus communis; *c* truncus pulmonalis; *d* lig. arteriosum (Botalli); *e* v. azygos sin.; *f, f* vv. pulmonales sin.; *g* v. cava cran.; *h* v. costocervicalis

1 a. coronaria sin., *2* its r. interventricularis paraconalis with branches to both ventricles, *3* its r. circumflexus (sin.); *4* r. and v. prox. ventriculi sin.; *5* r. marginis ventricularis sin.; *6* a. coni arteriosi; *7* r. and v. collateralis prox.; *8* r. and v. collateralis dist.; *9* a. and v. coni arteriosi; *10* r. prox. ventriculi dext.; *11* v. cordis magna, *12* its r. interventricularis paraconalis with branches to both ventricles; *13* v. cordis caud. with its branches to the left ventricle

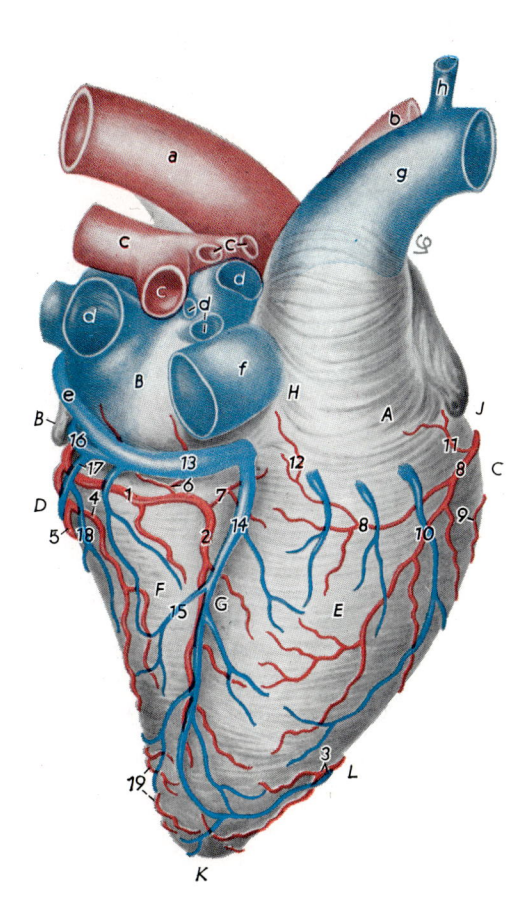

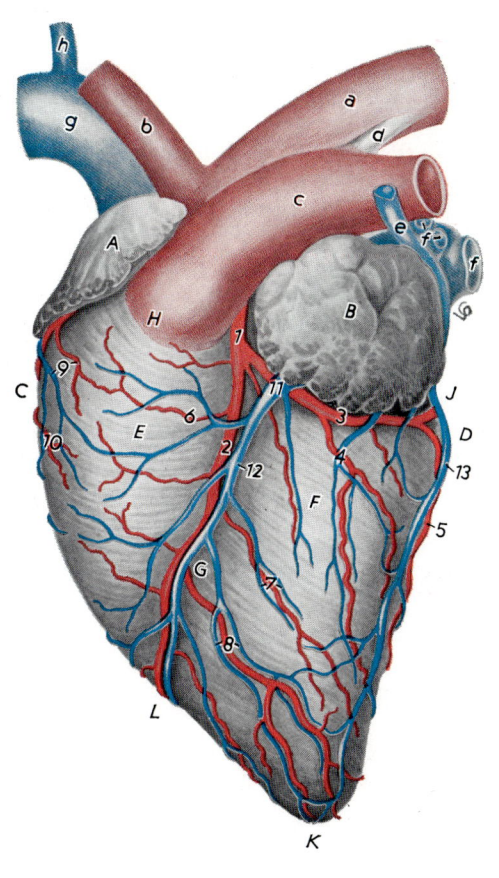

Fig. 45. Arteries and veins of the atrial surface of the heart of the goat. (After Hegazi, Diss. med. vet., Giessen, 1958.)

A atrium dext.; *B, B* atrium sin., *C* margo ventricularis dext.; *D* margo ventricularis sin.; *E* ventriculus dext.; *F* ventriculus sin.; *G* sulcus interventricularis subsinuosus; *H* sinus venarum cavarum; *J* sulcus coronarius dext.; *K* apex cordis; *L* incisura apicis

a arcus aortae; *b, b, b* truncus brachiocephalicus communis; *c* branches of the truncus pulmonalis; *d, d, d* vv. pulmonales; *e* v. azygos sin.; *f* v. cava caud.; *g* v. cava cran.; *h* v. costocervicalis

1 r. circumflexus of the a. coronaria sin.; *2* its r. interventricularis subsinuosus with branches to the right ventricle; *3* terminal branches of the r. interventricularis paraconalis of the a. coronaria sin. and the v. cordis magna; *4* r. dist. ventriculi sin.; *5* r. marginis ventricularis sin.; *6* r. dist. atrii sin.; *7* r. ventricularis dext.; *8, 8* r. circumflexus (dext.) of the a. coronaria dext., *9* its r. marginis ventricularis dext.; *10* r. and v. dist. ventriculi dext.; *11* r. intermed. atrii dext.; *12* r. dist. atrii dext.; *13* sinus coronarius; *14* v. cordis media s. interventricularis subsinuosa with its branches to the two ventricles, *15* its r. dist. ventriculi sin.; *16* v. cordis magna; *17* v. cordis caud., *18* its r. dist. ventriculi sin.; *19* terminal branches of the r. collateralis dist. of the a. coronaria sin.

Veins of the heart of the ox

The **sinus coronarius** (37/16; 39/13) is a collecting chamber preceeding the right atrium and it receives blood from the *v. cordis magna*, the *v. cordis media* and the *v. marginis ventriculi sin.*, the latter being a vessel which is peculiar to the ruminants. In ruminants, as in pigs, it also receives blood from the *v. azygos sin*. The coronary sinus of the ox is about 5 cm in length and its lumen is about 2 cm in diameter. It opens into the right atrium at the *ostium v. cavae caud.* which is provided with a valve.

The first large vein arising from the coronary sinus is the **v. cordis media** *s. v. interventricularis subsinuosa* (37/21; 39/14) which, together with the interventricular subsinuosal branch of the left coronary artery, follows the similarly named groove to the apex of the heart. There it divides and ultimately anastomoses with branches of the great coronary vein or the *v. marginis ventricularis sin*. It receives its blood from veins which drain the same region as that supplied by the arterial *r. interventricularis subsinuosus*.

The **v. cordis magna** (37/19; 38/11; 39/16) is the direct continuation of the coronary sinus. It runs first as the *r. circumflexus* in the left part of the coronary groove embedded in adipose tissue and covered by the left auricle. It then reaches the interventricular paraconal groove which it enters and is then known as the interventricular paraconal branch (37/20; 38/12), and accompanies the similarly named branch of the left coronary artery to the incisura apicis. There it links with the branches of the middle cardiac vein and forms the anastomoses mentioned above. From the area supplied by the circumflex and interventricular paraconal branches of the left coronary artery, the great cardiac vein collects blood in vessels of various sizes, the largest of them being named after the arteries which they accompany.

Of all domestic mammals, only ruminants have a *v. marginis ventricularis sin. s. v. cordis caud.* (37/18; 38/13 39/17). It is the most slender of the three great cardiac veins and it arises from the terminal portion of the coronary sinus, not far from the origin of the left azygos vein (39/e). It crosses the *r. circumflexus* of the left coronary artery and runs in the *sulcus intermedius* on the left ventricular border to the apex of the heart. Its branches, together with those of the great and middle cardiac veins, drain that part of the left ventricular wall which lies next to the *sulcus intermedius*.

The *vv. cordis dextt.* (parvae) spring directly from the right atrium and are responsible for draining the wall of the right half of the heart. They are indicated in figure 37 by the numbers 9 to 12 and 22.

The *vv. cordis minimae (Thebesii)* measure only a few millimetres in length. They arise directly from the myocardium and terminate in the corresponding chambers of the heart. They are numerous in both atria and less common in the ventricles.

Heart of the horse

In systole the heart of the horse has the form of a blunt cone only slightly longer than the breadth of its base. Its lateral surfaces, the *facies atrialis* and *auricularis,* are slightly flattened. The subepicardial adipose tissue is yellowish and its consistency is decidely soft because of its high content of unsaturated fatty acids. This adipose tissue fills the coronary and longitudinal grooves and in primitive breeds of horses, which are predisposed to fat deposition, it may extend well beyond these grooves.

Internal structure of the ventricles

The most typical of the three papillary muscles of the right ventricle is the *m. papillaris magnus* (10/f; 11/m) which is located on the outer wall. Its broad base is situated at the junction between the upper and middle thirds of the outer wall and it projects freely into the ventricle. It carries several protuberances from which tendinous chords go to the parietal and angular cusps. The *m. papillaris subarteriosus* (10/h; 12/k) has its broad base on the septum from which it projects only slightly as a flat swelling. Tendinous chords arise from it in irregular pattern and extend to the septal and angular cusps. The *mm. papillares parvi* (10/g; 11/l') arise from a broad base placed in that region of the septum which forms an acute angle with the subsinuosal part of the outer wall of the right ventricle. Tendinous chords spring from several wart-like excrescences and go to the septal and parietal cusps.

The *trabecula septomarginalis* (moderator band) (10/o; 11/p) of the right ventricle arises from the base of the subarterial papillary muscle, crosses the lumen of the ventricle and disappears into the base of the great papillary muscle. Nearer the apex of the heart there are a variable number of thin transverse bands (10/o').

The two papillary muscles of the outer wall of the left ventricle, the *m. papillaris subauricularis* (12/l) and the *m. papillaris subatrialis* (9/e; 11/o), are in the form of two massive muscular pillars which bulge into the ventricle, especially during systole. Their distal limit lies far towards the apex of the heart and, standing out from the wall, they run towards the base and reach about half the height of the ventricle. Here they make contact with neighbouring trabeculae carneae and give off chordae tendineae to both cusps. A number of delicate, branching *mm. transversi* cross the lumen of the ventricle to run between the septum and the base of the two papillary muscles.

Size and weight of the heart

Breed differences in both the absolute and relative weights of the heart are particularly obvious in the horse. The lowest relative heart weight is only 0.6% of the body weight and applies to heavy draft horses which are characterised by massive body structure. In comparison with this, the relative heart weight varies between 0.62 and 0.99% in the lighter breeds to the highest value of 1.04% in thoroughbreds.

Weight and size of the heart of the horse, age groups between 4 and 14 years*

Sex	Number	Live weight in kg range	Live weight in kg mean	Absolute heart weight in kg range	Absolute heart weight in kg mean	Relative heart weight in % range	Relative heart weight in % mean	Diameter of heart at base (cm) sagittal range	Diameter of heart at base (cm) sagittal mean
Gelding	42	190–480	375	1.36–3.82	2.98	0.62–0.94	0.78	13.5–21.0	18.1
Mare	62	250–510	324	1.78–4.18	2.79	0.63–0.99	0.78	15.0–21.0	16.2

Diameter of heart at base (cm) transverse range	Diameter of heart at base (cm) transverse mean	Circumference of the heart below the coronary groove (cm) range	Circumference of the heart below the coronary groove (cm) mean	Height of the margo ventricularis (cm) dext. range	Height of the margo ventricularis (cm) dext. mean	Height of the margo ventricularis (cm) sin. range	Height of the margo ventricularis (cm) sin. mean	Maximum thickness of the heart wall in cm left	Maximum thickness of the heart wall in cm right	Maximum thickness of the heart wall in cm septum
8.5–15.0	12.7	38.0–58.0	51	19.0–27.0	22.4	16.0–24.0	21.1	3.19	1.8	4.6
10.5–14.5	12.9	42.0–59.0	50.3	19.0–29.0	23.0	17.0–25.0	20.0	3.1	1.9	4.8

* After Blum (1925)

In a short report from Hoppegarten dated 1909 to 1910, the average absolute heart weight was given as 4.5 kg. This was based on seven thoroughbred horses housed at Hoppergarten which were 160–170 cm in height. The four year old racehorse "Faust", out of "Festa", measured 168 cm and had a heart weighing 5.75 kg.

This impressive value is dwarfed by the weight of a thoroughbred's heart which has been kept since 1927 in the Institute of Veterinary Anatomy of the University of Giessen. It belonged to the stallion "Fels" whose dam, like that of "Faust" was "Festa". Fels was killed at 24 because of old age and his formalin-preserved heart, empty of blood, weighs 8.9 kg.

Position of the heart
(7)

During diastole the cranial border of the heart extends up to the 2nd intercostal space while its caudal border is overlaid by the 6th rib. During systole the right ventricular (cranial) border is displaced to the

3rd intercostal space and the left ventricular (caudal) border to the 5th intercostal space. The axis of the heart points steeply to the sternum and its base lies at the transition between the middle and ventral third of the thoracic cavity. The apex of the heart is slightly deflected to the left and reaches the 6th to 7th costal cartilage, but does not make contact with the sternum. The right ventricular border initially follows the cranial border of the 3rd rib and then the internal contour of the sternum. The ventricular border is covered by the 6th rib as it drops almost vertically towards the sternum. The *linea anconaea* (caudal border of the long head of the triceps brachii muscle) leaves the caudal part of the left ventricle uncovered. Three fifths of the heart lies to the left of the midline. Its *facies auricularis* is therefore in direct contact with the left thoracic wall in the region of the 4th and 5th intercostal space and the 5th rib, where the left lung leaves a gap, the *cardiac notch*. On the right side the *facies subsinuosa* of the heart reaches the thoracic wall in the region of the 4th and 5th ribs (cf. vol. II. Figs 408 and 409).

As in the other domestic mammals, the foreleg of the horse has to be moved as far forward as possible during clinical examination of the heart.

The apex beat can be detected on the left side in the middle third of the thorax between the 3rd and 6th intercostal spaces and is most distinctly felt in the 5th space. On the right side it can be found in the region of the 3rd and 4th intercostal spaces.

By means of percussion a region of absolute cardiac dullness can be elicited on the left side between the 3rd and 5th intercostal spaces. This field is about equal in size to that of the palm of a hand and at the 4th intercostal space its upper border is in about the middle of the lower third of the chest. On the right side this area of dullness is occupied by the right ventricle and lies in the region of the 3rd and 4th intercostal spaces. These areas of absolute dullness merge gradually into a zone of relative dullness where the heart is covered by lung. The extent of these areas of dull percussion sound depends on breed differences, on heart size and on individual variation.

The most distinctly audible of all the heart sounds is that of the left ventricle which is best heard in the 4th and 5th intercostal spaces, that is to say, in the area of cardiac dullness. The right ventricular sound is most distinct on the right side in the 4th and 5th intercostal spaces at about half the height of the lower third of the thorax. The sound of the pulmonary valve is detected on the left side of the chest in the 3rd intercostal space, above the fourth rib in the middle of the ventral third of the chest. The aortic valve sound can be heard on the left in the 4th intercostal space.

Blood vessel
(46–49)

Arteries

The arterial supply to the equine heart is by the **a. coronaria sin.** and the **a. coronaria dext.** which latter is much stouter in this species and supplies a greater proportion of the heart (bilateral coronary type) (26).

The **a. coronaria sin.** (47/1) arises from the left sinus of the aortic bulbus. Between the pulmonary trunk and the left auricle it reaches the left part of the coronary groove where it forks into the *r. interventricularis paraconalis* and the *r. circumflexus*.

The *ramus interventricularis paraconalis* (47/2) is embedded in adipose tissue as it enters the longitudinal groove of the same name. It reaches the *incisura apicis* and, running past this, the atrial surface. It supplies those parts of the left ventricle, and to a less extent of the right ventricle, which are adjacent to the longitudinal groove through sideshoots of varying sizes. Branches also go to the interventricular septum (49/7). These shoots comprise seven or eight branches but in addition the interventricular paraconal ramus gives off two larger vessels. The first of these is the *r. collateralis sin. prox.* (47/8) which branches freely as it descends obliquely to the border of the left ventricle. The second, known as the *r. collateralis sin. dist.* (47/9), arises more distally but its branches also reach the left ventricular border. The most prominent of the arteries supplying the right ventricular wall is the *r. coni arteriosi* (/10) the name of which reflects its supply area.

The *r. circumflexus (sin.)* of the left coronary artery (46/3; 47/3) crosses the great coronary vein, which will be discussed below, and follows the coronary groove until it reaches the left ventricular border which it supplies through its terminal branches. In some cases its branches may also extend to the atrial surface of the left heart. The left circumflex ramus provides five to seven arteries of varying sizes for the supply of blood to the left ventricle, left atrium and the interatrial septum. The first branch artery of the left circumflex ramus is the *r. angularis* (47/4), followed by the stout *r. prox. ventriculi sin.* (47/5) and the *r. marginis ventricularis sin.* (47/6). The *r. prox. ventriculi sin.* and its branches lie between the other two rami.

The wall of the left atrium receives four to six branches from the left circumflex ramus. Two large branches, the *r. prox.* and the *r. intermed. atrii sin.* (46/8, 9), supply the major part of the wall of the left atrium while two smaller twigs, the *rr. auriculares dext. et sin.* (/8′, 8″), go to the wall of the left auricle.

The **a. coronaria dext.** (46/10) arises from the right cuspal sinus of the aortic bulbus and enters the right part of the coronary sinus as the *r. circumflexus (dext.)* (47/11; 48/1; 49/1). As it reaches the sulcus subsinuosus it becomes the *r. interventricularis subsinuosus* (46/15; 48/2; 49/2) which courses towards the apex of the heart. Along the way and below the right auricle, the circumflex ramus gives off a number of larger and smaller vessels to those parts of the right ventricle and atrium which lie next to the coronary groove. The named branches to the right ventricle are the *r. coni arteriosi* (47/12), the *r. prox. ventriculi dext.* (46/12; 47/13), the *r. marginis ventricularis dext.* (46/13; 48/3) and the *r. dist. ventriculi dext.* (48/4). The first of these four branches of the right circumflex ramus supplies the wall of the *conus arteriosus* and the *bulbus aortae*, the second and third the *margo ventricularis dext.* of the right ventricle and the fourth is distributed to part of the atrial surface of the right ventricle.

The *r. interventricularis subsinuosus* of the right coronary artery rests, as already mentioned, in the longitudinal groove of the same name without actually reaching the apex of the heart (48/2). By means of up to seven small vessels it supplies those parts of the atrial surfaces of the right and left ventricles which lie nearest the longitudinal groove. The *rr. collaterales dextt. prox. et dist.* (48/7, 8) are two further branches of the interventricular subsinuosal ramus which supply the right ventricle. The two larger vessels supply the right ventricular wall up to the *margo ventricularis dext.*

Two other large vessels arising from the same ramus play an important part in the arterial supply of the left ventricular wall. The first of these is the *r. coronarius sin.* (48/9) which arises at the point where the *r. interventricularis subsinuosus* itself branches from the circumflex ramus of the right coronary artery. This large artery is peculiar to the horse in this form. It runs in the right part of the coronary groove up to the left ventricular (caudal) border. The supply area of the left coronary ramus is inversely proportional to that of the *r. circumflexus (sin.)* which it meets from the opposite direction without, however, the terminal branches forming any anastomoses. The second and larger branch of the interventricular subsinuosal ramus is the *r. collateralis ventriculis sin.* (48/11) which sends several small vessels to the apical part of the left ventricular wall as far as the region of the left ventricular border. The circumflex branch of the right coronary artery gives off numerous small vessels and some larger arteries to the wall of the right atrium. The large vessels are the *r. prox.* (46/16), *intermedius* (46/17; 48/5) and *dist.* (/18; /6) *atrii dext.*

Although the arterial supply to the *papillary muscles* is variable, there is a basic pattern. The subauricular papillary muscle of the left ventricle receives branches from the *r. angularis* of the left circumflex artery (47/4) and from the *r. collateralis sin. prox.* (/8). The left ventricular subatrial papillary muscle receives arteries from the *r. prox. ventriculi sin.* (47/5) and from the *r. marginis ventricularis sin.* (/6) of the left coronary artery as well as from the *r. collateralis ventriculi sin.* (48/11) of the interventricular subsinuosal ramus.

In the right ventricle the *m. papillaris subarteriosus* is supplied by offshoots of the right coronary artery and septal branches of the interventricular paraconal ramus of the right coronary artery. The *mm. papillares parvi* receive septal branches from both the *rr. interventriculares* (49) while the large papillary muscle is in the supply area of the *r. marginis ventricularis dext.* (48/3).

The very thick interventricular septum (49) is supplied with 12 to 16 equally stout arteries arising at irregular intervals from the *rr. interventriculares paraconalis et subsinuosus*. Although these branches run towards each other from opposite directions, they do not anastomose. The first vessel, arising from the interventricular paraconal branch of the left coronary artery, is particularly large and in the horse is termed the *r. septi interventricularis* (49/8).

Veins

The **sinus coronarius** (46/20; 48/15), which is very short in the horse and has an indistinct *valvula sinus coronarius (Thebesii)* at its junction with the right atrium, acts as a collecting chamber for the blood

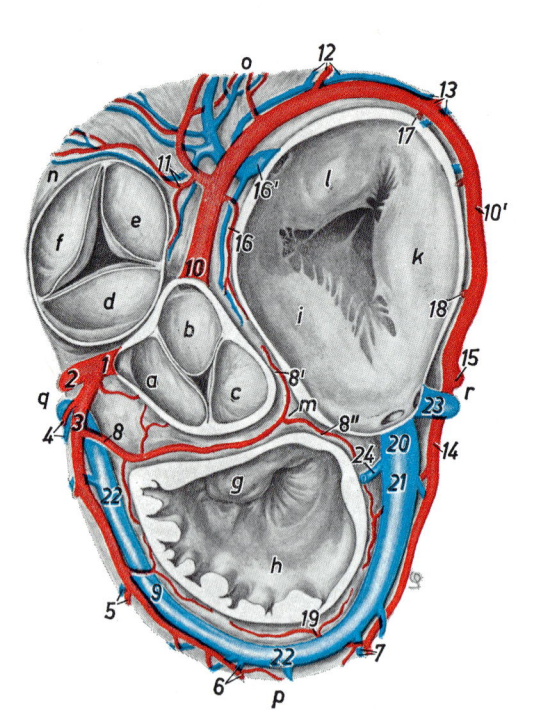

Fig. 46. Base of the heart of a horse after removal of the atria. (After Hoffmann, Diss. med. vet., Giessen, 1960.)

a, b, c valva aortae (*a* valvula semilunaris sin., *b* valvula semilunaris dext., *c* valvula semilunaris septalis); *d, e, f* valva trunci pulmonalis (*d* valvula semilunaris sin., *e* valvula semilunaris dext., *f* valvula semilunaris intermed.); *g, h* valva atrioventricularis sin. s. bicuspidalis (*g* cuspis septalis, *h* cuspis parietalis); *i, k, l* valva atrioventricularis dext. s. tricuspidalis (*i* cuspis septalis, *k* cuspis parietalis, *l* cuspis angularis); *m* septum interatriale; *n* conus arteriosus; *o* margo ventricularis dext.; *p* margo ventricularis sin.; *q* sulcus interventricularis paraconalis; *r* sulcus interventricularis subsinuosus

1 a. coronaria sin., *2* its r. interventricularis paraconalis, *3* its r. circumflexus; *4* r. and v. angularis; *5* r. and v. prox. ventriculi sin.; *6* r. and v. marginis ventriculi sin.; *7* v. dist. ventriculi sin.; *8* r. prox. atrii sin.; *8'* r. auricularis dext.; *8''* r. auricularis sin.; *9* r. intermed. atrii sin.; *10* a. coronaria dext., *10'* its r. circumflexus; *11* r. coni arteriosi and v. cordis parva; *12* r. prox. ventriculi dext. and vv. cordis parvae; *13* r. marginis ventricularis dext. and vv. cordis parvae; *14* r. coronarius sin.; *15* r. interventricularis subsinuosus; *16* r. prox. atrii dext.; *16'* v. coni arteriosi; *17* r. intermed. atrii dext.; *18* branch of the r. circumflexus to the wall of the right atrium; *19* branches of the r. coronarius sin. to the wall of the left atrium; *20* sinus coronarius; *21* v. cordis magna, *22* its r. circumflexus; *23* v. cordis media; *24* v. obliqua atrii sin.

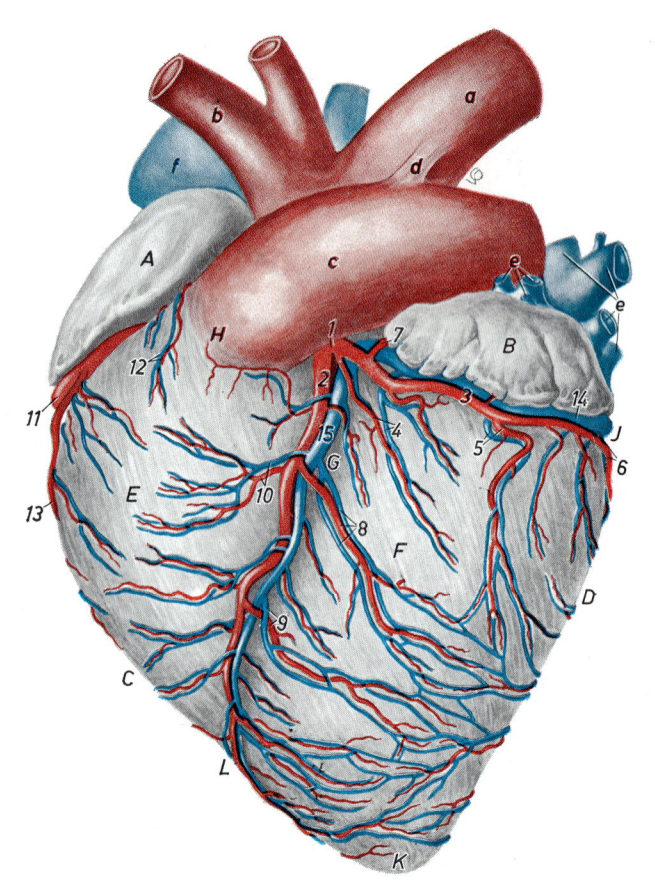

Fig. 47. Arteries and veins of the auricular surface of the heart of the horse. (After Hoffmann, Diss. med. vet., Giessen, 1960.)

A right auricle; *B* left auricle; *C* margo ventricularis dext.; *D* margo ventricularis sin.; *E* ventriculus dext.; *F* ventriculus sin.; *G* sulcus interventricularis paraconalis; *H* conus arteriosus; *I* sulcus coronarius, pars sin.; *K* apex cordis; *L* incisura apicis

a arcus aortae; *b* truncus brachiocephalicus communis; *c* truncus pulmonalis; *d* lig. arteriosum; *e* vv. pulmonales; *f* v. cava cran.

1 a. coronaria sin.; *2* its r. interventricularis paraconalis, *3* its r. circumflexus; *4* r. and v. angularis; *5* r. prox. ventriculi sin. and branch of the v. cordis magna; *6* r. marginis ventricularis sin. and branch of the v. cordis magna; *7* r. prox. atrii sin.; *8* r. collateralis sin. prox.; *9* r. collateralis sin. dist.; *10* r. and v. coni arteriosi; *11* r. circumflexus of the a. coronaria dext.; *12* r. coni arteriosi and v. cordis parva; *13* r. prox. ventriculi dext.; *14* r. circumflexus of the v. cordis magna; *15* v. interventricularis paraconalis

Fig. 48. Arteries and veins of the facies atrialis of the heart of the horse. (After Hoffmann, Diss. med. vet., Giessen, 1960.)

A atrium dext.; *B* atrium sin.; *C* margo ventricularis dext.; *D* margo ventricularis sin.; *E* ventriculus dext.; *F* ventriculus sin.; *G* sulcus interventricularis subsinuosus; *H* sinus venarum cavarum; *J* sulcus coronarius, pars dext.; *K* apex cordis

a arcus aortae; *b* truncus brachiocephalicus communis; *c,c* aa. pulmonales; *d* vv. pulmonales; *e* v. cava caud.; *f* v. cava cran.; *g* v. azygos dext.

1 r. circumflexus of the a. coronaria dext., *2* its r. interventricularis subsinuosus; *3* r. marginis ventricularis dext. and vv. cordis parvae; *4* r. dist. ventriculi dext. and vv. cordis parvae; *5* r. intermed. atrii dext.; *6* r. dist. atrii dext.; *7* r. collateralis dext. prox. and branch of the v. cordis media; *8* r. collateralis dext. dist. and branch of the v. cordis media; *9* r. coronarius sin. and branch of the v. cordis media; *10* v. paracoronaria; *11* r. and v. collateralis ventriculi sin.; *12* v. cordis media, *13* its parallel branch; *14* bypass vein of the vv. cordis parvae; *15* sinus coronarius; *16* v. obliqua atrii sin.; *17* v. cordis magna and transition into its pars circumflexa; *18* v. dist. ventriculi sin.

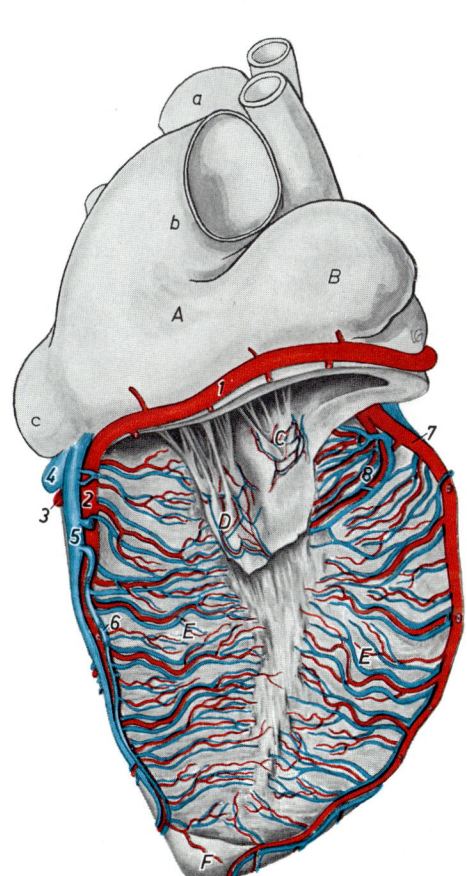

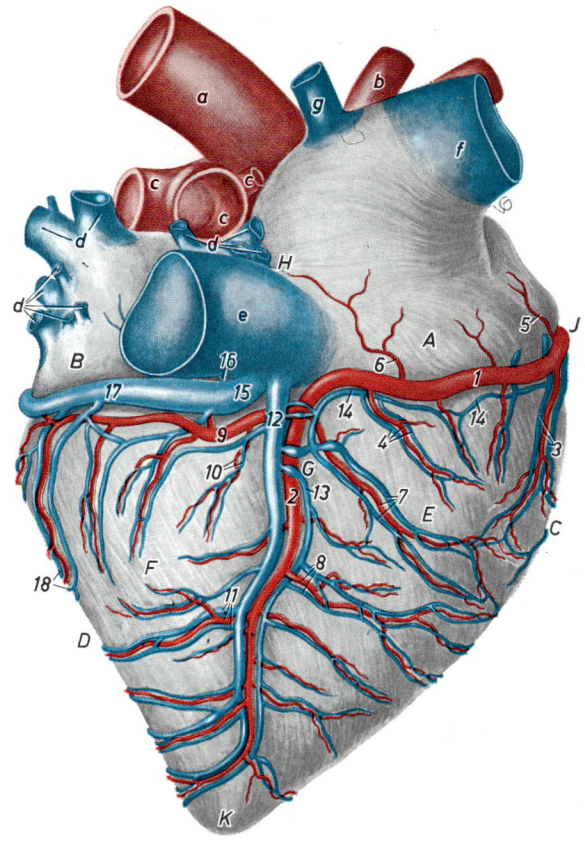

Fig. 49. Blood vessels of the interventricular septum and the mm. papillares subarteriosus et parvi of a horse's heart, right side. (After Hoffmann, Diss. med. vet., Giessen, 1960.)

A atrium dext.; *B* auriculum dext.; *C* m. papillaris subarteriosus; *D* mm. papillares parvi; *E* septum interventriculare; *F* apex cordis

a arcus aortae; *b* v. cava cran.; *c* v. cava caud.

1 r. circumflexus of the a. coronaria dext., *2* its r. interventricularis subsinuosus; *3* r. coronarius sin.; *4* sinus coronarius; *5* v. cordis media, *6* its parallel branch; *7* r. interventricularis paraconalis of the a. coronaria sin.; *8* r. and v. septi interventricularis

of the cardiac veins. It is a cylindrical dilatation of the right atrium lying in the coronary groove below the termination of the caudal vena cava, and it continues directly into the *v. cordis magna* (48/*17*) which equals it in diameter. In the horse the border between the two is located at the origin of the *v. obliqua atrii sin.* (/*16*). This latter vein is usually distinct in the horse; it drains the blood from part of the wall of the left atrium.

The large **v. cordis magna** commences at the coronary sinus. It enters the left part of the coronary groove and passes across the *margo ventricularis sin.* under the cover of the left auricle to the auricular surface of the heart. There it enters the left longitudinal groove as the *v. interventricularis paraconalis* (47/*15*) and accompanies the artery of that name to the *incisura apicis cordis*.

That part of the great coronary vein which runs in the coronary sinus is also known as the *v. circumflexa (sin.)* (46/*22*; 47/*14*). Its innominate branches accompany the collateral arteries to the wall of the left ventricle and atrium. Larger branches, which run with the arteries of the same name to the same supply areas, are the *v. angularis* (46/*4*), the *v. prox. ventriculi sin.* (/*5*), the *v. marginis ventricularis sin.* (/*6*) and the *v. dist. ventriculi sin.* (46/*7*; 48/*18*). Smaller, unnamed and sometimes paired branches of the interventricular paraconal vein (47/*15*) accompany offshoots of the arterial *r. interventricularis paraconalis* to those parts of the right and left ventricle which lie next to the left longitudinal groove. The *vv. collaterales prox. et dist.* (47/*8, 9*) correspond to arteries of similar names; they drain the wall of the left ventricle. The right atrial wall is drained by the *v. coni arteriosi* (47/*10*).

The **v. cordis media** *s. interventricularis subsinuosa* enters the right atrium (46/*23*; 48/*12*) near the termination of the coronary sinus and accompanies the similarly named branch of the left coronary artery in the subsinuosal groove. Like the artery, it divides into several veins before reaching the apex of the heart. Generally the interventricular paraconal vein gives rise to a collateral branch (48/*13*) with which it remains associated by cross-anastomoses. The interventricular paraconal vein gives off branches which, in company with small arteries, supply the left and right ventricular wall adjacent to the longitudinal groove. This vein, or its collateral, drains the right ventricle by means of the *vv. collaterales dext. prox. et dist.* (48/*7, 8*) and the left ventricle by the *v. paracoronaria sin.* (/*10*) and the *v. collateralis ventriculi sin.* (/*11*).

Finally one should mention the vessels which terminate in the middle cardiac vein and in the interventricular paraconal vein (49), and which run parallel to the septal branches of the two coronary arteries.

There are four to six *vv. cordis parvae* which enter the right atrium after having collected blood from the right ventricular wall in the region of the coronary groove. As a rule they are linked by continuous cross-anastomoses and this gives rise to a "shunting" vein (48/*14*) which runs parallel with the circumflex ramus of the right coronary artery and terminates in the middle cardiac vein. The four larger *vv. cordis parvae* are known respectively as the *v. coni arteriosi* (47/*12*), the *v. prox. ventriculi dext.* (/*13*), the *v. marginis ventricularis dext.* (48/*3*) and the *v. dist. ventriculi dext.* (/*4*).

The *vv. cordis minimae* are of very slender diameter and only a few millimeters in length. They carry blood from the walls of the atria and ventricles and open directly into these chambers. They are more numerous in the atria than in the ventricles.

Species-diagnostic features of the hearts of domestic mammals

The features by which the hearts of the different species of domestic mammals can be identified, particularly when these animals have about the same body size, will now be discussed.

Dog
(16, 17, 27–29)

The dog's heart is almost spherical and in cross section below the coronary groove it is circular. In large breeds it may weigh as much as 500 g. The borders of the auricles are smooth. The coronary and longitudinal grooves are bridged by strips of muscle tissue and only moderate amounts of yellow, soft adipose tissue are present in them. The smaller subepicardial arteries are generally accompanied by two collateral veins. Both the interventricular paraconal and subsinuosal rami are branches of the left coronary artery (27/*1, 2, 8*), so that the dog's heart is an example of a left coronary type of heart (25).

The great coronary and medial cardiac veins both arise from the coronary sinus (27/16, 17, 18), the latter shortly before the sinus enters the right atrium. Another distinguishing feature is the presence of the *v. obliqua atrii sin.* (/20) which is connected to the coronary sinus and represent a rudiment of the left azygos vein of the foetal heart. There are usually four small cardiac veins which enter the right atrium independently on the atrial surface (/10–13). An important feature distinguishing the dog from the pig, sheep and goat is that the former has only one *v. azygos dext.* and this enters the right atrium along with the cranial vena cava (29/10). If the aortic arch is retained on the organ then the hearts of the dog, the pig and the small ruminants can be identified by the pattern in which the arteries supplying the chest, forelimb, neck and head are given off. The branches of the cranial vena cava also arise in a distinctive manner in each species.

The base of the great papillary muscle is either entirely confined to the septum or is based on both the septum and the outer wall. The skeleton of the heart contains two cartilages of which one is very small.

Pig
(19, 34–36)

The pig's heart is in the form of a blunt cone with slightly flattened sides. Its greatest diameter at the coronary groove is about equal to the distance between this groove and the apex. It can weigh up to 500 g. The edges of both auricles, but especially the left, carry a few distinct notches. The adipose tissue of the coronary and longitudinal grooves is soft and white and it varies in amount according to the nutritional state but is not so abundant as one might expect from a species of animal which has such a tendency to fat storage. The blood vessels in the longitudinal groove are often bridged over by muscle bands. Both coronary arteries have an interventricular ramus. The left coronary artery (35/9) supplies the paraconal branch (/11) and the right coronary artery supplies the subsinuosal branch (36/14, 15); the pig, therefore, has a bilateral coronary type of heart (26). The coronary sinus (36/d) gives rise to the left azygos vein (/8) which is typical for both pigs and ruminants. The boundary between these two vessels is determined by the origin of the great coronary vein (/23) from the coronary sinus. Shortly thereafter the coronary sinus also receives the interventricular subsinuosal vein, also known as the medial cardiac vein (/21). The interventricular paraconal vein (35/21) divides into two collateral branches at the level of the coronary groove whereas its contralateral partner (36/21) only forks in the lower third of the subsinuosal groove. There are four *vv. cordis parvae* of which three arise from the right atrium by a common stem with the *v. circumflexa dext.* (34/20). As in the sheep and goat, but contrary to the situation in the dog, the great papillary muscle is always situated on the outer wall. The *trabecula septomarginalis* of the right ventricle is always very powerful and may measure up to 9 mm in diameter. Two cartilages, which can become ossified with advancing age, complete the skeleton of the heart.

Sheep and goat
(20, 41–45)

The heart of the sheep is cone-shaped and altogether more slender and pointed than that of the pig. In the goat it is in the shape of a pointed cone. The sheep's heart weighs up to 250 g. In both species the notches in the border of auricles, especially those of the left auricle, are more distinct than in the pig. The subepicardial adipose tissue is white, of tallowy consistency and not only fills the coronary groove but extends beyond it in well-nourished individuals. Characteristic for the heart of the sheep and the goat is the presence of subendocardial adipose tissue which appears as small islets. These islets are especially prominent on the apex of the papillary muscles (20).

The two species are of the left coronary type (25) in respect of the origin of both interventricular rami, that is to say both rami originate from the left coronary artery (43/1). As in the case of the pig, the coronary sinus of the small ruminants (42/12; 45/13) receives the left azygos vein (/e;/e). In the goat the interventricular subsinuosal vein (middle cardiac vein) (45/14) terminates in the coronary sinus, while in the sheep it enters directly into the right atrium (42/13). Unlike the dog and pig, both small ruminants have a *v. cordis caudalis* (41/13) which arises from the great coronary vein and runs to the *margo ventricularis sin.* Four to five *v. cordis parvae* arise independently and directly from the right atrium and are in part covered over by the auricle.

There are other differences between the sheep and the goat in respect of the cardiac vessels but since these vessels are small and prone to individual variation, they are unsuitable for diagnostic purposes.

Ox
(37–40)

Depending on its functional state, the heart of the ox is in the form of a squat, or rather more pointed cone with sides of equal length. It can weigh up to 3.3 kg. At the *margo interventricularis sin.* occurs the intermediate sulcus which is characteristic of the species. The borders of both auricles are very distinctly notched. One should also note the large amount of subepicardial adipose tissue which can form cushion-like structures extending beyond the limits of the grooves. Both interventricular rami stem from the left coronary artery (37/*1, 2, 3*; 38/*1, 2*; 39/*2*) so that the ox's heart belongs to the left coronary type (25). The coronary sinus (39/*13*) gives rise to the great coronary vein (38/*11*), the interventricular subsinuosal or middle cardiac vein (39/*14*) and the left azygos vein (37/*17*), which latter is typical for all the domestic ruminants. Also peculiar to this species is the caudal cardiac vein (37/*18*; 38/*13*) which arises from the coronary sinus; it runs in the *sulcus intermedius* which is present only in the ox. There are seven to eight *vv. cordis parvae* and they enter the right atrium separately. A particularly characteristic and easily determined feature of the bovine heart is the presence of the large and small bones which are part of the heart skeleton.

Horse
(46–49)

The heart of the horse is shaped like a blunt cone with slightly flattened sides. Its weight depends on the breed and varies between 1.3 and 4.2 kg, although in thoroughbreds it can far exceed even the larger figure. The border of the left auricle shows only indistinct notching. The subepicardial fat is remarkably yellow and soft, almost of a thickish oily consistency. The amount of adipose tissue present is obviously dependent on the breed and the heart of the more "primitive" breeds have so much fat that it extends beyond the grooves. The two interventricular arteries, the branches of which are usually accompanied by two collateral veins, both arise from the coronary arteries (46/*1*; *10*), the paraconal (/*2*) from the left and the subsinuosal (/*15*) from the right coronary artery. Unlike the ox, therefore, the horse's heart is of bilateral coronary type (26). Also characteristic of the equine heart is the presence of a right azygos vein which springs from the cranial vena cava (10/*2*). The coronary sinus (46/*20*; 48/*15*) becomes the great coronary vein (/*21*; /*17*) and at the transition it receives the *v. obliqua atrii sin.* (/*24*; /*16*). The interventricular subsinuosal, or medial cardiac vein, usually enters the coronary sinus a short distance before it terminates in the right atrium although it can empty directly into the atrium (48/*12*). The skeleton of the horse's heart is supplemented by small and large cardiac cartilages.

Arteries (arteriae)*

Truncus pulmonalis
(Pig: 96/*41*, 153/*46*; goat: 154/*28*; sheep: 99/*19*; ox: 102, 155/*1*; horse: 103/*30*)

The **truncus pulmonalis**, as the main artery of the pulmonary circulation, carries the venous blood to the lungs. It arises from the *conus arteriosus* of the right ventricle at the *ostium trunci pulmonalis*. The first part of the pulmonary trunk, which is flanked by the two auricles, has shallow depressions known as the *sinus trunci pulmonales* situated dorsal to each semilunar valve. Initially the pulmonary trunk runs dorsal within the pericardium, lying cranially and to the left of the aorta. Ventral to the brachiocephalic trunk it bends caudally, thus crossing the aortic arch on the left side, and it leaves the pericardium at a point dorsal to the left atrium. At this site the pulmonary trunk is joined to the aorta by the *ligamentum arteriosum*, which is the remnant of the *ductus arteriosus* (Botalli) which formed a direct connection between the pulmonary and systemic circulation during foetal life. A short distance beyond the ligament and ventral to the trachea, and to the right of the left azygos vein in the pig and ruminant, the pulmonary trunk divides into the *a. pulmonalis sinistra* and the *a. pulmonalis dextra*.

The **a. pulmonalis sinistra** curves caudolaterally to face the hilus of the left lung, thus crossing dorsally the left pulmonary veins. Together with the bronchial tree it divides into the *r. lobi caudalis* for the caudal lobe and into the *r. lobi cranialis* which latter, except in the horse, gives rise to the *r. ascendens* and the *r. descendens* to the divided cranial lobe of the lung.

The **a. pulmonalis dextra** goes to the hilus of the right lung passing ventrally to the trachea. The subdivision of the right pulmonary artery at the hilus varies according to the species. In carnivores it divides into the *r. lobi cranialis*, the *r. lobi medii* and *r. lobi caudalis*. In the pig and ruminant it gives rise to the *r. lobi cranialis* before entering the lung and this ramus runs outside the lung in a cranial direction along the right side of the trachea to the bronchus trachealis. In the ruminant, this ramus then forks like the corresponding bronchus, into the *r. ascendens* and the *r. descendens*. In both these species the continuation of the right pulmonary artery then divides at the hilus into a *r. lobi medii* and *r. lobi caudalis*. In the horse it divides into only a *r. lobi cranialis* and a *r. lobi caudalis*. In all the domestic mammals the *r. lobi caudalis* gives off the *r. lobi accessorii* for the accessory lobe of the right lung. The subsequent branching of the rami of the right pulmonary artery corresponds to that of the bronchi.

Aorta
(Comparative: 85–88/*1*, *31*, *39*; cat: 91/*1*, *1'*, *1"*, *30*; horse: 50/*1*, *5*, *20*, *25*)

The **aorta** arises from the left ventricle at the anulus fibrosus. It immediately enlarges to the *bulbus aortae* and gives off the right and left coronary arteries (see blood vessels of the heart) from the *sinus aortae* dorsal to the right or left semilunar valve. As the *aorta ascendens*, it rises craniodorsally on the right side of the pulmonary trunk and continues into the craniodorsally convex *arcus aortae*. The latter is enclosed by pericardium to an extent which varies according to the species. At the point of insertion of the pericardium the aorta receives the lig. arteriosum which, as the ductus arteriosus, forms a communication between the pulmonary trunk and the aorta in the foetal circulation. The aortic arch, enclosed within its mediastinum, reaches the vertebral column somewhat to the left of the midline at the level of the 5th, 6th or 7th thoracic vertebra and then continues caudally ventral to the column as the *aorta descendens*. Within the thoracic cavity it becomes the *aorta thoracica* and upon entry into the

---

* The topographic illustrations of the blood vessels are derived from various studies and therefore they are not uniformly annotated. Certain inessential details of lettering have been omitted in the legends of this book.

hiatus aorticus of the diaphragm and within the abdominal cavity, it is referred to as the *aorta abdominalis*. Its terminal bifurcation lies at the level of the last, or last but one, lumbar vertebra.

The cranially directed *truncus brachiocephalicus* arises from the aortic arch in all the domestic mammals. In the pig and carnivores the *a. subclavia sinistra* does not arise from the brachiocephalic trunk but also comes off the aortic arch.

Starting from between the 3rd and 6th thoracic vertebrae, depending on individual and species variation, the **aorta thoracica** gives off from its dorsal wall the *aa. intercostales dorsales*, which are segmentally distributed to both sides of the thorax. The *a. costoabdominalis dorsalis* goes to the caudal border of the last rib. The *a. broncho-oesophagea* arises dorsal to the base of the heart; in some animals it is paired but these two branches may be united close to their origin. It often has two branches, the *r. bronchalis* and *r. oesophageus*, but these may also arise directly from the thoracic aorta and, indeed, they may sometimes even originate from one of the dorsal intercostal arteries. The thoracic aorta also gives rise to the *rr. oesophagei, pericardiaci* and *mediastinales*. Only in the horse are the *aa. phrenicae craniales*, which supply the thoracic surface of the diaphragm, given off in the region of the *hiatus aorta*.

The **aorta abdominalis** lies to the left of the v. cava caudalis and contacts the thoracic duct and the inner lumbar muscles dorsally. From its dorsal wall issue segmentally the *aa. lumbales*. The *a. lumbalis I* arises bilaterally at the level of the aortic hiatus whereas the last lumbar artery issues from the *a. sacralis mediana* in carnivores, pigs and small ruminants and from the *a. iliolumbalis* in the ox. In the horse, the last two lumbar arteries originate from the *a. iliaca interna*.

On either side of the aorta arises an *a. phrenica caudalis* to the caudal surface of the diaphragm. In carnivores the caudal phrenic artery usually arises in company with the *a. abdominalis cranialis* and in pigs and ruminants it originates from the coeliac artery. In the horse, however, it is absent. The caudal phrenic artery infrequently arises from the last dorsal intercostal or one of the lumbar arteries. The *a. abdominalis cranialis*, which occurs only in carnivores and pigs, leaves the abdominal aorta at the level of the 2nd or 3rd lumbar vertebra. From the ventral wall of the abdominal aorta issues the unpaired *a. coeliaca* which supplies the abdominal viscera. In carnivores and ruminants this vessel arises at the level of the 1st lumbar vertebra and in the pig and horse at the level of the last thoracic vertebra. In all species the *a. mesenterica cranialis* originates ventrally at the level of the next vertebra while the *a. mesenterica caudalis* is given off ventral to the 5th lumbar vertebra in the carnivore, the pig and small ruminant, ventral to the 6th lumbar vertebra in the ox and to the 4th in the horse. To convey blood to the adrenal gland the abdominal aorta gives off an *a. suprarenalis media* in the carnivore and the *aa. suprarenales mediae* in the pig. The kidneys are supplied by the bilateral *a. renalis*, the origin of which depends on the species and the topography of the kidneys. As a rule the vessel to the right side arises somewhat further cranial than that to the left. The origin of the right renal artery is at the level of the 1st–2nd lumbar vertebrae in the dog, the 2nd–3rd lumbar vertebrae in the sheep and ox, the 3rd in the pig, the 3rd–4th in the cat and goat and at the level of the 1st lumbar vertebra in the horse. The *a. testicularis* in the male and the *a. ovarica* in the female are destined for the supply of the gonads. In the dog they arise bilaterally at the level of the 3rd–4th, in the horse at the 4th, the cat and sheep at the 4th–5th and the pig, goat and ox at the 5th lumbar vertebrae. In carnivores only the abdominal aorta give off the *a. circumflexa ilium* shortly before the origin of the external iliac artery. In the horse this vessel arises either in the angle of origin of the external iliac artery or, as in other domestic mammals, directly from this latter artery. The *a. iliaca externa* is a stout vessel which arises bilaterally from either side of the abdominal aorta at the level of the 7th lumbar vertebra in the cat, the 6th in the dog and ruminants and the 4th–5th lumbar vertebrae in the pig and horse. A short distance after the origin of the external iliac arteries but still cranially to the promontory and therefore within the abdominal cavity, the abdominal aorta divides into the stout left and right *aa. iliacae internae* and the *a. sacralis mediana*, which latter is very short in the horse or may be absent altogether.

Arcus aortae and truncus brachiocephalicus

(Comparative: 51–54, 85–88/1, 2; cat: 90, 91/1, 2; pig: 96/1, 2; sheep: 99/1, 2, 4; ox: 102/2'; 155/6; horse: 50/5, 6; 103/1, 3)

The **arcus aortae** gives rise to vessels which supply the head, the neck, the forelimb and the cranial region of the thorax as well as some of the thoracic organs. These vessels are the right and left *a. subclavia* and the right and left *a. carotis communis*. These two arteries are united into the *truncus*

Arcus aortae

brachiocephalicus except in carnivores and pigs in which the left subclavian artery is not included in the brachiocephalic trunk but arises directly from the aorta. In ruminants and horses the left subclavian artery arises from the brachiocephalic trunk before the right subclavian artery. The cranially directed carotid arteries are united into the *truncus bicaroticus* except in carnivores in which the *a. carotis communis sinistra* leaves the brachiocephalic trunk before the *a. carotis communis dextra*. At its origin

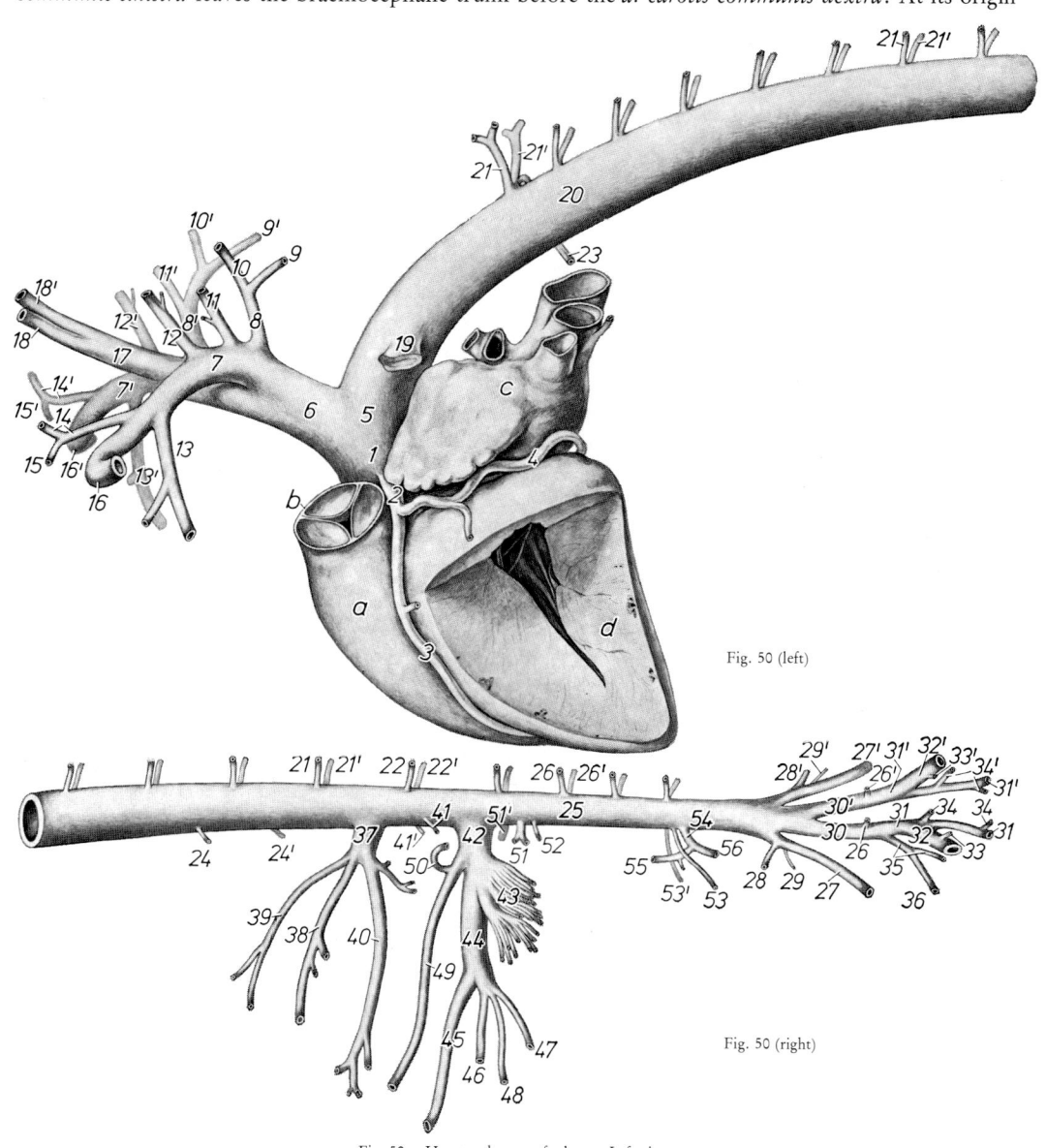

Fig. 50. Heart and aorta of a horse. Left view.
(After Schummer, unpublished). The arteries of the right side are identified by numbers with apostrophe.

a cor, ventriculus dexter; *b* ostium trunci pulmonalis with valva trunci pulmonalis; *c* atrium sinistrum with auricula sinistra and the terminating vv. pulmonales; ventriculus sinister, opened

1 aorta ascendens; *2* a. coronaria sinistra; *3* r. interventricularis paraconalis; *4* r. circumflexus; *5* arcus aortae; *6* truncus brachiocephalicus; *7* a. subclavia; *8* truncus costocervicalis; *9* a. intercostalis suprema; *10* a. scapularis dorsalis; *11* a. cervicalis profunda; *12* a. vertebralis; *13* a. thoracica interna; *14* a. cervicalis superficialis; *15* r. deltoideus; *16* a. axillaris; *17* truncus bicaroticus; *18* a. carotis communis; *19* lig. arteriosum (ductus arteriosus); *20* aorta descendens, aorta thoracica; *21* aa. intercostales dorsales; *22* a. costoabdominalis dorsalis; *23* a. broncho-oesophagea; *24* a. phrenica cranialis; *25* aorta descendens, abdominalis; *26* aa. lumbales; *27* a. iliaca externa; *28* a. circumflexa ilium profunda; *29* a. cremasterica or a. uterina; *30* a. iliaca interna; *31* a. glutaea caudalis; *32* a. glutaea cranialis before the origin of the a. obturatoria; *33* a. iliolumbalis; *34* rr. sacrales; *35* a. pudenda interna; *36* a. umbilicalis; *37* a. coeliaca; *38* a. lienalis; *39* a. gastrica sinistra; *40* a. hepatica; *41* a. suprarenalis; *42* a. mesenterica cranialis; *43* aa. jejunales and aa. ilei; *44* a. ileocolica; *45* r. colicus; *46* a. caecalis lateralis; *47* a. caecalis medialis; *48* r. ilei mesenterialis; *49* a. colica dextra; *50* a. colica media; *51* a. renalis; *52* r. suprarenalis; *53* a. testicularis or a. ovarica; *54* a. mesenterica caudalis; *55* a. colica sinistra; *56* a. rectalis cranialis

the brachiocephalic trunk is still encased within the pericardial sac. In carnivores, pigs, small ruminants and horses its origin is at the level of the 3rd rib whereas in the ox it is level with the 4th rib. After leaving the pericardium the trunk runs cranially and ventrolateral to the trachea within the mediastinum. It is accompanied on its course to the thoracic entrance by the *v. cava cranialis* which lies dorsal and to its right.

A. subclavia

(Comparative: 51–54, 85–88/*3*; 55–58/*1*; cat: 90, 91/*3*; pig: 96/*3*; sheep: 99/*3*; ox: 102/*6*; horse: 50/*7*; 103/*4*).

The **a. subclavia** turns in a cranial convex curve to the anterior border of the first rib and, because of its more dorsally situated origin, the left artery is tilted cranioventrally. From the subclavian artery arise the *a. vertebralis, a. cervicalis profunda, a. scapularis dorsalis* and *a. intercostalis suprema* or *a. vertebralis thoracica*. Two (pig and horse), three (carnivores) or all these arteries (ruminants) can be fused into a common stem of origin, the *truncus costocervicalis*. Since in the horse the right subclavian artery arises in a much more cranial position, the costocervical trunk, the deep cervical artery and the vertebral artery of the right side all originate directly from the brachiocephalic trunk. Before the subclavian artery continues into the axillary artery it gives off, at the thoracic entrance at the level of the 1st rib, the *a. thoracica interna* which runs in a caudoventral direction and the *a. cervicalis superficialis* which runs in a cranial direction. In the pig the right superficial cervical artery is fused with the *a. thyreoidea caudalis dextra* to form the *truncus thyreocervicalis*.

A. vertebralis

(Comparative: 51–54/*11*; 85–88/*5*; cat: 90, 91/*4*; pig: 96/*6*; sheep: 99/*12*; ox: 102, 155/*11*; horse: 50/*12*; 83/*49*; 103/*9*)

The **a. vertebralis** arises from the subclavian artery before the origin of the costocervical trunk in the carnivore, after the origin of that vessel in the horse and in the ox together with it. The vertebral artery turns craniodorsally towards the *foramen transversarium* of the 6th cervical vertebra, where it enters the transverse canal and follows it in a cranial direction. Except in the ox, it reaches the alar groove of the atlas and continues through the *incisura alaris* or the *for. alare*. In the dog, it always passes through the alar notch. In a manner similar to the dorsal intercostal and lumbar arteries, the vertebral artery gives off segmentally the *rr. spinales* which pass through the *forr. intervertebralia* or *forr. vertebralia lateralia* to vascularize the spinal cord and its meninges and the vertebral bodies. The vertebral artery itself then passes through the lateral vertebral foramen of the atlas in a similar manner to one of the spinal rami. It enters the vertebral canal and, together with the vertebral artery of the other side, it continues towards the cranium as the *a. basilaris*. The *rr. dorsales* and *rr. ventrales* supply the neighbouring musculature. In the region of the *incisura alaris* or the *foramen alare*, the *r. dorsalis* forms the *r. descendens* and is connected to the *a. cervicalis profunda*. The corresponding *r. ventralis* forms the *r. anastomoticus cum a. occipitali*. In the ox the vertebral artery terminates in the *r. spinalis III* before entering the transverse canal of the axis. Dorsal to the wing of the atlas there is a communication through the corresponding *r. dorsalis* with the *r. descendens* which is also present in the ox and also forms a connection with the *a. occipitalis* through the *r. anastomoticus*.

A. cervicalis profunda

(Comparative: 51–54/*10*; 85–88/*8*; cat: 90/*6′*; pig: 96/*4′*; sheep: 99/*11*; ox: 102, 155/*10*; horse: 50/*11*; 103/*8*)

In carnivores, pigs and ruminants the **a. cervicalis profunda** arises from the costocervical trunk. In the horse, on the other hand, the deep cervical artery of the left side stems from the subclavian artery and that of the right from the brachiocephalic trunk. It leaves the thoracic cavity in the carnivore and horse through the 1st, and in the pig through the 2nd, intercostal space. In ruminants it rises in front of the 1st rib. It runs towards the head and supplies, via dorsally directed branches, the cervical musculature from the withers to the nape. It forms numerous anastomoses with the vertebral artery's dorsal branches, which are destined for the muscles next to the cervical vertebrae, and also with their *r.*

descendens. In the small ruminants the field of supply of the deep cervical artery is confined to the neck and withers region, but the dorsal branches of the vertebral artery extend up to the ligamentum nuchae.

A. scapularis dorsalis
(Comparative: 51–54/*7*; 85–88/*9*; cat: 90, 91/*7*; pig: 96/*5*; sheep: 99/*10*; ox: 102, 155/*9*; horse: 50/*10*; 103/*6*)

In carnivores, ruminants and the horse the **a. scapularis dorsalis** arises from the costocervical trunk, but in the pig it arises independently from the subclavian artery. In carnivores and ruminants its origin is located cranial to the 1st rib, in the pig in the 1st intercostal space and in the horse in the 2nd intercostal space. Giving off craniodorsally and caudodorsally directed branches, it proceeds between the *m.*

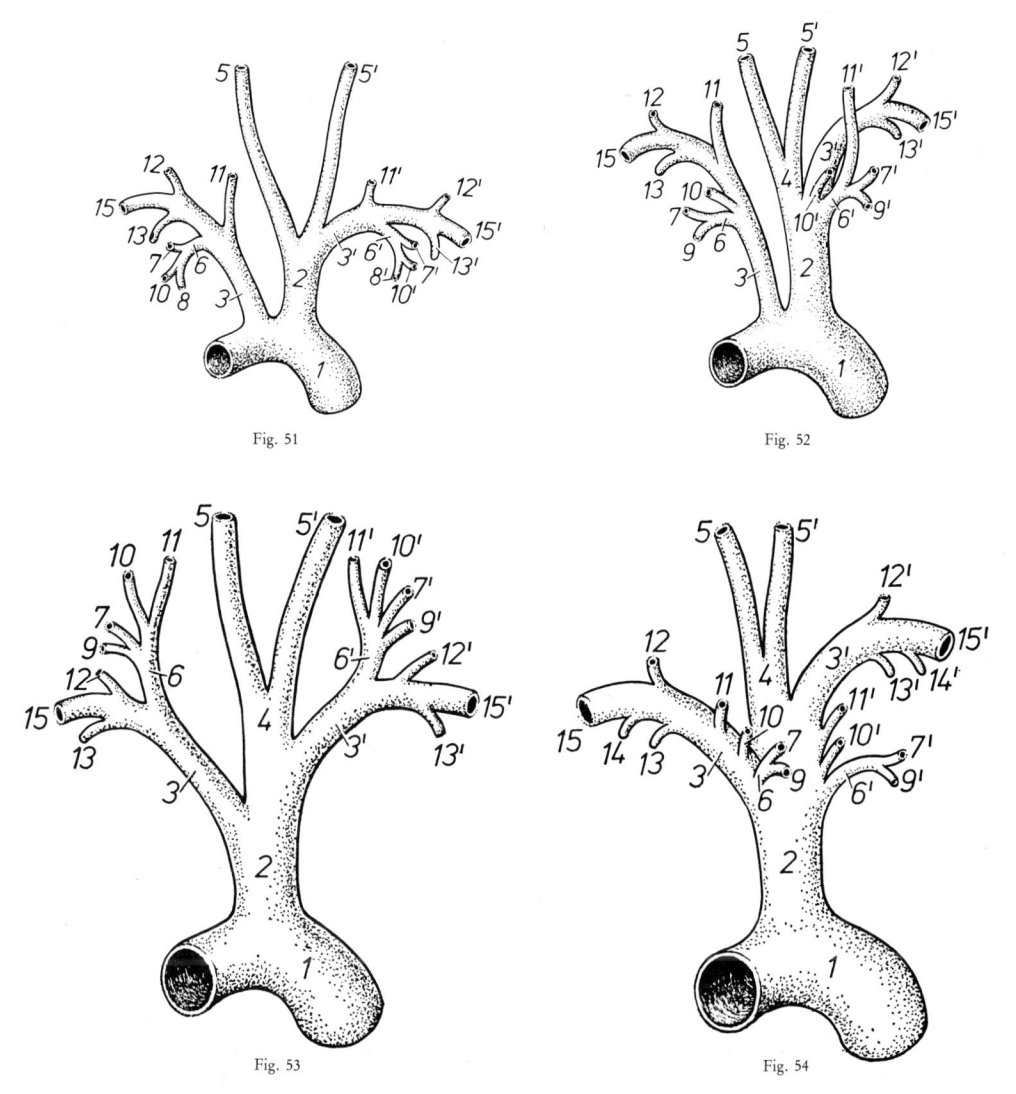

Figs 51, 52, 53, 54. Arcus aortae and truncus brachiocephalicus of the dog, pig, ox and horse. Dorsal view.

1 arcus aortae; *2* truncus brachiocephalicus; *3* a. subclavia sinistra; *3'* s. subclavia dextra; *4* truncus bicaroticus; *5* a. carotis communis sinistra; *5'* a. carotis communis dextra; *6* truncus costocervicalis sinister; *6'* truncus costocervicalis dexter; *7* a. scapularis dorsalis sinistra; *7'* a. scapularis dorsalis dextra; *8* a. vertebralis thoracica sinistra; *8'* a. vertebralis thoracica dextra; *9* a. intercostalis suprema sinistra; *9'* a. intercostalis suprema dextra; *10* a. cervicalis profunda sinistra; *10'* a. cervicalis profunda dextra; *11* a. vertebralis sinistra; *11'* a. vertebralis dextra; *12* a. cervicalis superficialis sinistra; *12'* a. cervicalis superficialis dextra; *13* a. thoracica interna sinistra; *13'* a. thoracica interna dextra; *14* a. thoracica externa sinistra; *14'* a. thoracica externa dextra, only shown in the horse where it arises more proximally; *15* a. axillaris sinistra; *15'* a. axillaris dextra

serratus ventralis cervicalis (or *thoracis*) and the longissimus dorsi muscle to the vertebral border of the scapula. There it ramifies in the muscles which are inserted at that site and also in the skin of the withers.

A. intercostalis suprema
(Comparative: 51–54/*9*; 85–88/*10*; cat: 90/6′; pig: 96/4‴; sheep: 99/9; ox: 102, 155/8; horse: 50/9; 103/7)

Up to four of the more cranial **aa. intercostales dorsales** are linked to the costocervical trunk in series, one after the other. In each case the succeeding artery arises lateral to the vertebral body from the preceding vessel. This paravertebral chain of anastomosing arteries, the *a. intercostalis suprema*, runs ventral to the rib head joints. This artery is absent in the dog where the leading segments of each of the dorsal intercostal arteries follow one behind the other dorsal to the necks of the ribs and ventral to the costotransverse articulations. This vessel is the *a. vertebralis thoracica.* The course and distribution of these dorsal intercostal arteries will be discussed together with the intercostal arteries arising from the thoracic aorta (p. 121).

A. thoracica interna
(Comparative: 51–54/*13*; 85–88/*12*; cat: 90, 91/*11*; dog: 93/*a*; pig: 96/8; sheep: 99/*13*; ox: 102, 155/*13*; horse: 50, 103/*13*)

The **a. thoracica interna** leaves the subclavian artery medial to the first rib. It then runs ventrocaudally in a subpleural position and dips at about the level of the 3rd sternebra on the floor of the thorax into the transversus thoracic muscle which it pervades to reach the diaphragm. Along its course it gives off at each segment a *r. intercostalis ventralis* which runs dorsad along the caudal border of the corresponding rib to anastomose with the *a. intercostalis dorsalis.* This arterial link is absent in the first two intercostal arteries of the pig; in the horse it is usually lacking in the first, and always in the second to fourth, intercostal arteries. Allowing for species and segmental differences, dorsally rising branches are also given off along the cranial borders of the ribs. These latter branches may originate together with the *rr. intercostales ventrales.* All these vessels supply the ventral part of the lateral wall of the thorax. The ventral thoracic wall is vascularized by the *rr. perforantes* which pass through the intercostal spaces close to the sternum, giving off *rr. sternales* and, in carnivores and pigs, the *rr. mammarii* to the thoracic mammary complex. The *rr. mediastinales* and, more cranially, the *rr. thymici,* run into the ventral mediastinum. An *a. pericardiacophrenica* corresponding to that of man can usually be traced only up to the pericardium in domestic animals. In company with the phrenic nerve it may reach the diaphragm or it may anastomose with the *a. phrenica* before reaching it. The internal thoracic artery divides into the *a. musculophrenica* and the *a. epigastrica cranialis* at the level of the 6th–8th intercostal spaces (6th in pigs, 7th in ruminants and 7th to 8th in carnivores and horses.)

A. musculophrenica
(Comparative: 85–88/*14*; pig: 96/*18*; 97/*31*; sheep: 101/*13*)

The **a. musculophrenica** follows caudodorsally the rib arch and perforates, at about the width of an intercostal space from its origin, the pars costalis of the diaphragm. Thereafter it runs subperitoneally between the digitations of the origin of the pars costalis of the diaphragm on the one hand and the transversus abdominis muscle on the other. In the carnivore this vessel extends to the 11th rib, in the pig and ruminant to the 10th and in the horse to the 11th and infrequently in the latter animal to the 12th, 13th or even 16th rib. Like the internal thoracic artery, it gives off *rr. intercostales ventrales* and, more irregularly, branches to the cranial borders of these ribs. Ventrally directed branches supply parts of the abdominal musculature in the regio hypochondriaca. The medially directed *rr. phrenici* vascularize the diaphragm.

A. epigastrica cranialis
(Comparative: 85–88/*15*; cat: 91/*31*; pig: 96, 98/*19*; 97/*14* sheep: 99/*14*)

The **a. epigastrica cranialis** is the second terminal limb of the internal thoracic artery. It perforates the diaphragm and, covered by the inner layer of the rectus sheath, it runs a paramedian course towards the pelvis, at first dorsally on the rectus abdominis muscle and later buried in that muscle. It ramifies in the ventral abdominal wall through lateral, medial and even segmentally arranged branches. The dorsally-directed, lateral branches anastomose in the thoracic region with corresponding branches of the *a. musculophrenica* or *aa. intercostales dorsales* in the pig and ruminants and in ruminants with those of the *a. costoabdominalis dorsalis*. Thus these dorsally-directed, lateral branches correspond to the *rr. intercostales ventrales* or the *r. costoabdominalis ventralis*. At the level of the umbilicus the diverging terminal branches make contact with those of the caudal epigastric artery. At the angle between the xyphoid process and the arch of the rib of carnivores and ruminants the cranial epigastric artery gives rise to the *a. epigastrica cranialis superficialis*. This latter vessel perforates the rectus abdominis muscle and the outer leaf of the rectus sheath to reach a subcutaneous position. It supplies the skin and in carnivores the caudal thoracic and cranial abdominal part of the mammary complex by means of the *rr. mammarii*. The terminal branches of the cranial superficial epigastric artery anastomose with those of the caudal superficial epigastric artery. In the pig the *rr. mammarii* arise from the cranial epigastric artery and perforate the superficial muscle layers.

A. cervicalis superficialis

(Comparative: 51–54/*12*; 55–58/*2*; 85–88/*19*; cat: 59/*24*; 90, 91/*8*; dog: 92/*18*; 19; pig: 96/*7*; sheep: 62/*20*; 99/*15*; ox: 63/*19*; 102, 155/*12*; horse: 50/*14*; 103/*10*)

The **a. cervicalis superficialis** springs from the subclavian artery medially to the 1st rib about opposite the origin of the internal thoracic artery. In the pig only this vessel is united on the right side with the *a. thyroidea caudalis* to form the *truncus thyreocervicalis*. Running in a cranial direction and giving off branches to the *lnn. cervicales profundi caudales*, it tilts slightly ventrad as it crosses the external jugular vein to reach the medial surface of the brachiocephalic muscle. It sends the *r. deltoideus* into the lateral pectoral groove. In the dog and the pig this deltoid branch may also arise from the axillary artery and in the ox it may originate as an additional *r. descendens* from the external thoracic artery. It accompanies the cephalic vein and supplies primarily the cleidobrachialis and the pectoralis descendens muscles.

The superficial cervical artery now gives off in a cranial direction the *r. ascendens* which then runs along the medial surface of the cleidocephalic muscle and supplies this and, in various species, the sternocephalicus, omohyoideus, omotransversarius and the scalenius muscles. The superficial cervical artery turns dorsally and gives off the *a. suprascapularis* in carnivores and small ruminants, the *r. suprascapularis* in the ox and in the pig the *r. acromialis*. The *r. acromialis* is described below with the axillary artery so is the *a. suprascapularis* which in the pig arises from the *a. circumflexa humeri* caudalis and in the ox and horse from the *a. axillaris*. The superficial cervical artery is continued, except in the horse, as the *r. praescapularis*, which runs dorsal and parallel to the *m. supraspinatus*. This prescapular ramus gives off branches to the superficial cervical lymph nodes and also supplies the omotransversarius muscle, the cervical part of the trapezius and the rhomboideus cervicis muscles. In the horse the lymph node branches arise directly from the superficial cervical artery or its r. ascendens, while a muscular branch turns into the cleidoscapularis muscle.

Arteries of the pectoral limb

A. axillaris

(Comparative: 51–54/*15*; 55–58/*8*; 85–88/*23*; cat: 59/*1*; 90, 91/*10*; pig: 61/*1*; 96/*13*; sheep: 62/*1*; 99/*3*'; ox: 63/*1*; 102, 155/*14*; horse: 50/*16*; 65/*1*; 103/*33*)

The **a. axillaris** arises from the subclavian artery at the cranial border of the 1st rib and it leaves the thoracic cavity through the ventral half of the thoracic outlet. Ventral to the medial scalenus muscle the axillary artery continues caudally the arc which began as the subclavian artery. It runs between the thoracic wall and the pectoral limb to reach medially the flexor aspect of the shoulder joint. It immediately gives off the *a. thoracica*.

78 Arteries

In the dog and pig the **r. deltoideum** may be given off even earlier. This is described under the superficial cervical artery. In carnivores the next branch is the *a. thoracica lateralis* which runs along the lateral wall of the chest. In the ox and horse the *a. suprascapularis* arises from the dorsal wall of the axillary artery at about the same level as the origin of the external thoracic. The suprascapular artery then takes a dorsal direction along the cranial border of the scapula. In all domestic animals the stout *a. subscapularis* also arises from the dorsal wall of the axillary artery and follows in a dorsal course the caudal border of the scapula. Still within the flexor region of the shoulder joint, the axillary artery curves distally and, except in the pig, it gives off the *a. circumflexa humeris* in the region of the collum humeri. Thereafter the axillary artery continues as the *a. brachialis*.

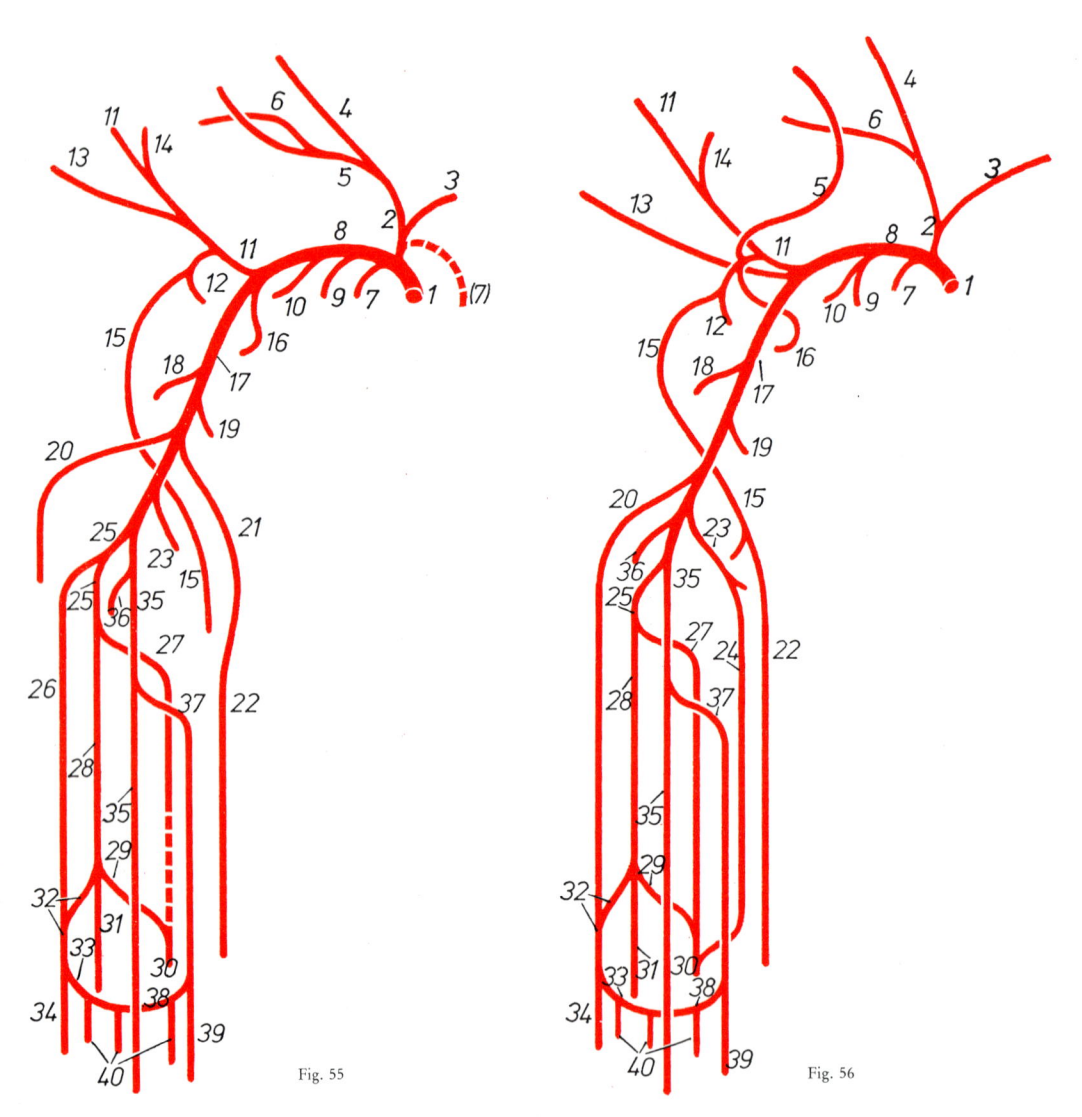

Figs 55, 56, 57, 58. Arteries of the left pectoral limb down to the carpal region of the dog, pig, ox and horse. Diagrammatic, medial view.

1 a. subclavia; *2* a. cervicalis superficialis; *3* r. ascendens; *4* r. praescapularis; *5* a. suprascapularis; *5'* r. suprascapularis; *6* r. acromialis; *7* r. deltoideus; *8* a. axillaris; *9* a. thoracica externa; *10* a. thoracica lateralis; *11* a. subscapularis; *12* a. circumflexa humeri caudalis; *13* a. thoracodorsalis; *14* a. circumflexa scapulae; *15* a. collateralis radialis; *16* a. circumflexa humeri cranialis; *17* a. brachialis; *18* a. profunda brachii; *19* a. bicipitalis; *20* a. collateralis ulnaris; *21* a. brachialis superficialis; *22* a. antebrachialis superficialis cranialis; *23* a. transversa cubiti, *24* its branch to the rete carpi dorsale; *25* a. interossea communis; *26* a. ulnaris; *27* a. interossea cranialis; *28* a. interossea caudalis; *29* r. interosseus; *30* r. carpeus dorsalis of *27* or, in the dog, of *29*; *31* r. carpeus palmaris of *28* or, in the ox, of *29*; *32* r. palmaris, *33* r. profundus, *34* r. superficialis; *35* a. mediana; *36* a. profunda antebrachii; *37* a. radialis; *37'* a. radialis proximalis of the horse, the r. carpeus palmaris is also shown; *38* r. profundus of *37*; *33* and *38* arcus palmaris profundus; *39* r. superficialis of *37*; *40* aa. metacarpei palmares

A. thoracica externa

(Comparative: 55–58/9; 85–88/24; cat: 59/2; 90/3'; pig: 96/9; sheep: 99/16''; ox: 102, 155/15; horse: 54/14; 103/19)

From its point of origin at the level of the 1st rib, the **a. thoracica externa** continues caudally and divides into a superficial and a deep branch. The superficial branch runs between the superficial and deep pectoral muscles, ramifying in both of these muscles. The deep branch sends twigs from the medial surface into the m. pectoralis profundus. In the pig the *a. thoracica lateralis* also arises from the external thoracic.

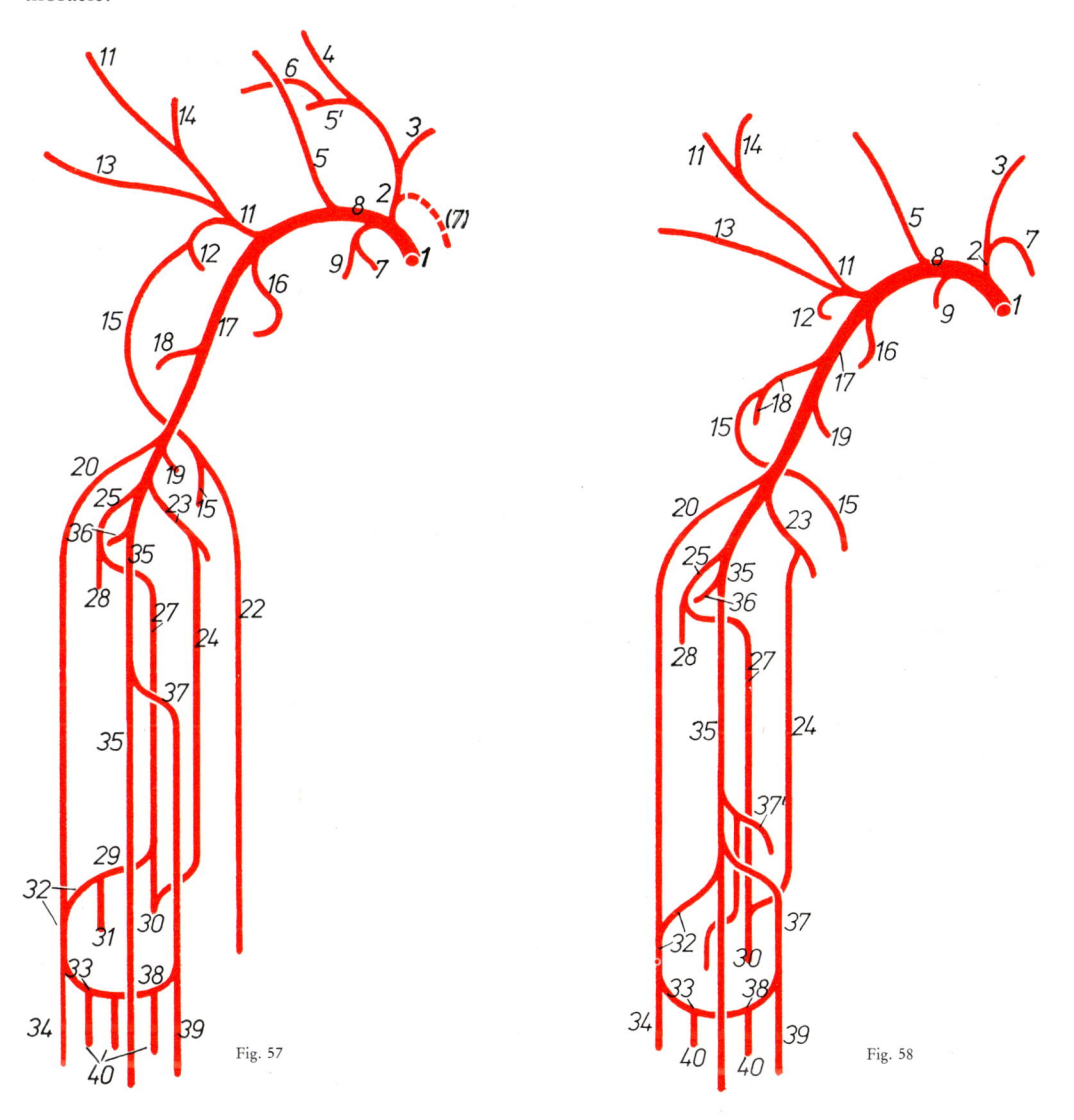

Fig. 57

Fig. 58

A. thoracica lateralis

(Comparative: 85–88/25; cat: 59/3; 90/9; dog: 92/22; 93/d; pig: 96/10)

The **a. thoracica lateralis** occurs only in carnivores and the pig. In the former species it arises from the axillary artery; in the pig from the external thoracic. The lateral thoracic artery proceeds caudally and reaches a superficial position in the angle between the deep pectoral and the latissimus dorsi muscles. It gives off branches to these muscles, to the m. cutaneus trunci and to the skin. In females there are also laterodorsally directed *r. mammarii laterales* which supply the thoracic mammary tissue.

A. suprascapularis

(Comparative: 55–58/5; cat: 59/27; pig: 61/7; sheep: 62/23; ox: 63/2; 64/1, 2; horse: 65/2; 66/1)

The **a. suprascapularis** of carnivores and small ruminants and the r. *suprascapularis* of the ox both arise from the superficial cervical artery. In the pig, on the other hand, the suprascapula artery stems from the *a. circumflexa humeri caudalis* and in the ox and horse from the axillary artery. The suprascapular ramus of the ox give off the r. *acromialis*. In accord with its variable origin, the course of this artery is caudal in carnivores and small ruminants, craniodorsal in the pig and dorsal in the ox and horse. Together with the suprascapular nerve, it travels between the subscapularis and supraspinatus muscles to reach the incisura scapulae. Here, as well as in the supraspinatus muscle, branches run to the margo dorsalis of the scapula to ramify in the muscles just mentioned. In the ox the caudally directed r. suprascapularis only just reaches the supraspinatus muscle with its smallest branches. The suprascapular artery also supplies the brachial plexus which in the horse usually receives additional branches from the *a. circumflexa scapulae*. Furthermore, the suprascapular artery anastomoses with the *a. circumflexa scapulae* medially at the collum scapulae and often also laterally along the suprascapular nerve. A distally directed branch of the suprascapularis turns lateral between the supraspinatus and coracobrachialis muscles to participate in the supply of the shoulder joint, the proximal extremity of the humerus and the muscles inserted there. It anastomoses with the *aa. circumflexae humeri*.

R. acromialis

(Comparative: 55–58/6; cat: 59/26; sheep: 62/22; ox: 63/22)

In carnivores and small ruminants the **r. acromialis** takes its origin from the suprascapular artery; in the ox it arises from the r. suprascapularis and in the pig from the superficial cervical artery. It curves round the cranial border of the supraspinatus

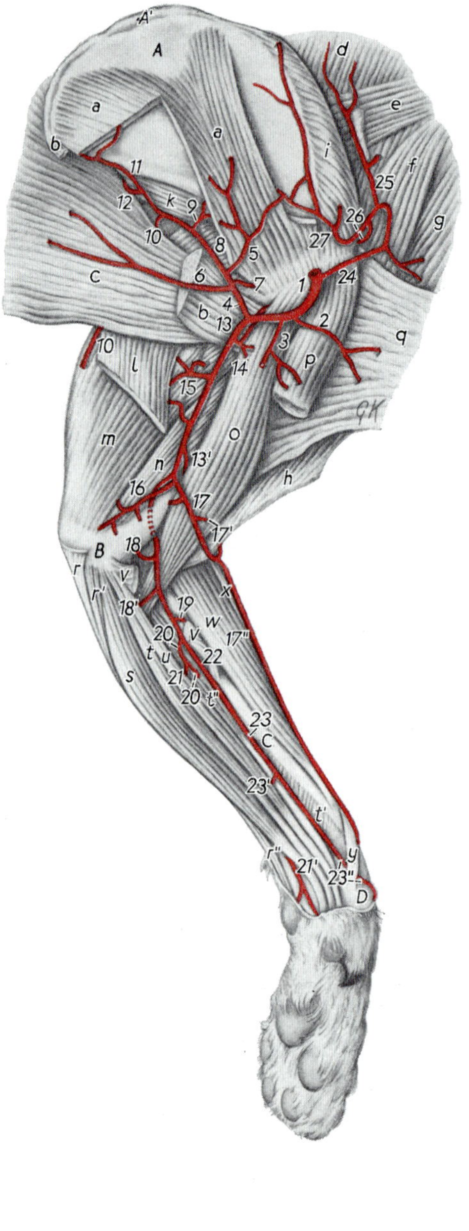

Fig. 59. Arteries of the left pectoral limb of a cat. Medial view.
(After Wissdorf, 1963. Study performed at the Institute of Veterinary Anatomy, Hanover).

A scapula; *A'* cartilago scapulae; *B* epicondylus medialis humeri; *C* radius; *D* os metacarpale I

a m. subscapularis; *b* m. teres major; *c* m. latissimus dorsi; *d* m. trapezius; *e* m. omotransversarius; *f* m. cleidomastoideus, *g* m. cleidocervicalis, *h* m. cleidobrachialis of the m. brachiocephalicus; *i* m. supraspinatus; *k* m. infraspinatus; *l* m. tensor fasciae antebrachii; *m* m. triceps brachii, caput longum, *n* caput mediale; *o* m. biceps brachii; *p* m. pectoralis profundus; *q* mm. pectorales superficiales; *r* m. flexor carpi ulnaris, caput ulnare, *r'* caput humerale, *r''* its terminal tendon; *s* m. flexor digitalis superficialis; *t* m. flexor digitalis profundus, caput humerale, *t'* caput radiale, *t''* caput ulnare; *u* m. flexor carpi radialis; *v* m. pronator teres; *w* m. extensor carpi radialis; *x* m. brachioradialis; *y* m. abductor pollicis longus

1 a. axillaris; *2* a. thoracica externa; *3* a. thoracica lateralis; *4, 8* a. subscapularis, *5* r. muscularis; *6* a. thoracodorsalis; *7* a. circumflexa humeri caudalis; *9* a. circumflexa scapulae; *10, 11, 12* terminal branches of the a. subscapularis; *13* a. brachialis; *13'* a. nutricia humeri; *14* a. circumflexa humeri cranialis; *15* a. profunda brachii; *16* a. collateralis ulnaris; *17* a. brachialis superficialis; *17'* a. bicipitalis; *17''* a. antebrachialis superficialis cranialis; *18* a. transversa cubiti; *18'* a. profunda antebrachii; *19* a. interossea cranialis; *20* a. interossea caudalis; *21* a. ulnaris; *21'* r. palmaris of the a. interossea caudalis; *22* a. mediana; *23* a. radialis, *23'* r. palmaris superficialis, *23''* r. carpeus dorsalis; *24* a. cervicalis superficialis, *25* r. praescapularis, *26* r. acromialis; *27* a. suprascapularis

Arteries of the pectoral limb 81

muscle, enters this muscle from lateral and continues laterally over the neck of the scapula. Here it anastomoses with branches from the suprascapular artery. No specific r. acromialis is present in the horse.

A. subscapularis

(Comparative: 55–58/*11*; cat: 59/*4, 8*; pig: 61/*2, 4*; sheep: 62/*2, 5*; ox: 63/*3, 7*; 64/*3*; horse: 65/*3*)

The **a. subscapularis** leaves the axillary artery in the flexor region of the shoulder joint. It goes between the subscapularis teres major muscles, thence on the medial surface of the long head of the biceps brachii muscle, and along the caudal border of the scapula to the caudal angle of the scapula. Immediately after its origin and while still within the flexor region of the shoulder joint, it gives rise caudodorsally to the *a. thoracodorsalis*. At about the same level, but with slight species differences, it gives off craniolaterally the *a. circumflexa humeri cranialis* and at the caudal border of the scapula in the region of the nutrient foramen, the *a. circumflexa scapulae* arises from it. The *a. circumflexa humeri cranialis* of the dog may be given off the subscapular artery prior to this. Along its course the subscapular artery sends out muscular branches, which are sometimes very stout, and which fork at the caudal border of the scapula to enter the muscles lying on either surface of the shoulder blade; the lateral branches perforate the long head of the triceps brachii muscle. Caudally directed offshoots supply especially the long head. One of these branches is fairly constant in all species and it runs

Fig. 60. Arteries of the left pectoral limb of a dog, distal to the upper arm. Medial view.
(After Zietzschmann, 1943.)

A humerus; *B* radius; *C* ulna; *D* os carpi accessorium

a m. triceps brachii; *b* m. brachiocephalicus; *c* m. biceps brachii and m. brachialis; *d* m. extensor carpi radialis; *e* m. pronator teres; *f* m. flexor carpi radialis; *g* m. flexor digitalis profundus; *h* m. flexor digitalis superficialis

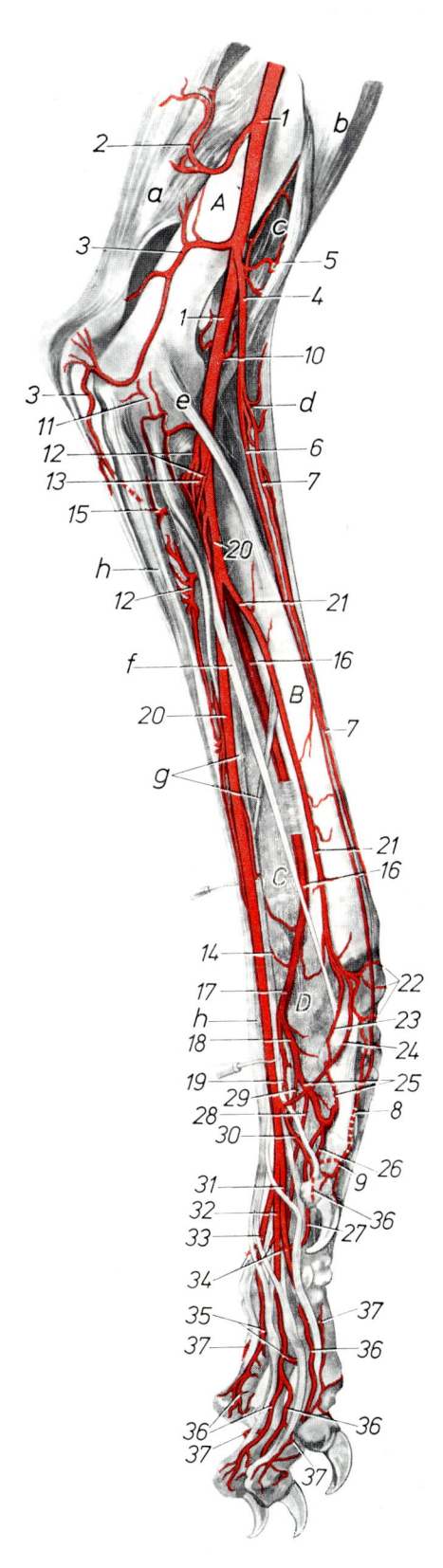

1 a. brachialis; *2* a. profunda brachii; *3* a. collateralis ulnaris; *4* a. brachialis superficialis; *5* a. bicipitalis; *6* a. antebrachialis superficialis cranialis, r. medialis; *7* r. lateralis; *8* a. digitalis dorsalis communis I; *9* a. digitalis dorsalis I axialis; *10* a. transversa cubiti; *11* rr. articulares; *12* a. profunda antebrachii; *13* a. interossea communis; *14* a. ulnaris; *15* a. recurrens ulnaris; *16* a. interossea caudalis; *17* r. palmaris; *18* r. profundus; *19* r. superficialis; *20* a. mediana; *21* a. radialis; *22* rr. carpei dorsales; *23* r. palmaris profundus; *24* r. palmaris superficialis; *25* arcus palmaris profundus; *26–29* aa. metacarpeae palmares I–IV; *30–33* aa. digitales palmares communes I–IV; *34* rr. tori metacarpei; *35* aa. interdigitales; *36* aa. digitales palmares propriae axiales; *37* aa. digitales palmares propriae abaxiales

distally as a large vessel in the caudal third of that muscle parallel to the fibres. Terminal branches reach the rhomboideus muscle and go past the caudal angle of the scapula to the trapezius muscle.

A. thoracodorsalis
(Comparative: 55–58/*13*; cat: 59/*6*; pig: 61/*3*; sheep: 62/*4*; ox: 63/*5*; horse: 65/*4*;)

The **a. thoracodorsalis** is usually the first vessel to arise from the subscapular artery; it does so in a caudodorsal direction. In carnivores, the goat and the ox it may also arise after the *a. circumflexa humeri caudalis* or together with it at the same level. It crosses the teres major muscle medially and then, accompanied by the thoracodorsal nerve, it runs along the medial surface of the latissimus dorsi muscle, all the while repeatedly dividing into divergent branches. In addition to supplying the two muscles mentioned, the thoracodorsal artery also provides branches to the lnn. axillares proprii and, in the dog, also the lnn. axillaris accessorii. Branches also go to the deep pectoralis, the ventral serratus, the long head of the triceps brachii and the tensor fasciae antebrachii muscles as well as to the cutaneus trunci muscle and the fascia and skin caudal to the scapula.

A. circumflexa humeri caudalis
(Comparative: 55–58/*12*; cat: 59/*7*; pig: 61/*6, 9*; sheep: 62/*3*; ox: 63, 64/*4*; horse: 65/*5*)

Immediately after its origin from the subscapular artery the **a. circumflexa humeri caudalis** turns laterally in the flexor region of the shoulder joint between the long head of the triceps brachii and the brachialis muscles where it is accompanied by the corresponding vein and the axillary nerve. Shortly after its origin it gives off the *a. collateralis radialis* (except in the horse) and anastomoses lateral to the neck of the humerus with the *a. circumflexa humeri cranialis*. In the pig the caudal circumflex humeral artery gives rise first to the *a. suprascapularis*, which has already been described, and then to the *a. circumflexa humeri cranialis*. In carnivores, ruminants and the horse the latter is the last vessel to branch from the axillary artery. Along its course the caudal circumflex humeral artery gives off branches to the shoulder joint, to all neighbouring muscles and, once it attains the lateral side, to the infraspinatus and deltoideus muscles. It finally anastomoses with a distal branch of the suprascapular artery.

A. collateralis radialis
(Comparative: 55–58/*15*; ox: 64/*5*; horse: 65/*10*; 66/*4*)

In carnivores, the pig and ruminants the **a. collateralis radialis** arises from the caudal circumflex humeral artery on the caudal surface of the brachialis muscle. In the horse it originates much further distally from the *a. profunda brachii*. While still caudal to the humerus it gives off the *a. nutricia humeri* (except in the horse) and the *a. collateralis media* which courses to the olecranon fossa to participate in the formation of the rete articulare cubiti. The collateral radial artery accompanies the radial nerve through the musculospiral groove (sulcus m. brachialis) and supplies branches to the neighbouring muscles. Its terminal branches vascularize the craniolateral group of muscles on the forearm. The collateral radial artery of pigs and ruminants also gives rise to the thin *a. antebrachialis superficialis cranialis*; in carnivores this latter is the continuation of the a. brachialis superficialis and it does not occur at all in the horse. It forms the point of origin for the dorsal superficial vessels of the toe.

A. circumflexa scapulae
(Comparative: 55–58/*14*; cat: 59/*9*; pig: 61/*5*; sheep: 62/*7*; ox: 63/*6*; horse: 65/*6*; 66/*2*)

The **a. circumflexa scapulae** originates from the subscapular artery in the ventral third of the shoulder blade at the level of the for. nutricium scapulae which is situated on the caudal border. Here it gives off the *a. nutricia scapulae* although this may arise independently from the subscapular artery. The circumflex scapular artery divides at the caudal border of the shoulderblade into a lateral and a medial branch, both of which can also arise independently from the subscapular artery. Their distribution is like that of the muscular branches of the subscapular artery, which have already been described.

A. circumflexa humeri cranialis
(Comparative: 55–58/*16*; cat: 59/*14*; pig: 61/*8*; sheep: 62/*10*; ox: 63/*9*; horse: 65/*7*)

The **a. circumflexa humeri cranialis** is the last vessel to arise from the axillary artery. However, this is rarely the case in the pig because in this animal it usually originates from the **a. circumflexa humeri caudalis** or it may, as it also may in the dog, arise from the subscapular artery. In the carnivores it takes a cranially directed course over the medial aspect of the coracobrachialis muscle but in the other domestic mammals it passes between the two parts of that muscle and only rarely does it lie directly against the humerus. The cranial circumflex humeral artery supplies the humerus and the shoulder joint and it contributes to the vascularization of the muscles attached in that region, especially the biceps brachii. It anastomoses with the caudal circumflex humeral artery above the cranial surface of the humerus and its proximally directed branches also unite with the suprascapular artery.

A. brachialis
(Comparative: 55–58/*17*; cat: 59/*13*; dog: 60/*1* pig: 61/*11* sheep: 62/*9*; ox: 63/*8*; horse: 65/*8*)

The **a. brachialis** is the continuation of the axillary artery distal to the shoulder joint. Transition into the brachial artery occurs after the origination of the cranial circumflex humeral artery or, if the circumflex vessel arises from another artery, from a similar position. The brachial artery takes a straight course to the elbow joint and traverses the supracondylar foramen, in the cat in a craniodistal direction. In so doing it crosses the distal half of the humerus medially and attains the cranial border of the pronator teres muscle. After giving off the *a. interossea communis*, or the *aa. interosseae* in the cat, at the level of the spatium interosseum antebrachii, the brachial artery becomes the *a. mediana*. Along its course it gives rise in a caudal direction to the *a. profunda brachii* and subsequently the *a. collateralis ulnaris*. In the cat, the latter vessel arises from the *a. brachialis superficialis*. In carnivores the superficial brachial artery issues from the brachial artery in a cranial direction and at the elbow joint the *a. transversa cubiti* is then given off the brachial artery in craniolateral direction. The *a. bicipitalis* is given off the brachial artery in a cranial direction proximal to the collateral ulnar artery in the dog, pig and horse. In ruminants the bicipital artery originates distal to the collateral ulnar artery although not infrequently it may spring from the transverse cubital artery. In the cat, and occasionally also in the dog, it arises from the superficial brachial artery. The bicipital artery is a stout muscular vessel which enters the distal half of the biceps brachii muscle and pervades it, especially in a proximal direction. Other unnamed branches go to the neighbouring muscles, particularly to the coracobrachialis muscle, and to the elbow joint. These vessels are particularly prominent in the carnivores where they are linked to the *a. recurrens ulnaris*. The brachial artery of the horse gives rise to the *a. nutricia humeri* distal to the bicipital artery.

A. profunda brachii
(Comparative: 55–58/*18*; cat: 59/*15* dog: 60/*2*; pig: 61/*12* sheep: 62/*11* ox: 63/*10* horse: 65/*9*)

The **a. profunda brachii** arises from the caudal aspect of the brachial artery at a point distal to the tuberosity teres. It immediately divides into several stout divergent muscular branches which are distributed, in company with branches of the radial nerve, in the triceps brachii muscle. In the horse it also gives off the *a. collateralis radialis*, which has already been described and with which the deep brachial artery of the other domestic mammals is linked.

A. collateralis ulnaris
(Comparative: 55–58/*20*; cat: 59/*16*; dog: 60/*3*; pig: 61/*13*; sheep: 62/*12*; ox: 63/*11*; 64/*10*; horse: 65/*12* 66/*9*)

The **a. collateralis ulnaris** leaves the brachial artery proximal to the medial condyle of the humerus except in the cat. In the latter it originates from the superficial brachial artery because in this species the brachial artery goes through the supracondylar foramen. The collateral ulnar artery runs along the

84 Arteries

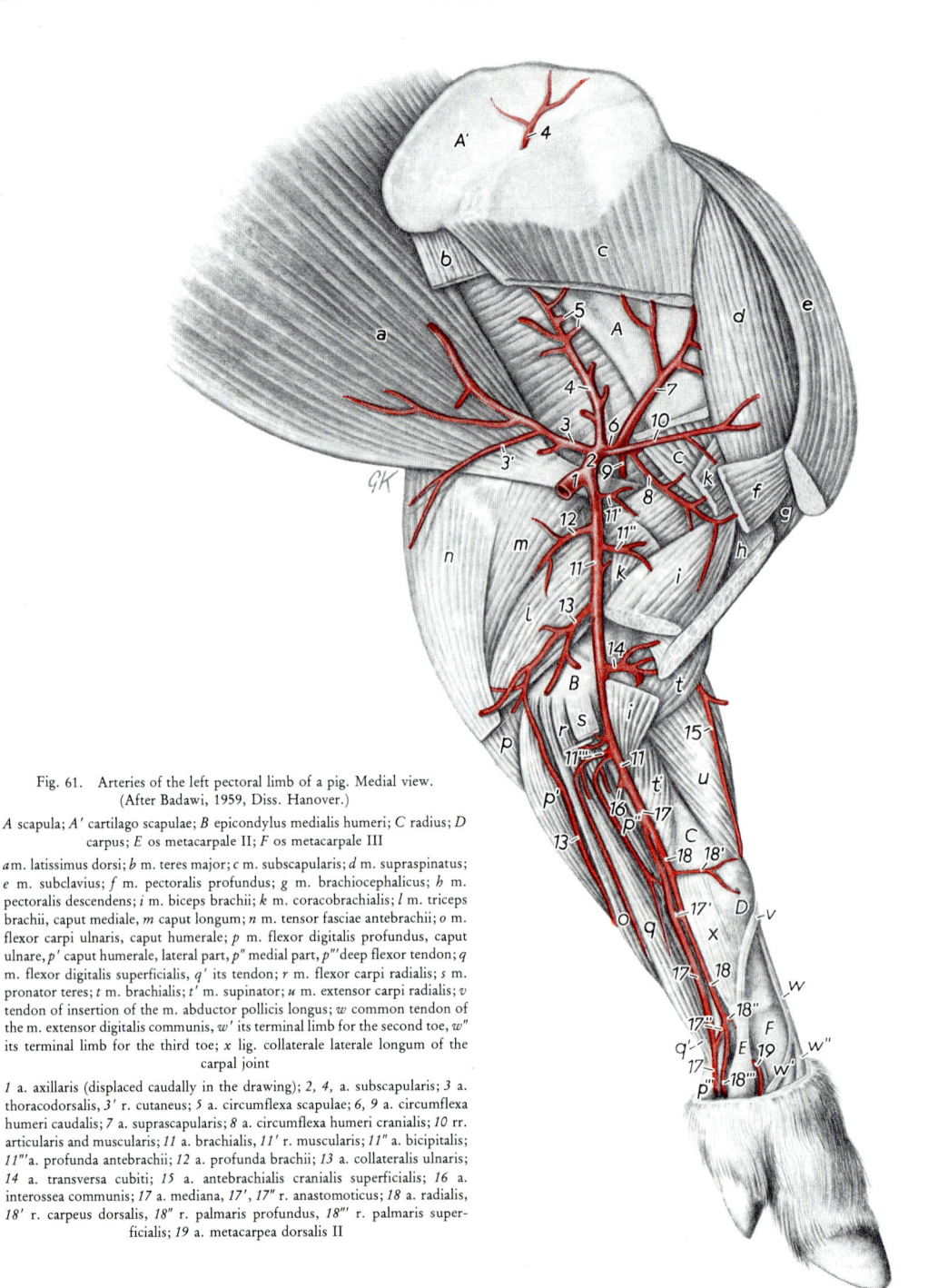

Fig. 61. Arteries of the left pectoral limb of a pig. Medial view. (After Badawi, 1959, Diss. Hanover.)

A scapula; *A'* cartilago scapulae; *B* epicondylus medialis humeri; *C* radius; *D* carpus; *E* os metacarpale II; *F* os metacarpale III

a m. latissimus dorsi; *b* m. teres major; *c* m. subscapularis; *d* m. supraspinatus; *e* m. subclavius; *f* m. pectoralis profundus; *g* m. brachiocephalicus; *h* m. pectoralis descendens; *i* m. biceps brachii; *k* m. coracobrachialis; *l* m. triceps brachii, caput mediale, *m* caput longum; *n* m. tensor fasciae antebrachii; *o* m. flexor carpi ulnaris, caput humerale; *p* m. flexor digitalis profundus, caput ulnare, *p'* caput humerale, lateral part, *p''* medial part, *p'''* deep flexor tendon; *q* m. flexor digitalis superficialis, *q'* its tendon; *r* m. flexor carpi radialis; *s* m. pronator teres; *t* m. brachialis; *t'* m. supinator; *u* m. extensor carpi radialis; *v* tendon of insertion of the m. abductor pollicis longus; *w* common tendon of the m. extensor digitalis communis, *w'* its terminal limb for the second toe, *w''* its terminal limb for the third toe; *x* lig. collaterale laterale longum of the carpal joint

1 a. axillaris (displaced caudally in the drawing); *2, 4,* a. subscapularis; *3* a. thoracodorsalis, *3'* r. cutaneus; *5* a. circumflexa scapulae; *6, 9* a. circumflexa humeri caudalis; *7* a. suprascapularis; *8* a. circumflexa humeri cranialis; *10* rr. articularis and muscularis; *11* a. brachialis, *11'* r. muscularis; *11''* a. bicipitalis; *11'''* a. profunda antebrachii; *12* a. profunda brachii; *13* a. collateralis ulnaris; *14* a. transversa cubiti; *15* a. antebrachialis cranialis superficialis; *16* a. interossea communis; *17* a. mediana, *17', 17''* r. anastomoticus; *18* a. radialis, *18'* r. carpeus dorsalis, *18''* r. palmaris profundus, *18'''* r. palmaris superficialis; *19* a. metacarpea dorsalis II

ventral border of the medial head of the triceps brachii muscle in the direction of the olecranon, accompanying the ulnar nerve en route. Together with this nerve it reaches the ulnar groove and, except in carnivores, it follows this in the direction of the carpus. Here it gives off the *r. carpeus dorsalis* and, except in the horse, the *r. carpeus palmaris* to the dorsal and palmar articular network respectively. In the pig and ruminant it then anastomoses with the *r. palmaris* of the a. interossea and with the same ramus of the a. mediana in the horse. While still in the upper arm region the collateral ulnar artery gives off muscular branches to the triceps brachii, the tensor fasciae antebrachii and the pectoralis transversus muscles. Thereafter it contributes to the formation of the *rete articulare cubiti* and in the lower arm to the supply of the flexors of the carpal and toe joints. In ruminants and the horse the r. carpeus dorsalis gives rise to a slender *r. dorsalis*; this branch arises from the *a. ulnaris* in carnivores. In the ox it continues into the very small dorsal common artery of the third toe and in the horse it accompanies the equally small *r. dorsalis* of the ulnar nerve.

A. brachialis superficialis

(Comparative: 55–58/*21*; cat: 59/*17*; dog: 60/*4*)

An **a. brachialis superficialis** is present only in carnivores in which species it arises proximal to the elbow from the medial aspect of the brachial artery. In the cat it immediately gives off the *a. collateralis ulnaris* and subsequently in this animal, and sometimes also in the dog, the *a. bicipitalis* which has already been described as a branch of the brachial artery. The superficial brachial artery crosses in a craniodistal direction the distal end of the biceps brachii muscle, medial and parallel to the vein of the same name. This vein anastomoses here with the *v. mediana cubiti*. The *aa. radiales superficiales* are then given off and they accompany branches of the n. cutaneus antebrachii on the fascia of the lower arm in the depression between the radius and the m. extensor carpi radialis. These superficial radial arteries finally terminate in the *r. carpeus dorsalis* of the radial artery. Distal to the elbow joint the superficial brachial artery becomes the cranial superficial antebrachial artery.

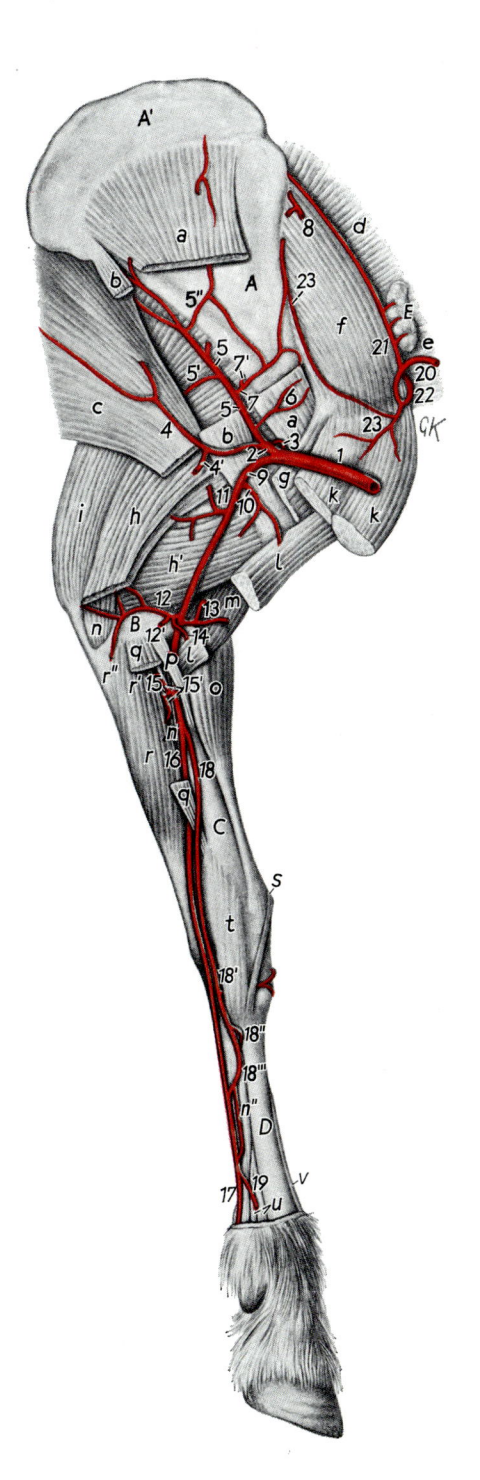

Fig. 62 Arteries of the left pectoral limb of a sheep. Medial view.
(After Wissdorf, 1961, Diss., Hanover.)

A scapula; *A'* cartilago scapulae; *B* epicondylus medialis humeri; *C* radius; *D* os metacarpale III + IV; *E* ln. cervicalis superficialis

a m. subscapularis; *b* m. teres major; *c* m. latissimus dorsi; *d* m. trapezius; *e* m. omotransversarius; *f* m. supraspinatus; *g* m. coracobrachialis; *h* m. triceps brachii, caput longum, *h'* caput mediale; *i* m. tensor fasciae antebrachii; *k* m. pectoralis profundus; *l* m. biceps brachii; *m* m. brachialis; *n* m. flexor digitalis profundus, caput ulnare, *n'* caput radiale, *n"* deep flexor tendon; *o* m. extensor carpi radialis; *p* m. pronator teres; *q* m. flexor carpi radialis; *r* m. flexor carpi ulnaris, *r'* caput humerale, *r"* caput ulnare; *s* m. abductor pollicis longus; *t* palmar supplementary band of the medial collateral ligaments; *u* m. interosseus medius; *v* tendon of the m. extensor digiti III proprius

1 a. axillaris; *2, 5* a. subscapularis; *3* a. circumflexa humeri caudalis; *4* a. thoracodorsalis, *4'* r. muscularis to the m. pectoralis profundus; *5', 5", 6* r. musculares; *7* a. circumflexa scapulae; *7'* a. nutricia scapulae; *8* branches of the a. scapularis dorsalis; *9* a. brachialis; *10* a. circumflexa humeri cranialis; *11* a. profunda brachii; *12* a. collateralis ulnaris, *12'* r. cutaneus; *13* a. transversa cubiti; *14* a. bicipitalis; *15* a. interossea communis; *15'* a. profunda antebrachii; *16* a. mediana; *17* a. digitalis palmaris communis III; *18* a. radialis, *18'* r. carpeus dorsalis, *18"* r. palmaris profundus, *18'"* r. palmaris superficialis; *19* a. digitalis palmaris communis II; *20* a. cervicalis superficialis, *21* r. praescapularis, *22* r. acromialis; *23* a. suprascapularis

Arteries

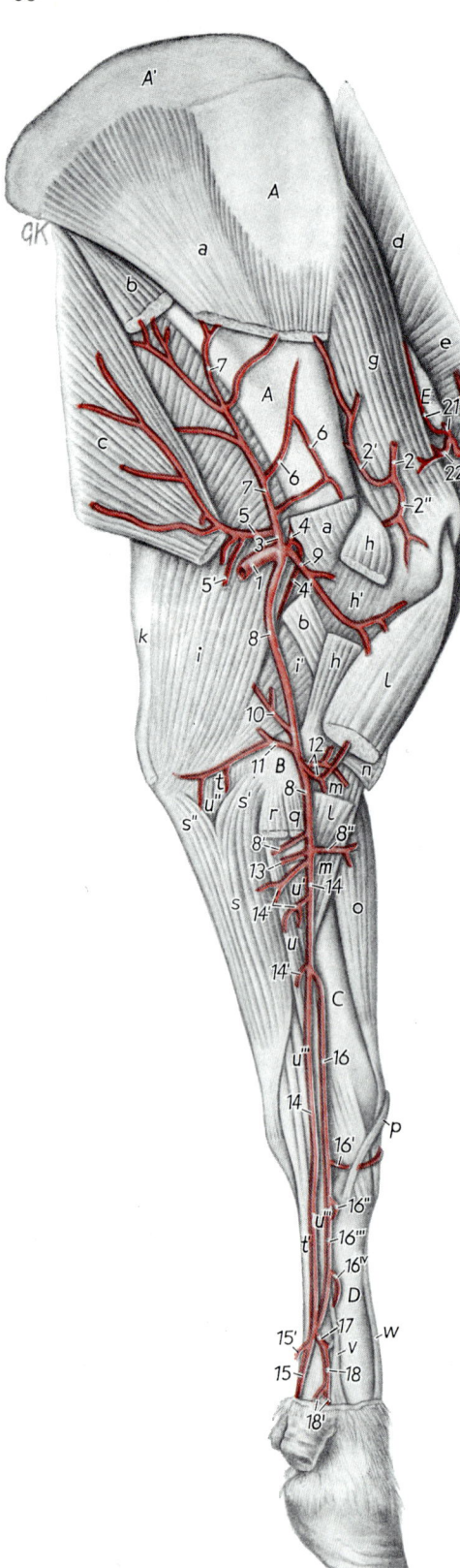

A. antebrachialis superficialis cranialis
(Comparative: 55–58/22; cat: 59/*17"*; dog: 60/6; 71/1, *1'*; pig: 61/*15*; 72/1; ox: 73/*1*)

This artery, which in carnivores is the continuation of the superficial brachial artery, in the pig and ruminant arises as a delicate vessel springing from the collateral radial artery. In the cat it runs distad with the r. lateralis of the r. superficialis of the radial nerve, joining with the *r. dorsalis* of the ulna artery in the metacarpal region and forming the *arcus dorsalis superficialis*. From this arch arise the *aa. digitalis dorsales communes I–IV* and the *a. digitalis dorsalis I abaxialis*.

Fig. 63. Arteries of the left pectoral limb of an ox. Medial view. (After Badawi and Wilkens, 1961, study performed at the Institute for Veterinary Anatomy, Hanover.)

A scapula; *A'* cartilago scapulae; *B* epicondylus medialis humeri; *C* radius; *D* os metacarpale III + IV; *E* ln. cervicalis superficialis

a m. subscapularis; *b* m. teres major; *c* m. latissimus dorsi; *d* m. trapezius; *e* m. omotransversarius; *f* m. brachiocephalicus; *g* m. supraspinatus; *h, h'* m. coracobrachialis; *i* m. triceps brachii, *i'* caput mediale; *k* m. tensor fasciae antebrachii; *l* m. biceps brachii; *m* m. brachialis; *n* mm. pectorales superficiales; *o* m. extensor carpi radialis; *p* m. abductor pollicis longus; *q* m. pronator teres; *r* m. flexor carpi radialis; *s* m. flexor carpi ulnaris, *s'* caput humerale, *s"* caput ulnare; *t* m. flexor digitalis superficialis, *t'* superficial flexor tendon; *u* m. flexor digitalis profundus, caput humerale, *u'* caput radiale, *u"* caput ulnare, *u'"* deep flexor tendon; *v* m. interosseus medius, medial branch; *w* tendon of the m. extensor digiti III proprius

1 a. axillaris (displaced caudally); *2, 2', 2"* a. suprascapularis; *3, 7* a. subscapularis; *4* a. circumflexa humeri caudalis; *4'* a. collateralis radialis; *5* a. thoracodorsalis, *5'* r. muscularis for the m. pectoralis profundus; *6* a. circumflexa humeri scapulae; *8* a. brachialis, *8', 8"* rr. musculares; *9* a. circumflexa humeri cranialis; *10* a. profunda brachii; *11* a. collateralis ulnaris; *12* a. bicipitalis and a. transversa cubiti; *13* a. interossea communis; *14* a. mediana; *14'* a. profunda antebrachii; *15* a. digitalis palmaris communis III; *15'* lateral part of the arcus palmaris superficialis; *16* a. radialis, *16'* r. carpeus dorsalis, *16"* r. palmaris profundus, *16'"* r. palmaris superficialis, *16(iv)* r. anastomoticus with the a. metacarpea palmaris II; *17* medial part of the arcus palmaris superficialis with connection to the a. metacarpea palmaris II; *18* a. digitalis palmaris communis II; *18'* aa. digitales palmares propriae; *19* a. cervicalis superficialis, *20* r. ascendens, *21* r. praescapularis, *22* r. suprascapularis with r. acromialis, *23* r. deltoideus

Arteries of the pectoral limb

In the dog the *a. antebrachialis superficialis cranialis* divides proximal to the m. extensor carpi radialis into a lateral and a medial branch which accompany respective branches of the r. superficialis of the radial nerve in the lower arm region. The medial branch continues at the metacarpus into the *a. digitalis dorsalis communis I* while the lateral branch gives off the *aa. digitales dorsales communes II–IV*. In the pig the a. antebrachialis superficialis cranialis gives rise to the delicate *a. digitalis dorsalis communis III* or, sometimes, to the *a. digitalis dorsalis communis II*. In ruminants, on the other hand, the thin *aa. digitales dorsales communes II* and *III* arise from it.

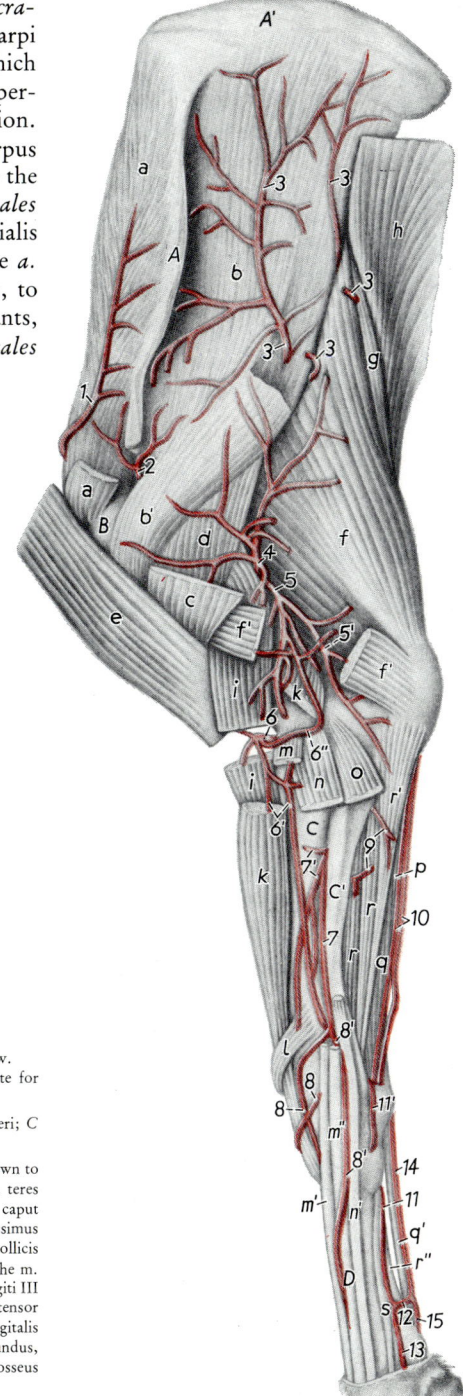

Fig. 64. Arteries of the left pectoral limb of an ox. Lateral view. (After Badawi and Wilkens, 1961, study performed at the Institute for Veterinary Anatomy, Hanover.)

A spina scapulae; *A'* cartilago scapulae; *B* tuberculum majus humeri; *C* radius; *C'* ulna; *D* os metacarpale III + IV

a m. supraspinatus, partly removed; *b* m. infraspinatus, removed down to its tendon; *b'* terminal tendon; *c* m. deltoideus, distal stump; *d* m. teres minor, distal stump; *e* m. brachiocephalicus; *f* m. triceps brachii, caput longum, *f'* caput laterale; *g* m. tensor fasciae antebrachii; *h* m. latissimus dorsi; *i* m. brachialis; *k* m. extensor carpi radialis; *l* m. abductor pollicis longus; *m* m. extensor digitalis communis; *m'* terminal tendon of the m. extensor digiti III proprius; *m"* terminal tendon of the m. extensor digiti III and IV; *n* m. extensor digitalis lateralis, *n'* terminal tendon; *o* m. extensor carpi ulnaris, proximal stump; *p* m. flexor carpi ulnaris; *q* m. flexor digitalis superficialis, *q'* superficial flexor tendon; *r* m. flexor digitalis profundus, caput humerale, *r'* caput ulnare, *r"* deep flexor tendon; *s* m. interosseus medius

1, 2 rr. musculares of the a. suprascapularis; *3* a. subscapularis; *4* a. circumflexa humeri caudalis; *5* a. collateralis radialis; *5'* a. collateralis media; *6, 6'* a. transversa cubiti; *6"* r. anastomoticus; *7* a. interossea cranialis, *7'* rr. musculares; *8* branches of the r. carpeus dorsalis of the a. interossea cranialis; *8'* superficial branch with connection to the a. metacarpea dorsalis III; *9* rr. musculares of the a. interossea communis; *10* a. collateralis ulnaris; *11* r. superficialis, *11'* lateral branch of the r. palmaris; *12* lateral part of the arcus palmaris superficialis; *13* a. digitalis palmaris communis IV; *14* a. mediana; *15* a. digitalis palmaris communis III

88   Arteries

A. transversa cubiti

(Comparative: 55–58/23; cat: 59/18; dog: 60/10; pig: 61/14; sheep: 62/13; ox: 63/12; 64/6, 6'; horse: 65/13; 66/5)

The **a. transversa cubiti** arises from the brachial artery proximal to the trochlea of the humerus. It immediately bends laterally, lying close against the humerus, and supplies the elbow joint. Below the extensors of the carpal and toe joints it reaches the deep branches of the radial nerve and supplies the above-mentioned extensor

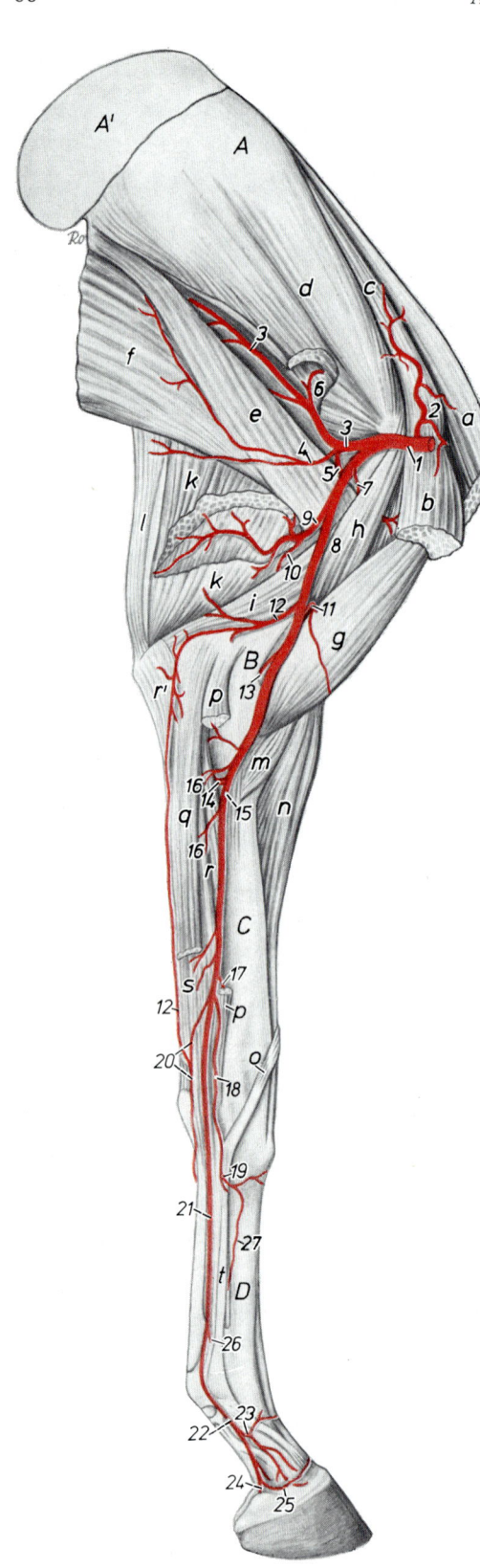

Fig. 65. Arteries of the left pectoral limb of a horse. Medial view.
(Redrawn after Ellenberger and Baum, 1932.)

A scapula; *A'* cartilago scapulae; *B* epicondylus medialis humeri; *C* radius; *D* os metacarpale III

a m. subclavius; *b* m. pectoralis profundus; *c* m. supraspinatus; *d* m. subscapularis; *e* m. teres major; *f* m. latissimus dorsi; *g* m. biceps brachii; *h* m. coracobrachialis; *i* m. triceps brachii, caput mediale, *k* caput longum; *l* m. tensor fasciae antebrachii; *m* m. brachialis; *n* m. extensor carpi radialis; *o* m. abductor pollicis longus; *p* m. flexor carpi radialis; *q* m. flexor carpi ulnaris; *r* m. flexor digitalis profundus, *r'* caput ulnare; *s* m. flexor digitalis superficiales; *t* m. interosseus medius

1 a. axillaris; *2* a. suprascapularis; *3* a. subscapularis; *4* a. thoracodorsalis; *5* a. circumflexa humeri caudalis; *6* a. circumflexa scapulae; *7* a. circumflexa humeri cranialis; *8* a. brachialis; *9* a. profunda brachii; *10* a. collateralis radialis; *11* a. bicipitalis; *12* a. collateralis ulnaris; *13* a. transversa cubiti; *14* a. interossea communis; *15* a. mediana; *16* a. profunda antebrachii; *17* a. radialis proximalis; *18* a. radialis, *19* r. palmaris profundus; *20* r. palmaris; *21* a. digitalis palmaris communis II; *22* a. digitalis palmaris (propria III) medialis; *23* r. dorsalis phalangis proximalis; *24* r. tori digitalis; *25* a. coronalis; *26* origin of the a. digitalis palmaris (propria III) lateralis in the absence of the a. digitalis palmaris communis III; *27* a. metacarpea dorsalis II

Arteries of the pectoral limb

muscles in company with these nerves. Before it terminates, vessels are also given off to supply the biceps brachii, brachialis, cleidobrachialis and pectoralis descendens muscles. In ruminants the *a. bicipitalis* sometimes also springs from the transvere cubital artery (see p. 83). Caudolaterally the transverse cubital artery anastomoses with the *a. interossea cranialis*. In its further distal course, lying close to the radius and crossing under the m. abductor pollicis longus, it reaches the *rete carpi dorsale* in all species except carnivores.

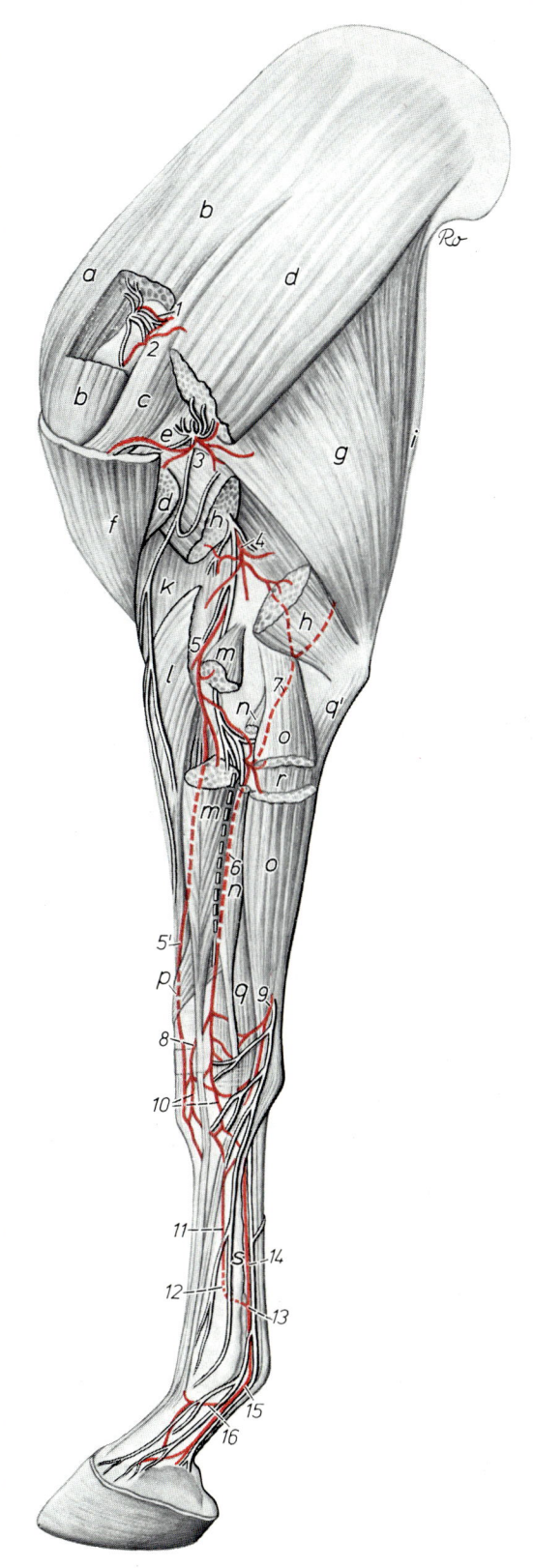

Fig. 66. Arteries of the left pectoral limb of a horse. Lateral view. (Redrawn after Ellenberger and Baum, 1932.)

a m. subclavius; *b* m. supraspinatus; *c* m. infraspinatus; *d* m. deltoideus; *e* m. teres minor; *f* m. brachiocephalicus; *g* m. triceps brachii, caput longum, *h* caput laterale; *i* m. tensor fasciae antebrachii; *k* m. brachialis; *l* m. extensor carpi radialis; *m* m. extensor digitalis communis; *n* m. extensor digitalis lateralis; *o* m. extensor carpi ulnaris; *p* m. abductor pollicis longus; *q* m. flexor digitalis profundus, *q'* caput ulnare; *r* m. flexor digitalis superficialis; *s* m. interosseus medius

1 a. suprascapularis with n. suprascapularis; *2* branches of the a. circumflexa scapulae; *3* a. circumflexa humeri caudalis with n. axillaris, which gives off the n. cutaneus antebrachii cranialis; *4* a. collateralis radialis with n. radialis; *5* a. transversa cubiti with *5'* connecting branch to the rete carpi dorsale; *6* a. interossea cranialis; *7* a. recurrens interossea; *8* r. carpeus dorsalis of the a. interossea cranialis; *9* r. carpeus dorsalis of the a. collateralis ulnaris with r. dorsalis of the n. ulnaris; *10* rete carpi dorsale; *11* a. metacarpea dorsalis III; *12* r. perforans distalis III; *13* junction of the aa. metacarpeae palmares with the aa. digitales palmares communes; *14* a. digitalis palmaris communis III with n. digitalis palmaris communis III; *15* a. digitalis palmaris (propria III) lateralis with n. digitalis palmaris (proprius III) lateralis; *16* r. dorsalis phalangis proximalis with r. dorsalis of the n. digitalis palmaris lateralis

A. interossea communis

(Comparative: 55–58/*25*; dog: 60/*13*; pig: 61/*16*; sheep: 62/*15*; ox: 63/*13*; horse: 65/*14*)

The **a. interossea communis** is the last vessel to leave the brachial artery before this becomes the median artery. It thus arises distal to the elbow joint in the region of the medial collateral ligament where, except in the horse, it is covered medially by the m. pronator teres. The common interosseous artery is absent in the cat but in its stead the *a. interossea cranialis* arises at the same site and, somewhat distal to it, the *a. interossea caudalis* originates. The common interosseous artery runs caudolaterally to the spatium interosseum antebrachii and then curves distad, dividing shortly afterwards into the *a. interossea cranialis* and the *a. interossea caudalis*. In addition to giving off branches to the elbow joint, the pronators and supinators, in the dog the common interosseous artery also gives off the *a. ulnaris*. It depends on the species whether the *aa. nutriciae* for the radius and ulna originate from the *a. interossea communis*, its branches or the *a. recurrens interossea*.

A. interossea cranialis

(Comparative: 55–58/*27*; 71–74/*14*; cat:59/*19*: ox: 64/*7*; horse: 66/*6*)

The **a. interossea cranialis** arises as a result of the division of the common interosseous artery. In the cat it may originate independently from the brachial artery. The cranial interosseous artery perforates the membrana interossea antebrachii and runs along it in a cranial direction towards the carpus. It is developed best in ruminants and most poorly in carnivores. In all domestic animals, shortly after it traverses the *spatium interosseum antebrachii proximale,* it gives off the *a. recurrens interossea* which is proximally directed and runs to the *rete articulare cubiti*. Here the cranial interosseous artery also anastomoses with the deep, caudally-directed branch of the a. transversea cubiti and gives off vessels to the extensors of the toe and the extensor carpi ulnaris muscle and, further distally, to the m. abductor policis longus. Except in the horse, the cranial interosseous artery is connected through the spatium interosseuum antebrachii distale via the *r. interosseous* with the *a. interossea caudalis* and together with the *r. carpeus dorsalis* it branches further and joins the *rete carpi dorsale*. In carnivores and the pig, in which species the distal part of the cranial interosseous artery is only weakly developed or may even be absent, the *r. carpeus dorsalis,* which is situated dorsal to the carpus, forms the continuation of the *r. interosseous*. The latter is invariably present but in carnivores and pigs it arises from the a. interossea caudalis.

A. interossea caudalis

(Comparative: 55–58/*28*; cat: 59/*20*; dog: 60, 67/*16*; pig: 68/*16*)

Only in the cat does the **a. interossea caudalis** arise from the brachial artery distal to the cranial interosseous artery. In the other domestic mammals it is the continuation of the *a. interossea communis* and it runs on the caudal surface of the membrana interossea antebrachii, being covered caudally in carnivores by the m. pronator quadratus. In carnivores and the pig it is joined through the spatium interosseum distale to the cranial interosseous artery by means of the *r. interosseous*. In these species the caudal interosseous artery is a stout vessel but in ruminants and the horse it is only slender and ramifies in the periosteum of the radius and ulna. In ruminants it not infrequently attains the r. interosseus. In the horse it sometimes connects with the r. carpeus palmaris of the collateral ulna artery. In the cat the caudal interosseous artery gives off the a. ulnaris, shortly after its origin, and in carnivores it supplies several branches, through the interosseous space, to the abductor pollicis longus muscle. In carnivores and pigs the *r. carpeus palmaris* to the palmar articular network stems from the a. interossea caudalis after its union with the r. interosseus. In ruminants it arises from the interosseus ramus itself. The caudal interosseous artery of carnivores and pigs and the r. interosseus of the ox, continue thereafter as the *r. palmaris*. Since in the horse, by virtue of the absence of a distal interosseous space, there is no interosseous ramus, the r. palmaris originates from the median artery. The r. palmaris runs in a caudomedial direction but medial to the accessory carpal bone and deep over the carpus. In so doing it receives the ulnar artery in carnivores and the collateral ulnar artery in the pig and ruminants. Distal to the carpus the r. palmaris divides into a *r. profundus* and a *r. superficialis*. The *r. profundus,* running in a transverse direction close to the bone, forms, together with the r. profundus of the radial artery, the *arcus palmaris profundus* from which the *aa. metacarpeae palmares* originate. The *r. superficialis*, which is usually lacking in the horse, participates in the formation of the arcus palmaris superficialis from which arise the palmar arteries of the toes.

A. ulnaris
(Comparative: 55–58/*26*; cat: 59/*21*; dog: 60/*14*; 67/*9*)

The **a. ulnaris** is peculiar to the carnivores. In the dog it arises from the common interosseous artery and in the cat somewhat more distally from the caudal interosseous artery as it branches from the brachial artery. The ulnar artery runs in caudodistal direction between the humeral head of the deep flexors of the toe and the ulna to reach the ulnar nerve. Here it is linked, by means of the proximally directed *a. recurrens ulnaris,* with the collateral ulnar artery. The ulnar artery is relatively a stouter vessel than the collateral ulnar artery of the pig, horse and ruminants. Within the ulnar groove it accompanies the ulnar nerve to the carpus where it terminates in the r. palmaris of the interosseous artery. Before this and proximal to the accessory carpal bone, it gives off the dorsal ramus which curves laterally round the distal end of the ulna to reach the carpus dorsally and, in the cat, it participates in the formation of the dorsal arch. In the dog it continues as the abaxial artery of the fifth digit. Subsequently it gives off the *r. carpeus dorsalis* and the *r. carpeus palmaris* to the dorsal and the palmar articular networks of the carpus respectively.

A. mediana
(Comparative: 55–58/*35*; 67–70/*22*; cat: 59/*22*; dog: 60/*20*; pig: 61/*17*; sheep: 62/*16*; ox: 63, 64/*14*; horse: 65/*15*)

After giving rise to the common interosseous artery or, in the cat, the caudal interosseous artery, the brachial artery continues as the **a. mediana**. In company with the vein of the same name and with the median nerve, it runs caudomedially along the radius in a distal direction where it is covered by the belly of the flexor carpi radialis muscle. In the groove between the tendon of the deep and superficial flexors of the toes or the deep part of the superficial flexors in pigs and ruminants, it continues over the flexor aspect of the carpal joint to the metacarpal region. Here it contributes, with some modifications in the different species, to the formation of the *arcus palmaris superficialis,* from which originate the palmar arteries of the toes. Along its course the median artery gives rise to a number of vessels: – shortly after its origin, the *a. profunda antebrachii* originates; distal to the insertion of the m. pronator teres, but at different levels in different species, the a. radialis is given off; in the horse only, the *a. radialis proximalis* arises by a separate origin from the *a. mediana* before the origin of the radial artery. Also in the horse, the median artery gives off, a little proximal to the carpus, the **r. palmaris.** In other domestic mammals the r. palmaris springs from the a. interossea caudalis, a vessel which is only rudimentary in the horse, but apart from this more superficial origin the equine r. palmaris corresponds to the same ramus of the other animals. Its *r. profundus* unites with that of the a. radialis to form the *arcus palmaris profundus.* Its *r. superficialis* is only rarely developed but, when present, it accompanies the *r. communicans* of the n. digitalis palmaris communis II and contributes to the *arcus palmaris superficialis.*

A. profunda antebrachii
(Comparative: 55–58/*36*; cat: 59/*18'*; dog: 60/*12*; pig: 61/*11'''*; sheep: 62/*15'*; ox: 63/*14'*; horse: 65/*16*)

Stout muscular branches arise from the first part of the median artery and often they have a common origin. In some species some of these may have already originated from the end of the brachial artery, the common interosseous or the caudal interosseous arteries. These vessels are collectively named the *a. profunda antebrachii.* They vascularize the flexors of the carpal and toe joints and run distally in these muscles.

A. radialis

(Comparative: 55–58/*37, 37'*; 67–70/*23*; cat: 59/*23*; dog: 60/*21*; pig: 61/*18*; sheep: 62/*18*; ox: 63/*16*; horse: 65/*17, 18*; 70/*23'*)

The **a. radialis** stems from the median artery. In the dog and pig the site of origin is located in the proximal-, in ruminants in the middle-, and in the cat and horse in the distal-third of the lower arm. In the horse there is first the small *a. radialis proximalis* and then, immediately proximal to the antebrachiocarpal joint, the a. radialis. Except in the cat and horse, the radial artery runs caudomedially to the median artery along the caudomedial edge of the radius. Immediately proximal to the carpus it gives rise to the *r. carpeus dorsalis,* which contributes to the formation of the *rete carpi dorsale,* and the *r. carpeus palmaris,* which goes to the palmar articular network. The radial artery then reaches the *retinaculum flexorum* in a palmar position. Along the medial insertion of the latter the radial artery crosses the carpus and divides proximally on the metacarpus into the *r. palmaris profundus* and the *r. palmaris superficialis.* In the distal third of the lower arm of the cat the radial artery takes over the function of the median artery which continues only as a slender vessel accompanying the median nerve. Immediately proximal to the antebrachiocarpal joint of the cat, the stout *r. carpeus dorsalis* of the r. radialis takes over as a direct continuation of the radial artery to the dorsal surface of the carpus. The *r. carpeus palmaris* goes, as in other domestic mammals, to the palmar articular network. The two terminal branches of the radial artery, the *r. palmaris profundus* and the *r. palmaris superficialis,* are only poorly developed. The *r. carpeus dorsalis* of the cat runs through the rete carpi dorsale and is continued directly by the *a. metacarpea dorsalis II* and its *r. perforans proximalis.* In the horse the slender *r. carpeus dorsalis* and the *r. carpeus palmaris* do not come off the radial artery but arise by an independent common stem, the *a. radialis proximalis.* Therefore the radial artery, which arises far distally, divides immediately into the deep and superficial palmar branches. In all domestic mammals the *r. palmaris profundus* is laterally directed lying proximally against the metacarpal bones and it participates in the formation of the deep palmar arch. The *r. palmaris superficialis* participates in the formation of the *arcus palmaris superficialis* but in ruminants and particularly in the horse, it may terminate in the median artery after only a short distance.

Comparative topography and nomenclature of the blood vessels of the autopodium

(Comparative: 55–58; 67–74; 105–108; 115–122; 156–159; 167–174; 190–193; 198–205)

Among the domestic mammals only in the dog are the blood vessels of the foot almost completely developed. As animals have changed their method of locomotion from one in which weight is born on the sole of the foot, to one in which it is born on the toe and on the point of the toe, there has been a concomitant regression of the pedal digits, a remodelling of both the active and passive locomotor apparatus and an associated reorganization of the vessels and nerves. Yet, despite such striking pedal specialization as has occurred, for example in the horse, the blood vessels still fit the scheme of the five-toes foot. There is thus a basis for a uniform homologous terminology. However, no allowance is made in such a scheme for the varying calibres of homologous vessels or for their functional importance in individual species.

The blood supply to the foot, the autopodium, is from the zeugopodium via cranial and caudal vessels. The participation of these vessels varies according to species because they have had to adapt to the phylogenetic differentiation of the passive and active locomotor apparatus. These vessels reach the basipodium and the proximal region of the metapodium. By means of interconnected deep and superficial branches they form the origin of the palmar, plantar, dorsal, deep and superficially located vessels of the metapodium.

Deep vessels of the metapodium

The linkage of the deep branches results in palmar and plantar, transversely-directed anastomoses which lie against the proximal extremities of the metacarpal or metatarsal bones and are known as the *arcus palmaris profundus* and *arcus plantaris profundus* respectively. From these arches arise the *aa. (vv.) metacarpeae palmares* and *aa. (vv.) metatarseae plantares* which run in a distal direction in palmar or plantar position in the groove between the neighbouring metacarpal or metatarsal bones. Depending on the number of digits present, there can be a maximum of four such vessels and they are identified as I–IV in the same direction as the toes themselves.

In the forefoot the dorsal connection of the deep vessels occurs at the carpus by means of net-like anastomoses, the dorsal articular network (*rete carpi dorsale*). From it arise the *aa. (vv.) metacarpeae dorsale I–II* which run dorsally in the groove between the neighbouring metacarpal bones. In the hind foot there is only a venous dorsal connection of the deep branches, and this is situated proximally on the metatarsus. There is no arterial arch since the transverse vessel is linked to only one deep branch and this link occurs solely in the dog in which it is known as the *a. arcuata*. The vessels continuing distal are the *aa.* and *vv. metatarseae dorsales I–IV*.

The palmar and plantar as well as the dorsal metacarpal and metatarsal vessels terminate in the superficially situated common vessels of the toe which have still to be discussed. In so doing, vessels designated by the same number are usually connected to each other. But since the terminal parts of both the palmar and plantar metacarpal and metatarsal vessels are frequently interconnected, forming on the venous side the *arcus palmaris* or *plantaris profundus distalis*, there results a common termination into the common palmar or plantar vessels of the toe. The palmar and plantar dorsal metacarpal and metatarsal vessels of the same number are connected proximally and distally between the neighbouring metacarpal or metatarsal bones by the *r. perforans proximalis* and the *r. perforans distalis*. These perforating rami are identified by the same numbers as those of the vessels they link. In the basipodium of the pelvic limb there is also a proximal *a. (v.) tarsea perforans proximalis* and a distal *a. (v.) tarsea perforans distalis* between the dorsal and plantar deep vessels. While both these are represented in the pig, the ruminants and the horse have only the distal connection and neither are present in carnivores. The deep vessels of the metapodium supply the central parts, the specialized toe muscles of that region and, in particular, the metacarpophalangeal joints.

Superficial vessels of the metapodium

The superficial branches of the vessels from the zeugopodium continue distal in the region of the metapodium as the deep branches. On the plantar (or palmar) and dorsal surfaces they are not only interconnected themselves but they are linked to the *arcus palmaris* or *plantaris superficialis* and the *arcus dorsalis superficialis*. If the superficial arch is missing, as happens particularly on the dorsal surface, then the superficial branches continue independently towards the toe. The common digital arteries arise directly from the superficial arches or the superficial branches. In the metapodium these digital arteries also run in the space between two neighbouring digits but, unlike the metacarpal and metatarsal vessels, they are superficially situated adjacent to the tendons leading to the distal phalanx. The vessels of the palmar and plantar side are the *aa. (vv.) digitales palmares* and *plantares communes I–IV* and, peripherally, the *aa. (vv.) digitales palmares* or *plantares abaxiales I* and *V*. On the dorsal side occur the *aa. (vv.) digitales dorsales communes I–IV* and peripherally the *aa. (vv.) digitales dorsales abaxiales I* and *V*. The termination of the metacarpal and metatarsal vessels in the common digital vessels on the distal part of the metapodium has already been described.

The superficial vessels of the metapodium vascularize the peripheral parts, including the metacarpal and metatarsal pads.

Vessels of the acropodium

Between the metacarpo- and metatarso-phalangeal joints and the middle of the proximal phalanx, each of the palmar or plantar and each dorsal common digital artery and vein divides into two vessels, the *aa. (vv.) digitales propriae*. The vessels supply and drain the two neighbouring toes. In the typical case, therefore, each toe receives for each quadrant one arterial and one venous blood vessel. The previously-mentioned *aa. (vv.) digitales abaxiales* continue peripherally on the first and fifth toes. For the complete identification of each of these vessels the names *aa.* and *vv. digitales propriae* are supplemented by the terms palmar, plantar or dorsal and the numerical suffices I (prima), II (secunda), III (tertia), IV (quarta), V (quinta). Consideration is also given to the concepts axial and abaxial to indicate whether the toe edges are turned towards or away from the foot axis. The abaxial vessels of the first and fifth toes which do not originate from the common digital vessels are not designated "propriae". The vessels of the third toe are listed below as an example:

a. (v.) digitalis palmaris/plantaris propria III abaxilis
a. (v.) digitalis palmaris/plantaris propria III axialis
a. (v.) digitalis dorsalis propria III abaxialis
a. (v.) digitalis dorsalis propria III axialis

Since in the horse only the third toe is developed, the terms axial and abaxial are replaced by lateral and medial. It is also unnecessary to use the designation "propria III" in this species.

As the common digital vessels divide into the proper ones, those having the same numbers are linked through the interdigital space by the *aa. (vv.) interdigitales I, II, III* and *IV*. These interdigital vessels may also be situated on the proximal part of the proper digital vessels. At about the middle of each phalanx each of the palmar or plantar proper digital vessels give off branches to the palmar or plantar surfaces respectively, these branches being the *r. palmaris* or *plantaris phalangis proximalis, mediae* and *distalis* as well as the dorsally directed branches known as the *r. dorsalis phalangis proximalis, mediae* and *distalis*. The origin of these branches can be located on either the common digital or the interdigital vessels in the region of the proximal phalanx. The rr. palmares or plantares of the same toe anastomose in the region of each phalanx with one another and the rr. dorsales are linked to the dorsal proper digital vessels which have the same numerical designation. Furthermore, each palmar and plantar proper digital vessel gives off at varying levels a **r. tori digitalis** vascularizing the appropriate pad (*torus digitalis*). They anastomose within the pads. From this branch, or sometimes from the r. dorsalis phalangis mediae, arises a vessel which goes to the coronary cushion, the *a. (v.) coronalis*. The terminal branches of the palmar and plantar proper vessels of each toe unite in a channel on the distal phalanx and form the *arcus terminalis*. Furthermore, the proper digital vessels also give off branches to all the central and peripheral parts of the toes and these are freely linked in anastomoses, especially in the hoofs or claws.

Arteries of the forefoot of carnivores

Palmar arteries
(cat: 59/*21'*, 22, *23'*; dog: 55; 60/*17–20*, 23–37; 67; 92)

In carnivores the **arcus palmaris profundus** is formed by the *r. palmaris profundus* of the radial artery and the *r. profundus* of the palmar branch of the caudal interosseous artery. In the cat these rami are only slender and the main tributary to this arch is from the dorsal side, via the *r. perforans proximalis II*. The deep palmar arch gives rise to the *aa. metacarpeae palmares I–IV* which are especially prominent in the cat. The *rr. perforantes proximales* connect the palmar with the dorsal metacarpal arteries. The palmar and dorsal metacarpal arteries are linked by the *rr. perforantes proximales* of which the cat has only one, the *r. perforans proximalis II*. In the dog these arteries are also linked by the *rr. perforantes distales*, while in the cat, where there is only a rudimentary dorsal metacarpal artery, the distal perforating ramus connects with the dorsal common digital artery instead. Distal to the metacarpus the palmar metacarpal artery unites with that palmar common digital artery which has the same number.

The **arcus palmaris superficialis** is formed by the r. palmaris superficialis of the radial artery and by the r. superficialis of the palmar ramus of the caudal interosseous artery. The median artery, which terminates in the arch, also contributes to its blood supply. In the cat the tributaries to this superficial arch are slender and sometimes even the arch itself may be lacking. The superficial palmar arch gives rise to the *aa. digitales palmares communes I–IV* and the *a. digitalis palmaris V abaxialis* and in the cat also to the *a. digitalis palmaris I abaxialis*. If this arch is absent, as is sometimes the case in cats, then the superficial palmar ramus of the radial artery is continued in the second palmar common digital artery, the median artery is continued in the third, and the r. superficialis of the palmar ramus of the caudal interosseous artery in the fourth palmar common digital artery and in the palmar abaxial artery of the fifth toe. In such cases the first toe receives its arterial supply from the deep arteries only. All the *aa. interdigitales* are fully developed in carnivores and they form the link between the palmar and dorsal common digital arteries of the same number in the region where the latter divide. The *aa. digitales palmares* are all present and arise from the point of division of the *aa. digitales palmares communes*, which in the cat acquire a substantial calibre only after they receive the *aa. metacarpeae palmares*. This, then, is the main blood supply from the dorsal side to the deep palmar arteries and from these via the terminal sections of the superficial arteries to the proper digital arteries.

Dorsal arteries
(cat: 59/*17"*, *19*, *23"*; dog: 55; 60/*6–9*, *22*; 71; 92)

The **rete carpi dorsale** is formed by the three dorsal carpal rami of the radial artery, of the interosseous ramus of the caudal interosseous artery and of the ulnar artery. This network is the source of the *aa. metacarpeae dorsales I–IV* which, in the cat, are only rudimentary and do not terminate in the aa. digitales dorsales communes. On the other hand, the first part of the *a. metacarpea dorsalis II* is a stout vessel in the cat and it represents the immediate continuation of the large r. carpeus dorsalis of the radial artery which traverses the dorsal carpal network. The deep palmar arch is supplied via the *r. perforans proximalis II*. As already mentioned, the remaining rr. perforantes proximales are absent in the cat but the distal perforating rami are represented in both the dog and the cat. Since in the cat the dorsal metacarpal arteries terminate more proximally, the *rr. perforantes distales* form the direct connection with the *aa. digitales dorsales communes*. In the dog the dorsal metacarpal artery unites in the distal part of the metacarpus with the dorsal common digital artery which has the same numerical designation.

Only the cat has an **arcus dorsalis superficialis**. This is formed by the *a. antebrachialis superficialis cranialis* and the *r. dorsalis* of the ulnar artery. Arising from this arch are the *aa. digitales communes I–IV* and the *a. digitalis dorsalis V abaxialis*. In the dog the *a. digitalis dorsalis communis I* arises from the medial branch and the *aa. digitales dorsales communes II–IV* from the lateral branch of the *a. antebrachialis superficialis cranialis*. The *a. digitalis dorsalis V abaxialis* arises from the r. dorsalis of the ulnar artery. In the dog the dorsal common digital arteries divide, after receiving the dorsal metacarpal arteries, into the *aa. digitales dorsales propriae*.

Arteries of the forefoot of the pig

Palmar arteries
(pig: 56; 61/*17"*, *18"*, *18"'*; 68)

In the pig the **arcus palmaris profundus** is formed by the *r. palmaris profundus* of the radial artery and by the *r. profundus* of the palmar ramus of the caudal interosseous artery. The deep palmar arch gives rise to the *aa. metacarpeae palmares II–IV*. The aa. metacarpeae palmares are linked to the aa. metacarpeae dorsales by the *rr. perforantes proximales* and the *r. perforans distalis III*, and occasionally also by the *rr. perforantes distales II and IV*. The palmar metacarpal arteries II and IV do not terminate in the palmar common digital arteries of corresponding number, because the latter do not arise until more distally on the metapodium. On the contrary, these two palmar metacarpal arteries unite with the *a. metacarpea palmaris III* shortly before it terminates in the *a. digitalis palmaris communis III*. The *arcus palmaris superficialis* is situated far distally on the metacarpus and it is formed by the r. superficialis of the radial artery and the r. superficialis of the palmar ramus of the causal interosseous artery. The stout median artery terminates in this arch and thus contributes to its supply of blood. The superficial palmar arch gives rise to the *aa. digitales palmares communes II–IV* which arise closely one after the other. The *aa. digitales palmares propriae* are developed on all the toes from the second to the fifth. The *a. digitalis palmaris propria II abaxialis* and, in the region of the toe, the *a. digitalis palmaris V abaxialis* are each supplied by the corresponding *rr. palmares phalangis proximalis*. The *a. interdigitalis III* links the common palmar and dorsal digital arteries of the same number, while the *aa. interdigitales II and IV* connect the appropriate abaxial proper digital arteries of the third and fourth toes.

96 Arteries

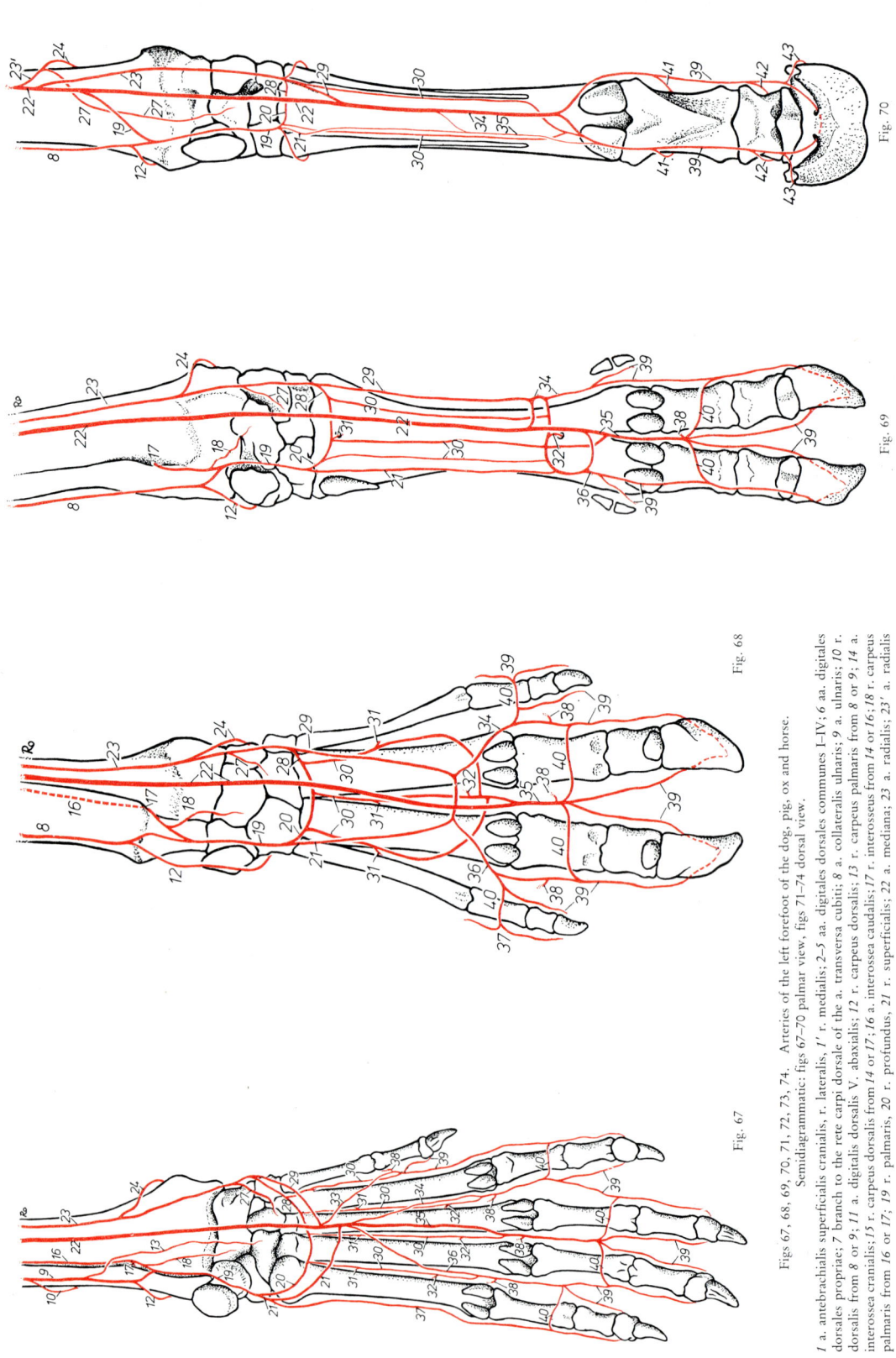

Figs 67, 68, 69, 70, 71, 72, 73, 74. Arteries of the left forefoot of the dog, pig, ox and horse. Semidiagrammatic: figs 67–70 palmar view, figs 71–74 dorsal view.

1 a. antebrachialis superficialis cranialis, r. lateralis; *1'* r. medialis; *2–5* aa. digitales dorsales communes I–IV; *6* aa. digitales dorsales propriae; *7* branch to the rete carpi dorsale of the a. transversa cubiti; *8* a. collateralis ulnaris; *9* a. ulnaris; *10* r. dorsalis from *8* or *9*; *11* a. digitalis dorsalis V. abaxialis; *12* r. carpeus dorsalis; *13* r. carpeus palmaris from *8* or *9*; *14* a. interossea cranialis; *15* r. carpeus dorsalis from *14* or *17*; *16* a. interossea caudalis; *17* r. interosseus from *14* or *16*; *18* r. carpeus palmaris from *16* or *17*; *19* r. palmaris, *20* r. profundus, *21* r. superficialis; *22* a. mediana; *23* r. radialis; *23'* a. radialis

Arteries of the forefoot 97

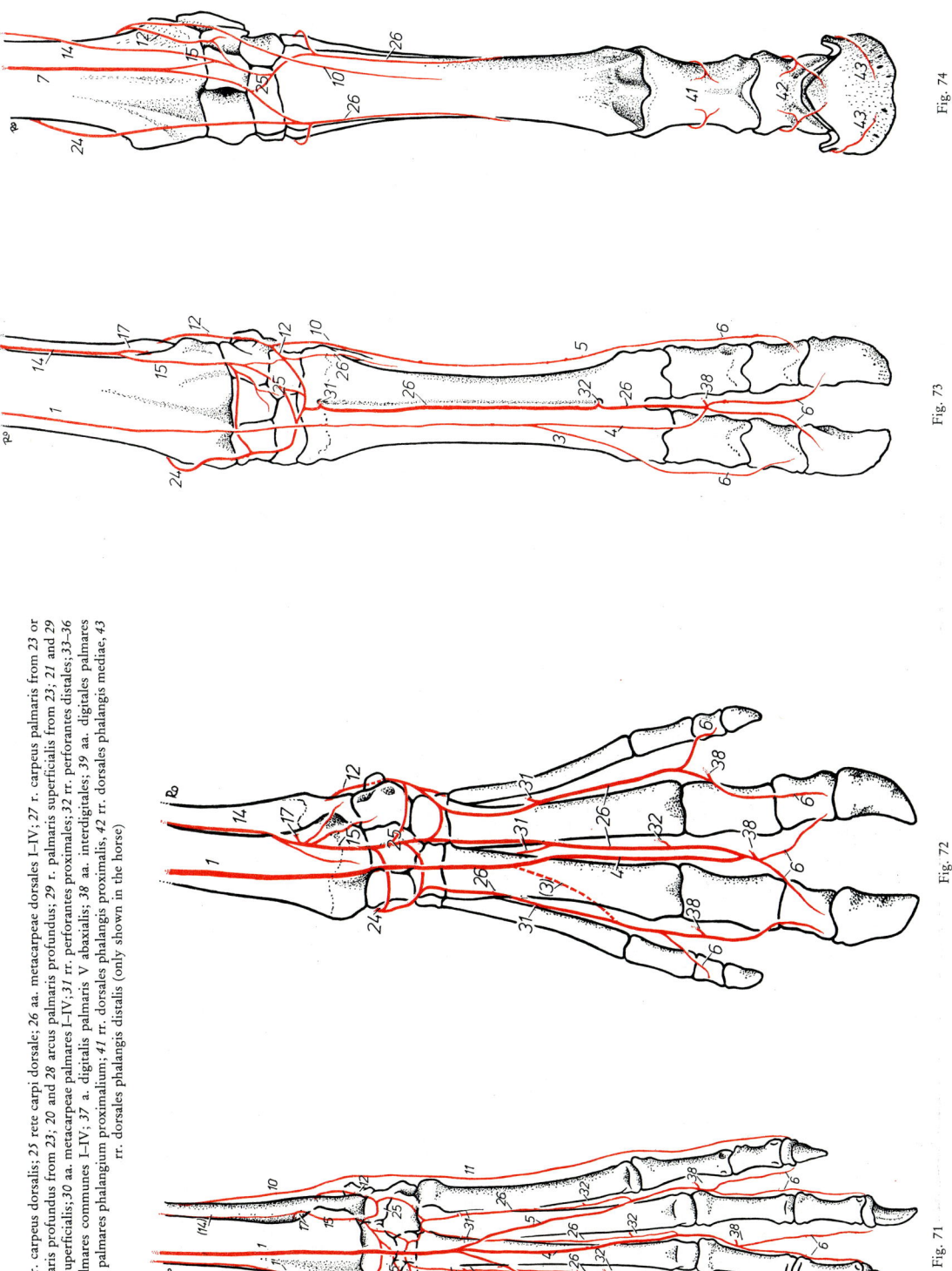

proximalis; 24 r. carpeus dorsalis; 25 rete carpi dorsale; 26 aa. metacarpeae dorsales I–IV; 27 r. carpeus palmaris from 23 or 23'; 28 r. palmaris profundus from 23; 20 and 28 arcus palmaris profundus; 29 r. palmaris superficialis from 23; 21 and 29 arcus palmaris superficialis; 30 aa. metacarpeae palmares I–IV; 31 rr. perforantes proximales; 32 rr. perforantes distales; 33–36 aa. digitales palmares communes I–IV; 37 a. digitalis palmaris V abaxialis; 38 aa. interdigitales; 39 aa. digitales palmares propriae; 40 rr. palmares phalangium proximalium; 41 rr. dorsales phalangis proximalis; 42 rr. dorsales phalangis mediae, 43 rr. dorsales phalangis distalis (only shown in the horse)

Fig. 71

Fig. 72

Fig. 73

Fig. 74

Dorsal arteries

(pig: 56; 61/*15, 18', 19*; 72)

The **rete carpi dorsale** is formed by the *r. carpeus dorsalis* of the cranial interosseous or the interosseous ramus of the caudal interosseous artery and by the dorsal carpal ramus of the collateral ulnar artery. From this network arise the *aa. metacarpeae dorsales II–IV*. The second and fourth of these are at first relatively slim but after receiving their proximal perforating ramus they become equal in size to the third. But in addition the third dorsal metacarpal artery invariably also receives a *r. perforans distalis III*. In the region of the metacarpophalangeal joints, the dorsal metacarpal artery III is linked to the thin *a. digitalis dorsalis communis III* which arises from the a. antebrachialis superficialis cranialis. However, this dorsal common digital artery III may be missing altogether. In such cases the equally delicate *a. digitalis dorsalis communis II* forms the continuation of the a. antebrachialis superficialis cranialis and it anastomoses with the *a. metacarpea dorsalis II*. The main supply vessels for the *aa. digitales dorsales propriae* are the dorsal metacarpal arteries and, in the case of the middle toes, the *aa. interdigitales* also contribute. The abaxial proper digital arteries are absent in the two smaller toes.

Arteries of the forefoot of ruminants

Palmar arteries

(sheep: 62/*16, 17, 18", 18''', 19*; ox: 57; 63/*14, 14", 15, 15', 16", 16''', 17, 18, 18'*; 64/*11–15*; 69)

In ruminants the **arcus palmaris profundus** is formed by the *r. palmaris profundus* of the radial artery and by the *r. profundus* of the palmar ramus of the interosseous ramus of the cranial interosseous artery. From the deep palmar arch arise the *aa. metacarpeae palmares II–IV* which form an arch-like anastomosis with one another in the distal part of the metacarpus. The a. metacarpea palmaris III is linked with the a. metacarpea dorsalis III by two vessels: firstly, in the region of the deep palmar arch by the *r. perforans proximalis III* which traverses the *can. metacarpi proximalis* and secondly, more distally in the region of the arch-like anastomosis through the distal metacarpal canal by the *r. perforans distalis III*. The arch-like anastomosis of the palmar metacarpal arteries is connected medially and laterally with the *aa. digitales palmares communes II* and *IV* and also, as a direct continuation of the *a. metacarpea palmaris III*, with the *a. digitalis palmaris communis III*.

In ruminants the **arcus palmaris superficialis** is formed by the *r. palmaris superficialis* of the radial artery and by the *r. superficialis* of the palmar ramus which arises from the interosseous ramus of the cranial interosseous artery. The median artery is the main vessel contributing to the arch and in the ox its junction with the medial part of the arch is always more proximal than with the lateral. The superficial palmar arch gives rise to the *aa. digitales palmares communes II–IV*. At their source the second and fourth of these vessels receive blood from the arch-like connections with the palmar metacarpal arteries, while the third palmar common digital artery, being the thickest vessel, forms the continuation of the median artery. The *a. interdigitalis III* connects the common palmar and dorsal digital arteries of the same numbers in the region of their division into the proper digital arteries. On the third and fourth toes, the *aa. digitales palmares propriae* are present on the axial and abaxial sides. On the second and fifth toes (dew claws), the axial vessel is always present and it sometimes gives rise to the appropriate abaxial vessel.

Dorsal arteries

(sheep: 62/*18'*; ox: 57; 63/*16'*; 64/*8, 8'*; 73)

The **rete carpi dorsale** is formed by the dorsal carpal rami of the radial, the cranial interosseous and the collateral ulnar arteries. This network gives rise, not only to the rudimentary *a. metacarpea dorsalis IV*, but also to the *a. metacarpea dorsalis III*. The latter is the only substantial vessel connected, as already described, with the palmar metacarpal arteries via the r. perforans proximalis III and the r. perforans distalis III. The *a. metacarpea dorsalis III* unites with the *a. digitalis dorsalis communis III* in the region of their terminal branches. In the lower third of the metacarpus the slender *a. antebrachialis superficialis cranialis* gives rise to the equally delicate *aa. digitales dorsales communes II* and *III* and from the *r. dorsalis* of the collateral ulnar artery originates the very thin *a. digitalis dorsalis communis IV*. As the dorsal common digital artery III subdivides, it anastomoses with both the dorsal metacarpal III and the interdigital III arteries. The *aa. digitales dorsales propriae* are developed only in the large third and fourth toes and of these arteries the axial ones receive the greatest supply of blood via the interdigital III artery.

Arteries of the forefoot of the horse

Palmar arteries
(horse: 58; 65/*15, 19–26*; 66/*12–16*; 70)

In the horse the **arcus palmaris profundus** is formed by the *r. palmaris profundus* of the radial artery and by the *r. profundus* of the palmar ramus which arises from the median artery. The deep palmar arch gives rise to the *aa. metacarpeae palmares II* and *III* which unite proximal to the fetlock joint and then terminate together by joining the lateral digital artery. *Rr. perforantes proximales* and *distales* can be present. Running peripherally round the heads of both medial and lateral splint bones are the two connecting branches, *rr. anastomotici*, to the dorsal metacarpal artery of the same number.

The superficial ramus of the radial artery terminates in the median artery on the proximal part of the metacarpus. The very slender *r. superficialis* of the palmar ramus, which latter stems from the median artery in the horse, only rarely connects with the median artery to form the *arcus palmaris superficialis*. If present this arch is located alongside the communicating ramus of the palmar nerves. It is more common for this superficial ramus to continue directly into the slender *a. digitalis palmaris communis III*. Whether there is or is not a superficial palmar arch, the median artery continues as the stout *a. digitalis palmaris communis II*. The latter gives off the *a. digitalis palmaris (propria III) medialis* and the main tributary to the *a. digitalis palmaris (propria III) lateralis*. This main tributary receives the united *aa. metacarpeae palmares II* and *III* and the *a. digitalis palmaris communis III*.

Dorsal arteries
(horse: 58; 65/*23*; 66/*5', 8–12, 16*; 74)

The **rete carpi dorsale** is formed by the r. carpeus dorsalis of the proximal radial artery, by the distally directed branch of the transverse cubital artery, the dorsal carpal rami of the cranial interosseous and by the collateral ulnar arteries. From this network arise the *aa. metacarpeae dorsales II* and *III* which end at the level of the heads of the splint bones. Here they anastomose with the palmar metacarpal arteries by means of the rr. anastomotici, which have already been described, or sometimes with the rr. perforantes as well. Only the slender r. dorsalis of the collateral ulnar artery runs dorsally to the metacarpus where it is present as a superficial vessel accompanying the dorsal branch of the dorsal ulnar nerve. The dorsal part of the toe is supplied only by the *rr. dorsales phalangis proximalis, mediae* and *distalis* of the two palmar proper digital arteries.

Arteries of the head and neck

A. carotis communis
(Comparative: 51–54/*5*; 77–82/*1*; 85–88/*27*; cat: 90/*13*; 91/*6*; dog: 75/*12*; pig: 96/*16*; 177/*8*; 183/*2*; sheep: 99/*7*; ox: 102, 155/*16*; horse: 50/*18*; 83/*1*; 103/*20*)

The **aa. carotides communes** arise from the truncus bicaroticus ventral to the trachea at the level of the 7th cervical vertebra. In carnivores they usually have a separate origin at the level of the 2nd rib. In the caudal part of the neck the left common carotid artery at first runs along the lateral aspect of the oesophagus. In its more cranial course it follows the oesophagus ventral to the longissimus colli muscle. The right common carotid artery, on the other hand, crosses the trachea to reach the groove between the trachea and the long muscle of the neck. Each of the common carotid arteries is related dorsally to the cervical part of the vagus and sympathetic nerves and ventrally to the recurrent laryngeal nerve and the truncus trachealis. In carnivores, especially cats, in pigs and ruminants, but rarely in horses, the internal jugular veins also lie ventral to the common carotid. In the cranial third of the neck these vessels and nerves are covered by the lateral omohyoideus muscle, except in carnivores in which this muscle is absent. The carotids supply dorsally- or ventrally-directed vessels to the trachea, the left side of the oesophagus, the cranial and medial deep cervical lymph nodes and the ventral muscles of the neck. In ruminants the **rr. sternocleidomastoidei** branch directly from the common carotid artery and, with certain modifications in the different species, it also gives off the *a. thyreoidea caudalis* and in all domestic mammals (except the pig on the left side) the *a. thyreoidea cranialis*. Subsequent branches of each common carotid are, in the pig and ruminants the *a. laryngea cranialis*, in ruminants alone the *a. pharyngea ascendens* and in the small ruminants the *a. palatina ascendens*, which latter will be described with the ascending palatine artery of the other domestic mammals as a branch of the lingual artery. Ventral to the wings of the atlas, the common carotid artery divides into the *a. carotis interna* and *a. carotis externa*.

A. thyreoidea caudalis
(dog: 75/9)

In carnivores and the pig the **a. thyreoid caudalis** arises in the same region as the carotids. In carnivores there is often a common stem for the left and right vessel from the brachiocephalic trunk whereas in the pig the right caudal thyroid artery arises from the thyrocervical trunk in common with the *a. cervicalis superficialis*. In ruminants and the horse its origin lies at the level of the caudal pole of the thyroid gland. In all the domestic mammals the caudal thyroid artery is smaller than the cranial artery and it may be absent on one or even both sides. The caudal thyroid artery, or its terminal branches, reach the caudal pole of the thyroid gland which they either enter directly or anastomose with branches of the cranial thyroid artery.

A. thyreoidea cranialis
(dog: 75/1; pig: 183/3; horse: 76/a; 83/5)

The **a. thyreoidea cranialis** arises at the level of the cranial pole of the thyroid gland. Only in carnivores does it give off the *r. sternocleidomastoideus* to the appropriate muscles. It then gives off the following branches although the sequence varies in the different species. The *r. pharyngeus* is cranially

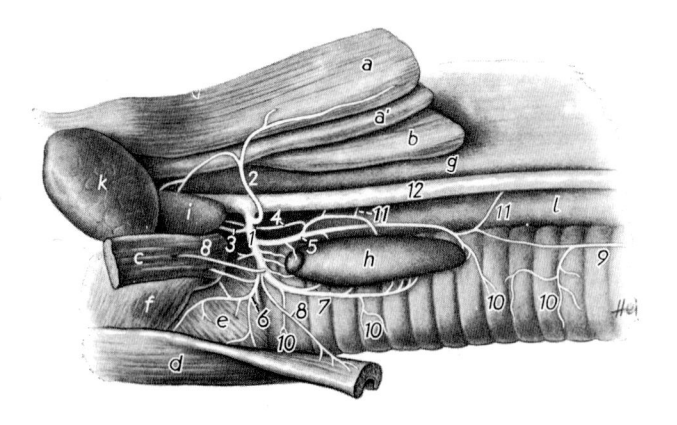

Fig. 75. Arteries of the larynx, trachea and thyroid gland of a dog. Left lateral view.
(After Loeffler, 1955, Diss., Hanover.)

a m. sternomastoideus; *a'* m. cleidomastoideus; *b* m. sternooccipitalis; *c* m. sternothyreoideus; *d* m. sternohyoideus; *e* m. cricothyreoideus; *f* m. thyreohyoideus; *g* m. longus capitis; *h* gl. thyreoidea; *i* ln. retropharyngeus medialis; *k* gl. mandibularis; *l* oesophagus

1 a. thyreoidea cranialis, *5* r. dorsalis, *7* r. ventralis; *2* r. sternocleidomastoideus; *3* r. laryngeus caudalis; *4* r. pharyngeus; *6* r. cricothyreoideus; *8* rr. musculares; *9* a. thyreoidea caudalis; *10* rr. tracheales; *11* rr. oesophagei; *12* a. carotis communis

directed and supplies the pharyngeal wall in the region of the caudal constrictors of the pharynx. The *r. cricothyreoideus*, which is absent in the goat, supplies the muscle of that name and the *r. laryngeus caudalis* enters the larynx dorsolaterally accompanied by the caudal laryngeal nerve. In the horse the cranial thyroid artery also gives off the *a. pharyngea ascendens* and the *a. laryngea cranialis*.

A. laryngea cranialis

(Comparative: 77–80/9; pig: 96/*16'*; 183/7; horse: 76/*c*; 83/7)

In the pig and ruminants the **a. laryngea cranialis** arises directly from the common carotid artery near the cranial part of the larynx. In the horse it originates from the cranial thyroid artery and in carnivores from the external carotid artery. In all the domestic mammals it gives off a *r. pharyngeus* and then continues as the *r. laryngeus* to the larynx. Except in the horse this branch then passes through the fiss. thyroidea in company with the cranial laryngeal nerve. In the horse it passes ventrolaterally through the cricothyroid muscle on the medial surface of the lam. thyroidea. It divides into a dorsal and a ventral branch on the ventriculus laryngis lateralis at the level of the vocalis muscle.

A. pharyngea ascendens

(Comparative: 77–80/7; horse: 76/*b*; 83/7')

The **a. pharyngea ascendens** originates as a branch of the common carotid artery in ruminants; in the horse it originates from the cranial thyroid artery and in carnivores it stems directly from the external carotid artery. In the pig it arises from the lingual artery. The ascending pharyngeal artery is

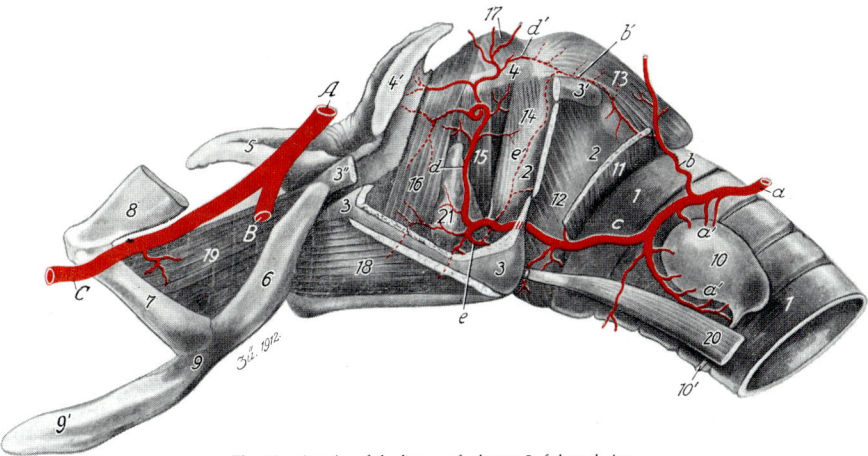

Fig. 76. Arteries of the larynx of a horse. Left lateral view.
(After Zietzschmann, 1943.)

A a. linguofacialis; *B* a. facialis; *C* a. lingualis

a a. thyreoidea cranialis; *a* rr. thyreoidei; *b* a. pharyngea ascendens; *b'* r. laryngeus caudalis; *c* a. laryngea cranialis lying on the larynx and continuing as the r. laryngeus; *d* dorsal, *e* ventral branches, *d'*, *e'* anastomoses with the r. laryngeus caudalis

1 trachea; *2* cartilago cricoidea; *3*, *3'*, *3"* cartilago thyreoidea; *4* cartilago arytaenoidea, *4'* proc. corniculatus; *5* epiglottis; *6*, *7*, *8*, *9*, *9'* apparatus hyoideus; *10* gl. thyreoidea, lobus sinister, *10'* isthmus fibrosus; *11* m. cricopharyngeus; *12* m. cricothyreoideus; *13* m. cricoarytaenoideus dorsalis; *14* m. cricoaryteanoideus lateralis; *15* m. vocalis; *16* m. ventricularis; *17* m. arytaenoideus transversus; *18* m. thyreohyoideus; *19* m. ceratohyoideus; *20* m. sternothyreoideus; *21* ventriculus laryngis lateralis

accompanied by the *rr. pharyngei* as it proceeds dorsally and laterally along the wall of the pharynx in the region of the medial constrictors of the pharynx. Except in the small ruminants, it gives off the *rr. palatini*. Finally, in the ox the *rr. tonsillares* are given off.

A. carotis interna

(Comparative: 77–82/2; ox: 87/28; horse: 83/8; 84/*a*; 88/28)

At the level of the larynx the common carotid artery gives off a more slender branch vessel, the **a. carotis interna**. In its course towards the skull the internal carotid artery of the horse is situated caudal and dorsal to the guttural pouch. To reach the cranial cavity in the cat the artery passes through the carotid canal and in the dog and pig through the carotid foramen. In the horse it traverses the sinus petrosus ventralis and then the carotid incisure. It is a relatively small vessel in the horse and carnivores and a stout one in the pig. In ruminants the situation is different in that prenatally the internal carotid artery goes through the for. jugulare into the cranial cavity but during the first months of extrauterine life the part outside the cranium degenerates and becomes merely a connective tissue strand. In the adult cat too, the internal carotid artery regresses. In pigs, ruminants, and usually also cats, the internal carotid gives off the *a. occipitalis* immediately after its origin. In the pig the occipital artery is followed by the *a. condylaris*. The course and distribution of the internal carotid artery within the cranium are described in conjunction with the blood supply to the brain (see. vol. IV).

A. occipitalis
(Comparative: 77–82/3; pig: 183/8; sheep: 184/3; ox: 87/29; horse: 83/9; 88/29)

The **a. occipitalis** arises in pigs, ruminants and usually in cats, from the region of origin of the internal carotid artery. In the dog and horse it arises close to the origin of the external carotid artery. Dorsally directed, it connects with the *r. anastomoticus cum a. occipitali* of the vertebral artery and, by means of its *r. occipitalis*, it ramifies in the musculature of the occipital region. In cattle the occipital artery gives off first the a. palatina ascendens (see. p. 103) and then the *a. stylomastoidea profunda* which passes through the stylomastoid foramen in the petrous temporal bone to the middle ear. In all ruminants it gives off the *a. meningea media*, although in the sheep this may originate from the condylar artery, whereas in all other domestic mammals it originates from the maxillary artery. Subsequently the occipital artery gives off the a. condylaris in carnivores, ruminants and the horse. From the occipital ramus arises the *a. meningea caudalis;* this latter vessel is absent in the cat and ox but after giving off muscular branches it passes through the temporal meatus in the dog, pig and horse and through openings in the occipital bone near the pars mastoidea in the small ruminants. It supplies the meninges. In the dog the caudal meningeal artery also gives rise to the *a. tympanica caudalis*.

A. condylaris
(Comparative: 77–82/4; horse: 83/11)

In carnivores, ruminants and horses the **a. condylaris** stems from the occipital artery; in the pig it arises from the internal carotid. The condylar artery, a stout vessel in ruminants, goes through the fossa condylaris ventralis and enters the cranial cavity through the canal for the hypoglossal nerve. In the pig, before entering the cranium it gives off the a. stylomastoidea which passes through the stylomastoid foramen to the middle ear.

A. carotis externa
(Comparative: 77–82/10; pig: 183/13; ox: 87/30; horse: 83/14; 88/30)

The **a. carotis externa** is the largest branch of the common carotid. It first bends in a dorsally directed curve covered laterally by the parotid gland, which it perforates obliquely in the sheep, and continues along the cervical border of the ramus of the mandible to the retromandibular fossa. In the pig it passes medially over the processus jugularis. It crosses laterally the stylohyoid and in the horse it also passes across the lateral bay of the guttural pouch. It then curves rostrally and continues as the maxillary artery. Along its course the external carotid gives off, immediately after its origin, the occipital artery in carnivores and horses. In carnivores the cranial laryngeal and ascending pharyngeal arteries are then given off. In carnivores, small ruminants and the pig the external carotid artery then sends off rostrally from the convexity of its dorsally directed arch, the *a. lingualis* and in carnivores and pigs shortly thereafter the *a. facialis*. In the ox and horse these two arteries arise as a common trunk, the *truncus linguofacialis* which, in the horse, also gives rise to the *a. palatina ascendens*. In all domestic mammals the external carotid artery gives rise to the *a. auricularis caudalis* from the caudal wall of its dorsally directed part. In carnivores the external carotid gives off the *a. parotidea* as an independent vessel and in the pig it provides several *rr. parotidei* which in this species form the main supply to the parotid gland. In the ox and horse there is a stout r. massetericus to the masseter muscles and in all domestic mammals the external carotid sends out, dorsally from its rostral curve, the *a. temporalis superficialis*.

A. lingualis
(Comparative: 77–82/*11*; pig: 183/*14*; sheep: 184/*63*; horse: 83/*18*)

In carnivores, small ruminants and the pig, the **a. lingualis** arises caudal to the ramus of the mandible from the external carotid artery whereas in the ox and horse it originates from the *truncus linguofacialis* medial to the pterygoideus medialis muscle. At first it accompanies the stylohyoid bone ventrally and, running medial to the hypoglossus muscle, it reaches the tongue. Here it becomes the *a. profunda linguae* which takes a more or less meandering course towards the tip of the tongue between the hypoglossus and genioglossus muscles. In so doing it gives off at short intervals the *rr. dorsales linguae* which form arborizations to the dorsum of the tongue. In the pig and ox the right and left deep lingual arteries anastomose in the tip of the tongue. Along its course to the tongue, the lingual artery gives off, only in ruminants, the *rr. glandulares* and these supply mainly the mandibular gland. In all the domestic mammals there next arises the *rr. perihyoidei;* these may be situated rostral, caudal or both rostral and caudal to the basihyoid and they unite in an arch. They provide branches to the epiglottis and the base of the tongue. The *a. palatina ascendens* arises from the lingual artery in carnivores before, and in the pig after, the perihyoid rami have been given off. In the pig there is also the ascending pharangeal artery, which has already been described. Shortly before entry into the tongue, at the transition into the deep lingual artery, the a. lingualis gives rise to the *a. sublingualis* in ruminants and pigs.

A. sublingualis
(Comparative: 77–82/*13*; sheep: 184/*65*; horse: 83/*19*)

In ruminants and the pig the **a. sublingualis** arises from the lingual artery while in the dog and the horse it stems from the submental artery. In the pig the latter vessels also give off an additional sublingual branch. The sublingual artery in the cat is replaced by several vessels from the submental artery. When it originates from the submental artery, the sublingual artery first perforates the mylohyoideus muscle and then, like its counterpart which originated from the lingual artery, it continues along the dorsal border of the geniohyoideus muscle to the point of the chin. It terminates superficially in the sublingual region of the floor of the mouth, where it also supplies the frenulum linguae, having given off branches to the neighbouring muscles and the sublingual glands.

A. palatina ascendens
(Comparative: 77–82/*8*; horse: 83/*17*)

The **a. palatina ascendens** arises in carnivores and pigs from the lingual artery. In small ruminants it springs from the common carotid, in the ox from the occipital artery and in the horse from the linguofacial trunk. It takes a course medial to the stylohyoid across the lateral wall of the pharynx to the soft palate and its muscles.

A. facialis
(Comparative: 77–82/*16*; pig: 182/*11*; horse: 83/*20*)

In carnivores and the pig the **a. facialis** stems from the external carotid artery and in the ox and the horse it arises from the truncus linguofacialis. There is no facial artery in small ruminants. Its initial course is along the medial aspect of the ventral border of the mandible to the inc. vasorum or the corresponding site. Here it turns onto the lateral surface of the lower jaw. In the pig it then gives off an additional branch to the face which, after a short course, ends in the masseter muscles and the skin of the mandibular space. In this animal the facial artery terminates soon after giving rise to this branch. In carnivores, ruminants and horses the facial artery follows the cranial border of the masseter muscle dorsad to an area caudal to the infraorbital foramen.

While in the mandibular space the facial artery gives off branches to the digastricus, pterygoideus and masseter muscles. In the pig and horse there is also a branch to the pharynx and in all species except the horse a *r. glandularis* to the mandibular gland. In the pig this glandular ramus also supplies the parotid

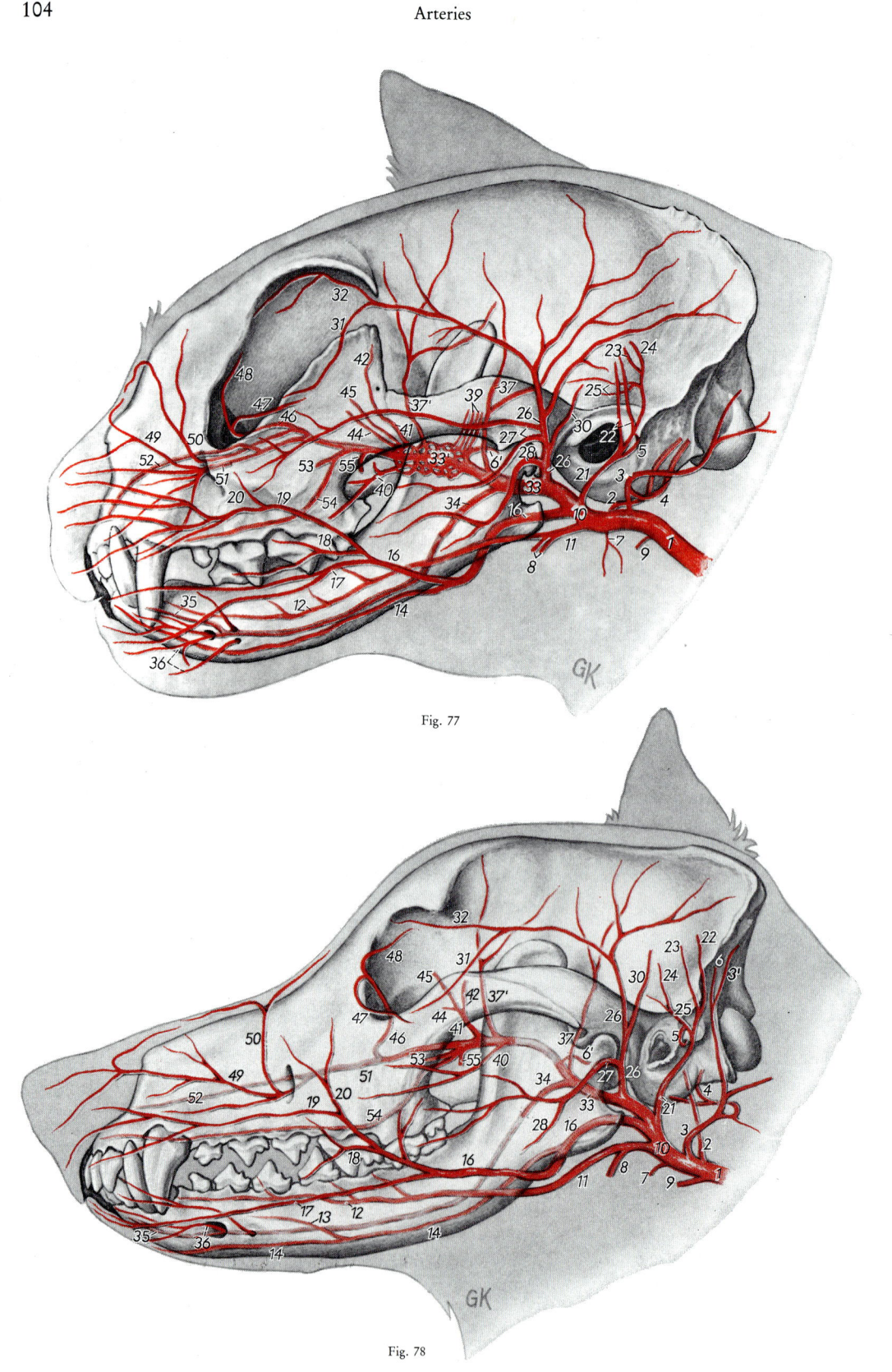

Arteries

Fig. 77

Fig. 78

Arteries of the head 105

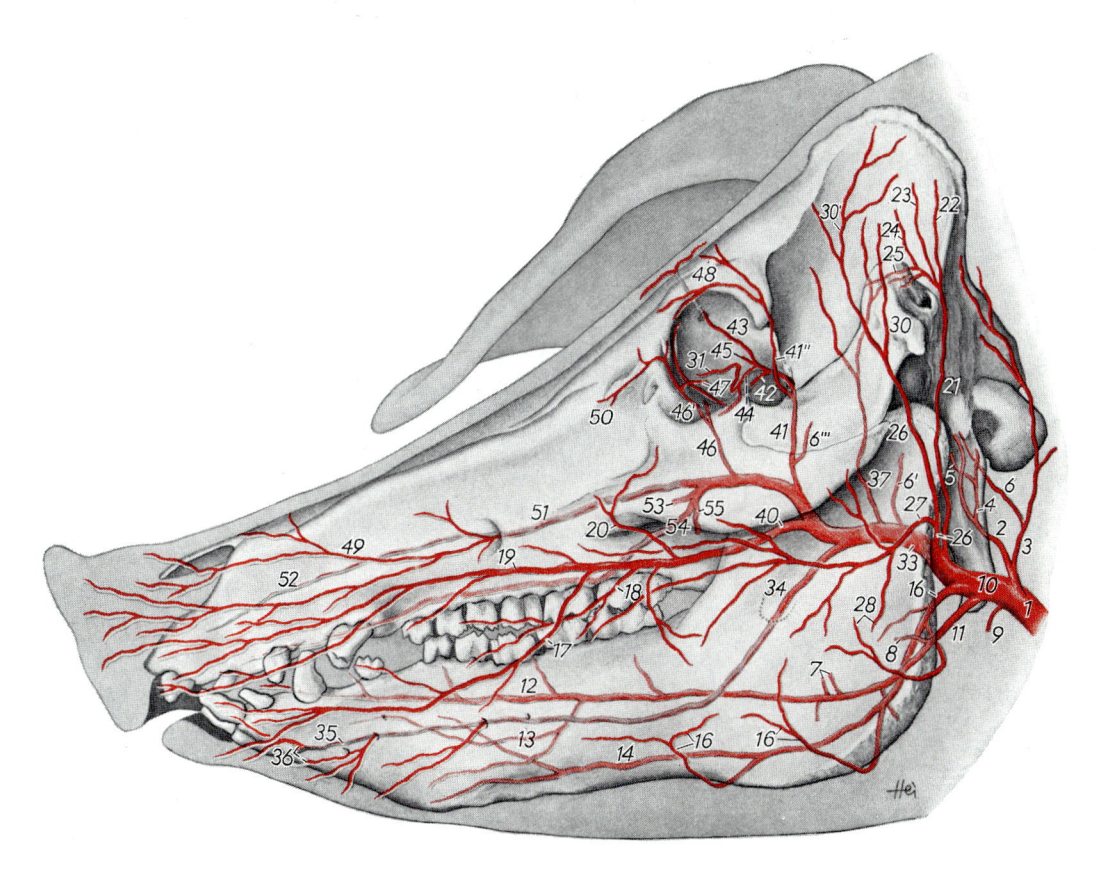

Fig. 79

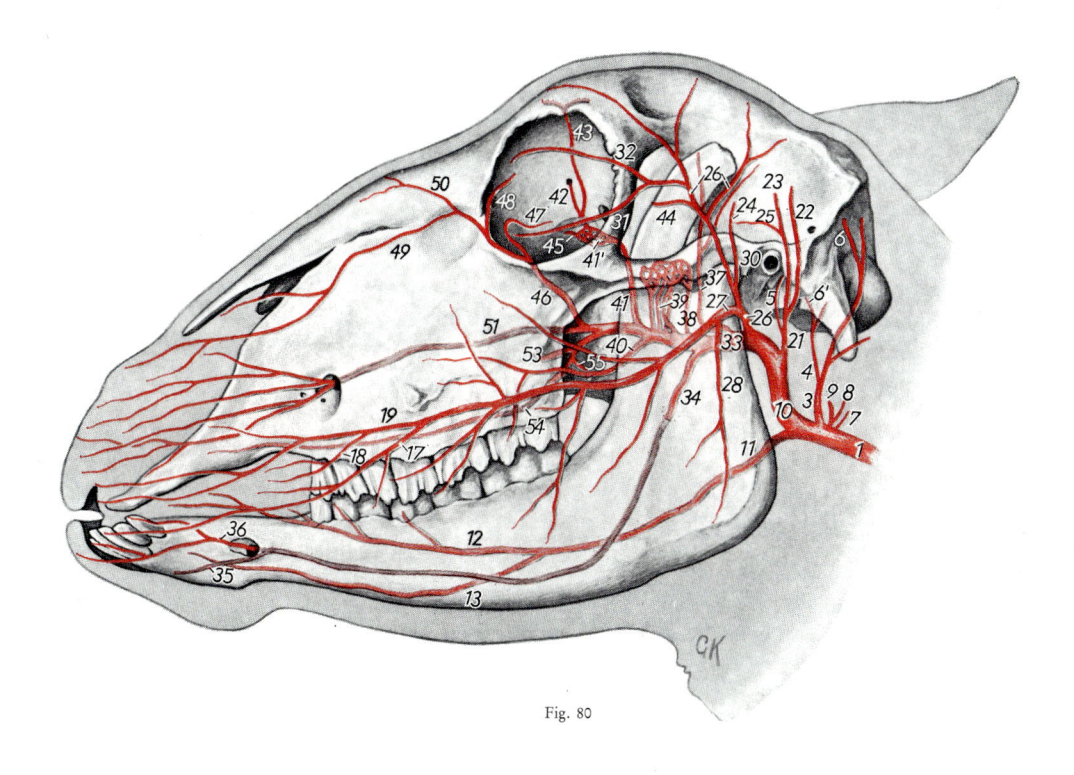

Fig. 80

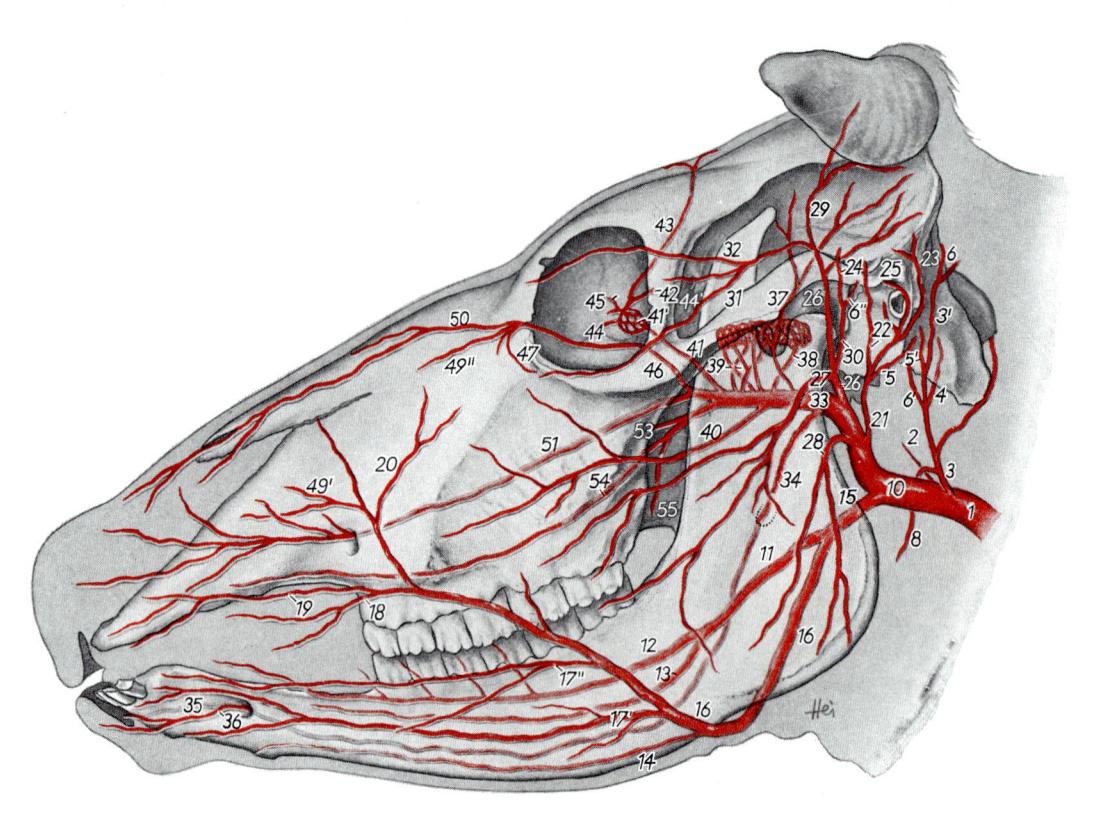

Fig. 81

gland. Except in the small ruminants, the facial artery also gives off the *a. submentalis* which courses medially along the mandible, ventrolateral to the mylohyoideus muscle, in a rostral direction. However, in neither the dog nor the ox does it attain the point of the mandible. As already described, in the dog and the horse the latter artery gives rise to the *a. sublingualis* and in the pig also there is a sublingual branch. In the cat, however, instead of this sublingual artery, there are several branches directed to the floor of the mouth.

On the surface of the face, the a. facialis gives rise to the *a. labialis mandibularis*, the *a. labialis maxillaris* in carnivores, the ox and the horse, the *a. angularis oris* only in carnivores, the *a. lateralis nasi rostralis* in the ox, the *a. lateralis nasi* and *a. dorsalis nasi* in the horse and finally the *a. angularis oculi* in carnivores, the ox and horse.

A. labialis mandibularis

(Comparative: *77–82/17, 17', 17"*; pig: 182/ *15;* horse: 83/*21*)

The **a. labialis mandibularis** of the carnivores, the ox and the horse is the first vessel to arise from the a. facialis on the surface of the face. In the pig it originates from the *a. buccalis* and in the small ruminants from the *a. transversa faciei*. It is destined to supply the upper lip. In the cat it divides into a dorsal and a ventral branch, in the ox into a superficial and a deep artery. In the horse the a. labialis mandibularis gives off the *a. angularis oris*.

A. angularis oris

(Comparative: *77–82/18*; pig: 182/*16*; sheep: 184/*61*; horse: 83/*21'*)

Only in carnivores does the **a. angularis oris** leave the facial artery after the labial mandibular artery. In the horse it springs from the labial mandibular artery, in the ox and small ruminants from the *a.*

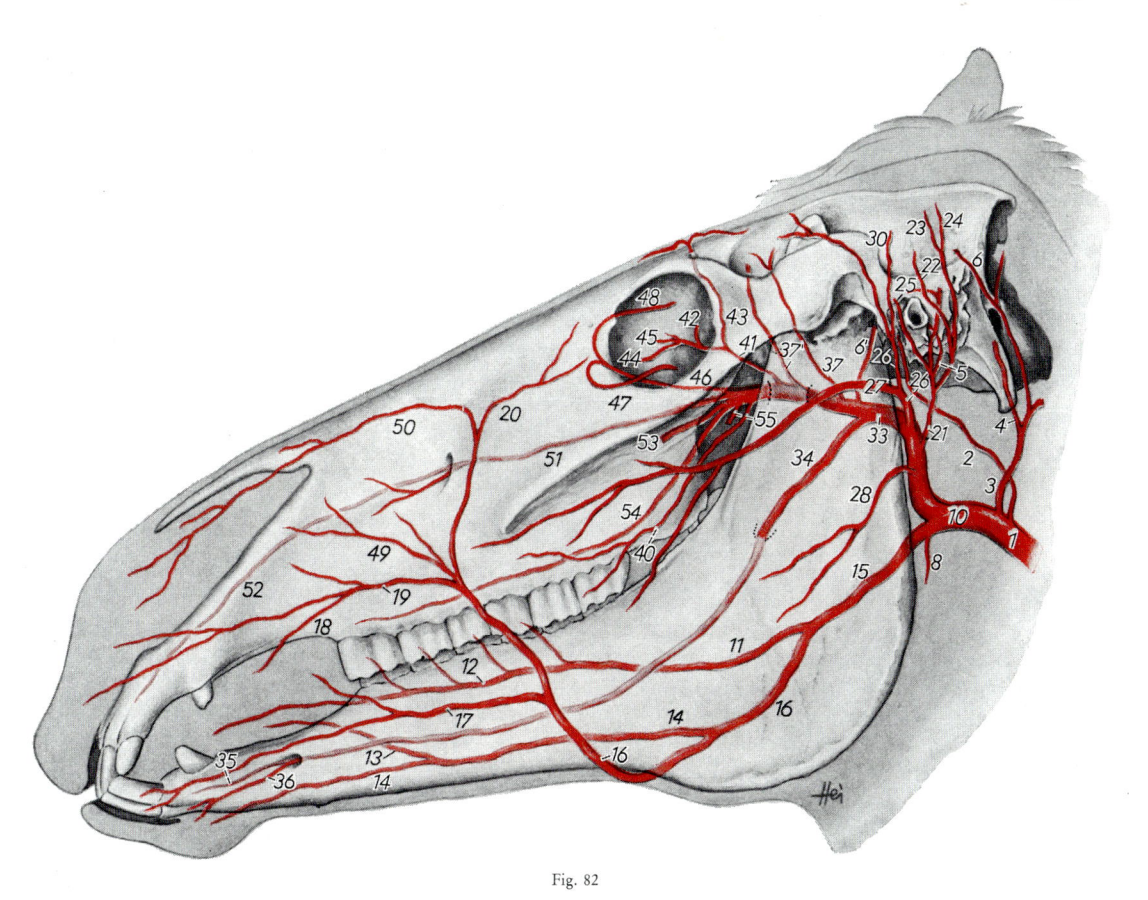

Fig. 82

Figs 77, 78, 79, 80, 81, 82. Arteries of the head of the cat, dog, pig, sheep, ox and horse.
Semidiagrammatic, left lateral view.
(After Nickel and Schwarz, 1961, study carried out at the Institute of Veterinary Anatomy, Hanover.)

1 a. carotis communis; *2* a. carotis interna; *3* a. occipitalis, *3'* r. occipitalis; *4* a. condylaris; *5* a. stylomastoidea; *5'* a. stylomastoidea profunda (ox); *6* a. meningea caudalis; *6'* a. meningea media; *6"* a. meningea accessoria (ruminants); *6'"* a. meningea rostralis (pig); *7* a. pharyngea ascendens; *8* a. palatina ascendens; *9* a. laryngea cranialis; *7* and *9* are not shown in the ox and the horse because their origin is situated further caudally, namely from the common carotid in the ox and from the cranial thyroid arteries in the horse; *10* a. carotis externa; *11* a. lingualis; *12* a. profunda linguae; *13* a. sublingualis; *14* a. submentalis; *15* truncus linguofacialis; *16* a. facialis; *17* a. labialis mandibularis; *17'* a. labialis mandibularis superficialis; *17"* a. labialis mandibularis profunda (ox); *18* a. angularis oris; *19* a. labialis maxillaris; *20* a. angularis oculi; *21* a. auricularis caudalis; *22* r. auricularis lateralis; *23* r. auricularis intermedius; *24* r. auricularis medialis; *25* a. auricularis caudalis; *26* a. temporalis superficialis; *27* a. transversa faciei; *28* r. massetericus; *29* a. cornualis; *30* a. auricularis rostralis; *30'* branch to the inner surface of the outer ear (pig); *31* a. palpebralis inferior lateralis; *32* a. palpebralis superior lateralis; *31* and *32* are not shown in the horse, being branches of the lacrimal artery; *33* a. maxillaris; *33'* rete mirabile a. maxillaris; *34* a. alveolaris mandibularis; *35* r. dentales from *34* to the incisor teeth; *36* a. mentalis or rr. mentales; *37* a. temporalis profunda caudalis; *37'* a. temporalis profunda rostralis (not shown in the pig, ox, being a branch of the buccal artery in these species); *38* r. caudalis ad rete mirabile epidurale rostrale; *39* rr. rostrales ad rete mirabile epidurale rostrale or rr. retis (cat); *40* a. buccalis; *41* a. ophthalmica; *41'* rete mirabile ophthalmicum; *41"* a. supratrochlearis; *42* a. ethmoidea externa; *43* a. supraorbitalis; *44* a. lacrimalis; *44'* r. lacrimalis from *26* (sheep, ox); *45* distribution of the a. ophthalmica on the bulbus of the eye; *46* a. malaris; *46'* r. frontalis; *47* a. palpebralis inferior medialis; *48* a. palpebralis superior medialis; *49* a. lateralis nasi; *49'* a. lateralis nasi rostralis (ox); *49"* a. lateralis nasi caudalis (ox); *50* a. dorsalis nasi or a. dorsalis nasi rostralis (dog); *51* a. infraorbitalis; *52* r. dentalis from *51* to the incisor teeth; *53–55* branches of the a. palatina descendens; *53* a. sphenopalatina, *54* a. palatina major, *55* a. palatina minor

labialis maxillaris, and in the pig it comes off the buccal artery. The branches of the angular artery of the mouth ramify in the angle of the mouth and the terminal dividing branches can arise independently from the parent vessel in the dog.

A. labialis maxillaris

(Comparative: 77–82/19; pig: 182/17; sheep: 184/60; horse: 83/22;)

The **a. labialis maxillaris** arises in carnivores, the ox and the horse from the facial artery at the alveolar border of the maxillary bone. In the pig it stems from the buccal artery and in the small ruminants from the transverse facial artery. The labial maxillar artery ramifies in the upper lip and in the ox also in the muzzle.

Aa. laterales nasi rostralis and caudalis or a. lateralis nasi
(Comparative: 77–82/49, 49', 49''; sheep: 184/56; horse: 83/24)

The **a. lateralis nasi rostralis** of the ox, or the corresponding **a. lateralis nasi** of the horse, is a branch of the facial artery. In the ox its origin is caudodorsal to the infraorbital foramen and in the horse it arises either a variable distance from the origin of the a. labialis maxillaris or from the latter vessel. However, the a. lateralis nasi of carnivores and pigs and the a. lateralis nasi rostralis of goats, arise from the infraorbital artery. In the sheep the a. lateralis nasi arises from the *a. malaris*. From the malar artery also arises the **a. lateralis nasi caudalis** of the goat and ox. The area supplied by the lateral nasal arteries in the ox and goat is the lateral wall of the nose up to the supply area of the artery of the upper lip.

A. dorsalis nasi
(Comparative: 77–82/50; sheep: 184/57; horse: 83/23)

The **a. dorsalis nasi** arises from the facial artery only in the horse in which its point of origin is caudodorsally to the infraorbital foramen. In carnivores it stems from the infraorbital artery and in the cat its origin precedes its entry into the infraorbital canal (see p. 115). In the sheep and ox it is given off the *a. malaris* and in the goat it comes off the *a. temporalis superficialis*. In the pig there is no such vessel to the dorsum of the nose but the rostral third of the nose is vascularized by ramifying branches of the *a. lateralis nasi*. The dorsal nasal artery runs rostrally on the nasal bone. In the sheep it barely attains the level of the fiss. nasomaxillaris while in the ox and horse it passes beyond the rostral end of the nasal bone. The dorsal nasal artery supplies the area of the bridge of the nose and, in the horse, the nasal diverticulum also.

A. angularis oculi
(Comparative: 77–82/20; horse: 83/25)

In carnivores, the ox and the horse the **a. angularis oculi** is the terminal branch of the facial artery. In the pig it arises from the buccal artery and it is absent in the small ruminants. It courses in a caudodorsal curve towards the medial canthus of the eye.

A. auricularis caudalis
(Comparative: 77–82/21; pig: 182/29, 183/22; sheep: 184/43; horse: 83/27)

The **a. auricularis caudalis** arises from the caudal wall of the dorsally-directed part of the external carotid artery and continues towards the base of the ear where it gives off branches, with certain modifications in the different species, to the auricle of the ear. Thereafter it curves round the base of the ear and runs between it and the temporal muscle. In carnivores, ruminants and the horse the caudal auricular artery gives rise to the *a. stylomastoidea*. In the pig the stylomastoid artery is a branch of the condylar artery and has already been described. In the other animals it continues alongside the facial nerve and passes through the stylomastoid foramen into the middle ear. There may be an additional delicate **a. tympanica caudalis** in the horse. The caudal auricular artery gives off to the parotid gland a *r. parotideus* in the pig and carnivores and several *rr. parotidei* in ruminants and the horse. Furthermore, in the dog, pig and goat it supplies a *r. sternocleidomastoideus* to the appropriate muscles and in the dog this ramus in turn has a branch to the salivary gland, the *r. glandularis*. The *r. meningeus* arises prior to the origin of the muscular branch in the goat and from a corresponding site in the sheep. This latter ramus enters the cranial cavity near the porus acusticus externus and it participates in the vascularization of the meninges of the brain.

At the base of the auricle the caudal auricular artery gives off the *r. auricularis lateralis*, which is usually duplicated in the cat and runs along the lateral border of the outer surface of the auricle towards the tip of the ear. It supplies the *r. auricularis intermedius* to the back of the ear. In the ox it is duplicated in the form of the *r. auricularis intermedius lateralis* and *r. auricularis intermedius medialis*. The next vessel to be given off, except in ruminants, is the *r. auricularis medialis* to the medial border of the outer surface of the ear. In ruminants, however, this branch arises from the *a. auricularis rostralis*. At the tip of the ear these arteries form anastomotic patterns which vary in the different species. There is yet another branch of the caudal auricular artery, the *a. auricularis profunda*, which varies in its origin from species to species. In the cat it arises after all the other auricular arteries, in the dog usually between the intermediate and medial auricular ramus or from one of these, and in the ox it is given off before the other auricular arteries. This deep auricular artery is but a small vessel which runs between the tragus and anthelix to attain the internal surface of the ear and supply the skin of the external auditory meatus. No such artery has been described in the other domestic mammals, although all the species have delicate vessels which perforate the ear cartilage or turn onto the internal surface round the base of the ear.

After giving off the auricular arteries, the caudal auricular artery supplies the *r. occipitalis* to the base of the skull and the temporal region and its branches penetrate down to the bone. The caudal auricular artery supplies several branches to the auricle of the ear and the temporalis muscle and it usually anastomoses with branches of the rostral auricular artery of the superficial temporal artery.

A. temporalis superficialis
(Comparative: 77–82/26; pig: 182/32; sheep: 184/49; horse: 83/32)

The dorsally directed **a. temporalis superficialis** arises at the caudal border of the lower jaw before the transition of the external carotid into the maxillary artery. It courses, either covered by or embedded in the parotid gland, rostral to the meatus acusticus externus and between the ear and the mandibular joint and then runs laterally across the zygomatic arch and into the temporal region. Shortly after its origin it gives off the *a. transversa faciei* dorsal to the facial nerve. However, the *a. auricularis rostralis* arises from the superficial temporal artery; in small ruminants it arises before the latter vessel and in the other domestic mammals it arises after it. In the horse the *r. auricularis temporomandibularis* to the mandibular joint is given off before the rostral auricular artery. In the pig and horse the terminal branches of the superficial temporal artery ramify superficially in the temporalis muscle but in carnivores and ruminants this artery continues in a rostral direction to the lateral canthus of the eye. Before reaching the canthus in horned ruminants, the *a. cornualis* is given off and this runs along the linea temporalis to the base of horn. At the lateral canthus of the eye the superficial temporal artery gives off, in the sheep and ox, the *r. lacrimalis* to the lacrimal gland. The superficial temporal artery divides in carnivores and ruminants into the *a. palpebralis superior lateralis* and the *a. palpebralis inferior lateralis* which terminate in the upper and lower eyelids. In the dog the lateral superior palpebral artery also gives rise to the *a. dorsalis nasi caudalis* which ramifies in the region of the forehead and the bridge of the nose. Only in the goat does a branch of the superficial temporal artery, the *a. dorsalis nasi*, supply the dorsum of the nose.

A. transversa faciei
(Comparative: 77–82/27; pig: 182/37; sheep: 184/38, 59; horse: 83/33)

The **a. transversa faciei** arises ventral to the proc. articularis of the mandible and attains the lateral surface of the masseter muscle dorsal to the facial nerve. In the cat it is duplicated. As it runs in a rostral direction the artery is accompanied by the vein of the same name, except in the cat in which species the vein is absent, and by branches of the auriculopalpebral nerve and of the auriculotemporal nerve. In the horse the transverse facial artery and its accompanying vein penetrate the masseter muscle superficially in a region ventral to the zygomatic arch. Its terminal branches extend barely beyond the masseter muscle except in the small ruminants where it is linked with the *a. labialis mandibularis*, the *a. labialis maxillaris*, and the *a. angularis oris* which have all been described in connection with the facial artery (see. p. 106). In addition to supplying branches to the neighbouring facial musculature and skin, in the pig and ox it gives the *r. articularis temporomandibularis* to the mandibular joint and in all the domestic mammals branches to the masseter muscle. There is a particularly stout *r. massetericus* in the small ruminants.

A. auricularis rostralis
(Comparative: 77–82/30; pig: 182/34; sheep: 184/48; horse: 83/32')

The *a. auricularis rostralis* arises from the superficial temporal artery. It reaches the base of the ear rostrally to the external auditory meatus and ramifies in the cleft angle of the auricle of the ear and the neighbouring muscles down to the scutulum. There it, or a branch of the superficial temporal artery itself, anastomoses with the caudal auricular artery. In ruminants only, the rostral auricular artery gives off the *r. auricularis medialis* which goes along the medial border of the outer surface of the auricle. Also in the ox, it gives off the *r. meningeus* which corresponds to that ramus in small ruminants which arises from the caudal auricular artery (see p. 108).

A. maxillaris
(Comparative: 77–82/32; pig: 183/24; sheep: 184/52; horse: 83/34; 84/b)

carnivores	pig	ruminants	horse
a. alveolaris mandibularis	a. meningea media	r. pterygoideus	a. alveolaris mandibularis
a. temporalis profunda caudalis	a. temporalis profunda caudalis	a. alveolaris mandibularis	rr. pterygoidei
a. tympanica rostralis	rr. pterygoidei	a. temporalis profunda (small ruminants)	a. tympanica rostralis
a. meningea media	a. alveolaris mandibularis	a. temporalis profunda caudalis (ox)	a. meningea media
rete mirabile a. maxillaris (cat)	a. buccalis	a. buccalis	a. temporalis profunda caudalis
a. temporalis profunda rostralis	a. temporalis profunda rostralis	a. temporalis profunda rostralis (ox)	a. temporalis profunda rostralis
rr. pterygoidei	a. ophthalmica externa	r. caudalis ad rete mirabile epidurale rostrale	a. ophthalmica externa
a. ophthalmica externa	a. malaris		a. buccalis
	a. infraorbitalis	rr. rostralis ad rete mirabile epidurale rostrale	a. infraorbitalis
a. temporalis profunda rostralis (dog)	a. palatina descendens		a. malaris
a. buccalis		a. ophthalmica externa	a. palatina descendens
a. infraorbitalis		a. malaris	
a. malaris		a. infraorbitalis	
a. palatina descendens		a. palatina descendens	

The **a. maxillaris** is the continuation towards the base of the skull of the external carotid artery after it has given off the superficial temporal artery. In the dog and horse it attains the fossa pterygopalatina after passing through the alar canal. In the cat the maxillary artery forms a network known as the *rete mirabile a. maxillaris* near the foramen ovale, the main artery itself being traceable through this network as a stouter vessel. This network extends dorsally and laterally to the apex of the periorbital region. In the cat the arteries for the bulbus and accessory structures arise from this network as do also the *rr. retis*, which pass through the fiss. orbitalis and go to the *circulus arteriosus cerebri*. The first vessel to leave the maxillary artery in carnivores is the *r. articularis temporomandibularis* destined for the mandibular joint.

There is considerable species variation in the sequence in which subsequent branches of the maxillary artery arise; this is shown in the table. The branch vessels are *a. alveolaris mandibularis, a. temporalis profunda* or *aa. temporales profundae caudalis* and *rostralis*, **rr. pterygoidei** for the muscles of that name, the *a. tympanica rostralis* in carnivores and the horse, the *a. meningea media* in all but ruminants, *rr. caudalis* and *rostrales ad rete mirabile epidurale ventrale* in ruminants only, *a. buccalis, a. ophthalmica externa, a. malaris* in pigs and ruminants, *a. infraorbitalis* and *a. palatina descendens*.

A. alveolaris mandibularis
(Comparative: 77–82/*34*; pig: 183/*25*; sheep: 184/*39*; horse: 83/*35*)

In all domestic mammals the **a. alveolaris mandibularis** arises in a rostrolateral direction from the first part of the maxillary artery. It runs towards the mandibular foramen through which it enters the mandibular canal. In ruminants it is more tortuous than in the other domestic mammals. Except in the horse, the *r. mylohyoideus* to the mylohyoid muscle is given off before entry into the mandibular canal. Within this canal the *rr. dentales* to the molar and premolar teeth are given off. Other branches pass through the alveolar canal to the canine and incisor teeth. In carnivores and pigs, the *rr. mentales* leave the mandibular canal through the mental foramina. In ruminants and the horse the *a. mentalis* emerges from the mental foramen. The branches of these arteries ramify in the region of the margo interalveolaris, in the gingiva of the incisor teeth and in the lower lip. In the pig there are anastomoses with the *a. submentalis* at the point of the mandible.

Aa. temporales profundae
(Comparative: 77–82/*37, 37'*; pig: 183/*26*; horse: 83/*37, 38*; 84/*e, f*)

The **a. temporalis profunda caudalis** branches from the maxillary artery to supply the temporal region and especially the temporalis muscle. In the small ruminants this is the only deep vessel to the temporal region and it is therefore known simply as the **a. temporalis profunda.** In the other domestic mammals there is also an **a. temporalis profunda rostralis** which, in the dog and horse stems from the maxillary artery, in the cat from the rete mirabile, and in the pig and ox from the buccal artery. The dorsally-directed deep temporal arteries enter the temporalis muscle rostral to the base of the zygomatic process of the temporal bone and anastomose within this muscle with branches of the superficial temporal artery. In carnivores, pigs and cattle the caudal deep temporal artery gives off beforehand the *a. masseterica.* In small ruminants the first part of the deep temporal artery is bound to the maxillary artery by fibrous tissue up to the point where the former rises dorsally to the temporal muscle and gives off the *r. articularis temporomandibularis* to the mandibular joint.

A. meningea media
(Horse: 83/*36*; 84/*d*)

In carnivores, the pig and horse the **a. meningea media** arises from the maxillary artery. In the dog and the horse this occurs before the maxillary artery enters the alar canal. In the cat it sometimes originates from the rete mirabile a. maxillaris; in ruminants it stems from the occipital artery. In the sheep this artery may also stem from the condylar artery. In carnivores and ruminants it traverses the for. ovale, in the pig and horse the for. lacerum orale, en route for the cranial cavity where it ramifies in

112 Arteries

the dura mater. In carnivores the middle meningeal artery has a *r. anastomoticus cum a. carotide interna* lateral to the middle cranial fossa, as well as another r. anastomoticus which passes through the orbital fissure to join the external ophthalmic artery. In the pig there is a *r. ad rete mirabile epidurale rostrale* to the extradural rete at the base of the skull.

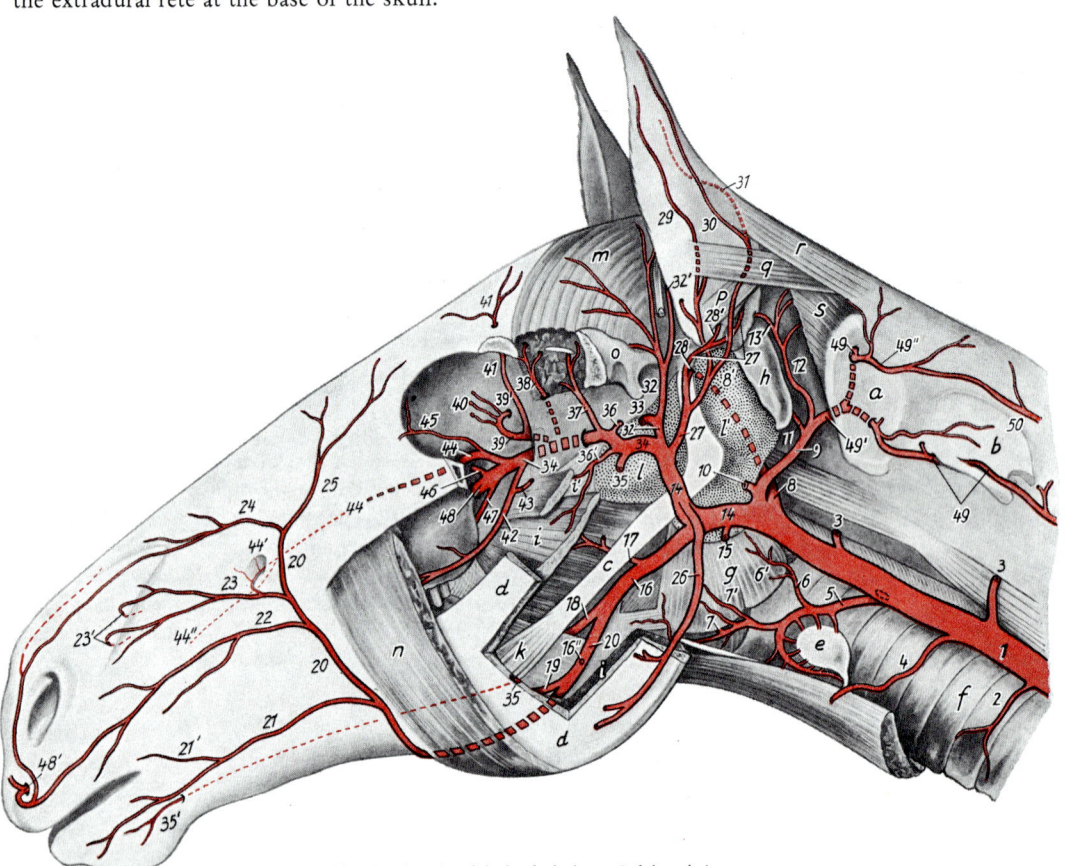

Fig. 83. Arteries of the head of a horse. Left lateral view.
(After Zietzschmann, 1943.)

a atlas; *b* axis; *c* stylohyoideum; *d* mandibula, partly removed; *e* gl. thyreoidea; *f* trachea; *g* mm. constrictores pharyngis caudalis; *h* proc. jugularis; *i* m. pterygoideus medialis; *i'* mm. tensor and levator veli palatini; *k* m. stylohyoideus; *l, l'* diverticulum tubae auditivae; *l* lateral, *l'* medial pouch; *m* m. temporalis; *n* m. masseter; *o* art. temporomandibularis; *p* m. cervicoauricularis profundus; *q* m. cervicoauricularis medius; *r* m. cervicoauricularis superficialis; *s* m. obliquus capitis cranialis

1 a. carotis communis, *2* r. trachealis, *3, 4* rr. musculares; *5* a. thyreoidea cranialis, *6* r. pharyngeus, *6'* r. laryngeus caudalis; *7* a. laryngea cranialis; *7'* a. pharyngea ascendens; *8* a. carotis interna, at *8'* placed into the guttural pouch; *9* a. occipitalis, *10* r. glandularis; *11* a. condylaris, *12* r. occipitalis, *13* a. meningea caudalis; *14* a. carotis externa, *15* r. glandularis; *16* a. linguofacialis; *17* a. palatina ascendens; *18* a. lingualis; *19* a. sublingualis; *20* a. facialis; *21* a. labialis mandibularis; *21'* a. angularis oris; *22* a. labialis maxillaris; *23* a. lateralis nasi, *23'* retrograde branches to the external nares; *24* a. dorsalis nasi; *25* a. angularis oculi; *26* r. massetericus; *27* a. auricularis caudalis; *28* a. stylomastoideus; *28'* a. auricularis profunda, *29* r. auricularis lateralis, *30* r. auricularis medius, *31* r. auricularis medialis; *32* a. temporalis superficialis; *32'* a. auricularis rostralis; *33* a. transversa faciei; *34* a. maxillaris; *35* a. alveolaris mandibularis; *35'* a. mentalis; *36* a. meningea media; *36'* r. pterygoideus; *37* a. temporalis profunda caudalis; *38* a. temporalis profunda rostralis; *39* a. ophthalmica externa, *40* its branches to the bulbus of the eye and its accessory organs; *39'* a. ethmoidalis externa; *41* a. supraorbitalis; *42* a. buccalis; *43* artery to the extraorbital adipose tissue; *44* a. infraorbitalis, *44'* its anastomosis to the a. lateralis nasi, *44"* rr. dentales; *45* a. malaris; *46* a. sphenopalatina; *47* a. palatina minor; *48* a. palatina major; *48'* its anastomosis with the a. labialis maxillaris; *49* a. vertebralis, *49'* r. anastomoticus cum a. occipitali, *49"* r. descendens; *50* a. cervicalis profunda

A. buccalis

(Comparative: 77–82/*40*; pig: 182/*18*; 183/*27*; horse: 83/*42*; 84/*o*)

The **a. buccalis** springs off the maxillary artery in a rostroventral direction. The former artery is, except in the pig, destined especially for the muscles of mastication and the glands of the cheek. In carnivores there are also *rr. glandulares zygomatici* for the zygomatic gland. As already described above, in the pig and ox the *a. temporalis profunda rostralis* is given off the buccal artery. Only in the pig does the buccal artery give rise to the *a. angularis oculi* which, in its turn, gives origin to the *a. palpebralis* *inferior medialis*, the *a. angularis oris*, the *a. labialis mandibularis* and the *a. labialis maxillaris*; these vessels have been described in detail in connection with the facial artery (see. p 107 ff.).

R. caudalis and rr. rostrales ad rete mirabile epidurale rostrale
(sheep: 80/*38*, *39*; ox: 81/*38*, *39*)

In ruminants the maxillary artery gives off dorsally directed rete branches which enter the cranial cavity through the for. ovale of the for. orbitorotundum. These branches link with the epidurally situated arterial network at the base of the skull, the *rete mirabile epidurale*.

The *r. caudalis ad rete mirabile epidurale rostrale* arises in the small ruminants at the level of the a. alveorlaris mandibularis and in the ox at the level of the buccal artery. After reaching the base of the skull in the ox, this branch bends caudally and then enters the oval foramen.

The *rr. rostrales ad rete mirabile epidurale rostrale* leave the maxillary artery at the level of the external ophthalmic artery, although isolated branches can also arise beforehand or, in the ox, originate from the buccal artery.

A. ophthalmica externa
(Comparative: 77–82/*41*; pig: 183/*28*; horse: 83/*39*)

In all the domestic mammals the **a. ophthalmica externa** arises from the maxillary artery; in the cat rostrodorsally from the rete mirabile. In the dog the site of origin is rostral to the alar canal and in the horse even within this canal. In the pig and ruminants its point of origin lies rostral to the crista pterygoidea. The external ophthalmic artery reaches the apex of the eye muscle pyramid which is surrounded by periorbita. It perforates this periorbital tissue and turns along the internal surface of the periorbita running dorsally over the ocular muscles to the medial side, thereby executing a rostrally convex curve.

In the domestic mammals the external ophthalmic artery forms the main supply to the bulbus oculi and its ancillary organs. It sends the *a. ethmoidalis externa* and, except in the cat and ruminants, the *a. meningea rostralis* into the cranial cavity. It supplies the frontal region by means of the *a. suborbitalis* and, in the pig, also the *a. supratrochlearis*. The bulbus is supplied by the *aa. ciliares posteriores breves*, the *aa. ciliares posteriores longae*, the *a. centralis retinae*, the *aa. episclerales* and the *aa. ciliares anteriores*. The accessory organs of the bulbus receive their blood supply through the *rr. musculares*, the *a. lacrimalis*, the *aa. conjunctivales posteriores*, the *aa. conjunctivales anteriores* and through some of the *aa. palpebrales*. There is considerable species and individual variation in the sequence with which these vessels arise.

In addition to the already-mentioned vessels, in the dog the external ophthalmic artery gives off, shortly after its origin, the *r. anastomoticus cum a. carotide interna* which is caudally directed and enters the cranial cavity through the orbital fissure where, lateral to the middle cranial fossa, it anastomoses with the internal carotid artery. Intracranially it also anastomoses with the middle meningeal artery via the *r. anastomoticus cum a. meningea media*. In ruminants the external ophthalmic artery forms the *rete mirabile opthhalmicum* within the periorbita at the site of origin of the eye muscles. In all domestic mammals the external ophthalmic artery gives off the *r. anastomoticus cum a. ophthalmica interna* which passes between the eye muscles and links up with the internal ophthalmic artery which accompanies the optic nerve.

In the domestic mammals the **a. ophthalmica interna** is only a slender vessel which arises from the *a. cerebri rostralis*, except in the ox, in which it arises from the rostral epidural rete mirabile or the *rete mirabile chiasmaticum*. The internal ophthalmic artery accompanies the optic nerve to the bulbus oculi. After joining the r. anastomoticus of the external ophthalmic artery, as noted above, and entering the optic bulb, the internal ophthalmic artery becomes the *a. centralis retinae*.

From this vessel junction arise in carnivores, the pig and horse, the *a. centralis retinae* to the optic papilla and the *aa. ciliares posteriores longae* which run between choroid and sclera to the ciliary body and the iris, giving off branches to the choroid. In ruminants the long posterior ciliary arteries are branches of the external ophthalmic artery and they give off the central retinal artery. In all the domestic mammals they are the source of the *aa. ciliares posteriores breves* which perforate the sclera near the optic

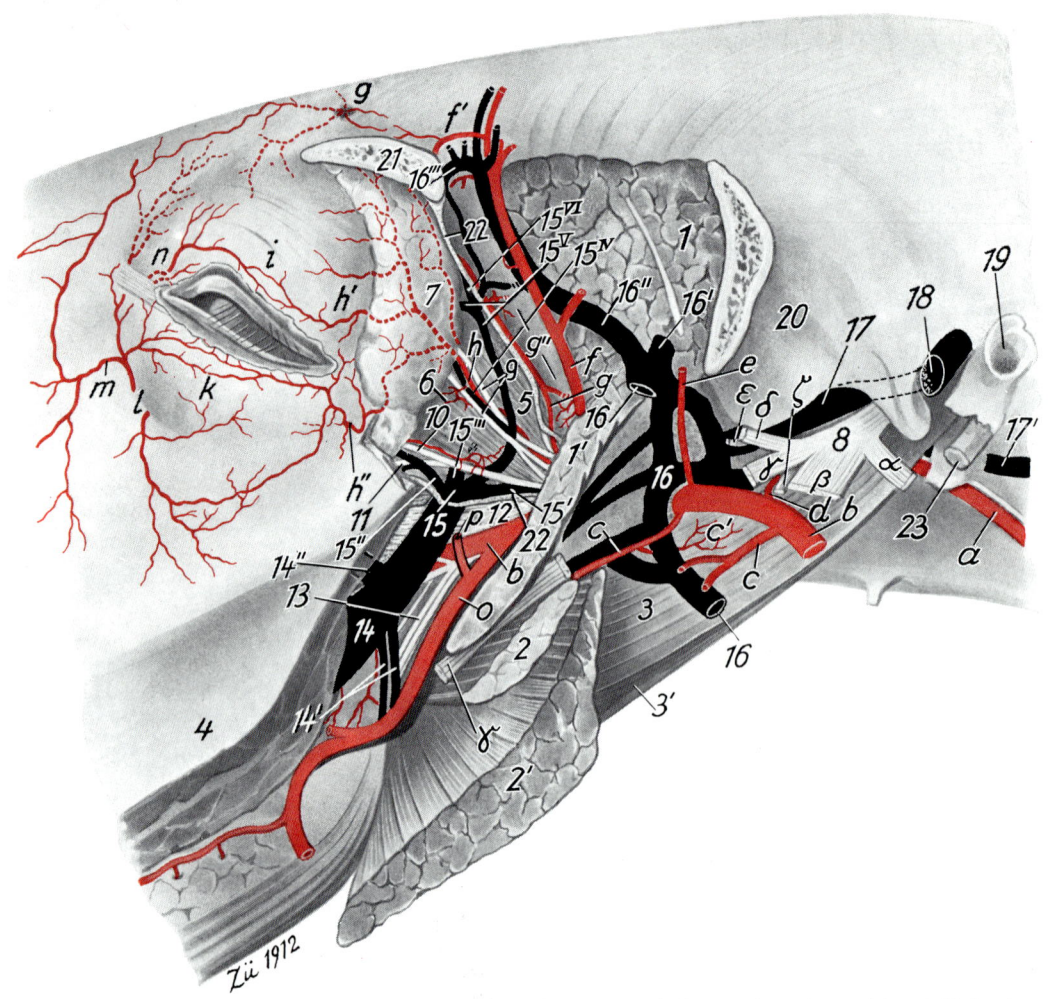

Fig. 84. Arteries and veins of the orbit and temporal fossa of a horse. (Part of the zygomatic arch, the temporal musculature and the periorbita have been removed. Left lateral view).
(After Zietzschmann, 1943.)

1, 1' m. temporalis; *2, 2'* mm. pterygoidei lateralis and medialis; *3* m. tensor veli palatini; *3'* m. levator veli palatini; *4* m. masseter; *5* m. rectus dorsalis; *6* m. rectus lateralis; *7* gl. lacrimalis; *8* n. mandibularis; *9* n. lacrimalis; *10* r. zygomaticofacialis from *12*; *11* branch of the n. oculomotorius to the m. obliquus ventralis; *12* n. maxillaris; *13* n. palatinus minor

Arteries: *a* a. carotis interna with n. sympathicus; *b* a. maxillaris; *c* rr. pterygoidei; *d* a. meningea media; *e* a. temporalis profunda caudalis; *f* a. temporalis profunda rostralis; *g* a. supraorbitalis; *h* a. lacrimalis; *h'* a. palpebralis superior lateralis; *h"* a. palpebralis inferior lateralis; *l, m* a. palpebralis inferior medialis; *n* a. palpebralis superior medialis; *o* a. buccalis; *p* artery to the orbital fat

Veins: *14* v. profunda faciei; *15* v. ophthalmica externa ventralis; *15'* v. emissaria fissurae orbitalis; *15"* v. malaris; *15'''* origin of the vv. ciliares; *15^{iv}* v. lacrimalis; *15^v* v. ophthalmica externa dorsalis; *15^{vi}* v. supraorbitalis; *16* plexus pterygoideus; *16'* v. temporalis profunda caudalis; *16"* v. temporalis profunda rostralis; *16'''* r. anastomoticus; *17* termination of the v. emissaria foraminis laceri into the sinus petrosus ventralis (*17'*); *18* v. emissaria foraminis retroarticularis

19 meatus acusticus externus; *20* facies articularis; *21* proc. zygomaticus of the os frontale, cut off; *22* orbita, cut edge; *23* proc. styloideus

nerve and the *aa. episclerales* which supply the sclera from the outside. Furthermore, the external ophthalmic artery gives off the *rr. musculares* to the muscles of the eye. In carnivores, ruminants and the horse, the *aa. ciliares anteriores* stem from the muscular branches, whereas in the pig they arise directly from the external ophthalmic artery. Except in the pig these muscular branches also supply other *aa. episclerales*. While these episcleral arteries participate in the vascularization of the sclera from the outside, the anterior ciliary arteries perforate the sclera near the corneo-scleral junction, unite with the posterior ciliary arteries and jointly vascularize the ciliary body and the iris. In carnivores and ruminants the rr. musculares also give off the *aa. conjunctivales posteriores*; in the horse these arteries originate from the external ophthalmic and in the pig from the anastomosing ramus with the internal ophthalmic artery. These arteries run along the sclera to reach the conjunctiva.

The **a. lacrimalis** to the lacrimal gland is a stout vessel which arises from the external opthalmic artery except in the cat, in which animal it derives from the maxillary artery or its rete. The lacrimal artery gives off in the dog, and especially in the cat, branches to the muscles of the bulb of the eye. In the pig and horse the lacrimal artery gives rise to the *a. palpebralis superior lateralis* and the *a. palpebralis inferior lateralis*, which supply, from the lateral canthus of the eye, the upper and lower eyelids respectively.

The *a. supraorbitalis* is absent in the dog. In the other animals it runs through the supraorbital canal and, in the cat, it leaves the orbit caudal to the zygomatic process of the frontal bone. It perforates the periorbita giving off branches to it, to the orbital periosteum and to the frontal sinus. Except in the small ruminants it extends to the frontal region. In the pig it divides into delicate twigs in this region, in the ox it ramifies in the frontal skin and musculature and in the horse it extends to the frontal and parietal regions and the dorsum of the nose. While still within the orbit, the supraorbital artery of the ox gives off both the *aa. conjunctivales anteriores* which enter the conjunctiva from the eyelids, and also the *a. ethmoidalis externa*. Only the pig has an *a. supratrochlearis* which stems from the first part of the external ophthalmic artery before the latter enters the periorbita. This supratrochlear artery also enters the periorbital region, giving off branches to the muscles of the eye before leaving the periorbita dorsally. Above the upper eyelid it lies on the zygomatic process where it gives off the *a. palpebralis superior medialis* and then ramifies in the scutular musculature.

Another stout vessel from the external ophthalmic which leaves the periorbita, is the *a. ethmoidalis externa*. In the ruminant it arises from the supraorbital artery. It courses to the ethmoid foramen through which it reaches the ethmoid fossa. Here it gives off, in the dog and horse, the *a. meningea rostralis*. In the pig the external ethmoidal artery stems directly from the external ophthalmic artery and gives off a *r. ad rete mirabile epidurale rostrale*. In the dog the external ethmoidal artery perforates the lamina cribrosa and participates with the *aa. septales caudales* in the vascularization of the nasal septum.

The *a. palpebrae tertiae* is a branch of the external ophthalmic artery only in the horse.

A. malaris
(Comparative: 77–82/46; sheep: 184/53; horse: 83/45)

The **a. malaris** rises ventral to the orbit, from the infraorbital artery in carnivores and the horse and from the maxillary artery in ruminants and in the pig. Running medial to the temporal process of the zygomatic bone and over the ventral surface of the orbit it reaches the medial canthus of the eye. Here it gives off the *a. palpebrae tertiae* to the nictitating membrane, which in the horse has already received branches of the external ophthalmic. It also gives off the *a. palpebralis inferior medialis* to the lower eyelid and, except in the pig and ox, the *a. palpebralis superior medialis* to the upper eyelid. The latter vessel arises in the pig from the supratrochlear artery but it is lacking altogether in the ox in which species the lateral superior palpebral artery supplies this area. In the pig the *r. frontalis* of the malar artery extends to the forehead and in the ox gives off the *r. angularis oculi*. This latter ramus runs to meet the a. angularis oculi. Only in the pig do *aa. conjunctivales anteriores* originate from the malar artery. The malar artery also gives rise in the sheep to the *a. lateralis nasi*, in the goat and ox to the *a. lateralis nasi caudalis* and in the pig, sheep and ox it also gives off the *a. dorsalis nasi*. These arteries have already been dealt with on a comparative basis (see p. 108).

A. infraorbitalis
(Comparative: 77–82/51; pig: 183/52′; sheep: 184/54; horse: 83/44)

As one of the terminal branches of the maxillary artery, the **a. infraorbitalis** passes through the maxillary foramen into the infraorbital canal. This canal is extremely short in the cat and therefore the initial part of this artery lies ventral in the orbit. In carnivores and horses the infraorbital artery gives off the malar artery, which has already been described, and then the *rr. dentales* which drain the molar teeth. In the cat these dental rami usually perforate the wall of the orbit ventrally. Before leaving the infraorbital canal the infraorbital artery, in all domestic mammals except ruminants, gives off the dental rami which pass through the alveolar canal to the anterior premolars, canines and incisor teeth. The *a. dorsalis nasi*, which has already been described on p. 108, originates from the infraorbital artery only

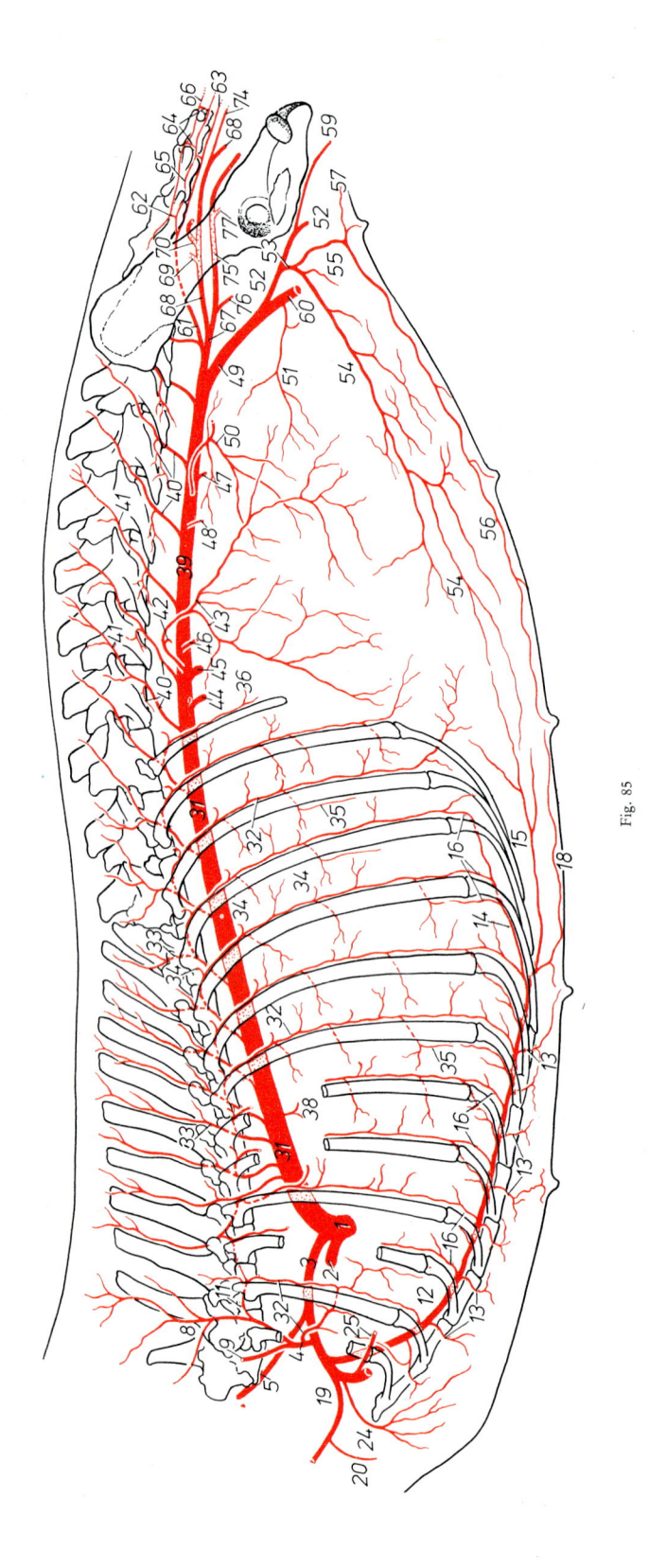

Figs 85, 86, 87, 88. Arteries of the trunk of the dog, pig, ox and horse. Semidiagrammatic, left lateral view. (After Marthen, 1939, Diss., Hanover; after Kähler, 1960, Diss., Hanover; after Seidler, 1966, Diss., Hanover; after Greiffenhagen, Diss., Hanover.

1 arcus aortae; *2* truncus brachiocephalicus; *3* a. subclavia sinistra; *4* truncus costocervicalis; *5* a. vertebralis; *6* rr. dorsales, *6'* r. descendens, *7* rr. ventrales, *7'* r. anastomoticus cum. a. occipitali; *8* a. cervicalis profunda; *9* a. scapularis dorsalis; *10* a. intercostalis suprema; *11* a. vertebralis thoracica (dog); *12* a. thoracica interna; *13* rr. perforantes with r. sternalis and, in the dog and pig, with rr. mammarii; *14* a. musculophrenica; *15* a. epigastrica cranialis; *16* rr. intercostales ventrales; *17* r. costoabdominalis ventralis; *18* a. epigastrica cranialis superficialis; *19* a. cervicalis superficialis; *20* r. deltoideus; *21* r. ascendens; *22* a. suprascapularis; *23* a. axillaris; *24* a. thoracica externa; *25* a. thoracica lateralis, cut off in the dog, and with the rr. mammarii in the pig; *26* truncus bicaroticus; *27* a. carotis communis sinistra; *28* a. carotis interna; *29* a. occipitalis; *30* a. carotis externa; *31* aorta thoracica; *32* aa. intercostales dorsales (branches to the intercostal muscles are shown only in the dog); *33* r. dorsalis, continuing as r. cutaneus medialis; *34* rr. cutanei laterales (except in the dog, it is shown in only one segment); *35* rr. collaterales; *36* a. costoabdominalis dorsalis; *37* a. phrenica cranialis (horse); *38* a. broncho-oesophagea, in the dog a. broncho-oeso- phagea sinistra; *39* aorta abdominalis; *40* aa. lumbales; *41* r. dorsalis; *42* a. phrenica caudalis; *43* a. abdominalis cranialis; *44* a. coeliaca; *45* a. mesenterica cranialis; *46* a. renalis sinistra; *47* a. mesenterica caudalis; *48* a. testicularis or a. ovarica sinistra; *49* a. iliaca externa; *50* a. circumflexa ilium profunda; *51* a. abdominalis caudalis; *52* a. profunda femoris; *53* truncus pudendoepigastricus; *54* a. epigastrica caudalis; *55* a. pudenda externa; *56* a. epigastrica caudalis superficialis (a. mammaria cranialis [female ox and horse]); *57* r. scrotalis ventralis or r. labialis ventralis (a. mammaria caudalis [female ox and horse]); *58* a. penis cranialis; *59* a. circumflexa femoris medialis; *60* a. femoralis; *61* a. sacralis mediana; *62* rr. sacrales; *63* a. caudalis mediana; *64* rr. caudales; *65* a. caudalis ventrolateralis; *66* a. caudalis dorsolateralis; *67* a. iliaca interna; *68* a. glutaea caudalis; *69* a. iliolumbalis; *70* a. glutaea cranialis; *71* a. obturatoria; *72* a. penis media or a. clitoris media; *73* a. caudalis lateralis medialis; *74* a. caudalis lateralis superficialis; *75* a. pudenda interna; *76* a. umbilicalis; *77* a. prostatica or a. vaginalis; *78* a. perinealis ventralis; *79* a. penis or a. bulbi vestibuli (horse)

Arteries of the trunk

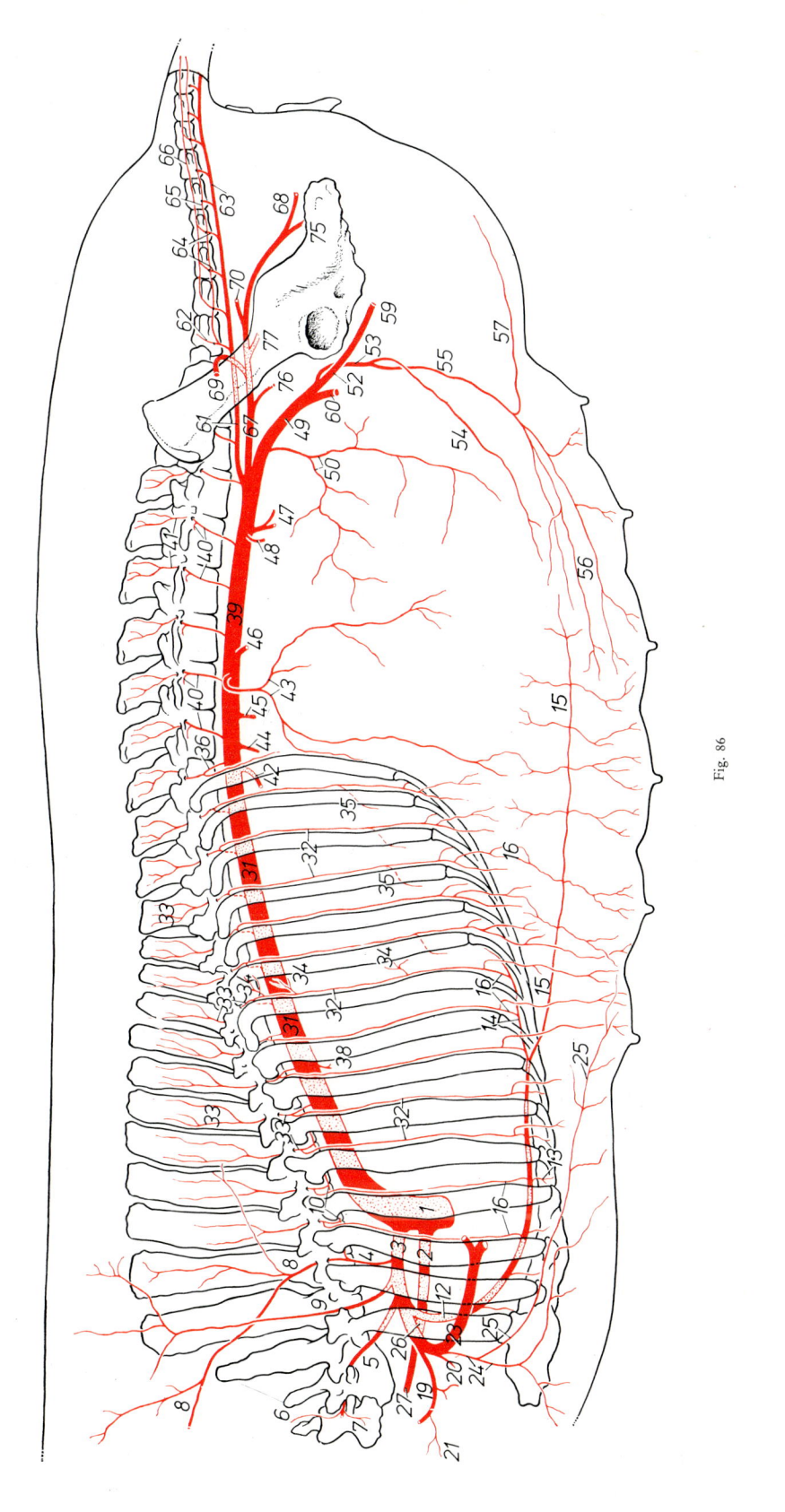

Fig. 86

118 Arteries

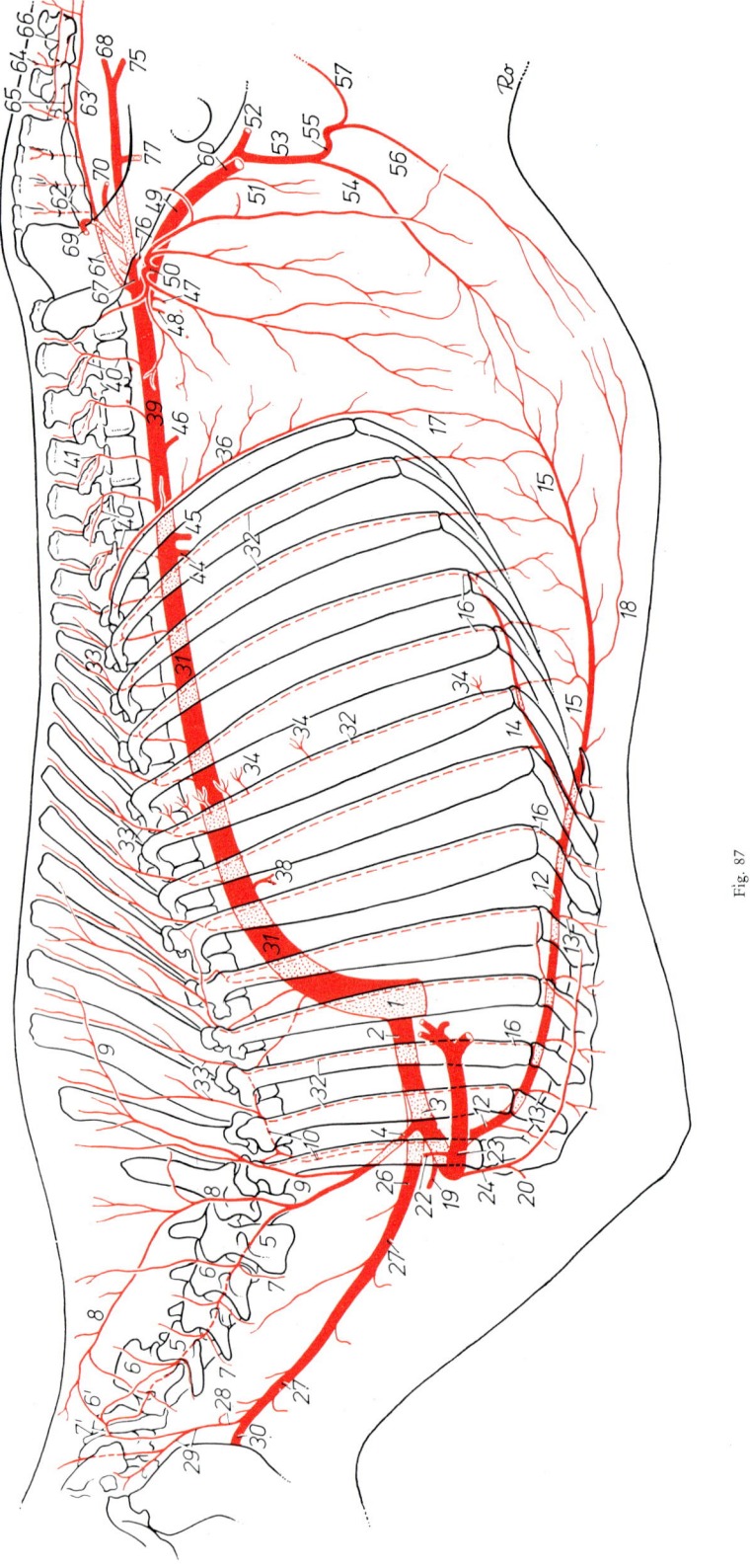

Fig. 87

Arteries of the trunk

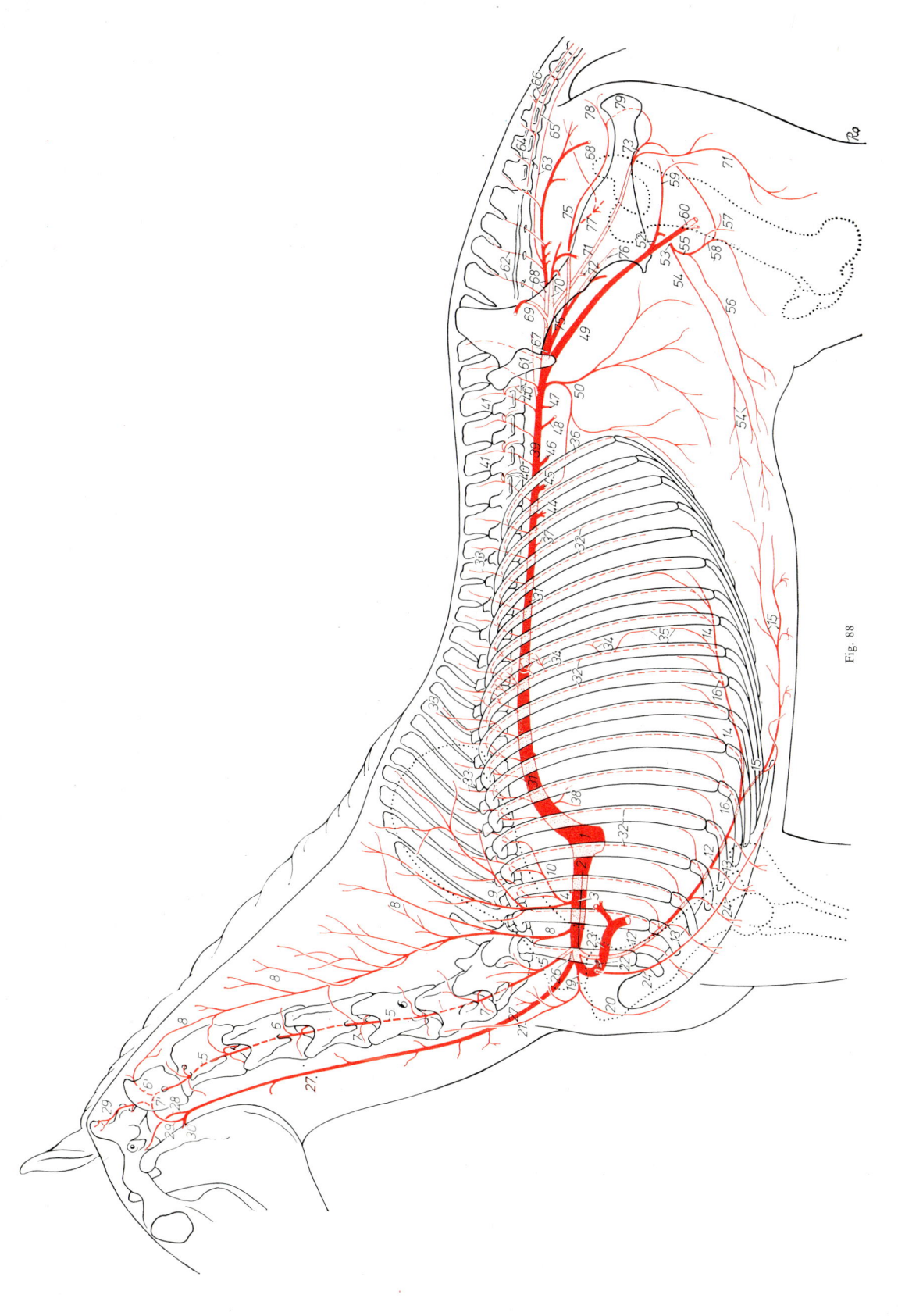

Fig. 88

in carnivores. In the cat it originates within the orbit and both it and its vessel of origin then pass through the infraorbital canal. In the dog, on the other hand, this artery, known in this species as the *a. dorsalis nasi rostralis,* arises only rostral to the infraorbital canal. The *a. lateralis nasi* of carnivores and the *aa. laterales nasi* of pigs also stem from the infraorbital artery (see p. 108).

A. palatina descendens
(Comparative: 77–82/*53–55*; pig: 183/*52*; sheep: 184/*22*)

The **a. palatina descendens** is the rostroventrally-directed terminal branch of the maxillary artery. In the fossa pterygopalatina it divides into the *a. sphenopalatina,* the *a. palatina minor* and the *a. palatina major.* In carnivores and the horse the sphenopalatine artery is the last and in the pig and ruminants the first vessel. In the cat the lesser palatine artery usually arises independently from the maxillary artery before the descending palatine artery is given off. The *a. sphenopalatina* runs through the sphenopalatine foramen and reaches the nasal cavity caudally and then ramifies with its *aa. nasales caudales, laterales* and *septales* in the mucosa of the ventral meatus and of the caudal part of the ventral nasal turbinate and the nasal septum. The *a. palatina minor* courses lateral to the pterygoid process to supply the velum palatinum. The *a. palatina major* goes through the major palatine canal and along the sulcus palatinus rostralis. In the region of the palatine fissure it unites with the artery of the other side to form an arch. Along its course through the palatine groove it gives off branches to the hard palate and, by way of the palatine fissure, sends branches to the mucosa of the rostral part of the floor of the ventral nasal meatus where it joins branches of the sphenopalatine artery.

Aorta thoracica
(Comparative: 85–88/*31*; cat: 91/*1'*; dog: 94, 95/*1*; pig: 96/*1'*; 153/*45*; goat: 154/*29*; sheep: 99/*1'*; ox: 102, 155/*2*; horse: 50/*20*; 89/*1*; 103/*2*; 211/*1*)

A summary of the course of the thoracic aorta and its branches has already been given (see p. 72)

Aa. intercostales dorsales
(Comparative: 85–88/*32*; cat: 90/*1'*, *14*; 91/*13*, *14*; dog: 92/*31*, *32*; 94, 95/*2*, *6*; pig: 96/*17*; 97/*21–25*; 98/*17'*; sheep: 99/*17*; 101/*17"*; ox: 102, 155/*5*; horse: 50/*21*; 89/*2*; 103/*22*)

Those **aa. intercostales dorsales** which do not originate from the a. intercostalis suprema or, the a. vertebralis thoracica in the dog, leave the thoracic aorta in a segmental pattern. In the domestic mammals they correspond to the number of intercostal spaces present. The species variations in the origin of the dorsal intercostal arteries are shown in the following table although every possible variation is not listed.

Vessels of origin of the first and subsequent aa. intercostales dorsales

There are no fundamental differences in the course and subsequent branching of the intercostal arteries whether they originate from the a. intercostalis suprema, the a. vertebralis thoracica or the aorta thoracica. However, the left and right branches of any one segment may arise as a common stem. The arteries which are destined for the cranial intercostal spaces and which do not arise from the vessels of origin recorded above, are only of rudimentary development. It should be pointed out that the *truncus costocervicalis,* the *a. cervicalis profunda* and the *a. scapularis dorsalis* are homologous, all being very stout dorsal or lateral branches of these segmental vessels.

Initially the dorsal intercostal artery courses towards the body of the vertebra which has the same numerical designation. It then crosses the lateral aspect of the vertebral body and gives off the *r. dorsalis* caudoventral to the transverse process. The artery itself continues into the intercostal space where at first it runs for a short distance between the intercostal muscles. It then lies subpleurally close to the caudal border of the rib and continues ventrad in the sulcus costae in company with the corresponding nerve and the homonymous vein, lying caudally to the former and cranially to the latter. In carnivores and the pig it sends several *rr. collaterales* across the rib to its cranial border. In the horse, similar branches go through the intercostal space to the cranial border of the following rib. Allowing for species and regional differences, there are up to seven *rr. cutanei laterales*, the *rr. mammarii* to the thoracic mammary complex and the *rr. phrenici* in the region of the asternal ribs. With the exception of the cranial rudimentary vessels, the dorsal intercostal arteries anastomose at about the level of the costochondral junction with the *rr. intercostales ventrales* of the internal thoracic and, where applicable, the musculophrenic artery. In the pig and ruminants ventral intercostal branches in the more caudal region stem from the cranial epigastric artery.

The *r. dorsalis* traverses the intercostal space, giving off a *r. interspinosus* to the spinous processes and their ligaments and muscles and then, at the level of the for. intervertebrale, it gives off the *r. spinalis* which passes through either the intervertebral foramen or the lateral vertebral foramen and enters the vertebral canal. The spinal ramus divides into the *r. canalis vertebralis* and the *a. nervomedullaris*. The latter is not constantly present at every segment, expecially in pigs. The dorsal ramus now ascends caudal to the transverse process where, in the pig, it is bridged by a bony lamella, and proceeds lateral to the m. multifidus to reach the skin as the *r. cutaneus medialis*.

In their course the dorsal intercostal arteries supply the bodies of the thoracic vertebrae, the vertebral canal and its contents, the muscles of the trunk, that part of the thoracic wall which is supported by the ribs, the thoracic part of the musculature of the pectoral girdle and the skin except over the shoulder blade. The *rr. cutanei laterales* and the muscle branches are arranged in series, especially in the region of the long back muscles. Two or three of these lateral vessels enter the longissimus dorsi and some run between it and the iliocostalis muscle. These lateral cutaneous rami from the sequential dorsal intercostal arteries progress towards the surface along with the lateral cutaneous rami of the dorsal spinal nerve branches, while the dorsal rami of the intercostal arteries continue as cutaneous vessels in company with the cutaneous branches of these dorsal spinal nerve branches.

Vessels of origin of the first and subsequent aa. intercostales dorsales

cat	I truncus costocervicalis	II + III a. intercostalis suprema	IV–XII aorta thoracica
dog	I truncus costocervicalis	II and on the right also III a. vertebralis thoracica	III (left), IV–XII aorta thoracica
pig	I + II Generally absent or represented by a slender branch of the artery which passes through the 1st or 2nd intercostal space	III–V a. intercostalis suprema	VI–XIV aorta thoracica
ruminants	I–III a. intercostalis suprema		IV–XII aorta thoracica
horse	I a. cervicalis profunda	II a. scapularis dorsalis	III + IV (V) a. intercostalis suprema	V–XVII aorta thoracica

A. costoabdominalis dorsalis

(Comparative: 85–88/36; cat: 90/15; pig: 97/20; horse: 50/22)

The thoracic aorta sends the **a. costoabdominalis dorsalis** to the last rib, the branches of this artery being typical of a dorsal intercostal artery. The name of this vessel indicates that it runs along the border between the thoracic and abdominal wall but that it is no longer situated in an intercostal space. Its area of supply extends into the lateral abdominal wall. In the dog and pig the dorsal costoabdominal artery is developed only in the proximal part of the last rib. In its place the pig has a branch of the cranial

122   Arteries

Fig. 89. A. intercostalis dorsalis and r. intercostalis ventralis of the horse. Transverse section through the thorax, diagrammatic. Caudal view.

A corpus vertebrae; *B* proc. spinosus; *C* costa; *D* sternum

a m. multifidus; *b* m. spinalis thoracis, m. longissimus thoracis; *c* m. iliocostalis; *d* m. serratus dorsalis; *e* m. serratus ventralis; *f* m. latissimus dorsi; *g* m. cutaneus trunci; *h* m. serratus ventralis; *i* m. pectoralis profundus, *k* m. transversus thoracis

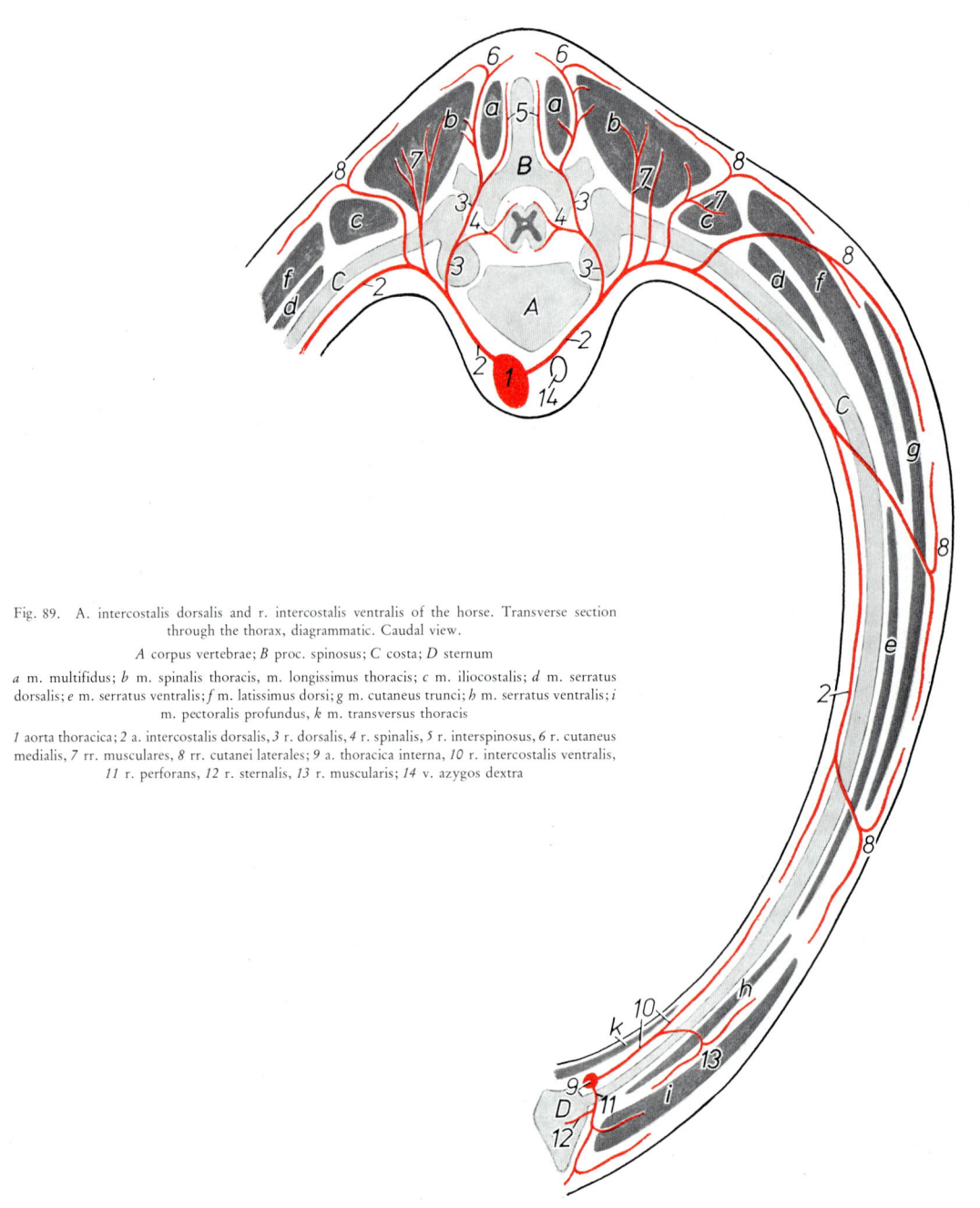

1 aorta thoracica; *2* a. intercostalis dorsalis, *3* r. dorsalis, *4* r. spinalis, *5* r. interspinosus, *6* r. cutaneus medialis, *7* rr. musculares; *8* rr. cutanei laterales; *9* a. thoracica interna, *10* r. intercostalis ventralis, *11* r. perforans, *12* r. sternalis, *13* r. muscularis; *14* v. azygos dextra

abdominal artery which vascularizes the distal part of the last rib. In the cat, ruminants and the horse, on the other hand, the dorsal costoabdominal artery continues beyond the last rib; in the ox it anastomoses with the *r. costoabdominalis ventralis* of the cranial epigastric artery.

A. phrenica cranialis

(horse: 50/24; 88, 103/37)

The **a. phrenica cranialis** occurs only in the horse. It arises at the level of the 16th thoracic vertebra as a slender vessel from the ventral wall of the thoracic aorta and immediately enters either the right or left crura of the diaphragm.

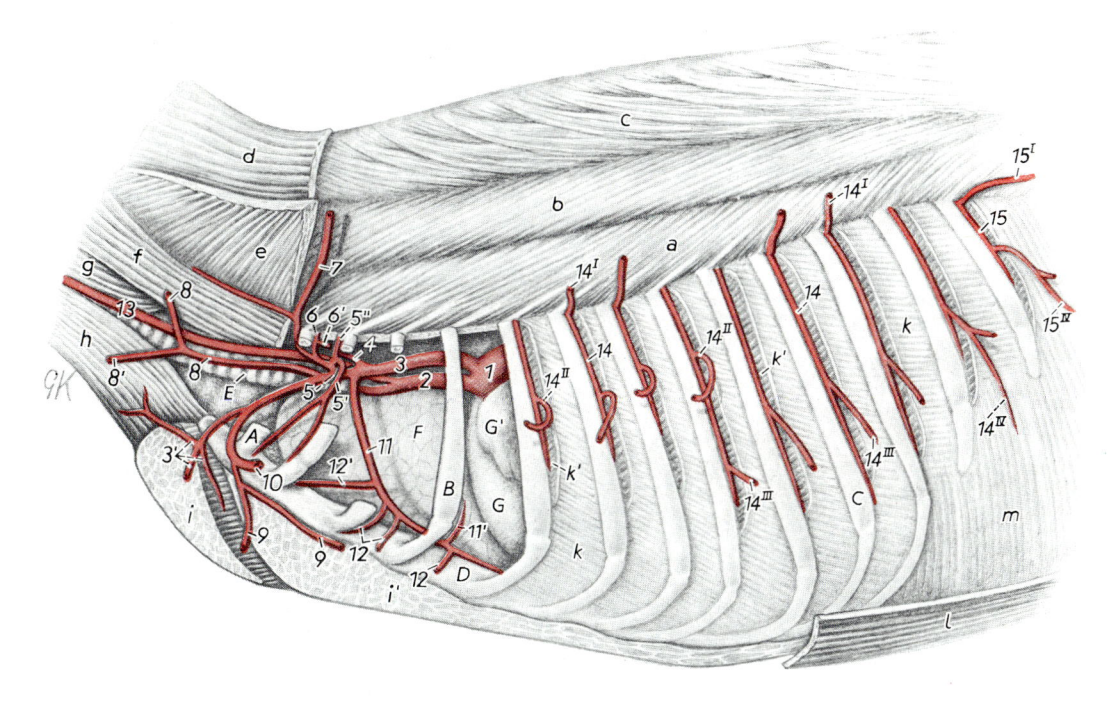

Fig. 90. Arteries of the thoracic inlet and of the thoracic wall of a cat. Left lateral view.
(After Opitz, 1961, Diss., Hanover.)

A I., *B* IV., *C* X. costa; *D* sternum; *E* trachea; *F* lobus cranialis pulmonis dextri; *G* cor; *G'* auricula sinistra

a m. iliocostalis thoracis; *b* m. longissimus thoracis; *c* mm. spinales et semispinales thoracis; *d* m. splenius; *e* m. serratus ventralis cervicis; *f* m. scalenus; *g* m. longus capitis; *h* m. sternocephalicus; *i* mm. pectorales superficiales; *i'* m. pectoralis profundus; *k* mm. intercostales externi; *k'* mm. intercostales interni; *l* m. rectus abdominis; *m* m. transversus abdominis

1 arcus aortae; *2* truncus brachiocephalicus; *3* a. subclavia sinistra; *3'* a. thoracica externa; *4* a. vertebralis; *5* truncus costocervicalis; *5'* a. intercostalis dorsalis I with r. collateralis; *5''* r. dorsalis; *6* a. cervicalis profunda; *6'* a. intercostalis suprema; *7* a. scapularis dorsalis; *8* a. cervicalis superficialis; *8'* r. ascendens; *9* a. thoracica lateralis; *10* a. axillaris; *11* a. thoracica interna; *11'* a. intercostalis ventralis; *12* rr. perforantes; *12'* common vessel of origin for the aa. intercostales ventrales I and II; *13* a. carotis communis; *14* aa. intercostales dorsales; *14'*, *14''*, *14'''*, *14^{iv}* rr. cutanei laterales; *15* a. costoabdominalis, *15'*, *15^{iv}* rr. cutanei laterales

Visceral arteries of the thoracic aorta

A. broncho-oesophagea

(Comparative: 85–88/38; dog: 94, 95/3, 7; sheep: 99/18; 100/1; ox: 155/3, 4; horse: 50/23; 103/27)

The **a. broncho-oesophagea** arises from the thoracic aorta or from one of the first three dorsal intercostal arteries which themselves stem from the thoracic aorta. It may be a paired or but a single vessel and the *r. bronchalis* and the *r. oesophageus* may each arise independently. In the cat both bronchial rami arise at the level of the 4th intercostal space from the thoracic aorta or the 5th dorsal intercostal artery and the oesophageal rami have variable points of origin. The dog has a right and a left broncho-oesophageal artery which arise from the 4th, 5th or 6th dorsal intercostal artery close to the thoracic aorta or, indeed, they may spring from the aorta itself. In the pig the thoracic aorta gives off a single broncho-oesophageal artery. In the small ruminants the origin of the unpaired broncho-oesophageal artery is at the level of the 6th and in the ox at the level of the 7th thoracic vertebra. The bronchial and oesophageal rami can also spring from the aorta independently. The unpaired and very short broncho-oesophageal artery of the horse arises, as in the ox, from the thoracic aorta or rarely the 5th or 6th dorsal intercostal artery at the level of the 6th thoracic vertebra. In the carnivore the bronchial ramus reaches the radix pulmonis on each side and subdivides in company with the bronchi as the nutritive vessels of the lung. In all the other domestic mammals the corresponding division of the bronchial ramus to each lung occurs in the region of the bronchial bifurcation. The oesophageal ramus and its branches supply the intrathoracic part of the oesophagus. In the pig, however, the oesophageal branch vascularizes that organ no further than the base of the heart.

124 Arteries

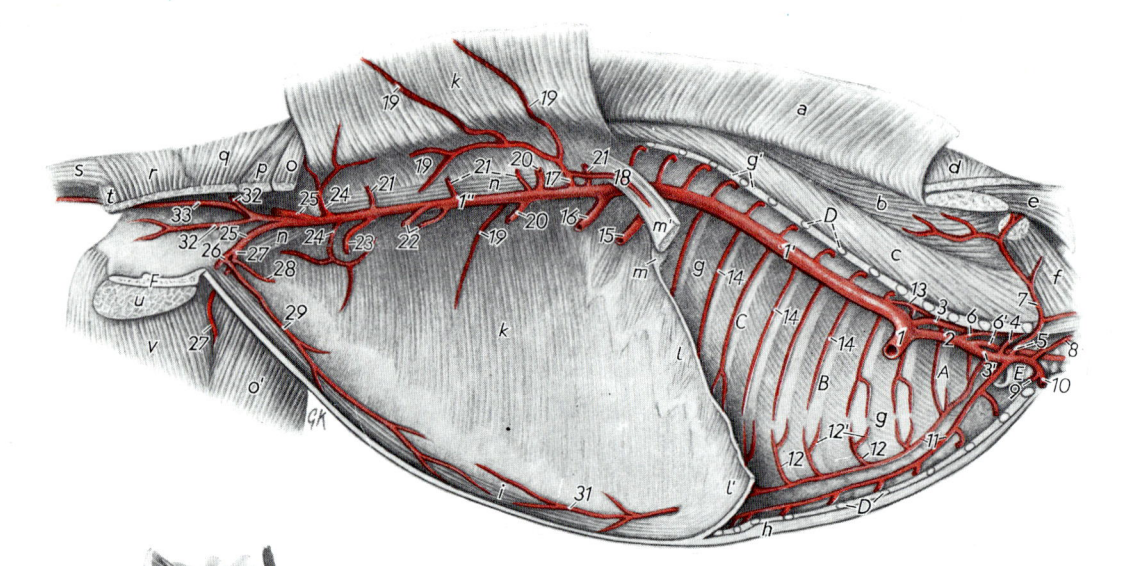

Fig. 91. Branches of the aorta and arteries to the body wall of a cat. View from the right and ventromedial.
(After Opitz, 1961, Diss., Hanover.)

A III., *B* VI., *C* IX. costa; *D* stumps of the right ribs or costal cartilages; *E* trachea; *F* symphysis pelvina

a m. latissimus dorsi; *b* mm. spinales et semispinales thoracis et cervicis; *c* mm. longissimi thoracis et cervicis; *d* m. trapezius; *e* mm. rhomboidei cervicis et capitis; *f* m. serratus ventralis cervicis; *g* mm. intercostales interni; *g'* mm. intercostales, cut surface; *h* m. pectoralis profundus; *i* m. rectus abdominis; *k* m. transversus abdominis; *l* diaphragma, pars costalis, *l'* pars sternalis, *m, m'* pars lumbalis; *n* m. psoas minor; *o* m. sartorius of the right, *o'* of the left pelvic limb; *p* m. tensor fasciae latae; *q* m. glutaeus medius; *r* m. glutaeus superficialis; *s* m. sacrocaudalis dorsalis lateralis; *t* m. abductor cruris cranialis; *u* mm. abductores, cut surface; *v* m. gracilis

1 arcus aortae; *1'* aorta thoracica; *1", 30* aorta abdominalis; *2* truncus brachiocephalicus; *3* a. subclavia sinistra; *3'* a. subclavia dextra; *4* a. vertebralis; *5* truncus costocervicalis; *6* a. carotis communis sinistra; *6'* a. carotis communis dextra; *7* a. scapularis dorsalis; *8* a. cervicalis superficialis; *9* a. thoracica externa; *10* a. axillaris; *11* a. thoracica interna sinistra or dextra; *12* aa. intercostales ventrales, *12'* rr. collaterales; *13* common vessel of origin for the aa. intercostales dorsales III, IV and V; *14* aa. intercostales dorsales; *15* a. coeliaca; *16* a. mesenterica cranialis; *17* common vessel of origin for *18* a. phrenica caudalis and *19* a. abdominalis cranialis; *20* aa. renales; *21* aa. lumbales; *22* aa. ovaricae; *23* a. mesenterica caudalis; *24* aa. circumflexae ilium profundae; *25* aa. iliacae externae; *26* a. profunda femoris; *27* a. femoralis; *28* a. abdominalis caudalis; *29* a. epigastrica caudalis; *30* aorta abdominalis; *31* a. epigastrica cranialis; *32* aa. iliacae internae; *33* a. sacralis mediana

Fig. 93. Arteries and veins of the ventral body wall of a bitch. Ventral view.
(After Zietzschmann, 1943.)

I, II, III, IV gll. mammariae

a a. and v. thoracica interna, rr. sternales and rr. mammarii of the rr. perforantes; *b* a. and v. epigastrica cranialis superficialis, rr. mammarii; *c* a. and v. epigastrica caudalis superficialis with the rr. mammarii; *c'* r. labialis ventralis of the a. and v. pudenda externa; *d* a. and v. thoracica lateralis with rr. mammarii

1 mm. pectorales superficiales; *2* m. pectoralis profundus; *3* proc. vaginalis; *4* vulva

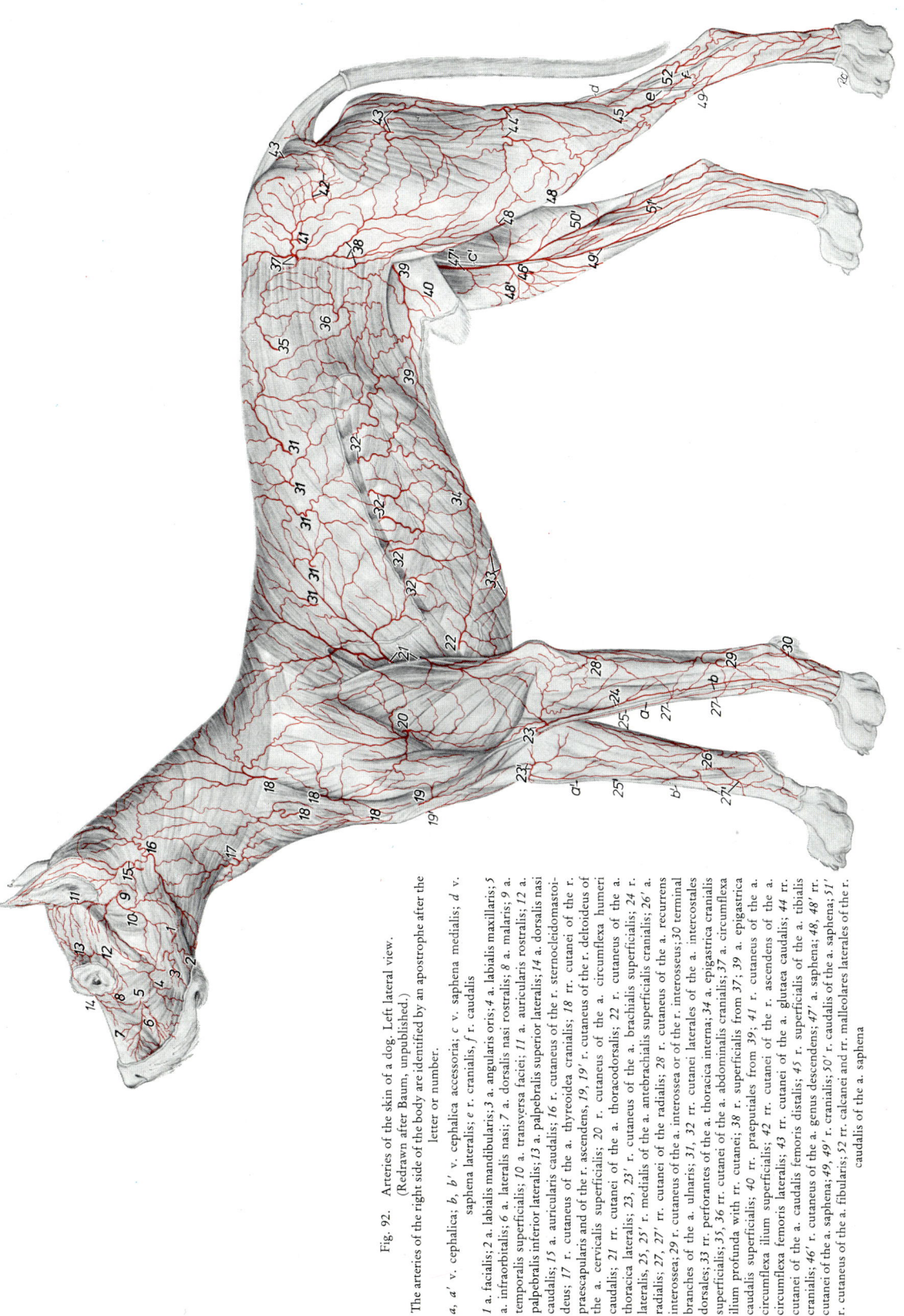

Arteries of the thorax and abdomen

Fig. 92. Arteries of the skin of a dog. Left lateral view.
(Redrawn after Baum, unpublished.)

The arteries of the right side of the body are identified by an apostrophe after the letter or number.

a, a' v. cephalica; *b, b'* v. cephalica accessoria; *c* v. saphena medialis; *d* v. saphena lateralis; *e* r. cranialis; *f* r. caudalis

1 a. facialis; *2* a. labialis mandibularis; *3* a. angularis oris; *4* a. labialis maxillaris; *5* a. infraorbitalis; *6* a. lateralis nasi; *7* a. dorsalis nasi rostralis; *8* a. malaris; *9* a. temporalis superficialis; *10* a. transversa faciei; *11* a. auricularis rostralis; *12* a. palpebralis inferior lateralis; *13* a. palpebralis superior lateralis; *14* a. dorsalis nasi caudalis; *15* a. auricularis caudalis; *16* r. cutaneus of the r. sternocleidomastoideus; *17* r. cutaneus of the a. thyreoidea cranialis; *18* rr. cutanei of the r. praescapularis and of the r. ascendens, *19, 19'* r. cutaneus of the r. deltoideus of the a. cervicalis superficialis; *20* r. cutaneus of the a. circumflexa humeri caudalis; *21* rr. cutanei of the a. thoracodorsalis; *22* r. cutaneus of the a. thoracica lateralis; *23, 23'* r. cutaneus of the a. brachialis superficialis; *24* r. lateralis, *25, 25'* r. medialis of the a. antebrachialis superficialis cranialis; *26'* a. radialis; *27, 27'* rr. cutanei of the r. radialis; *28* r. cutaneus of the a. recurrens interossea; *29* r. cutaneus of the a. interossea or of the r. interosseus; *30* terminal branches of the a. ulnaris; *31, 32* rr. cutanei laterales of the a. intercostales dorsales; *33* rr. perforantes of the a. thoracica interna; *34* a. epigastrica cranialis superficialis; *35, 36* rr. cutanei of the a. abdominalis cranialis; *37* a. circumflexa ilium profunda with rr. cutanei; *38* r. superficialis from *37*; *39* a. epigastrica caudalis superficialis; *40* rr. praeputiales from *39*; *41* rr. cutanei of the a. circumflexa ilium superficialis; *42* rr. cutanei of the r. ascendens of the a. circumflexa femoris lateralis; *43* rr. cutanei of the a. glutaea caudalis; *44* rr. cutanei of the a. caudalis femoris distalis; *45* r. superficialis of the a. tibialis cranialis; *46* r. cutaneus of the a. genus descendens; *47'* a. saphena; *48, 48'* rr. cutanei of the a. saphena; *49, 49'* r. cranialis; *50'* r. caudalis of the a. saphena; *51'* r. cutaneus of the a. fibularis; *52* rr. calcanei and rr. malleolares laterales of the r. caudalis of the a. saphena

Fig. 94. Arteria and vena broncho-oesophagea sinistra of a dog.
(After Stitz, 1936, Diss., Hanover.)

a trachea; *b* oesophagus

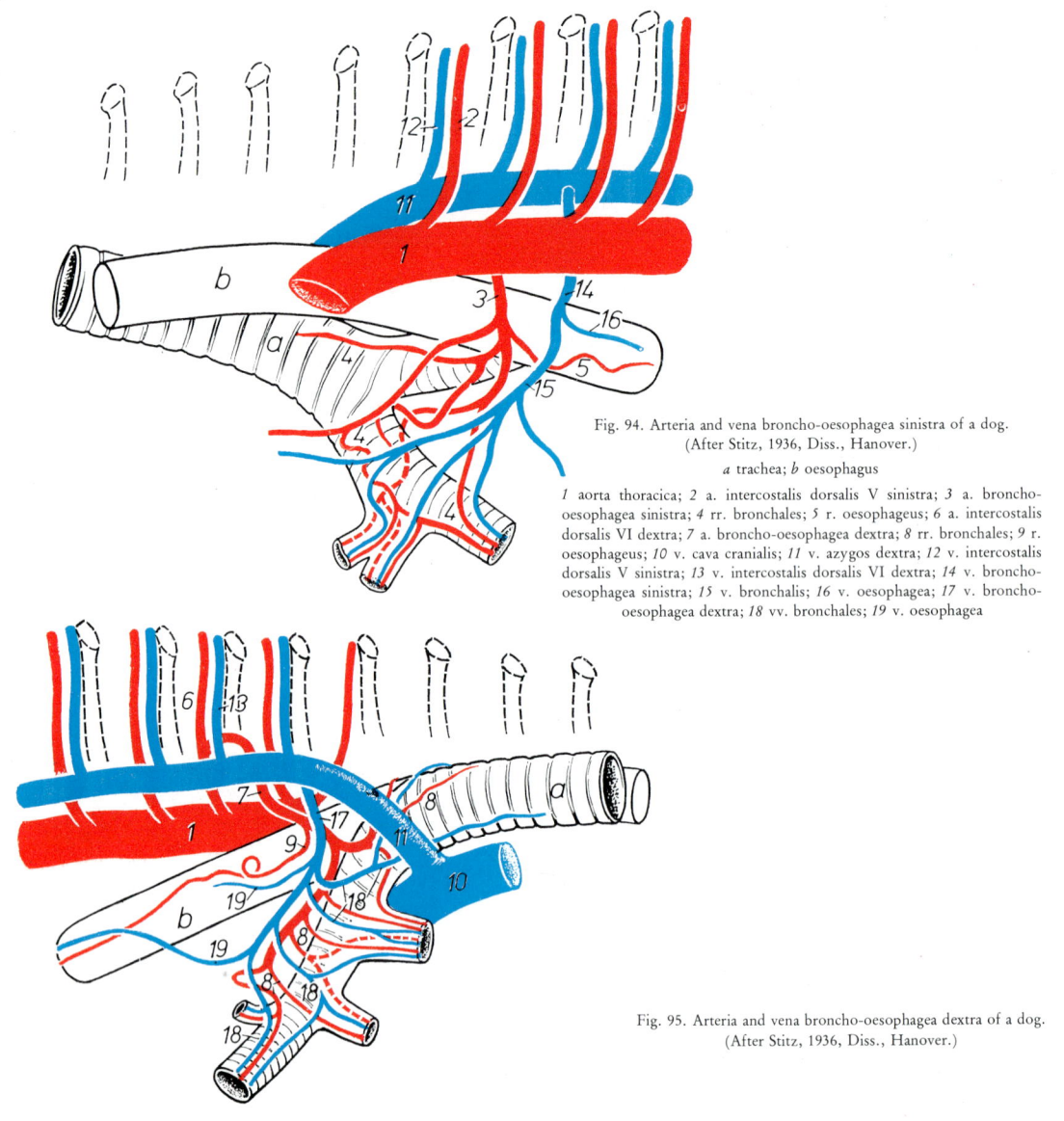

1 aorta thoracica; *2* a. intercostalis dorsalis V sinistra; *3* a. broncho-oesophagea sinistra; *4* rr. bronchales; *5* r. oesophageus; *6* a. intercostalis dorsalis VI dextra; *7* a. broncho-oesophagea dextra; *8* rr. bronchales; *9* r. oesophageus; *10* v. cava cranialis; *11* v. azygos dextra; *12* v. intercostalis dorsalis V sinistra; *13* v. intercostalis dorsalis VI dextra; *14* v. broncho-oesophagea sinistra; *15* v. bronchalis; *16* v. oesophagea; *17* v. broncho-oesophagea dextra; *18* vv. bronchales; *19* v. oesophagea

Fig. 95. Arteria and vena broncho-oesophagea dextra of a dog.
(After Stitz, 1936, Diss., Hanover.)

In all animals the thoracic aorta gives off further *rr. oesophagei*. In the pig, these vascularize only the caudal part of the oesophagus. The *rr. pericardiaci* and *mediastinales* also stem from the aorta. All the above-mentioned branches of the thoracic aorta participate in the blood supply to the lymph nodes which are situated within their distribution area.

Aorta abdominalis

(Comparative: 85–88/*39*; 105–108, 136–143/*1*; cat: 91/*1″*, 30; 109/*1*; dog: 110/*1*; pig: 97, 111/*1*; 98/*1″*; sheep: 101/*1″*; 112/*1*; ox: 113/*1*; horse: 50/*25*; 104, 114/*1*; 211/*1′*)

From the point of view of comparative anatomy, the place where the thoracic aorta becomes the abdominal aorta is located at the thoracic side of the *hiatus aorticus*. For this reason the arteries supplying the lumbar region, the lateral abdominal wall and the abdominal viscera are all tributaries of the aorta abdominalis. The reader is referred to the summary of the aorta on page 72.

Aa. lumbales

(Comparative: 85–88/*40*; cat: 91/*21*; 109/*5*; dog: 110/*2*; pig: 97/*18*; 98/*20*; 111/*2, 2'*; sheep: 101/*21*; 112/*4, 6*; ox: 113/*1', 1"*; horse: 50/*26*)

In the various domestic mammals the paired **aa. lumbales** correspond in number to the lumbar vertebrae and the majority leave the dorsal wall of the abdominal aorta as segmental vessels. In carnivores, small ruminants and the pig the last lumbar artery arises from the *a. sacralis mediana,* in the ox it comes off the *a. iliolumbalis* and in the horse the last two lumbar arteries branch from the *a. iliaca*

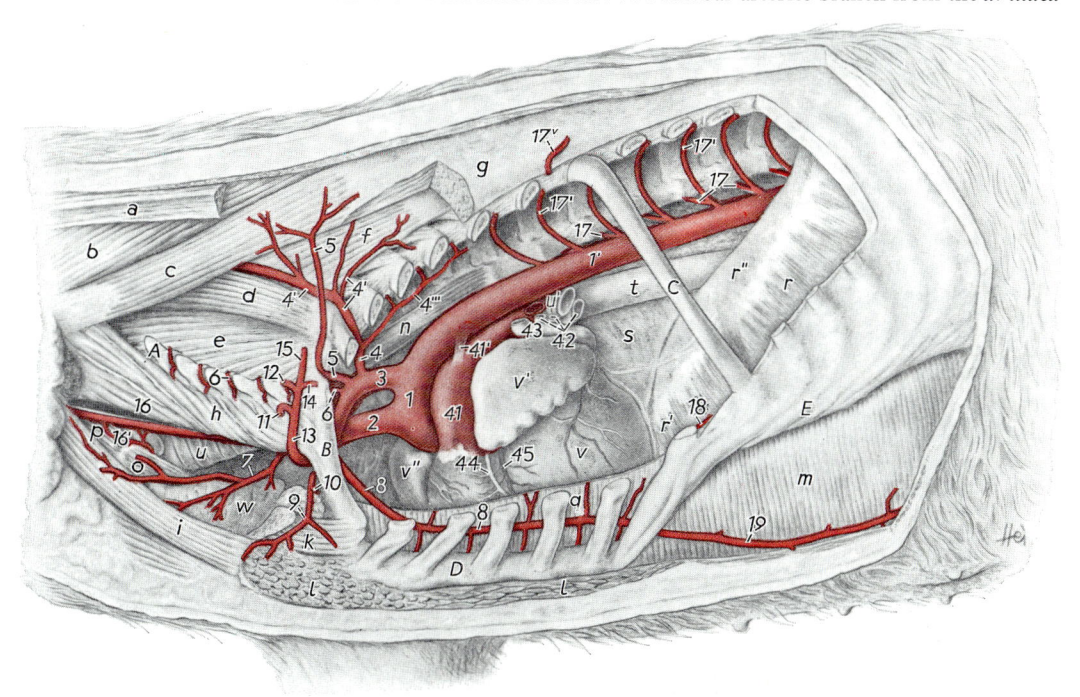

Fig. 96. Arteries of the thoracic cavity of a pig. Left lateral view.
(After Kähler, 1960, Diss., Hanover.)

A vertebra cervicalis III, proc. transversus; *B* costa I; *C* costa VIII; *D* sternum; *E* arcus costalis

a m. rhomboideus; *b* m. splenius capitis; *c* m. splenius cervicis; *d* m. complexus; *e* mm. spinales thoracis et cervicis; *f* m. multifidus; *g* m. longissimus thoracis; *h* m. iliocostalis cervicis; *i* m. sternomastoideus; *k* m. scalenus ventralis; *l* mm. pectorales superficiales and m. pectoralis profundus; *m* m. transversus abdominis; *n* m. longus colli; *o* m. sternothyreoideus; *p* m. sternohyoideus; *q* m. transversus thoracis; *r–r"* diaphragma: *r* pars costalis, *r'* pars sternalis, *r"* centrum tendineum; *s* mediastinum; *t* oesophagus; *u* trachea; *u'* bronchus principalis; *v* ventriculus sinister; *v'* auricula sinistra; *v"* auricula dextra; *w* thymus

1 arcus aortae; *1'* aorta thoracica; *2* truncus brachiocephalicus; *3* a. subclavia sinistra; *4* truncus costocervicalis; *4'* a. cervicalis profunda; *4"* a. intercostalis suprema; *5* a. scapularis dorsalis; *6* a. vertebralis; *7* a. cervicalis superficialis; *8* a. thoracica interna; *9* a. thoracica externa; *10* a. thoracica lateralis; *11* a. brachialis; *12* a. suprascapularis; *13* a. axillaris (dorsally displaced); *14* a. subscapularis; *15* a. thoracodorsalis; *16* a. carotis communis; *16'* a. thyreoidea cranialis; *17* aa. intercostales dorsales sinistrae; *17'* a. intercostalis dorsalis dextra; *17ᵛ* r. cutaneus lateralis; *18* a. musculophrenica; *19* a. epigastrica cranialis; *41* truncus pulmonales; *41'* lig. arteriosum; *42* vv. pulmonales; *43* v. azygos sinistra; *44* r. interventricularis paraconalis of the a. coronaria sinistra; *45* v. cordis magna

interna. The arteries for one and the same segment can have a common origin. The pattern of branching of the lumbar artery resembles that of the dorsal intercostalis.

Lateral to each appropriate lumbar vertebra, the a. lumbalis curves to the caudal border of the transverse process and immediately gives off a branch to the body of the vertebra. This branch is followed by the *r. spinalis* which supplies the spinal canal and cord, and the *r. dorsalis* which courses through the musculature of the back, to which it supplies branches, and finally ends as a cutaneous branch. The main trunk of the lumbar artery, which follows the caudal border of the lumbar transverse process, supplies dorsally-directed branches to the trunk muscles and these branches, like the dorsal intercostal arteries, are arranged in rows corresponding to the course of the long muscles of the back. Some of these branches participate in the vascularization of the skin of the back. Ventrally directed branches go to the inner lumbar musculature. Only in the horse is it possible to follow the lumbar arteries beyond the transverse processes of the lumbar vertebrae between the transverse and internal

128   Arteries

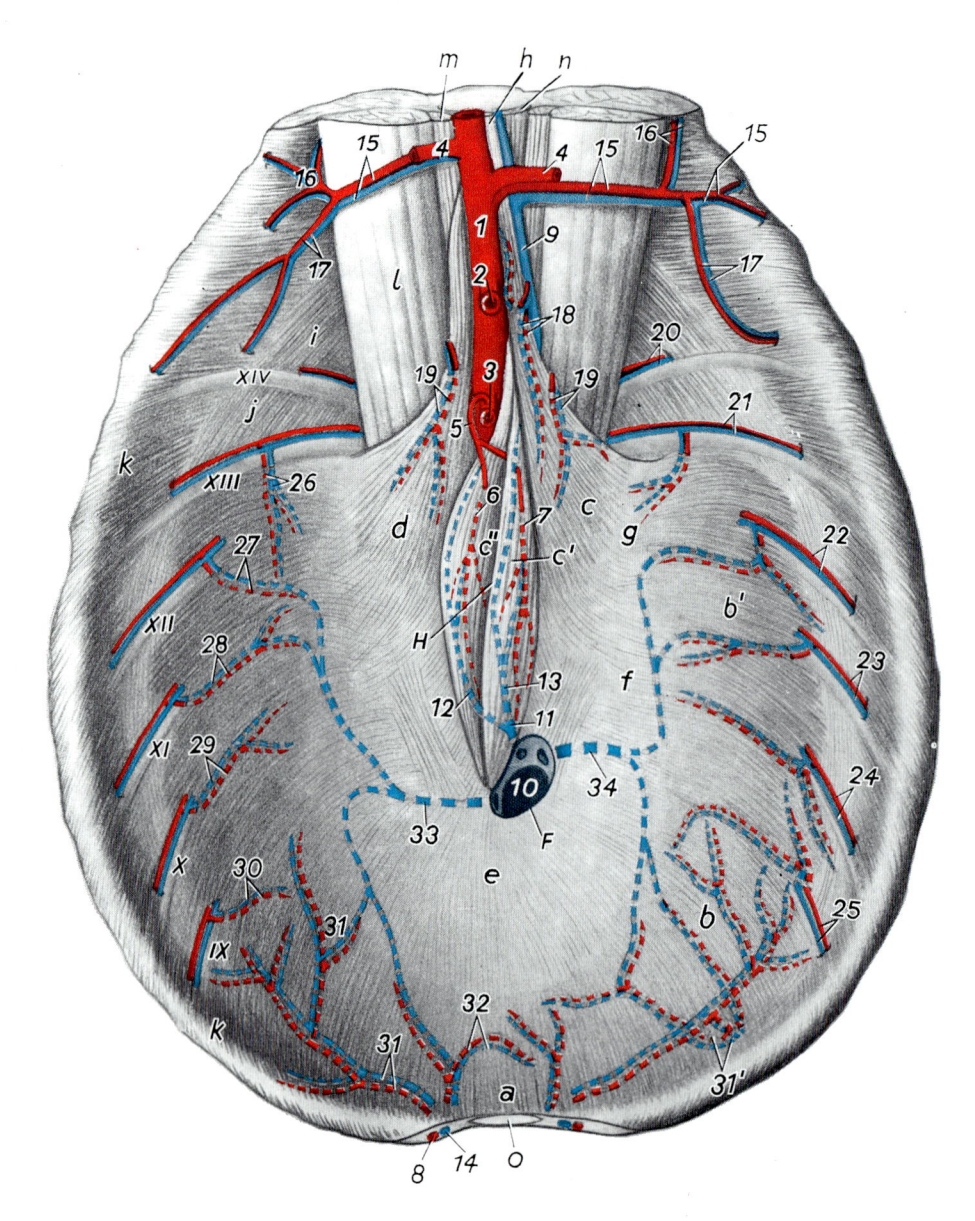

Fig. 97. Arteries and veins of the diaphragm of a pig. Caudal view.
(After Biermann, 1953, Diss., Hanover.)
F for. venae cavae; *H* hiatus oesophageus

a–h diaphragma: *a* pars sternalis, *b*, *b'* pars costalis, *c*, *c'*, *c''* crus dextrum, *d* crus sinistrum of the pars lumbalis, *e*, *f*, *g* centrum tendineum, *h* tendon of origin of the pars lumbalis; *i* m. retractor costae; *j* m. intercostalis internus; *k* m. transversus abdominis; *l* m. psoas major; *m* m. psoas minor; *n* m. quadratus lumborum; *o* proc. xiphoideus; IX–XIV costae IX–XIV

1 aorta abdominalis; *2* a. mesenterica cranialis; *3* a. coeliaca; *4* a. renalis; *5* a. phrenica caudalis, *6* branch to the crus mediale sinistrum, *7* branch to the crus mediale dextrum; *8* a. epigastrica cranialis; *9* v. hemiazygos dextra; *10* v. cava caudalis; *11* v. phrenica cranialis from the crura medialia, *12* branch from the crus mediale sinistrum, *13* branch from the crus mediale dextrum; *14* v. epigastrica cranialis; *15* a. and v. abdominalis cranialis, *16* r. caudalis, *17* r. cranialis; *18* rr. phrenici of the a. and v. lumbalis I; *19* rr. phrenici from *20* a. and v. costoabdominalis; *21–25* aa. and vv. intercostales dorsales XIII–IX, *26–30* rr. phrenici; *31* a. and v. musculophrenica, *31'* rr. phrenici; *32* r. phrenicus of the a. and v. epigastrica cranialis; *33* v. phrenica cranialis sinistra; *34* v. phrenica cranialis dextra

oblique abdominal muscles, to which muscles they supply branches. In the pig and ruminants the first pair of lumbar arteries send *rr. phrenici* to the crura of the diaphragm. The *rr. suprarenales* to the adrenal glands are given off the 1st and 2nd lumbar arteries in the small ruminants and the 2nd lumbar artery in the ox. In the dog, also, the adrenal glands receive branches from the lumbar arteries.

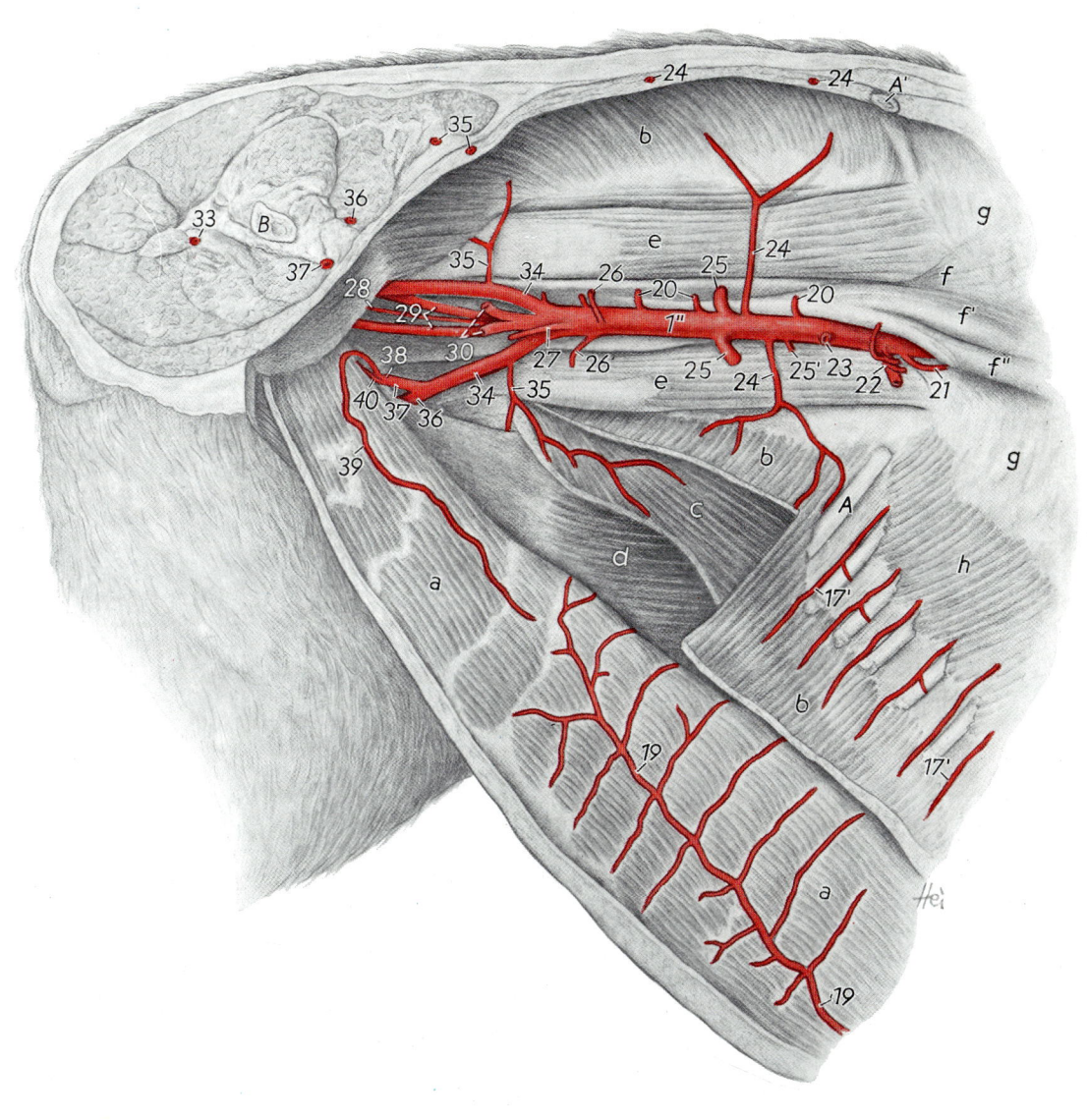

Fig. 98. Arteries of the abdominal cavity and wall of a pig. Left ventrolateral view.
(After Kähler, 1960, Diss., Hanover.)

A, A' costa XIV sinistra and dextra; *B* os femoris, transected distal to the greater trochanter

a m. rectus abdominis; *b* m. transversus abdominis; *c* m. obliquus internus abdominis; *d* m. obliquus externus abdominis; *e* m. psoas major; *f–h* diaphragma: *f* crus laterale dextrum, *f'* crus mediale dextrum, *f''* crus mediale sinistrum, *g* centrum tendineum, *h* pars costalis

1'' aorta abdominalis; *17'* aa. intercostales dorsales; *19* a. epigastrica cranialis; *20* aa. lumbales; *21* a. phrenica caudalis; *22* a. coeliaca; *23* a. mesenterica cranialis; *24* a. abdominalis cranialis; *25* a. renalis; *25'* a. suprarenalis media; *26* a. ovarica; *27* a. mesenterica caudalis; *28* a. sacralis mediana; *29* a. iliaca interna; *30* a. umbilicalis; *33* a. glutaea caudalis; *34* a. iliaca externa; *35* a. circumflexa ilium profunda; *36* a. femoralis; *37* a. profunda femoris; *38* truncus pudendoepigastricus; *39* a. epigastrica caudalis; *40* a. pudenda externa

A. phrenica caudalis

(Comparative: 85–87/*42*; cat: 91/*18*; dog: 125/*2*; pig: 97/*5*; 98/*21*; 126/*2*; sheep: 101/*19'*, *19''*; ox: 127/*2*)

The **a. phrenica caudalis** is absent in the horse. In carnivores it arises, together with the *a. abdominalis cranialis*, at the level of the 2nd lumbar vertebra either from the angle between the abdominal aorta and the renal artery or from the renal artery itself. Sometimes in the dog the caudal phrenic artery may arise from the thoracic aorta in the region of the aortic hiatus. In the pig and ruminants, and occasionally also the cat, this artery arises as a single branch from the coeliac, but in the ox there may be separate branches to the right and left diaphragmatic crura respectively. In the pig and the ox it may leave the abdominal aorta directly. The caudal phrenic artery runs dorsal to the adrenal gland, giving off *rr. suprarenales craniales* to it, and continuing in a cranial direction it enters the crus of the diaphragm where it ramifies. This completes the arterial blood supply to the pars muscularis of the diaphragm up to the centrum tendineum.

A. abdominalis cranialis
(cat: 91/*19*; dog: 85/*43*; 92/*35, 36*; pig: 96/*43*; 97/*15*; 98/*24*)

In carnivores the **a. abdominalis cranialis** and the a. phrenica caudalis arise by a common trunk from the abdominal aorta. The cranial abdominal artery turns towards the lateral wall of the abdomen, thereby crossing the inner lumbar musculature. After giving off the cranial suprarenal rami and branches to the inner lumbar musculature and to the iliocostalis muscle, it passes through the transverse

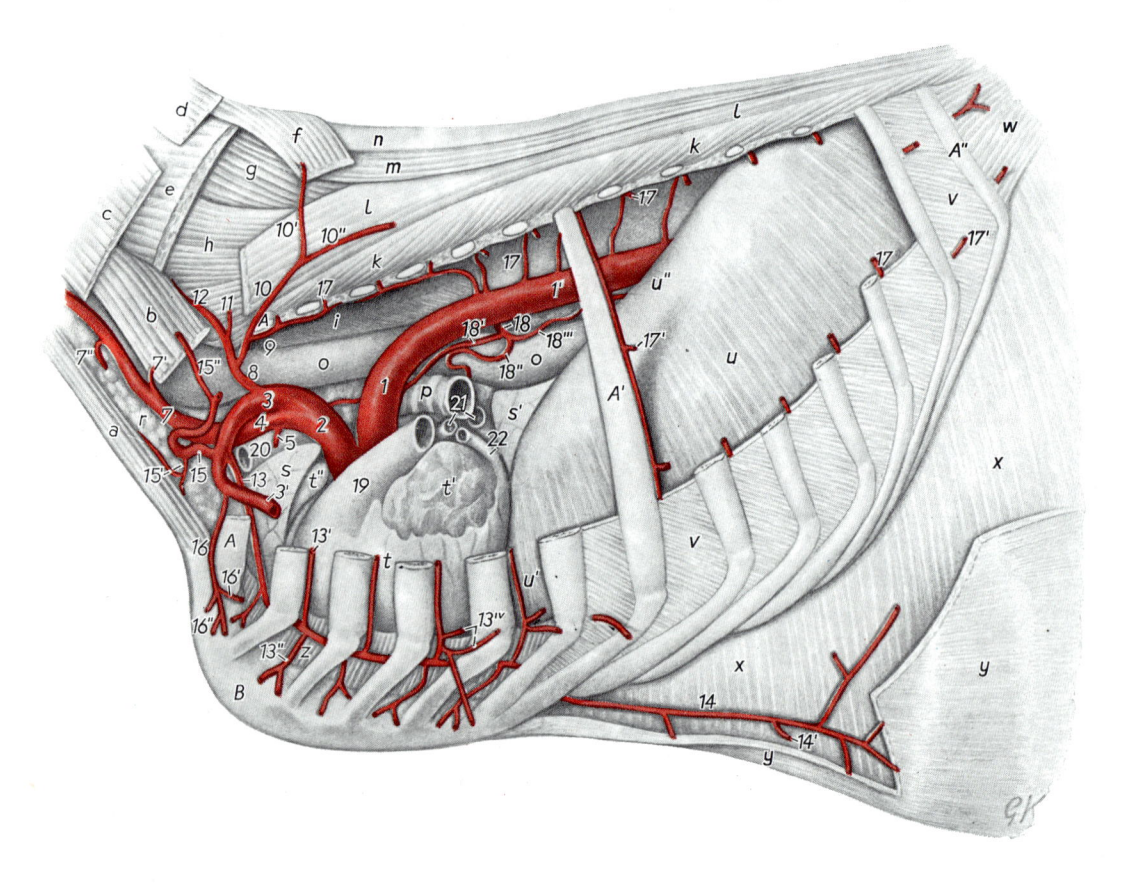

Fig. 99. Arteries of the thoracic cavity of a sheep. Left lateral view.
(After Münter, 1962, Diss., Hanover.)

A costa I; *A'* costa VII; *A"* costa XIII; *B* sternum

a m. sternomastoideus; *b* m. scalenus ventralis; *c* m. brachiocephalicus; *d* m. trapezius, pars cervicalis; *e* m. serratus ventralis cervicis; *f* m. rhomboideus cervicis; *g* m. semispinalis capitis; *h* m. longissimus cervicis; *i* m. longus colli; *k* m. iliocostalis thoracis; *l* m. longissimus thoracis; *m* mm. spinalis et semispinalis thoracis et cervicis; *n* expansion of nuchal ligament at withers; *o* oesophagus; *p* trachea; *r* thymus, cervical part; *s* lobus cranialis, *s'* lobus accessorius of the right lung; *t* cor; *t'* auricula sinistra; *t"* auricula dextra; *u–u"* diaphragma: *u* pars costalis, *u'* pars sternalis, *u"* centrum tendineum; *v* mm. intercostales externi; *w* m. retractor costae; *x* m. transversus abdominis; *y* m. rectus abdominis; *z* m. transversus thoracis

1 arcus aortae; *1'* aorta thoracica; *2, 4* truncus brachiocephalicus; *3* a. subclavia sinistra; *3'* a. axillaris; *5* r. thymicus; *7* a. carotis communis sinistra, *7'* r. muscularis, *7"* r. trachealis; *8* truncus costocervicalis; *9* a. intercostalis suprema; *10, 10', 10"* a. scapularis dorsalis; *11* a. cervicalis profunda; *12* a. vertebralis; *13* a. thoracica interna, *13'* rr. intercostales ventrales, *13"* rr. perforantes, *13^{iv}* rr. musculares; *14* a. epigastrica cranialis, *14'* a. epigastrica cranialis superficialis; *15* a. cervicalis superficialis, *15'* r. deltoideus, *15"* r. ascendens; *16, 16', 16"* a. thoracica externa; *17* aa. intercostales dorsales, *17'* r. cutaneus lateralis; *18* a. broncho-oesophagea, *18', 18"* r. bronchialis, *18'''* r. oesophageus; *19* truncus pulmonalis; *20* v. cava cranialis; *21* vv. pulmonales; *22* v. azygos sinistra

Fig. 100. A. bronchialis of a sheep. Dorsal view.
(After Härtl, 1942, Diss., Hanover.)

A aorta thoracica; *B* oesophagus; *C* trachea; *D* bronchus lobaris caudalis sinister; *E* bronchus lobaris caudalis dexter; *F* bronchus trachealis (Bronchus lobaris cranialis dexter); *G* bronchus lobaris cranialis sinister; *H* bronchus lobaris intermedius; *J* bronchus lobaris accessorius; I–V bronchi segmentales dorsales and ventrales

1 a. broncho-oesophagea; *2, 5–9* rr. bronchales; *3* branch to the lymph node; *4* r. oesophageus

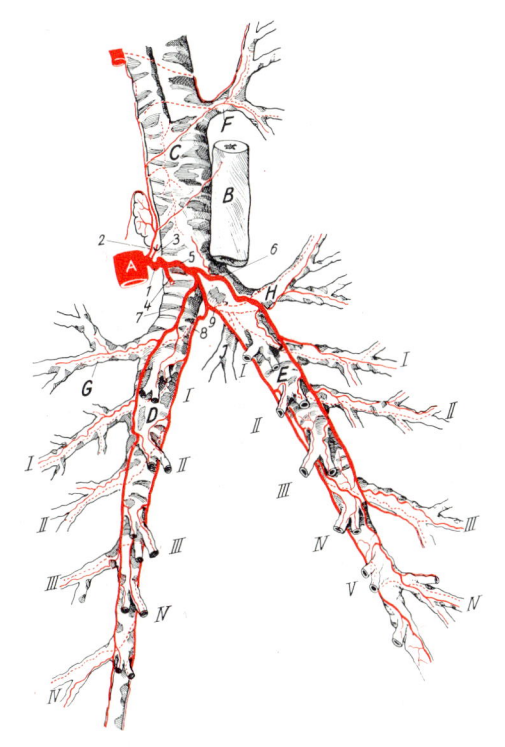

abdominis muscle and courses between it and the internal oblique abdominis muscle. It divides into two diverging branches of roughly equal calibre which convey blood to the cranial part of the abdominal wall and also perforate the superficial muscles as far as the skin. In the cat its branches attain the level of the stifle fold. In the pig the cranial abdominal artery springs from the abdominal aorta at the level of the 3rd lumbar vertebra; it runs over the inner lumbar muscles into the lateral abdominal wall and here it divides into two divergent branches. One limb of the cranial branch runs along the distal part of the caudal border of the last rib. There are anastomoses between the cranial abdominal and neighbouring arteries in the lateral and ventral abdominal wall of the pig and carnivores.

A. circumflexa ilium profunda

(Comparative: 85–88/*50*; 105–108/*10*; 136–143/*8*; cat: 91/*24*; 109/*4*; dog: 92/*41*; 110/*4*; pig: 98/*35*; 111/*6*; sheep: 101/*28*; 112/*8*; ox: 113/*20*; 144/*8*; horse: 50/*28*; 104/*13*; 114/*3*)

The **a. circumflexa ilium profunda** arises in carnivores from the abdominal aorta at the level of the 6th lumbar vertebra. In the other domestic animals, and occasionally even in the dog, it originates from the external iliac artery. In the ox and especially in the horse it may also arise from the angle at the origin of the external iliac artery. In all the domestic animals it crosses the inner lumbar muscles ventrally and perforates the transverse abdominis muscle and then divides into a *r. cranialis* and *r. caudalis*. These two rami proceed between the m. transversus abdominis and the m. obliquus internus abdominis which they supply with branches. The lnn. iliaci laterales are situated in the bifurcation of these rami. The caudal ramus gives off the *r. superficialis* which perforates the external oblique abdominis muscle in a lateral direction and meets the n. cutaneus femoris lateralis with which it continues to the tensor fasciae latae muscle and the stifle fold. There it supplies blood to the lnn. subiliaci in all the domestic mammals except carnivores in which these lymph nodes are absent.

In carnivores the division is less typical and the r. cranialis is the thinner of the two branches. In these species the caudal ramus participates to only an insignificant degree in the supply of the abdominal musculature. On the other hand, its superficial ramus is by far the most prominent of the branches of the deep circumflex iliac artery in the dog. This ramus gives off branches not only to the stifle fold and the lateral surface on the thigh but also branches running in the cutaneus trunci muscle to the lateral

132   Arteries

abdominal wall, and dorsally directed branches to the skin of the lumbar and gluteal regions. In the pig, too, the caudal branch runs immediately peripherally as the superficial ramus and divides as in the dog although the dorsal branches do not extend as far as the lumbar and gluteal regions. In ruminants and the horse, which do not have an a. abdominalis cranialis, the *a. circumflexa ilium profunda* supplies the lateral wall of the abdomen by means of its cranial and caudal rami. In the horse these extend

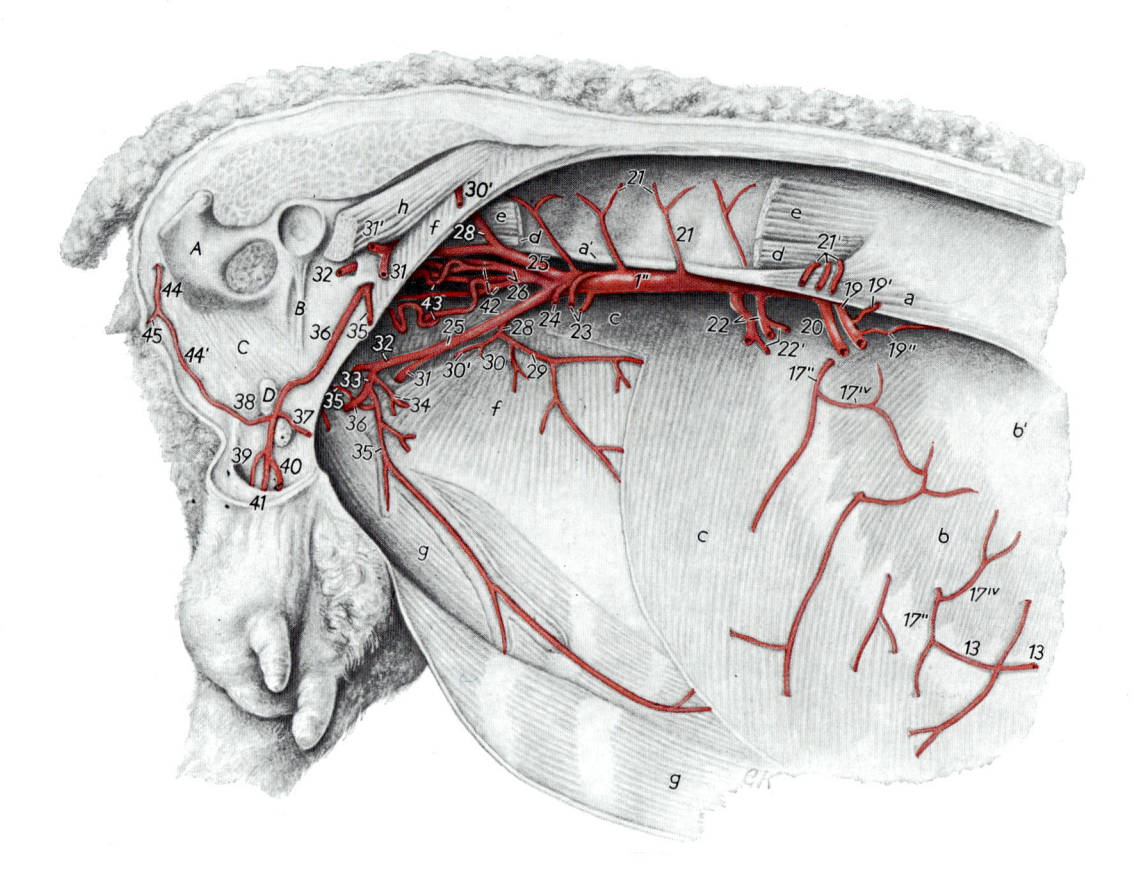

Fig. 101. Arteries of the abdominal and pelvic cavities and of the abdominal wall of a sheep. Right and medial view.
(After Münter, 1962, Diss., Hanover.)

A os ischii; *B* tendo praepubicus; *C* tendo symphysialis; *D* lnn. mammarii

a–b' diaphragma; *a* crus dextrum, *a'* tendon of origin, *b* pars costalis, *b'* centrum tendineum; *c* m. transversus abdominalis (caudal part of the muscle removed); *d* m. psoas minor; *e* m. psoas major (middle part of both muscles has been excised); *f* m. obliquus internus abdominis; *g* m. rectus abdominis; *h* m. iliacus

1" aorta abdominalis; *13* a. musculophrenica; *17"* aa. intercostales dorsales, *17^iv* r. phrenicus; *19* a. coeliaca; *19', 19"* aa. phrenicae caudales; *20* a. mesenterica cranialis; *21* aa. lumbales; *21'* rr. suprarenales craniales; *22* a. renalis; *22'* rr. suprarenales caudales; *23* a. ovarica; *24* a. mesenterica caudalis; *25* a. iliaca externa; *26* a. iliaca interna; *28* a. circumflexa ilium profunda, *29* r. cranialis, *30* r. caudalis, *30'* r. superficialis; *31* a. femoralis; *31'* a. circumflexa femoris lateralis; *32* a. profunda femoris; *33* truncus pudendoepigastricus; *34* a. abdominalis caudalis; *35* a. epigastrica caudalis; *36* a. pudenda externa; *37* a. epigastrica caudalis superficialis (a. mammaria cranialis); *38* r. labialis ventralis (a. mammaria caudalis); *39, 40, 41* rr. mammarii; *42* a. umbilicalis; *43* a. uterina; *44* a. perinealis ventralis, *44'* r. mammarius *45* r. labialis dorsalis

craniomedially to beyond the costal arch. The superficial ramus in the ox, and especially the horse, is confined to the regions of the stifle fold and the upper thigh. The peripheral branches of the deep circumflex iliac artery can anastomose with neighbouring vessels and in this context special mention should be made of the possible connection of the superficial ramus with the *a. epigastrica caudalis superficialis*, the mammary artery in females.

The visceral arteries of the abdominal aorta will be discussed together with the visceral arteries of the pelvic cavity (see p. 159).

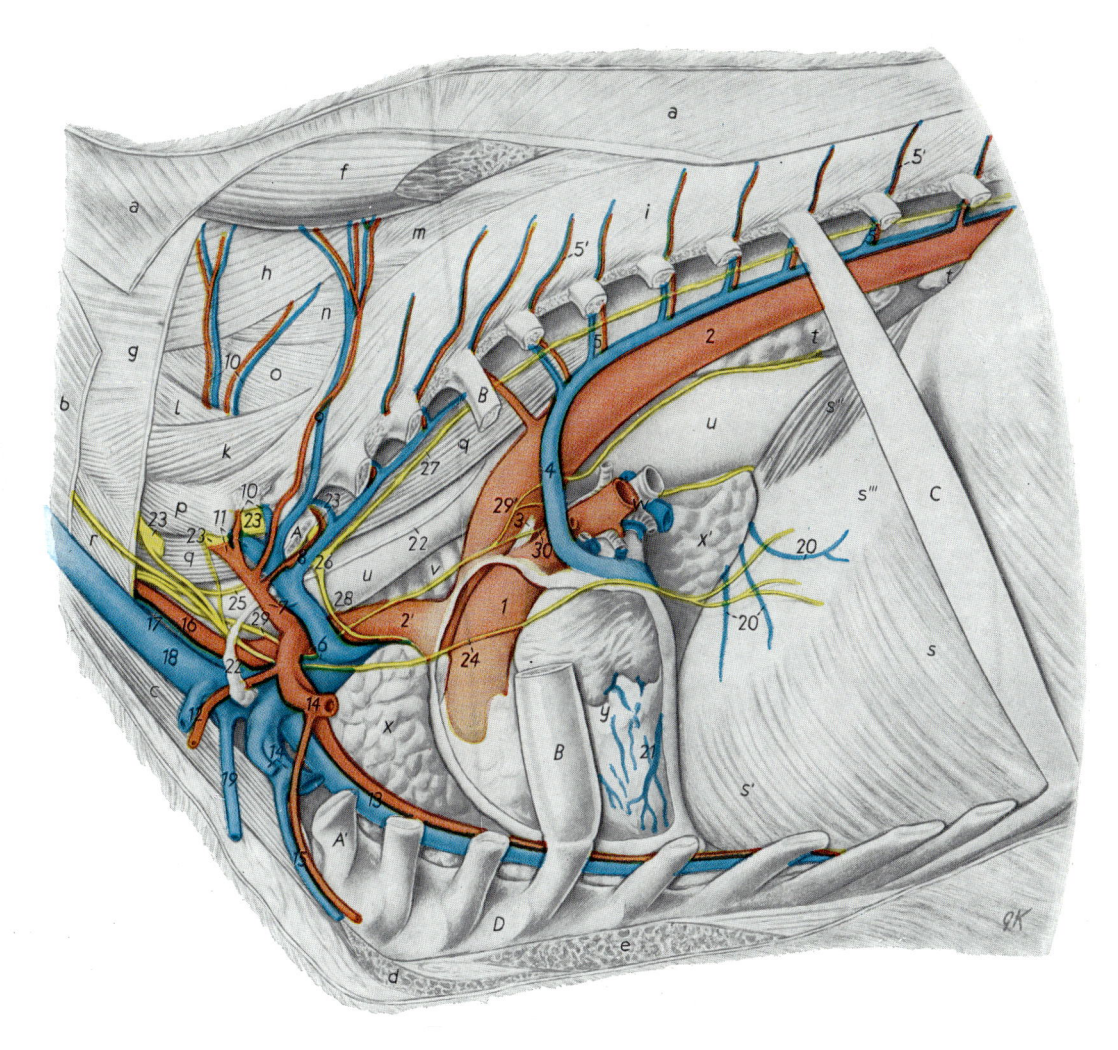

Fig. 102. Arteries and veins of the thoracic cavity of an ox. Pleural mediastinum has been removed. Left lateral view.
A, A' costa I; *B* costa IV; *C* costa IX; *D* sternum

a m. trapezius; *b* m. brachiocephalicus; *c* m. sternocephalicus; *d* mm. pectorales superficiales; *e* m. pectoralis profundus; *f* m. rhomboideus cervicis; *g* m. serratus ventralis cervicis; *h* m. splenius; *i* m. longissimus thoracis; *k* m. longissimus cervicis; *l* mm. longissimi capitis et atlantis; *m* mm. spinales et semispinales thoracis et cervicis; *n* m. biventer cervicis; *o* m. complexus of the m. semispinalis capitis; *p* m. intertransversarius between vertebrae cervicales VI and VII; *q* m. longus colli; *r* m. scalenus; *s* diaphragma, pars costalis, *s'* pars sternalis, *s"* crus sinistrum, *s'''* centrum tendineum; *t* ln. mediastinalis caudalis longissimus; *u* oesophagus; *v* trachea; *w* radix pulmonis; *x* pulmo dexter, lobus cranialis, *x'* lobus accessorius; *y* cor, pericardium removed

1 truncus pulmonalis; *2* aorta thoracica; *2'* truncus brachiocephalicus; *3* lig. arteriosum; *4* v. azygos sinistra; *5* aa. and vv. intercostales dorsales, *5'* rr. cutanei laterales; *6* a. and v. subclavia sinistra; *7* truncus and v. costocervicalis; *8* a. and v. intercostalis suprema; *9* a. and v. scapularis dorsalis; *10* a. and v. cervicalis profunda; *11* a. and v. vertebralis; *12* a. and v. cervicalis superficialis; *13* a. and v. thoracica interna; *14* a. axillaris (dorsally displaced) and *14'* vv. axillares; *15* a. and v. thoracica externa; *16* a. carotis communis; *17* v. jugularis interna; *18* v. jugularis externa; *19* v. cephalica; *20* v. phrenica cranialis; *21* r. intermedius of the v. cordis magna; *22* ductus thoracicus; *23* radices plexus brachialis; *24* n. phrenicus; *25* cervical part of the n. sympathicus; *26* ggl. stellatum; *27* truncus sympathicus, pars thoracica; *28* cervical branches of the n. sympathicus; *29* n. vagus; *29'* bifurcation into trunci vagales dorsalis et ventralis; *30* n. laryngeus recurrens

A. iliaca externa

(Comparative: 85–88/49; 105–108/9; 136–143/7; cat: 91/25; 109/6; dog: 110/5; pig: 98/34; 111/5; sheep: 101/25; 112/5; ox: 113/3; 144/7; horse: 50/27; 104/14; 114/2)

The **a. iliaca externa** is a stout vessel which issues from the abdominal aorta, in the cat at the level of the 7th, in the dog and ruminants at the 6th and in the pig and horse at the 4th to 5th lumbar vertebrae. Its course is initially directed ventrad over the inner lumbar musculature and then, lying craniomedial to the body of the ilium and medial to the fascia iliaca, it continues to the lacuna vasorum. It becomes the

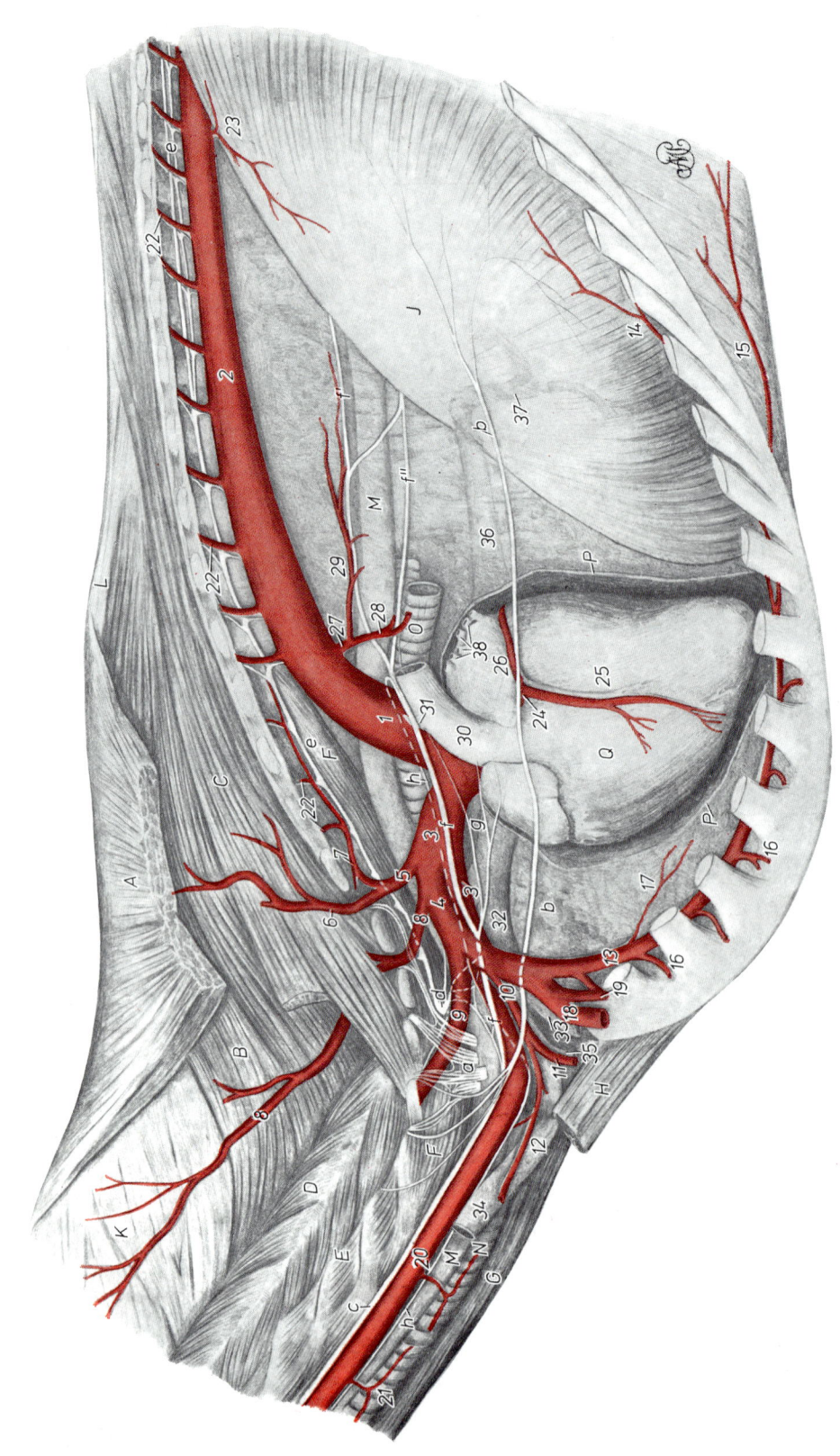

Fig. 103. Arteries of the thoracic cavity of a horse. Left lateral view. (After Martin, 1915.)

A mm. rhomboidei; B m. spinalis cervicis; C mm. longissimi; D mm. multifidi; E mm. intertransversarii; F m. longus colli; G mm. sternohyoideus and sternothyreoideus; H m. sternomandibularis; J diaphragma; K lam. nuchae; L lig. supraspinale; M oesophagus; N trachea; O bifurcatio tracheae; P pericardium, line of incision; Q cor a plexus brachialis; b n. phrenicus; c truncus vagosympathicus; d ggl. stellatum; e truncus sympathicus, pars thoracica; f n. vagus; f' truncus vagalis dorsalis; f'' truncus vagalis ventralis; g n. depressor and plexus cardiacus; h n. laryngeus recurrens

1 arcus aortae; 2 aorta thoracica; 3 truncus brachiocephalicus; 4 a. subclavia sinistra; 5 truncus costocervicalis; 6 a. scapularis dorsalis; 7 a. intercostalis suprema; 8 a. cervicalis profunda; 9 a. vertebralis; 10 a. cervicalis superficialis; 11 r. deltoideus; 12 r. ascendens; 13 a. thoracica interna; 14 a. musculophrenica; 15 a. epigastrica cranialis; 16 rr. perforantes; 17 r. mediastinalis; 18 a. axillaris; 19 a. thoracica externa; 20 a. carotis communis; 21 rr. tracheales; 22 aa. intercostales dorsales; 23 a. phrenica cranialis; 24 a. coronaria sinistra; 25 r. interventricularis paraconalis; 26 r. circumflexus; 27 a. bronchoesophagea; 28 r. bronchialis; 29 r. oesophageus; 30 truncus pulmonalis; 31 lig. arteriosum; 32 v. cava cranialis; 33 v. axillaris; 34 v. jugularis externa; 35 v. cephalica; 36 v. cava caudalis; overlaid by mediastinum; 37 v. phrenica cranialis; 38 vv. pulmonales

femoral artery as it enters the femoral canal. Except in carnivores, it first gives off the deep circumflex iliac artery which has already been described. In the horse only, the *a. cremasterica* (in males) or the *a. uterina* (in females) are given off a short distance later (see below & p. 177). Even before entry into the femoral canal the external iliac artery gives rise to the caudoventrally directed *a. profunda femoris*. The *a. abdominalis caudalis* arises proximal to this artery in the ox and distally to it in carnivores. Occasionally in the horse the *truncus pudendoepigastricus* arises from the external iliac proximal to the origin of the deep femoral artery; in other instances its origin is, as in other domestic mammals, from the first part of the deep femoral artery, whence it runs cranioventrally.

A. abdominalis caudalis
(cat: 91/*28*; 109/*18*; dog: 85/*51*; 105/*17*; 110/*6*; sheep: 101/*34*; 112/*11'''*; ox: 87/*51*; 107/*17*)

Only carnivores, sheep and cattle have an **a. abdominalis caudalis.** It arises from the external iliac artery. in carnivores distal and in the ox proximal to the origin of the deep femoral, while in the sheep it stems from the deep femoral or the pudendoepigastric trunk. The latter may occasionally be the source in the dog and the ox. Unlike the cranial abdominal artery, the caudal artery is but a slender vessel running in a cranioventral direction, at first medial to the internal oblique abdominal muscle and then within this muscle, parallel to the lateral border on the rectus abdominis. It gives off branches to the external oblique abdominal muscle. In the dog there are connections with the deep branch of the caudal epigastric and the deep circumflex iliac arteries.

A. profunda femoris
(Comparative: 85–88/*52*; 105–108/*11*; cat: 91/*26*; 109/*14*; dog: 110/*7*; pig: 98/*37*; 111/*8*; sheep: 101/*32*; 112/*9*; ox: 113/*21*; horse: 114/*5*)

Before it enters the femoral canal, the external iliac artery gives off the deep femoral artery and from the initial section of the latter arises the *truncus pudendoepigastricus*. The deep femoral artery passes caudally through the lacuna vasorum and turns lateroventral to the iliopubic eminence between the iliopsoas and pectineus muscles. Progressing caudodistally it reaches the abductor muscles where it gives rise to the *a. circumflexa femoris medialis*. Only in the dog and the pig does it continue distally on the caudal surface of the fenur; in this location it is a stout vessel in the dog but slender in the pig. It supplies a nutrient branch to the femur and, in the dog, several caudodistally directed muscular branches to the mm. adductores, one of which vessels perforates these muscles. In the pig, too, there are small branches to the adductor muscles but they do not perforate them. These muscular branches correspond to the initial part of the aa. perforantes of man.

Truncus pudendoepigastricus
(Comparative: 85–88/*53*; 105–108/*13*; 136–143/*9*; dog: 110/*8*; pig: 98/*38*; 111/*9*; sheep: 101/*33*; 112/*11*; ox: 113/*22*; horse: 114/*6*)

The short **truncus pudendoepigastricus** originates from the deep femoral artery although in the horse it may occasionally arise from the external iliac artery. It is the vessel of origin of the *a. epigastrica caudalis* and the *a. pudenda externa*. From the pudendoepigastric trunk, or from one of these two bifurcating branches, arises the *a. cremasterica* in males, except in the horse where this artery branches from the first part of the external iliac artery. It supplies the m. cremaster externus and the proc. vaginalis. A further branch in carnivores and pigs is the *a. vesicalis media* which runs from the ventral body wall to the middle part of the urinary bladder.

A. epigastrica caudalis
(Comparative: 85–88/*54*; 105–108/*14*; 136–143/*10*; cat: 91/*29*; 109/*15*; dog: 110/*9*; pig: 98/*39*; sheep: 101/*35*; 112/*11''*; ox: 113/*22'*; horse: 114/*7*)

At the caudal border of the anulus inguinalis profundus the **a. epigastrica caudalis** issues from either the pudendoepigastric trunk or, often in the cat and less frequently in the dog, from the deep femoral

136   Arteries

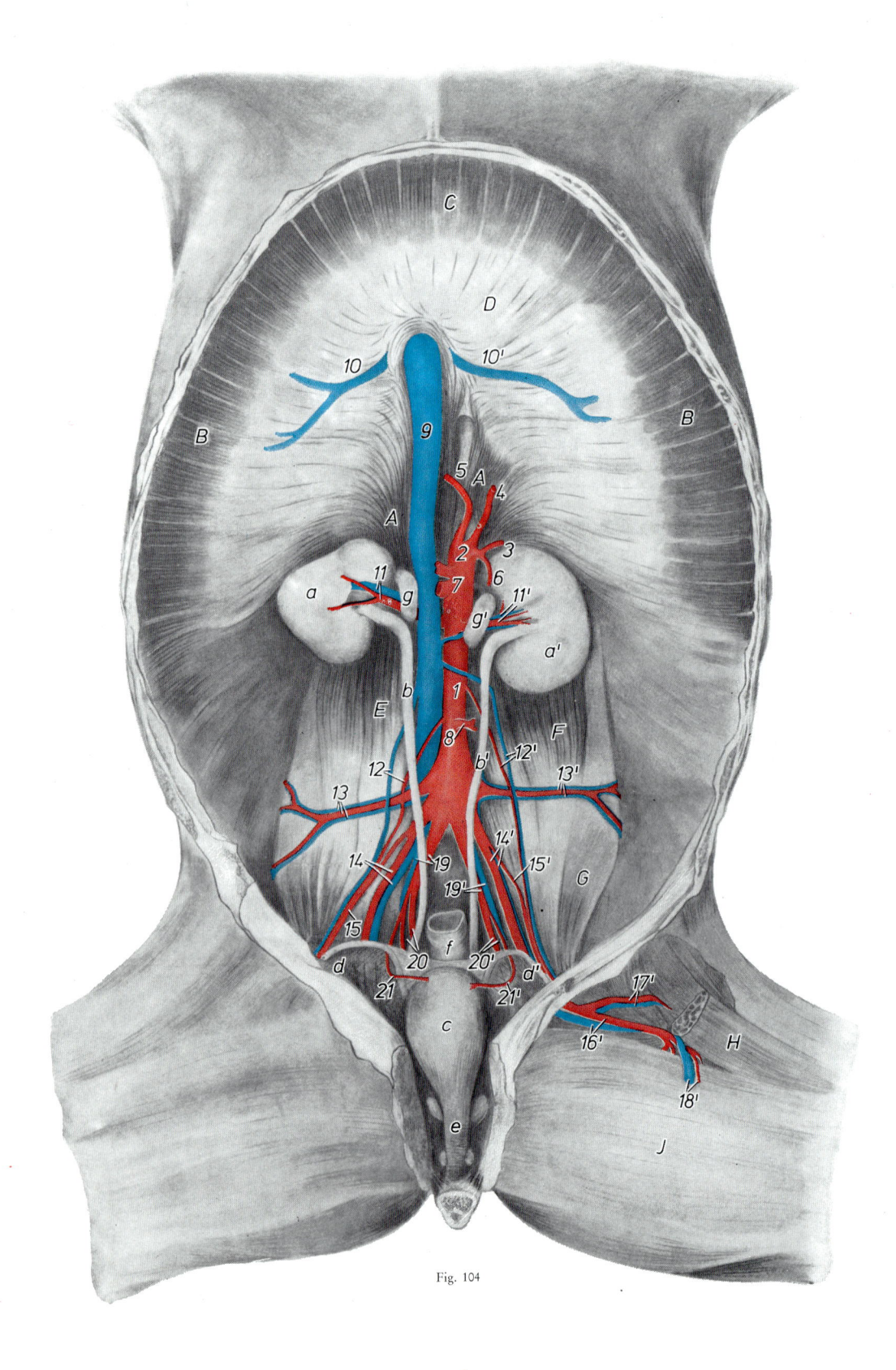

Fig. 104

artery. It runs in a cranial direction medial to the internal inguinal ring, crosses the lateral border of the rectus abdominis muscle and dips into the dorsal surface of this muscle which it vascularizes together with the internal oblique abdominis muscle. At the level of the umbilicus its diverging terminal branches link with those of the cranial epigastric artery and there are further anastomoses with the neighbouring arteries of the lateral abdominal wall.

A. pudenda externa

(Comparative: 85–88/*55*; 105–108/*15*; 136–143/*12*; cat: 109/*16*; dog: 110/*10*; pig: 98/*40*; sheep: 101/*36*; 112/*11'*; ox: 113/*22"*; 114/*25*; horse: 114/*8*)

The **a. pudenda externa** is the second vessel branching from the pudendoepigastric trunk. Sometimes in the cat and, more rarely, in the dog the external pudendal stems from the deep femoral artery. It passes through the inguinal canal and is accompanied caudomedially in the male by the m. cremaster externus. Thus this artery attains a superficial position in the inguinal region where it divides into the cranially directed *a. epigastrica caudalis superficialis* and either the *r. scrotalis ventralis* to the scrotum or the *r. labialis ventralis* to the vulva. In male horses the external pudendal artery also gives off a stout vessel, the **a. penis cranialis,** which participates in the blood supply to the penis.

The **a. epigastrica caudalis superficialis** runs towards the umbilicus along the sheath of the rectus abdominis where it is situated superficially on the ventral abdominal wall. It supplies the skin and the cutaneous muscles. It anastomoses with branches of the *a. epigastrica cranialis superficialis* in the region of the umbilicus in ruminants and caudal to the umbilicus in carnivores. Branches are also supplied to the lnn. inguinales superficiales, in so far as the latter lie within its ramification area. In males it sends branches to the prepuce. In females, on the other hand, its distribution depends on the arrangement of the mammary complex of the particular species. Its branches supply the abdominal and inguinal mammary complexes. In the udder region of ruminants and the mare it becomes known as the **a. mammaria cranialis** and its calibre here exceeds that of its preuberous part.

The course and distribution of the caudally directed branch of the external pudendal artery is also dependent on species and sex. Its terminal branches usually link with corresponding branches of the internal pudendal artery in the perineal region. As the **r. scrotalis ventralis** it supplies the scrotum in males and, depending on the position of the scrotum, it subsequently has to travel a varying distance in towards the perineum. In the female the **r. labialis ventralis** always runs superficially between the thighs to the vulva. In the udder region of ruminants and horses it is present as the stout **a. mammaria caudalis** and it also supplies the lnn. inguinales superficiales s. mammaria.

Arteries of the pelvic limb

The a. profunda femoris has already been described as a branch of the a. iliaca externa (see p. 135).

A. circumflexa femoris medialis

(Comparative: 85–88/*59*; 105–108/*12*; dog: 110/*11*; pig: 111/*10*; sheep: 112/*13*; ox: 113/*24*; horse: 114/*9*)

The **a. circumflexa femoris medialis** arises from the deep femoral artery cranial to the adductor muscles and runs in these muscles ventral to the pelvic floor to the long ischiatic muscles. In a sequence which varies according to the species, it gives off the r. obturatorius, the r. acetabularis, r. profundus, r.

Fig. 104. Aorta abdominalis and vena cava caudalis of a horse. Ventral view.
(After Martin, 1915.)
The organs and vessels of the left half of the body are marked by an apostrophe after the letter or number.

A–D diaphragma: *A* pars lumbalis, *B* pars costalis, *C* pars sternalis, *D* centrum tendineum; *E* m. psoas minor; *F* m. psoas major; *G* m. iliacus; *H* m. sartorius; *J* m. gracilis

a ren; *b* ureter; *c* vesica urinaria; *d* ductus deferens; *e* pars pelvina urethrae masculinae; *f* rectum; *g* gl. suprarenalis

1 aorta abdominalis; *2* a. coeliaca; *3* a. lienalis; *4* a. gastrica sinistra; *5* a. hepatica; *6* r. pancreaticus; *7* a. mesenterica cranialis; *8* a. mesenterica caudalis; *9* v. cava caudalis; *10* v. phrenica cranialis; *11* a. and v. renalis; *12* a. and v. testicularis; *13* a. and v. circumflexa ilium profunda; *14* a. and v. iliaca externa; *15* a. cremasterica; *16'* a. and v. femoralis; *17'* a. and v. circumflexa femoris lateralis; *18'* a. saphena and v. saphena medialis; *19* a. and v. iliaca interna; *20* a. and v. pudenda interna; *21* a. umbilicalis

138 Arteries

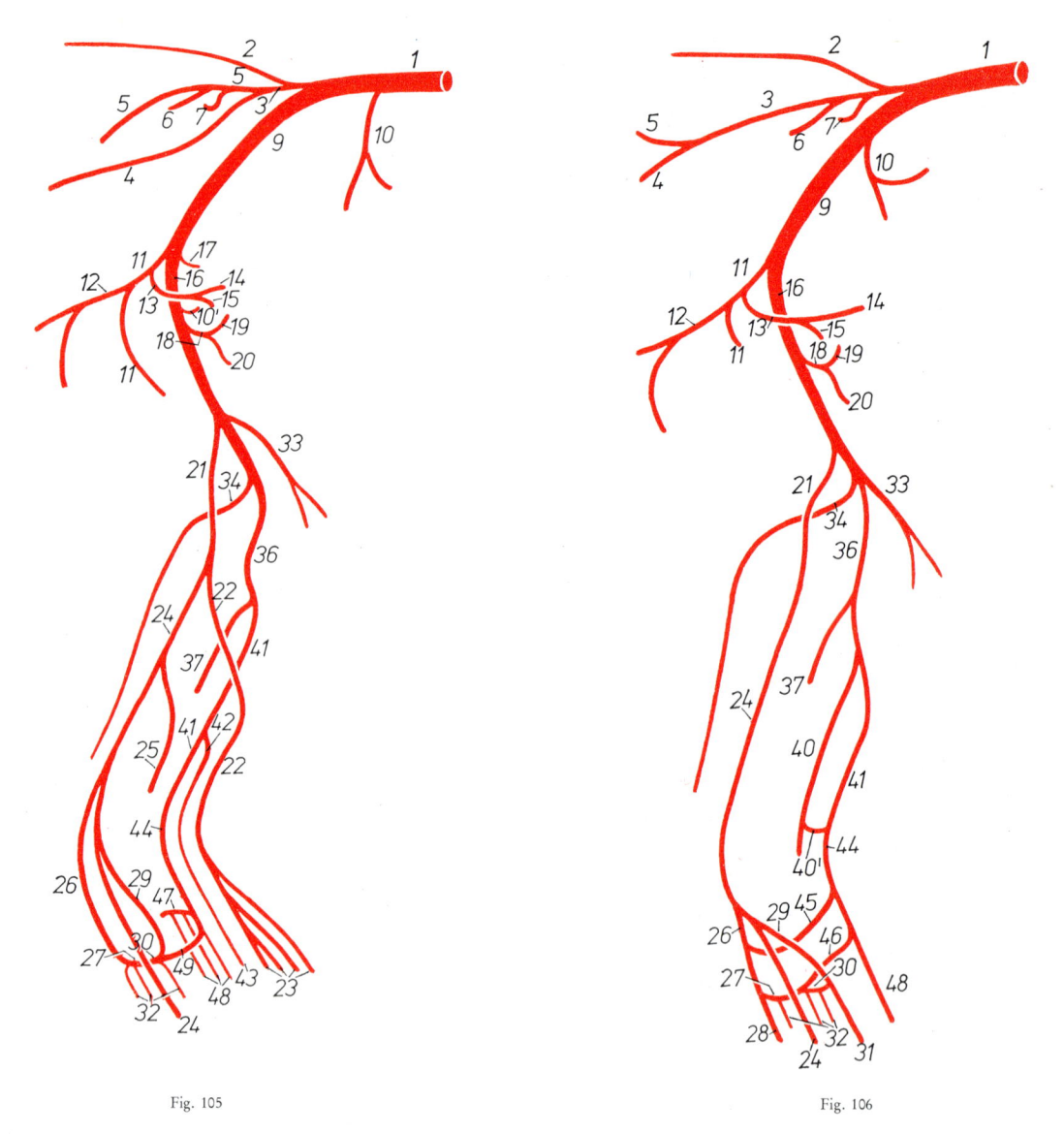

Fig. 105

Fig. 106

ascendens and r. transversus. This nomenclature was adopted in veterinary anatomy from the corresponding branches of the medial circumflex femoral artery of man in which this artery has a less extensive supply area. In man the distally directed deep femoral artery, which runs caudally on the upper thigh, is a stout vessel, the muscular branches of which, the aa. perforantes, go through the adductor muscles and supply only the musculature situated on the caudal part of the upper thigh. In the domestic mammals, on the other hand, the deep femoral artery continues further distal only in the dog and to some extent in the pig and still participates in supplying the caudal muscles of the thigh. In domestic mammals this supply region extends from the proximocaudal part of the thigh towards the flexor aspect of the knee for a distance which increases progressively in carnivores, pigs and ruminants. This region is supplied not only by the *aa. femoris caudales,* which will be described under the branches of the femoral artery, and which are represented in man in the distal part only by slender vessels, but also by the *a. circumflexa femoris medialis* with its *r. transversus.* In domestic mammals, however, the r. transversus is a descending vessel and would thus be better termed the *r. descendens.* It is the thickest branch of the medial circumflex femoral artery and is its functional continuation. In the horse the medial circumflex femoral artery itself is but a slender vessel and the ramification area of the r. transversus, or descendens, follows that of the obturator artery (q. v.). The other branches of the medial femoral

Fig. 107

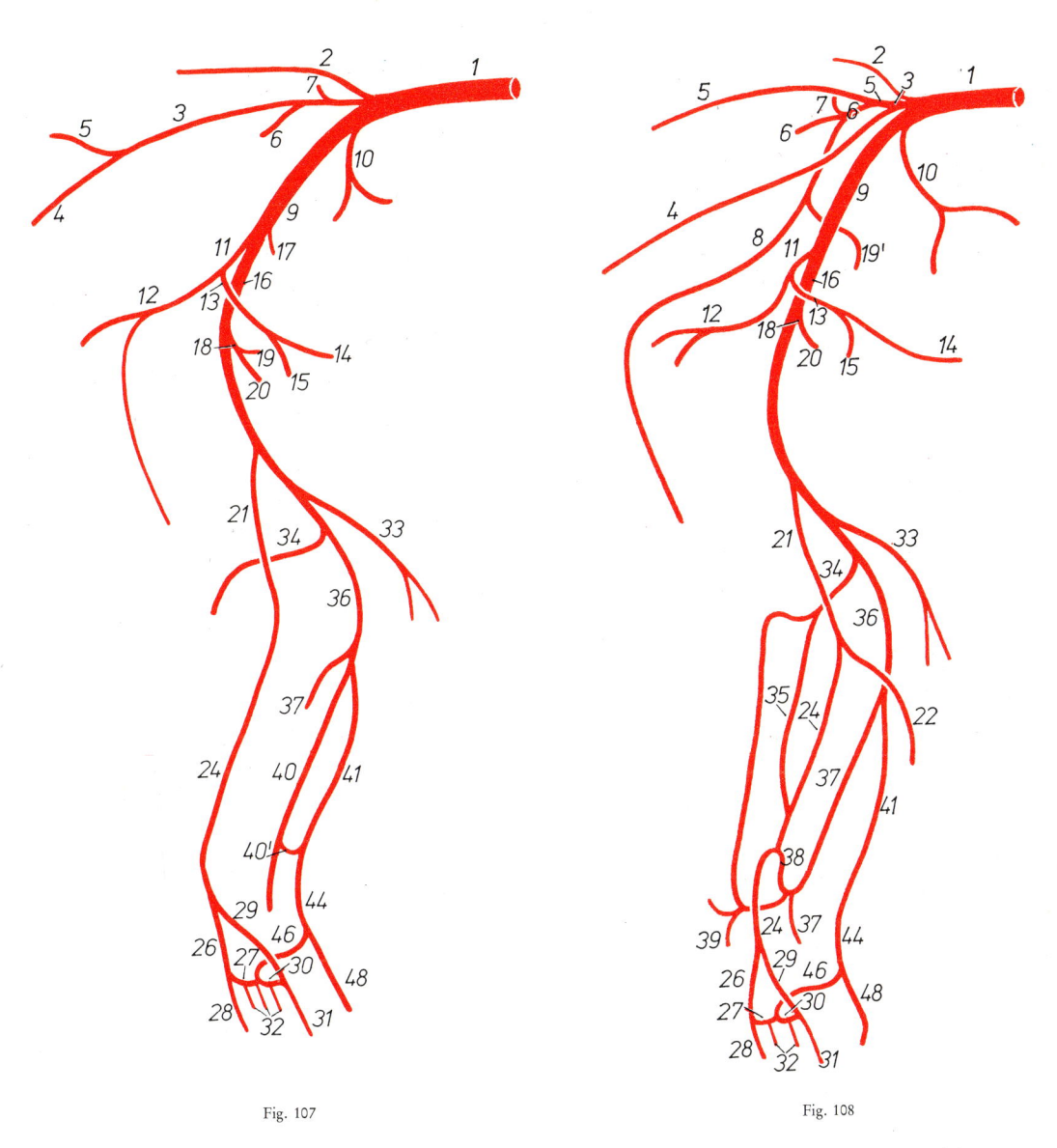

Fig. 108

Figs. 105, 106, 107, 108. Arteries of the left pelvic limb supplying the tarsal region of the dog, pig, ox and horse. Diagrammatic, medial view.
1 aorta abdominalis; *2* a. sacralis mediana; *3* a. iliaca interna; *4* a. pudenda interna; *5* a. glutaea caudalis; *6* a. glutaea cranialis; *7* a. iliolumbalis; *8* a. obturatoria; *9* a. iliaca externa; *10* a. circumflexa ilium profunda; *10'* a. circumflexa ilium superficialis; *11* a. profunda femoris; *12* a. circumflexa femoris medialis; *13* truncus pudendoepigastricus; *14* a. epigastrica caudalis; *15* a. pudenda externa; *16* a. femoralis; *17* a. abdominalis caudalis; *18* a. circumflexa femoris lateralis; *19* r. ascendens; *19'* a. iliacofemoralis; *20* r. descendens; *21* a. saphena, *22* r. cranialis; *23* aa. digitales dorsales communes I–IV; *24* r. caudalis from *21*; *25* branch of *24*. Its terminology has not yet been standardized: in the literature it is referred to as either a. peronea or a. fibularis; *26* a. plantaris lateralis, *27* r. profundus, *28* r. superficialis; *29* a. plantaris medialis, *30* r. profundus, *31* r. superficialis; *27* and *30* arcus plantaris profundus; *32* aa. metatarseae plantares II–IV; *33* a. genus descendens; *34* r. caudalis femoris distalis; *35* a. comitans n. tibialis; *36* a. poplitea; *37* a. tibialis caudalis; *38* r. anastomoticus cum a. saphena; *39* a. malleolaris caudalis lateralis; *40* a. interossea cruris; *40'* r. interosseus s. perforans; *41* a. tibialis cranialis; *42* r. superficialis; *43* a. digitalis dorsalis V abaxialis; *44* a. dorsalis pedis; *45* a. tarsea perforans proximalis; *46* a. tarsea perforans distalis; *47* a. arcuata; *48* aa. metatarseae dorsales II–IV; *49* r. perforans proximalis II

circumflex artery are not very large in any of the domestic mammals. The *r. obturatorius* runs in a dorsal direction through the cranial part of the obturator foramen to vascularize the intrapelvic parts of the obturator muscles. The *r. acetabularis* gives off branches which pass through the inc. acetabuli to the hip joint and it also reaches the rotators of the hip. The *r. ascendens* courses ventral to the floor of the pelvis to reach the tuber ischiadicum and ramifies in the adductor and long ischiatic muscles. The *r. profundus* is the true terminal branch of the artery and it passes caudal to the femur between the external obturator

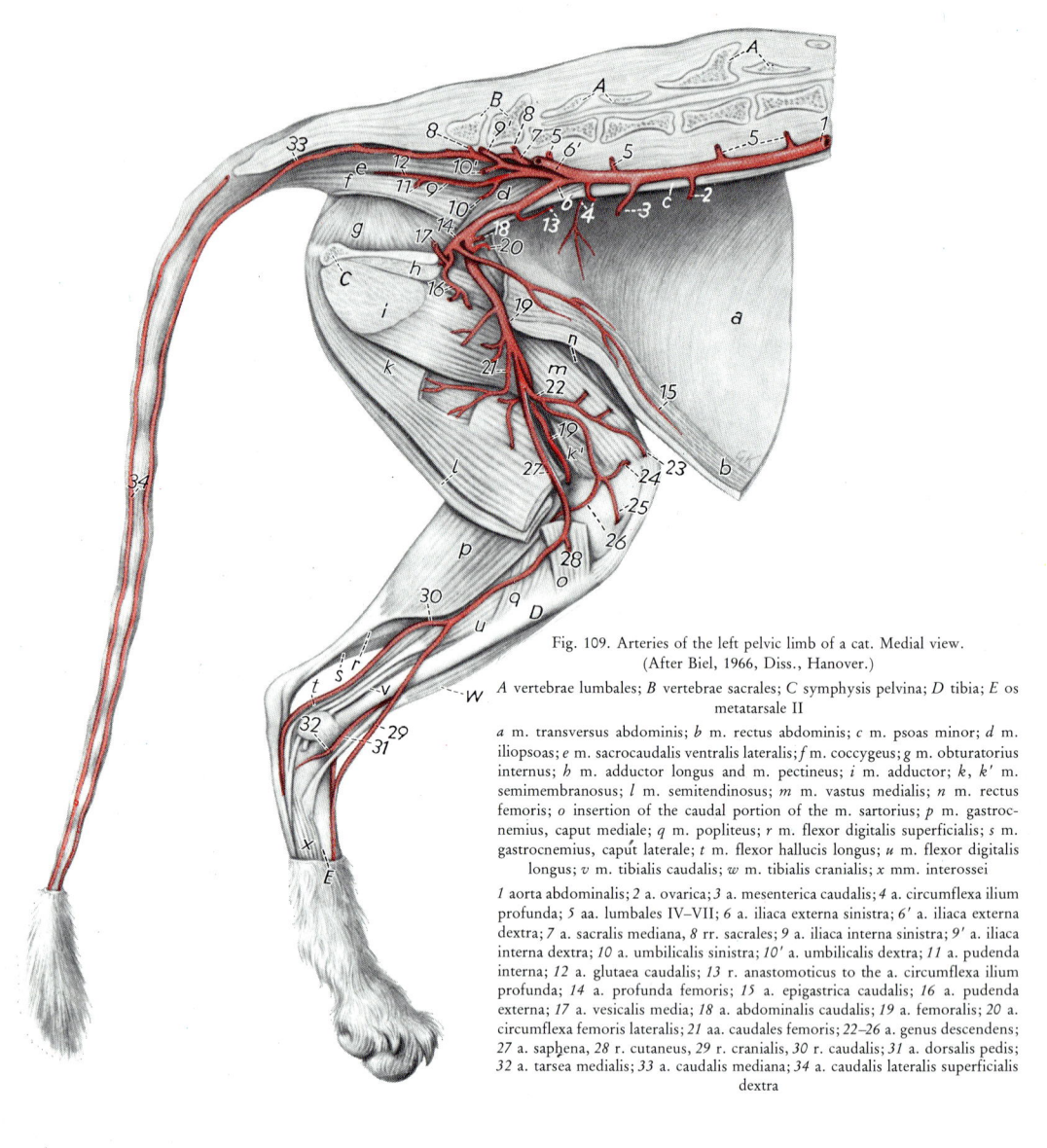

Fig. 109. Arteries of the left pelvic limb of a cat. Medial view.
(After Biel, 1966, Diss., Hanover.)

A vertebrae lumbales; *B* vertebrae sacrales; *C* symphysis pelvina; *D* tibia; *E* os metatarsale II

a m. transversus abdominis; *b* m. rectus abdominis; *c* m. psoas minor; *d* m. iliopsoas; *e* m. sacrocaudalis ventralis lateralis; *f* m. coccygeus; *g* m. obturatorius internus; *h* m. adductor longus and m. pectineus; *i* m. adductor; *k*, *k'* m. semimembranosus; *l* m. semitendinosus; *m* m. vastus medialis; *n* m. rectus femoris; *o* insertion of the caudal portion of the m. sartorius; *p* m. gastrocnemius, caput mediale; *q* m. popliteus; *r* m. flexor digitalis superficialis; *s* m. gastrocnemius, caput laterale; *t* m. flexor hallucis longus; *u* m. flexor digitalis longus; *v* m. tibialis caudalis; *w* m. tibialis cranialis; *x* mm. interossei

1 aorta abdominalis; *2* a. ovarica; *3* a. mesenterica caudalis; *4* a. circumflexa ilium profunda; *5* aa. lumbales IV–VII; *6* a. iliaca externa sinistra; *6'* a. iliaca externa dextra; *7* a. sacralis mediana, *8* rr. sacrales; *9* a. iliaca interna sinistra; *9'* a. iliaca interna dextra; *10* a. umbilicalis sinistra; *10'* a. umbilicalis dextra; *11* a. pudenda interna; *12* a. glutaea caudalis; *13* r. anastomoticus to the a. circumflexa ilium profunda; *14* a. profunda femoris; *15* a. epigastrica caudalis; *16* a. pudenda externa; *17* a. vesicalis media; *18* a. abdominalis caudalis; *19* a. femoralis; *20* a. circumflexa femoris lateralis; *21* aa. caudales femoris; *22–26* a. genus descendens; *27* a. saphena, *28* r. cutaneus, *29* r. cranialis, *30* r. caudalis; *31* a. dorsalis pedis; *32* a. tarsea medialis; *33* a. caudalis mediana; *34* a. caudalis lateralis superficialis dextra

and quadratus femoris muscles to the lateral side. Here it anastomoses with the lateral circumflex femoral artery or, in the horse, the iliacofemoral artery.

A. femoralis

(Comparative: 85–88/*49*; 105–108/*16*; cat: 109/*19*; dog: 110/*12*; pig: 98/*36*; sheep: 101/*31*; 112/*10*; ox: 113/*25*; horse: 104/*16*; 114/*10*)

The **a. femoralis** is the continuation of the external iliac artery after it enters the lacuna vasorum. In the pig and ruminants the artery and its accompanying vein pass between the heads of origin of the sartorius muscle. The femoral artery runs in a distal direction cranial to the femoral vein in the femoral canal. It crosses the femur medially over the medial vastus muscle and reaches the flexor aspect of the knee by passing through or distal to the adductor muscle. Between the heads of the gastrocnemius it becomes the *a. poplitea*. The *a. circumflexa ilium superficialis,* which is present only in carnivores, is given off the femoral artery before the entrance to the pelvic cavity. This is followed by the *a.*

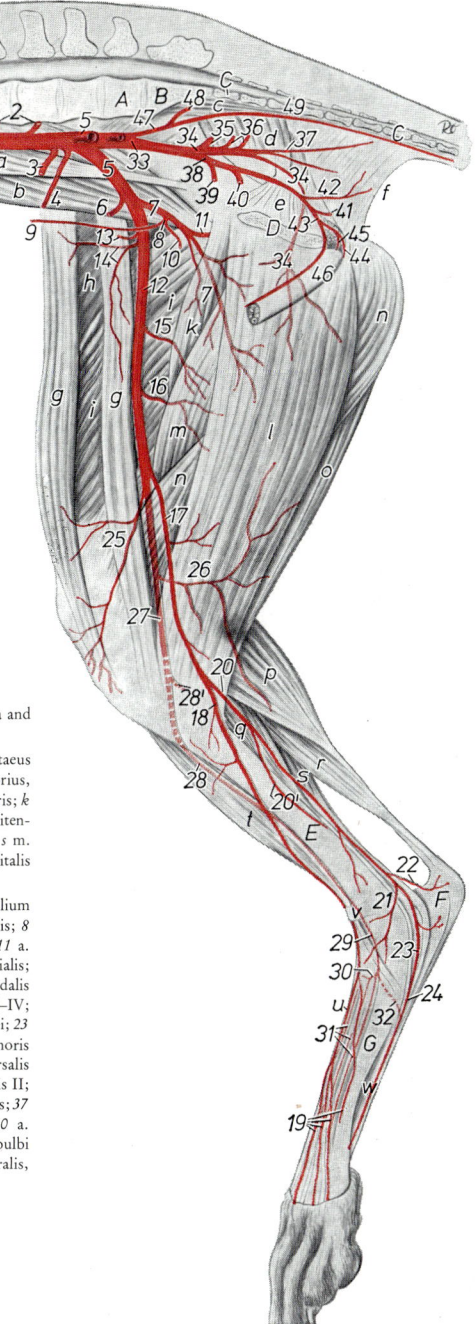

Fig. 110. Arteries of the right pelvic limb of a dog. Medial view. (Redrawn after Martin, 1915.)

A vertebrae lumbales; *B* os sacrum; *C* vertebrae caudales; *D* symphysis pelvina and root of the penis; *E* tibia; *F* tuber calcanei; *G* ossa metatarsalia

a m. psoas minor; *b* m. iliopsoas; *c* mm. sacrocaudales ventrales; *d* m. glutaeus medius; *e* m. obturatorius internus; *f* m. coccygeus, caudal border; *g* m. sartorius, pars cranialis and pars caudalis; *h* m. tensor fasciae latae; *i* m. quadriceps femoris; *k* m. pectineus; *l* m. gracilis; *m* m. adductor; *n* m. semimembranosus; *o* m. semitendinosus; *p* m. gastrocnemius; *q* m. popliteus; *r* m. flexor digitalis superficialis; *s* m. flexor digitalis profundus; *t* m. tibialis craniales; *u* tendon of the m. extensor digitalis longus; *v* retinaculum extensorum; *w* mm. interossei

1 aorta abdominalis; *2* aa. lumbales; *3* a. mesenterica caudalis; *4* a. circumflexa ilium profunda; *5* a. iliaca externa; *6* a. abdominalis caudalis; *7* a. profunda femoris; *8* truncus pudendoepigastricus; *9* a. epigastrica caudalis; *10* a. pudenda externa; *11* a. circumflexa femoris medialis; *12* a. femoralis; *13* a. circumflexa femoris superficialis; *14* a. circumflexa femoris lateralis; *15* a. caudalis femoris proximalis; *16* a. caudalis femoris media; *17* a. saphena, *18* r. cranialis; *19* aa. digitales dorsales communes I–IV; *20* r. caudalis from *17*; *20'* a. fibularis; *21* rr. malleolares mediales; *22* rr. calcanei; *23* a. plantaris medialis, *24* r. profundus; *25* a. genus descendens; *26* a. caudalis femoris distalis; *27* a. poplitea; *28* a. tibialis cranialis; *28'* a. tibialis caudalis; *29* a. dorsalis pedis; *30* a. arcuata; *31* aa. metatarseae dorsales II–IV; *32* r. perforans proximalis II; *33* a. iliaca interna; *34* a. glutaea caudalis; *35* a. iliolumbalis; *36* a. glutaea cranialis; *37* a. caudalis lateralis superficialis; *38* a. pudenda interna; *39* a. umbilicalis; *40* a. prostatica; *41* a. perinealis ventralis; *42* a. rectalis caudalis; *43* a. penis; *44* a. bulbi penis; *45* a. profunda penis; *46* a. dorsalis penis; *47* a. sacralis mediana; *48* r. sacralis, *49* a. caudalis mediana

circumflexa femoris lateralis. At the distal end of the femoral canal the distally directed *a. saphena* arises from the medial wall of the femoral artery and a short distance later the *a. genus descendens* comes off and continues craniodistally. In carnivores the latter may also arise proximal to the saphenous artery. Three muscular branches, the *aa. caudales femoris proximalis*, *media* and *distalis* which vary in calibre in the different species of domestic mammals, leave the femoral artery in a caudal direction one after the other. The last named, the distal artery, is the largest of the three in all the domestic mammals and is the last branch of the femoral artery. In carnivores the femoral artery can be palpated through the skin where it lies in the shallow, broad femoral canal so that the pulse can be taken on this vessel.

A. circumflexa ilium superficialis
(dog: 92/41; 105/10'; 110/13)

An **a. circumflexa ilium superficialis** is found only in carnivores. It is a relatively slender vessel which arises from the femoral artery proximal to the a. circumflexa femoris lateralis or, as occurs normally in the cat, from the latter vessel itself. It runs in a craniodorsal direction, medially over the *m. rectus femoris* and between the *m. tensor fasciae* latae and the m. sartorius. It gives off branches to these three muscles and reaches the skin over the spina iliaca ventralis. In the other domestic mammals this area is supplied by branches of the a. circumflexa femoris lateralis or the a. iliacofemoralis as well as the r. superficialis of the deep circumflex artery.

A. circumflexa femoris lateralis
(Comparative: 105–108/18; cat: 109/20; dog: 92/42; 110/14; pig: 111/13'; sheep: 101/31'; ox: 113/27; horse: 88/72; 104/17; 108/19'; 114/11)

The **a. circumflexa femoralis lateralis** arises from the femoral artery while it is still within the femoral canal and continues between the medial vastus and the rectus femoris muscles. It gives off an ascending ramus (except in the horse), a descending and a transverse ramus. The *r. transversus* is only a slender vessel which forms the continuation of the lateral circumflex femoral artery along the lateral surface of the femur where it anastomoses with the medial circumflex femoral artery and supplies branches to the intermediate and lateral vastus muscles. The *r. ascendens* is directed towards the pelvis and contributes in the supply of the iliopsoas and gluteus muscles. Branches run medial to the tensor fasciae latae muscle in the direction of the tuber coxae, except in the horse and in carnivores which have a special superficial circumflex iliac artery which can arise from the lateral circumflex femoral artery. Arising independently or from one of the branches already mentioned, there are arteries to the hip joint and the femur. In the horse the supply area of the transverse and ascending rami is taken over by the iliacofemoral artery (see p. 157). The *r. descendens* is distally directed and ramifies in the various parts of the quadriceps femoris muscle. It represents the largest supply vessel of this group of muscles.

A. saphena
(Comparative: 105–108/21; 115–118/7; cat: 109/27; dog: 92/47; 110/17; 119/1; pig: 111/14; sheep: 112/13; ox: 113/28; horse: 104/18; 114/12)

The **a. saphena** originates from the femoral artery at the distal end of the femoral canal. It continues superficially, together with the homonymous vein and saphenous nerve, in a caudodistal direction over the tendon of insertion of the gracilis muscle and it divides into a cranial and a caudal ramus. The point of division varies in different species; in the cat it is distal to the popliteus muscle about half way down the thigh, in the dog in the region of insertion of the gracilis muscle and in the horse in the area where the semitandinosus muscle is inserted. In the pig and ox the vessel does not divide. During its course the saphenous artery gives off muscular branches to the insertions of the medial thigh muscles and cutaneous branches to the knee and the cranial shank region.

The *r. cranialis* is only a slender vessel in the cat and the horse. It crosses, in a craniodistal direction, the medial aspect of the tibia and continues in a superficial position past the flexor aspect of the tarsal joint. In carnivores it reaches as far as the dorsal metatarsal region but in the horse it terminates at the tarsal joint. In carnivores the cranial ramus is the origin of the dorsal common digital artery. In the cat the latter is only a slight vessel even though it has been joined by the superficial ramus of the cranial tibial artery.

The *r. caudalis* takes up a subfascial position and crosses, accompanied by the corresponding vein, the medial aspect of the *m. flexor digitalis pedis longus* in a caudal direction. Proximal to the tarsal joint the caudal ramus reaches the tibial nerve at the craniomedial part of the flexor tendons. In company with this nerve and the corresponding vein, it continues over the sustentaculum tali. In carnivores a vessel arises, generally from the caudal ramus although in the cat it also frequently springs from the cranial ramus, which continues laterodistally for about half the length of the tibia between this bone and the long digital flexor and posterior tibial muscles. In the cat this vessel links, caudal to the interosseous

Arteries of the pelvic limb

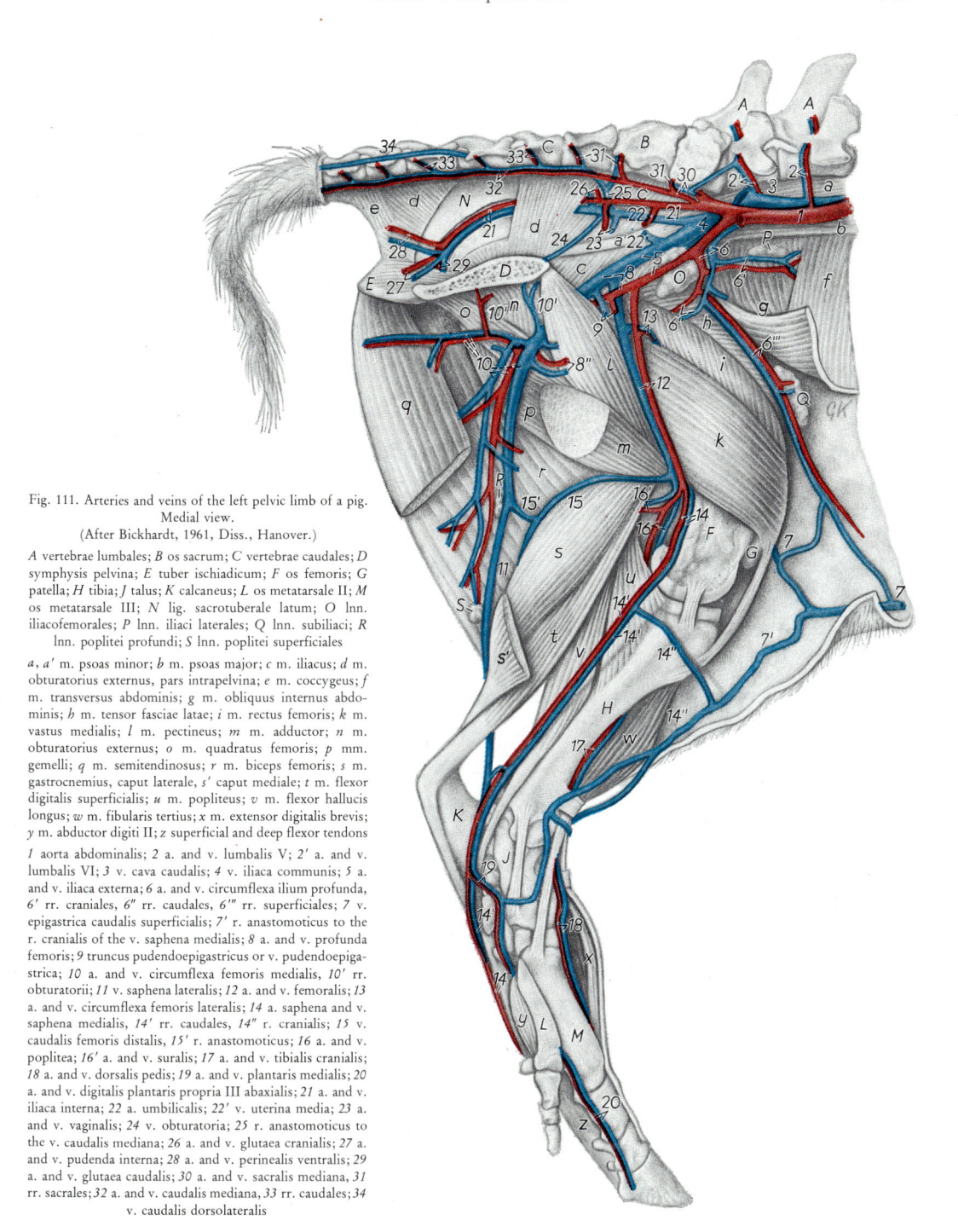

Fig. 111. Arteries and veins of the left pelvic limb of a pig. Medial view.
(After Bickhardt, 1961, Diss., Hanover.)

A vertebrae lumbales; *B* os sacrum; *C* vertebrae caudales; *D* symphysis pelvina; *E* tuber ischiadicum; *F* os femoris; *G* patella; *H* tibia; *J* talus; *K* calcaneus; *L* os metatarsale II; *M* os metatarsale III; *N* lig. sacrotuberale latum; *O* lnn. iliacofemorales; *P* lnn. iliaci laterales; *Q* lnn. subiliaci; *R* lnn. poplitei profundi; *S* lnn. poplitei superficiales

a, a' m. psoas minor; *b* m. psoas major; *c* m. iliacus; *d* m. obturatorius externus, pars intrapelvina; *e* m. coccygeus; *f* m. transversus abdominis; *g* m. obliquus internus abdominis; *h* m. tensor fasciae latae; *i* m. rectus femoris; *k* m. vastus medialis; *l* m. pectineus; *m* m. adductor; *n* m. obturatorius externus; *o* m. quadratus femoris; *p* mm. gemelli; *q* m. semitendinosus; *r* m. biceps femoris; *s* m. gastrocnemius, caput laterale, *s'* caput mediale; *t* m. flexor digitalis superficialis; *u* m. popliteus; *v* m. flexor hallucis longus; *w* m. fibularis tertius; *x* m. extensor digitalis brevis; *y* m. abductor digiti II; *z* superficial and deep flexor tendons

1 aorta abdominalis; *2* a. and v. lumbalis V; *2'* a. and v. lumbalis VI; *3* v. cava caudalis; *4* v. iliaca communis; *5* a. and v. iliaca externa; *6* a. and v. circumflexa ilium profunda, *6'* rr. craniales, *6"* rr. caudales, *6'''* rr. superficiales; *7* v. epigastrica caudalis superficialis; *7'* r. anastomoticus to the r. cranialis of the v. saphena medialis; *8* a. and v. profunda femoris; *9* truncus pudendoepigastricus or v. pudendoepigastrica; *10* a. and v. circumflexa femoris medialis, *10'* rr. obturatorii; *11* v. saphena lateralis; *12* a. and v. femoralis; *13* a. and v. circumflexa femoris lateralis; *14* a. saphena and v. saphena medialis, *14'* rr. caudales, *14"* r. cranialis; *15* v. caudalis femoris distalis, *15'* r. anastomoticus; *16* a. and v. poplitea; *16'* a. and v. suralis; *17* a. and v. tibialis cranialis; *18* a. and v. dorsalis pedis; *19* a. and v. plantaris medialis; *20* a. and v. digitalis plantaris propria III abaxialis; *21* a. and v. iliaca interna; *22* a. umbilicalis; *22'* v. uterina media; *23* a. and v. vaginalis; *24* v. obturatoria; *25* r. anastomoticus to the v. caudalis mediana; *26* a. and v. glutaea cranialis; *27* a. and v. pudenda interna; *28* a. and v. perinealis ventralis; *29* a. and v. glutaea caudalis; *30* a. and v. sacralis mediana, *31* rr. sacrales; *32* a. and v. caudalis mediana, *33* rr. caudales; *34* v. caudalis dorsolateralis

membrane of the leg (*membrana interossea cruris*), with the interosseous or perforating ramus which pierces this membrane and the vessel formed by this union continues in the region of the tarsal joint between the cranial tibial artery and the distal end of the distal caudal femoral artery. In the dog this vessel ends plantar to the tarsal joint. Although the terminology is still undecided, this vessel is usually referred to in the dog as the *a. fibularis*. Proximal to the hock joint the caudal ramus gives off, except in the horse, the *rr. malleolares mediales* and *rr. calcanei* which form the *rete calcanei*. At the level of the tarsocrural joint the caudal ramus gives off, except in the cat, the *a. plantaris lateralis,* and the *a. plantaris medialis* and it then continues in carnivores and the pig as an independent vessel to the planta.

Except in the cat, in which it is absent, the **a. plantaris medialis** divides into a *r. profundus* and a *r. superficialis.* In the dog the latter is represented only as a slender vessel in association with the first digit. The **a. plantaris lateralis** divides into a deep and a superficial ramus, except in carnivores which only have a deep ramus. The *r. profundus* of both the lateral and medial plantar arteries participate in the formation of the *arcus plantaris profundus* from which originate the *aa. metatarseae plantares.* The *r. superficialis* and the superficially continuing *r. caudalis* form the origin of the *aa. digitales plantares.*

A. genus descendens
(Comparative: 105–108/*33*; cat: 109/*22–26*; dog: 110/*25*; sheep: 112/*14*; ox: 113/*29*; horse: 114/*14*)

The **a. genus descendens** arises from the femoral artery a short distance before the origin of the saphenous artery. In carnivores it may arise in common with the latter vessel. Stout muscular branches to the deep parts of the quadriceps femoris muscle arise from both the first part of the genicular artery and the femoral artery. Sometimes they may arise directly from the femoral artery alone. The descending genicular artery continues thereafter along the border between the medial vastus and semimembranosus muscles, covered medially by the sartorius muscle, to the knee joint, giving off branches to the neighbouring muscles. At the knee it divides into its terminal branches which supply mainly the medial regions of the patellar and femerotibial joints and the *corpus adiposum infrapatellare.*

Aa. caudales femoris
(Comparative: 105–108/*34*; cat: 109/*21*; dog: 110/*15*; *16, 26*; sheep: 112/*15*; ox: 113/*25', 25"*; horse: 114/*15*)

The **aa. caudales femoris** are large muscular vessels which arise in a caudal direction from the femoral artery. In all the domestic mammals there are several such muscular vessels, the most proximally situated of which leaves the femoral artery a short distance before the saphenous artery. The most distally situated branch leaves the femoral artery shortly before its transition to the popliteal artery. This latter distal branch is of constant origin in all the domestic mammals and it is termed the *a. caudalis femoris distalis.* Of all the other branches we differentiate by name only two which occur in carnivores, the *a. caudalis femoris proximalis* and the *a. caudalis femoris media*, the latter arising only a short distance proximal to the distal caudal femoral artery. In addition to these the femoral artery of carnivores gives off other smaller, unnamed muscular branches which go to the caudal and medial muscles of the thigh. It should also be mentioned here that there are unnamend, cranially-directed branches of the femoral artery supplying the quadriceps muscle.

The **a. caudalis femoris proximalis** of carnivores arises either from the saphenous artery or together with this vessel within the femoral canal. It crosses medially over the belly of the pectineus muscle and the adductor muscle and then, caudodistally directed, it enters the semimembranosus muscle. It ramifies in all these muscles as well as the gracilis which covers it medially.

The **a. caudalis femoris media** of carnivores leaves the femoral artery distal to the descending genicular artery and mainly supplies the gracilis, adductor and semimembranosus muscles.

In all the other domestic mammals the topography of the caudal femoral arteries in the thigh is similar. They are not specially mentioned since their origin is variable and because their distribution area is restricted due to the more prominent development of the medial circumflex femoral artery. The caudal femoral arteries anastomose not only with the medial circumflex femoral artery but also among themselves.

The **a. caudalis femoris distalis** is the most prominent of these arteries in all the domestic mammals and, compared with the preceding ones, it curves more laterally. It courses over the lateral belly of the gastrocnemius muscle which it supplies with branches as it does the medial belly. The artery divides into caudally and proximally directed branches which ramify in the biceps femoris and gluteobiceps muscles and supply the deep popliteal lymph nodes. It also gives off a stout distally-directed branch. In the horse the distal caudal femoral artery gives off, shortly before the bifurcation, where the tibial nerve crosses, a vessel which runs parallel to the vein and follows the tibial nerve distad to anastomose with the caudal ramus of the saphenous artery. This used to be termed the *a. recurrens tibialis* in the older nomenclature but it is now known as the *a. comitans n. tibialis*. The distally directed branch of the distal caudal femoral artery follows the caudal surface of the lateral head of the gastrocnemius and, in company with the lateral saphenous vein and the n. cutaneous surae caudalis, it follows the tendons to the hock joint. This does not apply to the ruminants. It also gives off branches to the gastrocnemius muscle and the superficial flexors of the toe, where it ends in ruminants. In the pig it also supplies the superficial popliteal lymph nodes. In carnivores and the pig this branch anastomoses proximal to the calcaneus with the *r. calcanei* of the *r. caudalis* of the saphenous artery and in the horse with those of the *a. malleolaris caudalis lateralis*. In the cat it reaches as far as the *a. tarsea lateralis*.

A. poplitea
(Comparative: 105–108/*36*; dog: 110/*27*; pig: 111/*16*; sheep: 112/*16*; ox: 113/*31*; horse: 114/*17*)

While in the lower animals the **a. poplitea** forms the continuation of the ischiatic artery, in the domestic mammals it runs caudally along the femur as the continuation of the femoral artery after the origin of the distal caudal femoral artery. It continues between the two heads of the gastrocnemius, medial to the superficial flexor of the toes, across the flexor aspect of the knee joint and between the tibia and the popliteal muscle. Cranial to the popliteal muscle, but in the cat at its proximal border, it gives rise to the *a. tibialis caudalis* and, as has been shown in the pig and ox, it can give off the *a. interossea cruris*, caudodistally to the lateral condyle of the tibia. The popliteal artery then becomes the *a. tibialis cranialis*, which passes craniolaterally through the interosseous membrane of the leg to reach the tibia. Along its course the popliteal artery gives rise to the *aa. surales* which permeate the gastrocnemius and the long flexor muscles of the toes.

The popliteal artery is also the vessel of origin for numerous arteries supplying the knee joint. Thus it gives off a proximal and a distal pair of vessels to the sides of the knee joint, the *aa. genus proximales* and *distales laterales* and *mediales* and an unpaired middle artery, the *a. genus media* which passes between the two joint capsules. In the cat there are no distal genicular arteries and the medial proximal genicular artery arises from the cranial tibial artery. In ruminants the medial and lateral proximal genicular arteries arise from the distal caudal femoral artery. Together with the *a. genus descendens* these arteries of the knee joint form the *rete articulare genus* and the *rete patellae*.

A. tibialis caudalis
(Comparative: 105–108/*37*; sheep: 112/*17*; ox: 113/*30*; horse: 114/*18*; 118/*25*)

The **a. tibialis caudalis** is a smaller vessel than the cranial tibial artery. After its origin from the popliteal artery it curves round the proximal border of the popliteal muscle to attain its caudal surface. The caudal tibial artery ramifies in the caudal muscles of the shank, especially the deep flexors of the toes. It may, however, also participate in vascularizing the muscles of the lateral part of the shank, as in the pig where the *r. circumflexus fibulae* curves round the neck of the fibula to the lateral side. In the horse the caudal tibial artery gives off the *a. nutricia tibiae* at the level of the proximal third of the tibia. In the pig and ox it links with the *r. anastomoticus* of the *a. interossea cruris*. In the ox and the horse the caudal tibial artery continues even further distad and in the ox it gives off the *rr. malleolares mediales* and in the horse the *a. malleolaris caudalis lateralis*. These are the articular branches for the tarsal joint. Only in the horse does the caudal tibial artery anastomose with the caudal ramus of the saphenous artery and thus contribute to the vascularization of the foot.

A. interossea cruris
(pig: 106/*40*; ox: 107/*40*; 113/*32*)

The **a. interossea cruris** is phylogenetically an old vessel which, unlike the cranial tibial artery, runs caudally along the interosseous membrane of the leg in a distal direction. This slender vessel is found only in the pig and ox where it participates in the supply of blood to the deep flexors of the toes. In the pig it gives rise to the *aa. nutriciae tibiae* and *fibulae*. The *a. interossea cruris* is connected to the caudal

146   Arteries

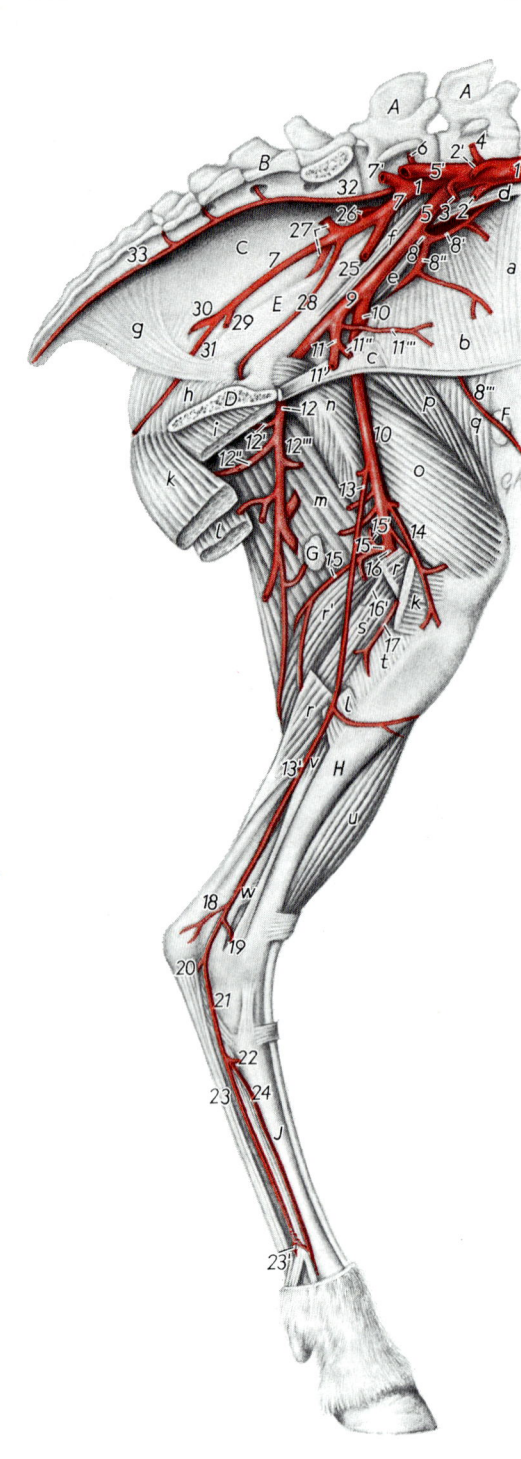

Fig. 112. Arteries of the left pelvic limb of a sheep. Medial view.
(After Freytag, 1962, Diss., Hanover.)

A vertebrae lumbales; *B* os sacrum; *C* lig. sacrotuberale latum; *D* symphysis pelvina; *E* os ilium; *F* ln. subiliacus; *G* ln. popliteus; *H* tibia; *J* os metatarsale III + IV

a m. transversus abdominis; *b* m. obliquus internus abdominis; *c* pelvic tendon of the m. obliquus externus abdominis; *d* m. psoas major; *e* m. iliacus; *f* m. psoas minor; *g* m. coccygeus; *h* m. obturatorius externus, pars intrapelvina; *i* m. adductor; *k* m. semimembranosus; *l* m. semitendinosus; *m* m. glutaeobiceps; *n* m. pectineus; *o* m. vastus medialis; *p* m. rectus femoris; *q* m. tensor fasciae latae; *r* m. gastrocnemius, caput mediale, *r'* caput laterale; *s* m. flexor digitalis superficialis; *t* m. popliteus; *u* m. fibularis tertius; *v* m. flexor digitalis longus; *w* m. tibialis caudalis

1 aorta abdominalis; *2* a. ovarica sinistra; *2'* a. ovarica dextra; *3* a. mesenterica caudalis; *4* a. lumbalis V; *5* a. iliaca externa sinistra; *5'* a. iliaca externa dextra; *6* a. lumbalis VI; *7* a. iliaca interna sinistra; *7'* a. iliaca interna dextra; *8* a. circumflexa ilium profunda, *8'* r. cranialis, *8''* r. caudalis, *8'''* r. superficialis; *9* a. profunda femoris; *10* a. femoralis; *11* truncus pudendoepigastricus; *11'* a. pudenda externa; *11''* a. epigastrica caudalis; *11'''* a. abdominalis caudalis; *12* a. circumflexa femoris medialis, *12'* r. caudalis, *12''* r. ascendens, *12'''* r. transversus (descendens); *13* a. saphena, *13'* r. caudalis; *14* a. genus descendens; *15* a. caudalis femoris distalis; *15'* a. genus proximalis lateralis; *16* a. poplitea; *16'* a. suralis; *17* a. tibialis caudalis; *18* rr. calcanei, *19* r. articularis of the r. caudalis of the a. saphena; *20* a. plantaris lateralis; *21* a. plantaris medialis, *22* r. profundus, *23* r. superficialis; *23'* a. digitalis plantaris communis II; *24* a. metatarsea plantaris II; *25* a. umbilicalis; *26* a. iliolumbalis; *27* a. glutaea cranialis; *28* a. obturatoria; *29* a. vaginalis; *30* a. glutaea caudalis; *31* a. pudenda interna; *32* a. sacralis mediana with rr. sacrales; *33* a. caudalis mediana

tibial by means of the *r. anastomoticus*. The r. interosseus s. perforans links the interosseous crural and cranial tibial arteries through the interosseous membrane of the leg. At about the same level it gives off the *rr. malleolares laterales* and *mediales* to the tarsal joint.

Arteries of the pelvic limb 147

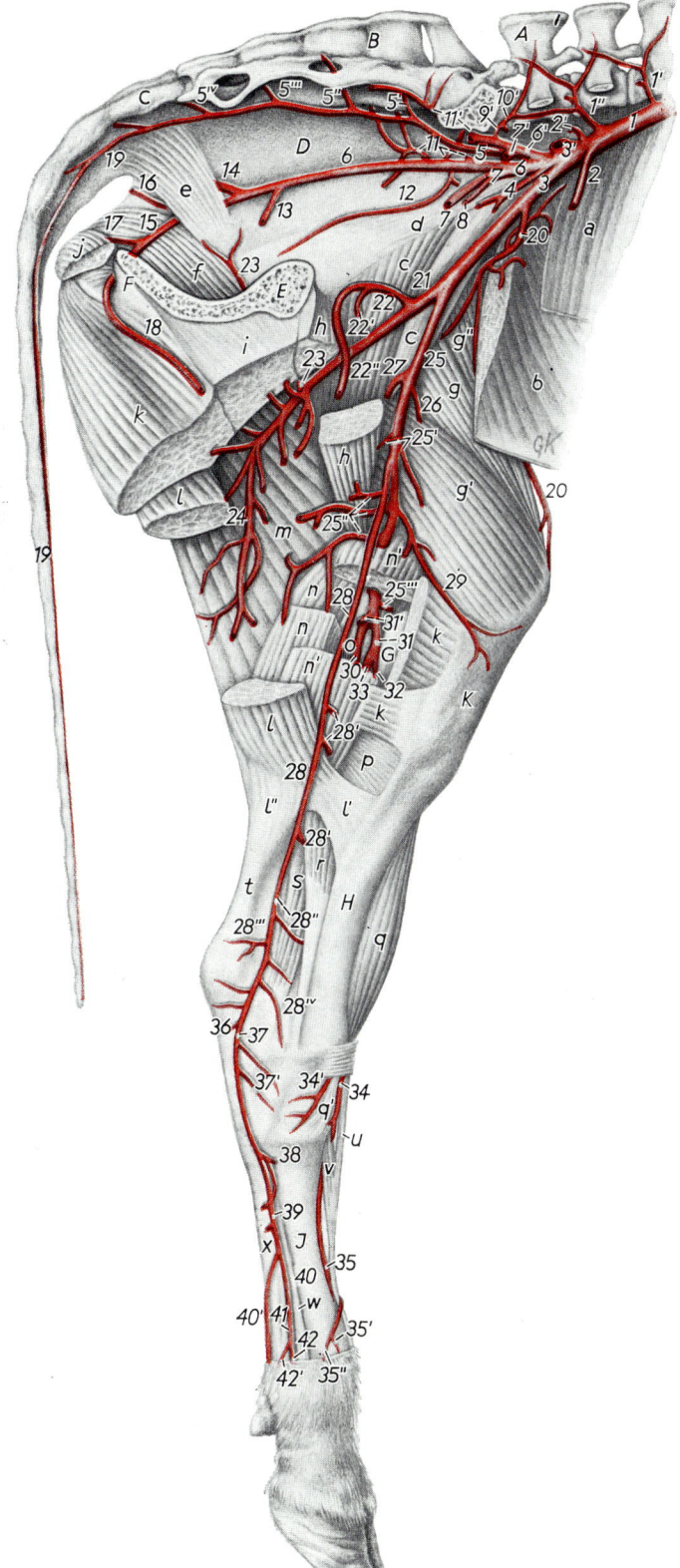

Fig. 113. Arteries of the left pelvic limb of an ox. Medial view.
(After Wilkens and Badawi, 1962, at the Institute of Veterinary Anatomy, Hanover.)

A vertebra lumbalis VI; *B* os sacrum; *C* vertebra caudalis I; *D* lig. sacrotuberale latum; *E* os pubis; *F* os ischii; *G* condylus medialis ossis femoris; *H* tibia; *J* os metatarsale III + IV; *K* fascia genus

a m. transversus abdominis; *b* m. obliquus internus abdominis; *c* m. iliopsoas; *d* m. psoas minor; *e* m. coccygeus; *f* m. obturatorius externus, pars intrapelvina; *g*, *g'* m. quadriceps femoris; *g* m. rectus femoris, *g'* m. vastus medialis; *g''* m. tensor fasciae latae; *h* m. pectineus; *i* mm. gracilis and adductor; *j* m. ischiocavernosus; *k* m. semimembranosus; *l* m. semitendinosus, *l'*, *l''* its tendons; *m* m. biceps femoris; *n* m. gastrocnemius, lateral, *n'* medial portion; *o* m. flexor digitalis superficialis; *p* m. popliteus; *q* m. fibularis tertius, *q'* its terminal tendon; *r* m. flexor digitalis longus; *s* mm. flexor hallucis longus and tibialis caudalis; *t* tendo calcaneus communis; *u* tendons of the m. extensor digitalis longus; *v* m. extensor digitalis brevis; *w* m. interosseus medius; *x* tendons of the flexor digitalis superficialis and profundus muscles

1 aorta abdominalis; *1'* a. lumbalis IV dextra; *1''* a. lumbalis V dextra; *2* a. testicularis sinistra; *2''* a. testicularis dextra; *3* a. iliaca externa sinistra; *3'* a. iliaca externa dextra; *4* a. mesenterica caudalis; *5* a. sacralis mediana, *5'–5^{iv}* rr. sacrales; *6* a. iliaca interna sinistra; *6'* a. iliaca interna dextra; *7* a. umbilicalis sinistra; *7'* a. umbilicalis dextra; *8* a. ductus deferentis; *9'* a. iliolumbalis dextra; *10'* a. lumbalis VI dextra; *11* a. glutaea cranialis sinistra; *11'* a. glutaea cranialis dextra; *12* a. obturatoria; *13* a. prostatica; *14* a. glutaea caudalis; *15* a. penis and *16* a. perinealis ventralis, the terminal branches of the a. pudenda interna; *17* a. bulbi penis; *18* a. dorsalis penis; *19* a. caudalis mediana with rr. caudales; *20* a. circumflexa ilium profunda; *21* a. profunda femoris; *22* truncus pudendoepigastricus; *22'* a. epigastrica caudalis; *22''* a. pudenda externa; *23* r. obturatorius; *24* a. circumflexa femoris medialis; *25* a. femoralis; *25'* a. caudalis femoris proximalis and r. muscularis to the quadriceps femoris; *25''* rr. musculares of the a. saphena, a. caudalis femoris media and a. caudalis femoris distalis; *25'''* a. genus media; *26* a. circumflexa femoris lateralis, r. descendens, *27* r. ascendens with r. transversus; *28* a. saphena, *28'* rr. cutanei, *28''* r. caudalis, *28'''* rr. calcanei, *28^{iv}* rr. malleolaris medialis; *29* a. genus descendens; *30* a. tibialis caudalis; *31* a. poplitea; *31'* a. suralis; *32* a. interossea cruris; *33* a. tibialis cranialis; *34* a. dorsalis pedis; *34'* a. tarsea medialis; *35* a. metatarsea dorsalis III; *35'* a. digitalis dorsalis communis III; *35''* a. digitalis dorsalis communis II; *36* a. plantaris lateralis; *37* a. plantaris medialis; *37'* rr. articulares; *38* r. profundus, *39* r. superficialis; *40* a. digitalis plantaris communis II; *40'* a. digitalis plantaris communis III; *41* junction of the transverse anastomosis of the aa. metatarseae plantares; *42* a. digitalis plantaris propria III abaxialis; *42'* a. digitalis plantaris propria II axialis

A. tibialis cranialis
(Comparative: 105–108/*41*; 119–122/*28*; dog: 110/*28*; pig: 111/*17*; ox: 113/*33*)

The largest of the terminal branches of the popliteal artery is the **a. tibialis cranialis** and in domestic mammals it forms the continuation of that vessel, passing through the interosseous membrane craniolaterally to reach the tibia. In the distal third of the tibia it turns, still closely applied to the bone, onto the cranial surface of the tibia, except in the horse in which species it continues craniolaterally. The cranial tibial artery lies medial to the tendon of the long extensor of the toes, being covered by it in the horse, and courses to the flexor aspect of the tarsal joint where it becomes the *a. dorsalis pedis*. Immediately after its passage through the interosseous membrane the cranial tibial artery gives off, except in the horse, the *a. recurrens tibialis cranialis*. In ruminants the latter may also arise in common with the muscular branches to be mentioned below. The recurrent cranial tibial artery is proximally directed and contributes to the plexus of the knee joint. In the cat the recurrent cranial tibial artery gives off the *a. genus proximalis medialis*, in carnivores the *a. nutricia tibiae et fibulae* and in ruminants the *a. nutricia tibiae*. In all the domestic mammals at the level of the proximal part of the crural bones, stout muscular branches are given off which vascularize the group of muscles lying craniolaterally on the shank. The *ramus superficialis* arises, except in the pig, at about the middle of the tibia. Lateral to the long extensors of the toes this vessel attains a superficial position and continues distally. Except in the horse it contributes to the formation of the dorsal superficial plexus of the toes and in the cat it terminates, still in the tarsal region, in the *r. cranialis* of the *a. saphena medialis*. At the distal part of the shank the *r. interosseus s. perforans* connects the cranial tibial artery with the interosseous crural artery through the interosseous membrane and in the cat it joins it to the malleolar branches of the distal caudal femoral artery. In the pig and the ox the terminal part of the cranial tibial artery also gives off the *aa. malleolares craniales lateralis* and *medialis*.

A. dorsalis pedis
(Comparative: 105–108/*44*; 119–122/*31*; cat: 109/*31*; dog: 110/*29*; pig: 111/*18*; ox: 113/*34*)

The **a. dorsalis pedis** is the continuation of the cranial tibial artery as it crosses the flexor aspect of the tarsal joint. Accompanied by the vein of the same name and the deep fibular nerve, it runs to the metatarsus. Except in the horse it gives off the *a. tarsea lateralis* and the *a. tarsea medialis* each of which run almost transversally to the appropriate side of the tarsal joint and, in so doing, in the cat the lateral artery connects with the distal caudal femoral artery. In the pig the lateral tarsal artery gives rise to the *a. tarsea perforans proximalis* which anastomoses with the *a. plantaris lateralis* between the talus and calcaneus. Except in carnivores the dorsal pedal artery gives rise to either the *a. tarsea perforans* or, in the case of the pig, the *a. tarsea perforans distalis*. This perforating tarsal artery runs through the tarsal canal to the plantar aspect of the foot where it links with the *arcus plantaris profundus*. In the ox it passes out of the tarsal canal and between the proximal articular surfaces of the fused third and fourth metatarsal bones to continue to the plantar surface between these two bones. Thus it seems that in the ox this perforating vessel is the *a. tarsea perforans* which has fused with the *r. perforans proximalis III*. In carnivores the dorsal pedal artery reaches the metatarsus dorsomedially and terminates by giving off the transversally directed *a. arcuata* which, in turn, gives rise to the *aa. metatarseae dorsales*. In the pig, ruminants, and the horse the dorsal pedal artery continues as the *a. metatarsea dorsalis III*.

Arteries of the hindfoot of carnivores*
Plantar arteries
(cat: 109/*30*; dog: 92; 105; 110/*20–24, 32*; 115)

In carnivores the **r. caudalis** of the *a. saphena* gives rise in the proximal tarsal region to the *a. plantaris lateralis* and in the dog only, it also gives off the *a. plantaris medialis* a short distance afterwards. It then continues distad on the plantar aspect. The medial plantar artery divides, in the dog, into a slender *r.*

---

* The topography and nomenclature of the blood vessels of the autopodium have already been described in general terms on page 92.

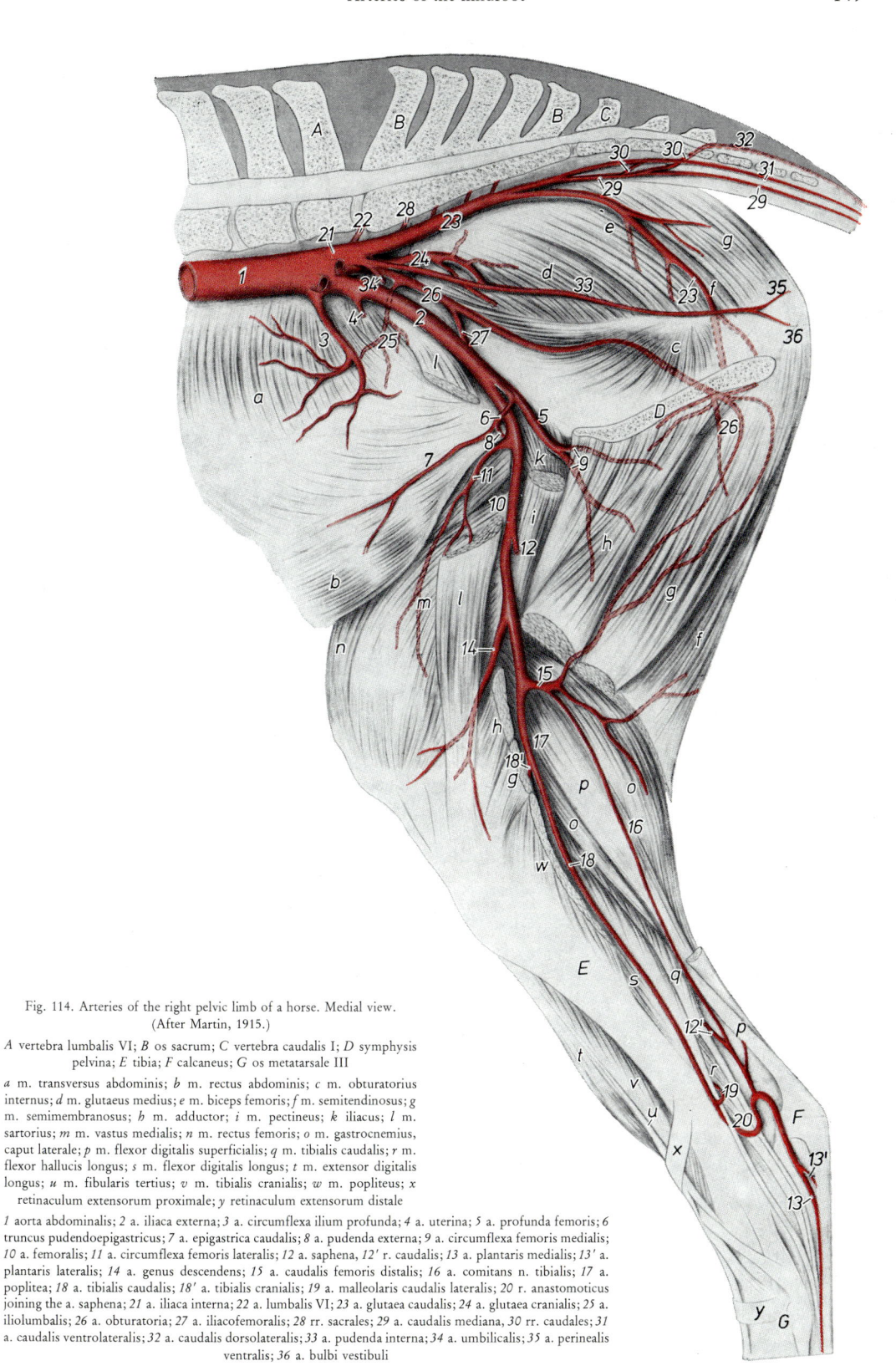

Arteries of the hindfoot

Fig. 114. Arteries of the right pelvic limb of a horse. Medial view. (After Martin, 1915.)

A vertebra lumbalis VI; *B* os sacrum; *C* vertebra caudalis I; *D* symphysis pelvina; *E* tibia; *F* calcaneus; *G* os metatarsale III

a m. transversus abdominis; *b* m. rectus abdominis; *c* m. obturatorius internus; *d* m. glutaeus medius; *e* m. biceps femoris; *f* m. semitendinosus; *g* m. semimembranosus; *h* m. adductor; *i* m. pectineus; *k* iliacus; *l* m. sartorius; *m* m. vastus medialis; *n* m. rectus femoris; *o* m. gastrocnemius, caput laterale; *p* m. flexor digitalis superficialis; *q* m. tibialis caudalis; *r* m. flexor hallucis longus; *s* m. flexor digitalis longus; *t* m. extensor digitalis longus; *u* m. fibularis tertius; *v* m. tibialis cranialis; *w* m. popliteus; *x* retinaculum extensorum proximale; *y* retinaculum extensorum distale

1 aorta abdominalis; *2* a. iliaca externa; *3* a. circumflexa ilium profunda; *4* a. uterina; *5* a. profunda femoris; *6* truncus pudendoepigastricus; *7* a. epigastrica caudalis; *8* a. pudenda externa; *9* a. circumflexa femoris medialis; *10* a. femoralis; *11* a. circumflexa femoris lateralis; *12* a. saphena, *12'* r. caudalis; *13* a. plantaris medialis; *13'* a. plantaris lateralis; *14* a. genus descendens; *15* a. caudalis femoris distalis; *16* a. comitans n. tibialis; *17* a. poplitea; *18* a. tibialis caudalis; *18'* a. tibialis cranialis; *19* a. malleolaris caudalis lateralis; *20* r. anastomoticus joining the a. saphena; *21* a. iliaca interna; *22* a. lumbalis VI; *23* a. glutaea caudalis; *24* a. glutaea cranialis; *25* a. iliolumbalis; *26* a. obturatoria; *27* a. iliacofemoralis; *28* rr. sacrales; *29* a. caudalis mediana, *30* rr. caudales; *31* a. caudalis ventrolateralis; *32* a. caudalis dorsolateralis; *33* a. pudenda interna; *34* a. umbilicalis; *35* a. perinealis ventralis; *36* a. bulbi vestibuli

superficialis and a more robust *r. profundus*. The lateral plantar artery continues in both the cat and dog as the *r. profundus* without giving off a superficial ramus. In the dog the *rr. profundi* unite to form the *arcus plantaris* to which the large *r. perforans proximalis II* also contributes. In the cat, on the other hand, the deep plantar arch is formed only by the *r. profundus* of the lateral plantar artery and the *r. perforans proximalis II*. In both the cat and the dog this arch gives rise to the *aa. metatarseae plantares II–IV* which are connected with the dorsal metatarsal arteries via the *rr. perforantes distales,* and terminate in the plantar common digital arteries of the same number.

The superficial ramus of the medial plantar artery, which, as noted above, is present only in the dog, continues as the *a. digitalis plantaris communis I*. This vessel in turn gives off the slender *a. digitalis plantaris propria II* and, if the first toe is present, the *a. digitalis plantaris propria I axialis*. The caudal ramus of the saphenous artery runs medially between the flexor tendons and divides at the distal half of the metatarsus into the *aa. digitales plantares communes II–IV*. Proximal to the metatarsophalangeal joints these vessels unite with plantar metatarsal arteries and, distal to this joint, they link via the *aa. interdigitales* with the dorsal common digital arteries of the same number. Shortly thereafter they give off the axial *aa. digitales plantares propriae*. The abaxial plantar proper digital arteries arise in each case from the *rr. plantares,* especially on the proximal phalanges. These arteries are only rarely given off by plantar common digital arteries.

Dorsal arteries
(cat: 109/29, *31, 32;* dog: 92; 105; 110/*18, 19, 29–32;* 119)

In carnivores the dorsal pedal artery gives off, in the region of the tarsometatarsal joint, the transversally directed *a. arcuata* which lies close to the bone. In the cat the latter vessel anastomoses with the distal caudal femoral artery. The arcuate artery gives rise to the *aa. metatarseae dorsales II–IV*. Of these the a. metatarsea dorsalis II forms the main supply from the dorsal pedal artery via the *r. perforans proximalis II* to the deep plantar arch. The *rr. perforantes distales* are all present. The dorsal metatarsal arteries terminate distally on the metatarsus in the dorsal common digital arteries of the same numbers.

The cranial ramus of the saphenous artery gives off, from two branch vessels in the cat and one after the other in the dog, the *aa. digitales dorsales communes I–IV*. After receiving the dorsal metatarsal arteries and linking with the *aa. interdigitales* these common digital arteries give off the *aa. digitales dorsales propriae*. From the common dorsal digital artery IV arises in the cat the *a. digitalis dorsalis V abaxialis;* in the dog this stems from the superficial ramus of the cranial tibial artery.

Arteries of the hindfoot of the pig

Plantar arteries
(pig: 106; 111/*14;* 19, 20; 116)

In the pig the caudal ramus of the saphenous artery gives off, distally to the sustentaculum tali, the *a. plantaris lateralis* and, a short distance thereafter, the *a. plantaris medialis*. It then continues distally on the plantar aspect. At the level of the tarsometatarsal joint each plantar artery divides into a *r. profundus* and a *r. superficialis*. The deep rami unite proximally on the metatarsus to form the *arcus plantaris profundus* which also receives the *a. tarsea perforans distalis*. From this arch arise the *aa. metatarseae plantares II–IV*. On the dorsum of the foot the IInd and IVth dorsal metatarsal arteries arise from the *rr. perforantes proximales II* and *IV*. The single *ramus perforans distalis III* links up with the IIIrd dorsal metatarsal artery. The second and fourth plantar metatarsal arteries do not connect with the plantar common digital arteries of the same number but they unite distally on the metatarsus with the third plantar metatarsal artery. They terminate in the third plantar common digital artery.

The caudal ramus of the saphenous artery continues distally along the superficial flexor tendon and links up with the superficial rami of both the medial and lateral plantar arteries in the distal part of the metatarsus where it forms a type of superficial arch. From this arise the *aa. digitales plantares communes II–IV* which, a short distance afterwards, give rise to the axial *aa. digitales plantares propriae*. The abaxial plantar proper digital arteries arise in each case via the *rr. plantares,* especially at the proximal phalanges. The interdigital connections are made by the *rr. dorsales* of the appropriate proximal phalanx.

Dorsal arteries
(pig: 106; 111/*14″, 18*; 120)

In the pig the dorsal pedal artery, after giving off the distal perforating tarsal artery to the deep plantar arch, continues as the *a. metatarsea dorsalis III* which is connected to the plantar metatarsal artery of the same number by the *r. perforans distalis III*. The *aa. metatarseae dorsales II* and *IV* arise from the appropriate proximal perforating rami without receiving proximal tributaries on the dorsum of the foot.

There are no superficial arteries on the dorsum of the foot and, therefore, the *aa. digitales dorsales propriae* arise directly from the dorsal metatarsal arteries. The abaxial arteries of the third and fourth toes extend only to the middle phalanx; distal to that phalanx they are represented, like the abaxial arteries of the second and fifth toes, by the dorsal rami of the plantar proper digital arteries.

Arteries of the hindfoot of ruminants

Plantar arteries
(sheep: 112/*13′, 18–24*; ox: 107; 113/*28″, 28‴, 28^{iv}, 36–42′*; 117)

In ruminants the **r. caudalis** of the saphenous artery forks proximal to the sustentaculum tali into the *a. plantaris medialis* and *a. plantaris lateralis*. Over the proximal extremity of the metatarsus each of these plantar arteries then divides into a *r. profundus* and a *r. superficialis*. At the level of the proximal metatarsal canal the deep rami unite to form the *arcus plantaris profundus* which in the small ruminants receives blood via the *a. tarsea perforans* and in the ox via the *r. perforans proximalis III* which is linked to the *a. tarsea perforans (distales)*. From the arch arise the *aa. metatarseae plantares II–IV*. The latter are connected with one another at the distal part of the metatarsus by means of a transverse anastomosis which also joins them laterally to the third and fourth plantar common digital arteries. Passing through the distal metatarsal canal the *r. perforans distalis III* links the transverse anastomosis with the third dorsal metatarsal artery.

At a variable level in the distal half of the metatarsus, the superficial ramus of the medial plantar artery divides into the *aa. digitales plantares communes II* and *III*. In the ox this division may sometimes be more proximal and it can even occur from the medial plantar artery. The lateral plantar artery runs distad on the metatarsus where it becomes the *a. digitalis plantaris communis IV*. The transverse anastomosis of the plantar metatarsal artery terminates in the second and fourth plantar common digital artery. The third plantar common digital artery receives a large volume of blood from the third common dorsal digital artery via the *a. interdigitalis III*. The common plantar digital arteries divide into the *aa. digitales plantares propriae*.

Dorsal arteries
(ox: 107; 113/*34–35″*; 121)

The dorsal pedal artery of ruminants gives off the *a. tarsea perforans (distalis)* and then becomes the *a. metatarsea dorsalis III,* which is the largest artery of the foot. It is linked to the transverse anastomosis of the plantar metatarsal artery by means of the *r. perforans distalis* and, distal to the metatarsophalangeal joint, it unites with the slender *a. digitalis dorsalis communis III*.

The *a. digitalis dorsalis communis III* arises about half way down the metatarsus from the slender superficial ramus of the cranial tibial artery together with the *aa. digitales dorsales communes II* and *IV*. The latter are only rudimentary vessels in the ox. The third dorsal common digital artery, which is augmented by the third dorsal metatarsal artery, gives rise to the large *a. interdigitalis III* and the rudimentary *aa. digitales dorsales propriae III* and *IV axiales*.

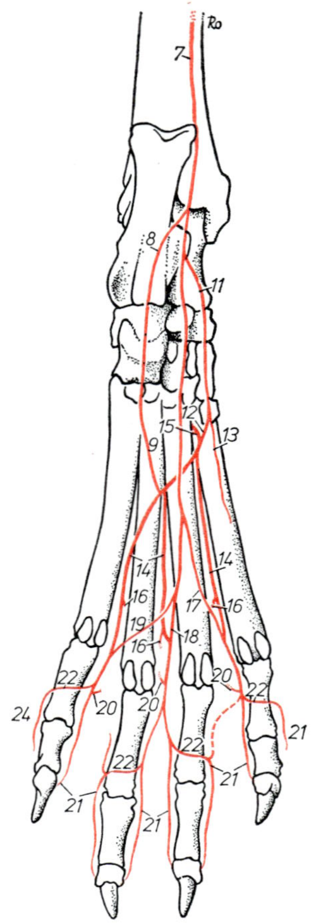

152 Arteries

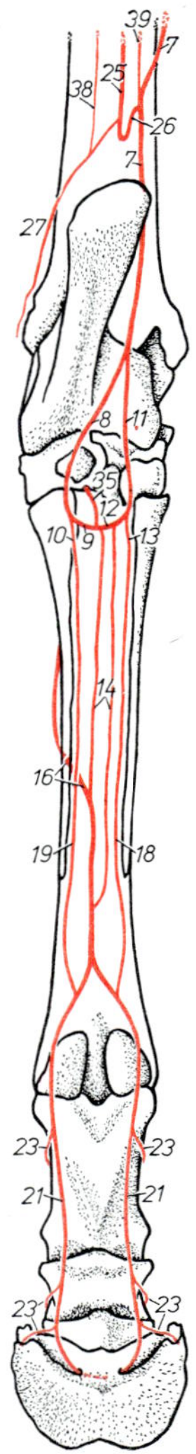

Figs 115, 116, 117, 118, 119, 120, 121, 122. Arteries of the left hind foot of the dog, pig, ox and horse. Semidiagrammatic.
Figs 115–118: plantar view; Figs 119–122: dorsal view.

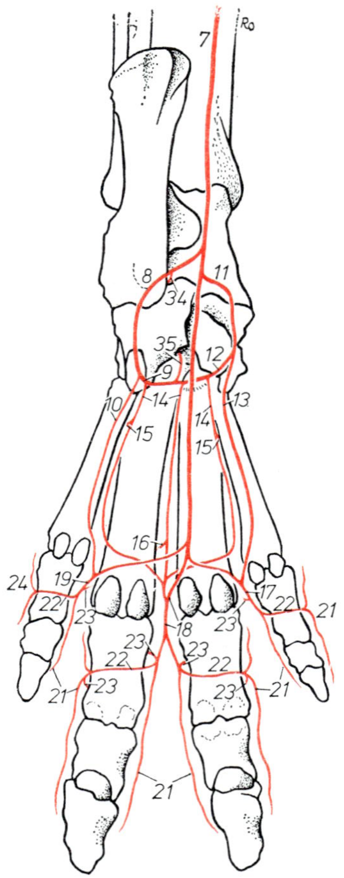

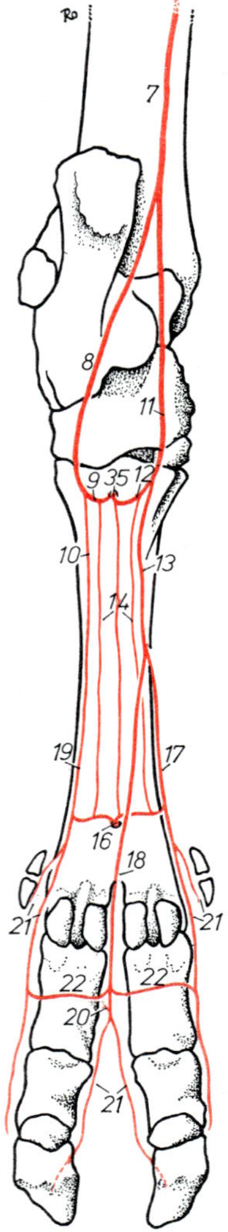

1 r. cranialis of the a. saphena; *2–5* aa. digitales dorsales communes I–IV; *6* aa. digitales dorsales propriae; *7* r. caudalis of the a. saphena; *8* a. plantaris lateralis; *9* r. profundus; *10* r. superficialis; *11* a. plantaris medialis; *12* r. profundus; *13* r. superficialis; *9* and *12* arcus plantaris profundus; *14* aa. metatarseae plantares II–IV; *15* rr. perforantes proximales; *16* rr. perforantes distales; *17–19* aa. digitales plantares communes

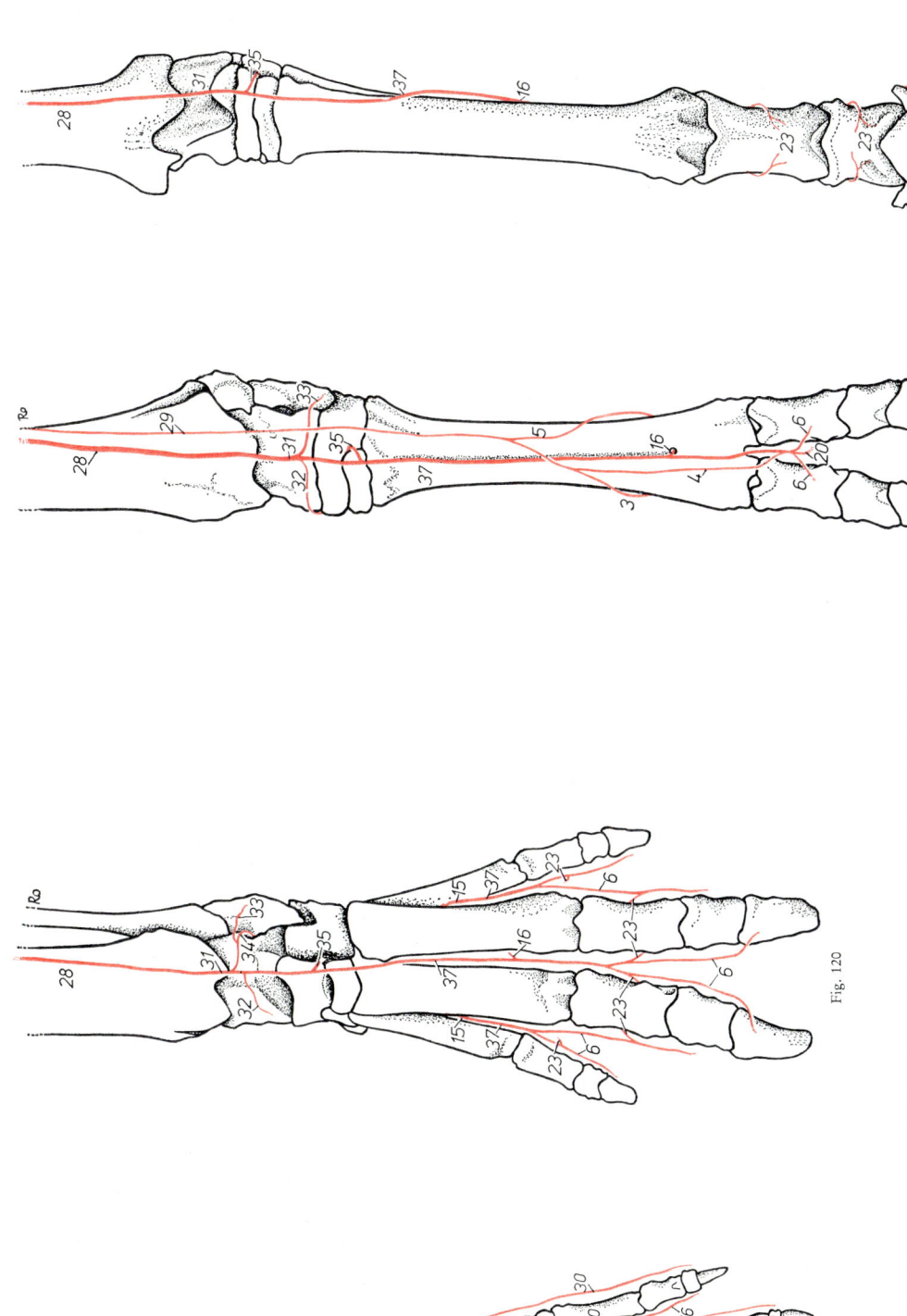

Arteries of the hindfoot

II–IV: *20* aa. interdigitales; *21* aa. digitales plantares propriae; *22* rr. palmares phalangium proximalium; *23* rr. dorsales phalangium proximalium, or in the horse, phalangis proximalis, mediae and distalis; *24* a. digitalis plantaris V abaxialis; *25* a. tibialis caudalis; *26* r. anastomoticus cum a. saphena; *27* a. malleolaris caudalis lateralis; *28* a. tibialis cranialis; *29* r. superficialis; *30* a. digitalis dorsalis V abaxialis; *31* a. dorsalis pedis; *32* a. tarsea medialis; *33* a. tarsea lateralis; *34* a. tarsea perforans proximalis; *35* a. tarsea perforans distalis; *36* a. arcuata; *37* aa. metatarseae dorsales II–IV; *38* anastomose of the a. caudalis femoris distalis; *39* a. comitans n. tibialis

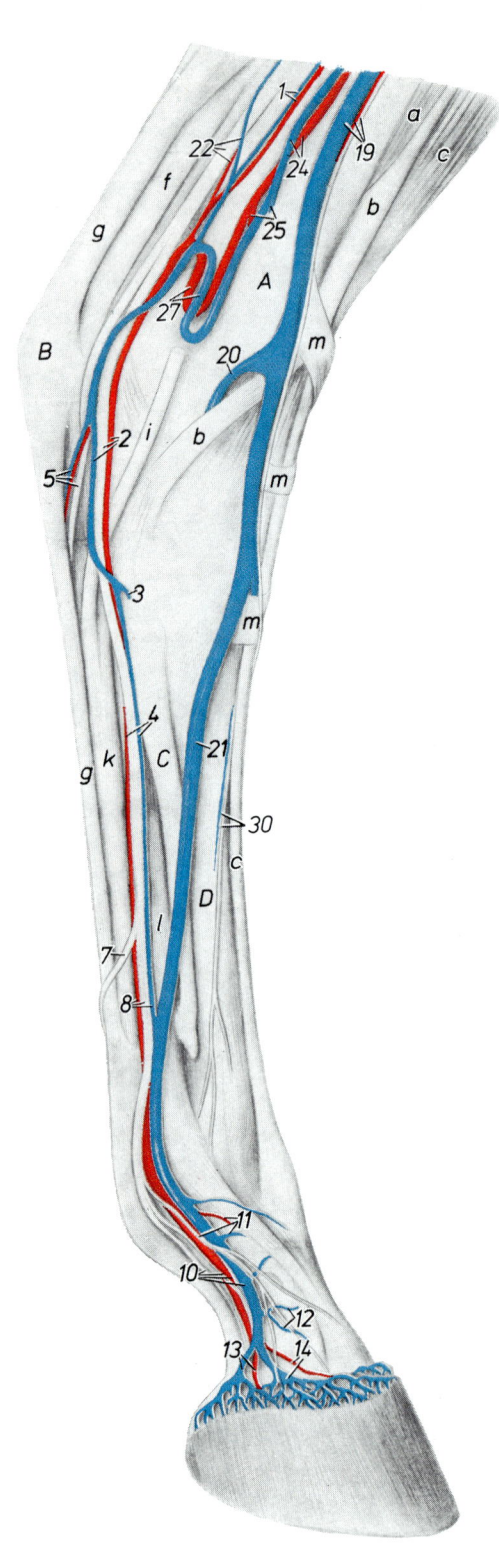

Arteries of the hindfoot of the horse

Plantar arteries
(horse: 108; 118/*12–13′, 19, 20*; 123; 124)

The caudal ramus of the saphenous artery receives, proximal to the tarsal joint, the *a. comitans n. tibialis* as a tributary from the distal caudal femoral artery and it is connected by an S-shaped anastomosis with the caudal tibial artery. At the level of the sustentaculum tali the caudal ramus of the saphenous artery forks into the medial and lateral plantar arteries. Each of these plantar arteries divides at the proximal part of the metatarsus into a deep and superficial ramus. The deep rami unite, receive the *a. tarsea perforans* (*distalis*) and form the *arcus plantaris profundus*. Out of this arch arise the *aa. metatarseae plantares II* and *III*. In the lower half of the metatarsus the two plantar metatarsal arteries link up with the stout *r. perforans distalis III*. This arterial vascular union forks proximal to the sesamoid bones and these branches link respectively with the *a. digitalis plantaris communis II* and the *a. digitalis plantaris communis III* which represent a continuation of the superficial ramus of the lateral plantar artery. The *a. digitalis plantaris* (*propria III*) *medialis* and the *a. digitalis plantaris* (*propria III*) *lateralis* arise from this ramification.

Dorsal arteries
(horse: 108; 122; 123; 124; 206/2)

The dorsal pedal artery gives off the distal perforating tarsal artery and then becomes the *a. metatarsea dorsalis III*. This vessel in turn is continued by the *r. perforans distalis III* which carries blood to the plantar system. During its course the perforating ramus III passes gradually and obliquely in a distoplantar direction between the third and second metatarsal bones. It is possible to feel the pulse beat in the a. metatarsea dorsalis III proximal to this perforating site and in the groove between these two bones. The dorsal part of the toe is only supplied, as in the forelimb, by the *rr. dorsales phalangis proximalis, mediae* and *distalis* of the two plantar digital arteries.

Fig. 123. Arteries and veins of the left hind foot of a horse. Medial view. (After Martin, 1915.)
For legends see fig. 124.

Pelvic and tail arteries

Fig. 124. Arteries and veins of the left hind foot of a horse. Lateral view.
(After Martin, 1915.)

A. tibia; *B* tuber calcanei; *C* os metatarsale II; *D* os metatarsale III; *E* os metatarsale IV

a m. tibialis cranialis; *b* m. fibularis tertius; *c* m. extensor digitalis longus; *d* m. extensor digitalis lateralis; *e* m. extensor digitalis brevis; *f* tendon of the gastrocnemius muscle; *g* m. flexor digitalis superficialis; *h* m. flexor hallucis longus and m. tibialis caudalis; *i* tendon of the m. flexor digitalis longus; *k* tendon of the m. flexor digitalis profundus; *l* m. interosseus medius; *m* retinacula extensoria

1 a. saphena, r. caudalis, and v. saphena medialis, r. caudalis; *2* a. and v. plantaris medialis with n. plantaris medialis, *3* r. profundus, *4* r. superficialis; *5* a. and v. plantaris lateralis with n. plantaris lateralis, *6* r. superficialis, *7* r. communicans; *8* a. and v. digitalis plantaris communis III with n. digitalis plantaris communis II; *9* a. and v. digitalis plantaris communis II with n. digitalis plantaris communis III; *10* a. and v. digitalis plantaris propria III medialis with n. digitalis plantaris proprius III medialis, *11* r. dorsalis phalangis proximalis with r. dorsalis, *12* r. dorsalis phalangis mediae, *13* r. tori digitalis; *14* a. and v. coronalis; *15* a. and v. digitalis plantaris propria III lateralis with n. digitalis plantaris propria III lateralis, *16* r. dorsalis phalangis proximalis with r. dorsalis, *17* r. tori digitalis; *18* a. and v. coronalis; *19* a. saphena, r. cranialis, and v. saphena medialis, r. cranialis, with n. saphenus; *20* r. anastomoticus; *21* v. digitalis dorsalis communis II; *22* a. and v. comitans n. tibialis with n. tibialis; *23* v. saphena lateralis, r. caudalis with accompanying artery and n. cutaneus surae caudalis; *24* a. and v. tibialis caudalis; *25* a. and v. malleolaris caudalis lateralis, *26* rr. calcanei, *27* r. anastomoticus; *28* a. and v. tibialis cranialis with n. fibularis profundus; *29* a. and v. dorsalis pedis; *30* v. metatarsea dorsalis II with n. metatarseus dorsalis II; *31* a. metatarsea dorsalis III with n. metatarseus dorsalis III, *32* r. perforans distalis; *33* n. fibularis superficialis

Arteries of the pelvic and tail regions

A. iliaca interna

(Comparative: 85–88/*67*; 105–108/*3*; 136–143/*19*; cat: 91/*32*; 109/*9*; dog: 110/*33*; pig: 98/*29*; 111/*21*; sheep: 101/*26*; 112/*7*; ox: 113/*6*; 114/*9*; horse: 50/*30*; 104/*19*; 114/*21*)

The **a. iliaca interna** arises from the abdominal aorta while the latter is still cranial to the promontory. In carnivores this occurs ventral to the 7th, in pigs and ruminants ventral to the 6th and in the horse ventral to the 4th–5th lumbar vertebrae. Thence it passes over the medial surface of the iliopsoas muscle into the pelvic cavity. In the horse it gives off the *aa. lumbales* V and VI and divides a short distance afterwards at the level of the 5th and 6th lumbar vertebrae into the *a. glutea caudalis* and the *a. pudenda interna.* In carnivores the internal iliac first gives off the *a. umbilicalis* and it then divides. In the dog this division takes place immediately cranial to the base of the sacrum and it gives rise to the caudal gluteal and internal pudendal arteries. In the cat the *a. glutea cranialis* is given off before the bifurcation which occurs at the level of the greater ischiatic notch. In the pig and ruminants the internal iliac artery gives off the a. umbilicalis as it enters the pelvis. The internal iliac now crosses the shaft of the ilium and gives rise to the *a. iliolumbalis* in a medial direction. Also arising from the parent artery in the pig are either the *a. prosta-*

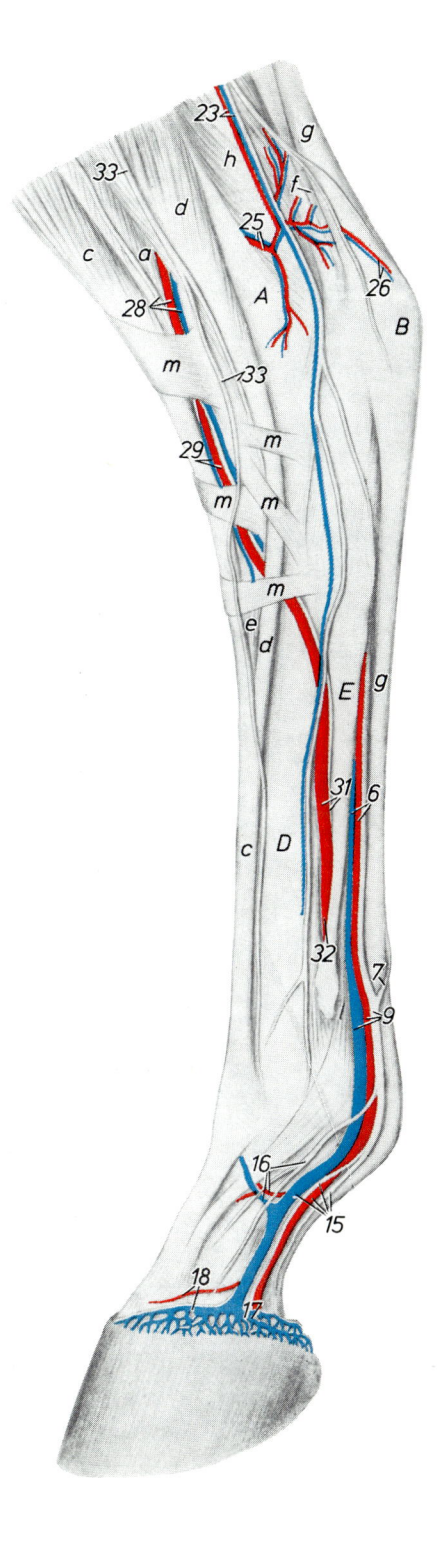

tica or the *a. vaginalis*. In ruminants the *a. glutea cranialis* arises caudal to the shaft of the ilium. In the sheep the *a. obturatoris* also originates from the internal iliac artery. Thereafter, in the pig and ox, the internal iliac artery perforates the broad sacrotuberal ligament in the region of the greater ischiatic notch and so gains the lateral surface of that ligament. Here the cranial gluteal artery is given off in the pig. At the level of the hip joint the prostatic or vaginal artery is given off in ruminants and, in the ox, it perforates the broad sacrotuberal ligament to enter the pelvic cavity. In the region of the lesser ischiatic notch the internal iliac arteries of the pig and ruminants give off branches to the rotators of the hip joint and then divides into the caudal gluteal and internal pudendal arteries.

The end of the internal iliac artery and the start of the internal pudendal artery are thus determined phylogenetically by the origin of the caudal gluteal artery because the latter is homologous with the initial section of the *a. ischiadica*. The a. ischiadica is still fully developed in birds. It will be seen from the above that in carnivores and the horse the internal iliac is only short and its further course corresponds to the internal pudendal artery. This brings about a long "pudendal type" in carnivores and the horse and a short "pudendal type" in the pig and ruminants. Thus while the site of origin of "visceral arteries" such as the umbilical artery in the horse and the prostatic or vaginal arteries in carnivores and the horse, is comparable to that of other domestic mammals, these vessels stem from the internal pudendal artery. Similarly the "parietal vessel", the a. iliolumbalis, arises from the caudal gluteal artery directly in the dog and indirectly via the cranial gluteal artery in the horse. In the cat it also arises from this artery but prior to the bifurcation of the internal iliac artery.

A. glutea cranialis

(Comparative: 85–88/*70*; 105–108/*6*; 136–143/*26*; dog: 110/*36*; pig: 111/*26*; sheep: 112/*27*; ox: 113/*11*; 144/*15*; horse: 50/*32*; 114/*24*)

In all domestic mammals the **a. glutea cranialis** arises on the medial surface of the ilium. In the cat, pig and ruminants it springs from the internal iliac artery and in the dog and horse from the caudal gluteal artery. In the cat and also usually in the horse it gives off the *a. obturatoria* and the *a. iliolumbalis*. In the dorsal part of the greater ischiatic notch the cranial gluteal artery curves laterally round the caudal border of the ilium and, by means of numerous diverging branches, it ramifies in the gluteal musculature. In ruminants it also supplies the gluteobiceps muscle and in the pig it passes over the lumbar part of the gluteus medius muscle into the longissimus dorsi.

A. iliolumbalis

(Comparative: 85–88/*69*; 105–108/*7*; 136–143/*25*; dog: 110/*35*; sheep: 112/*26*; ox: 113/*10*; horse: 50/*33*; 144/*25*)

In the cat and horse the **a. iliolumbalis** arises from the cranial gluteal artery but in the dog it stems from the caudal gluteal and in the pig and ruminants form the internal iliac artery. But in all the domestic mammals the origin of the iliolumbar artery can vary and, in fact, this vessel may occasionally arise from any of these three arteries. The iliolumbar artery then runs between the ilium and the iliopsoas muscle in the direction of the tuber coxae, giving off on its course branches to the iliopsoas and the psoas minor muscles and to the ilium. Caudoventrally to the tuber coxae it bends round the lateral border of the ilium, providing branches for the m. tensor fasciae latae in the horse and carnivores and for the sartorius muscles in carnivores. In the cat there are also branches to the rectus femoris and lateral vastus muscles. Only in the horse and carnivores does this vessel then continue on the lateral side of the wing of the ilium, to ramify in the gluteus medius muscle. In the horse its branches can be traced to the lumbar part of this muscle and in the dog to the same muscle and also to the deep gluteal muscle. In the pig and ruminants the slender iliolumbar artery supplies only the sublumbar musculature.

A. obturatoria

(Comparative: 105–108/*8*; 136–143/*27*; sheep: 112/*28*; ox: 113/*12*; horse: 88/*71*; 114/*26*)

In the cat and the horse the **a. obturatoria** arises as a slender vessel from the cranial gluteal artery. In the goat too, and sometimes in the ox, it has a similar origin, while in the pig it stems as a slender vessel from the iliolumbar artery and in the sheep from the internal iliac. In the dog and, generally, in the ox this artery is absent. The obturator artery, in company with the obturator nerve, runs along the body of the ilium. In the pig and horse it follows the iliac head of the pars intrapelvina m. obturatorii externi or the same head of the m. obturatorius internus, to the cranial border of the obturator foramen. It rarely reaches the obturator foramen in the goat. In the horse it gives off, while still dorsal to the tuberc. m. psoas minoris, the *a. iliofemoralis*. Following the lateral border of the obturator foramen, the obturator artery leaves the pelvic cavity to anastomose in the cat, pig and sheep with the *r. obturatorius* of the deep femoral artery. In the sheep this junction lies at the craniolateral border of the intrapelvic part of the external obturator muscle. In this region the vessel primarily supplies this and the lateral ventral sacrocaudal muscle. In the horse it gives off, ventral to the tabula ischiadica, the *a. penis media* or, in females, the *a. clitoridis media*, and runs distad to the level of the knee joint between the rotators of the hip joint and the long ischiatic muscles giving off branches to these muscle groups.

A. iliacofemoralis
(horse: 88/*72*; 108/*19'*; 114/*27*)

The **a. iliacofemoralis** is present only in the horse in which it substitutes for the *r. transversus* and the *r. ascendens* of the lateral circumflex femoris artery. It arises from the obturator artery, dorsal to the tuberc. m. psoas minoris, and continues in company with the paired veins of the same name over the cranial surface of the body of the ilium onto its craniolateral ridge. It gives off several branches to the iliopsoas muscle, a nutritive vessel to the iliac body and branches to the hip joint. Finally it anastomoses, like the transverse ramus of the lateral circumflex femoral artery of the other domestic mammals, with the medial circumflex femoral artery around the shaft of the femur. Before this anastomosis, however, the iliacofemoral artery gives off the *r. ascendens* which vascularizes the tensor fasciae latae, quadriceps femoris, middle and superficial gluteal and, by passing through the latter, the triceps femoris muscles.

A. glutea caudalis
(Comparative: 85–88/*68*; 105–108/*5*; 136–143/*26*; cat: 109/*12*; dog: 110/*34*; pig: 98/*33*; 111/*29*; sheep: 112/*30*; ox: 113/*14*; 144/*16*; horse: 50/*31*; 114/*23*)

The **a. glutea caudalis** arises as one of the terminal branches of the internal iliac artery. In the dog its site of origin lies at the base of the sacrum, in the cat at the level of the greater ischiatic notch, in the pig and ruminants at the lesser ischiatic notch and in the horse at the 5th to 6th lumbar vertebrae.

In the dog and cat it runs in a caudal direction ventral to the sacrum, crosses medially the piriformis and superficial gluteal muscles and curves laterally at the lesser ischiatic notch, in the dog cranioventral to the sacrotuberal ligament. In the dog the caudal gluteal artery gives off the *a. iliolumbalis* cranial to the wing of the sacrum and the *a. glutea cranialis* medial to it. Before curving off laterally it gives rise in the dog to the *a. caudalis lateralis superficialis* and the *a. perinealis dorsalis*. Other branches arise here which ramify in the rotators of the hip joint and there is a special collateral artery for the ischiatic nerve, the *a. comitans n. ischiadici*.

In the pig and ruminants the caudal gluteal artery runs laterally immediately after its origin near the lesser ischiatic notch. In small ruminants, however, it has first to pass through the small vascular foramen in the broad pelvic ligament. In the pig it may give off the *a. rectalis caudalis*.

The caudal gluteal artery of the horse gives origin to the *a. glutea cranialis* shortly after its own origin and ventral to the iliosacral joint. The *a. iliolumbalis* and the *a. obturatoria* can also occasionally arise at this location. Passing the wing of the sacrum ventrally, the caudal gluteal artery reaches the broad pelvic ligament which it perforates in a lateral direction ventral to the 2nd or 3rd sacral segment. It provides three to four *rr. sacrales* to the sacrum. The *a. caudalis mediana* arises ventral to the third sacral segment from either the left or the right caudal gluteal artery. At the level of the 4th to 5th sacral segment the *a. caudalis ventrolateralis* is given off on each side and it goes to form the 5th, or 4th and 5th, sacral ramus or rami.

Muscular branches of the caudal gluteal artery ramify in the ventral and lateral muscles of the tail in all the domestic mammals with only minor variations. In the horse they also supply the multifidus and rectococcygeus muscles and large diverging muscular branches go to the gluteal muscles. In the cat the cranial abductor cruris muscle, the vertebral and pelvic heads of the long ischiatic muscles and the skin of

A. pudenda interna

(Comparative: 85–88/*75*; 105–108/*4*; 136–143/*29*; cat: 109/*11*; dog: 110/*38*; pig: 111/*27*; sheep: 112/*31*; ox: 113/*15, 16*, 144/*21*; horse: 50/*35*; 104/*20*; 114/*33*)

The **a. pudenda interna** is the second terminal branch of the internal iliac artery, the caudal gluteal being the other branch as recorded above. It has already been mentioned (see p. 156) that we differentiate between a long "pudendal type" in carnivores and the horse, and a short "pudendal type" in pigs and ruminants. In carnivores and the horse the internal pudendal has the same course within the pelvic cavity as the internal iliac has in pigs and ruminants. The internal pudendal artery gives off the *a. umbilicalis* only in the horse and it gives off an *a. prostatica* or *vaginalis* only in carnivores and the horse.

In the caudal part of the pelvic cavity the internal pudendal artery gives off the *a. urethralis* which is absent in the horse. The internal pudendal artery ends at the pelvic exit by dividing into the *a. perinealis ventralis* and the *a. penis* or *a. clitoris* as the case may be. Instead of the last vessel the mare has the *a. bulbi vestibuli*. Before the terminal bifurcation, the internal pudendal artery also gives off the *a. vestibularis* in the ox and the *r. vestibularis* in the horse.

A. perinealis ventralis

(Comparative: 85–88/*78*; 136–143/*39*; dog: 110/*41*; pig: 111/*28*; sheep: 101/*44*; ox: 113/*16*; 144/*23, 24*; horse: 114/*35*)

The **a. perinealis ventralis** is one of the terminal branches of the internal pudendal artery which originate in the pelvic exit. The ventral perineal artery gives off the *a. rectalis caudalis* in a caudodorsal direction to the anus. In the female pig and ox, however, this vessel arises from the dorsal perineal artery and in the male pig the caudal rectal artery can arise from either the dorsal perineal or from the caudal gluteal artery. The terminal branches of the ventral perineal artery supply the perineum. In carnivores and pigs, in which the scrotum is in an inguinal position, the *r. scrotalis dorsalis* goes to the wall of the scrotum. In females the *r. labialis dorsalis* goes to the labia of the vulva but in female ruminants the *r. labialis dorsalis et mammarius* extends to the interthigh region. Here it anastomoses with the r. labialis ventralis or the caudal mammary artery from the external pudendal artery.

A. penis

(Comparative: 85–88/*79*; 136–139/*42*; dog: 110/*43*; ox: 113/*15*)

In male domestic mammals the *a. penis* is another terminal branch of the internal pudendal artery which latter also gives off the artery of the bulb, the deep artery of the penis and the dorsal artery of the penis. The *a. bulbi penis* supplies the corpus spongiosum penis. The *a. profunda* passes through the tunica albuginea at the root of the penis and ramifies in the corpus cavernosum. The *a. dorsalis penis* runs along the dorsum of the penis towards the tip of the organ. In the dog this vessel anastomoses with the *r. praeputialis* of the external pudendal artery. In the horse the dorsal artery of the penis is initially only slender but in the interthigh region it receives a stout tributary, the *a. penis media*, and in the inguinal region it is joined by another vessel, the *a. penis cranialis*, from the external pudendal artery.

A. clitoridis

(Comparative: 85–88/*79*; 140–143/*42*)

The **a. clitoridis** of female mammals is a terminal branch of the internal pudendal artery which is analogous with the *a. penis* of the male. The artery of the clitoris gives off the a. bulbi vestibuli and, except in the horse, the deep artery of the clitoris and also the dorsal artery of the clitoris. The *a. bulbi vestibuli*, which in the ox is represented by the a. vestibularis from the internal pudendal, arises lateral to the vestibule of the vagina and courses caudoventrally to the vestibular bulb. The *a. profunda clitoridis* and the *a. dorsalis clitoridis*, which in the horse stem from the *a. clitoridis media*, a branch vessel of the obturator artery, enter the erectile tissue of the clitoris.

The visceral terminal branches of the internal iliac and the internal pudendal arteries will be discussed in connection with the branches of the abdominal aorta (see p. 176).

A. sacralis mediana and a. caudalis mediana

(Comparative: 85–88/*61, 63*; 105–108/2, 136–143/6; cat: 91, 109/*33*; dog: 110/*47, 49*; pig: 111/*30*; *32*; sheep: 112/*32, 33*; ox: 113/*5*; 19; horse: 114/*29*)

The **a. sacralis mediana** is the direct continuation of the abdominal aorta subsequent to the origin of the internal iliac arteries. It runs ventral to the sacrum from the last or penultimate lumbar vertebra. In the horse the median sacral artery is only poorly developed or completely absent. In the other domestic mammals this vessel runs beyond the sacrum, passing ventrally along the coccygeal vertebrae and continuing as the *a. caudalis media*. The latter vessel is usually present in the horse but in that animal it arises from either the left or right caudal gluteal artery, one of the terminal branches of the internal iliac artery. These two parts of the median vessel, the sacral and caudal, are much smaller than the aorta and they give rise to segmental vessels, the *rr. sacrales* or *rr. caudales*. They vascularize the sacrum and the coccygeal vertebrae respectively. They ramify in the musculature lying next to the sacrum and the tail muscles and in the sacral region they give rise to the *rr. spinales* which enter the vertebral canal. Between these segmental vessels there are also several longitudinally directed arteries. In the cat, and occasionally also in the dog, a bilateral vessel is formed, ventral to the sacrum and immediately dorsolateral to the median sacral artery, by the anastomosis of either the sacral ramus and the first caudal ramus. This vessel continues in the tail region and lies closely dorsolateral to the median caudal artery. In the sacral region this vessel corresponds to the a. sacralis lateralis of man and in the tail region in carnivores it is occasionally termed the *a. caudalis ventralis*, but so far no exact name has been decided upon. Usually only the first caudal ramus arising from the median caudal artery remains independent. The subsequent caudal rami are linked to two anastomotic chains, the *a. caudalis ventrolateralis* and the *a. caudalis dorsolateralis* which lie respectively ventral and dorsal to the rudimentary transverse processes. In the ox the sacral rami I and II stem from the cranial gluteal artery. In the horse three to four sacral rami stem from the caudal gluteal artery and the fourth or the fifth becomes the ventrolateral caudal artery. It should be pointed out that in carnivores the caudal gluteal artery gives off the *a. caudalis lateralis* which runs superficially and laterally towards the point of the tail and should correctly be termed the *a. caudalis lateralis superficialis*. This is particularly pertinent in view of the paramedian and ventrally situated sacral and tail arteries which have just been described.

Visceral arteries of the abdominal aorta

A. coeliaca

(Comparative: 85–88/*44*; 125–128/*1*; cat: 91/*15*; pig: 97/*3*; 98/*22*; 130/*1*; sheep: 101/*19*; Horse: 50/*37*; 104/*2*)

The **a. coeliaca** is the first visceral branch and it leaves the ventral wall of the abdominal aorta to gain the mesogastrium dorsale. In carnivores and the ox it arises at the level of the 1st lumbar vertebra whereas in the horse it arises at the level of the 17th to 18th thoracic vertebrae still within the aortic hiatus. In pigs, ruminants and occasionally the cat, it gives off the initially unpaired caudal phrenic artery (see p. 129). In the ox there may be a separate caudal phrenic artery for each diaphragmatic crus in which case each artery arises from the coeliac artery independently. In ruminants and occasionally the dog, the coeliac artery also releases the *rr. suprarenales craniales*. The further subdivisions of the coeliac artery into branches to the stomach, liver, spleen, pancreas and the first part of the duodenum, depend on the structure and position of these organs in the respective domestic animals. In carnivores and especially the horse, the coeliac is short and shows a characteristic division into the following three vessels; the *a. lienalis* which branches to the left and remains in the dorsal mesogastrium, the cranially directed *a. gastrica sinistra* and the *a. hepatica* which runs to the right. These are situated at first in the dorsal mesogastrium and then enter the ventral mesogastrium. In those cases where the coeliac artery is extremely short, the branch vessels may spring from the abdominal aorta. Only the splenic and hepatic arteries arise from the coeliac artery in the pig. In ruminants the relatively long coeliac artery gives rise

A. coeliaca

Carnivores	Pig	Ruminants	Horse
(a. phrenica caudalis) (cat)	a. phrenica caudalis	aa. phrenicae caudales rr. suprarenales craniales	

a. lienalis
  rr. pancreatici
  aa. gastricae breves
  a. gastroepiploica
    sinistra
	a. lienalis	**a. lienalis**
		  rr. pancreatici
		  a. ruminalis dextra
		    r. epiploicus
			a. lienalis
			  rr. pancreatici
			  aa. gastricae breves
			  a. gastroepiploica sinistra

a. gastrica sinistra
  rr. oesophagei
	a. gastrica sinistra
	  rr. oesophagei
	  a. diverticuli
	  r. pancreaticus
	  r. gastrolienalis
	  a. gastroepiploica sinistra
		a. gastrica sinistra
		  a. gastroepiploica sinistra
		  a. reticularis accessoria
		  a. ruminalis sinistra
		  a. reticularis
		    rr. phrenici
		    rr. oesophagei
			a. gastricasinistra
			  r. visceralis
			  r. parietalis
			  r. oesophageus

a. hepatica
  r. dexter lateralis
    a. lobi caudati
  r. dexter medialis
  r. sinister
    rr. sinistri mediales
      a. cystica
    rr. sinistri laterales
  a. gastrica dextra
  a. gastroduodenalis
    a. pancreaticoduodenalis
      cranialis
    a. gastroepiploica dextra
	a. hepatica
	  rr. pancreatici
	  r. dexter lateralis
	    a. lobi caudati
	  a. gastroduodenalis
	    a. pancreaticoduodenalis
	      cranialis
	    a. gastroepiploica dextra
	  r. dexter medialis
	    a. cystica
	  r. sinister
	    rr. sinistri laterales
	    rr. sinistri mediales
	  a. gastrica dextra
		a. hepatica
		  rr. pancreatici
		  r. dexter
		    a. lobi caudati
		    a. cystica
		  r. sinister
		  a. gastrica dextra
		  a. gastroduodenalis
		    a. pancreaticoduodenalis
		      cranialis
		    a. gastroepiploica
		      dextra
			a. hepatica
			  rr. pancreatici
			  a. gastrica dextra
			  a. gastroduodenalis
			    a. pancreaticoduodenalis
			      cranialis
			    a. gastroepiploica
			      dextra
			  r. dexter
			  r. sinister

to only the three arteries as in carnivores and the horse or it may also give off the *a. ruminalis sinistra* and, rarely, the *a. ruminalis dextra*.

A. lienalis
(Comparative: 125–128/*3*; dog: 129/*D*, *15*; pig: 130/*15*; horse: 50/*38*; 104/*3*)

In all the domestic mammals the **a. lienalis** originates from the coeliac artery. In carnivores the splenic artery curves to the left round the cranial border on the left pancreatic lobe, to which it gives off branches, and continues ventrad towards the centre of the splenic hilus. About half way along its length the artery provides the dorsal trunk vessel for the *rr. lienales* of the spleen. Continuing ventrad, it supplies two to three further trunks for the *rr. lienales* to the central and ventral region of the spleen. It then continues as the *a. gastroepiploica sinistra* which makes a large curve to the right to reach the greater curvature of the stomach. Before entering the splenic parenchyma the artery sends the *aa. gastricae breves* to the fundic region of the greater curvature of the stomach and the *rr. epiploici* to the splenic omentum. Besides, the branches to the ventral region of the spleen give rise to several *rr. epiploici* for the omental veil and other epiploic rami go over the ventral extremity of the spleen to the omental bursa.

There are particularly prominent visceral and parietal branches to the plicature of the omental bursa. In the cat two special branches to the visceral surface of the stomach arise near the origin of the dorsal splenic trunk artery. One of these immediately splits into diverging branches while the other releases several secondary branches to the angulus ventriculi.

Shortly after its origin the splenic artery of the pig gives rise to the *a. gastrica sinistra* to the lesser curvature of the stomach and immediately thereafter the *a. diverticuli* which reaches the medial part of the annular groove of the diverticulum and continues craniad therein. It supplies branches to both the diverticulum and the fundic region. The splenic artery runs along the cranial border of the left lobe of the pancreas, for which it provides the stout *r. pancreaticus,* and it continues to the dorsal extremity of the spleen. Before reaching the hilus of the spleen, the *r. gastrolienalis* branches off and provides several *rr. lienales* to the dorsal part of the spleen and the *aa. gastricae breves* which usually originate from a common vessel. From the visceral surface of the stomach the latter enter the annular groove of the diverticulum, supplying not only the diverticulum itself but also ramifying in the fundic region along the greater curvature. Only rarely does one find anastomoses with the left gastroepiploic artery and these run towards the body of the stomach. After giving rise to the *r. gastrolienalis* the splenic artery runs along the hilus of the spleen and at about halfway along its length the *a. gastroepiploica sinistra* arises. The splenic artery sends numerous rr. lienales into the splenic parenchyma along the entire length of the hilus and it provides fine *rr. epiploici* for the greater omentum. Finally it continues as a small vessel past the ventral extremity of the spleen to the greater omentum.

In ruminants, in the majority of cases, the *a. ruminalis dextra,* and frequently also the *a. ruminalis sinistra,* leave the splenic artery immediatly after the origin of the *rr. pancreatici*. The splenic artery then courses to the left and dorsally over the rumen, past its area of contact with the dorsal abdominal wall and reaches the dorsal extremity of the spleen. Thence it descends, close to the cranial border of that organ, to the more expansive hilus where it divides into three *rr. lienales* in small ruminants and into four or five *rr. lienales* in the ox. In the small ruminants this division of the splenic artery into its branches can give the impression of a duplication of the artery. In the ox one of these splenic rami runs within the spleen, close to the visceral surface, to reach the ventral extremity.

In the horse the splenic artery passes cranial to the pancreas and caudodorsal to the saccus caecus of the stomach to attain the dorsal extremity of the spleen. In so doing it provides the *rr. pancreatici* and, on its course along the hilus of the spleen, it supplies numerous *rr. lineales* and *aa. gastricae breves* to the left side of the greater curvature of the stomach. Finally it continues past the ventral extremity of the spleen as the left gastroepiploic artery to the greater omentum.

A. gastrica sinistra
(Comparative: 125–128/*8*; pig: 130/*16*; horse: 50/*39*; 104/*4*)

In the cat, and rarely also in the dog, the **a. gastrica sinistra** arises from the coeliac artery. In the dog it usually originates from the splenic artery and in this species it can also occur as a paired vessel. It attains the cardia in the lig. gastrophrenicum. Here it gives off branches to the oesophagus in both the cat and the dog. The *r. oesophageus* anastomoses with the oesophageal ramus of the *a. broncho-oesophagea*. The left gastric artery follows the lesser curvature of the stomach in the region of insertion of the mesogastrium to reach the incisura angularis where it anastomoses with the a. gastrica dextra. Along this course it gives rise to the *rr. gastrici* to the parietal surface and smaller vessels to the visceral surface of the stomach. These vessels run towards the *aa. gastricae breves* or, in the cat, towards the special branches of the splenic artery which have been described above as occurring on the visceral surface.

In the pig the left gastric artery stems from the splenic artery and continues to the incisura angularis and, forming a network, it ramifies in only the middle third of the visceral surface. Only rarely does one encounter a *r. oesophageus*. Branches to the parietal surface are also infrequent as are anastomoses with the right gastric artery and with the vessels from the greater curvature. Sometimes the left gastric artery may give origin to the *a. diverticuli*.

In ruminants the a. gastrica sinistra is generally an offshoot from the coeliac artery although in the goat it often arises from the hepatic artery. In these species the left gastric artery follows a cranioventral course over the right side of the atrium of the rumen giving off the left gastroepiploic artery dorsal to the omasum. It continues over the convexity of the caudal surface of the omasum to the lesser curvature of the abomasum. In this latter region it is duplicated in its entire length in small ruminants and in part of its length in the ox. At the site of insertion of the omentum it anastomoses with the right gastric artery, in the small ruminants at the level of the incisura angularis and in the ox near the pylorus. It supplies branches to the cranial region of the rumen and the omasum. In the majority of cases in sheep the *a. reticularis* is also an offshoot. In the small ruminants the *a. reticularis accessoria* arises shortly after the origin of the left gastroepiploic artery. This artery supplies the right wall of the omasum and the right and cranial wall of the reticulum up to the cardia. It forms connections with all the neighbouring vessels. In the region of the lesser curvature the left gastric artery gives off *rr. gastrici* to both surfaces of the abomasum. These in their turn give rise to particularly stout branches coursing in the groove between the omasum and abomasum and anastomose with similar branches of the left gastroepiploic artery.

The left gastric artery of the horse is a branch of the coeliac artery and it gives rise to the *rr. pancreatici*, dividing shortly afterwards into the *r. visceralis* and the *r. parietalis*. These vessels passing from the lesser curvature to the appropriate surface of the stomach ramify and run towards the *aa. gastricae breves* with which they anastomose. Similarly they connect with the rr. gastrici and the right gastric artery. The *r. oesophageus* to the dorsal surface of the oesophagus derives either from the left gastric artery itself or one of its limbs or, in rare instances, even from the splenic artery. It anastomoses with the oesophageal ramus of the broncho-oesophageal artery.

A. hepatica
(Comparative: 125–128/*11*; pig: 130/*2*; horse: 50/*40*; 104/*5*)

The **a. hepatica** is a branch of the coeliac artery. It turns towards the liver and gives rise to the hepatic branches, the *rr. pancreatici* (which are not present in carnivores), the *a. gastrica dextra* and the *a. gastroduodenalis*, the parent vessel of the *a. pancreaticoduodenalis cranialis* and the *a. gastroepiploica dextra*. There are species differences in the sequence of the origin of these vessels which result from the varying topography of their internal organs.

In carnivores the hepatic artery first gives off to the liver the *r. dexter lateralis*, the *r. dexter medialis* and the *r. sinister*. Thereafter it divides into the *a. gastrica dextra* and the *a. gastroduodenalis*.

The hepatic artery of the pig first gives rise to the *rr. pancreatici* which are caudoventrally directed and supply the body of the pancreas. Then liver and intestinal branches are given off and these alternate thus: *r. dexter lateralis*, *a. gastroduodenalis*, *r. dexter medialis*, *a. gastrica dextra* and the *r. sinister*.

In the ruminants the hepatic artery gives off first the *rr. pancreatici*, then to the liver it gives off the *r. dexter* which usually arises together with the *a. cystica*. On the other side the *r. sinister* usually comes off simultaneously with the *a. gastrica dexter*. Thereafter the hepatic artery is continued as the *a. gastroduodenalis*.

The hepatic artery of the horse gives rise to the *rr. pancreatici*, the right gastric and gastroduodenal arteries and, to the liver, the *r. dexter* and the *r. sinister*.

The distribution of the hepatic branches supplying the lobes in the domestic mammals is shown in the table although this does not record the numerous variations.

Coeliac artery

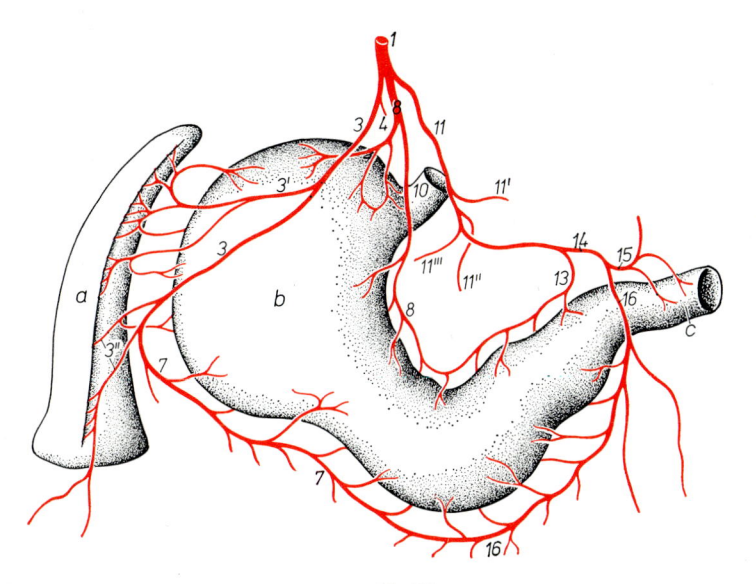

Fig. 125

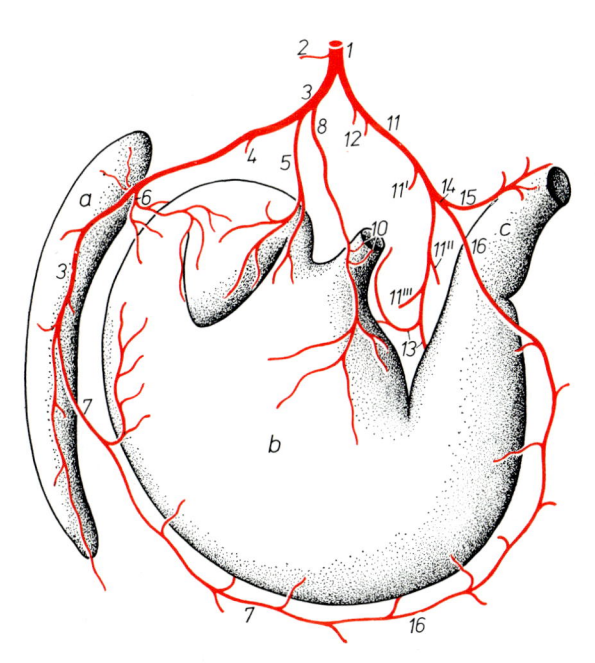

Fig. 126

Figs 125, 126, 127, 128. A. coeliaca of the dog, pig, ox and horse. Semidiagrammatic.

a spleen; *b* stomach; *b′* rumen; *b″* reticulum; *b‴* omasum; b^{iv} abomasum; *c* duodenum

1 a. coeliaca; *2* a. phrenica caudalis or aa. phrenicae caudales; *3* a. lienalis with rr. lienales and aa. gastricae breves; *3′* proximal parent branch, *3″* distal parent branches of the rr. lienales; *4* rr. pancreatici; *5* a. diverticuli; *6* r. gastrolienalis with rr. lienales and aa. gastricae breves; *7* a. gastroepiploica sinistra with rr. gastrici and rr. epiploici; *8* a. gastrica sinistra, *8′* r. visceralis, *8″* r. parietalis; *9* rr. pancreatici; *10* rr. eosophagei; *11* a. hepatica, *11′* r. dexter lateralis, *11″* r. dexter medialis, *11‴* r. sinister; *12* rr. pancreatici; *13* a. gastrica dextra with anastomosis of the r. oesophageus of the broncho-oesophageal artery in the pig; *14* a. gastroduodenalis; *15* a. pancreaticoduodenalis cranialis with rr. pancreatici and rr. duodenales; *16* a. gastroepiploica dextra with rr. gastrici and rr. epiploici; *17* a. ruminalis dextra; *18* a. ruminalis sinistra; *19* a. reticularis; *20* rr. phrenici; *21* rr. oesophagei

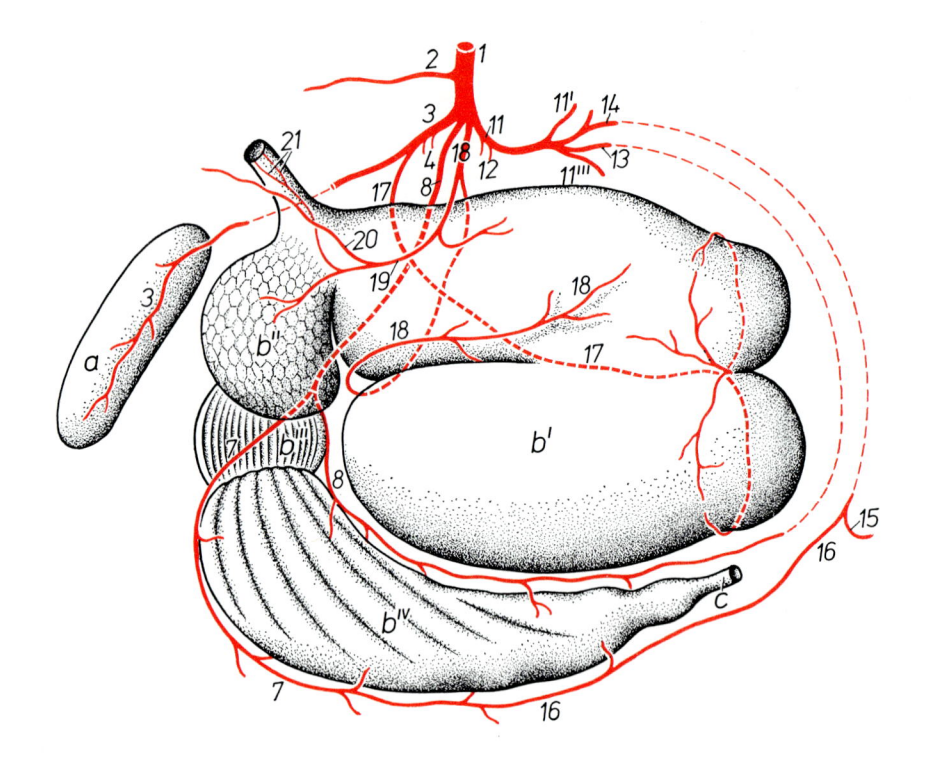

Fig. 127

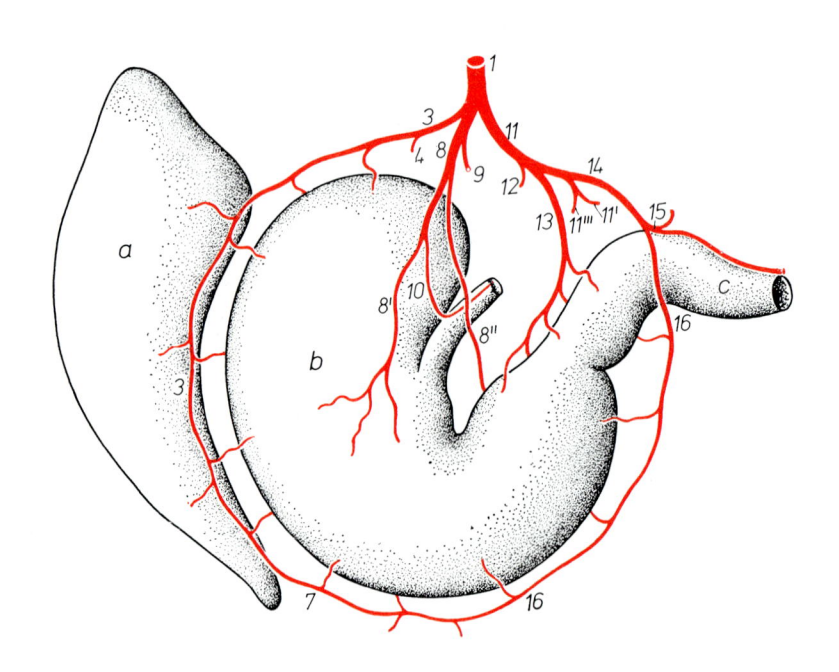

Fig. 128

A. hepatica (hepatic branches only)

Carnivores	Pig	Ruminants	Horse
r. dexter lateralis 　a. lobi caudati r. dexter medialis r. sinister 　rr. sinistri 　　mediales 　　　a. cystica 　rr. sinistri 　　laterales	r. dexter lateralis 　a. lobi caudati r. dexter medialis 　a. cystica r. sinister 　rr. sinistri 　　laterales 　rr. sinistri 　　mediales	r. dexter 　a. lobi caudati 　a. cystica r. sinister	r. dexter r. sinister

A. gastrica dextra
(Comparative: 125–128/*13*; pig: 130/*13*)

In all the domestic animals the **a. gastrica dextra** arises from the hepatic artery but, as already mentioned, the sequence in which its origin is related to the other vessels varies among the species.

Running in the lesser omentum, the slender right gastric artery of the carnivores attains the pyloric region, follows the lesser curvature and anastomoses in the region of the incisura angularis with the left gastric artery. In the cat it gives rise to a special *r. pancreaticus*. From the right part of the stomach it sends the *rr. gastrici* to both gastric surfaces; these do not make any visible connections with the aa. gastricae breves. Branches also go to the lesser omentum.

In the pig the right gastric artery also runs in the lesser omentum to the parietal surface of the stomach. Before reaching the latter it gives off the r. oesophageus which anastomoses with a similarly-named branch of the broncho-oesophageal artery. In the same manner as the left gastric artery is distributed to the visceral surface of the stomach, so the right gastric artery supplies the middle third of the parietal surface.

In ruminants this artery travels in the hepatoduodenal ligament from the first part of the duodenum to the pylorus. Here it issues vessels to the duodenum and the pylorus. As it runs along the lesser curvature it is invariably duplicated in the small ruminants but in the ox only certain parts are double. At the incisura angularis it anastomoses with the left artery of the stomach. The *rr. gastrici* go to both surfaces of the pyloric part of the abomasum and they link up with the short gastric arteries. Branches also enter the lesser omentum.

In the horse the right gastric artery courses in the lesser omentum, ventral to the body of the pancreas, to the pylorus, giving off branches to it and the first part of the duodenum. From the lesser curvature it supplies several gastric rami to both surfaces of the right part of the stomach. The right and left gastric arteries link up along the lesser curvature.

A. gastroduodenalis
(Comparative: 125–128/*14*; dog: 129/*K, 1*; pig: 130/*5*)

As a branch of the hepatic artery (see. p. 162), the **a. gastroduodenalis** goes to the pars cranialis duodeni which it reaches in either the neighbourhood of the pylorus or, in ruminants, at the first part of the ansa sigmoidea. In the ox it is remarkably short. In all domestic animals it divides at the duodenum into the *a. pancreaticoduodenalis cranialis* and the *a. gastroepiploica dextra*.

A. pancreaticoduodenalis cranialis
(Comparative: 125–128/*15*; dog: 129/*G, 3–12*; pig: 130/*7*)

The **a. pancreaticoduodenalis cranialis** is one of the bifurcating limbs of the gastroduodenal artery. It runs in the mesoduodenum along the cranial and descending parts of the duodenum and is embedded to a variable extent, according to the species, in the right lobe of the pancreas. At the level of the caudal

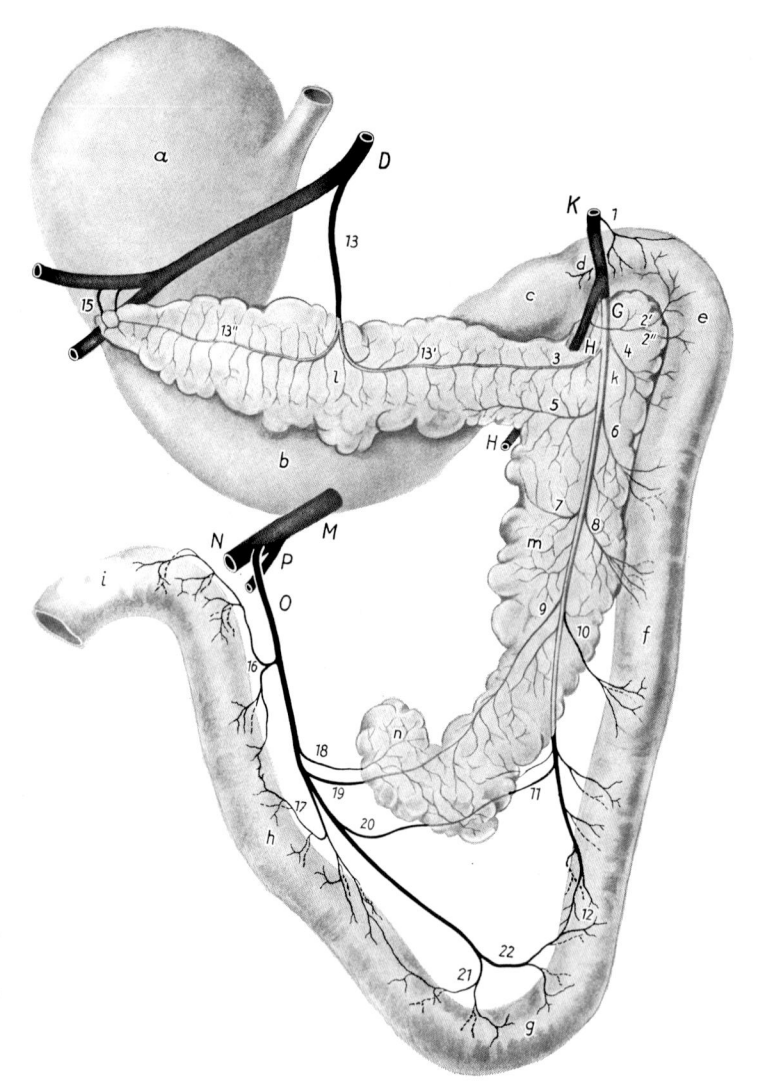

Fig. 129. Arteries of the duodenum and pancreas of a dog. Semidiagrammatic. (After Thamm, 1941, Diss., Hanover.)

a–d stomach; *e–i* duodenum: *e* flexura duodeni cranialis, *f* pars descendens, *g* flexura duodeni caudalis, *h* pars ascendens, *i* flexura duodenojejunalis; *k–n* pancreas: *k* corpus pancreatis, *l* lobus pancreatis sinister, *m* lobus pancreatis dexter, *n* processus uncinatus

D a. lienalis; *G* a. pancreaticoduodenalis cranialis; *H* a. gastroepiploica dextra; *K* a. gastroduodenalis; *M, N* a. mesenterica cranialis; *O* a. pancreaticoduodenalis caudalis; *P* a. ileocolica

1 r. pyloricus of the a. gastroduodenalis; *2* r. pancreaticoduodenalis of the a. gastroepiploica dextra; *3, 5, 7, 9, 11* rr. pancreatici, *4, 6, 8* rr. pancreaticoduodenales, *10, 12* rr. duodenales of the a. pancreaticoduodenalis cranialis; *13, 15* rr. pancreatici of the a. lienalis; *16, 17, 21, 22* rr. duodenales, *18, 19, 20* rr. pancreatici of the a. pancreaticoduodenalis caudalis

flexure of the duodenum it anastomoses with the caudal pancreaticoduodenal artery, which latter is a branch of the cranial mesenteric artery. Along its course the cranial pancreaticoduodenal artery gives rise to *rr. pancreatici* and *rr. duodenales*.

A. gastroepiploica dextra
(Comparative: 125–128/*16*; dog: 129/*H, 2*; pig: 130/*6*)

The **a. gastroepiploica dextra** is the other terminal limb of the gastroduodenal artery and it reaches the parietal layer of the greater omentum caudal to the pars cranialis of the duodenum. The artery runs close to the greater curvature of the stomach or, in ruminants, at first along the pars cranialis to the pylorus and then along the greater curvature of the abomasum. At the level of the incisura angularis it anastomoses with the left gastroepiploic artery. In the pig this connection is made by several parallel branches. The right gastroepiploic artery gives off the *aa. gastricae breves* to the two surfaces of the right half of the stomach and these can anastomoses with the *rr. gastrici*. The *rr. epiploici* go to the greater omentum and in carnivores one particularly stout ramus, forming the border vessel of the omental bursa, anastomoses with corresponding branches of the splenic artery.

A. gastroepiploica sinistra
(Comparative: 125–128/7)

In carnivores, the pig and horse the **a. gastroepiploica sinistra** stems from the splenic artery. In ruminants, on the other hand, it arises, dorsal to the omasum, from the left gastric artery and, giving off branches to the atrium of the rumen, the omasum and the reticulum, it passes through the groove between the reticulum and the omasum to reach the greater curvature of the abomasum and thus the greater omentum. In all the domestic mammals it runs within the parietal sheet of the greater omentum along the greater curvature of the stomach or abomasum, where it anastomose with the right gastroepiploic artery. In the pig this junction is accomplished by several parallel branches. It supplies both surfaces of the left half of the stomach or abomasum by means of short gastric arteries which may link with the gastric rami. The epiploic rami supply the greater omentum.

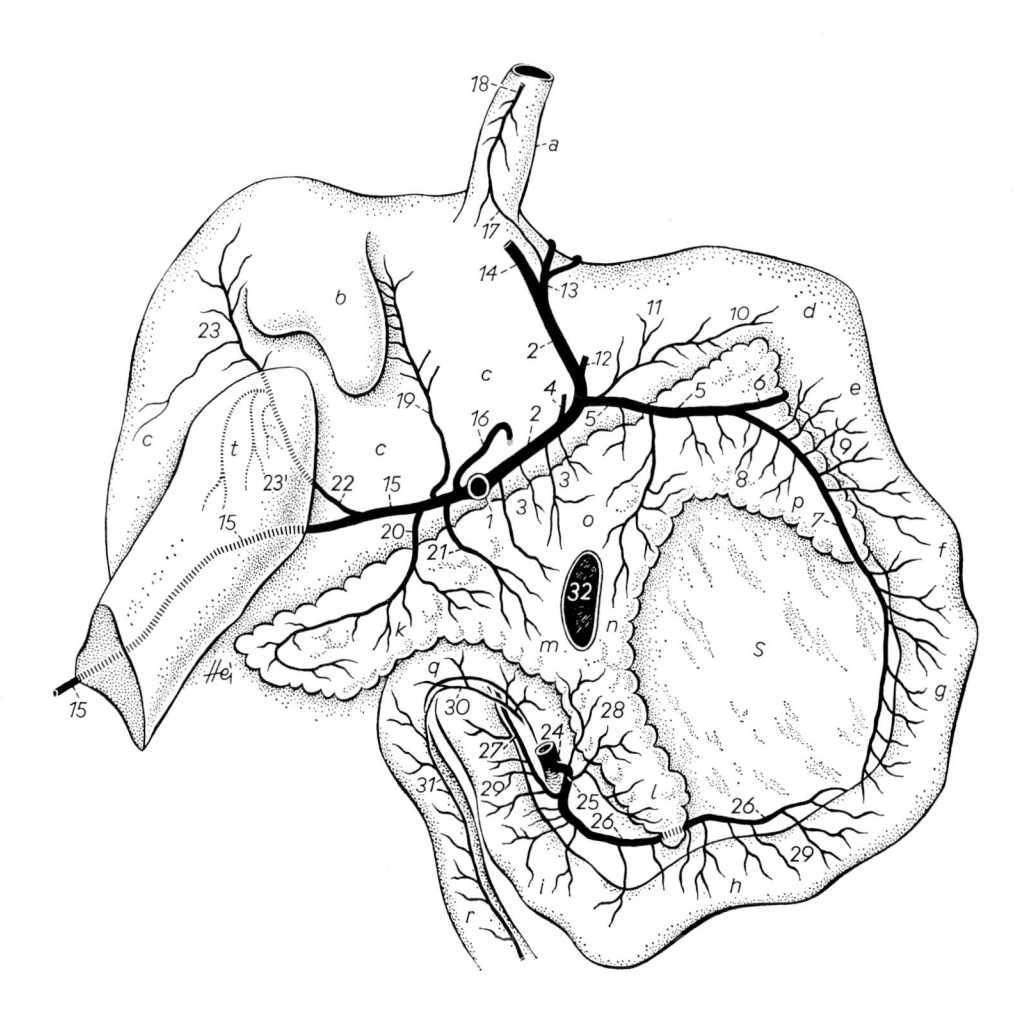

Fig. 130. Arteries of the stomach, duodenum, transverse colon, descending colon and pancreas of a pig. Semidiagrammatic.
(After Schiltsky, 1966, Diss., Hanover.)

a oesophagus; *b* diverticulum ventriculi; *c* stomach; *d* pylorus; *e–i* duodenum: *e* pars cranialis, *f* flexura duodeni cranialis, *g* pars descendens, *h* flexura duodeni caudalis, *i* pars ascendens; *k, l, m, n, o, p* pancreas: *k* lobus pancreatis sinister, *l, m, n* corpus pancreatis, *p* lobus pancreatis dexter; *q* colon transversum; *r* colon descendens; *s* mesoduodenum; *t* lien

1 a. coeliaca; *2* a. hepatica; *3* rr. pancreatici; *4* r. dexter lateralis; *5* a. gastroduodenalis; *6* a. gastroepiploica dextra; *7* a. pancreaticoduodenalis cranialis; *8* rr. pancreatici; *9* rr. duodenales; *10* rr. pylorici; *11* branches to the lesser curvature of the stomach; *12* r. dexter medialis; *13* a. gastrica dextra; *14* r. sinister; *15* a. lienalis; *16* a. gastrica sinistra; *17* r. oesophageus; *18* r. oesophageus of the a. broncho-oesophagea; *19* a. diverticuli; *20, 21* r. pancreatici; *22* r. gastrolienalis; *23* aa. gastricae breves; *23'* rr. lienalis; *24* a. mesenterica cranialis; *25, 26, 27* a. pancreaticoduodenalis caudalis; *28* rr. pancreatici; *29* rr. duodenales; *30* a. colica media; *31* a. colica sinistra; *32* v. portae, cut off in the anulus pancreaticus

A. ruminalis dextra
(ox: 127/*17*)

Usually the **a. ruminalis dextra** arises from the splenic artery, rarely from the coeliac. It represents the main supply to the rumen. It runs caudoventrally along the visceral surface of the cranial sac of the rumen to the right accessory groove. There it gives off dorsally and ventrally directed ruminal branches as well as the *aa. coronaria dextrae dorsalis* and *ventralis* to the appropriate sulci, and continues to the caudal groove. Passing through this latter groove it gains the parietal surface where it gives rise to the *aa. coronariae sinistrae dorsalis* and *ventralis* to the appropriate coronary grooves. In the ox it then anastomoses with the left ruminal artery. Since the dorsal coronary grooves are only indistinctly developed in the small ruminants, the dorsal coronary arteries are correspondingly inconspicuous. The visceral layer of the greater omentum is supplied by branches which arise from the *r. epiploicus*, a parallel vessel to the right ruminal artery. This parallel vessel can originate from either the right ruminal, the splenic or the coeliac arteries.

A. ruminalis sinistra
(ox: 127/*18*)

The **a. ruminalis sinistra** stems from the coeliac, splenic or left gastric arteries. It runs on the right side of the atrium of the rumen to the cranial groove, but before reaching it the *a. reticularis* is usually given off in the goat and ox but rarely in the sheep. It gains the parietal surface through the sulcus cranialis. Here it provides a small branch to the left longitudinal groove which in the ox links with the right ruminal artery. It also gives off dorsal and ventral branches. A particularly large, dorsally-directed branch runs in the left accessory groove to the dorsal sac of the rumen. Haemorrhage may arise from this latter branch during rumenotomy operations. The ventral branches which come from the cranial groove also supply the right side of the recessus ruminis and a very large vessel is distributed over the parietal surface of the ventral sac of the rumen. *Rr. epiploici* go to the parietal layer of the greater omentum.

A. reticularis
(ox: 127/*19*)

The **a. reticularis** takes its origin from the left ruminal artery. In small ruminants it sometimes stems from the left gastric or the splenic arteries and it courses over the craniodorsal surface of the cranial sac of the rumen to the left and into the ruminoreticular groove. It gives off a *r. oesophageus* which anastomoses with the oesophageal ramus of the broncho-oesophageal artery. There are also vessels to the cranial surface of the reticulum and to the cranial sac. In the goat and ox there are one or two additional *rr. phrenici* to the crura of the diaphragm.

A. mesenterica cranialis
(Comparative: 85–88/*45*; 131–134/*1*; cat: 91/*16*; dog: 129/*M, N*; pig: 97/*2*; 98/*23*; 130/*24*; sheep: 101/*20*; horse: 50/*42*; 104/*7*; 135/*1*)

The **a. mesenterica cranialis** arises caudal to the coeliac artery as the unpaired second visceral branch from the ventral wall of the abdominal aorta. Its origin is at the level of the 2nd lumbar vertebra in ruminants and carnivores and at the level of the 1st lumbar vertebra in pigs and horses. It immediately enters the cranial mesentery thus forming the root of the mesentery. During embryonic development the gut twists round the cranial mesenteric artery with the result that this artery, being the axis of rotation, has a cord-like character. In all domestic mammals it lies caudal to the transverse colon and is flanked on the right by the descending limb of the duodenum and the ascending colon and on the left by the ascending limb of the duodenum and the descending colon. In the horse this vessel subdivides here but in the other domestic mammals it continues caudoventrally so gaining the plate-like mesojejunum.

In carnivores it runs more centrally in the mesojejunum but in the pig more peripherally. In small ruminants it lies next to the colonic convolution at a level between the first centripetal and the last centrifugal coil. In the ox it runs near the jejunum and in a wide arch round the loops of the colon, where it is accompanied by the more centrally situated *r. collateralis* with which it forms multiple anastomotic links. It also supplies branches to the neighbouring part of the last centrifugal coil of the ascending colon.

The cranial mesenteric artery supplies all those parts of the digestive tract which are attached to this mesentery and which participate in the embryonic gut rotation. As is shown in the table below, the branches arising from the cranial mesenteric artery vary according to the morphological and topographical differences of the various intestinal segments of the different animal species.

A. mesenterica cranialis

- rr. pancreatici (ruminants)
- a. pancreaticoduodenalis caudalis
- aa. jejunales
    - rr. colici (small ruminants)
- r. collateralis (ox)
- aa. ilei
- a. ileocolica
    - r. colicus (carnivores, pig, horse)
    - rr. colici (ruminants)
    - aa. colicae dextrae (ruminants)
    - a. caecalis (carnivores, pig, ruminants)
        - r. ilei antimesenterialis (carnivores, ruminants)
    - a. caecalis medialis (horse)
    - a. caecalis lateralis (horse)
    - r. ilei mesenterialis
- a. colica dextra
- a. colica media

The species differences in the origin of these vessels are shown in the illustrations which represent the most common findings.

Rr. pancreatici

Only in ruminants do the **rr. pancreatici** derive directly from the cranial mesenteric artery and supply the right lobe of the pancreas. Some branches even supply the greater omentum. Two of these pancreatic rami are particularly large in small ruminants and they are sometimes termed the *a. pancreatica magna* and the *a. pancreaticoepiloica*.

A. pancreaticoduodenalis caudalis

(Comparative: 131–134/2; dog: 129/0, *16–22*; pig: 130/*25–29*; horse: 135/2)

The **a. pancreaticoduodenalis caudalis** leaves the cranial mesenteric artery in caudal direction and courses in the mesentery of the ascending limb of the duodenum to the caudal duodenal flexure. Shortly after its origin it sends a branch to the ascending limb of the duodenum and this branch continues to the duodenojejunal flexure where it links with the jejunal artery. The caudal pancreaticoduodenal artery, giving off the *rr. pancreatici* and *rr. duodenales*, follows the duodenum to the caudal flexure where it anastomoses with the cranial artery of the same name. In the pig this anastomosis takes place in the region of the descending duodenum.

Aa. jejunales
(Comparative: 131–134/3; horse: 50/43; 135/3)

The number of **aa. jejunales** varies from species to species but they leave the cranial mesenteric artery at regular intervals. In the horse these jejunal arteries leave the cranial mesenteric artery as a bundle of vessels in the region of the mesenteric root. The jejunal arteries run in the mesojejunum at first radially towards the jejunal loops and then connecting with one another by means of vascular arches which become progressively smaller as they get closer to the intestine. From the smallest arches of the resultant vascular net a large number of vessels emerge which finally reach the jejunum. In the small ruminants the jejunal arteries also supply the outer centrifugal loop of the ascending colon.

Aa. ilei
(Comparative: 131–134/4; horse: 50/43; 135/3')

The **aa. ilei** originate from the terminal part of the cranial mesenteric artery. In the horse they arise together with the bundle of jejunal arteries. They run in the fold of mesentery, known here as the mesoileum, towards the ileum where they are arranged in a similar pattern to the jejunal arteries with which they form arch-like connections. In the ox they give off branches to the neighbouring part of the last centrifugal coil of the ascending colon. They also anastomose in the mesentery with the *r. ileus mesenterialis* of the ileocolic artery.

A. ileocolica
(Comparative: 131–134/5; dog: 129/P; horse: 50/44; 135/6)

In all domestic mammals the **a. ileocolica** arises from the cranial mesenteric artery and, caudoventrally directed, it courses to the caecocolic junction. In carnivores the iliocolic artery gives off first the *a. colica media* to the first part of the transverse colon, while in the dog it also gives rise to a second middle colic artery supplying the terminal part of the transverse colon (see p. 174). Other offshoots from the ileocolic artery are the *a. colica dextra* in carnivores and also the right colic arteries of ruminants which supply the terminal part of the ascending colon. It shows species and individual variation in the pattern of its branch vessels which are the *r. colicus* or, in ruminants, the *rr. colici*, the *r. ilei mesenteralis* and the *a. caecalis* or, in carnivores and the horse, the *aa. caecales*.

The *r. colicus* supplies the first part of the ascending colon and in ruminants it is represented by the *rr. colici*. In the cat the colic ramus arises by a common stem with the dorsal a. caecalis. The colic ramus of the pig runs in wide spiral coils in the colonic cone, giving off numerous vessels to the centripetal coils. In the ruminants only one colic ramus arises directly from the ileocolic artery to terminate in the proximal loop. The remaining rr. colici stem, together with the right colic arteries, from a special side shoot of the ileocolic artery. This offshoot leaves the ileocolic artery near its origin. The colic rami of the sidebranch are wound together with the right colic arteries as they course from the right side of the colon disc to the terminal part of the proximal loop and on to the individual centripetal coils. In the horse the colic ramus supplies the ventral layers of the ascending colon and runs in the root of the ascending mesocolon. The colic ramus and the right colic artery anastomose, in the dog at about half the length of the ascending colon, in the pig at the central flexure and in the horse at the pelvic flexure. In ruminants the colic rami link up with the right colic arteries, often via neighbouring secondary branches.

The *r. ilei mesenterialis* follows the mesenteric insertion along the ileum from the caecocolic junction. It supplies the ileum and links with branches of the last ileal artery.

In the cat, as already mentioned, the dorsal caecal artery arises in common with the colic ramus, sending branches to the dorsal surface of the caecum and giving rise to the *r. ilei antimesenterialis*. The almost equally thick ventral caecal artery which springs from the r. ilei mesenterialis, crosses the end of the ileum ventrally and disseminates its branches from the ventral surface of the caecum. This causes a circular anastomosis to be formed round the orifice of the ileum.

The *a. caecalis* of the dog crosses the end of the ileum dorsally and runs central to the caecal coils to which it supplies arch-like branches. It gives rise to the *r. ilei antimesenterialis* which runs in the ileocaecal ligament towards the jejunum and initially also provides branches to the caecum. It anastomoses with the *r. ilei mesenterialis* of the last ileal artery. In the dog, too, there is another, though thinner, *a. caecalis* from the *r. ilei mesenterialis* which courses ventrally past the junction between the

Cranial mesenteric artery 171

Figs 131, 132, 133, 134. A. mesenterica cranialis and a. mesenterica caudalis of the dog, pig, ox and horse. Semidiagrammatic.

a stomach or, in the ox, abomasum; *b* duodenum; *c* jejunum; *d* ileum; *e* caecum; *f* colon ascendens; *g* colon transversum; *h* colon descendens; *i* colon sigmoideum; *k* rectum

1 a. mesenterica cranialis; *1'* r. collateralis (ox); *2* a. pancreaticoduodenalis caudalis; *3* aa. jejunales; *4* aa. ilei; *5* a. ileocolica; *6* r. colicus (dog, pig, horse) or rr. colici (ox); *7* a. caecalis (dog, pig ox); *7'* a. caecalis medialis (horse); *7"* a. caecalis lateralis (horse); *8* r. ilei antimesenterialis (dog, ox); *9* r. ilei mesenterialis; *10* a. colica dextra (dog, pig, horse) or aa. colicae dextrae (ox); *11* a. colica media; *12* a. mesenterica caudalis; *13* a. colica sinistra; *14* aa. sigmoideae; *15* a. rectalis cranialis

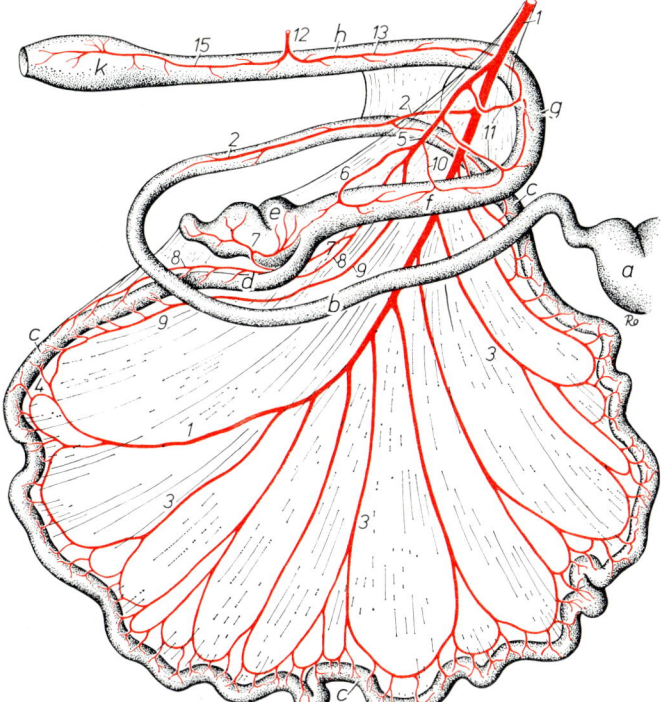

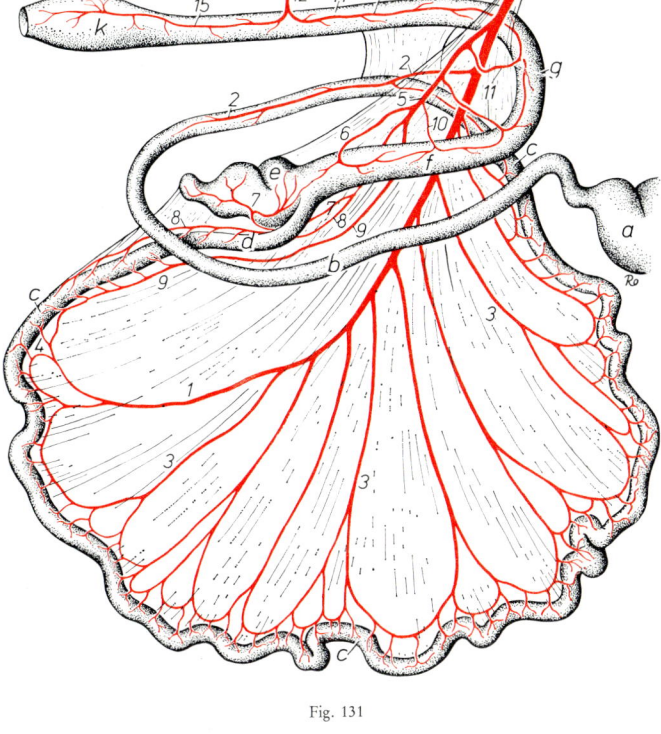

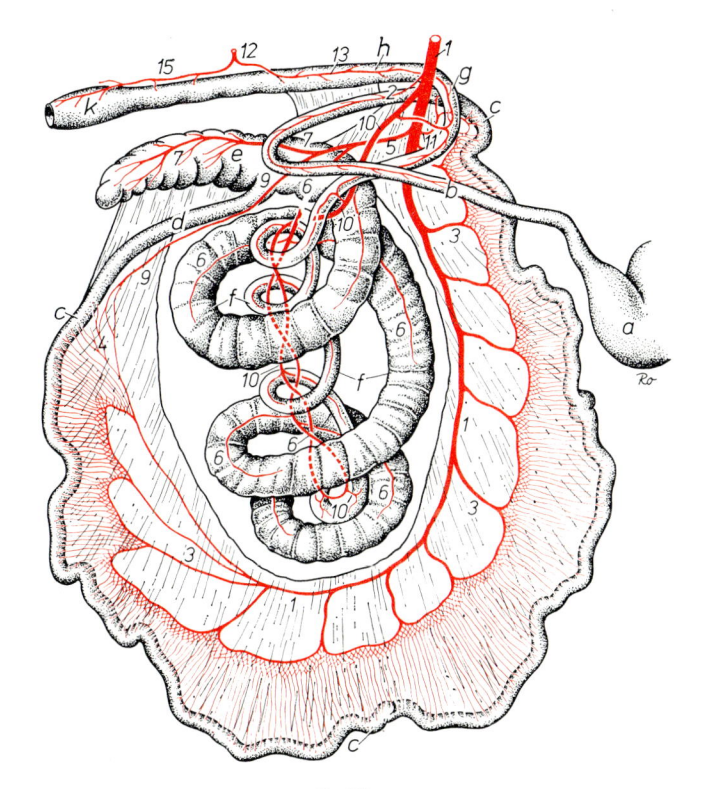

Fig. 131

Fig. 132

172 Arteries

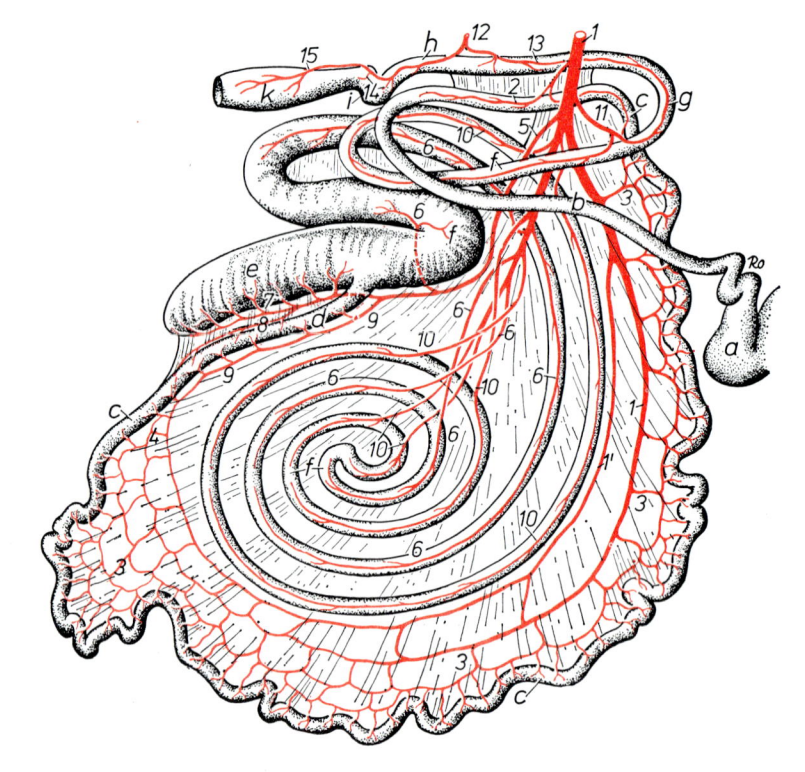

Fig. 133

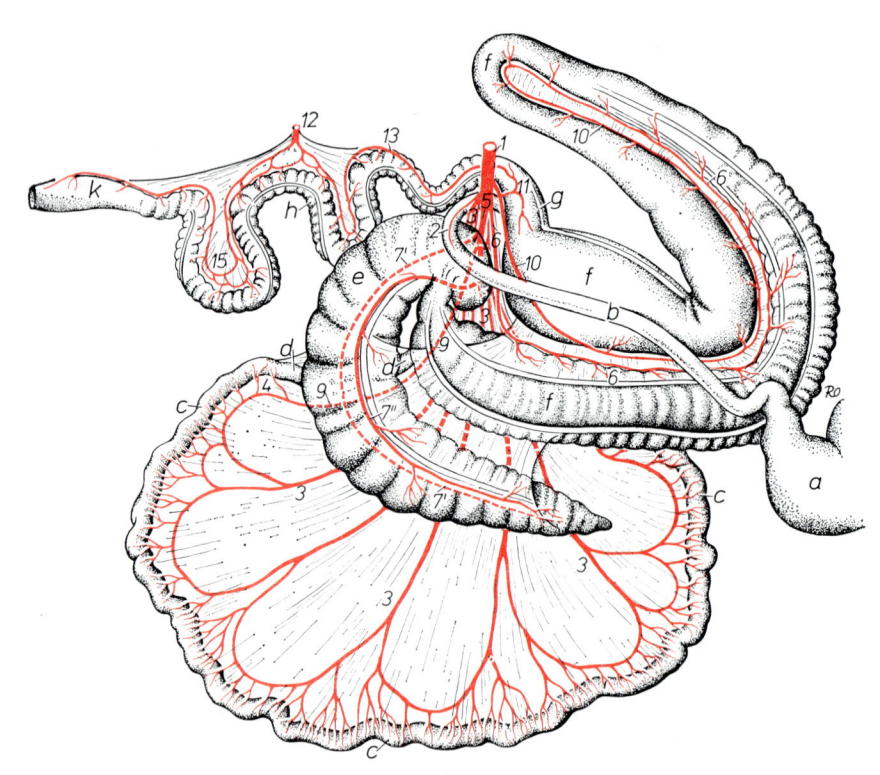

Fig. 134

small and large intestines where its branches are distributed to neighbouring parts of the large intestine, even onto the antimesenteric surface. It then links with the larger caecal artery or the colic ramus.

In the pig the *a. caecalis* passes on the right over the ileal orifice into the ileocaecal ligament and towards the apex of the caecum, thereby coming close to the ventral band. The caecal artery is represented by a bundle of vessels which sends secondary branches over the lateral and medial bands to the antimesenteric border of the caecum.

The *a. caecalis* of ruminants passes on the left of the ileal orifice, which is surrounded by a vascular ring, goes into the ileocaecal ligament and gives off branches to both sides of the caecum as well as antimesenteric vessels to the ileum. Except in sheep, the latter form connecting links which run parallel to the gut in the neighbourhood of the ileum and are referred to collectively as the *r. ilei antimesenterialis*. The caecal artery anastomoses with the ileal arteries across the free border of the ileocaecal ligament.

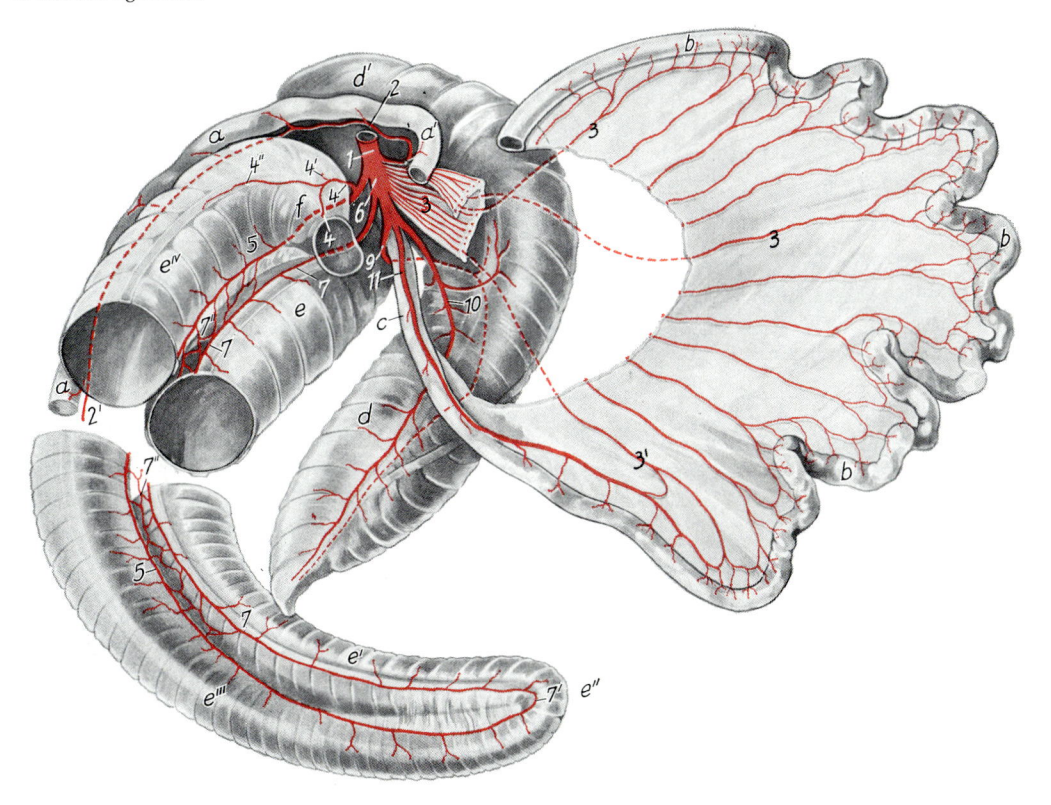

Fig. 135. A. mesenterica cranialis of the horse.
(After Zietzschmann, 1943.)

a duodenum, pars descendens, *a'* pars ascendens; *b* jejunum; *c* ileum; *d* corpus caeci; *d'* basis caeci; *e–e^{iv}* colon ascendens: *e* colon ventrale dextrum, *e'* colon ventrale sinistrum, *e"* flexura pelvina, *e'''* colon dorsale sinistrum, *e^{iv}* colon dorsale dextrum with ampulla coli; *f* colon transversum

1 a. mesenterica cranialis; *2* a. pancreaticoduodenalis caudalis; *2'* a. pancreaticoduodenalis cranialis; *3* aa. jejunales; *3'* aa. ilei; *4* a. colica media, *4'* r. pancreaticus, *4"* branch to the ampulla coli; *5* a. colica dextra; *6* a. ileocolica, *7* r. colicus, *7'* terminal anastomosis, *7"* further net-like anastomoses of the r. colicus with the a. colica dextra, *9* a. caecalis lateralis, *10* a. caecalis medialis, *11* r. ilei mesenterialis

The *aa. caecales lateralis* and *medialis* of the horse originate from the ileocolic artery to the left of the ileal orifice. The lateral caecal artery surrounds the ileum cranially and passes over the lesser curvature of the base of the caecum to the right between the first part of the colon and the body of the caecum near the insertion of the caecocolic ligament. It reaches the lateral band which it follows to the caecal apex. A dorsal offshoot embraces the caecocolic orifice laterally and extends to the first part of the right ventral colon at the insertion of the caecocolic ligament. An anastomotic arch links the medial caecal artery with the colic ramus and this arch issues radial branches to the base of the caecum. Caudal to the ileal orifice the caecal artery reaches the medial band and accompanies it to the apex of the caecum.

A. colica dextra

(Comparative: 131–134/*10*; horse: 50/*49*; 135/*5*)

The **a. colica dextra** arises from the ileocolic artery in carnivores whereas in the pig and horse it stems from the cranial mesenteric together with the middle colic artery. In ruminants this vessel is represented by the *aa. colicae dextrae* which arise, in common with the *rr. colici*, from a secondary branch of the ileocolic artery. The right colic artery of all domestic mammals runs towards the distal part of the ascending colon. In carnivores this artery passes between, and links up with, the colic ramus and the middle colic artery which bends to the right and reaches the ascending colon. In the pig it is coiled in narrow spirals as it passes ventrad within the colonic cone. It gives off branches to those inner centrifugal coils of the ascending colon which are without sacculations. At the tip of the cone it anastomoses with the colic ramus. The right colic arteries of the ruminants behave like the colic rami (see p. 170). The artery to the distal loop anastomoses with the middle colic artery. Each subsequent right colic artery goes to the next half of a centrifugal coil of the colonic disc. An exception to this is that part of the last centrifugal coil of small ruminants which is supplied by the jejunal arteries. The right colic artery of the horse runs near the insertion of the ascending mesocolon, along the dorsal colon, giving off branches to this part of the ascending colon, down to the pelvic flexure, where it anastomoses with the colic ramus.

A. colica media

(Comparative: 131–134/*11*; pig: 130/*30*; horse: 50/*50*; 135/*4*)

In carnivores the **a. colica media** is usually supplemented by a second vessel which lies next to the right colic artery. In the dog these arteries arise from the ileocolic artery but in the cat the vessel which is directed more to the left stems from the cranial mesenteric artery. In the pig and the horse the middle colic artery shares a common stem of origin with the right colic artery. In ruminants it arises directly from the cranial mesenteric artery.

In carnivores both vessels run craniad in the mesentery towards the transverse colon. Here they form arch-like connections both to each other and to the right colic artery and to the left with the left colic artery. In the other domestic mammals the middle colic artery reaches the transverse colon where the latter is fused to the dorsal abdominal wall, and here the vessel forms connections with the right and left colic arteries.

A. mesenterica caudalis

(Comparative: 85–88/*47*; 131–134/*12*; 136–143/*5*; cat: 91/*23*; dog: 110/*3*; sheep: 101/*24*; 112/*3*; horse: 50/*54*; 104/*8*)

The **a. mesenterica caudalis** is the third unpaired visceral branch to spring from the ventral wall of the abdominal aorta. In carnivores, the pig and small ruminants its origin is located at the level of the 5th, in the ox at the 6th and in the horse at the level of the 4th lumbar vertebrae. This artery enters the caudal mesentery immediately and then divides into the *a. colica sinistra* and the *a. rectalis cranialis*. The vessels known as the *aa. sigmoideae* go to that part of the intestine known by the comparative term *colon sigmoideum*, but which is distinct only in ruminants.

A. mesenterica caudalis

    A. colica sinistra
    Aa. sigmoideae
    A. rectalis cranialis

A. colica sinistra

(Comparative: 131–134/*13*; pig: 130/*31*; horse: 50/*55*)

The **a. colica sinistra** is a branch of the caudal mesenteric and it supplies the greater part of the descending colon and anastomoses with the middle colic artery. In carnivores, pigs and ruminants the artery, immediately after its origin, takes an arched, cranially-directed course and gives off short vessels to the gut. In the horse, on the other hand, it splits into several long branches which diverge like the jejunal arteries and enter the extensive mesentery of the garland-like coils of the descending colon.

A. rectalis cranialis
(Comparative: 131–134/*15*; horse: 50/*56*)

The **a. rectalis cranialis** is the caudally-directed branch of the caudal mesenteric artery. Immediately after its origin, it turns dorsad within the mesentery towards the intestinal wall. In carnivores, pigs and horses it first reaches the colon and then extends to the rectum. In ruminants it goes directly to the rectum. In carnivores and pigs it divides at the rectum into two equal limbs which run to the left and right along the intestinal wall. It is confined to the dorsal part of the wall in regions to which the middle rectal artery is distributed but in the pig and ruminants it extends to the anus. It has anastomotic connection with the left colic, the middle rectal and especially the caudal rectal arteries.

A. suprarenalis media or aa. suprarenales mediae
(pig: 98/*25'*; ox: 114/*2*; horse: 50/*41*)

In carnivores the abdominal aorta gives off the **a. suprarenalis media** caudal to the origin of the cranial mesenteric artery. In the pig, however, there are several **aa. suprarenales mediae** arising from the aorta. They are laterally directed and go to the middle region of the adrenal gland. The gland is supplied by several other adrenal vessels which arise from neighbouring parietal and/or visceral arteries; these vessels and their sources are shown in the following table.

Possible sources of the arteries supplying the adrenal glands

		cat	dog	pig	goat	sheep	ox	horse
rr.	suprarenales craniales							
	from a. phrenica caudalis	+	+	+	+	+	+	+
	from a. abdominalis		+					
	from a. coeliaca		+		+	+	+	
	from a. mesenterica cranialis		+					
rr.	suprarenales							
	from aa. lumbales I or II		+		+	+	+	
a.	suprarenalis media							
	from aorta abdominalis	+	+					
aa.	suprarenales mediae							
	from aorta abdominalis			+				
rr.	suprarenales caudales							
	from aa. renales	+	+	+	+	+	+	+

A. renalis
(Comparative: 85–88/*46*; cat: 91/*20*; pig: 98/*25*; sheep: 101/*22*; ox: 144/*1*; horse: 50/*51*; 104/*11*)

The sites of origin of the **aa. renales dextra** and **sinistra** from the abdominal aorta vary according to the renal topography of the different species. Thus, in the cat they arise at the level of the 3rd–4th lumbar vertebrae, in the dog at the 1st–2nd, in the pig at the 3rd, the sheep at the 2nd–3rd, the goat at the 3rd–4th, the ox at the 2nd–3rd and the horse at the 1st lumbar vertebrae. As a rule the right artery arises more cranially than the left. Each of the two renal arteries courses towards the hilus and in doing so the right renal artery crosses the caudal vena cava dorsally. Each artery divides in the hilar region into two or more branches which, in their turn, give rise to the *aa. interlobares* and these latter penetrate into the organ.

Further subdivisions of the renal arteries are discussed in volume II. However, before dividing each renal artery gives off the *rr. suprarenales caudales* to the adrenal gland, a *r. uretericus* to the ureters and also branches to the capsula adiposa.

A. testicularis or a. ovarica

(Comparative: 85–88/*48*; 136–143/*2*; cat: 91/*22*; sheep: 101/*23*; 112/*2′*; ox: 113/*2*; 144/*4*; horse: 50/*53*; 104/*12*)

Another paired visceral vessel arising laterally from the abdominal aorta and supplying the gonads is the **a. testicularis** in the male and the **a. ovarica** in the female. The origin of this artery in the cat is at the level of the 4th–5th, in the dog the 3rd–4th, the pig the 5th, the sheep the 4th–5th, the goat and ox the 5th and the horse the 4th lumbar vertebrae. In rare instances the gonadal artery may take its origin from the renal artery.

The **a. testicularis** runs initially ventrad over the inner lumbar muscles and then passes along the lateral abdominal wall in the proximal mesorchium, the plica vasculosa, to the internal inguinal ring. Continuing in the plica vasculosa, and thus as part of the spermatic cord, it reaches the head extremity of the testis. It gives off the *rr. epididymales* which, together with the *rr. ductus deferentis*, is involved in the vascular supply to the ductus deferens.

The **a. ovarica** runs along the dorsal abdominal wall into the mesovarium and the right artery crosses the caudal vena cava ventrally. The artery continues towards the ovary, close to the cranial border of the mesentery, becoming more and more contorted. It gives rise to the *r. tubarius* which lies in the mesosalpinx, and supplies the uterine or Fallopian tube by means of several meandering branches. It also supplies the ovarian bursa. The ovarian artery provides blood for the horn of the uterus via the *r. uterinus* which generally arises before the tubarius branch. In the pig, carnivores and the ox there are several uterine rami. The uterine ramus anastomoses in the mesometrium with the uterine artery and gives off branches to the horn of the uterus; in the ox branches are also sent to the isthmus of the uterine tube. The extremely twisted terminal branches form a cone-shaped vascular bundle, the base of which is related to the ovary. These terminal vessels enter the zona vasculosa at the insertion of the mesovarium.

Visceral arteries of the a. iliaca interna and the a. pudenda interna

A. umbilicalis

(Comparative: 85–88/*76*; 136–143/*20*; cat: 109/*10*; dog: 110/*39*; sheep: 112/*25*; ox: 113/*7, 8*; 144/*10*; horse: 50/*36*; 104/*21*; 114/*34*)

In the region of the pelvic entrance the **a. umbilicalis** arises from the internal iliac artery in carnivores, pig and the ox and from the internal pudendal artery in the horse. The artery enters the lateral ligament of the bladder and runs near its cranial border towards the apex of the bladder. In the foetal circulation and also for a short time after birth, the left and right umbilical arteries accompany the urachus to the umbilical opening. At that time these are stout arteries but during the first weeks they regress from the navel towards the bladder. The part of the vessel lying in the lateral ligament of the bladder is known, in all the domestic mammals, as the *lig. teres vesicae*. Except in carnivores, the male umbilical artery gives rise to the *a. ductus deferentis* while that of females forms the *a. uterina*. The latter vessel has a different origin in the horse. Subsequently the *r. uretericus* is given off the umbilical artery although in females it sometimes springs from the uterine artery. In the ewe a stout *r. uterinus* is sometimes described as an additional branch. The last vessel originating from the umbilical artery is the *a. vesicalis cranialis*; this is usually lacking in the dog and is very slim, or may be absent, in the ox. In the sheep, this cranial vesicular artery reaches to the neck of the bladder and in rams it gives rise to the *r. ductus deferentis* which, in males of other domestic mammals, stems from the *a. prostatica*.

A. ductus deferentis
(Comparative: 136–139/*21*; ox: 113/*9*)

In pigs, ruminants and horses the **a. ductus deferentis** is the first branch vessel of the umbilical artery. It enters the plica genitalis and supplies the ductus deferens while following it towards the tail of the epididymis. Here it anastomoses with the *rr. ductus deferentis* from the epididymal rami of the testicular artery. Nearer the pelvic cavity it anastomoses with the *r. ductus deferentis* of the prostatic artery. In carnivores, however, this branch of the prostatic artery becomes the *a. ductus deferentis*.

A. uterina
(Comparative: 140–143/*21*; sheep: 101/*43*; horse: 50/*29*)

In the pig and ruminant the **a. uterina** is the first vessel emerging from the umbilical artery. In the horse, on the other hand, the uterine artery stems from the external iliac. The uterine artery divides in the broad ligament (lig. latum uteri) into several consecutive branches which diverge and supply the mesometrial border of the ipselateral horn of the uterus. Here these vessels form arched anastomoses between one another, while the cranially directed branches link up with the *r. uterinus* of the ovarian artery and the caudally directed branches join the *r. uterinus* of the vaginal artery. Arteries are given off which supply both surfaces of the uterine horn. In carnivores the uterine ramus of the vaginal artery actually becomes the *a. uterina*. This latter artery courses from the vagina close to the mesometrial border of the uterus towards the tip of the uterine horn where it anastomoses with the uterine ramus of the ovarian artery. Along its course it gives off secondary arteries to both sides of the uterine horn and also fine branches to the mesometrium and the round ligament (lig. teres uteri). The uterine vessels are very tortuous but this decreases with advancing pregnancy and at the same time there is a marked increase in thickness of the uterine artery. The diameter of its lumen enlarges and the muscular media becomes thicker. From the third month of pregnancy onwards the uterine artery of the cow can be palpated by rectal examination in which pulsations are felt as a typical "whirring" of the uterine artery. The morphological changes in the arterial wall persist *post partum* even after involution of the uterus and they indicate that the animal has previously been pregnant.

A. prostatica
(Comparative: 85–88/*77*; 136–139/*30*; dog: 140/*40*; ox: 113/*13*)

In carnivores and horses the **a. prostatica** arises from the internal pudendal artery in the region of the greater ischiatic notch cranial to the ischiatic spine. In pigs it originates from the internal iliac artery medial to the body of the ilium and in ruminants from the same vessel but at the level of the hip joint. In the ox the internal iliac lies in this region within the broad pelvic ligament so that the prostatic artery can gain access to the pelvic cavity only after it has penetrated this broad ligament. The prostatic artery runs laterally along the pelvic peritoneum in the direction of the prostate. While doing so it gives off, except in the sheep (see below), the *r. ductus deferentis*. The latter vessel is known as the *a. ductus deferentis* in the dog. The *a. rectalis media* is also a branch of the prostatic artery in several species but in the cat, sheep and ox it has a different origin; in the cat it arises further caudally from the *r. prostaticus* of the internal pudendal artery and in the sheep and ox it stems from the internal pudendal artery itself. In all domestic mammals the middle rectal artery supplies the ventrolateral region of the rectal ampulla. A *r. urethralis* to the pelvic part of the urethra arises from the terminal portion of the prostatic artery in the dog, pig and ruminant and in the cat it stems from the above-mentioned prostatic ramus.

R. ductus deferentis
(Comparative: 136–139/*31*)

The **r. ductus deferentis**, a branch of the prostatic artery, goes to the terminal part of the ductus deferens. In carnivores this vessel also supplies those areas which in the other domestic mammals are nourished by the *a. ductus deferentis*; the latter is a branch of the umbilical artery and therefore, in

178 Arteries

Figs 136, 137, 138, 139. Arteries of the pelvic organs of the male dog, pig, ox and horse. Semidiagrammatic.
(based on Ackerknecht, 1943.)

A vertebrae lumbales; *B* os sacrum; *C* vertebrae caudales; *D* symphysis pelvis

a rectum; *b* ureter; *c* vesica urinaria; *d* urethra; *e* testis; *f* epididymis; *g* ductus deferens; *h* gl. prostatica; *h'* gl. vesiculosa; *h"* gl. bulbourethralis, *i* can. urogenitalis; *k* penis; *l* scrotum; *m* proc. vaginalis; *n* praeputium; *o* m. retractor penis; *p* lnn. inguinales superficiales

1 aorta abdominalis; *2* a. testicularis; *5* a. mesenterica caudalis; *6* a. sacralis mediana continuing, except in the horse, as the a. caudalis mediana; *7* a. iliaca externa; *8* a. circumflexa ilium profunda; *9* truncus pudendoepigastricus; *10* a. epigastrica caudalis; *11* a. vesicalis media; *12* a. pudenda externa; *13* r. scrotalis ventralis; *14* a. epigastrica caudalis superficialis; *16* rr. praeputiales; *17* a. cremasterica; *18* a. penis cranialis; *19* a. iliaca interna; *20* a. umbilicalis; *21* a. ductus deferentis; *22* r. uretericus; *23* a. vesicalis cranialis; *24* a. glutaea caudalis; *25* a. iliolumbalis; *26* a. glutaea cranialis; *27* a. obturatoria; *28* a. penis media; *29* a. pudenda interna; *30* a. prostatica; *31* r. ductus deferentis or, in the dog, a. ductus deferentis; *32* a. vesicalis caudalis; *33* r. uretericus; *34* r. urethralis; *35* a. rectalis media; *37* a. urethralis; *39* a. perinealis ventralis; *40* a. rectalis caudalis; *41* r. scrotalis dorsalis; *42* a. penis; *43* a. bulbi penis; *44* a. profunda penis; *45* a. dorsalis penis

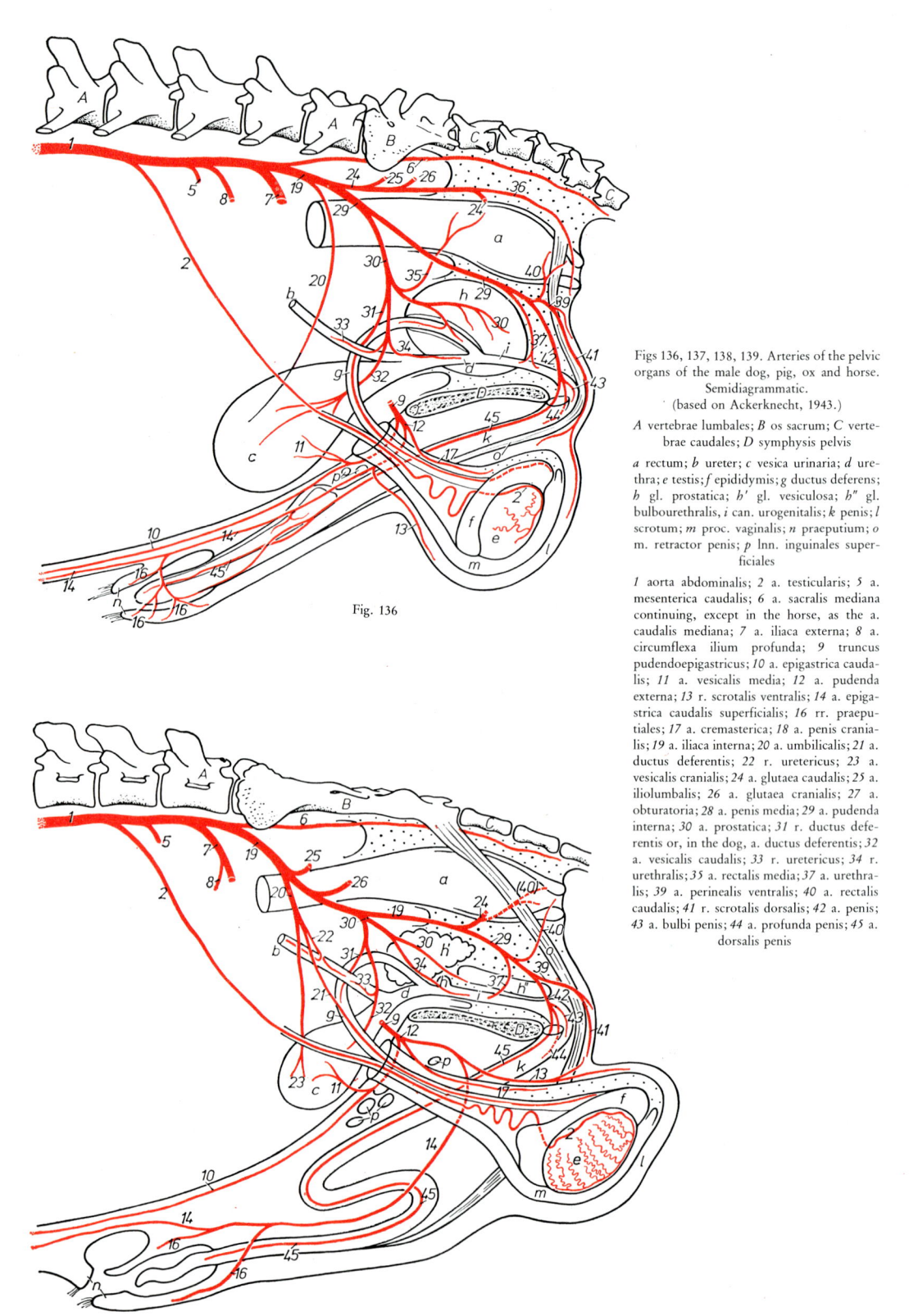

Fig. 136

Fig. 137

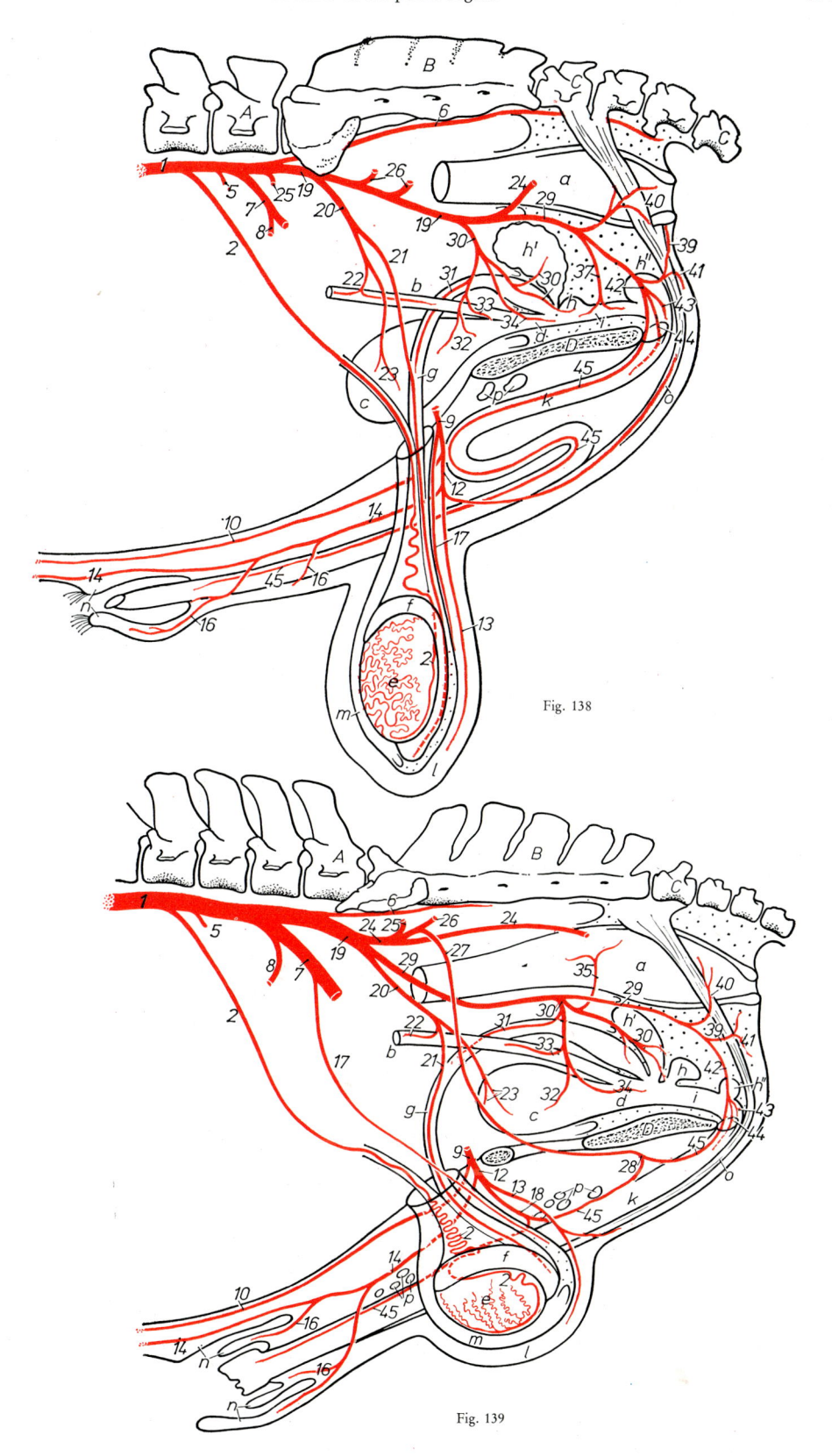

Arteries of the pelvic organs

Fig. 138

Fig. 139

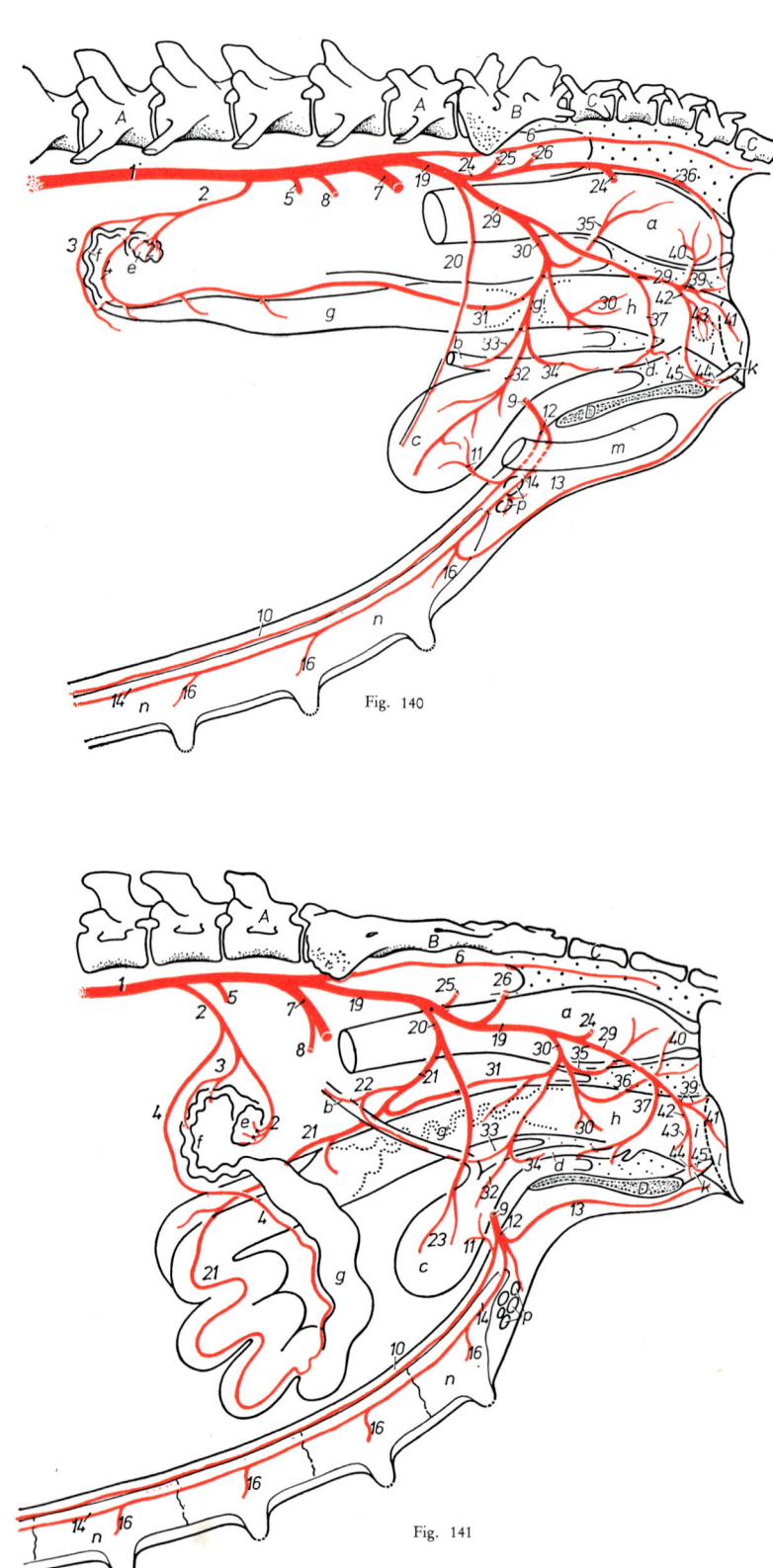

Figs 140, 141, 142, 143. Arteries of the pelvic organs of the female dog, pig, ox and horse. Semidiagrammatic. (based on Ackerknecht, 1943.)

A vertebrae lumbales; *B* os sacrum; *C* vertebrae caudales; *D* symphysis pelvis

a rectum; *b* ureter; *c* vesica urinaria; *d* urethra; *e* ovar; *f* tuba uterina; *g* uterus; *g'* cervix uteri; *h* vagina; *i* vestibulum vaginae; *k* clitoris; *l* vulva; *m* proc. vaginalis; *n* mamma; *p* lnn. inguinales superficiales

1 aorta abdominalis; *2* a. ovarica, *3* r. tubarius; *4* r. uterinus; *5* a. mesenterica caudalis; *6* a. sacralis mediana continuing, except in the mare, as the a. caudalis mediana; *7* a. iliaca externa; *8* a. circumflexa ilium profunda; *9* truncus pudendoepigastricus; *10* a. epigastrica caudalis; *11* a. vesicalis media; *12* a. pudenda externa; *13* r. labialis ventralis or, in ruminants and the horse, a. mammaria caudalis; *14* a. epigastrica caudalis superficialis or, in ruminants and the horse, a. mammaria cranialis; *14'* anastomosis of the r. superficialis of the a. circumflexa ilium profunda; *15* a. mammaria medialis; *16* rr. mammarii; *19* a. iliaca interna; *20* a. umbilicalis; *21* a. uterina; *22* r. uretericus; *23* a. vesicalis cranialis; *24* a. glutaea caudalis; *25* a. iliolumbalis; *26* a. glutaea cranialis; *27* a. obturatoria; *28* a. clitoridis media; *29* a. pudenda interna; *30* a. vaginalis; *31* r. uterinus or, in the dog, a. uterina; *32* a. vesicalis caudalis; *33* r. uretericus; *34* r. urethralis; *35* a. rectalis media; *36* a. perinealis dorsalis; *37* a. urethralis; *38* a. vestibularis; *38'* r. vestibularis; *39* a. perinealis ventralis; *40* a. rectalis caudalis; *41* r. labialis dorsalis or r. labialis dorsalis et mammarius; *42* a. clitoridis; *43* a. bulbi vestibuli; *44* a. profunda clitoridis; *45* a. dorsalis clitoridis

Fig. 142

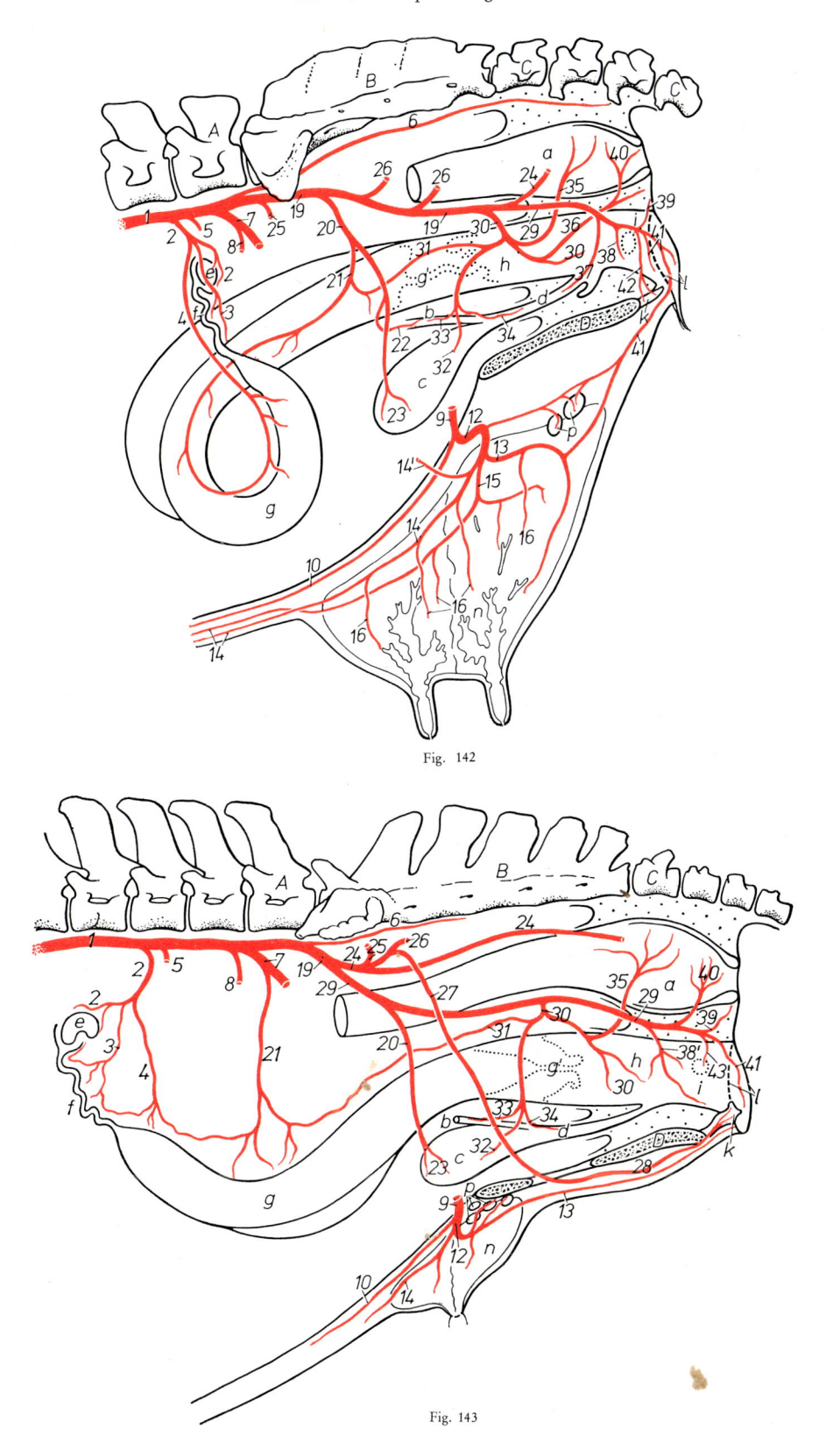

Fig. 143

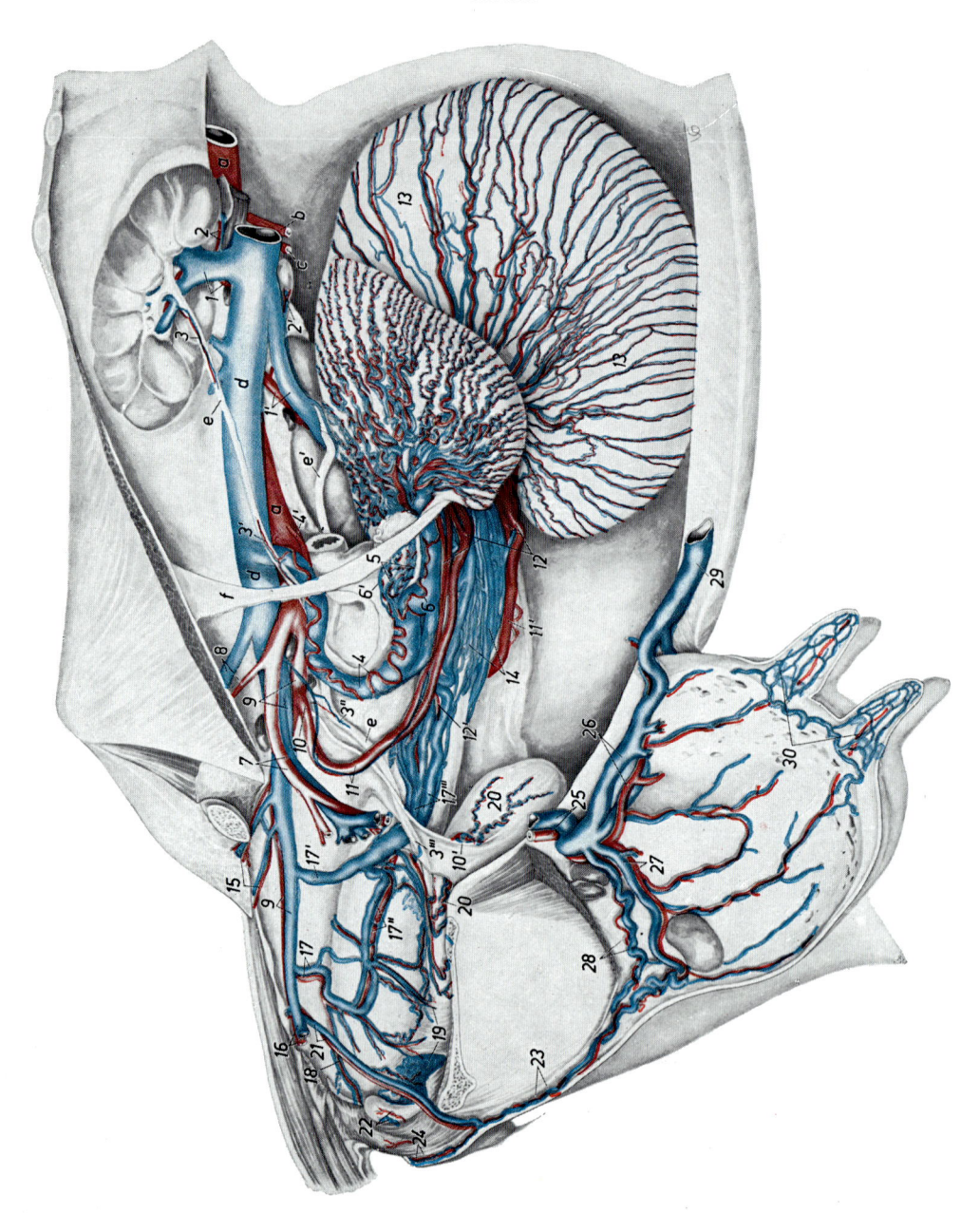

Fig. 144. Arteries and veins of the urogenital system of a cow in the 5th month of pregnancy. Right and ventrolateral view. (After Vollmerhaus, 1964, Institute of Veterinary Anatomy, Giessen.)

a aorta abdominalis; *b* a. coeliaca; *c* a. mesenterica cranialis; *d* v. cava caudalis; *e* ureter dexter; *e′* ureter sinister; *f* origin of the plica urogenitalis

1 a. and v. renalis dextra; *1′* a. and v. renalis sinistra; *2* a. and v. suprarenalis dextra; *2′* a. and v. suprarenalis sinistra; *3–3′′′* rr. ureterici; *3* from the a. or v. renalis, *3′* from the a. or v. ovarica, *3′′* from the a. umbilicalis or v. uterina, *3′′′* from the a. or v. vaginalis; *4* a. and v. ovarica dextra; *4′* a. ovarica sinistra; *5* plexus of ovarian vessels; *6* r. uterinus; *6′* r. tubarius; *7* a. and v. iliaca externa; *8* a. and v. circumflexa ilium profunda; *9* a. and v. iliaca interna; *10* a. umbilicalis; *10′* lig. teres vesicae; *11* a. and v. uterina dextra, *11′* a. and v. uterina sinistra, *12* rr. uterini; *12′* anastomosis between a. uterina and r. uterinus of the a. vaginalis; *13* ramification of the uterine vessels; *14* plexus of the uterine veins; *15* a. and v. glutaea cranialis; *16* a. and v. glutaea caudalis; *17* a. and v. vaginalis; *17′* v. vaginalis accessoria; *17′′* r. uterinus from *17*; *17′′′* plexus from *17′*; *18* a. and v. perinealis dorsalis; *19* r. urethralis of the a. or v. vaginalis and the a. and v. urethralis; *20* a. and v. vesicalis caudalis; *21* a. and v. pudenda interna; *22* a. and v. vestibularis; *23* r. mammarius; *24* r. labialis dorsalis; *25* a. and v. pudenda externa; *26* a. and v. epigastrica caudalis superficialis (a. and v. mammaria cranialis); *27*, *28* r. or v. labialis ventralis (a. and v. mammaria caudalis); *29* v. epigastrica caudalis superficialis; *30* vessels of the teats

carnivores, the ramus is termed the *arteria ductus deferentis* (see above). The ramus or, as the case may be, the artery of the ductus deferens gives off the *a. vesicalis caudalis* to the urinary bladder. In the dog the latter vessel also supplies the cranial region of the bladder because in this species the umbilical artery becomes so completely obliterated postnatally that there is no cranial vesicular artery. In all domestic mammals the caudal vesicular artery supplies the ureter via the *r. uretericus* while in carnivores and horses the initial part of the urethra has an additional provision of blood from the *r. urethralis*.

A. vaginalis
(Comparative: 85–88/77; 140–143/30; ox: 144/17)

The **a. vaginalis** of the female is analogous to, and corresponds in origin to, the prostatic artery of the male. It supplies the vagina giving off the *r. uterinus* which in carnivores is designated the *a. uterina*. In all the domestic mammals it is the parent vessel of the *a. rectalis media* and, in the pig, goat and ox, is also the source of the *a. perinealis dorsalis*. In females it also supplies the ventrolateral region of the ampulla recti. The dorsal perineal artery of the female pig, goat and ox is caudodorsally directed and supplies the perineum, giving off the *a. rectalis caudalis* to the anus.

R. uterinus
(Comparative: 140–143/31; ox: 144/17″)

The **r. uterinus** is a branch of the vaginal artery which runs from the lateral wall of the vagina to the cervix of the uterus. It anastomoses with the uterine artery in the mesometrium. In carnivores this vessel undertakes the supply of the region served by the uterine artery in the other domestic mammals with the result that it is known as the arteria uterina. From the uterine ramus, or the uterine artery of carnivores, arises the *a. vesicalis caudalis*. In males of the domestic mammals it runs to the bladder, supplying the *r. ureticus* to the terminal part of the ureter and the *r. urethralis* to the proximal part of the urethra.

A. urethralis
(pig: 137, 141/37; ox: 138, 142/37; 144/19)

The **a. urethralis** springs from the internal pudendal artery caudal to the origin of the vaginal artery. The horse has no urethral artery. In the small ruminants its origin is more caudally situated. This artery supplies the caudal part of the pelvic segment of the urethra in males and its terminal portion in females.

A. vestibularis – r. vestibularis
(ox: 142/38; 144/22; horse: 143/38′)

In cows and heifers the **a. vestibularis** is a strong vessel which arises from the internal pudendal artery and supplies the lateral wall of the vestibule of the vagina, especially the gll. vestibulares majores. In female horses the internal pudendal artery gives off the *r. vestibularis* which runs parallel with the dorsal nerve of the clitoris to the ventrolateral region of the vestibule of the vagina, although it does not extend as far as the clitoris.

Veins (venae)

In the following account the veins will be described in a centrifugal direction, as suggested by Schmaltz (1898), thus providing a better overall view and allowing comparison with the arteries.

Venae pulmonales
(pig: 96/*42*; 153/*47*; sheep: 99/*21*; ox: 155/*1*; horse: 103/*38*)

The **vv. pulmonales**, the veins of the small or pulmonary circulation are devoid of valves and carry arterial blood from the lungs to the left atrium of the heart. Arising from the roof of the left atrium, ventral to the hilus of the lung where the truncus pulmonalis divides into its branches, these veins are invariably multiple, the number depending on the species. Their number usually corresponds to the number of pulmonary lobes and the veins are arranged almost symmetrically into a left and a right group. This is especially the case in the dog. In the cat, on the other hand, the veins arise in an asymmetrical manner in three groups, each group being composed of two or three veins originating from corresponding depressions on the roof of the right atrium. One of these drains the bipartite left cranial lobe, the other drains the middle and cranial lobe of the right side and the last the caudal lobes of both sides. In pigs, small ruminants and horses the roof of the atrium carries a larger right and a smaller left depression from which a number of veins of different diameter arise and these supply the left and right lungs. In the ox there are usually only one large and two or three small pulmonary veins.

In the ox the pulmonary veins accompany the branches of the pulmonary arteries along the bronchi. A similar method of distribution occurs in carnivores and pigs only in the cranial and middle lobes. In the caudal lobes of the latter animals the branches of the pulmonary veins are distributed exclusively intersegmentally, as they are in sheep and horses, and they always give off their branches to two neighbouring pulmonary segments. Since in carnivores, small ruminants and horses the bronchial veins only reach to the hilus, the pulmonary veins are responsible in these species for drainage of the major part of the bronchial tree.

Vena cava cranialis
(Comparative: 145–152/*1*; pig: 153, 176/*1*; goat: 154/*1*; sheep: 99/*20*; ox: 155/*6*; horse: 103/*32*)

The **v. cava cranialis** arises from the craniodorsal part of the sinus venosus of the right atrium. Although there are some species differences, its origin lies on a transverse plane passing through about the 4th pair of ribs. It is the vein which corresponds to the brachiocephalic trunk. It runs towards the thoracic inlet in the cranial mediastinum to the right of the midline and ventral to the trachea. At first it is situated to the left of the brachiocephalic trunk but by the thoracic inlet is reached it has become ventral to it. In carnivores, ruminants and horses the *v. azygos dextra* arises from this segment of the cranial vena cava which also gives rise to the v. broncho-oesophagea in cats. The next branch is the *v. costocervicalis* which occurs only on the right in the dog but bilaterally in the other domestic mammals. Then follows the *vv. thoracicae internae dextra* and *sinistra,* which in carnivores usually arise by a common stem. In the horse only, the cranial vena cava gives rise to the *v. vertebralis* on the right side. In carnivores and pigs, rarely in goats, the cranial vena cava then divides at the thoracic inlet into the *vv. brachiocephalicae dextra* and *sinistra*. In ruminants and horses it first gives rise at this level to the *vv. subclaviae dextra* and *sinistra* and only then does it fork into the *vv. jugulares dextra* and *sinistra* immediately cranial to the apertura thoracic cranialis.

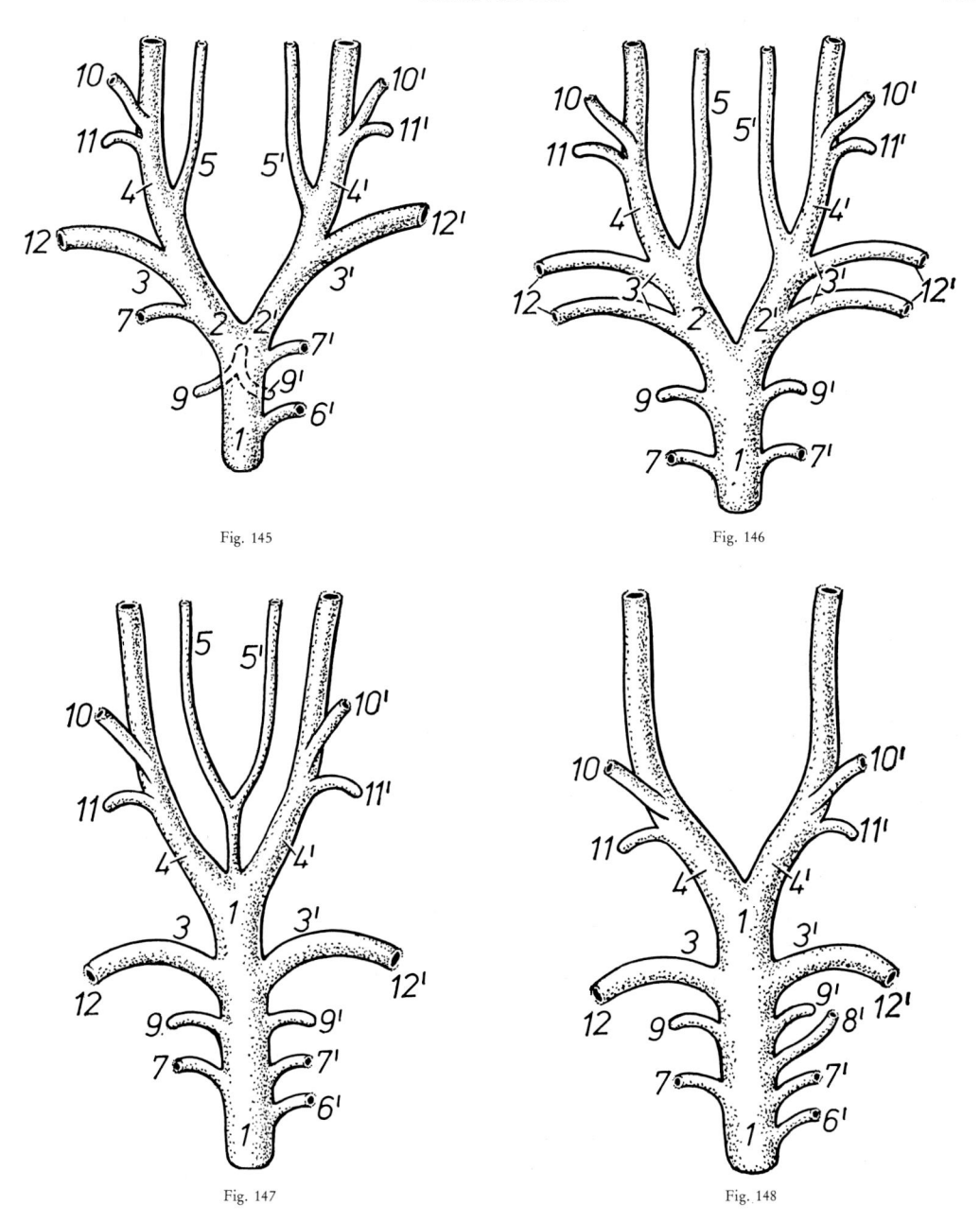

Figs 145, 146, 147, 148. Vena cava cranialis of the dog, pig, ox and horse. Dorsal view.

1 v. cava cranilis; *2* v. brachiocephalica sinistra; *2'* v. brachiocephalica dextra; *3* v. subclavia sinistra; *3'* v. subclavia dextra; *4* v. jugularis externa sinistra; *4'* v. jugularis externa dextra; *5* v. jugularis interna sinistra; *5'* v. jugularis interna dextra; *6'* v. azygos dextra; *7* v. costocervicalis sinistra; *7'* v. costocervicalis dextra; *8'* v. vertebralis dextra; *9* v. thoracica interna sinistra; *9'* v. thoracica interna dextra; *10* v. cervicalis superficialis sinistra; *10'* v. cervicalis superficialis dextra; *11* v. cephalica sinistra; *11'* v. cephalica dextra; *12* v. axillaris sinistra; *12'* v. axillaris dextra

V. azygos dextra – v. azygos sinistra

(dog: 94, 95/*11*; 145/*6'*; 149/*2*; pig: 97/*9*; 150/*31*; 153/*43*; goat: 154/*2, 24*; sheep: 99/*22*; ox: 102/*4*; 147/*6'*; 151/*2, 31*; 155/*21*; horse: 148/*6'*; 152/*2*)

The **v. azygos dextra,** which is missing in the pig, arises in carnivores, ruminants and horses from that part of the cranial vena cava which lies close to the insertion of the pericardium and still contains heart muscle tissue. In carnivores and horses it rises in a cranially convex curve to the thoracic vertebral column, crossing the trachea and oesophagus on their right side. Then, lying to the right and dorsal of the thoracic aorta, it accompanies this vessel and the thoracic duct through the hiatus aorticus. In the horse it occasionally ends in the thoracic cavity. The right azygos vein of carnivores and horses may give off a *v. hemiazygos sinistra* in the caudal half of the thorax. After passing through the aortic hiatus it terminates in one of the first lumbar veins, their common vessel of origin or in the caudal vena cava. In ruminants the right azygos vein runs vertically in dorsal direction, immediately cranial to the tracheal bronchus, continues over the lateral surface of the right longus colli muscle to the 2nd or 3rd intercostal space and then swings caudad. In most cases the right azygos vein of ruminants behaves as a *v. intercostalis suprema dextra* extending from the 2nd or 3rd to the 5th, 6th or 7th intercostal space. Only in exceptional cases is its course similar to that of the right azygos vein of carnivores and horses; rarely it extends to the last thoracic vertebra where it joins with the left azygos vein.

The **v. azygos sinistra** is present only in pigs and ruminants. It arises from the sinus coronarius of the heart and is rudimentarily represented in the horse and carnivores as the *v. obliqua atrii sinistri*. It runs dorsally over the left atrium, caudally around the pulmonary veins and along the dorsal border of the left auricle. It then swings to the left of the pulmonary artery and dorsal to the aorta. Curving caudad it accompanies the thoracic aorta along the origins of the intercostal arteries from the 5th or 6th thoracic vertebra onwards. Together with the aorta it passes through the aortic hiatus to join the first lumbar veins, their common vessel of origin or, in the pig, directly with the caudal vena cava. However, it often terminates in the caudal half of the thorax. Before then, or sometimes even from its terminal part, it gives off a *v. hemiazygos dextra*. The latter vessel may, however, already have been given off the continuation of the right azygos vein.

The **v. hemiazygos dextra** of pigs and ruminants and the **v. hemiazygos sinistra** of carnivores and horses can arise from the left or right azygos vein in the caudal part of the thorax. The hemiazygos vein crosses to the other side of the vertebral column along which it then continues caudad. Each hemiazygos vein supplements, or substitutes for, the azygos vein.

The segmental veins to the body wall show considerable species variation in their origin. In carnivores and horses they arise from the right azygos vein, in pigs and ruminants from the left, or in ruminants from both since in that species both left and right azygos veins may occasionally exist simultaneously. In all domestic mammals they may also arise from the hemiazygos vein in those areas where this substitutes for the azygos vein. Allowing for species variations and peculiarities these segmental veins to the body wall are the cranial lumbar veins, the dorsal costoabdominal vein and the dorsal intercostal veins. In the case of the latter the cranial dorsal intercostal veins do not arise from the azygos system but from the *vv. costocervicalis, intercostalis suprema* and *vertebralis thoracica*. Although it is, of course, impossible to consider all the variations, the segmental veins arising from the azygos veins, and the species peculiarities, are shown in the table on p. 194. Attention is drawn to the fact that these azygos veins are usually valveless and form a functional connection between the cranial and caudal vena cavae.

In the dog and horse the right azygos vein gives off a visceral vein, the *v. broncho-oesophagea*, which in the cat is present only on the right side and derives from the cranial vena cava or sometimes even from the right supreme intercostal vein. In the pig and ox the right azygos vein gives rise to the *vv. oesophageae* and *vv. bronchales*. While in all the domestic mammals the oesophageal veins are distributed in company with the arteries, the bronchial vein reaches only the hilus in carnivores, small ruminants and the horse. The remainder of the bronchial tree receives its nutritive supply from the pulmonary veins (see p. 184).

Vv intercostales dorsales and v. costoabdominalis dorsalis

(Comparative: 149–152/*32, 33*; dog: *94, 95/12, 13*; pig: 97/*20, 21–25*; 153, 188/*8*; goat: 154/*3, 4, 25*; ox: 102, 155/*5*)

The vessels from which the **vv. intercostales dorsales** and *v. costoabdominalis dorsalis* originate are shown in the table on p. 193. The dorsal intercostal veins of an individual thoracic segment can arise by a common trunk. Each dorsal intercostal and dorsal costoabdominal vein gives off a *r. dorsalis*. Thereafter both dorsal intercostal and costoabdominal veins run cranially along the corresponding arteries and branch with them.

In the cranial thoracic part of all domestic mammals except the horse the *v. cervicalis profunda* and the neighbouring dorsal rami of the dorsal intercostal arteries are joined, immediately after their origin, by

Segmental vessels of the azygos veins

	Vv. intercostales dorsales		V. costoabdominalis dorsalis	Vv. lumbales
cat	right III–V v. azygos dextra	VI–XII v. azygos dextra	v. azygos dextra	I + II v. azygos dextra
dog		(III left) IV–XII v. azygos dextra left IX–XI also from v. hemiazygos sinistra	v. azygos dextra	I + II (III) v. azygos dextra
pig		right (V) VI–XIV (XV) left (IV) V–XIV (XV) v. azygos sinistra or in the caudal part of the thorax from v. hemiazygos dextra	v. azygos sinistra or v. hemiazygos dextra	I + II (III) v. azygos sinistra or v. hemiazygos dextra
ruminants	right II–V v. azygos dextra	right VI–XII v. azygos sinistra or in the caudal part of the thorax v. hemiazygos dextra rarely v. azygos dextra left (IV) V–XII v. azygos sinistra	common vessel of origin from the v. azygos for the first vv. lumbales	I + II (III) common vessel of origin from the v. azygos
horse		right V (VI)–XVII left (VI) VII–XVII v. azygos dextra or in the caudal part of the thorax v. hemiazygos sinistra	v. azygos dextra or v. hemiazygos sinistra	

vascular bridges running between the neck and tubercle of the ribs. These anastomoses are the *v. vertebralis thoracica* which can extend a variable distance beyond the cranial thoracic segments, depending on the species and individual. In the dog this thoracic vertebral vein forms the vessel of origin for the dorsal intercostal veins if the supreme intercostal vein is absent.

The **r. dorsalis** gives off the *v. intervertebralis* which participates in forming the *plexus vertebralis externi ventralis* and *dorsalis*. In the pig especially, the ventral plexus also receives direct connections from the dorsal intercostal veins. The intervertebral vein gains entry to the vertebral canal through the lateral vertebral foramen or the intervertebral foramen. In the vertebral canal it forms the *plexus vertebralis internus ventralis*. From this ventral internal vertebral venous plexus branch the *rr. interarcuales* which, so far, have been described only in the dog and are absent in the pig. The interarcuate rami give off the *vv. interspinosae* which anastomose with the dorsal external vertebral venous plexus. The veins running in the vertebral canal give off the *rr. spinales*, but these do not arise regularly at every segment. The spinal rami continue as the *vv. spinales* to the spinal cord and its meninges. Some segments of these vessels are referred to as *vv. nervomedullares* and *vv. radiculares dorsales* or *ventrales*. From the ventral internal vertebral plexus issue the *vv. basivertebrales* which pass to either side of the middle of the vertebral body. These veins ramify in the vertebral body and

Fig. 149

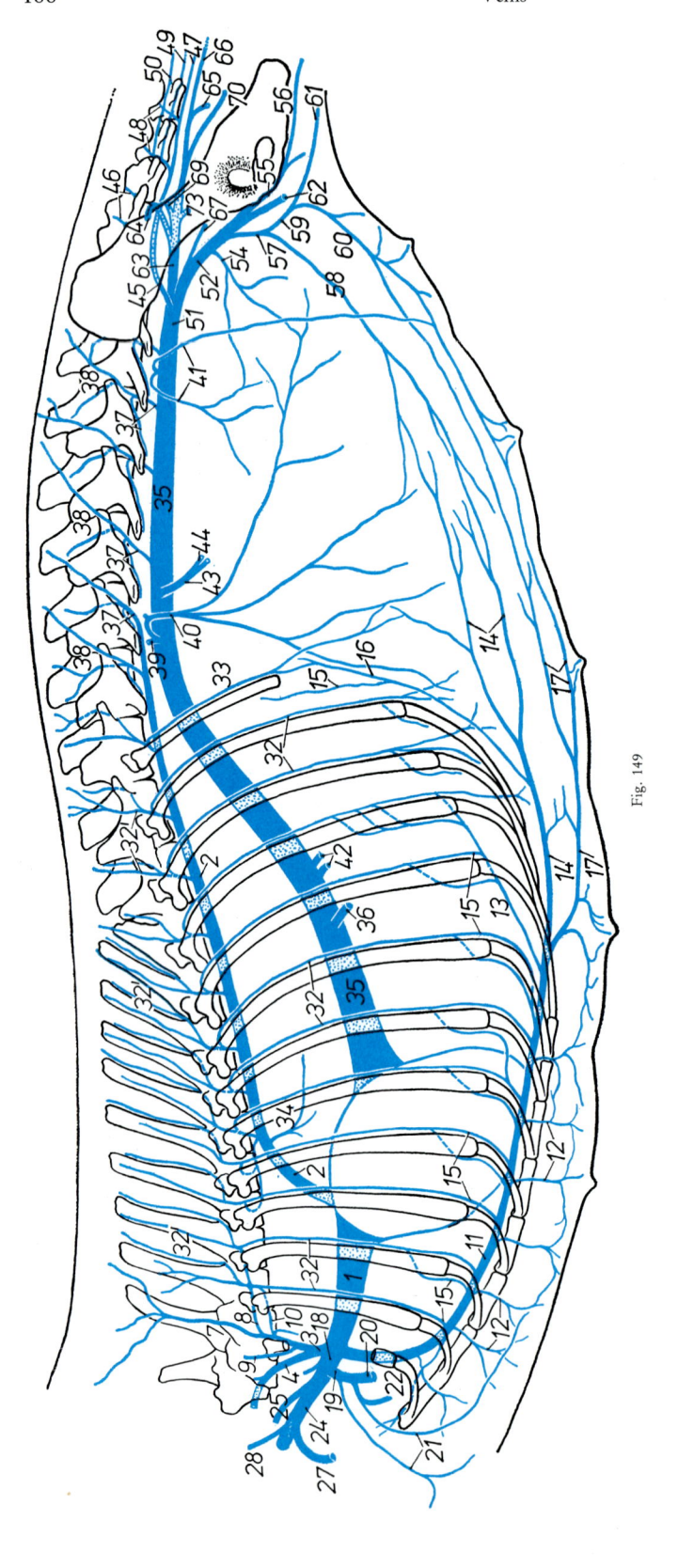

Figs 149, 150, 151, 152. Veins of the trunk of the dog, pig, ox and horse. Semidiagrammatic. Left lateral view.
(After Wieboldt, 1966, Diss., Hannover; after Wolff, 1963, Diss., Hannover; after Seidler, 1966, Diss., Hannover; after Leschke, in preparation, Diss., Hannover.)

1 v. cava cranialis; *2* v. azygos dextra; *3* v. costocervicalis; *4* v. vertebralis with *5* rr. dorsales, *5'* r. descendens, *6* rr. ventrales, *6'* r. anastomoticus cum v. occipitali; *7* v. cervicalis profunda; *8* v. vertebralis thoracica; *9* v. scapularis dorsalis; *10* v. intercostalis suprema; *11* v. thoracica interna; *12* vv. perforantes with rr. sternales and in the dog with rr. mammarii; *13* v. musculophrenica; *14* v. epigastrica cranialis; *15* vv. intercostales ventrales; *16* v. costoabdominalis ventralis; *17* v. epigastrica cranialis superficialis; *18* v. brachiocephalica; *19* v. subclavia; *20* v. axillaris; *21* v. thoracica externa; *22* v. thoracica lateralis; *23* v. thoracica superficialis (in the horse from the v. thoracodorsalis); *24* v. jugularis externa; *25* v. jugularis interna; *26* v. occipitalis; *27* v. cephalica; *28* v. cervicalis superficialis; *29* v. linguofacialis; *30* v. maxillaris; *30'* v. auricularis caudalis; *31* v. azygos sinistra; *32* vv. intercostales dorsales with *32'* r. dorsalis, continuing as r. cutaneus medialis (the remaining branches, which behave like the corresponding arteries, are not shown); *33* v. costoabdominalis dorsalis; *34* v. broncho-oesophagea or vv. bronchales and vv. oesophageae; *35* v. cava caudalis; *36* v. phrenica cranialis; *37* vv. lumbales with *38* r. dorsalis; *39* v. phrenica caudalis; *40* v. abdominalis cranialis; *41* v. circumflexa ilium profunda; *42* vv. hepaticae; *43* v. renalis; *44* v. testicularis/v. ovarica; *45* v. sacralis mediana; *46* rr. sacrales; *47* v. caudalis mediana; *48* rr. caudales; *49* v. caudalis ventrolateralis; *50* v. caudalis dorsolateralis; *51* v. iliaca communis; *52* v. iliaca externa; *53* v. iliacofemoralis; *54* v. abdominalis caudalis; *55* v. profunda femoris; *56* v. circumflexa femoris medialis; *57* v. pudendoepigastrica; *58* v. epigastrica caudalis; *59* v. pudenda externa; *60* v. epigastrica caudalis superficialis (in female ruminants and horses v. mammaria cranialis); *61* v. scrotalis ventralis/v. labialis ventralis (in female ruminants and horses v. mammaria caudalis); *61'* v. penis cranialis; *62* v. femoralis; *63* v. iliaca interna; *64* v. iliolumbalis; *65* v. glutaea caudalis; *66* v. caudalis lateralis superficialis; *67* v. obturatoria; *68* v. penis media/v. clitoridis media; *69* v. glutaea cranialis; *70* v. pudenda interna; *71* v. uterina; *72* v. vaginalis accessoria; *73* v. prostatica/v. vaginalis; *74* v. perinealis ventralis; *75* v. penis/v. clitoridis

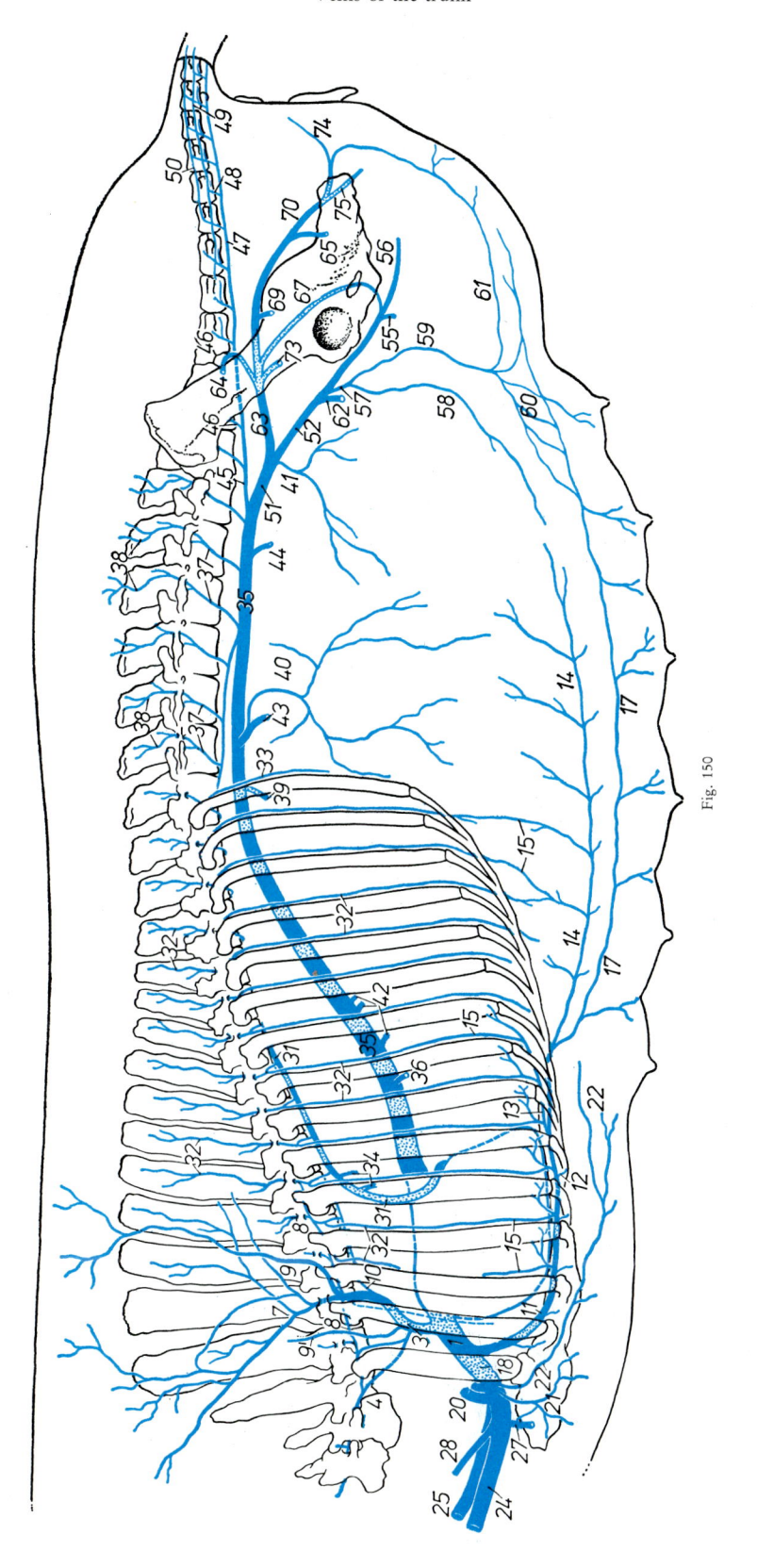

Veins of the trunk

Fig. 150

Fig. 151

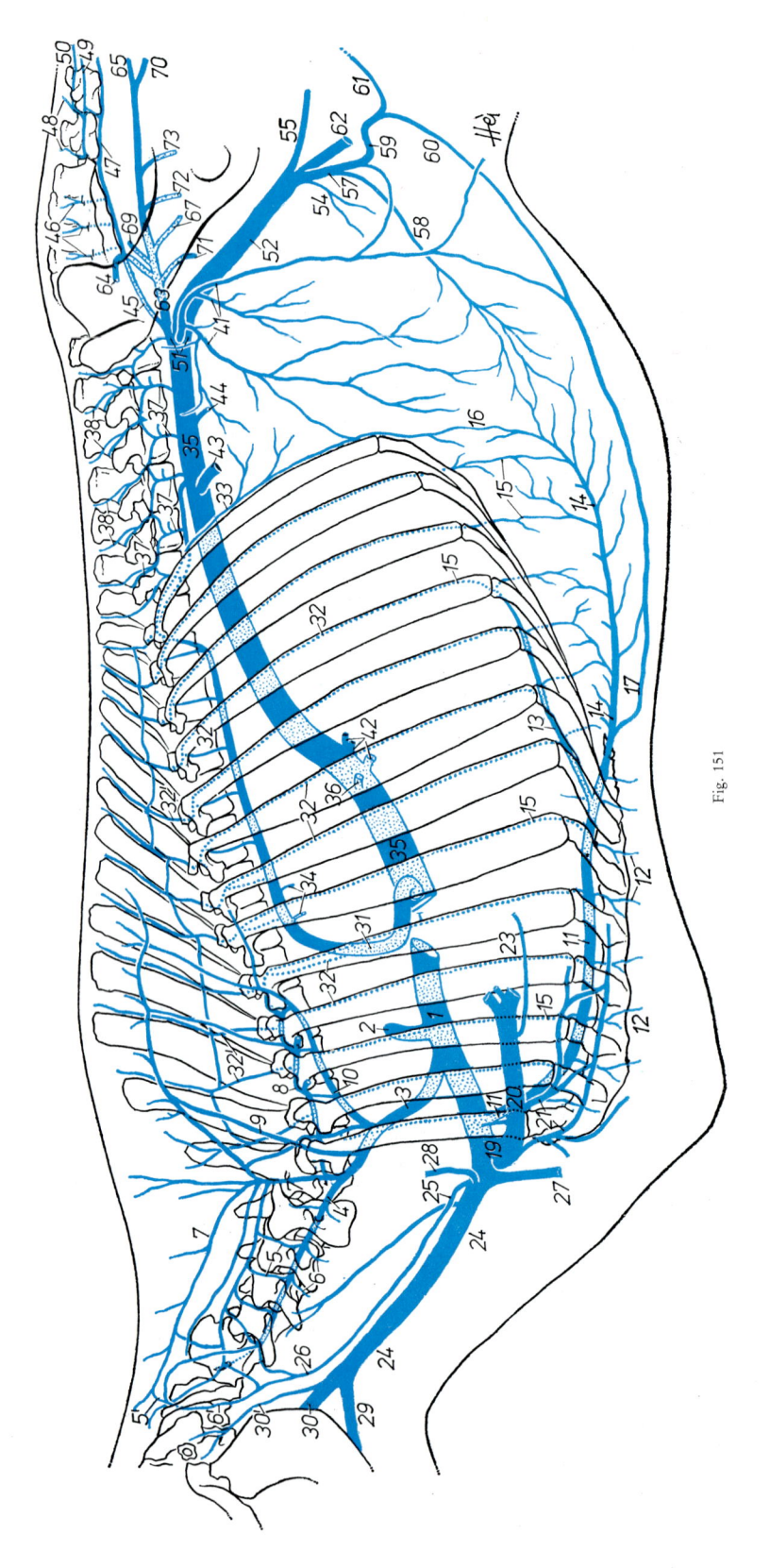

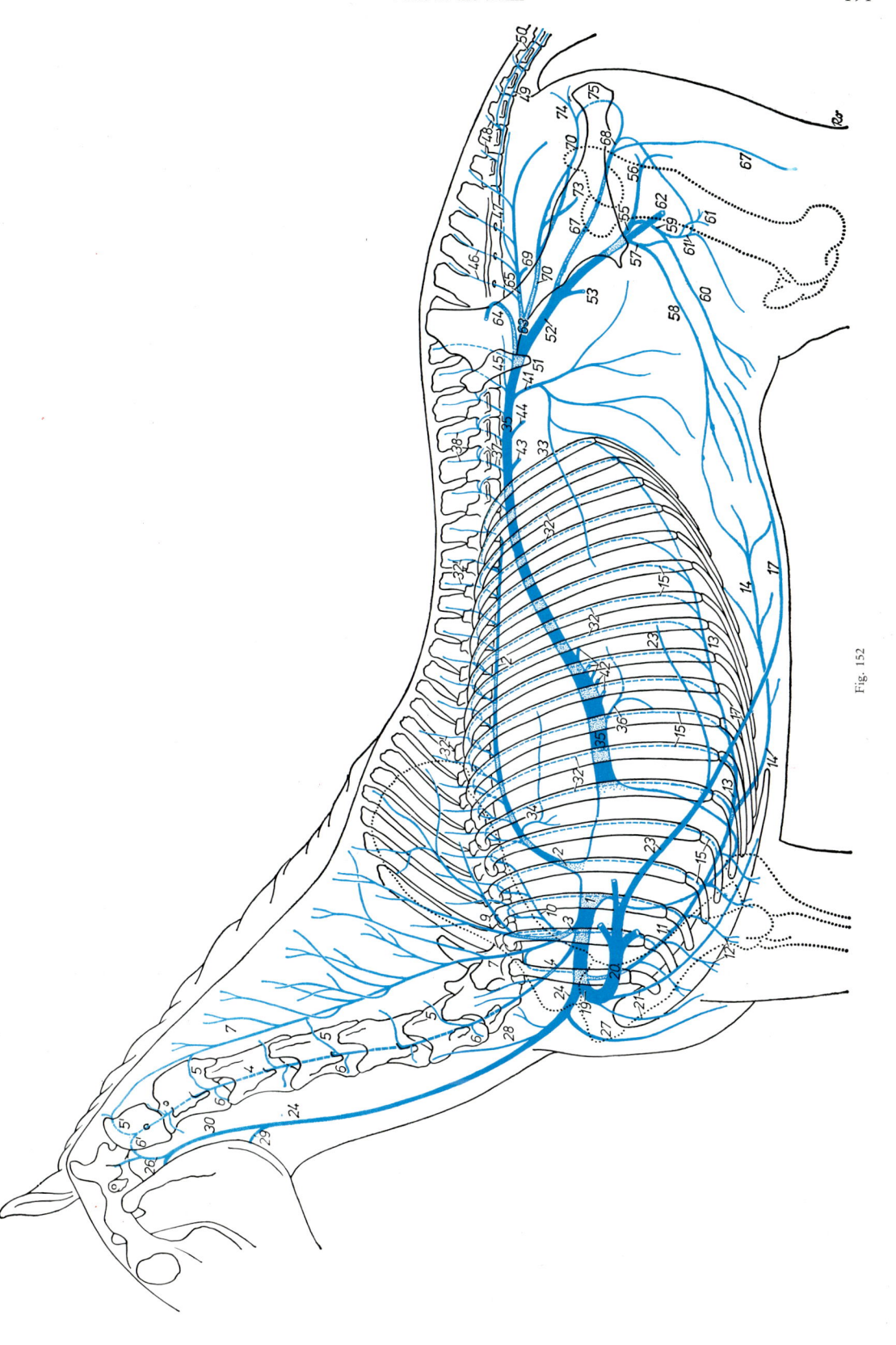

Veins of the trunk

Fig. 152

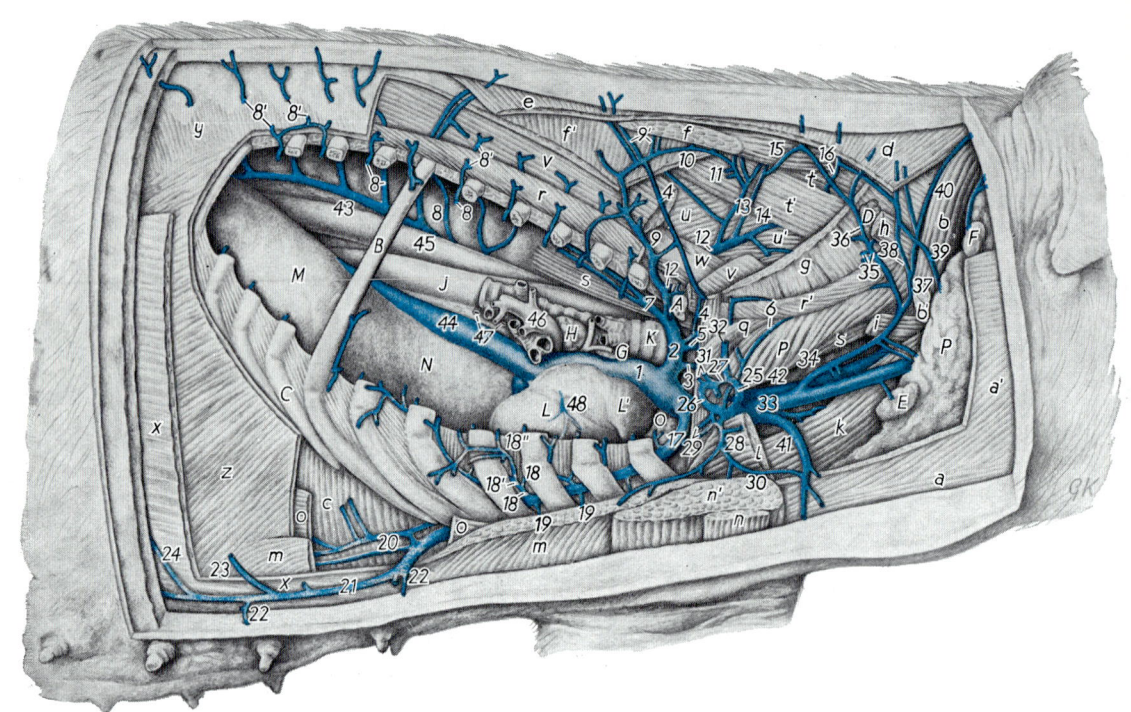

Fig. 153. Veins of the thoracic cavity and neck of the pig. Right lateral view.
(After Wolff, 1963, Diss., Hanover.)

A costa II; *B* costa VIII; *C* arcus costalis; *D* lnn. cervicales superficiales dorsales; *E* lnn. cervicales superficiales ventrales; *F* lnn. retropharyngei laterales; *G* lnn. tracheobronchales craniales; *H* lnn. bifurcationes dextri; *J* oesophagus; *K* trachea; *L* cor (pericardium has been removed); *L'* auricula dextra; *M* diaphragma; *N* membrane of the vena cava; *O* thymus; *P* gl. parotis

a, a' platysma; *b* m. cleido-occipitalis; *b'* m. cleidomastoideus; *c* m. transversus abdominis; *d* m. trapezius, pars cervicalis, *e* pars thoracica; *f* m. rhomboideus cervicis; *f'* m. rhomboideus thoracis; *g* m. serratus ventralis cervicis; *h* m. omotransversarius; *i* m. omohyoideus; *k* m. sternomastoideus; *l* m. subclavius; *m* m. pectoralis profundus; *n, n'* mm. pectorales superficiales; *o* m. rectus abdominis; *p, q* m. scalenus; *r* m. iliocostalis thoracis; *r'* m. iliocostalis cervicis; *s* m. longus colli; *t, t'* m. splenius; *u* m. biventer cervicis; *u'* m. complexus major; *v* m. longissimus thoracis; *w* m. multifidus; *x* m. cutaneus trunci; *y* m. serratus dorsalis caudalis; *z* m. obliquus externus abdominis

1 v. cava cranialis; *2* v. costocervicalis; *3* r. muscularis for m. longus colli; *4* collateral vein of the a. scapularis dorsalis; *5* v. vertebralis, *6* rr. ventrales with anastomosis; *7* v. intercostalis suprema; *8* vv. intercostales dorsales, *8'* rr. cutanei laterales; *9, 9'* v. scapularis dorsalis; *10* r. anastomoticus; *11* r. anastomoticus cum v. suprascapulari; *12* v. cervicalis profunda, *13* its superficial, *14* its deep part; *15, 16* rr. anastomotici cum v. cervicali superficiali; *17* v. thoracica interna; *18* vv. intercostales ventrales, *18'* rr. collaterales, *18"* rr. musculares; *19* rr. perforantes; *20* v. epigastrica cranialis; *21* v. epigastrica cranialis superficialis; *22* rr. mammarii, *23, 24* rr. cutanei; *25, 26* v. axillaris; *27* r. anastomoticus; *28* r. thoracica externa; *29* v. thoracica lateralis; *30* r. deltoideus; *31* v. subscapularis and v. thoracodorsalis; *32* v. suprascapularis; *33* v. jugularis externa; *34* v. cervicalis superficialis, *35* r. acromialis, *36* r. praescapularis, *37, 38* r. ascendens, *39* r. anastomoticus, *40* r. auricularis; *41* v. cephalica; *42* v. jugularis interna; *43* v. azygos sinistra; *44* v. cava caudalis; *45* aorta thoracica; *46* a. pulmonalis dextra; *47* vv. pulmonales; *48* v. cordis media

anastomose on its outer surface with the ventral external vertebral venous plexus. The subsequent distribution of the dorsal ramus in the trunk region corresponds to its accompanying arterial dorsal ramus. There are species peculiarities only in the region lying medial to the scapula and these will be described in connection with the costocervical vein.

Vessels of origin of:

	Vv. intercostales dorsales				V. costoabdominales dorsalis
cat	I v. costocervicalis	II v. intercostalis suprema or v. vertebralis thoracica	right III–V v. azygos dextra left III–V common parent vessel from the v. cava cranialis	VI–XII v. azygos dextra	v. azygos dextra
dog	I v. costocervicalis	II + III v. intercostalis suprema or v. vertrebralis thoracica		(III left) IV–XII v. azygos dextra left IX–XI and from the v. hemiazygos sinistra	v. azygos dextra
pig	I v. vertebralis thoracica	II v. costocervicalis	III, IV, V v. intercostalis suprema	right (V) VI–XIV (XV) left (IV) V–XIV (XV) v. azygos sinistra or in the caudal part of the thorax from the v. hemiazygos dextra	v. azygos sinistra or v. hemiazygos dextra
ruminants	right I absent or v. intercostalis suprema	II–V v. azygos dextra		VI–XII v. azygos sinistra or in the caudal part of the thorax v. hemiazygos dextra, rarely v. azygos dextra (IV) V–XII v. azygos sinistra	common parent vessel from the v. azygos for the first vv. lumbales
horse	I v. cervicalis profunda	right II–IV (V) left II–(V) VI v. intercostalis suprema		right V (VI)–XVII left (VI) VII–XVII v. azygos dextra or in the caudal part of the thorax v. hemiazygos sinistra	v. azygos dextra or v. hemiazygos sinistra

V. costocervicalis
(Comparative: 145–148/7; 149–152/3; pig: 153, 176/2; goat: 154/5; ox: 102,155/7)

The **vv. costocervicales dextra** and **sinistra** arise from the cranial vena cava. An exception to this is found in carnivores where in the cat frequently and in the dog almost invariably, the left costocervical vein arises from the left brachiocephalic vein. In the cat the right costocervical arises only after the internal thoracic veins have been given off and sometimes it, like the vessel of the left side, comes off the right brachiocephalic vein.

The costocervical vein gives off the *v. vertebralis*, except in the horse in which this vessel arises from the right side, frequently also from the left side, of the cranial vena cava. The costocervical vein also gives rise to the *v. cervicalis profunda*, the *v. scapularis dorsalis*, the *v. intercostalis suprema*, in carnivores the *v. intercostalis dorsalis I* and in the pig the *v. intercostalis dorsalis II*. The sequence in which these veins issue from the costocervical vein is shown in the table on page 195. The listed veins accompany, sometimes in pairs, the arteries of the same name and branch with these. Less well developed as a collateral vein is the dorsal scapular vein which, except in the horse, is supplemented by the stout lateral branches of the more caudally situated intercostal veins. By contrast, the latter are larger than the arteries they accompany. The deep cervical vein is the vessel of origin of the *v. vertebralis thoracica* which has already been described with the intercostal veins and which is accompanied by an artery only in the dog.

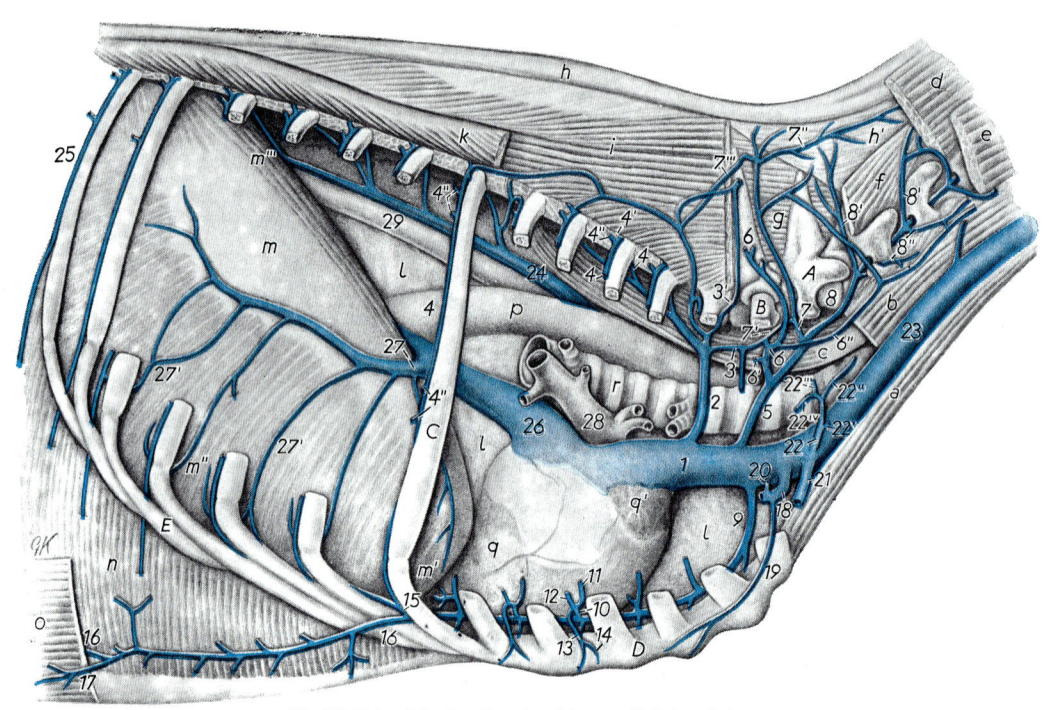

Fig. 154. Veins of the thoracic cavity of the goat. Right lateral view.
(After Rauhut, 1962, Diss., Hanover.)

A vertebra cervicalis VII; *B* costa I; *C* costa VII; *D* sternum; *E* arcus costalis

a m. sternomandibularis; *b* m. scalenus; *c* m. longus colli; *d*, *e* m. semispinalis capitis; *d* m. biventer cervicis, *e* m. complexus; *f* m. multifidus cervicis; *g* mm. interspinales; *h* lig. supraspinale; *h'* lam. nuchae; *i* mm. spinales et semispinales thoracis et cervicis; *k* m. longissimus thoracis; *l* mediastinum; *m–m'''* diaphragma: m. centrum tendineum, *m'* pars sternalis, *m''* pars costalis, *m'''* pars lumbalis; *n* m. transversus abdominis; *o* m. rectus abdominis; *p* oesophagus; *q* cor (pericardium has been removed); *q'* auricula dextra; *r* trachea

1 v. cava cranialis; *2* v. azygos dextra; *3* v. intercostalis suprema with v. intercostalis dorsalis I; *3'* r. dorsalis I; *4* vv. intercostales dorsales, *4'* r. dorsalis, *4''* rr. cutanei laterales; *5* v. costocervicalis; *6* v. scapularis dorsalis; *7*, *7'* v. cervicalis profunda, *7''*, *7'''* its branches; *8* v. vertebralis, *8'* rr. dorsales, *8''* rr. ventrales; *9* v. thoracica interna; *10*, *11* vv. intercostales ventrales, *12* r. collateralis, *13* r. perforans, *14* r. sternalis; *15* v. musculophrenica; *16* v. epigastrica cranialis; *17* v. epigastrica cranialis superficialis; *18* v. subclavia, v. axillaris; *19* v. thoracica externa; *20* v. suprascapularis; *21* v. cephalica; *22* v. cervicalis superficialis, *22'* r. muscularis, *22''* r. ascendens, *22'''* r. praescapularis, *22*[iv] v. suprascapularis; *23* v. jugularis externa; *24* v. azygos sinistra; *25* v. costoabdominalis dorsalis; *26* v. cava caudalis; *27* v. phrenica cranialis, *27'* anastomoses with rr. phrenici of the vv. intercostales; *28* a. pulmonalis gdextra; *29* aorta thoracia

V. costocervicalis

carnivores	pig	ruminants	horse
v. vertebralis	v. vertebralis	v. intercostalis suprema	v. cervicalis profunda
v. scapularis dorsalis	v. intercostalis suprema	v. scapularis dorsalis	v. intercostalis suprema
v. intercostalis dorsalis I	v. intercostalis dorsalis II	v. cervicalis profunda	v. scapularis dorsalis
v. cervicalis profunda	v. scapularis dorsalis	v. vertebralis	v. vertebralis (left)
v. intercostalis suprema	v. cervicalis profunda		

V. thoracica interna
(Comparative: 145–148/9; 149–152/11; pig: 153/17; 176/3; goat: 154/9; ox: 102, 155/13)

In the cat the **v. thoracica interna** arises from the cranial vena cava at the level of the 2nd intercostal space, in the dog and pig at the 1st intercostal space and in ruminants and in horses at the level of the 1st rib. In the cat, and usually in the dog, the vessels of the two sides originate from a common stem. When the left internal thoracic vein arises independently in the dog, it stems from the brachiocephalic vein. The internal thoracic runs ventromedial to the homologous artery up to the diaphragm and, like the artery, it is overlaid dorsally from the 2nd costal cartilage onwards by the transversus thoracis muscle. In the thoracic cavity the internal thoracic vein gives off the *vv. intercostales ventrales* and the *vv. perforantes* which latter have *rr. sternales* and, in carnivores and pigs, *rr. mammarii* draining the thoracic mammary complex. Also originating from the internal thoracic vein are the *vv. mediastinales*, to the mediastinum and, in young animals, the *vv. thymicae* and the *v. pericardiacophrenica*. These veins branch with the corresponding arteries. Some are not accompanied by arteries and these include those which follow the caudal and cranial borders of two consecutive ribs and also those which arise by a common stem and supply several segments. Thus, in the cat the veins destined for the first and second segments spring from a cranially directed branch of the internal thoracic vein. When it reaches the diaphragm the internal thoracic vein divides, with the corresponding artery, into the *v. musculophrenica* and the *v. epigastrica cranialis*.

During its course along the origin of the pars costalis of the diaphragm, the musculophrenic vein gives off further *vv. intercostales ventrales*, which in the pig are delicate vessels. On those asternal ribs which no longer receive ventral intercostal veins from the musculophrenic vein, the dorsal intercostal veins extend to the costal arch or even beyond that to the ventral abdominal wall.

The *v. epigastrica cranialis* gains access to the ventral wall of the abdomen through the diaphragm. Here it ramifies along with the corresponding artery and usually anastomoses through its terminal branches with the terminal branches of the caudal epigastric vein. Except in the horse, the *v. epigastrica cranialis superficialis* springs from the initial part of the cranial epigastric vein.

The *v. epigastrica cranialis superficialis*, also known as the *v. subcutanea abdominis*, passes through the abdominal musculature after its origin from the internal thoracic vein. However, the horse is again an exception in that here this vein arises on the lateral wall of the thorax from the superficial thoracic vein, a branch of the thoracodorsal. The superficial cranial epigastric vein runs subcutaneously caudad, covered by the cutaneus trunci muscle. It gives off the *rr. mammarii* to the neighbouring mammary complexes in carnivores and pigs and anastomoses with the superficial caudal epigastric vein (see. p. 240). In female ruminants and mares, which have inguinally situated mammary glands, the latter vein is the *v. mammaria cranialis*. Thus, especially in ruminants, the superficial cranial epigastric and the superficial caudal epigastric are together responsible for the bulk of the venous drainage from the udder. In lactating mammary glands this stout, meandering vessel bulges the skin on the ventrolateral wall of the abdomen. In ruminants this extends from the point where it perforates the abdominal wall at a depression (the "milk well") which lies in the angle between the costal arch and the xyphoid process.

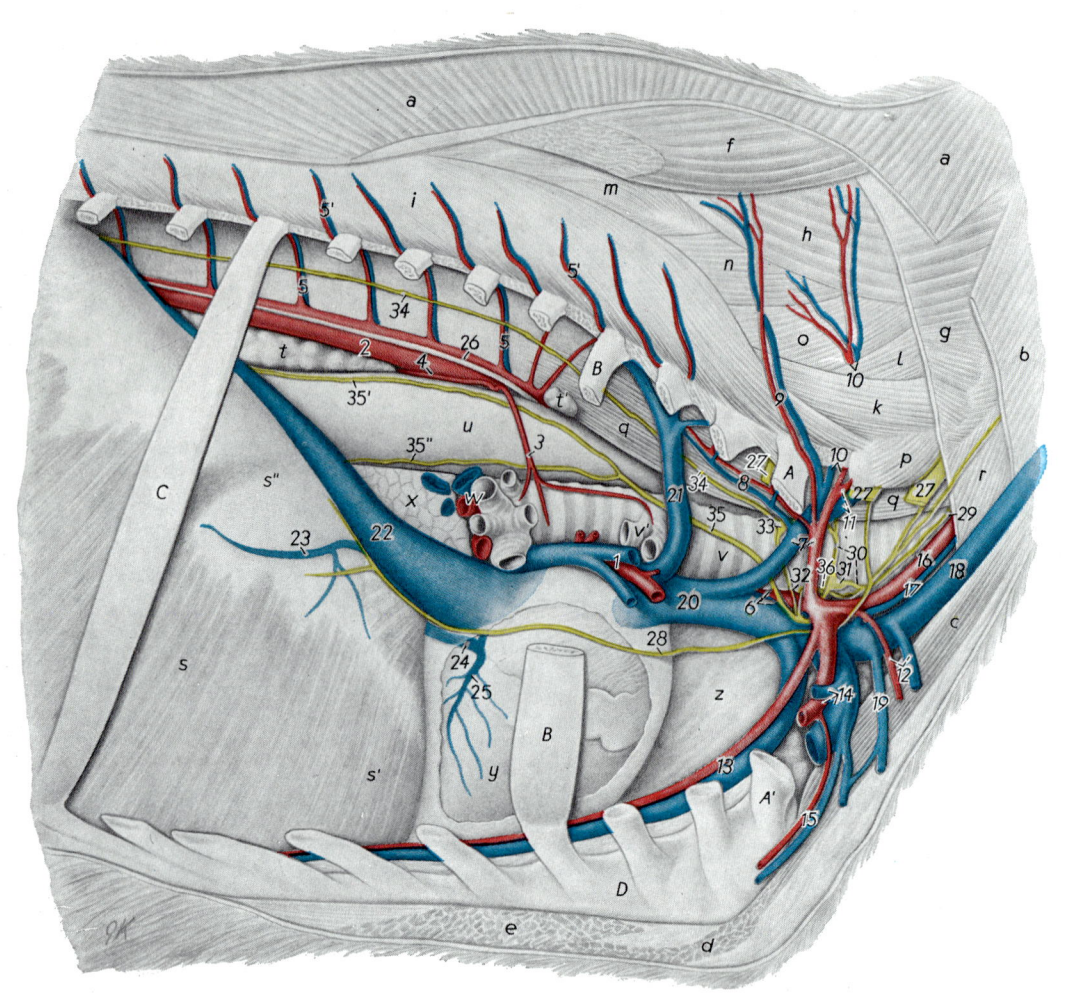

Fig. 155. Veins and arteries of the thoracic cavity of an ox. The plura mediastinalis has been removed. Right lateral view.
(After Wilkens and Rosenberger, 1957, study performed at the Institute of Veterinary Anatomy, Hanover.)

A, A' costa I; *B* costa IV; *C* costa IX; *D* sternum

a m. trapezius; *b* m. brachiocephalicus; *c* m. sternocephalicus; *d* mm. pectorales superficiales; *e* m. pectoralis profundus; *f* m. rhomboideus cervicis; *g* m. serratus ventralis cervicis; *h* m. splenius; *i* m. longissimus thoracis; *k* m. longissimus cervicis; *l* mm. longissimi capitis et atlantis; *m* mm. spinales et semispinales dorsi et cervicis; *n* m. biventer cervicis, *o* m. complexus of the m. semispinalis capitis; *p* m. intertransversarius; *q* m. longus colli; *r* m. scalenus; *s* diaphragma, pars costalis, *s'* pars sternalis, *s''* centrum tendineum; *t* ln. mediastinalis caudalis longissimus; *t'* ln. thoracicus aorticus; *u* oesophagus; *v* trachea; *v'* bronchus trachealis; *w* radix pulmonis; *x* pulmo dexter, lobus accessorius; *y* cor (pericardium partly removed); *z* mediastinum craniale

1 a. and v. pulmonalis, branches to the right apical lobe; *2* aorta thoracica; *3* r. bronchalis, *4* r. oesophageus of the a. broncho-oesophagea; *5* aa. and vv. intercostales dorsales, *5'* rr. cutanei laterales; *6* truncus brachiocephalicus and v. cava cranialis; *7* truncus and v. costocervicalis; *8* a. and v. intercostalis suprema; *9* a. and v. scapularis dorsalis; *10* a. and v. cervicalis profunda; *11* a. and v. vertebralis; *12* a. and v. cervicalis superficialis; *13* a. and v. thoracica interna; *14* a. axillaris and vv. axillares; *15* a. and v. thoracica externa; *16* a. carotis communis; *17* v. jugularis interna; *18* v. jugularis externa; *19* v. cephalica; *20* v. cava cranialis; *21* v. azygos dextra; *22* v. cava caudalis; *23* v. phrenica cranialis; *24* sinus coronarius; *25* v. cordis media; *26* ductus thoracicus; *27* radices plexus brachialis; *28* n. phrenicus; *29* truncus vagosympathicus; *30* cervical part of the n. sympathicus; *31* ggl. cervicale medium; *32* ansa subclavia; *33* ggl. stellatum; *34* truncus sympathicus, pars thoracica; *35* n. vagus; *35'* truncus vagalis dorsalis; *35''* truncus vagalis ventralis; *36* n. laryngeus recurrens

V. brachiocephalica

(cat: 160/*1*; dog: 145/*2*; 149/*18*; 156, 161/*1*; 175/*9*; pig: 146/*2*; 150/*18*; 157, 163/*1*)

The *vv. brachiocephalicae dextra* and *sinistra* are the two terminal branches of the cranial vena cava in carnivores, pigs and, very occasionally, in goats. Each brachiocephalic vein in turn divides into a *v.*

subclavia, which is double in the pig, and a *v. jugularis externa.* The left brachiocephalic vein gives off, frequently in the cat and almost invariably in the dog, the *v. costocervicalis sinistra* and, rarely in dog, the *v. thoracica interna sinistra* and the *v. jugularis interna sinistra.* In exceptional cases in the cat the right brachiocephalic vein gives rise to the *v. costocervicalis dextra.* Furthermore, in the dog and usually also in the cat, the left and sometimes the right brachiocephalic vein gives rise to the *v. thyreoidea caudalis.*

V. thyreoidea caudalis s. v. thyreoidea ima
(cat: 181/2; dog: 175/4)

The unpaired **v. thyreoidea caudalis** is present only in carnivores in which it usually arises from the left, rarely the right, brachiocephalic vein. It runs ventrally along the neck between the sternohyoid and sternothyroid muscles and the trachea. It supplies branches to these muscles and the thyroid gland, usually only the left lobe, and it anastomoses with the cranial thyroid vein. It thus links up with the veins of the larynx, this being accomplished in the dog by means of a special branch.

V. subclavia
(Comparative: 145–148/3; 149–152/19; 156–159/2; cat: 160/11; dog: 161/15; pig: 163/2, 2'; goat: 154/18; ox: 102/6)

The **v. subclavia** arises in carnivores and pigs from the division of the brachiocephalic and in ruminants and horses at the thoracic inlet from the cranial vena cava. On each side of the body the subclavian vein lies ventral to the homonymous artery but in the pig it is duplicated so that one vessel lies ventral, the other dorsal to the artery. In company with the artery it curves laterally round the cranial border of the first rib and then continues as the caudally directed *v. axillaris.* The subclavian vein of the goat often gives off the *v. cervicalis superficialis* at the thoracic inlet.

Veins of the pectoral limb

The v. cephalica together with the v. mediana cubiti and the v. cephalica accessoria are described as branches of the v. jugularis externa (see p. 216 and 217).

V. axillaris
(Comparative: 145–148/12; 156–159/3; cat: 160/12; dog: 161/16; 175/10; pig: 153/25, 26; 163/2, 2'; 176/4, 5; goat: 154/18; sheep: 164/1; ox: 102, 155/14; 165/1; horse: 103/33; 166/a)

At the cranial border of the first rib the **v. axillaris** arises from the subclavian vein and then runs, medial to the homonymous artery, towards the shoulder joint. There are two axillary veins in the pig, one running proximally and the other distally to the axillary artery. First the axillary vein gives off the ventrolaterally directed *v. thoracica externa;* in the horse and pig this arises in the region of the thoracic inlet and could thus be classed as a branch of the subclavian. Shortly thereafter the *v. thoracica lateralis* is given off, although such a vessel is lacking in ruminants and horses. In the ox the axillary vein gives off the *v. thoracica superficialis* in a caudal direction but in the horse this latter vein stems from the thoracodorsal vein. The axillary vein, in the pig the proximal of the two veins, sends the *v. suprascapularis* to the cranial border of the shoulder blade, except in carnivores, and it also gives off the *v. subscapularis* to the caudal scapular border. Then, curving distad, the axillary vein turns onto the medial side of the forearm giving off the double *v. thoracodorsalis* during this part of its course. The thoracodorsal vein does not originate from this source in the sheep. In the region of the neck of the humerus, the axillary vein gives off the *v. circumflexa humeri cranialis,* except in ruminants, and then continues as the *v. brachialis.*

V. thoracica externa

(Comparative: 149–152/*21*; 156–159/*4*; cat: 160/*21*; pig: 153/*28*; goat: 154/*19*; sheep: 164/2; ox: 102, 155/*15*; 165/2, *2'*; horse: 166/*f*)

The **v. thoracica externa** arises from the axillary vein at the level of the first rib. It mainly ramifies in the pectoralis musculature, one branch running between the superficial and deep pectorals and another distal to the deep pectoral. In the ox, horse and carnivores the latter branch arises, unlike its arterial collateral, independently from the axillary vein.

V. thoracica lateralis

(Comparative: 149–152/22; cat: 160/22; dog: 156/*5*; pig: 153/*29*; 157/*5*)

The **v. thoracica lateralis** of carnivores and pigs takes its origin from the axillary vein a short distance after the external thoracic arises from that vessel. It runs in a caudal direction and, for a variable distance along the lateral thoracic wall, in the angle between the ascending pectoralis and latissimus dorsi muscles. In female animals it vascularizes the thoracic mammary complex.

V. thoracica superficialis

(ox: 151/*23*; 158/*6*; 165/*4*; horse: 152/*23*; 159/*6*; 166/*f'*)

The **v. thoracica superficialis** of the ox branches from the axillary vein at the caudal border of the 2nd rib. It runs laterally, without arterial accompaniment, along the serratus ventralis thoracic muscle in a caudodorsal direction. It then perforates the cutaneus trunci muscle, continues subcutaneously to the 10th rib and branches on the lateral chest wall. In the horse this vein arises from the thoracodorsal vein. It runs medially on the ventral border of the cutaneus maximus muscle and continues medial to the pectoralis ascendens to reach the lateral chest wall. Here it gives rise to the cranial epigastric vein, also known as the "spur vein".

V. suprascapularis

(Comparative: 156–159/*7*; cat: 160/*9*; dog: 161/*6*; 162/*9*; pig: 153/*32*; 163/*3*; goat: 154/*20*; sheep: 164/*10*; ox: 165/*3*, *3'*, *3"*; horse: 166/*c*)

In carnivores the **v. suprascapularis** arises from the v. cervicalis superficialis whereas in the other domestic mammals it stems from the axillary vein. In the pig it comes off the proximal vessel. In the ox it originates by two equally stout roots. The vein goes between the subscapularis and supraspinatus muscles and it unites, at the level of the incisura scapulae, with the *r. suprascapularis* of the v. subscapularis in the pig and with the *r. suprascapularis* of the v. cervicalis superficialis in ruminants (see p. 215). In ruminants the r. suprascapularis gives off the *r. acromialis* which in carnivores and pigs arises directly from the superficial cervical vein. The acromial ramus runs caudad and laterally into the supraspinatus muscle. It then passes distal to the acromion over the neck of the scapula to the infraspinatus muscle and joins with the neighbouring vessels. The suprascapular vein gives off strong branches to the medial aspect of the scapula. In the pig corresponding branches arise independently from the proximal portion of the axillary vein. There they form a net-like anastomosis with branches of the subscapular vein, with the v. circumflexa scapulae and also with the segmental vessels of the region of the shoulder girdle. This net forms the supply of the subscapularis and serratus ventralis muscles. Through the incisura scapulae a branch crosses to the lateral side and anastomoses with the acromial ramus. Another branch rises dorsally along the border of the shoulder blade to supply vessels to the neighbouring musculature.

V. subscapularis

(Comparative: 156–159/*8*; cat: 160/*16*, *16'*, *16"*; dog: 161/*17*; 162/*12*; pig: 153/*31*; 163/*5*; sheep: 164/*3*, *4*, *8*; ox: 165/*5*; horse: 166/*b*)

The **v. subscapularis** arises from the axillary vein, or its proximal vessel in the pig, before the vein bends distad. It courses between the scapularis and teres major muscles to the medial surface of the caput longum of the biceps brachii and further on this surface it reaches and passes along the caudal border of

Veins of the pectoral limb

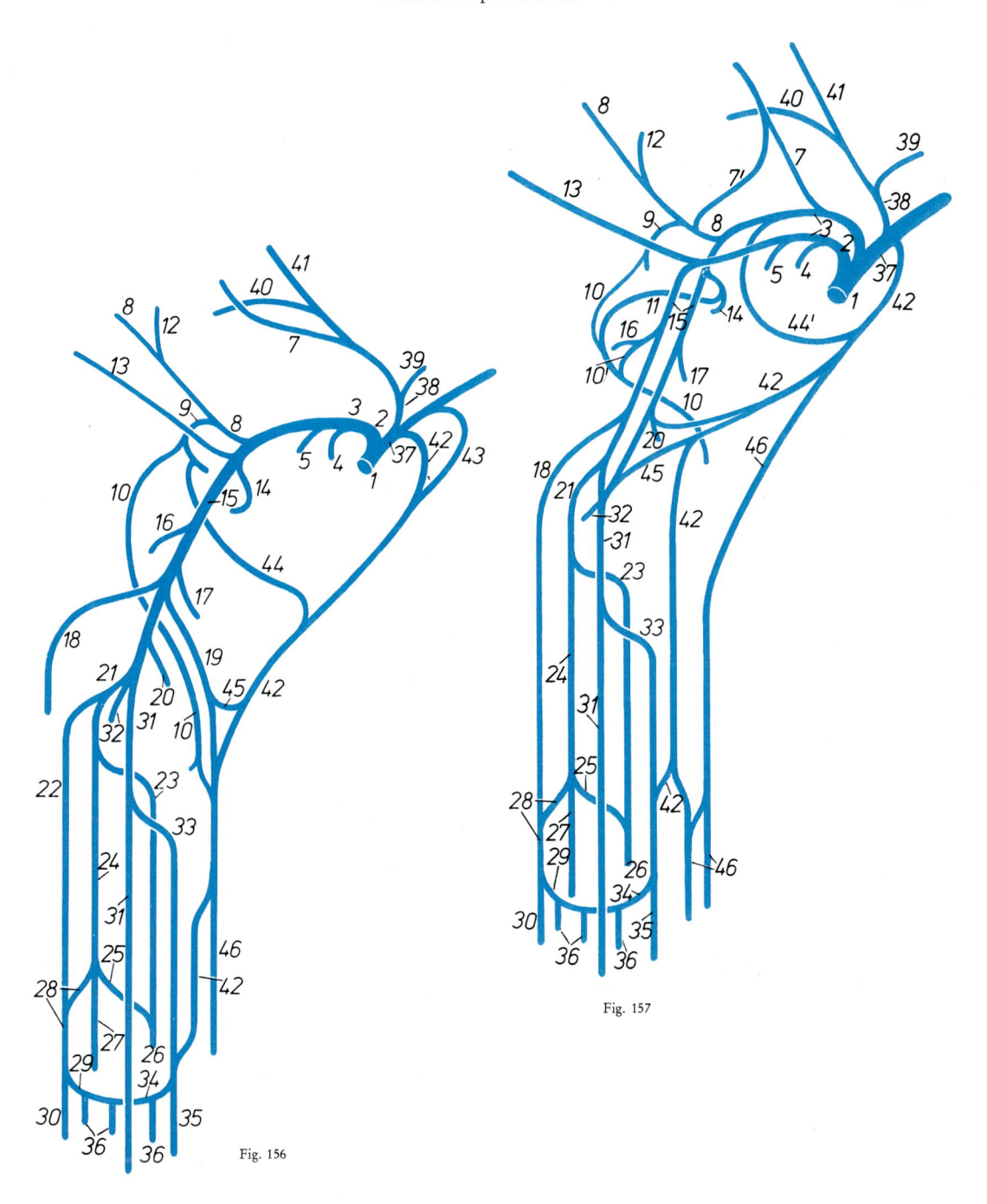

Figs 156, 157, 158, 159. Veins of the left pectoral limb down to the carpal region in the dog, pig, ox and horse. Diagrammatic. Medial view. (After Badawi, Münster and Wilkens, in preparation, work carried out at the Institute of Veterinary Anatomy, Hanover.)

1 v. brachiocephalica; *2* v. subclavia; *3* v. axillaris; *4* v. thoracica externa; *5* v. thoracica lateralis; *6* v. thoracica superficialis; *7* v. suprascapularis; *7'* r. suprascapularis; *8* v. subscapularis; *9* v. circumflexa humeri caudalis; *10* v. collateralis radialis; *10'* anastomosis of 10; *11* anastomosis of 10 in the pig; *12* v. circumflexa scapulae; *13* v. thoracodorsalis; *14* v. circumflexa humeri cranialis; *15* v. brachialis; *16* v. profunda brachii; *17* v. bicipitalis; *18* v. collateralis ulnaris; *19* v. brachialis superficialis; *20* v. transversa cubiti, in the pig with anastomosis to 42, in the ox to 45; *21* v. interossea communis; *22* v. ulnaris; *23* v. interossea cranialis; *24* v. interossea caudalis; *25* r. interosseus; *26* r. carpeus dorsalis of 23; *27* r. carpeus palmaris of 24 or in the ox of 25; *28* r. palmaris, *29* r. profundus, *30* r. superficialis; *31* v. mediana; *32* v. profunda antebrachii; *33* v. radialis; *33'* v. radialis proximalis, in the horse with r. carpeus palmaris; *34* r. profundus of 33; *29* and *34* arcus palmaris profundus; *35* r. superficialis of 33; *36* vv. metacarpeae palmares; *37* v. jugularis externa; *38* v. cervicalis superficialis; *39* r. ascendens; *40* r. acromialis; *41* r. praescapularis; *42* v. cephalica; *43* v. omobrachialis; *44* v. axillobrachialis; *44'* connecting vein of the v. cephalica with the proximal vessel of the v. axillaris in the pig; *45* v. mediana cubiti; *46* v. cephalica accessoria, in the pig as medial and lateral vein

Fig. 158

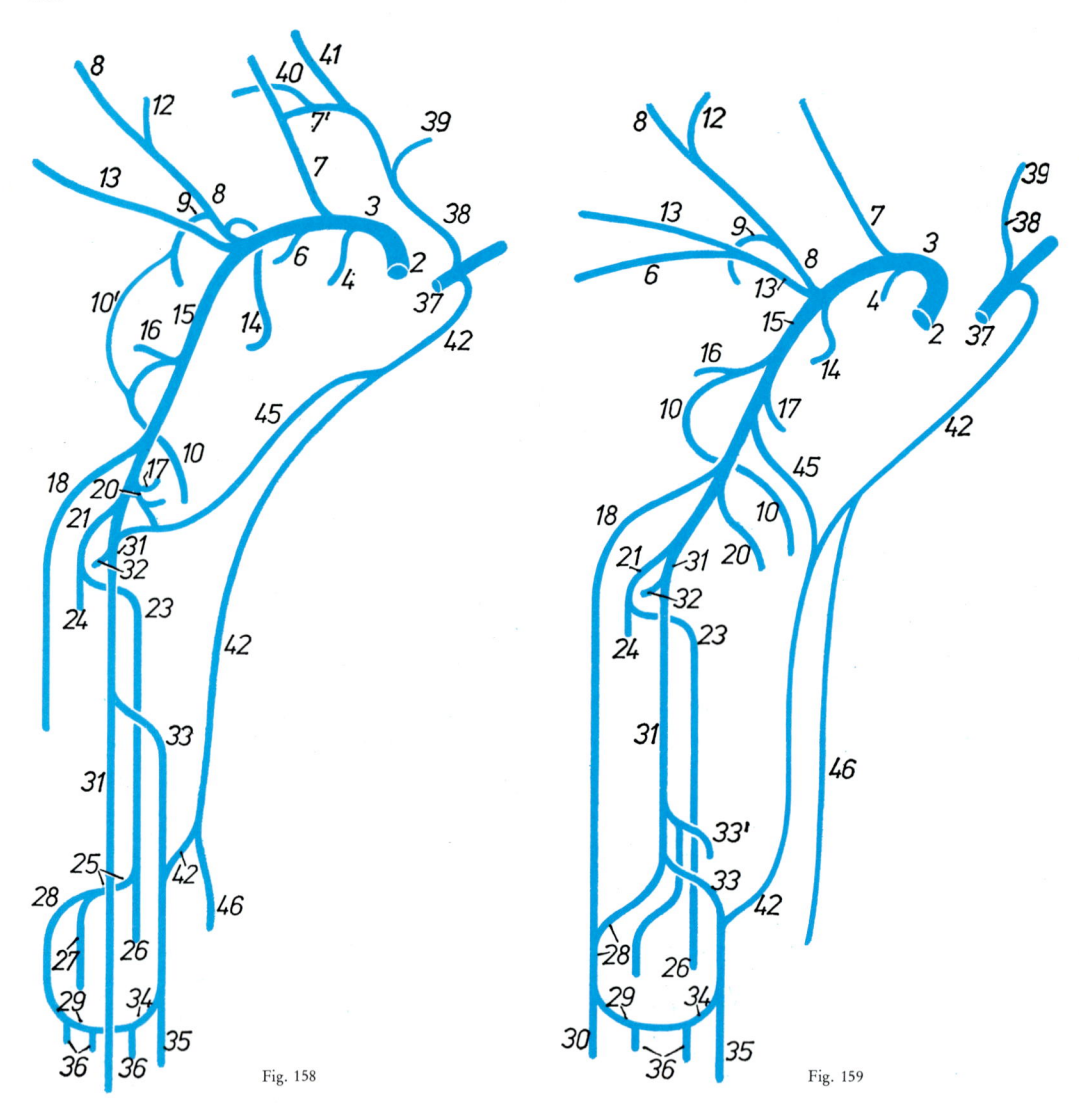

Fig. 159

the scapula. Immediately after its origin it gives off the *v. circumflexa humeri caudalis*. In some species, however, the *v. circumflexa humeri cranialis* may be given off first; this is invariably the case in the ox, occasionally in the pig but rarely in the dog. Sometimes in the dog, and always in the sheep, the *v. thoracodorsalis* also arises from the subscapular vein. This latter vessel gives off the *r. suprascapularis* in the pig and this runs parallel to the suprascapular artery. Finally, at the level of the nutrient foramen of the scapula, the *v. circumflexa scapulae*, which behaves in a similar manner to the homonymous artery, and a nutritive vessel penetrating the scapula, are given off. Thereafter the subscapular vein divides into several muscular branches which, together with the circumflex scapular vein, vascularize the long head of the triceps brachii, the tensor fasciae antebrachii and the muscles of the shoulder joint. These muscular branches participate in the formation of the network which lies on both sides of the scapula.

V. circumflexa humeri caudalis

(Comparative: 156–159/9; cat: 160/15; dog: 161/18; 162/15; ox: 165/7)

In all the domestic mammals the **v. circumflexa humeri caudalis** springs from the subscapular vein at the level of the flexor aspect of the shoulder joint. Rarely in the pig and ox the cranial circumflex humeral vein arises with it. In carnivores, pigs and the small ruminants it gives off the *v. collateralis radialis*. The caudal circumflex humeral vein anastomoses around the neck of the humerus with the cranial circumflex humeral vein and gives off branches to the shoulder joint and the neighbouring musculature.

V. circumflexa humeri cranialis

(Comparative: 156–159/*14*; cat: 160/*14, 14'*; dog: 161/*21*; pig: 163/*19*; sheep: 164/*15*; ox: 165/*6*)

In domestic mammals the origin of the **v. circumflexa humeri cranialis** does not correspond to that of the artery. It usually arises in carnivores, pigs and horses from the axillary vein. Only rarely in the dog, more often in the pig and invariably in the ox is it given off from the subscapular vein. It courses medially over the cranial part of the humerus and anastomoses with the caudal circumflex humeral vein. It mainly drains the biceps brachii and coracobrachialis but also the pectoralis profundus and triceps brachii muscles and the humerus.

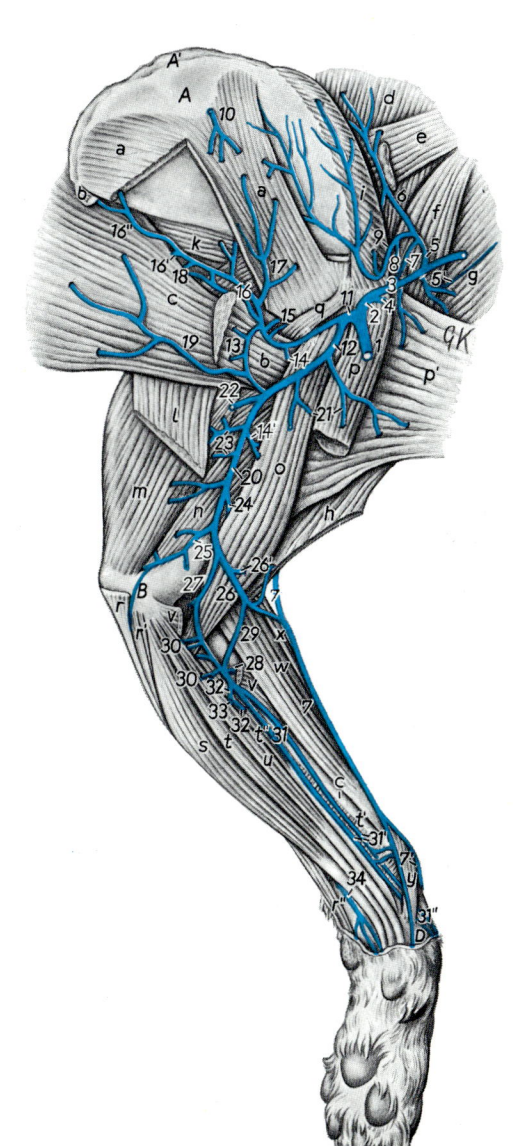

Fig. 160. Veins of the left pectoral limb of a cat. Medial view.
(After Wissdorf, 1965, work carried out at the Institute of Veterinary Anatomy, Hanover.)

A scapula; *A'* cartilago scapulae; *B* epicondylus medialis humeri; *C* radius; *D* os metacarpale I

a m. subscapularis; *b* m. teres major; *c* m. latissimus dorsi; *d* m. trapezius; *e* m. omotransversarius; *f* m. cleidomastoideus; *g* m. cleidocervicalis, *h* m. cleidobrachialis of the m. brachiocephalicus; *i* m. supraspinatus; *k* m. infraspinatus; *l* m. tensor fasciae antebrachii; *m* m. triceps brachii, caput longum, *n* caput mediale; *o* m. biceps brachii; *p* m. pectoralis profundus; *p'* mm. pectorales superficiales; *q* m. coracobrachialis; *r* m. flexor carpi ulnaris, caput ulnare, *r'* caput humerale, *r"* tendon of insertion; *s* m. flexor digitalis superficialis; *t* m. flexor digitalis profundus, caput humerale, *t'* caput radiale, *t"* caput ulnare; *u* m. flexor carpi radialis; *v* m. pronator teres; *w* m. extensor carpi radialis; *x* m. brachioradialis; *y* m. abductor pollicis longus

1 v. brachiocephalica; *2* v. jugularis communis; *3* v. jugularis externa; *4* v. jugularis interna; *5* v. cervicalis superficialis, *5'* r. ascendens, *6* r. praescapularis; *7* v. cephalica; *7'* v. cephalica accessoria; *8* r. acromialis; *9* v. suprascapularis; *10* branch of the v. intercostalis dorsalis III; *11* v. subclavia; *12* v. axillaris; *13* r. anastomoticus of *16* and *19*; *14, 14'* branches of origin of the v. circumflexa humeri cranialis; *15* v. circumflexa humeri caudalis; *16, 16', 16"* v. subscapularis; *17* v. circumflexa scapulae, *18* rr. musculares; *19* v. thoracodorsalis; *20* v. brachialis; *21* v. thoracica externa; *22* v. thoracica lateralis; *23* v. profunda brachii; *24* v. nutricia humeri; *25* v. collateralis ulnaris; *26* v. brachialis superficialis; *26'* v. bicipitalis; *27* v. transversa cubiti; *28* v. interossea cranialis; *29* v. mediana cubiti; *30* v. profunda antebrachii; *31* v. mediana; *31'* v. radialis; *31"* r. carpeus dorsalis; *32* v. interossea caudalis; *33* v. ulnaris; *34* r. palmaris

V. thoracodorsalis

(Comparative: 156–159/*13*; cat: 160/*19*; dog: 161/*20*; pig: 163/*9*; sheep: 164/*9*; ox: 151/*31*; 165/*10*; horse: 166/*d*)

The **v. thoracodorsalis** takes its origin from the axillary vein, except in the sheep in which it stems from the subscapular vein and this latter vessel is on rare occasions its source in the dog and goat. After supplying branches to the teres major and the pectoralis profundus it follows the direction of the fibres of the latissimus dorsi and, continuing to give off further branches, it reaches the skin in the region of the lumbodorsal fascia. Shortly after its origin in the horse, this vein gives rise to the *v. thoracica superficialis*.

V. collateralis radialis

(Comparative: 156–159/*10*; dog: 162/*16*; ox: 165/*12*)

The **v. collateralis radialis** arises in carnivores, pigs and goats from the caudal circumflex humeral vein and in the sheep, ox and horse from the v. profunda brachii. In the pig this vein has an additional stout connection with either the axillary or cranial circumflex humeral vein and in the sheep and ox a branch joining the caudal circumflex humeral is present. The collateral radial vein and the homonymous artery accompany the radial nerve. At the transition of the middle to the distal third of the humerus it gives off the *v. collateralis media* which goes to the olecranon and supplies branches to the extensor muscles of the elbow and it then contributes to the formation of the *rete articulare cubiti*. The collateral radial vein supplies branches to the muscles of the elbow joint and to the extensors of the carpal and toe joints, finally making a connection with the cephalic vein in dogs and ruminants and also with the transverse cubital vein of the ox.

V. brachialis

(Comparative: 156–159/*15*; cat: 160/*20*; dog: 161/*22*; pig: 163/*17, 18*; sheep: 164/*16*; ox: 165/*11*; horse: 166/*e*)

The **v. brachialis** forms the distal continuation of the axillary vein. Usually present in duplicate, it courses from the medial side of the flexor aspect of the shoulder joint diagonally across the medial side of the humerus to the medial collateral ligament of the elbow joint. In so doing it crosses, except in the horse, the pronator teres muscle. At the level of the proximal interosseous space of the forearm it gives off the *v. interossea communis* and becomes the *v. mediana*. Along its course it gives rise to the *v. transversa cubiti* and in carnivores, shortly before this, the *v. brachialis superficialis*.

The *v. bicipitalis* arises in the distal third of the forearm. It is given off from the brachial vein in a cranial direction and ramifies, proximally directed, in the biceps brachii muscle. In the cat it stems from the superficial brachial vein and in ruminants usually from the transverse cubital vein.

V. profunda brachii

(Comparative: 156–159/*16*; cat: 160/*23*; dog: 161/*23*; sheep: 164/*17*; ox: 165/*13*; horse: 166/*g*)

The **v. profunda brachii** arises from the brachial vein about half way down the forearm and runs in a caudal direction.

Its diverging branches mainly vascularize the triceps brachii. In the sheep, ox and horse it gives off the *v. collateralis radialis*.

V. collateralis ulnaris

(Comparative: 156–159/*18*; 167–170/*10*; cat: 160/*25*; dog: 161/*25*; pig: 163/*21*; sheep: 164/*18*; ox: 165/*14*; horse: 166/*h*)

The **v. collateralis ulnaris** arises from the brachial vein at the level of the proximal edge of the olecranon fossa. In the pig and ox there is a second root situated more proximally. Being caudodistally directed, it runs medially over the olecranon giving off branches to the anconaean muscles, the flexors of

Veins of the pectoral limb

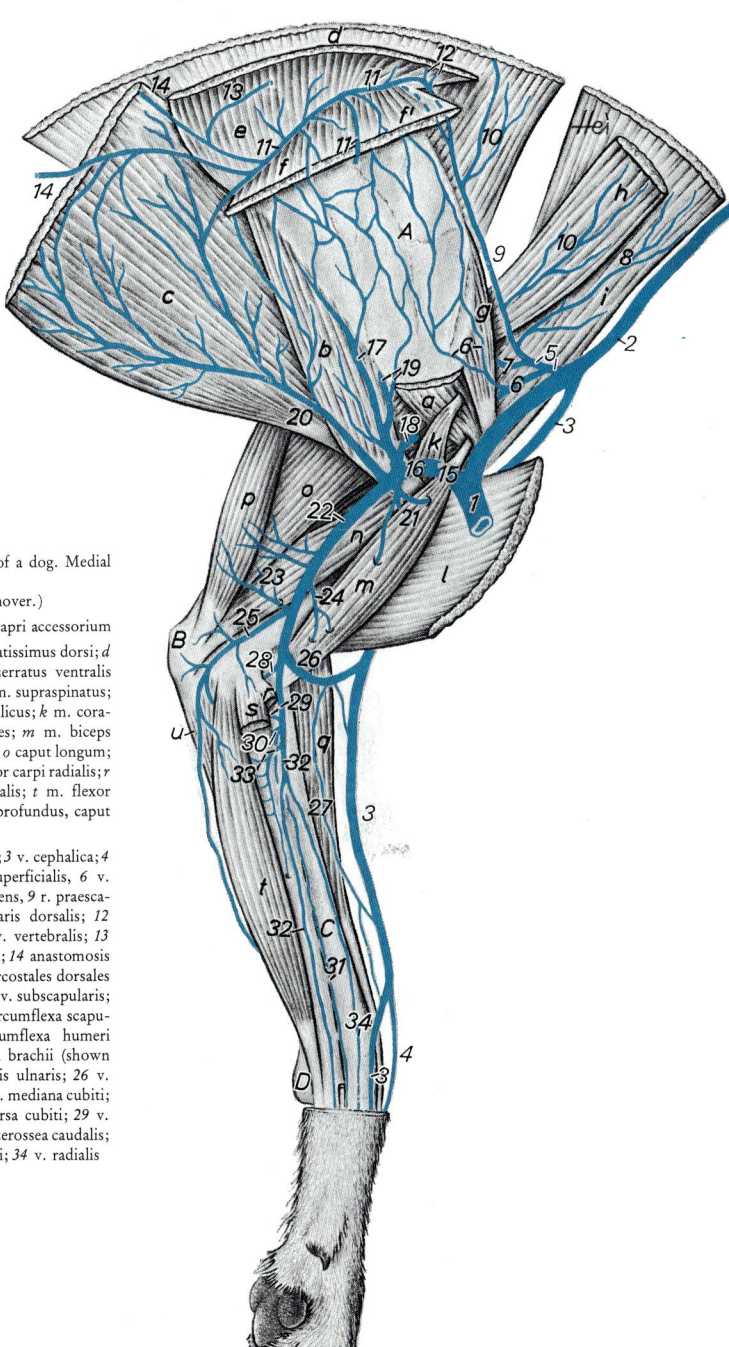

Fig. 161. Veins of the left pectoral limb of a dog. Medial view.
(After Paulick, 1967, Diss., Hanover.)

A humerus; *B* olecranon; *C* radius; *D* os capri accessorium

a m. subscapularis; *b* m. teres major; *c* m. latissimus dorsi; *d* m. trapezius; *e* m. rhomboideus; *f* m. serratus ventralis thoracis; *f'* m. serratus ventralis cervicis; *g* m. supraspinatus; *h* m. omotransversarius; *i* m. brachiocephalicus; *k* m. coracobrachialis; *l* mm. pectorales superficiales; *m* m. biceps brachii; *n* m. triceps brachii, caput mediale, *o* caput longum; *p* m. tensor fasciae antebrachii; *q* m. extensor carpi radialis; *r* m. pronator teres; *s* m. flexor carpi radialis; *t* m. flexor digitalis superficialis; *u* m. flexor digitalis profundus, caput ulnare

1 v. brachiocephalica; *2* v. jugularis externa; *3* v. cephalica; *4* v. cephalica accessoria; *5* v. cervicalis superficialis; *6* v. suprascapularis; *7* r. acromialis; *8* r. ascendens; *9* r. praescapularis; *10* rr. musculares; *11* v. scapularis dorsalis; *12* anastomosis with the rr. dorsales of the v. vertebralis; *13* anastomosis with the v. cervicalis profunda; *14* anastomosis with the rr. cutanei laterales of the vv. intercostales dorsales IV and V; *15* v. subclavia; *16* v. axillaris; *17* v. subscapularis; *18* v. circumflexa humeri caudalis; *19* v. circumflexa scapulae; *20* v. thoracodorsalis; *21* v. circumflexa humeri cranialis; *22* v. brachialis; *23* v. profunda brachii (shown double); *24* v. bicipitalis; *25* v. collateralis ulnaris; *26* v. brachialis superficialis with transition into v. mediana cubiti; *27* vv. radiales superficiales; *28* v. transversa cubiti; *29* v. ulnaris; *30* v. interossea communis; *31* v. interossea caudalis; *32* v. mediana; *33* v. profunda antebrachii; *34* v. radialis

the carpal and toe joints and to the elbow joint. Here it anastomoses with the *v. recurrens ulnaris* and, sometimes, with the *v. collateralis media*. Except in ruminants it accompanies the ulnar nerve along the ulnar groove. In carnivores the collateral ulnar vein terminates in the ulnar vein, in pigs and ruminants it terminates in the r. palmaris of the caudal interosseous vein and in the horse in the *r. palmaris* of the median vein. In the pig, however, before it terminates it gives off the *r. dorsalis* which continues as the *v. digitalis dorsalis V abaxialis*.

V brachialis superficialis
(cat: 160/26; dog: 156/19; 161/26)

The **v. brachialis superficialis** of carnivores accompanies the homonymous artery and, as with that vessel, muscular branches are sent to the biceps brachii. In the cat the *v. bicipitalis* is given off to the brachioradialis and extensor carpi radialis muscles; the *vv. radiales superficiales* are also present in this animal and these run parallel to the arteries. The superficial brachial vein is joined by the so-called *v. mediana cubiti*.

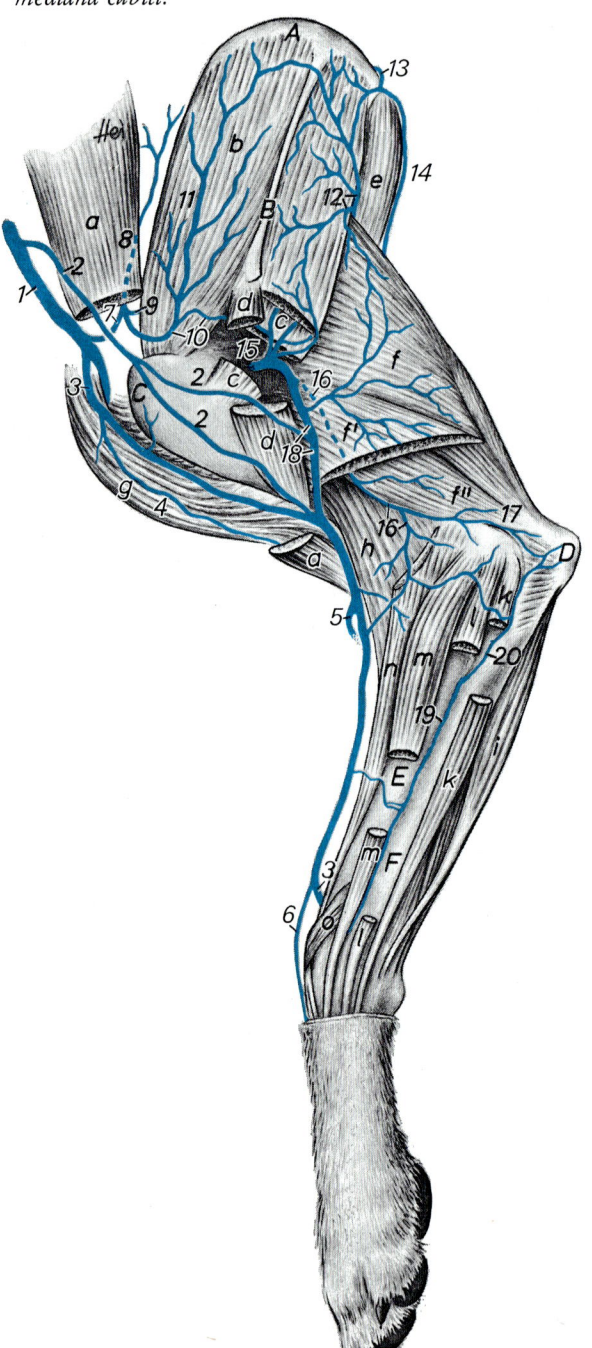

V. transversa cubiti
(Comparative: 156–159/20; cat: 160/27; dog: 161/28; pig: 163/22; sheep: 164/19; ox: 165/15; horse: 166/i)

The **v. transversa cubiti** arises at the flexor aspect of the elbow joint, turns laterally and ramifies in the neighbouring flexors of the elbow joint and in the extensors of the forearm. Its branches anastomose with almost all the veins lying proximal and distal to the elbow joint. In ruminants this vein usually gives off the *v. bicipitalis*.

V. interossea communis
(Comparative: 156–159/21; cat: 160/28; dog: 161/30; pig: 163/26; sheep: 164/21; ox: 165/16; horse: 166/n)

The **v. interossea communis**, which is lacking in the cat, arises in the other animals from the brachial vein in the proximal region of the interosseous space of the forearm. It gives off the *v. ulnaris* in the

Fig. 162. Veins of the left pectoral limb of a dog. Lateral view. (After Paulick, 1967, Diss., Hanover.)

A margo dorsalis scapulae or cartilago scapulae; *B* spina scapulae; *C* tuberculum majus humeri; *D* olecranon; *E* radius;

a m. brachiocephalicus; *b* m. supraspinatus; *c* m. infraspinatus; *d* m. deltoideus; *e* m. teres major; *f* m. triceps brachii, caput longum, *f'* caput laterale, *f"* caput accessorium; *g* mm. pectorales superficiales; *h* m. brachialis; *i* m. flexor carpi ulnaris, caput ulnare; *k* m. extensor carpi ulnaris; *l* m. extensor digitalis lateralis; *m* m. extensor digitalis communis; *n* m. extensor carpi radialis; *o* m. abductor pollicis longus

1 v. jugularis externa; *2* v. omobrachialis; *3* v. cephalica, *4* r. muscularis; *5* v. mediana cubiti; *6* v. cephalica accessoria; *7* v. cervicalis superficialis, *8* r. praescapularis, *9* v. suprascapularis, *10* r. acromialis, *11* rr. musculares; *12* v. subscapularis; *13* v. scapularis dorsalis; *14* branch of the v. thoracodorsalis; *15* v. circumflexa humeri caudalis; *16* v. collateralis radialis; *17* v. collateralis media; *18* v. axillobrachialis; *19* v. interossea cranialis; *20* v. recurrens interossea

Veins of the pectoral limb

dog and the *v. recurrens ulnaris* in ruminants, and then divides into the *v. interossea cranialis* and the *v. interossea caudalis*. These latter two vessels arise in the cat directly from the brachial vein.

Fig. 163. Veins of the left pectoral limb of the pig. Medial view. (After Badawi, 1959, Diss., Hanover.)

A scapula; A' cartilago scapulae; B epicondylus medialis humeri; C radius; D carpus; E os metacarpale III; F os metacarpale II

a m. latissimus dorsi; b m. teres major; c m. subscapularis; d m. supraspinatus; e m. trapezius; f m. rhomboideus cervicis et capitis; g m. pectoralis profundus; g' m. subclavius; h m. cleidobrachialis; i mm. pectorales superficiales; k m. biceps brachii; l m. coracobrachialis; m m. triceps brachii, caput mediale, n caput longum; o m. tensor fasciae antebrachii; p m. flexor carpi ulnaris, caput ulnare, p' caput humerale; q m. flexor digitalis profundus, caput ulnare, q' caput humerale, lateral mass, q'' caput humerale, medial mass, q''' deep flexor tendon; r m. flexor digitalis superficialis, superficial mass, r' its tendon; s m. flexor carpi radialis; t m. pronator teres; u m. brachialis; v m. extensor carpi radialis; w m. abductor pollicis longus; x common tendon of the m. extensor digitalis communis, x' terminal limb for the 2nd toe, x'' terminal limb for the 3rd toe; y lig. collaterale mediale longum of the carpal joint

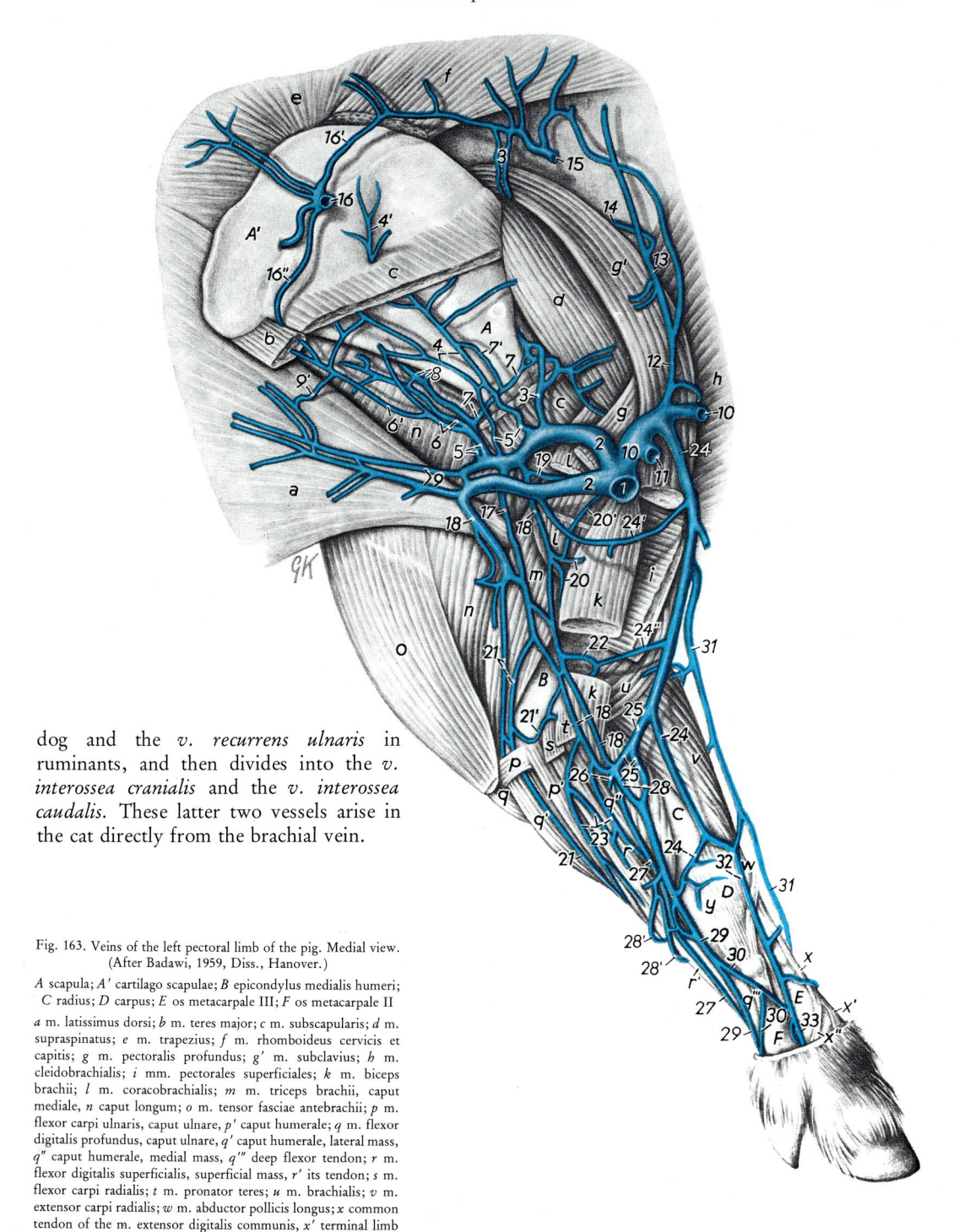

1 v. brachiocephalica; *2* v. subclavia, immediately merging into the v. axillaris; *3* v. suprascapularis; *5* v. subscapularis with *4, 4', 6, 6', 7, 7'* reticulating branches; *8* v. circumflexa scapulae; *9* v. thoracodorsalis, *9'* r. anastomoticus; *10* v. jugularis externa; *11* v. jugularis interna; *12* v. cervicalis superficialis, *13* r. praescapularis, *14* branch to the lymph node; *15* branch to the v. cervicalis profunda; *16, 16', 16''* v. scapularis dorsalis; *17, 18* v. brachialis; *19* v. circumflexa humeri cranialis; *20* v. bicipitalis, *20'* r. anastomoticus; *21* v. collateralis ulnaris, *21'* r. articularis; *22* v. transversa cubiti; *23* v. profunda antebrachii; *24* v. cephalica, *24', 24''* rr. anastomotici; *25* v. mediana cubiti; *26* v. interossea communis; *27* v. mediana; *28* v. radialis, *28'* rr. cutanei, *29* r. palmaris superficialis; *30* v. digitalis palmaris communis I; *31* v. cephalica accessoria, lateral vessel, *32* medial vessel; *33* v. digitalis dorsalis communis II

V. interossea cranialis
(Comparative: 156–159/*23*; 171–174/*15*; dog: 162/*19*)

The **v. interossea cranialis** runs on the extensor aspect in the groove between the two bones of the forearm. Proximally it gives off the *v. recurrens interossea* as a branch which communicates with the *v. collateralis media* or the *rete articulare cubiti*; it also supplies branches to the extensor muscles. In the distal part of the forearm it gives off the *r. carpeus dorsalis* to the *rete carpi dorsale*. In carnivores and pigs it is distally linked to the *v. interossea caudalis* by means of the r. interosseus which passes through the interosseous space of the forearm. In ruminants it gives off the *r. interosseus* from which arise those vessels which in carnivores and pigs stem from the caudal interosseous vein; they supply the palmar aspect of the carpal region.

V. interossea caudalis
(Comparative: 156–158/*24*; cat: 160/*32*; dog: 161/*31*; 167/*17*; pig: 168/*17*)

The **v. interossea caudalis** is only rudimentary in ruminants and usually completely absent in the horse. It runs caudally between the two bones of the forearm to the carpus. In carnivores and pigs it is a larger vessel than the cranial interosseous vein. In cats the *v. ulnaris* is given off immediately by the caudal interosseous vein. In carnivores and pigs it is connected with the cranial interosseous vein through the distal part of the interosseous space by means of the *r. interosseus* and it supplies the *r. carpeus palmaris* which vascularizes the flexor aspect of the carpal joint. Further, a large, medially-directed anastomosis links the caudal interosseous vein, or in ruminants the interosseous ramus, with the *v. radialis*. In carnivores and pigs the anastomosis also joins it to the *v. cephalica*. Subsequently the caudal interosseous vein, or the interosseous ramus, continues as the *r. palmaris*. In the horse this ramus is connected with the median vein. The palmar ramus crosses the carpus in a distal direction running to the accessory carpal bone. In so doing it receives the ulnar vein in carnivores and the collateral ulnar vein in ruminants. In the proximal metacarpal region it divides into the *r. profundus* and the *r. superficialis* which contribute to the formation of the deep and superficial arch respectively.

V. mediana
(Comparative: 156–159/*31*; 167–170/*23*; cat: 160/*31*; dog: 161/*32*; pig: 163/*27*; sheep: 164/*23*; ox: 165/*17*; horse: 166/*o*)

After giving off the common interosseous vein, the brachial vein continues in the antebrachium as the **v. mediana,** which is usually duplicated. It accompanies the median artery and nerve and initially is situated subfascially on the medial aspect of the radius covered by the flexor carpi radialis muscle. In the carpal region it is applied medially to the long flexors of the toes and, in the region of the metacarpus, it participates in the formation of the superficial palmar arch, when that arch is present, or in forming the common veins of the toes. Along its course the median vein gives off, in the forearm region, the *v. profunda antebrachii* and subsequently the *v. radialis*. In the cat the median vein continues directly into the radial vein which is also duplicated. In the distal third of the forearm of the horse the *v. radialis proximalis* is given off and the radial vein itself arises only immediately proximal to the carpus. At the same level as the origin of the radial vein, the median vein of the horse becomes the *r. palmaris*. The palmar ramus first receives the *v. collateralis ulnaris* and is then deflected medially towards the accessory carpal bone. It divides in the proximal metacarpal region, like the palmar ramus of the caudal interosseous vein of the other domestic mammals, into the *r. profundus* which helps to form the deep arch and the *r. superficialis* which is the origin of the lateral (palmar common) vein of the toe.

The muscular branches of the proximal part of the forearm are collectively known as the **v. profunda antebrachii** but they do not always have a common stem of origin. Usually they arise proximally from the median vein but sometimes even stem from the brachial vein. They run caudodistally to supply the flexors of the carpal joints and the toe joints.

V. ulnaris
(cat: 160/*33*; dog: 156/*22*; 161/*29*; 167/*11*)

The **v. ulnaris** arises in the cat from the caudal interosseous vein and in the dog from the common interosseous vein; it is lacking in all the other domestic mammals. Immediately after its origin it gives off the *v. recurrens ulnaris*, a proximally directed anastomosis with the collateral ulnar vein. The ulnar vein runs deep in the ulnar groove and contributes to the vascularization of the deep flexor of the toes. In the region of the carpus it gives off the *rr. carpei dorsales* and, in the cat, the *r. dorsalis* which participate in the formation of the superficial dorsal arch. Subsequently it terminates in the r. palmaris of the caudal interosseous vein.

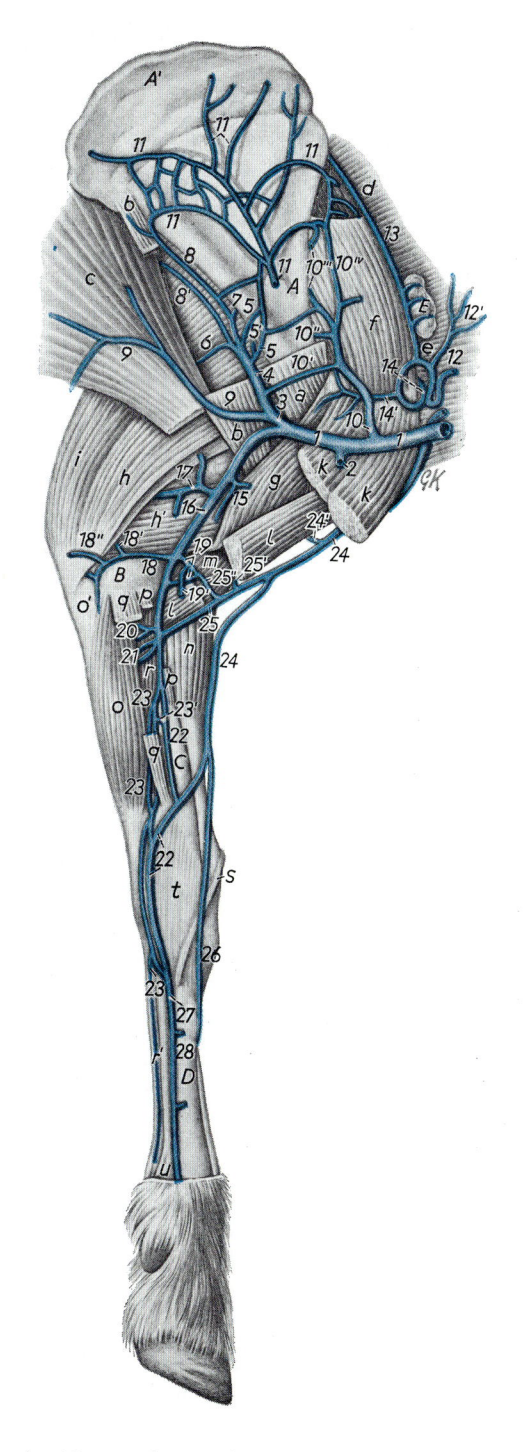

Fig. 164. Veins of the left pectoral limb of the sheep. Medial view. (After Wissdorf, 1961, Diss., Hanover.)

A scapula; *A'* cartilago scapulae; *B* epicondylus medialis humeri; *C* radius; *D* os metacarpale III + IV; *E* ln. cervicalis superficialis

a m. subscapularis; *b* m. teres major; *c* m. latissimus dorsi; *d* m. trapezius; *e* m. omotransversarius; *f* m. supraspinatus; *g* m. coracobrachialis; *h* m. triceps brachii, caput longum, *h'* caput mediale; *i* m. tensor fasciae antebrachii; *k* m. pectoralis profundus; *l* m. biceps brachii; *m* m. brachialis; *n* m. extensor carpi radialis; *o* m. flexor carpi ulnaris, caput humerale, *o'* caput ulnare; *p* m. pronator teres; *q* m. flexor carpi radialis; *r* m. flexor digitalis profundus, *r'* deep flexor tendon; *s* m. abductor pollicis longus; *t* palmar reinforcing band of the medial collateral ligament; *u* m. interosseus medius

1 v. axillaris; *2* v. thoracica externa; *3, 4, 8* v. subscapularis; *5, 5'* v. circumflexa scapulae, *6, 7* rr. musculares; *9* v. thoracodorsalis; *10* v. suprascapularis, *10'–10^{iv}* its branches; *11* network at the scapula with anastomoses of the v. scapularis dorsalis and the vv. intercostales dorsales; *12* v. cervicalis superficialis, *12'* r. ascendens, *13* r. praescapularis, *14* r. acromialis, *14'* r. suprascapularis; *15* v. circumflexa humeri cranialis; *16* v. brachialis; *17* v. profunda brachii; *18* v. collateralis ulnaris, *18'* r. muscularis, *18"* r. cutaneus; *19* v. transversa cubiti; *19'* v. bicipitalis; *20* v. profunda antebrachii; *21* rr. musculares of the v. interossea communis; *22* v. radialis; *23* v. mediana, *23'* r. anastomoticus; *24* v. cephalica, *24'* r. muscularis; *25* v. mediana cubiti, *25', 25"* rr. anastomotici; *26* v. cephalica accessoria, *27* r. palmaris profundus; *28* v. metacarpea palmaris II

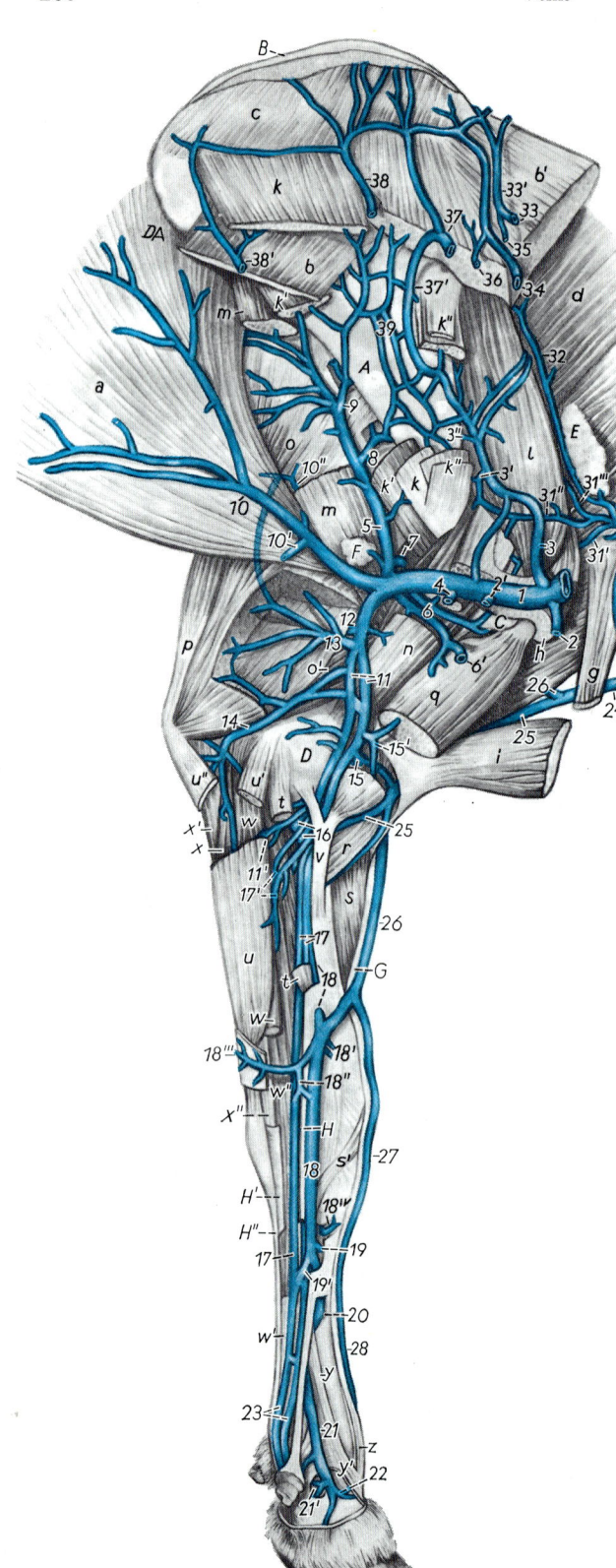

Fig. 165. Veins of the left pectoral limb of the ox. Medial view.
(After Münster and Schwarz, 1968, work carried out at the Institute for Veterinary Anatomy, Hanover.)

A scapula; *B* cartilago scapulae; *C* tuberculum minus humeri; *D* trochlea humeri; *E* lnn. cervicales superficiales; *F* lnn. axillares proprii; *G* fascia antebrachii; *H–H″* cut edges of the deep parts of the palmar fascia, between which the tendon of the superficial belly of the m. flexor digitalis superficialis is situated, *H* cut edge of the retinaculum flexorum and of the deep leaf of the palmar fascia which is here still closely applied to the retinaculum, *H′* cut edge of the retinaculum flexorum, *H″* cut edge of the deep leaf of the palmar fascia

a m. latissimus dorsi; *b* m. serratus ventralis thoracis; *b′* m. serratus ventralis cervicis; *c* m. rhomboideus thoracis (m. rhomboideus cervicis, removed entirely); *d* m. trapezius, pars cervicalis; *e* m. omotransversarius; *f* m. brachiocephalicus; *g* m. subclavius; *h* m. pectoralis profundus; *i* m. pectoralis descendens; *k–k″* m. subscapularis; *l* m. supraspinatus; *m* m. teres major; *n* m. coracobrachialis; *o* m. triceps brachii, caput longum, *o′* caput mediale; *p* m. tensor fasciae antebrachii; *q* m. biceps brachii; *r* m. brachialis; *s* m. extensor carpi radialis; *s′* m. abductor pollicis longus; *t* m. flexor carpi radialis; *u* m. flexor carpi ulnaris, *u′* caput humerale, *u″* caput ulnare; *v* m. pronator teres; *w* m. flexor digitalis superficialis, superficial mass, *w′* its tendon, *w″* deep mass; *x* m. flexor digitalis profundus, caput humerale, *x′* caput ulnare, *x″* deep flexor tendon; *y* m. interosseus medius, *y′* its branch to the m. extensor digitalis communis (digiti III proprius); *z* tendon of the m. extensor digitalis communis (digiti III proprius)

1 v. axillaris; *2, 2′* v. thoracica externa; *3, 3′, 3″* v. suprascapularis; *4* v. thoracica superficialis; *5* v. subscapularis; *6* v. circumflexa humeri cranialis, *6′* r. muscularis to the m. pectoralis profundus; *7* v. circumflexa humeri caudalis; *8* v. circumflexa scapulae; *9* branch to the venous network of the scapula; *10* v. thoracodorsalis, *10′, 10″* rr. musculares; *11* v. brachialis, *11′* r. muscularis; *12* v. collateralis radialis; *13* v. profunda brachii; *14* v. collateralis ulnaris; *15* v. transversa cubiti; *15′* v. bicipitalis; *16* v. interossea communis; *17* v. mediana; *17′* v. profunda antebrachii; *18* v. radialis, *18′* r. carpeus dorsalis, *18″* r. anastomoticus, *18‴* r. cutaneus, *18^iv* r. articularis; *19* r. palmaris profundus, *19′* r. palmaris superficialis; *20* v. metacarpea palmaris II; *21* v. digitalis palmaris communis II, *21′* r. palmaris phalangis proximalis, *22* r. dorsalis phalangis proximalis; *23* v. digitalis palmaris communis III; *24, 26* v. cephalica; *25* v. mediana cubiti; *27* v. cephalica accessoria; *28* v. digitalis dorsalis communis III; *29, 31* v. cervicalis superficialis, *30* r. ascendens, *31* r. anastomoticus with the v. circumflexa humeri cranialis, *31″* r. suprascapularis, *31‴* r. acromialis, *32* r. praescapularis; *33* branch of the v. cervicalis profunda, *33′* its r. anastomoticus with *34* v. scapularis dorsalis; *35–38′* rr. anastomotici with the vv. intercostales dorsales I–IV; *39* venous network on the scapula

V. radialis

(Comparative: 156–158/*33*; 167–169/*24*; cat: 160/*31'*; dog: 161/*34*; pig: 163/*28*; sheep: 164/*22*; ox: 165/*18*; horse: 166/*q, r*; 170/*24, 24'*)

The **v. radialis** is usually duplicated. In the cat it is a direct continuation of the median vein and in the dog it arises from this vessel at the level of the insertion of the pronator teres muscle. In company with the artery of that name it courses distad. It unites with the cephalic vein proximally to the carpus and anastomoses at about the same level with the caudal interosseous vein. Thereafter it gives off the *r. carpeus palmaris* and the *r. carpeus dorsalis* to the palmar and dorsal articular network respectively. In the cat the dorsal carpal ramus is stout and courses medially round the carpus to reach the rete carpi dorsale. It passes through the venous network and continues through the *v. metacarpea dorsalis II* into the *r. perforans proximalis II*. The latter links with the deep palmar arch. In the distal carpal region the radial vein of the dog divides into the deep and superficial palmar rami. In the cat the deep ramus is absent and only the superficial palmar ramus is represented. The *r. palmaris profundus* of the dog participates in the formation of the deep palmar arch and in both carnivores the *r. palmaris superficialis* receives the terminal part of the cephalic vein. Proximal to the metacarpophalangeal joint and palmar to the flexor tendon, the superficial palmar branch joins the superficial branch of the palmar ramus of the caudal interosseous vein and this union forms the superficial palmar arch. Additionally, in the proximal half of the metacarpus there is, parallel to the arteries, a superficial palmar arch in which terminates the slender median vein of the dog. This arch is partly situated between the two limbs of the flexor tendon.

In the pig the radial vein arises from the median near the termination of the median cubital vein. Often it consists of two to three collateral veins of the radial artery, one of which has already linked up with the cephalic vein proximal to the carpal joint while the other components of the radial vein join the cephalic vein in the carpal region. Rete branches are given off to the carpus in a dorsal and palmar direction. At the proximal part of the metacarpus the radial artery divides into the *r. palmaris profundus* and *r. palmaris superficialis* which respectively contribute to the deep and superficial palmar arches.

In ruminants the radial vein is duplicated. It arises from the median vein half-way down the forearm. Accompanied by the radial artery it courses subfascially towards the carpus and joins the cephalic vein immediately proximal to the carpus. Distally to the carpus the radial vein divides into the deep palmar arch and the superficial palmar ramus which latter, after a short course or sometimes further distally, terminates in either the median vein or its communicating branch to the arcus palmaris profundus distalis.

In the horse the *v. radialis proximalis* arises in the lower third of the forearm and in parallel with the homonymous artery it divides into a *r. carpeus palmaris* and a *r. carpeus dorsalis*. Proximal to the carpus, at about the same level as the palmaris ramus, the radial vein arises from the median vein and, having received the cephalic vein, runs subfascially and laterally along the tendon of the flexor carpi radialis muscle. Progressing parallel to the radial artery but separated from it by the retinaculum flexorum, the radial vein passes over the carpus and divides into the deep and superficial palmar rami, the former joining the deep palmar arch and the latter forming the source of the medial (palmar common) vein of the toes.

Veins of the forefoot of carnivores*

Palmar veins
(cat: 160/*34*; dog: 156; 167)

The **arcus palmaris profundus** of the cat derives from the r. perforans proximalis II which is formed through the dorsal carpal rete directly from the dorsal carpal ramus of the radial vein and from the deep ramus of the palmar ramus of the caudal interosseous vein. In the dog the deep palmar ramus of the radial vein and the deep ramus of the palmar ramus of the caudal interosseous vein unite to form the deep palmar arch. In carnivores the *vv. metacarpeae palmares I–IV* spring from this arch although the first of these vessels may be absent in the cat. The *rr. perforantes* behave as their corresponding arterial

---

* General accounts of the topography and nomenclature of the blood vessels of the autopodium have already been given on page 92 and the reader is referred to these.

210   Veins

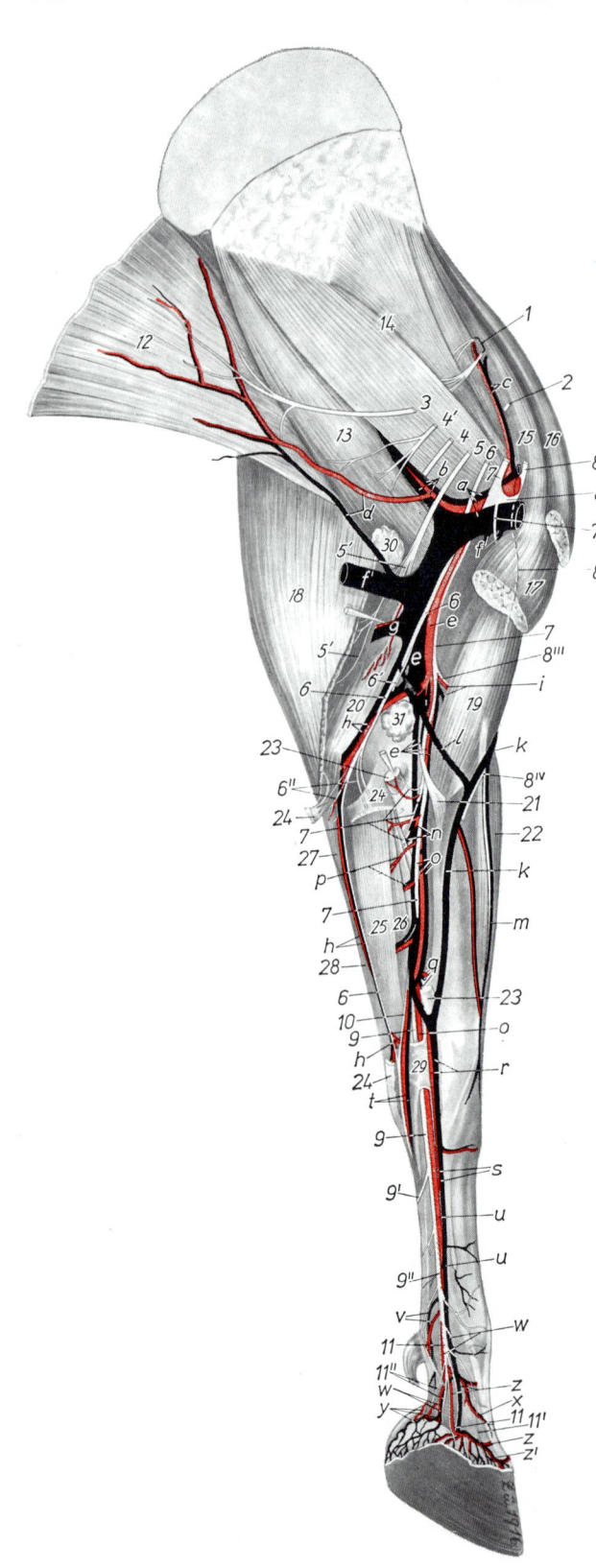

Fig. 166. Veins and arteries of the left pectoral limb of the horse. Medial view.
(After Zietzschmann, 1943.)

1 nn. subscapulares; *2* n. suprascapularis; *3* n. thoracodorsalis; *4* n. axillaris, *4'* branches to the m. teres major with one n. pectoralis caudalis; *5*, *5'* n. radialis; *6*, *6'*, *6"* n. ulnaris; *7* n. medianus, *7'* one n. pectoralis cranialis; *8* n. musculocutaneus, *8'* ansa axillaris, *8"* r. muscularis proximalis, *8'''* r. muscularis distalis; *8^{iv}* n. cutaneus antebrachii medialis; *9* n. palmaris medialis, *9'* r. communicans; *9"* n. digitalis palmaris communis II; *10* n. palmaris lateralis; *11* n. digitalis palmaris proprius III medialis, *11'* r. dorsalis, *11"* rr. tori digitalis; *12* m. latissimus dorsi; *13* m. teres major; *14* m. subscapularis; *15* m. supraspinatus; *16* m. subclavius; *17* m. pectoralis profundus; *18* m. tensor fasciae antebrachii; *19* m. biceps brachii; *20* m. triceps brachii, caput mediale; *21* m. pronator teres; *22* m. extensor carpi radialis; *23* m. flexor carpi radialis; *24* m. flexor carpi ulnaris; *25* m. flexor digitalis superficialis; *26* m. flexor digitalis profundus, caput humerale, *27* caput ulnare; *28* m. extensor carpi ulnaris; *29* retinaculum flexorum; *30* lnn. axillares; *31* lnn. cubitales

a v. and a. axillaris; *b* v. and a. subscapularis; *c* v. and a. suprascapularis; *d* v. and a. thoracodorsalis; *e* v. and a. brachialis; *f* v. thoracica externa; *f'* v. thoracica superficialis; *g* v. and a. profunda brachii; *h* v. and a. collateralis ulnaris; *i* v. and a. transversa cubiti; *k* v. cephalica; *l* v. mediana cubiti; *m* v. cephalica accessoria; *n* v. and a. interossea communis; *o* v. and a. mediana; *p* v. and a. profunda antebrachii; *q* v. and a. radialis proximalis; *r* v. and a. radialis, *s* r. palmaris superficialis, *t* r. palmaris; *u* v. and a. digitalis palmaris communis II, *v* r. tori metacarpei; *w* v. and a. digitalis palmaris (propria III) medialis, *x* r. dorsalis phalangis proximalis, *y* rr. tori digitalis, *z* r. dorsalis phalangis mediae; *z'* v. and a. coronalis

branches. In the distal part of the metacarpus the palmar metacarpal veins unite with the common digital veins which are designated by the same number, but in the dog they first form arch-like anastomoses.

The **arcus palmaris superficialis** arises in carnivores in the distal third of the metacarpus, palmar to the flexor tendon. It is formed by the union between the superficial ramus of the radial vein, after its junction with the cephalic vein, and the superficial ramus of the palmar ramus of the caudal interosseous vein. In the dog an additional wider arch is formed half way down the metacarpus by the union of the two superficial palmar rami and the slender median vein. This subsidiary arch lies parallel to the arterial arcus palmaris superficialis and, like this arterial arch, part of its course lies between the two limbs of the flexor tendons. From the superficial palmar arch arise the *vv.*

digitales palmares communes I–IV and, in the cat, the *v. digitalis palmaris V abaxialis*. Each of these common digital veins receives the isonumerical palmar metacarpal vein and subsequently divides into the *vv. digitales palmares propriae*. In their distribution area the latter are connected through the *v. interdigitalis* with the isonumerical common dorsal digital vein or with one of the proper digital veins. Certain proper palmar digital veins may also originate directly from the superficial palmar arch. The *v. digitalis palmaris I abaxialis* arises from the cephalic vein where it unites with the superficial ramus of the radial vein.

Dorsal veins
(cat: 160/7', *31''*; dog: 156; 161/4; 162/6; 171)

The **rete carpi dorsale** is formed in carnivores by the *rr. carpei dorsales* of the radial, the cephalic and the accessory cephalic veins. Furthermore, in the cat the dorsal carpal branch of the interosseous ramus also contributes to this network and in the dog there are contributory dorsal carpal rami from the cranial interosseous and ulnar veins. From this network issue the *vv. metacarpeae dorsales I–IV* which in the cat are only rudimentary like the corresponding arteries, except for the first part of the dorsal metacarpal vein II. This last vessel represents the continuation of the dorsal carpal ramus of the radial vein and it immediately becomes the *r. perforans proximalis II* which contributes to the formation of the deep palmar arch. The other perforating rami behave like their arterial counterparts. The dorsal metacarpal veins, or, in the cat, the distal perforating rami, terminate in the corresponding *vv. digitales dorsales communes*.

In the cat the superficial vein is the accessory cephalic vein which crosses the carpus dorsomedially and the metacarpus in a laterodistally directed arch and then links up with the more slender dorsal ramus of the ulnar vein. From this arch arise the *vv. digitales dorsales communes I–IV* which split into the *vv. digitales dorsales propriae*. Some of the latter may also arise directly from the arch. In the dog too, the accessory cephalic vein runs across the carpus, medial to the cranial superficial antebrachial artery. In the distal part of the forearm it gives off a medial branch which accompanies the medial branch of the cranial superficial artery of the forearm, and finally becomes the *v. digitalis dorsalis communis I*. In the proximal metacarpal region the accessory cephalic vein gives off the *v. digitalis dorsalis V abaxialis* and halfway down the metacarpus it divides into the *vv. digitales dorsales communes II–IV*. In the dog the dorsal ramus of the ulnar vein also joins with the Vth abaxial dorsal digital vein and there is an arch-like anastomosis between the medial branch of the accessory vein and its terminal branches. Thus, even in the dog there is a rudimentary arcus dorsalis superficialis.

Veins of the forefoot of the pig

Palmar veins
(pig: 157; 163/27, *29, 30*; 168)

In the pig the **arcus palmaris profundus** consists of the deep palmar ramus of the radial vein and the deep ramus of the palmar ramus of the caudal interosseous vein. From this arch arise the *vv. metacarpeae palmares II–IV*. In the distal metacarpal region the three palmar metacarpal veins unite to form the *arcus palmaris profundus distalis*. This joins with the first part of the *v. digitalis palmaris communis III* as it arises from the superficial palmar arch. Only the *II*nd to the *IV*th *rr. perforantes proximales* are developed in the pig.

The **arcus palmaris superficialis** is formed, in the distal third of the metacarpus palmar to the flexor tendon, by the union between the superficial palmar ramus of the radial vein, after the junction with the cephalic vein, and the superficial branch of the palmar ramus of the caudal interosseous vein. The superficial palmar arch has a lateral anastomosis with the Vth abaxial dorsal digital vein which arises from the dorsal ramus of the collateral ulnar vein. From the superficial palmar arch arise the *vv. digitales palmares communes I–IV* and the *v. digitalis palmaris V abaxialis*. The Ist common palmar digital vein arises medially from the first part of the arch and it has a stout anastomosis to this arch at the level of the origin of the IInd common palmar digital vein. The IIIrd common palmar digital vein is joined, immediately after its origin, by the median vein.

212 Veins

While the Ist common palmar digital vein gives off only the *v. digitalis palmaris propria II abaxialis*, the other common palmar digital veins divide into the *vv. digitales palmares propriae*. The common digital veins of the same number are linked near the point where they divide by the *vv. interdigitales II–IV*.

Dorsal veins
(pig: 157; 163/*31–33*; 172)

The **rete carpi dorsale** is formed by the dorsal carpal rami of the radial, cephalic, accessory cephalic, cranial interosseous and collateral ulnar veins. The *vv. metacarpeae dorsales II–IV* do not stem from this network but from the *rr. perforantes proximales II–IV* and they unite with the dorsal common digital veins.

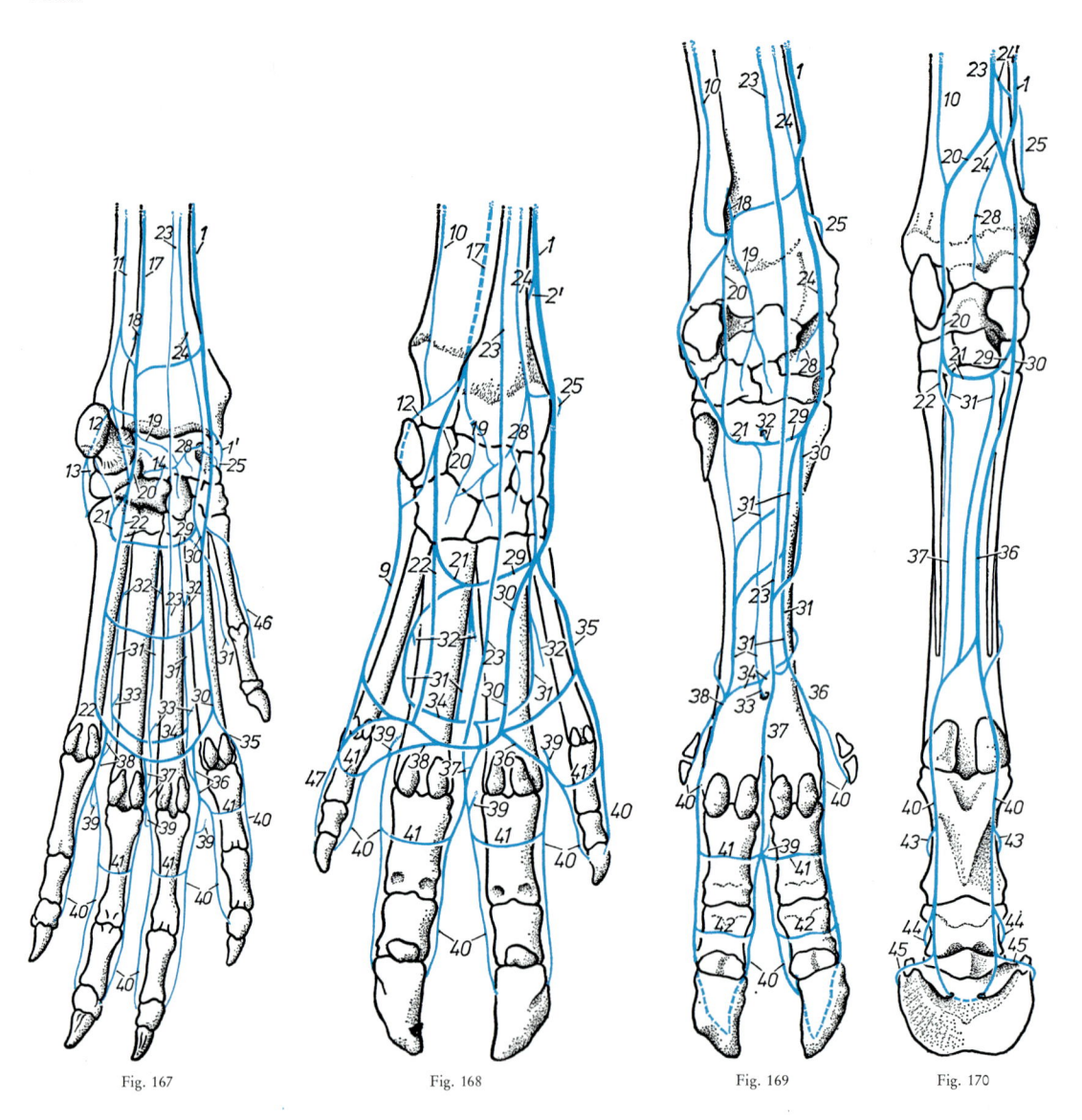

Fig. 167   Fig. 168   Fig. 169   Fig. 170

Figs 167, 168, 169, 170, 171, 172, 173, 174. Veins of the left fore-foot of the dog, pig, ox and horse. Semidiagrammatic. (After Münster, Badawi and Wilkens, in preparation, work carried out at the Institute of Veterinary Anatomy, Hanover.)

Figs 167–170: palmar view, Figs 171–174: dorsal view

1 v. cephalica; *1'* branch to the rete carpi dorsale; *2* v. cephalica accessoria; *2'* v. cephalica accessoria, medial vein (pig); *2"* v. cephalica accessoria, lateral vein (pig); *3* r. carpeus dorsalis of *2*; *4–7* vv. digitales dorsales communes; *8* vv. digitales dorsales propriae; *9* v. digitalis dorsalis V abaxialis; *10* v. collateralis ulnaris; *11* v. ulnaris, *12* r. dorsalis; *13* r. carpeus dorsalis of *10* or *11*; *14* r. carpeus palmaris of *11*; *15* v. interossea cranialis, *16* r. carpeus

Veins of the forefoot

The accessory cephalic vein, sends a lateral and a medial vessel to the dorsum of the foot as does the superficial rami of the radial nerve. Immediately proximal to the carpus these two vessels anastomose with one another and with the cephalic vein. From the medial vessel arises the *v. digitalis dorsalis communis II* and from the latter vessel branch the *vv. digitales dorsales communis III* and *IV*. In those cases where either the medial or lateral vessel terminates in one of the anastomoses, all the common dorsal digital veins originate from one only of these two vessels. After receiving the dorsal metacarpal veins, the dorsal common digital veins divide into the *vv. digitales dorsales propriae* at about the level where the interdigital veins join. The *v. digitalis dorsalis V abaxialis* arises from the dorsal ramus of the collateral ulnar vein and terminates from a lateral direction in the superficial palmar arch, but it also links with the *v. digitalis palmaris V abaxialis*.

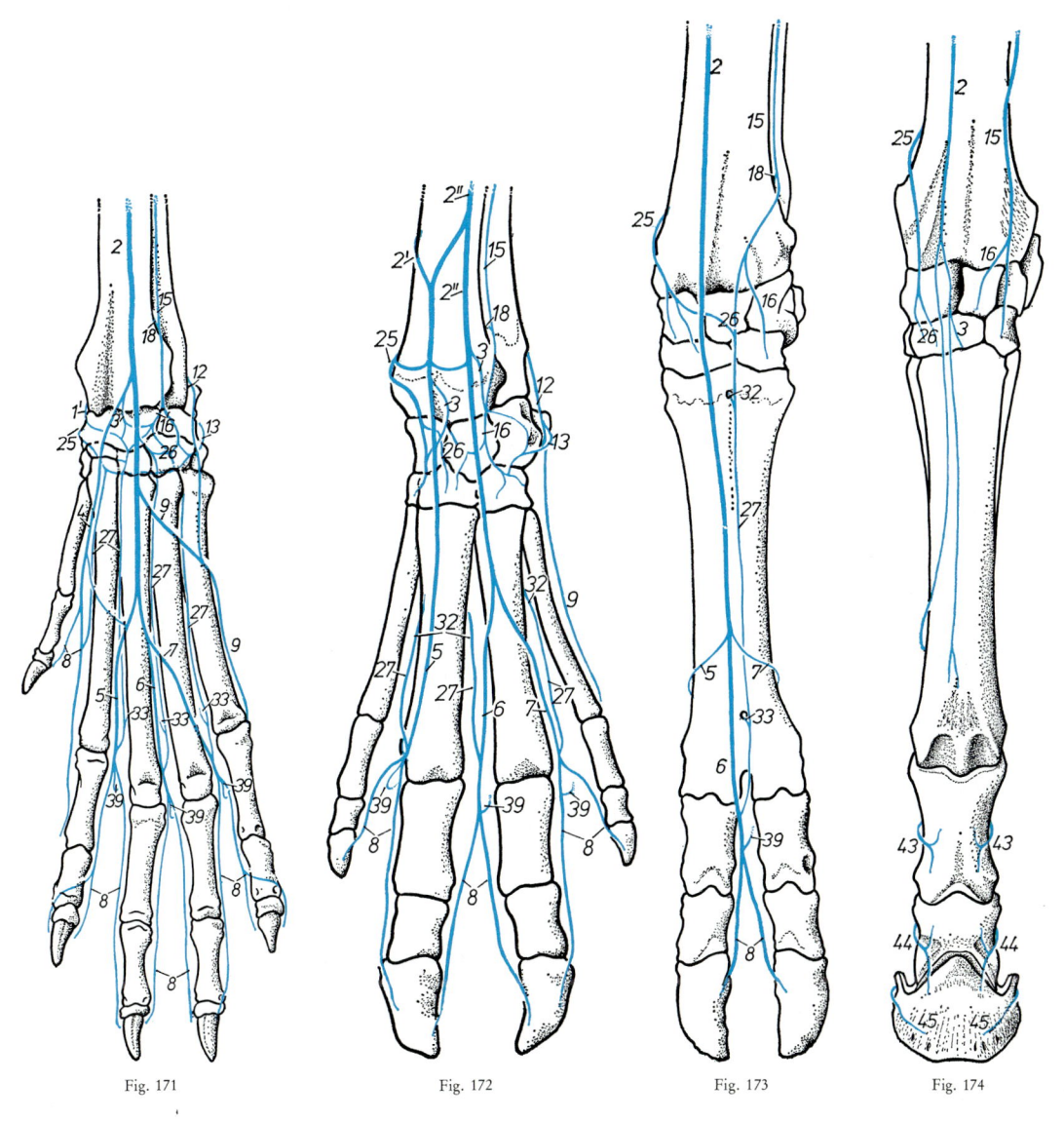

Fig. 171 Fig. 172 Fig. 173 Fig. 174

dorsalis; *17* v. interossea caudalis; *18* r. interosseus; *19* r. carpeus palmaris of *17*; *20* r. palmaris, *21* r. profundus, *22* r. superficialis; *23* v. mediana; *24* v. radialis; *24'* v. radialis proximalis; *25* r. carpeus dorsalis of *24* or in the horse of *24'*; *26* rete carpi dorsale; *27* vv. metacarpeae dorsales; *28* r. capeus palmaris of *24* or in the horse of *24'*; *29* r. palmaris profundus; *21* and *29* arcus palmaris profundus; *30* r. palmaris superficialis; *22* and *30* arcus palmaris superficialis; *31* vv. metacarpeae palmares; *32* rr. perforantes proximales; *33* rr. perforantes distales; *34* arcus palmaris profundus distalis; *35–38* vv. digitales palmares communes; *39* vv. interdigitales; *40* vv. digitales palmares propriae; *41* rr. palmares phalangium proximalium; *42* rr. palmares phalangium mediarum; *43* rr. dorsales phalangis proximalis, *44* rr. dorsales phalangis mediae, *45* rr. dorsales phalangis distales (shown only in the horse); *46* v. digitalis palmaris I abaxialis; *47* v. digitalis palmaris V abaxialis

Veins of the forefoot of ruminants

Palmar veins
(sheep: 164/23, 27, 28; ox: 158; 165/17, 19–22; 169)

The **arcus palmaris profundus** is formed firstly by the deep palmar ramus of the radial vein, which is a slender, often double vein which has joined with the cephalic vein proximally to the carpus, and secondly by the deep branch of the palmar ramus of the interosseous ramus of the cranial interosseous vein. From this arch arise the *vv. metacarpeae palmares II–IV*. These vessels give rise to the *v. metacarpea palmaris II* which originates at the commencement of the deep ramus, and therefore at the beginning of the arch, and it forms the functional continuation of the radial vein. Laterodistally-directed cross anastomoses interconnect the palmar metacarpal veins, thus strenthening distally the IIIrd and IVth palmar metacarpal veins which are weak in their proximal part. A particularly strong transverse anastomosis forms the *arcus palmaris profundus distalis* proximal to the metacarpophalangeal joint. The *rr. perforantes proximales III* and *distalis III* arise from deep palmar and distal deep palmar arches respectively.

Whereas the distal arch-like anastomosis of the palmar metacarpal arteries forms medially a junction with the IInd and laterally a junction with the IVth common palmar digital arteries, the venous distal deep palmar arch serves as origin for the *vv. digitales palmares communes II* and *IV*. The first part of the IInd common palmar digital vein is linked by a medial semicircular arch with the median vein and in the sheep the IVth also forms a lateral semicircular arch which joins that vein. At this level the median vein becomes the *v. digitalis palmaris communis III*. It is only in rare cases that the superficial palmar ramus of the radial vein reaches the medial semicircular arch; usualy it ends more proximally at a variable level in the median vein. The IIIrd common palmar digital vein is connected by the robust *v. interdigitalis III* with the dorsal common digital vein of the same number. Each of the palmar common digital veins divides into the *vv. digitales palmares propriae*. The axial veins of the second and of the fifth toes are only small since they supply the dew claw.

Dorsal veins
(sheep: 164/26; ox: 158; 165/22, 28; 173)

The **rete carpi dorsale** is formed by the dorsal carpal rami of the radial and cranial interosseous veins. From this network arises the slender *v. metacarpea dorsalis III* which receives the proximal and distal perforating rami and then terminates in the third dorsal common digital vein at the level of the proximal phalanx.

At the distal half of the metacarpus the accessory cephalic vein becomes the *v. digitalis dorsalis communis III*. Here it gives off the *vv. digitales dorsales communes II* and *IV*, which merely act as anastomoses to the initial part of the appropriately numbered palmar common digital veins. The medial of these anastomoses is strongly developed and connects the medial semicircular arch of the median vein and the distal deep palmar arch. The IIIrd dorsal common digital vein receives the IIIrd interdigital vein and then divides into the *vv. digitales dorsales propriae III* and *IV axiales*.

Veins of the forefoot of the horse

Palmar veins
(horse: 159; 166/s–z'; 170)

The **deep palmar arch** is formed by the deep palmar ramus of the radial vein and the deep branch of the palmar ramus of the median vein. From this arch arise the *vv. metacarpeae palmares II* and *III* which unite in the distal part of the metacarpus and form the *arcus palmaris profundus distalis*. The second palmar metacarpal vein runs laterally to the corresponding artery and almost medial to the third metacarpal bone. The third palmar metacarpal vein is usually rudimentary and this results in an equally insignificant distal deep arch. The two palmar metacarpal veins and the distal deep arch unite with the arch-like link of the palmar common digital veins II and III. The superficial palmar ramus of the radial vein, which has united with the cephalic vein immediately after its origin, becomes the *v. digitalis palmaris communis II* at the point where the communicating branch of the medial palmar nerve originates. The superficial branch of the palmar ramus of the median vein becomes the *v. digitalis palmaris communis II* at the level where the communicating ramus ends in the lateral palmar nerve. Proximal to the pastern joint, the palmar common digital veins form an arch-like anastomosis between the median interosseous muscle and the deep flexor tendon and give off the *vv. digitales palmares (propria III) medialis* and *(propria III) lateralis*.

Dorsal veins
(horse : 159; 166/x, z, z'; 174)

The **rete carpi dorsale** is formed by the dorsal carpal rami of the radial, accessory cephalic and cranial interosseous veins. The dorsal metacarpal veins are lacking.

In addition to the rete branches, the accessory cephalic vein gives off only skin branches which extend just proximal to the pastern joint. A more medially directed skin branch connects with the palmar common digital vein II over the distal end of the second metacarpal bone. For this reason the superficial venous links of the dorsal part of the forefoot are lacking. The dorsal part of the toe is supplied by *rr. dorsales, phalangis proximalis, phalangis mediae* and *phalangis distalis* in a similar manner to the arterial system.

Veins of the head and neck

V. jugularis externa
(Comparative: 145–148/4; 149–152/24; 156–159/37; cat: 160/3; 178/7; 181/1; dog: 161/2; 162/1; 175/11; 179/7; pig: 153/23; 163/10; 176/7; 177, 182/1; ox: 102, 155/18; 185, 186/1; horse: 180/7)

In carnivores and pigs the **v. jugularis externa** is the second branch of the division of the brachiocephalic vein, the other branch being the subclavian vein. In ruminants and horses the external jugular veins of the two sides represent the terminal divisions of the cranial vena cava. In ruminants the common stem for the left and right *v. jugularis interna* arises from this angle of bifurcation whereas in the other domestic mammals the internal jugular vein originates independently from the first part of the external jugular, although it is only present in the goat and the horse in very exceptional cases. Up to the point of origin of the internal jugular vein the external jugular can be looked upon as a *v. jugularis communis*. The external jugular vein reaches the jugular groove between the scalenus medius and the sternohyoideus and sternothyreoideus muscles. In the lower third of the neck it is covered by the cutaneus colli muscle. The superficially situated vein progresses craniad in the jugular groove and, in the upper third of the neck, it crosses the lateral face of the omohyoideus muscle. This muscle is lacking in carnivores. At this site it is accessible for intravenous injections, especially in ruminants and horses. Near the thoracic inlet the external jugular vein gives rise, at the same level, to the *v. cervicalis superficialis* and the *v. cephalica*, which vessels have a common stem in the cat, and also to the *v. omobrachialis* in the dog. The omobrachialis vein is a second root of the cephalic vein. The external jugular divides into the *v. linguofacialis* and the *v. maxillaris* ventral to the wings of the atlas. However, in small ruminants and also sometimes in the ox it gives off the *v. occipitalis* prior to this division.

V. cervicalis superficialis
(Comparative: 145–148/10; 149–152/28; 156–159/38; cat: 160/5; dog: 161/5; 162/7; pig: 153/34; 163/12; 177/9; 182/2; goat: 154/22; sheep: 164/12; ox: 102, 155/12; 165/29, 31)

In all domestic mammals the **v. cervicalis superficialis** arises from the external jugular vein at the level of the thoracic inlet. In the cat only it immediately gives off the *v. cephalica*. Above the shoulder joint the *r. ascendens* leaves the superficial cervical vein and runs towards the head, medial to the cleidocephalicus, and it anastomoses with the *v. auricularis caudalis*. In the pig this anastomosis is accomplished through the *r. auricularis*. In carnivores the *v. suprascapularis* is given off and runs towards in the inc. scapulae. In ruminants a *r. suprascapularis* supplies branches to the omotransversarius muscle and the cervical part of the trapezius before anastomosing with the suprascapular vein. The *r. acromialis* originates from the suprascapular ramus in ruminants and directly from the superficial cervical vein in carnivores and pigs. This acromial ramus turns into the supraspinous fossa (see p. 198). Except in the horse the superficial cervical vein continues along the cranial border of the supraspinatus muscle, or the subclavius muscle in the pig, as the *r. praescapularis*. This latter ramus gives off branches to the superficial cervical lymph nodes and, progressing in the direction of the muscle fibres, branches medial to the omotransversarius muscle and the cervical part of the trapezius. At the cranial angle of the scapula it anastomoses with branches of the *v. scapularis dorsalis* or the *v. cervicalis profunda*. In the horse the branches to the lymph nodes derive from the *r. ascendens*.

V. cephalica

(Comparative: 145–148/*11*; 149–152/*29*; 156–159/*42*; 167–170/*1*; cat: 160/*7*; dog: 161, 162/*3*; pig: 153/*41*; 163/*24*; 177/*2, 3*; 182/*7*; goat: 154/*21*; sheep: 164/*24*; ox: 102, 155/*19*; 165/*24, 26*; horse: 166/*k*)

The v. cephalica, v. mediana cubiti and v. cephalica accessoria are here considered as part of the veins of the pectoral limb only in respect of their origin from the external jugular vein.

The **v. cephalica** generally arises from the external jugular vein although in the dog it always has a second vein of origin, the *v. omobrachialis*, which branches from the external jugular further cranially. The omobrachial vein runs in a caudoventral direction over the cleidocephalicus muscle and it frequently unites also, or exclusively, with the *v. axillobrachialis*. Only in the cat does the cephalic vein stem from the superficial cervical vein which itself is given off the external jugular vein. In carnivores there is an additional lateral link between the cephalic vein and the caudal circumflex humeral vein namely the *v. axillobrachialis*. This vessel can also be found in the ox in a similar situation but it is more slender in that animal. In the pig the connecting vein is associated with the proximal vessel of the axillary vein. While at first the cephalic vein of the dog is overlaid by the brachiocephalicus muscle, in all other domestic mammals except the ox this vessel runs subcutaneously in the lateral thoracic groove to the flexor aspect of the elbow joint. Only in the ox does it follow the border of the brachiocephalicus muscle. At the elbow, or in the ox more proximally, it gives off the *v. mediana cubiti* which runs through the fascia along the medial aspect of the leg and joins with the brachial vein. In the region of the forearm and medial to the extensor carpi radialis, the cephalic vein continues along in a subcutaneous position, giving off several cutaneous and muscular branches as well as the accessory cephalic vein. The point of origin of the latter vessel varies in the different species. Proximally to the carpus the cephalic vein joins, through the fascia, with the radial vein at a point where the latter receives the stout anastomosing branch with the caudal interosseous vein. Thus it terminates in the pig, ruminants and horse while in carnivores it unites with the radial vein and participates in the formation of the palmar vascular arches. The cephalic vein of the dog runs parallel to the radial vein in mediopalmar direction and passes over the carpus to unite with the superficial palmar ramus of the radial vein distal to the carpal joint (see p. 209). Proximal to the flexor aspect of the elbow joint, the pig has a connecting vessel between the cephalic and transverse cubital veins. In the distal third of the forearm the cephalic vein gives off a second root to the assessory cephalic vein.

V. mediana cubiti

(Comparative: 156–159/*45*; cat: 160/*29*; dog: 161/*26*; 162/*5*; pig: 163/*25*; sheep: 164/*25*; ox: 165/*25*; horse: 166/*l*)

In veterinary anatomy the term **v. mediana cubiti** is applied to the large vessel joining the subcutaneously situated cephalic vein to the more deeply placed brachial vein. In carnivores the *v. brachialis superficialis* forms part of this connecting link. The origin of the median cubital vein from the cephalic vein is situated a variable distance proximal to the elbow joint depending on the species and, except in the horse, it is caudodistally directed. In carnivores it terminates in the superficial brachial vein through which it communicates in the cat with the brachial vein. In the pig the median cubital vein is very short, being connected to the end of the caudal vessels of the paired brachial vein. In the ox, however, it is very long, running distally in the lateral thoracic groove, bending mediodistally about half way down the elbow joint and perforating the fascia of the forearm. At the site of the brachialis and biceps brachii muscles the median cubital vein joins with the brachial vein at the point of transition into the median vein. The v. mediana cubiti supplies muscular branches and has an anastomosis with the *v. transversa cubiti*. In the horse the median cubital vein forms a caudoproximally-directed junction with the brachial vein.

V. cephalica accessoria

(Comparative: 156–159/46; cat: 160/7'; dog: 161/4; 162/6; 171/2; pig: 163/31, 32; 172/2', 2"; sheep: 164/26; ox: 165/27; 173/2; horse: 166/m; 174/2)

In carnivores the **v. cephalica accessoria** arises from the cephalic vein at the border between the middle and distal two thirds of the forearm. It courses cranially and subcutaneously along the forearm in a distal direction. At the rete carpi dorsale it gives rise to branches which perforate the fascia as they change from a superficial to a deep position. At the dorsum of the foot they form the origin for the dorsal digital vessels and in the cat they link up with the dorsal ramus of the ulnar vein (see p. 206). In the pig the accessory cephalic vein is replaced by lateral and medial vessels. The lateral vessel arises from the cephalic vein at the level of the middle third of the upper arm whereas the medial vessel has two roots, one stemming from the cephalic vein proximal to the carpal joint, and the other arising from the lateral vessel. These lateral and medial vessels of the porcine accessory cephalic vein supply branches to the rete carpi dorsale and also give off the common digital veins to the dorsal surface of the foot (see p. 212). In ruminants the accessory cephalic vein arises in the lower third of the forearm and follows distally the medial border of the tendon of the extensor carpi radialis. At about the middle of the metacarpus it attains the dorsal surface in the proximity of the extensor tendons. It ends in this location in the goat, in which species the accessory cephalic vein is but a slender vessel. In the other species it becomes the *v. digitalis dorsalis communis III* in the metacarpal region. The *rr. anastomotici* link the accessory cephalic and the radial veins (see p. 209). In the horse, the accessory cephalic vein arises on the flexor aspect of the elbow joint immediately before the median cubital vein is given off and it runs distad along the craniomedial aspect of the extensor carpi radialis muscle. At the carpus it divides into two branches. One of these continues in the same direction along the metacarpus giving off branches to the dorsal carpal network; it terminates in the skin region a hand's breadth proximal to the pastern joint. The other, more medially-directed, branch in the horse gives off medial and palmar cutaneous branches in the metacarpal region. This branch is linked with the palmar common digital vein II across the distal end of the second metacarpal bone (see p. 214).

V. jugularis interna

(Comparative: 145–147/5; 149–151/25; cat: 160/4; 178, 181/3; dog: 175/12; 179/3; pig: 153/42; 163/11; 176/6; 177/7; 183/1; ox: 102, 155/17; 186/53)

The **v. jugularis interna** is absent in the small ruminants and, usually, in the horse. It arises from the first part of the external jugular vein which can therefore be termed the *v. jugularis communis*. In the ox the right and left internal jugular veins arise together from the bifurcation of the external jugular veins. The internal jugular courses craniad in company with, and ventral to, the common carotid artery. Ventral to the alar groove of the atlas, or the axis in the pig, it gives off the *v. occipitalis* and then passes through the jugular foramen in company with the *v. emissaria foraminis jugularis*. In the ox the latter is only a slender vessel. In carnivores and pigs it gives off the *v. comitans a. carotidis externae* which accompanies the external carotid artery. In the ox the *v. pharyngea ascendens* is also given off by the internal jugular.

V. thyreoidea media

(cat: 181/4; 175/6, 6'; sheep: 184/2; ox: 186/54)

The **v. thyreoidea media** originates from the internal jugular vein a variable distance caudal to the thyroid gland. In the horse it may occasionally arise as a branch of the cranial thyroid vein. The middle thyroid vein reaches the caudal pole of the gland.

Fig. 176. Veins in the region of the cervical vertebrae of a pig. Left lateral view. The transverse canal of the 4th cervical vertebra has been opened.
(After Wissdorf, 1970, habil. thesis, Hanover.)

a atlas; *b* vertebra cervicalis VII; *c* vertebra thoracica I

1 v. cava cranialis; *2* v. costocervicalis; *3* v. thoracica interna; *4* v. axillaris proximalis; *5* v. axillaris distalis; *6* v. jugularis interna; *7* v. jugularis externa; *8* v. occipitalis; *9* v. comitans a. carotidis externa; *10* v. emissaria foraminis jugularis; *11* v. vertebralis (cervicalis); *12–24* branches of the v. vertebralis; *12* r. dorsalis at the axis and another r. descendens, *13* r. anastomoticus cum v. occipitali, *14* r. ventralis at the axis and another r. anastomoticus cum v. occipitali, *15* r. descendens, *16* v. intervertebralis, *17, 18* rr. dorsales, *19* r. muscularis, *20* rr. ventrales, *21* connection with the v. vertebralis thoracica, *22* r. muscularis, *23* r. dorsalis, *24* r. spinalis; *25* v. vertebralis thoracica; *27* collateral vein of the a. scapularis dorsalis; *28, 29* r. dorsalis; *31* v. intercostalis suprema; *32, 35, 36* v. cervicalis profunda; *33* v. scapularis dorsalis; *34* v. intercostalis dorsalis II

Fig. 175. Veins of the larynx, trachea and thyroid of a dog. Ventral view.
(After Loeffler, 1955, Diss., Hanover.)

a gl. thyreoidea; *b* m. sternohyoideus; *c* m. sternothyreoideus; *d* m. sternocephalicus; *e* m. cricothyreoideus; *f* m. thyreohyoideus

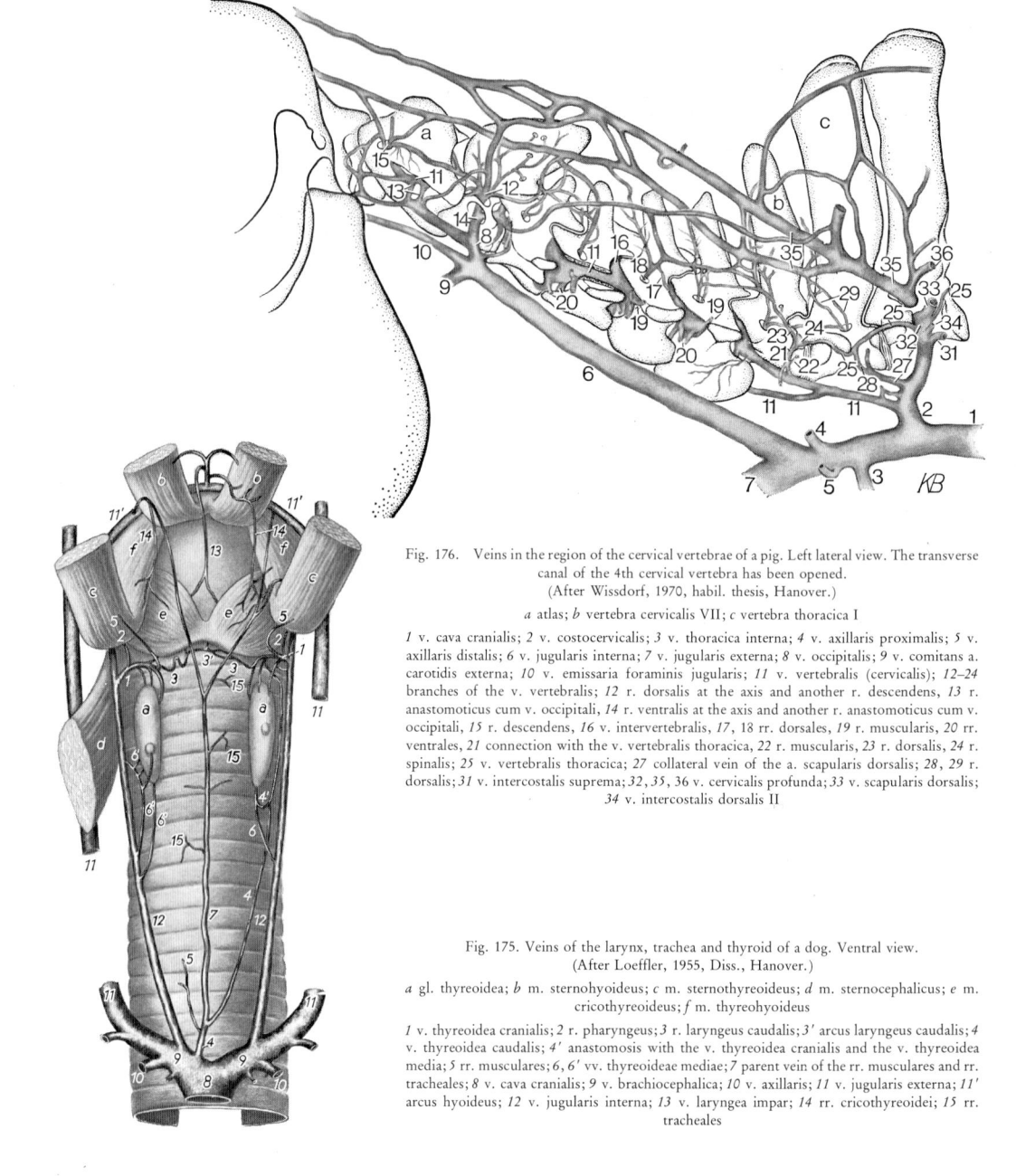

1 v. thyreoidea cranialis; *2* r. pharyngeus; *3* r. laryngeus caudalis; *3'* arcus laryngeus caudalis; *4* v. thyreoidea caudalis; *4'* anastomosis with the v. thyreoidea cranialis and the v. thyreoidea media; *5* rr. musculares; *6, 6'* vv. thyreoideae mediae; *7* parent vein of the rr. musculares and rr. tracheales; *8* v. cava cranialis; *9* v. brachiocephalica; *10* v. axillaris; *11* v. jugularis externa; *11'* arcus hyoideus; *12* v. jugularis interna; *13* v. laryngea impar; *14* rr. cricothyreoidei; *15* rr. tracheales

V. thyreoidea cranialis

(cat: 181/5; dog: 175/1; pig: 183/3; sheep: 184/2; ox: 186/56, 57)

The **v. thyreoidea cranialis** usually arises from the internal jugular near the cranial pole of the thyroid gland. In small ruminants, however, it stems from the external jugular and in the horse it originates either from the maxillary or the linguofacial veins. Branches enter at the cranial pole of the thyroid gland. The *v. cricothyreoidea* is given off to the cricothyroid muscle and a *r. laryngeus caudalis* enters the larynx in company with the caudal laryngeal nerve. In carnivores this caudal laryngeal ramus gives issue to a ventrally directed branch which unites immediately caudal to the larynx with the branch of the other side, thus forming the *arcus laryngeus caudalis*. In the ox the cranial thyroid vein also gives rise to

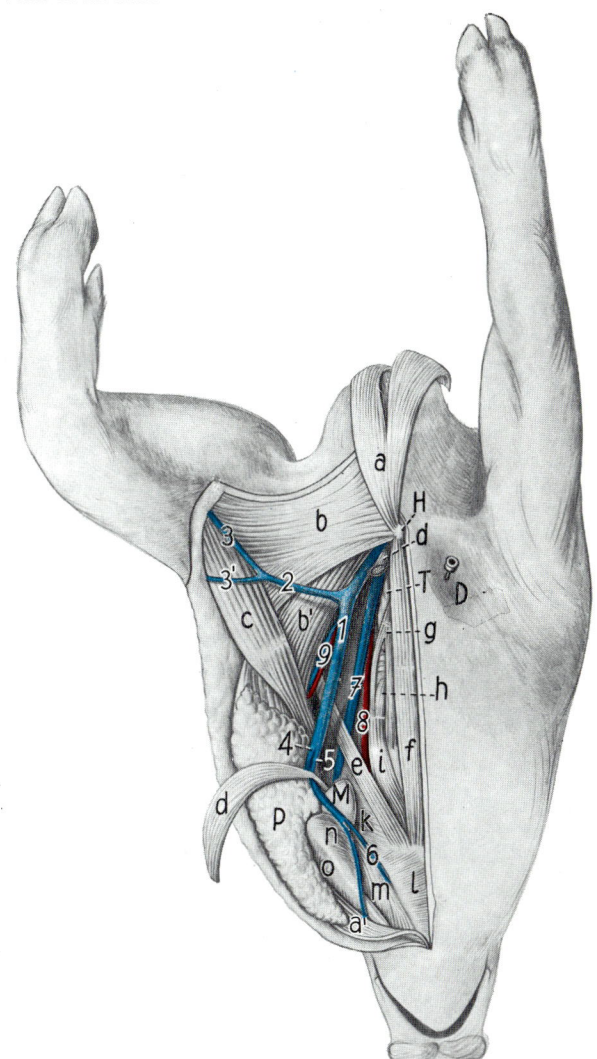

Fig. 177. V. jugularis externa, v. jugularis interna and a. carotis communis of a pig. Topographical. Ventral view. (After Hütten and Preuss, 1953, work carried out at the Institute for Veterinary Anatomy, Hanover.)

D fossa jugularis; *H* manubrium sterni; *M* gl. mandibularis; *P* gl. parotis; *T* gl. thyreoidea

a m. cutaneus colli; *a'* mm. cutaneus faciei et labiorum; *b* mm. pectorales superficiales; *b'* m. subclavius; *c* m. brachiocephalicus; *d* m. sternomastoideus; *e* m. omohyoideus; *f* m. sternohyoideus; *g* m. sternothyreoideus; *h* m. cricothyreoideus; *i* m. thyreohyoideus; *k* m. occipitohyoideus; *l* m. mylohyoideus; *m* m. digastricus; *n* m. pterygoideus medialis; *o* masseter

1 v. jugularis externa; *2, 3* v. cephalica; *3'* v. cephalica accessoria, lateral vessel; *4* v. maxillaris; *5* v. linguofacialis; *6* v. lingualis; *7* v. jugularis interna; *8* a. carotis communis; *9* a. and v. cervicalis superficialis

the *v. laryngea cranialis*. The cranial thyroid vein of the horse gives off the *v. pharyngea ascendens* and sometimes the *v. thyreoidea media*.

V. occipitalis

(cat: 178/4; dog: 179/4; pig: 176, 183/8; sheep: 184/3; ox: 151/26; 186/55; horse: 152/26; 180/4)

In the cat, the pig and sometimes the ox, the **v. occipitalis** stems from the internal jugular vein; in the small ruminants it stems from the external jugular vein. In all these animals except the pig, the point of origin lies ventral to the wing of the atlas. In the pig the occipital vein leaves the internal jugular vein at the level of the axis and here the occipital vein has additionally an anastomosis with the vertebral vein. In individual cattle which have a very short internal jugular vein, the occipital vein arises from the external jugular. In the horse it originates from the maxillary vein. As with the artery of that name, the occipital vein links with the *r. anastomoticus cum v. occipitalis* of the vertebral vein. In the ox this union occurs at the level of the axis. The *r. occipitalis* when present reaches the base of the skull, but this ramus is lacking in dogs, small ruminants and horses. The occipital vein gives rise to the *v. emissaria occipitalis* in all the domestic mammals and to the *v. stylomastoidea* in the pig and horse. In those bovines in which it arises from the external jugular, the occipital vein gives off a common stem for the *v. pharyngea ascendens* and the slender *v. emissaria foraminis jugularis*.

220 Veins

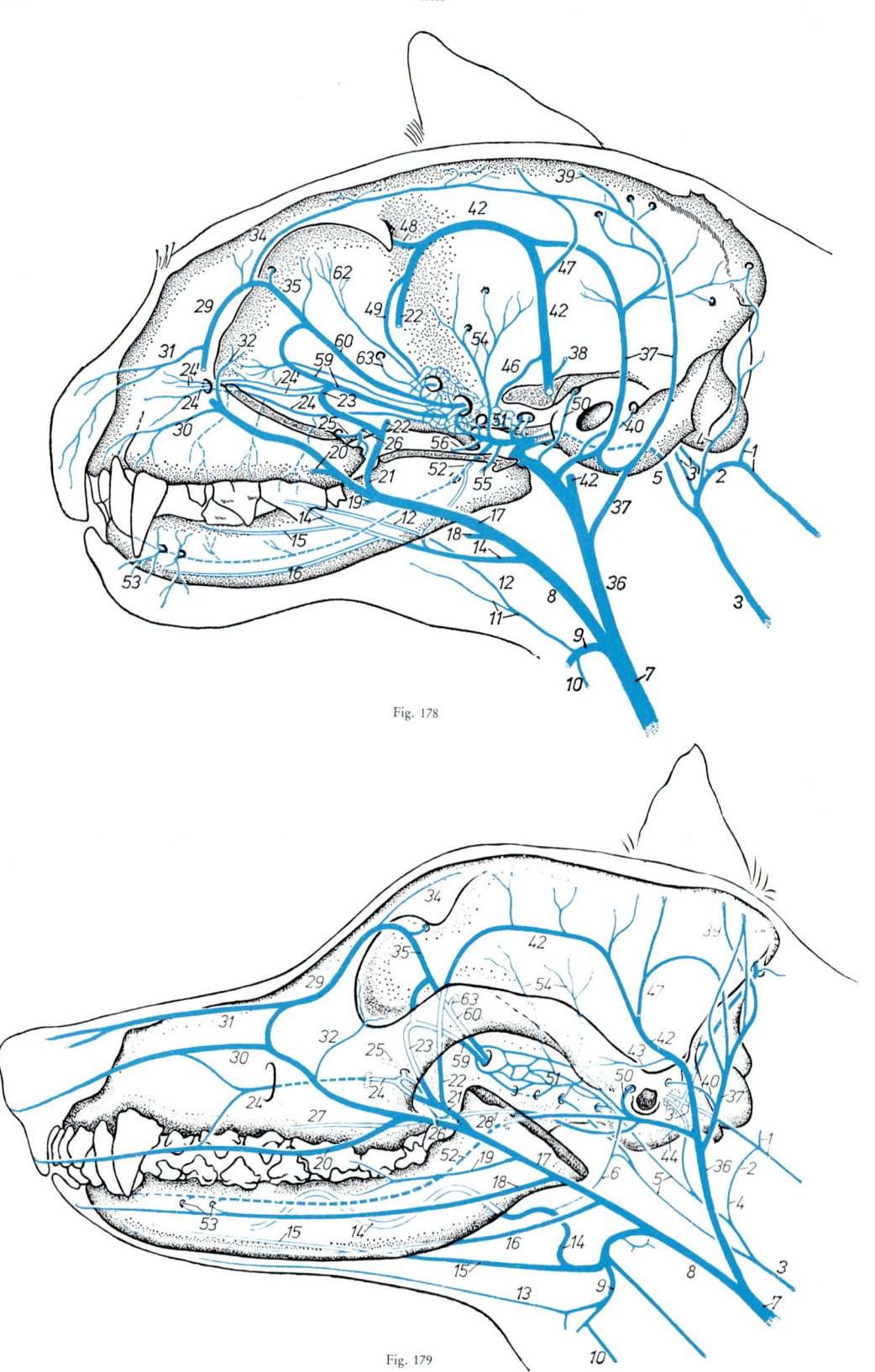

Fig. 178

Fig. 179

Fig. 180

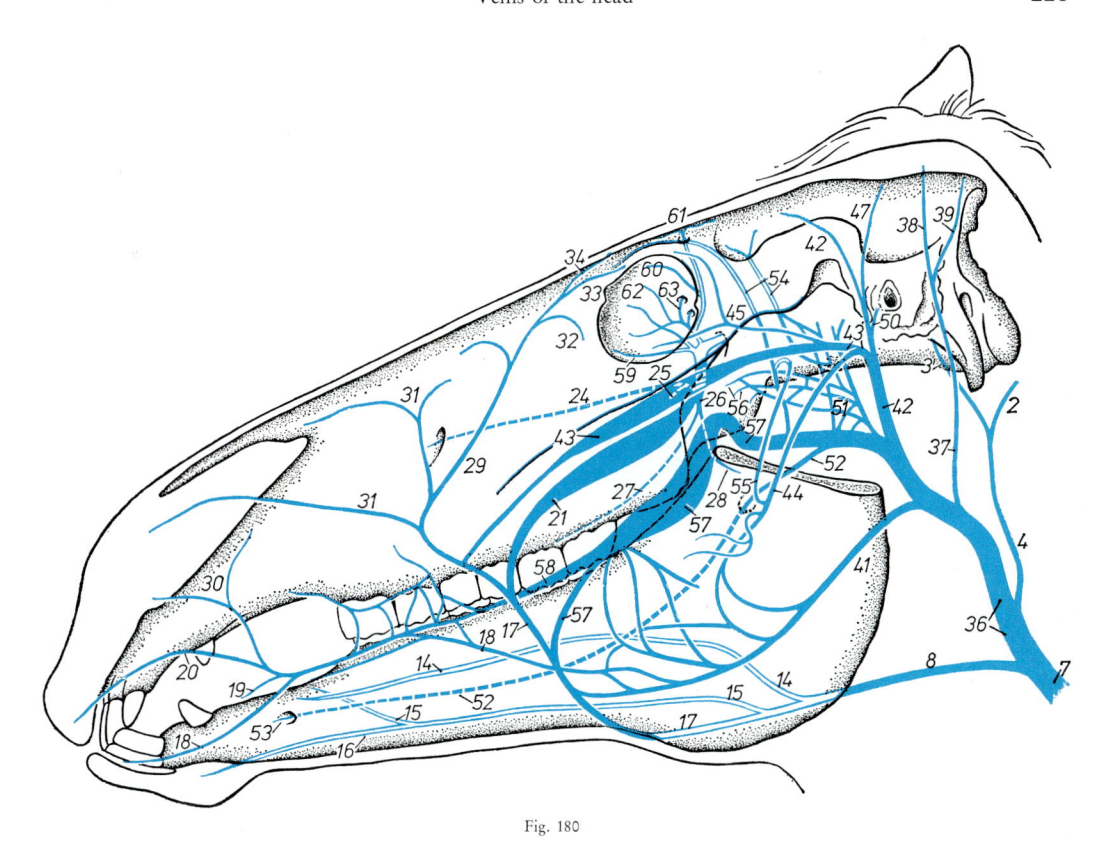

Figs 178, 179, 180. Veins of the head of the cat, dog and horse. Semidiagrammatic. Left lateral view. (After Frenzel, 1967, Diss., Hanover; after Rümpler, 1967, Diss., Hanover, after Münster et al., in preparation, work carried out at the Institute for Veterinary Anatomy, Hanover.)

1 v. vertebralis with *2* r. anastomoticus cum v. occipitali; *3* v. jugularis interna; *3'* v. emissaria foraminis jugularis; *4* v. occipitalis; *5* v. comitans a. carotidis externae; *6* v. comitans a. lingualis, not shown in the cat; *7* v. jugularis externa; *8* v. linguofacialis; *9* arcus hyoideus; *10* v. laryngea impar; *11* v. lingualis impar; *12* r. lingualis; *13* r. submentalis; *14* v. lingualis; *15* v. sublingualis; *16* v. submentalis; *17* v. facialis; *18* v. labialis mandibularis; *19* v. angularis oris; *20* v. labialis maxillaris; *21* v. profunda faciei, in the horse with sinus venae profundae faciei; *22* r. anastomoticus cum v. temporali superficiali; *23* r. anastomoticus cum v. ophthalmica externa ventrali; *24* v. infraorbitalis, in the cat rr. dentales are also shown; *24'* r. infraorbitalis; *25* v. sphenopalatina; *26* v. palatina descendens; *27* v. palatina major; *28* v. palatina minor; *29* v. angularis oculi; *30* v. lateralis nasi; *31* v. dorsalis nasi; *32* v. palpebralis inferior (carnivores) or v. palpebralis inferior medialis (horse); *33* v. palpebralis superior medialis, only shown in the horse; *34* v. frontalis; *35* r. anastomoticus cum v. ophthalmica externa dorsali with v. diploica frontalis; *36* v. maxillaris; *37* v. auricularis caudalis; *38* v. auricularis lateralis; *39* v. auricularis intermedia; *40* v. stylomastoidea; *41* v. masseterica ventralis; *42* v. temporalis superficialis; *43* v. transversa faciei, in the horse with sinus venae transversae faciei; *44* v. masseterica dorsalis; *45* common parent vessel of the v. palpebralis inferior lateralis and the v. palpebralis superior lateralis; *46* r. anastomoticus cum plexu pterygoideo; *47* v. auricularis rostralis with v. auricularis medialis; *48* v. diploica frontalis; *49* r. anastomoticus cum plexu opthalmico; *50* v. emissaria foraminis retroarticularis; *51* plexus pterygoideus; *52* v. alveolaris mandibularis, in the cat with anastomosis to the v. lingualis, in the cat the rr. dentales are also shown; *53* v. mentalis or vv. mentales; *54* vv. temporales profundae; *55* v. masseterica, not shown in the dog; *56* vv. pterygoideae, not shown in the dog; *57* v. buccalis, in the horse with sinus venae buccalis; *58* r. labialis; *59* v. ophthalmica externa ventralis with v. emissaria fissurae orbitalis; *60* v. ophthalmica externa dorsalis; *61* v. supraorbitalis; *62* v. lacrimalis, not shown in the dog; *63* v. emissaria foraminis ethmoidalis

V. comitans a. carotidis externae
(cat: 178/5; dog: 179/5; pig: 176/9; 183/5)

The **v. comitans a. carotidis externae** is present only in carnivores and pigs and it corresponds to the external carotid artery. It originates from the internal jugular vein as the second terminal branch, the other branch being the jugular emissary vein. In pigs it gives off the cranial laryngeal vein and in both carnivores and pigs it also gives rise to the pharyngeal vein and the *v. comitans a. lingualis*. The latter accompanies the first part of the lingual artery and unites in the lingual region with the lingual vein. In the cat the concomitant vein of the external carotid artery also gives rise to the *v. palatina* which is connected to the *plexus palatinus*. The veins recorded here will be described with the corresponding vessels in the other species.

V. linguofacialis

(cat: 178/8; dog: 179/8; pig: 177/5; 182/8; sheep: 184/12; ox: 151/29; 185/19; 186/23; horse: 152/29; 180/8)

The **v. linguofacialis** arises from the external jugular ventral to the wing of the atlas in superficial situation. Unaccompanied by an artery, it runs towards the mandibular angle, crossing the tendon of the sternomandibularis muscle in the goat, ox and horse, and then dividing into the *v. lingualis* to the mandibular space and the *v. facialis* to the face. Except in the dog the linguofacial vein also gives rise to the *vv. glandulares* which supply branches to, especially, the mandibular gland. The cranial laryngeal vein is given off the linguofacial vein only in the sheep. In the cat the linguofacial veins of the left and right sides connect through the *arcus hyoideus* at the level of the basihyoid.

V. lingualis

(cat: 178/14; 181/26; dog: 179/14; pig: 177/6; 183/15, 16; sheep: 184/14; ox: 186/27; horse: 180/14)

The **v. lingualis** arises from the linguofacial vein in the mandibular space, caudal to the inc. vasorum in the region of the mandibular lymph glands. In dogs, pigs and ruminants the lingual vein unites with the vein of the other side at the level of the basihyoid and this union forms the superficially-situated hyoid arch. Prior to this junction it gives off in the dog the *v. pharyngea ascendens* and the *v. glandularis*, the latter passing to the mandibular gland. From its superficial position in the caudal part of the mandibular space, the lingual vein of the cat gives off the *v. submentalis* and then reaches the medial surface of the mylohyoid muscle. The *v. sublingualis* originates at the ventral border of the styloglossus but its rostral position varies between species. Then, curving mediad, it lies next to the sublingual artery and in carnivores and pigs receives the v. comitans a. lingualis. Together with the artery, the lingual vein enters the tongue and continues as the *v. profunda linguae* on a tortuous route towards the tip of the tongue. All the way along its course this vein gives off the *vv. dorsales linguae* which are grouped in bundles and supply a dense network to the dorsum of the tongue. In the dog the deep vein of the tongue is joined through the *arcus hyoideus profundus* to its companion from the other side.

Arcus hyoideus

(cat: 178/9; 181/17; dog: 175/11'; 179/9; pig: 182/13'; 183/18)

The **arcus hyoideus** is situated superficially in the region of the basihyoid and it consists of a stout transverse connection between the right and left linguofacial veins in the cat and between the right and left lingual veins in the dog, pig and ruminant. The *v. laryngea impar* arises from this arch only in the carnivore and it takes a caudal course passing between the two sternohyoideus muscles and ventrally over the body of the thyroid cartilage. While so doing it gives off branches to the cricothyroid muscle and, passing between the thyroid and cricoid cartilage, to the laryngeal mucosa. Finally it anastomoses with the other veins of the larynx. In the dog the hyoid arch gives rise to the robust unpaired, superficially situated and rostrally directed *r. submentalis,* the branches of which anastomose in the chin region with the vv. submentales, vv. mentales and vv. labiales mandibulares. In the cat, on the other hand, the large *v. lingualis impar* stems from this arch. This latter vein gives origin to a *v. pharyngea ascendens* to each side. Then it gives off the *r. lingualis*, the largest of the veins of the tongue, and finally turns onto the dorsal surface of the mylohyoideus muscle and reaches a median position in the depth of the tongue. Near the hyoid bone this ramus unites with the v. comitans a. lingualis and gives off the vv. dorsales linguae.

V. sublingualis

(cat: 178/15; 181/29; dog: 179/15; pig: 183/17; sheep: 184/15; ox: 186/29; horse: 180/15)

In carnivores, pigs and ruminants the **v. sublingualis** is a branch of the lingual vein but in the horse it usually arises independently from the facial vein. It attains the dorsal surface of the mylohyoideus muscle and vascularizes the sublingual floor of the mouth. In the dog it also gives off, caudal to the

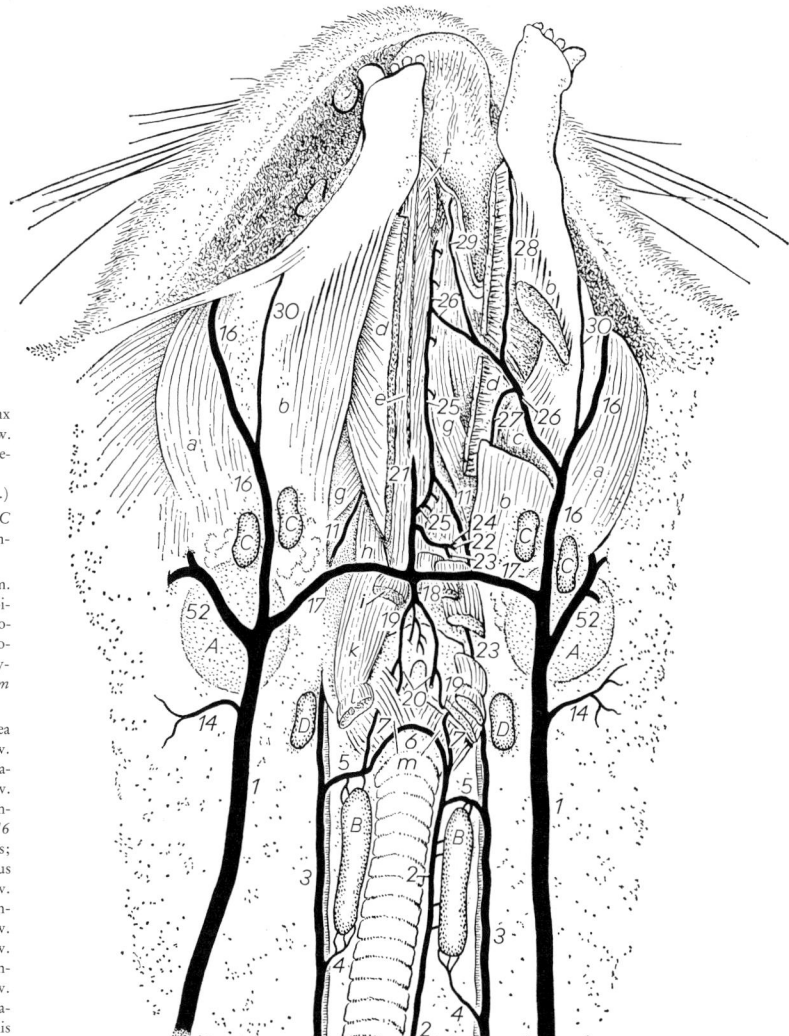

Fig. 181. Veins of the tongue, larynx and thyroid of the cat. Ventral view. Left mandible has been displaced laterally.
(After Frenzel, 1967, Diss., Hanover.)

A gl. mandibularis; *B* gl. thyreoidea; *C* lnn. mandibulares; *D* lnn. retropharyngei

a m. masseter; *b* m. digastricus; *c* m. pterygoideus medialis; *d* m. mylohyoideus; *e* m. geniohyoideus; *f* m. genioglossus; *g* m. styloglossus; *h* m. hyoglossus; *i* m. sternohyoideus; *k* m. thyreohyoideus; *l* m. sternothyreoideus; *m* m. cricothyreoideus

1 v. jugularis externa; *2* v. thyreoidea caudalis; *3* v. jugularis interna; *4* v. thyreoidea media; *5* v. thyreoidea cranialis; *6* arcus laryngeus caudalis; *7* v. cricothyreoidea; *11* v. comitans a. lingualis; *14* v. sternocleidomastoidea; *16* v. facialis; *17* arcus venosus hyoideus; *18* v. laryngea impar; *19* r. laryngeus caudalis; *20* r. cricothyreoideus; *21* v. lingualis impar; *22* v. pharyngea ascendens; *23* v. laryngea cranialis; *24* v. palatina ascendens; *25* r. lingualis; *26* v. lingualis with transition into v. profunda linguae; *27* r. anastomoticus cum v. alveolari mandibulari; *28* v. submentalis; *29* v. sublingualis; *30* v. labialis mandibularis; *52* v. maxillaris

frenulum, the *v. superficialis ventralis linguae*. This vessel runs in a paramedian position along the ventral surface of the tongue to the apex, which it vascularizes.

V. submentalis
(cat: 176/16; 181/28; dog: 179/16; pig: 183/20; ox: 185/22; 186/30; horse: 180/16)

In the cat the **v. submentalis** leaves the lingual vein before the origin of the sublingual vein but in pigs, small ruminants and horses it originates from the latter, and in the dog and ox from the facial vein. The submental vein courses along the ventral surface of the mylohyoid muscle in the mandibular space passing towards the chin. At the chin it links up with the neighbouring veins and forms a network.

V. pharyngea ascendens
(cat: 181/22)

Only in the dog does the **v. pharyngea ascendens** arise from the lingual vein. In the cat it is a branch of the v. lingualis impar and its first part is also unpaired. In the pig it comes from the sublingual, in the ox from the occipital and in the horse from the cranial thyroid vein. The ascending pharyngeal vein of carnivores and pigs passes dorsally to the lateral pharyngeal wall. In the ox and horse this vein is rostrally directed and runs to the pharynx along a course which is determined by the site of its origin. It forms anastomoses with neighbouring veins and contributes to the formation of the *plexus pharyngeus*. In carnivores it also gives off the *v. laryngea cranialis* and the *v. palatina ascendens*.

V. laryngea cranialis
(cat: 181/*23*; pig: 183/*7*; ox: 186/*58*)

In carnivores the **v. laryngea cranialis** stems from the ascending pharyngeal, in the pig from the v. comitans a. carotidis externae, in the sheep from the linguofacial and in the ox from the cranial thyroid vein. This vein has not been described in the horse. The cranial laryngeal vein passes through the thyroid fissure to the larynx.

V. palatina ascendens
(cat: 181/*24*)

The **v. palatina ascendens** occurs only in carnivores. It arises from the ascending pharyngeal vein and runs dorsad to the soft palate. It participates in the formation of the palatine plexus.

V. facialis
(cat: 178/*17*; 181/*16*; dog: 179/*17*; pig: 182/*13*; 183/*32, 33*; sheep: 184/*16*; ox: 185/*23*; 186/*31*; horse: 180/*17*)

The **v. facialis** is the terminal branch of the linguofacial vein which goes to the face. The facial vein leaves the madibular space through either the inc. vasorum or the corresponding place on the ventral border of the body of the mandible. It runs caudal to the facial artery or, in the pig, caudal to one of the short facial vessels; this topographical relationship does not apply to small ruminants because there is no facial artery. On the facial surface the facial vein follows the cranial border of the masseter muscle dorsally. In the dog and ox the *v. submentalis* is first given off. In all domestic mammals it supplies the *v. labialis mandibularis*, which may be represented by both a superficial and a deep vessel in ruminants and which, also in ruminants, give rise to the *v. angularis oris*. In the horse the v. angularis oris and the *v. labialis maxillaris* leave the facial vein here and both the former vessels are linked in their initial portions with the *v. labialis mandibularis*. In the horse at the same level the facial vein receives the *v. buccalis* which protrudes at the rostral border of the masseter muscle. In carnivores the v. angularis oris leaves the facial vein a short distance after the origin of the mandibular labial vein. In the pig the facial vein is joined by the wide buccal vein at the level of the angle of the mouth and in this species the buccal vein usually gives off the v. angularis oris a short distance before its termination. Dorsal to the angle of the mouth the facial vein gives rise, except in the horse, to the *v. labialis maxillaris* from which, in the pig, the v. angularis oris arises and which in ruminants consists of a superficial and a deep vessel. The veins of the lips whose origins have been described above, namely the v. labialis mandibularis, v. angularis oris and the v. labialis maxillaris, branch and ramify as do their corresponding arteries.

At the rostral border of the masseter muscle the facial vein also gives rise to the *v. profunda facei*. In carnivores and ruminants the site of origin is at the level of the mandibular body whereas in the pig and horse it is ventral to the facial crest. In carnivores and ruminants this vein is directed dorsomedially; in the pig and horse it is caudomedially directed. Caudal to the infraorbital foramen the facial vein of carnivores gives off the *v. palpebralis inferior* which drains the lower eyelid. In all the domestic mammals the rostrally directed *v. lateralis nasi* goes to the lateral wall of the nose and the *v. dorsalis nasi* to the bridge of the nose. The *v. palpebralis inferior medialis* draining the lower eyelid arises between the nasal veins in the pig and distal to them in the ox. Finally, the *v. angularis oculi* is the terminal branch of the facial vein and it continues the course of that vessel around the medial angle of the eye and towards the frontal region.

In the frontal region the facial vein gives off the *v. frontalis* (*v. supratrochlearis*) which courses on the caudal part of the forehead along the border of the orbit. It anastomoses with the supraorbital vein or branches of the superficial temporal vein in a pattern which varies in the different species. Except in the pig, the horse and small ruminants the v. angularis oris anastomoses over the supraorbital border with the *v. ophthalmica externa dorsalis*. Thus the large *r. anastomoticus cum v. ophthalmica externa dorsali* becomes a connection between the facial vein and the veins of the orbit. The *v. palpebralis superior medialis* arises from the *v. angularis oculi* in all the domestic mammals; it supplies the upper eyelid from the medial angle of the eye. In the cat it also supplies the *v. palpebralis inferior medialis* which runs to the lower eyelid from the medial canthus of the eye.

V. profunda faciei
(cat: 178/*21*; dog: 179/*21*; pig: 182/*19*; 183/*34*; sheep: 184/*18*; ox: 185/*25*; 186/*18, 33, 35*; horse: 180/*21*)

The **v. profunda faciei** leaves the facial vein at the rostral border of the masseter muscle. Under cover of this muscle the vein continues, in the horse, ventrally along the facial crest, over the maxillary tuber to the pterygopalatine fossa. Along its course it forms the *plexus v. profundae faciei* in the ox and ventral to the malar tuber this latter plexus gives off the *r. labialis* to the *v. labialis maxillaris superficialis*. In the region of the malaris muscle, the plexus forms another stout anastomosis with the branches of the facial vein. In the horse the deep facial vein dilates to form the *sinus v. profundae faciei*. In carnivores the deep facial vein joins with the superficial temporal vein through the *r. anastomoticus cum. v. temporali superficiali* which runs in a convex curve to the temporal groove passing medial to the zygomatic arch and lateral over the periorbita. In the dog this anastomosing ramus supplies branches to the zygomatic gland and the upper molar teeth. The deep facial vein of carnivores also supplies the *r. anastomoticus cum v. ophthalmica externa ventrale* which unites with the ventral external ophthalmic vein in the periorbital region. In the pig and horse the deep facial vein itself forms the main drainage vessel for the ophthalmic sinus or plexus, as the case may be. In ruminants the deep facial vein receives the buccal vein in the region of the maxillary tuber and, furthermore, there are robust anstomoses to the masseteric branches of the maxillary or transverse facial veins in both ruminants and horses. The deep facial vein also gives off the *v. infraorbitalis*, except in the cat, and the *v. palatina descendens* or, in the pig, the *v. sphenopalatina*. In the cat only the *r. infraorbitalis* arises in this area. This ramus crosses the floor of the orbit without, at first, giving rise to any dental rami but then it also passes through the short infraorbital foramen. This infraorbital ramus participates in the vascularization of the nose and upper lip.

V. infraorbitalis
(cat: 178/*24*; dog: 179/*24*; pig: 183/*52, 52'*; sheep: 184/*24*; horse: 180/*24*)

In the cat the **v. infraorbitalis** arises from the pterygoid plexus of the maxillary vein. It then runs laterally along the pterygoid process, across the floor of the orbit and, with the infraorbital ramus of the deep facial vein, passes through the infraorbital canal. In none of the domestic mammals does the first part of the infraorbital vein follow the infraorbital artery. The infraorbital artery is a branch of the maxillary artery but the vein is a terminal branch of the deep facial vein. In its subsequent course however, it accompanies the infraorbital artery through the infraorbital canal onto the surface of the face and participates in the vascularization of the nose and upper lip. It sends the *rr. dentales* to the upper teeth. In the dog it gives off the *v. malaris* with branches to the third eyelid and the lacrimal gland and it then anastomoses with veins of the lower eyelid.

V. palatina descendens
(cat: 178/*26*; dog: 179/*26*; sheep: 184/*22*; horse: 180/*26*)

The **v. palatina descendens** is, except in pigs, the second terminal branch of the deep facial vein and it in turn divides in the pterygopalatine fossa into three veins, the v. palatina minor and major and the v. sphenopalatina. In the pig the sphenopalatine vein is the second terminal branch of the deep facial vein, while the descending palatine and the buccal veins are the two terminal branches of the maxillary vein. The descending palatine vein in the pig thus divides into only the minor and major palatine veins.

The *v. palatina minor* supplies the soft palate. The *v. palatina major* runs, parallel to the artery, through the palatine canal only in the small ruminants. In the other domestic mammals a small branch

226 Veins

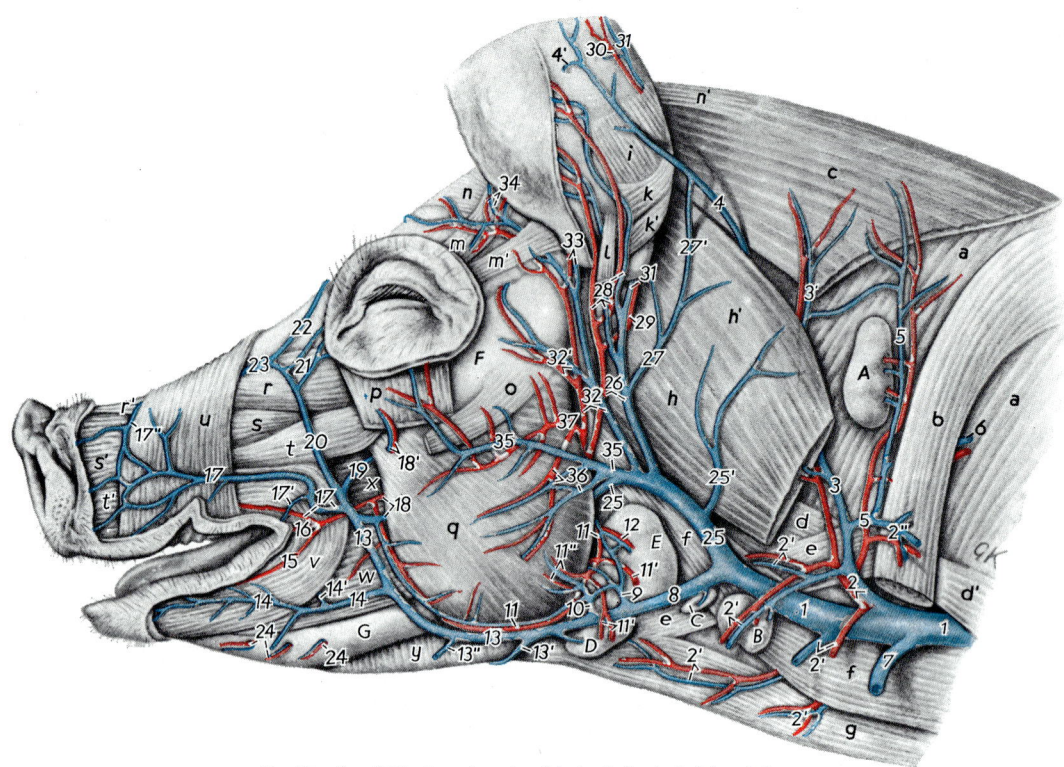

Fig. 182. Superficial veins and arteries of the head of a pig. Left lateral view.
(After Becker, 1960, Diss., Hanover.)

A ln. cervicalis superficialis dorsalis; *B* ln. cervicalis superficialis ventralis; *C* ln. mandibularis accessorius; *D* ln. mandibularis; *E* gl. mandibularis; *F* arcus zygomaticus; *G* mandibula

a m. serratus ventralis cervicis; *b* m. subclavius; *c* m. trapezius, pars cervicalis; *d* m. longus capitis; *d'* m. longus colli; *e* m. omohyoideus; *f* m. sternomastoideus; *g* m. sternohyoideus; *h* m. cleidomastoideus; *h'* m. cleido-occipitalis; *k* m. cervicoauricularis profundus major; *k'* m. cervicoauricularis profundus minor; *l* m. auricularis ventralis; *m, m'* m. frontoscutularis; *n* m. interscutularis; *n'* m. cervicoscutularis; *o* m. zygomaticus; *p* m. malaris; *q* m. masseter; *r, r'* m. levator labii maxillaris; *s, s'* m. caninus; *t, t'* m. depressor labii maxillaris; *u* m. levator nasolabialis; *v* m. orbicularis oris; *w* m. depressor labii mandibularis; *x* m. buccinator; *y* m. mylohyoideus

1 v. jugularis externa; *2* a. and v. cervicalis superficialis, *2"* r. acromialis, *3, 3'* r. ascendens, *4* r. auricularis, *5* r. praescapularis; *7* v. cephalica; *8* v. linguofacialis; *9* v. glandularis; *11* a. facialis; *12* rr. glandulares; *13* v. facialis; *13'* arcus hyoideus, origin of the v. lingualis obscured; *14* v. labialis mandibularis; *15* a. labialis mandibularis; *16* a. angularis oris; *17* a. and v. labialis maxillaris; *17'* v. angularis oris; *17"* v. lateralis nasi; *18* a. and v. buccalis; *19* v. profunda faciei; *20* v. facialis before its transition into the v. angularis oculi; *21* v. palpebralis inferior medialis and v. palpebralis superior medialis; *22* v. frontalis; *23* v. dorsalis nasi; *24* aa. and vv. mentales; *25* v. maxillaris; *25'* v. sternocleidomastoidea; *26* a. and v. auricularis caudalis; *27* r. muscularis with *27'* r. anastomoticus of the v. auricularis caudalis; *28* r. and v. auricularis lateralis; *29* a. auricularis caudalis; *30* r. auricularis intermedius; *31* v. auricularis intermedia; *32* a. and v. temporalis superficialis; *33* a. and v. to the inner surface of the outer ear; *34* a. and v. auricularis rostralis; *35* v. transversa faciei; *36* a. and v. masseterica dorsalis; *37* a. transversa faciei

may accompany the artery but the main part of the vein passes over the ventral border of the pterygopalatine fossa into the palatine groove. Its branches form a tight venous network in the mucosa of the hard palate and this network anastomoses with the venous nets of the nasal cavity in the region of the palatine fissure. The *v. sphenopalatina* passes through the sphenopalatine foramen into the caudal part of the nasal cavity and the branches of this vein also form extensive venous networks in the mucosa of the septum and conchae.

V. maxillaris

(cat: 178/*36*; 181/*52*; dog: 179/*36*; pig: 177/*4*; 182/*25*; 183/*24*; sheep: 184/*11*; ox: 151/*30*; 185, 186/*2*; horse: 152/*30*; 180/*36*)

The **v. maxillaris** and the linguofacial vein are the two terminal branches of the external jugular. They arise caudoventral to the parotid gland or, in carnivores, caudal to the mandibular gland. The maxillary

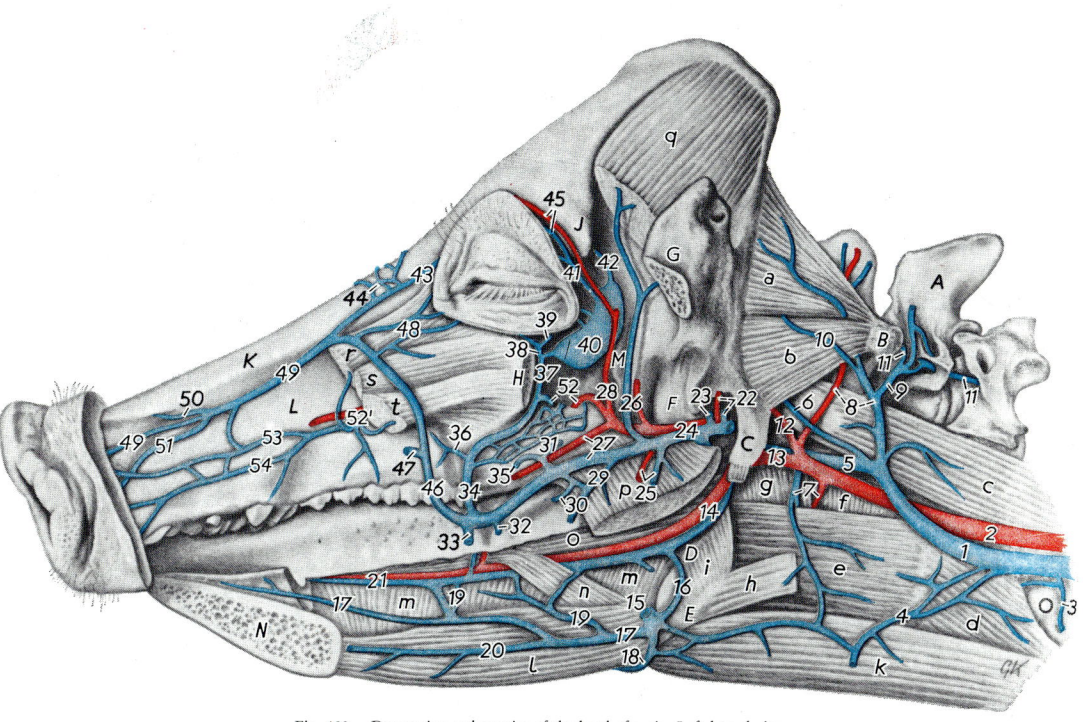

Fig. 183. Deep veins and arteries of the head of a pig. Left lateral view.
(After Becker, 1960, Diss., Hanover.)

A proc. spinosus of the axis; *B* ala atlantis; *C* proc. jugularis (with tendon of origin of the m. biventer mandibulae); *D* stylohyoideum; *E* thyreohyoideum; *F* bulla tympanica; *G* proc. zygomaticus of the os temporale (cut off); *H* os zygomaticum (cut off); *J* proc. zygomaticus of the os frontale; *K* os nasale; *L* os maxillare; *M* crista pterygoidea; *N* mandibula; *O* gl. thyreoidea

a m. obliquus capitis cranialis; *b* m. rectus capitis ventralis; *c* m. longus capitis; *d* m. sternothyreoideus; *e* m. hyothyreoideus; *f* m. cricopharyngeus; *g* m. thyreopharyngeus; *h* m. omohyoideus; *i* m. stylohyoideus; *k* m. sternohyoideus; *l* m. geniohyoideus; *m* m. genioglossus; *n* m. hyoglossus; *o* m. styloglossus; *p* m. pterygoideus medialis; *q* m. temporalis; *r* m. levator labii maxillaris; *s* m. caninus; *t* m. depressor labii maxillaris

1 v. jugularis interna; *2* a. carotis communis; *3* v. thyreoidea cranialis; *5* v. comitans a. carotidis externae; *6* v. emissaria foraminis jugularis; *7* a. and v. laryngea cranialis; *8* a. and v. occipitalis; *9* r. ventralis of the v. vertebralis at the axis, anastomoses like r. anastomoticus cum v. occipitali at the atlas; *10* r. occipitalis; *11* v. vertebralis; *12* a. carotis interna; *13* a. carotis externa; *14* a. lingualis with v. comitans a. lingualis; *15, 16* v. lingualis; *17* v. sublingualis; *18* arcus hyoideus; *19* rr. anastomotici; *20* v. submentalis; *21* a. and v. profunda linguae; *22* a. and v. auricularis caudalis; *23* v. temporalis superficialis; *24* a. and v. maxillaris; *25* a. and v. alveolaris mandibularis; *26* a. and v. temporalis profunda; *27* a. buccalis and sinus pterygoideus with transition to the v. buccalis; *28* a. ophthalmica externa; *29* v. pterygoidea; *30* vv. pharyngeae; *31* v. emissaria foraminis orbitorotundi; *32* parallel vein to the v. facialis with branches to the m. masseter; *33* v. facialis; *34* v. profunda faciei; *35* v. palatina descendens; *37* transition of the v. profunda faciei into the sinus ophthalmicus; *38* v. ophthalmica externa ventralis; *39* v. conjunctivalis; *40* sinus ophthalmicus; *41* v. ophthalmica externa dorsalis; *42* v. supraorbitalis; *43* v. frontalis; *44* plexus venosus frontalis; *45* a. and v. lacrimalis; *46* v. facialis; *47* v. labialis maxillaris; *48* vv. palpebrales mediales; *49, 50* v. dorsalis nasi; *51, 53, 54* v. lateralis nasi; *52* a. palatina descendens and v. infraorbitalis; *52'* a. and v. infraorbitalis

vein runs in a dorsorostral direction to the retromandibular fossa passing laterally over the digastricus muscle except in the pig in which it runs laterally over the jugular process. In the cat it dips into the parotid gland but remains ventral to this in the dog. It is completely covered by the parotid gland in the pig and in ruminants it reaches the medial surface of the gland. In the horse it at first follows the caudal border of this gland, then perforates its lateral surface and passes through the gland at the caudal border of the ramus of the mandible. Laterally to the pterygoideus medialis muscle it forms the *plexus pterygoideus* except in the pig in which animal it dilates and forms the *sinus pterygoideus*. Only the parts of the network which lie against the base of the skull accompany the maxillary artery and in the dog and horse a slender venous branch may also pass through the alar canal. In the pig the pterygoid sinus, which lies immediately ventrolateral to the maxillary artery, is continued as the buccal vein. In the horse the pterygoid plexus divides into a bundle of veins which accompany the artery and a large vein which takes a more ventrolateral course to reach the rostral border of the ramus of the mandible and then continues as the buccal vein. There are numerous connections between the two parts of the network. In carnivores and pigs the initial part of the maxillary vein gives off the *v. sternocleidomastoidea* which, in company

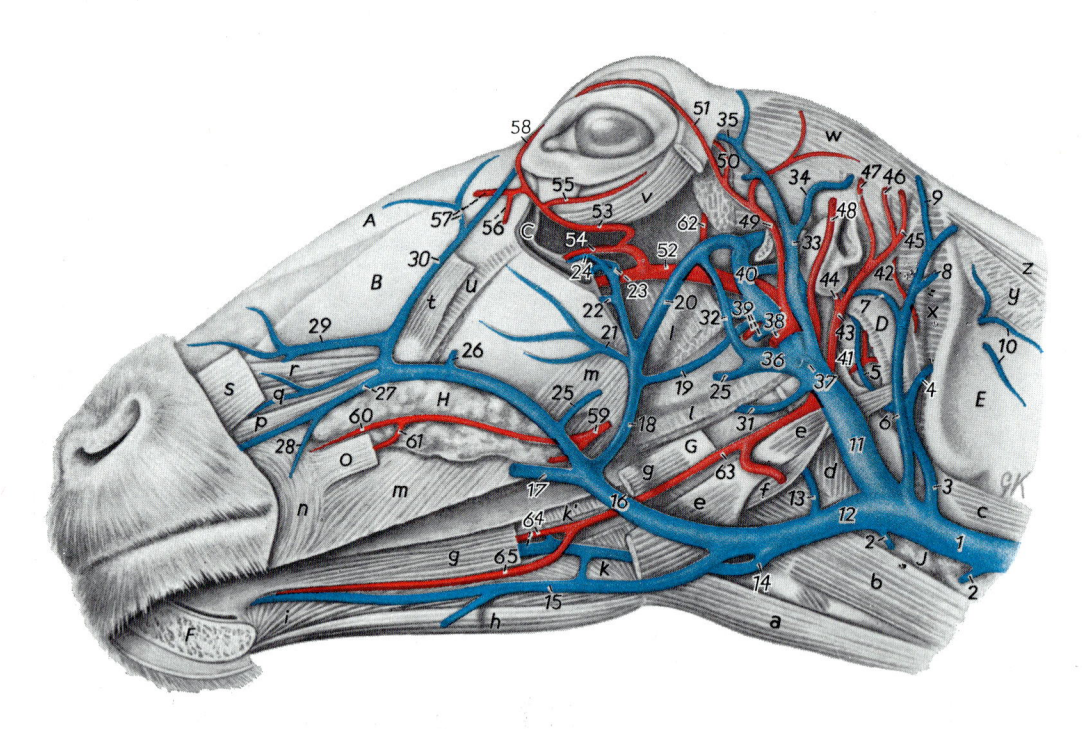

Fig. 184. Deep veins and arteries of the head of a sheep. Left lateral view.
(After Heeschen, 1958, Diss., Hanover.)

A os nasale; *B* os maxillare; *C* sinus maxillaris; *D* proc. jugularis; *E* ala atlantis; *F* mandibula; *G* os hyoideum; *H* gll. buccales dorsales; *J* gl. thyreoidea
a m. sternohyoideus; *b* m. sternothyreoideus; *c* cleidomastoideus; *d* mm. constrictores pharyngis caudales; *e* m. biventer mandibulae; *f* m. stylohyoideus; *g* m. styloglossus; *h* m. geniohyoideus; *i* m. genioglossus; *k, k'* m. hyoglossus; *l* m. pterygoideus; *m* m. buccinator; *n* m. orbicularis oris; *o* m. zygomaticus; *p* m. depressor labii maxillaris; *q* m. caninus; *r* m. levator labii maxillaris; *s* m. levator nasolabialis; *t* m. malaris; *u* m. masseter; *v* m. obliquus bulbi ventralis; *w* m. temporalis; *x* m. obliquus capitis cranialis; *y* m. obliquus capitis caudalis; *z* m. rectus capitis dorsalis major

1 v. jugularis externa; *2* vv. thyreoideae; *3* v. occipitalis; *4* r. anastomoticus; *5* v. emissaria foraminis jugularis; *6* v. auricularis caudalis; *7* v. stylomastoideus; *8* v. auricularis lateralis; *9* v. auricularis intermedia; *11* v. maxillaris; *12* v. linguofacialis; *13* v. laryngea cranialis; *14* v. lingualis; *15* v. sublingualis; *16* v. facialis; *17* v. labialis mandibularis; *18* v. profunda faciei; *19* v. buccalis; *20, 32* branches of the v. masseterica; *22* v. palatina descendens; *23* v. sphenopalatina; *24* v. infraorbitalis; *25, 36* masseterica ventralis; *26* v. palpebralis inferior medialis; *27* v. labialis maxillaris; *28* v. angularis oris; *29* v. lateralis nasi; *30* v. angularis oculi; *31* v. pharyngea; *32* branch of the v. masseterica; *33* v. temporalis superficialis; *34* v. auricularis rostralis; *35* v. ophthalmica externa dorsalis; *37* v. transversa faciei; *38, 59* a. transversa faciei; *39* a. and v. alveolaris mandibularis; *40* v. temporalis profunda; *41* a. occipitalis; *42* r. occipitalis; *43* a. auricularis caudalis; *44* a. stylomastoidea; *45* r. auricularis lateralis; *46* r. auricularis intermedius; *47* r. meningeus; *48* a. auricularis rostralis; *49* a. temporalis superficialis; *50* a. lacrimalis; *51* a. palpebralis superior lateralis; *52* a. maxillaris; *53* a. malaris; *54* a. infraorbitalis; *55* a. palpebralis inferior medialis; *56* a. lateralis nasi; *57* a. and v. dorsalis nasi; *58* a. palpebralis superior medialis; *60* a. labialis maxillaris; *61* a. angularis oris; *62* a. temporalis profunda; *63* a. lingualis; *64* a. and v. profunda linguae; *65* a. sublingualis

with other muscular branches, ramifies in the muscle of that name. In carnivores a *v. glandularis* to the mandibular gland is also derived from the maxillary vein. Shortly after its origin the maxillary vein of the horse gives off the *v. thyreoidea cranialis* and then, while still on the caudal border of the parotid gland and ventral to the wing of the atlas, the *v. occipitalis* (see p. 219). The *v. auricularis caudalis* arises from the maxillary vein of ruminants immediately at the latter's origin. In carnivores and pigs it originates at the level of the dorsal border of the mandibular gland and in the horse it usually appears shortly after the origin of the occipital vein. In some horses the occipital and caudal auricular veins may have a common origin. The caudal auricular vein lies laterally and superficially in the parotid gland and then runs dorsally, caudal to the base of the ear. In ruminants and horses the *v. masseterica ventralis* branches from the maxillary vein at the caudal border of the mandible and then follows, within the masseter muscle, the caudal border of the lower jaw in a rostral direction. Its branches generally anastomose with neighbouring veins in the masseter muscle but in the horse one particularly stout branch connects it with the buccal vein. Caudoventrally to the temporomandibular joint the maxillary vein gives off the *v. temporalis superficialis* which passes in a dorsal direction rostral to the base of the ear and lateral to the base of the zygomatic process. In the cat, and usually also in the horse, another separate vein is given off the maxillary vein rostroventrally to the base of the ear; this vessel corresponds to the deep branch of the caudal auricular vein of the other domestic mammals.

The following veins leave the pterygoid plexus or sinus in a sequence which varies in the different species:

The *v. masseterica* corresponds to the homonymous artery and ramifies in the masseter muscle.

The *vv. articulares temporomandibulares* run to the temporomandibular joint.

The *vv. pharyngeae* pass to the dorsal and lateral walls of the pharynx, except in the pig and carnivores where these veins are branches of the v. comitans a. carotidis externae (see p. 221).

The *vv. palatinae* are rostrally directed and pass into the palatine plexus. Only in the cat do these veins arise from the v. comitans a. carotidis externae.

The *v. alveolaris mandibularis* which enters the mandibular canal and then divides like the artery of the same name. It also gives off the *v. mentalis* or *vv. mentales* which link up with the veins of the chin region.

The *vv. temporales profundae* of carnivores, pigs and horses and the *v. temporalis profunda* of ruminants arise either as a cranial and caudal vessel, or alternatively, as a single trunk initially and they accompany the homonymous artery into the depth of the temporal fossa. There are links with their neighbouring veins of which the *r. anastomoticus cum plexu ophthalmico* of the horse should receive especial mention. Besides this there a connections through the skull to the diploic veins (*vv. diploica temporales et parietales*) and also to the sinus system.

The *r. sublingualis* of the horse accompanies the lingual nerve over the lateral aspect of the stylohyoideus and styloglossus muscles to the base of the tongue where it joins with the sublingual vein.

The *v. buccalis*, which in carnivores is only an insignificant slender vessel. In the pig it represents the rostral continuation of the wide pterygoid sinus. In this animal it passes round the rostral border of the masseter muscle and so moves onto the surface of the face to terminate in the facial vein a variable distance ventral to the origin of the deep facial vein. Shortly before its termination the buccal vein usually gives off the *v. angularis oris* and a connecting vein to the mandibular labial vein. In ruminants the buccal vein has only a short course and terminates in the transverse facial vein. In the horse the buccal vein stems from the stout ventrolateral vein of the pterygoid plexus, curves round the rostral border of the mandibular ramus where it dilates to form the sinus *v. buccalis* and then, becoming narrower again, it continues, overlaid laterally by the masseter muscle, in a rostral direction along the ventral border of the molar part of the buccinator muscle. At the level of the origin of the labial mandibular vein it ends in the facial vein. In the region of its sinus it receives the already-mentioned connecting branch from the ventral masseteric vein. Thereafter it gives off in a ventral direction the stout *r. labialis* which crosses the facial artery and vein medially to join with the labial mandibular vein. The *vv. pterygoidae* vascularize the lateral and medial pterygoid muscles.

The *v. infraorbitalis* of the cat (see p. 225).

The *v. palatina descendens* of the pig curves immediately caudal to the pterygopalatine fossa towards the hard palate (see p. 225). The *plexus ophthalmicus* of carnivores is the direct continuation of the pterygoid plexus in an orbital direction.

The *vv. emissariae* for the cranial cavity are: the *v. emissaria foraminis retroarticularis*, the *v. emissaria canalis carotici*, the *v. emissaria foraminis ovalis*, the *v. emissaria foraminis laceri* and the *v. emissaria foraminis rotundi*. These vessels pass through the appropriate foramina and make connections with the *sinus durae matris* (see vol. IV).

V. auricularis caudalis

(cat: 178/37; dog: 179/37; pig: 182/26; 183/22; sheep: 184/6; ox: 151/30'; 185/3, 5; 186/3; horse: 152/30'; 180/37)

From its origin out of the maxillary vein the **v. auricularis caudalis** courses in a caudodorsal direction to the base of the concha of the ear. Thence it continues ventral to the auricle in a medial curve round the ear, giving off branches to the temporalis muscle. In the cat these latter branches give rise to the *vv. diploicae parietalis*. The caudal auricular vein then joins with either the *v. auricularis rostralis* or with the *v. temporalis superficialis*. In the cat and horse the caudal auricular vein is often formed by the union of two vessels both of which stem from the maxillary vein. In the dog the caudal auricular vein receives a

230   Veins

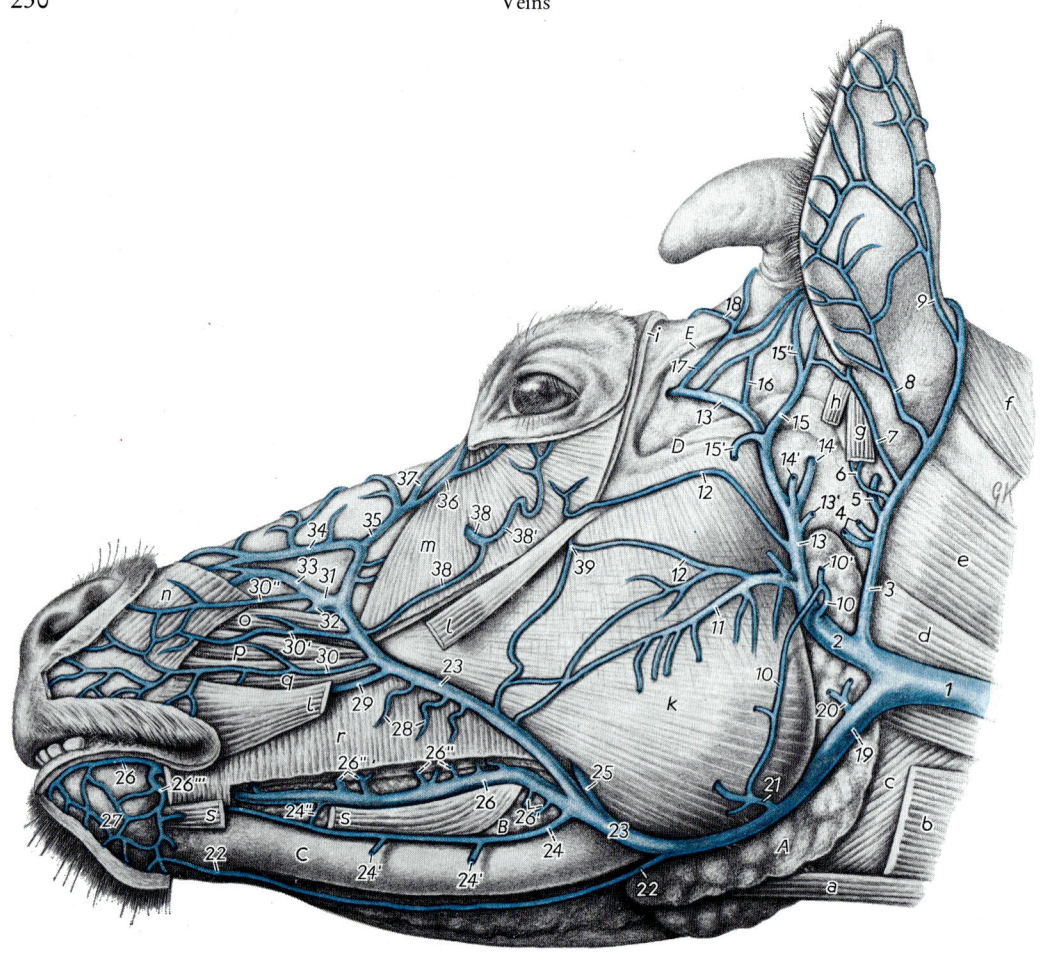

Fig. 185. Superficial veins of the head of an ox. Left lateral view.
(After Le Roux, 1959, Diss., Hanover.)

A gl. mandibularis; *B* gll. buccales ventrales; *C* mandibula; *D* arcus zygomaticus; *E* crista frontalis externa

a m. sternohyoideus; *b* m. sternomandibularis; *c* m. omohyoideus; *d* m. sternomastoideus; *e* m. cleidomastoideus; *f* m. cleido-occipitalis; *g* m. auricularis ventralis; *h* m. zygomaticoauricularis; *i* m. cutaneus frontalis (cut surface); *k* m. masseter; *l* m. zygomaticus; *m* m. malaris; *n* m. nasolabialis; *o* m. levator labii maxillaris; *p* m. caninus; *q* m. depressor labii maxillaris; *r* m. buccinator; *s* m. depressor labii mandibularis

1 v. jugularis externa; *2* v. maxillaris; *3* v. auricularis caudalis; *4, 10', 13', 14', 15', 20* vv. glandulares et rr. parotidei; *5* v. auricularis caudalis, running around the base of the ear; *7* vein to the inner surface of the ear trumpet; *8* v. auricularis lateralis; *9* v. auricularis intermedia; *10, 11* v. masseterica ventralis; *12* v. transversa faciei; *13* v. temporalis superficialis; *14* v. emissaria foraminis retroarticularis; *15* v. auricularis rostralis; *15''* branch to the base of the horn; *17* v. cornualis; *18* anastomosis to *37*; *19* v. linguofacialis; *21* r. massetericus; *22* v. submentalis; *23* v. facialis; *24* v. labialis mandibularis superficialis; *25* v. profunda faciei; *26* v. labialis mandibularis profunda; *27* plexus mentalis; *29, 32* v. labialis maxillaris profunda; *30* v. labialis maxillaris superficialis; *30', 30'', 33* vv. laterales nasi; *34* v. dorsalis nasi; *35* v. angularis oculi; *36* vv. palpebrales mediales; *37* v. frontalis; *38* anastomosis with the plexus v. profundae faciei; *38'* branch to the lower eye lid; *39* anastomosis with the v. masseterica

stout anastomosis from the stylomastoid vein and in both carnivores and pigs it gives off a *r. muscularis* to those superficial muscles of the neck nearest the head. In the pig this muscular ramus anastomoses especially with the auricular ramus of the superficial cervical vein. Caudoventrally to the base of the ear the caudal auricular vein of carnivores, pigs and horses gives off the *rr. parotidei* to the parotid gland and of ruminants it gives off the *vv. glandulares* to the parotid and mandibular glands. In dogs and ruminants the caudal auricular vein gives rise to the *v. stylomastoidea* which passes through the stylomastoid foramen to the tympanic cavity. This latter vessel arises in pigs and horses from the occipital vein (see p. 219). Thereafter the caudal auricular vein gives off the *v. auricularis lateralis*, except in the cat, and the *v. auricularis intermedia* which course along either the lateral border or the middle part of the external ear towards its tip. The intermediate auricular vein, running parallel with the artery, often forks into two branches in the pig. In the pig the supply area of this vein receives another

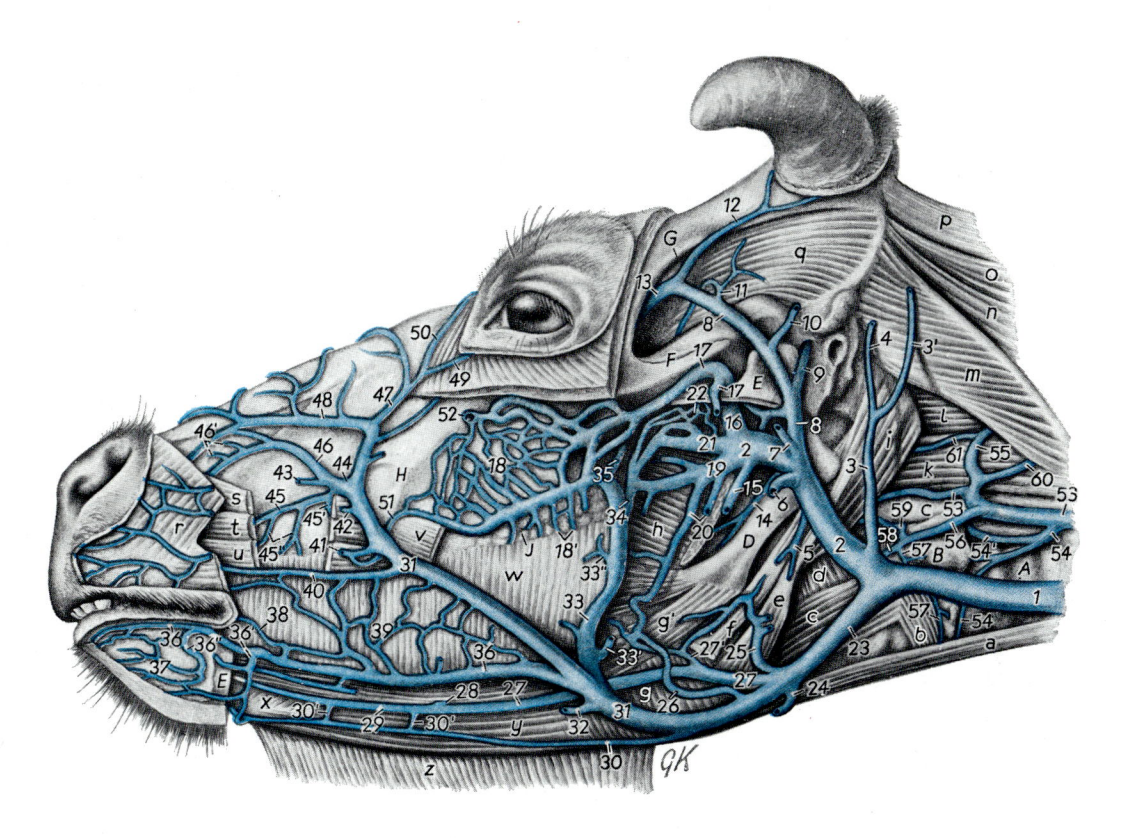

Fig. 186. Deep veins of the head of the ox. Left lateral view.
(After Le Roux, 1959, Diss., Hanover.)

A trachea; *B* gl. thyreoidea; *C* oesophagus; *D* stylohyoideum; *E* mandibula; *F* arcus zygomaticus; *G* crista frontalis externa; *H* tuber malare; *J* gll. buccales dorsales

a m. sternohyoideus; *b* m. cricothyreoideus; *c* m. hyothyreoideus; *d* m. thyreopharyngeus; *e* m. stylohyoideus; *f* m. digastricus; *g* m. hyoglossus; *g'* m. styloglossus; *h* m. pterygoideus medialis; *i* m. occipitostyloideus; *k* m. longus capitis; *l* m. rectus capitis lateralis; *m* m. obliquus capitis cranialis; *n* m. rectus capitis dorsalis minor; *o* m. rectus capitis dorsalis major; *p* lig. nuchae; *q* m. temporalis; *r* m. nasolabialis; *s* m. levator labii maxillaris; *t* m. caninus; *u* m. depressor labii maxillaris; *v* m. masseter; *w* m. buccinator; *x* m. genioglossus; *y* m. geniohyoideus; *z* m. mylohyoideus

1 v. jugularis externa; *2* v. maxillaris; *3* v. auricularis caudalis; *3'* v. auricularis lateralis; *4* continuation of *3* around tha base of the ear; *5* r. pterygoideus; *6* v. masseterica ventralis; *7* v. transversa faciei; *8* v. temporalis superficialis; *9* v. emissaria foraminis retroarticularis; *10* v. auricularis rostralis; *12* v. cornualis; *13* transition to the v. ophthalmica externa dorsalis; *14* v. pharyngea; *15* v. alveolaris mandibularis; *16* v. temporalis profunda; *17* v. masseterica with connection to *18* plexus v. profundae faciei; *19–22* plexus pterygoideus; *23* v. linguofacialis; *24* r. massetericus; *25, 26, 27'* rr. pterygoidei; *27* v. lingualis; *28* r. dorsalis linguae; *29* v. sublingualis; *30* v. submentalis; *31* v. facialis; *32* v. labialis mandibularis superficialis; *33* v. profunda faciei; *33'* r. massetericus; *34* v. buccalis; *35* v. profunda faciei before its subdivision in the pterygopalatine fossa; *36* v. labialis mandibularis profunda; *37* plexus mentalis; *38* v. angularis oris; *40, 45* vv. labiales maxillares profundae; *41* v. labialis maxillaris superficialis; *42, 43, 46* vv. laterales nasi; *47* v. angularis oculi; *48* v. dorsalis nasi; *49* vv. palpebrales mediales; *50* v. frontalis; *51* r. labialis of *18*; *52* anastomosis to a branch of the v. facialis; *53* v. jugularis interna; *54* v. thyreoidea media; *54'* r. oesophageus; *55* v. occipitalis; *56, 57* v. thyreoidea cranialis; *58* v. laryngea cranialis; *59* r. pharyngeus; *60* r. anastomoticus cum v. occipitali of the v. vertebralis; *61* r. muscularis

and considerably stouter *r. auricularis* of the ascending ramus of the superficial cervical vein which anastomoses in a very variable manner with the neighbouring veins. The caudal auricular vein gives rise to the *v. auricularis medialis* only in the horse and this vessel runs along the medial border of the ear to its tip.

V. temporalis superficialis
(cat: 178/*42*; dog: 179/*42*; pig: 182/*32*; 183/*23*; sheep: 184/*33*; ox: 185/*13*; 186/*8*; horse: 180/*42*)

The **v. temporalis superficialis** passes over the base of the zygomatic process of the temporal bone to reach the lateral aspect of the temporal muscle. It makes a curve to gain the zygomatic process of the frontal bone. With certain variations depending on the different species, it gives off branches to the parotid gland. In the cat the *v. auricularis lateralis,* which drains the lateral border of the external surface of the outer ear, and the *v. auricularis profunda,* which is distributed in the wall of the external auditory meatus, are given off here. The *v. transversa faciei* is not developed in the cat but in the other species it arises from the superficial temporal vein a variable distance ventral to the zygomatic arch. In the horse the transverse facial vein is embedded in the masseter muscle; sometimes it is distended to form the *sinus transversus faciei* in this animal. The transverse facial vein accompanies, and branches in a similar manner to, the artery and in ruminants and horses it joins the facial vein at the rostral border of the masseter. In ruminants it gives off the *v. palpebralis inferior lateralis*. In the pig too, this vessel sometimes arises from the transverse facial but generally it is the next branch of the superficial temporal. The *v. emissaria foraminis retroarticularis* stems from the superficial temporal in the ox but in the other domestic mammals it generally originates from the pterygoid plexus. Thereafter the superficial temporal vein gives off the *v. auricularis rostralis* which in ruminants and horses is the vessel of origin of the *v. auricularis profunda*. The latter is the sole terminal branch of the rostral auricular vein in the horse and, in both the ruminant and the horse, it is distributed on the inner surface of the outer ear and the external auditory meatus to its inner limits. The rostral auricular vein of the pig has two additional branches to the inner surface of the auricle and these extend towards the tip of the ear. Except in the horse, the *v. auricularis medialis* forms the continuation of the rostral auricular vein. The former follows the medial border of the auricle to the tip of the ear. The *v. palpebralis superior lateralis* is another branch of the superficial temporal vein of pigs and ruminants; it drains the upper eyelid. In horned ruminants the *v. cornualis* to the base of the horn is yet a further branch of this vessel. Finally numerous muscular branches of the superficial temporal vein are distributed in the temporal muscle and in carnivores the vein is continued, medial to the orbital ligamtnt, to the deep facial vein via the stout *r. anastomoticus*. In carnivores there is also a *r. anastomoticus cum plexu ophthalmico*. In the ruminants the superficial temporal vein goes directly into the *v. ophthalmica externa dorsalis*.

Plexus ophthalmicus and Sinus ophthalmicus
(cat: 178/59, 60; dog: 179/59; pig: 183/37, 38, 40; sheep: 184/35; ox: 186/13; horse: 180/59, 60)

The **plexus ophthalmicus** consists of the *v. ophthalmica externa dorsalis* and the *v. ophthalmica externa ventralis* as well as their numerous interconnecting anastomoses. In the pig these veins show sinus-like dilatations and together they appear as a uniform sinus ophthalmicus in which the walls of what were originally neighbouring vessels have been reduced to mere bridges of tissue. Surrounded by the periorbita, the two external ophthalmic veins run one dorsal and the other ventral to the cone of ocular muscles. The ventral external ophthalmic vein also penetrates this cone to some extent. The two veins unite towards the periorbital apex and they communicate with the sinus cavernosus, in carnivores and horses via the v. emissaria fissurae orbitalis and in pigs and ruminants via the v. emissaria foraminis orbitorotundi. The drainage area of the two ophthalmic veins corresponds to the supply area of the external ophthalmic artery.

Apart from these communications with the intracranial sinus system, there are other connecting vessels which perforate the periorbite and reach the cranial veins lying in the neighbourhood of the orbit. These include the following.

(1) In carnivores, the pterygoid plexus of the maxillary vein which passes into the ophthalmic plexus near the apex of the periorbita.

(2) In carnivores, pigs and horses, the deep facial vein which, after giving off its branches in the pterygopalatine fossa, anastomoses with the ventral external ophthalmic vein. This is the most important connection in the pig and horse.

(3) In carnivores and the ox, the angularis oculi vein which anastomoses dorsal to the medial angle of the eye with the dorsal external ophthalmic vein.

(4) In the pig, the v. frontalis which is linked with the supraorbital vein and therefore with the ophthalmic plexus.

(5) In carnivores and ruminants, the superficial temporal vein which in ruminants passes directly into the dorsal external ophthalmic vein.

In pigs, ruminants and horses the *v. supraorbitalis* (which is absent in carnivores) arises from the ophthalmic sinus or plexus. This vein also perforates the periorbita, passes through the supraorbital canal or foramen and is disseminated, like the supraorbital artery, on the dorsal part of the forehead and nose. In the pig it makes the already-mentioned connection with the frontal vein. In carnivores, on the other hand, the *v. diploica frontalis* arises from the plexus which links with the diploic vein through an opening which in the cat lies caudal and in the dog rostral to the zygomatic process of the frontal bone. The *v. ethmoidalis externa* also leaves the ophthalmic plexus or sinus, perforates the periorbita and passes, in company with the artery, through the ethmoid foramen into the cranial cavity to the lamina cribrosa. It also connects with the sinus system. Further connections between the ophthalmic plexus or sinus and the veins outside the orbit are established by these veins.

Apart from branches to the ocular muscles, the ophthalmic plexus or sinus also supplies veins to the bulbus oculi and its accessory organs. These are the vv. vorticosae, vv. ciliares, vv. conjunctivales, v. lacrimalis and, except in the dog, the v. malaris. The four *vv. vorticosae* turn towards the four quadrants of the eye where, in the equatorial region, they contribute a ray-like system of veins to the choroid. The *vv. ciliares* behave like the arteries and form the *plexus venosus sclerae*. The *vv. conjunctivales* are disseminated in the conjunctive. The *v. lacrimalis* is dorsally directed and drains the lacrimal glands. The *v. malaris*, in the dog a branch of the infraortibal vein, perforates the periorbita, curves round the margo infraorbitalis and branches in the lower eyelid. In the pig it also ramifies in the upper eyelid and the surface of the face. In the pig and ruminant the *v. palpebrae tertiae* to the nictitating membrane and the accessory lacrimal gland also arises from the malar vein.

Vena cava caudalis
(Comparative: 149–152/*35*; 187; 190–193, 212–215/*1*; cat: 194/*1*; pig: 97/*10*; 111/*3*; 153/*44*; 188/*9*; goat: 154/*26*; sheep: 189, 195/*1*; ox: 144/*d*; 155/*22*; 196/*1*; horse: 103/*36*; 104/*9*; 197/*1*; 211/*8*)

The **v. cava caudalis** arises from the caudal part of the sinus venosus of the right atrium. It runs in the plica venae cavae through the right pleural cavity to the for. venae cavae in the tendinous centre of the diaphragm. As it enters the abdominal cavity it turns dorsad between the right crus and the liver. In so doing it creates an impression, the sulcus venae cavae, on the diaphragmatic surface of the liver which varies in depth according to species and individual. It passes over the dorsal border of the liver, at first still applied to the diaphragmatic crus, to reach a location ventral to the vertebral column and to the right of the abdominal aorta. It follows the aorta in a caudal direction along the lumbar vertebral column. The final bifurcation of the caudal vena cava into the two *vv. iliacae communes* lies at the level of the 6th to 7th lumbar vertebrae in the cat. In the dog, pig and small ruminants the bifurcation is at the 6th and in the horse at the 5th lumbar vertebra whereas in the ox it is at the level of the 1st sacral vertebra. From the angle of bifurcation or from the one of the two common iliac veins, arises the *v. sacralis mediana*. In the horse this latter is either absent or only a slender vessel.

The caudal vena cava gives off the following vessels: vv. phrenicae craniales, v. phrenica caudalis, in carnivores and pigs the v. abdominalis cranialis, the vv. lumbales and, except in the pig, the v. circumflexa ilium profunda. The visceral branches of the caudal vena cava are the vv. hepaticae, the v. renalis, the v. testicularis or v. ovarica and, in the ox and horse, the vv. suprarenales.

Vv. phrenicae craniales
(Comparative: 149–152/*36*; pig: 97/*11*, *12*, *13*, *33*, *34*; horse: 103/*37*; 104/*10*)

The **vv. phrenicae craniales** leave the caudal vena cava in the vena caval foramen of the tendinous centre of the diaphragm. Each of these cranial phrenic veins gives rise to a laterally directed vessel to the costal and sternal parts of the diaphragm. Other veins to the crura medialia of the lumbar part arise in a dorsal direction from the laterally directed veins or from the vena cava itself. These veins are given off singly or in groups depending on the species and they form anastomoses with the rr. phrenicae of the segmental vessels.

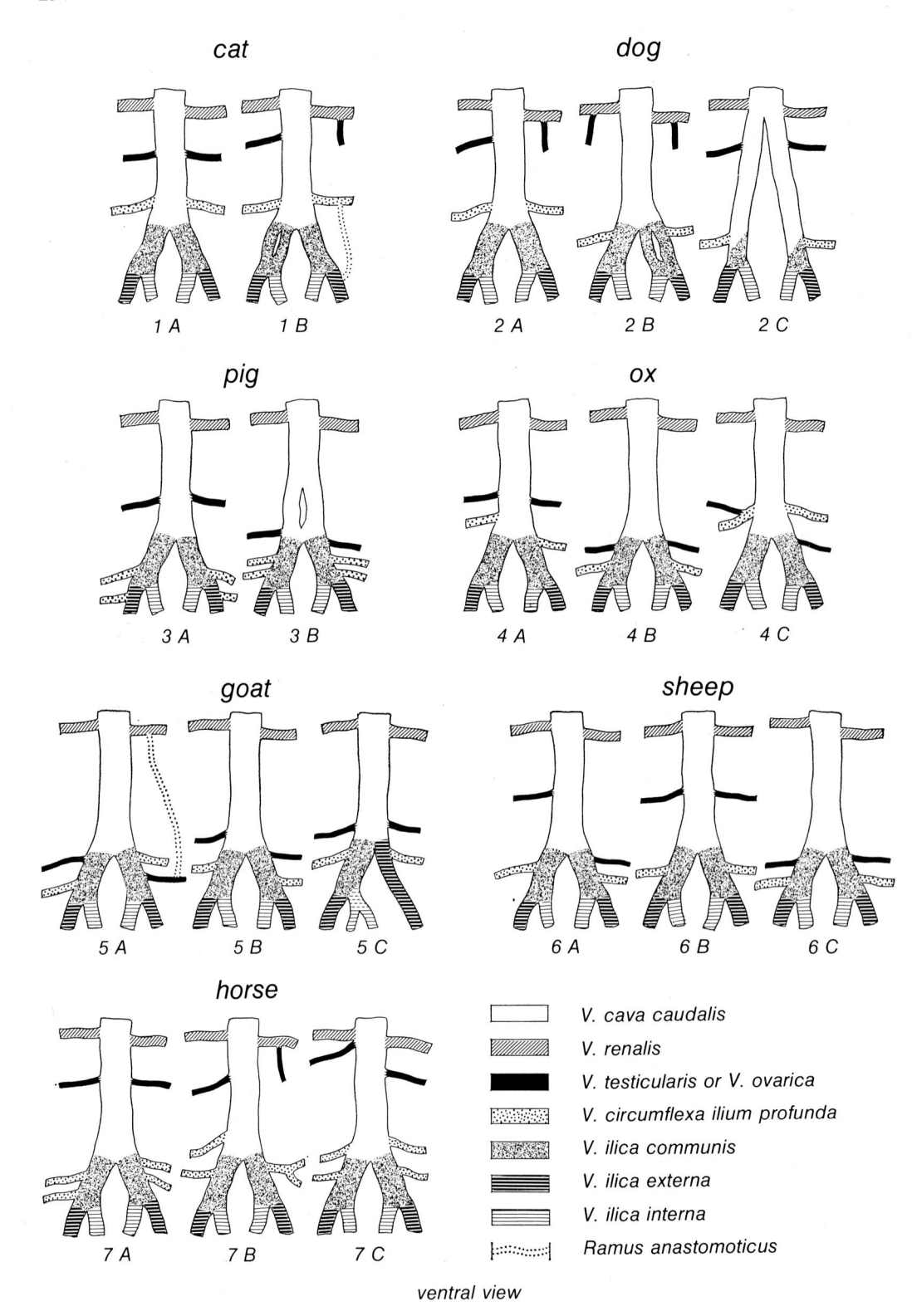

Fig. 187. Terminal sub-division of the caudal vena cava with its variations in the cat, dog, pig, ox, goat, sheep and horse. Diagrammatic. Ventral view. (After Schwarz and Badawi, 1962, work carried out at the Institute for Veterinary Anatomy, Hanover.)

V. phrenica caudalis
(Comparative: 149–152/39)

The **vena phrenica caudalis** arises, one on each side, from the caudal vena cava in the region of the crura of the diaphragm. In carnivores it has a common stem with the cranial abdominal vein. It vascularizes the lateral crus and, in carnivores, the crus intermedium. In exceptional cases in the cat the left vein may arise from the renal vein. In carnivores the caudal phrenic vein gives rise to the *rr. suprarenales craniales* to the adrenal gland.

V. abdominalis cranialis
(dog: 149/40; pig: 97/15; 150/40; 188/12)

In the pig the caudal vena cava gives off the **v. abdominalis cranialis** immediately caudal to the caudal phrenic vein. The cranial abdominal vein is absent in ruminants and horses and in carnivores it arises from a common stem with the caudal phrenic vein. The left cranial abdominal vein of the pig is a branch of the renal vein. The cranial abdominal vein branches in the same manner as the artery and it supplies the cranial part of the abdominal wall.

Vv. lumbales
(Comparative: 149–152/37; cat: 194/4; pig: 111/2, 2'; 188/13; sheep: 189/3–6; 195/7, 8; ox: 196/6; horse: 197/3)

Parent vessels of the Vv. lumbales

cat	I and II v. azygos dextra	III–VI v. cava caudalis		VII v. iliaca communis
dog	I and II, rarely III v. azygos dextra	III–V (VI) v. cava caudalis	VI v. circumflexa ilium profunda v. cava caudalis v. iliaca communis	VII v. cava caudalis v. sacralis mediana v. iliaca communis v. iliaca interna
pig	I–III v. azygos sinistra	(III) IV and V v. cava caudalis	VI and VII v. iliaca communis right: v. iliaca communis dextra left: v. cava caudalis v. sacralis mediana	
small ruminants	I–III common vessel of origin from the v. azygos	(III) IV and V (VI) v. cava caudalis	VI v. iliaca communis v. sacralis mediana	VII v. sacralis mediana (sheep)
ox	I and II (III) common vessel of origin from the v. azygos	III–V v. cava caudalis	VI v. iliaca communis v. iliaca interna	
horse		I–IV (V) v. cava caudalis	(V) VI v. iliaca communis	

Despite the fact that the **vv. lumbales** take their origin from several different veins, they will be described here as a group. The number of pairs of lumbar veins corresponds to the number of lumbar vertebrae. It is not only possible for the left and right vein of one segment to arise from a common stem, but also for veins of consecutive segments to have a common vessel of origin. Except in the horse, the cranial pairs of lumbar veins arise from the azygos vein, which itself is subject to species variation. The subsequent pairs of veins, and in the horse also the cranial pairs, originate from the caudal vena cava. The caudal lumbar veins stem from the bifurcating branches of the caudal vena cava. The species peculiarities of the lumbar veins are shown in the table. Each lumbar vein accompanies the corresponding artery in its cranial course and subdivides in unison and it, and the venous *r. dorsalis*, behaves like a dorsal intercostal vein.

V. circumflexailium profunda

(Comparative: 149–152/*41*; 187; 190–193, 212–215/4; cat: 194/3; pig: 111/6; 188/*16*; sheep: 189/7; 195/4; ox: 196/3; horse: 197/*41*)

A short distance before its final bifurcation the caudal vena cava gives rise to the **v. circumflexa ilium profunda**. This is often duplicated in carnivores, the ox and the horse. Species differences in the origin of this vessel are illustrated in fig. 187. Along with the homonymous artery this vein ramifies in the lateral abdominal wall, extending to the costal arch in ruminants and horses. In pigs and ruminants the *r. superficialis* of this vein's *r. caudalis* is particularly prominent and extends to the stifle fold where it anastomoses with the superficial caudal epigastric vein.

V. iliaca communis

(Comparative: 149–152/*51*; 187; 190–193, 212–215/3; cat: 194/5; pig: 111/*4*; 188/*15*; sheep: 189/*15*; 195/3; ox: 196/5; horse: 197/2)

The **vv. iliacae communes dextra** and **sinistra** form the terminal branches of the caudal vena cava. On each side of the body the common iliac gives off dorsally the last lumbar veins, namely the 5th in the horse, the 6th in pigs, cattle and horses and the 7th in carnivores. The deep circumflex iliac vein is given off to the lateral abdominal wall in the pig, ruminant and horse as well as the *v. iliolumbalis* in the horse. The *v. testicularis sinistra* arises from the common iliac in the male sheep and ox and the *v. ovarica sinistra* is given off in the female goat and ox. Each common iliac divides medial to the ilium into the *v. iliaca interna* and *externa*.

V. iliaca externa

(Comparative: 149–152/*52*; 187, 190–193/*12*; 212–215/5; cat: 194/*12*; pig: 111/*5*; 188/*26*; sheep: 189/*28*; 195/9; ox: 196/*14*; horse: 197/4)

The **v. iliaca externa** is the direct continuation of the common iliac and it runs along the shaft of the ilium to the lacuna vasorum, in the pig and ruminant passing between the two origins of the sartorius muscle. In the pig and horse it gives off the *v. ductus deferentis* in males and the *v. uterina* in females. In the horse it also gives rise to the *v. iliacofemoralis* and the *v. obturatoria* (see p. 258). Furthermore,

Fig. 188. Veins of the abdominal and pelvic cavities and of the abdominal wall of a pig. Ventral view.
(After Wolff, 1963, Diss., Hanover.)

A cartilago xiphoidea; *B* lnn. iliaci mediales; *C* lnn. iliaci laterales; *D* lnn. inguinales superficiales; *E* oesophagus

a m. pectoralis profundus; *b* m. cutaneus trunci; *c* m. rectus abdominis; *d* m. transversus abdominis; *e* diaphragma, centrum tendineun; *g* pars lumbalis, crus sinistrum, *g'* crus dextrum; *f* m. psoas major; *h* m. quadratus lumborum; *i* m. psoas minor; *k* m. iliacus; *l* m. obturatorius internus; *m* m. obliquus internus abdominis; *n* m. gracilis; *o* m. sartorius; *p* m. semimembranosus; *q* m. vastus medialis; *r* m. rectus femoris

1 v. epigastrica cranialis superficialis; *2* r. superficialis of *16*; *3* r. anastomoticus between *2* and *1*; *4* r. mammarius; *5* v. epigastrica caudalis superficialis; *6* branches to the lymph nodes; *6 '* r. anastomoticus; *7* vv. hepaticae, freed of hepatic parenchyma; *8* vv. intercostales dorsales; *9* v. cava caudalis; *10* v. renalis sinistra; *11* v. renalis dextra; *12* v. abdominalis cranialis; *13* vv. lumbales; *14* v. ovarica; *15* v. iliaca communis; *16* v. circumflexa ilium profunda; *16'* r. cranialis, *16"* r. caudalis; *17* v. sacralis mediana; *17'* rr. sacrales; *18* v. iliaca interna; *19* v. vaginalis; *20* v. pudenda interna; *21* v. perinealis ventralis; *22* v. bulbi vestibuli; *23* vv. dorsalis and profunda clitoridis; *24, 25* v. labialis dorsalis; *26* v. iliaca externa; *27* v. pudendoepigastrica; *28* v. epigastrica caudalis; *29* v. pudenda externa, *29'* v. labialis ventralis; *30* v. saphena medialis, *30'* rr. anastomotici; *31* v. epigastrica cranialis; *32* v. caudalis mediana, *32'* rr. caudales

Common iliac vein

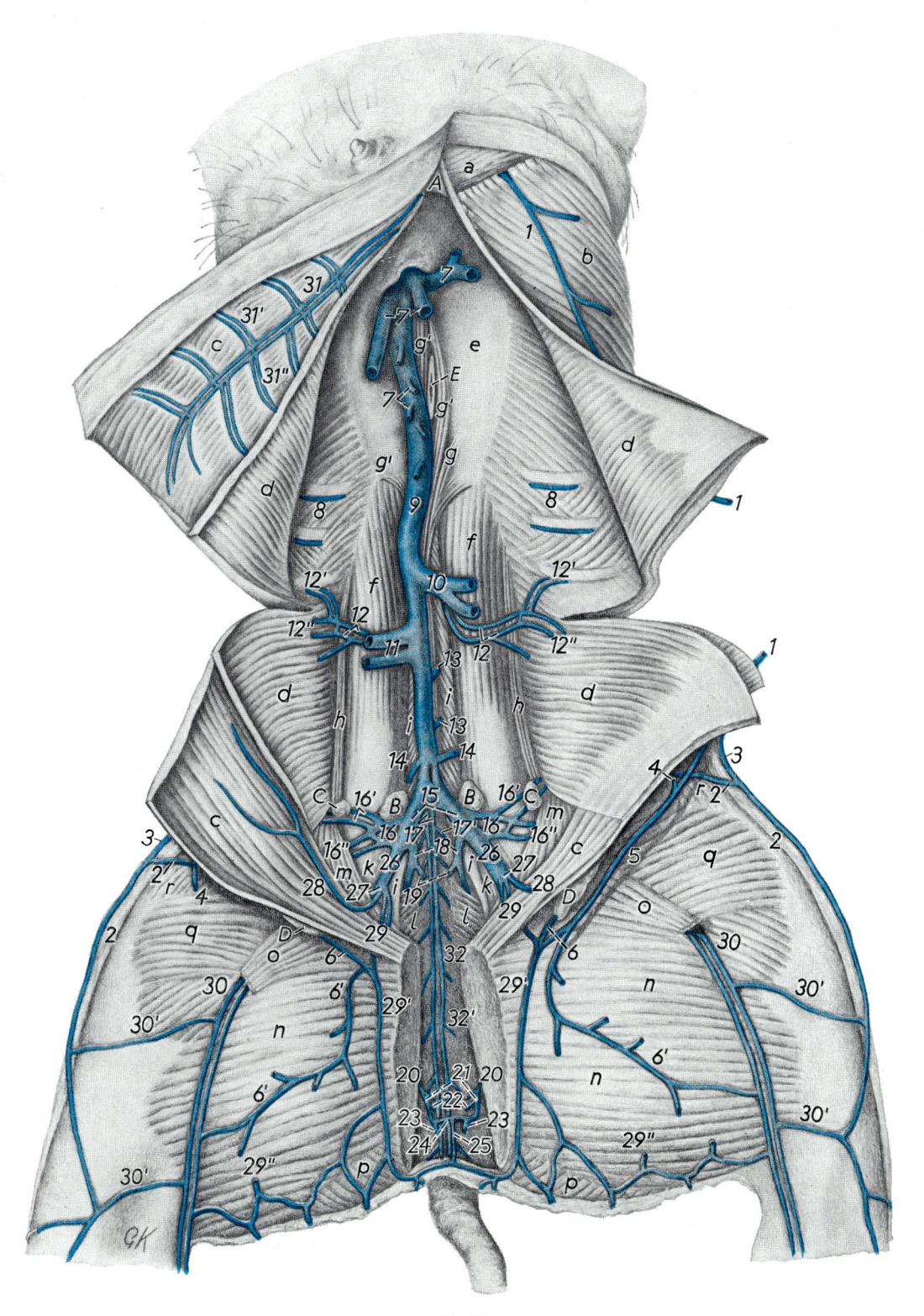

Fig. 188

shortly before its entry into the femoral canal, the external iliac of carnivores gives rise to the *v. abdominalis caudalis* and, in both carnivores and the ox, the *v. pudendoepigastrica*. The terminal branch vessels of the latter arise separately in the cat. At the entrance of the femoral canal the external iliac vein of all animals gives rise to the caudally-directed *v. profunda femoris*. Subsequently the external iliac is continued distally as the *v. femoralis*.

V. iliacofemoralis
(horse: 152/*53*; 193/*22'*; 215/*7*)

In the horse the **v. iliacofemoralis** is usually paired and arises from the external iliac vein, whereas the homonymous artery takes its origin from the obturator artery. Corresponding to the latter then, the iliacofemoral vein takes over the drainage area of the ascending ramus of the lateral circumflex femoral vein. In company with the artery the iliacofemoral vein courses cranial to the body of the ilium and along its lateral border. It divides into a laterally directed branch to the iliopsoas muscle and another branch to the tensor fasciae latae, the quadriceps femoris and, through the superficial gluteal muscle, to the biceps femoris.

V. profunda femoris
(Comparative: 149–152/*55*; 190–193/*17*; 212–215/*9*; cat: 194/*18*; pig: 111/*8*; sheep: 189/*30*; 195/*11*; ox: 196/*15*; horse: 197/*9*)

In all domestic mammals the **v. profunda femoris** arises from the external iliac proximal to the femoral canal and, except in carnivores and the ox, it gives off the *v. pudendoepigastrica*. Accompanied by the homonymous artery, the deep femoral vein passes between the pectineus and iliopsoas muscles to the adductors, thereafter giving off, in a caudal direction and distal to the hip joint, the *v. circumflexa femoris medialis*. In the dog the deep femoral vein continues distad as a large vessel which lies caudomedial to the femur and it gives off caudodistally directed muscular branches to the adductor muscles. These correspond to the initial part of the *vv. perforantes* of man; they ramify in the adductors but, except for one branch in the dog, they do not perforate the long ischiatic muscles.

V. pudendoepigastrica
(Comparative: 149–152/*57*; 190–193/*14*; 212–215/*10*; pig: 111/*9*; 188/*27*; sheep: 189/*31*; 195/*12*; ox: 196/*37*)

The **v. pudendoepigastrica** springs from the deep femoral, except in carnivores and the ox in which animals it has already arisen from the external iliac shortly before the latter enters the femoral canal. In ruminants the pudendoepigastric vein first gives off the *v. abdominalis caudalis* and then in this and the other domestic mammals except cats, it divides into the *v. epigastrica caudalis* and the *v. pudenda externa*. In the cat the caudal epigastric and external pudendal veins arise independently from the external iliac.

V. abdominalis caudalis
(cat: 194/*15*; dog: 149/*54*; 190/*13*; 212/*8*; sheep: 189/*32*; 195/*12'''*; ox: 151/*54*; 192/*13*; 214/*8*)

The **v. abdominalis caudalis** is invariably present only in the carnivore and the ox; it occasionally occurs in the small ruminants. In carnivores it arises from the external iliac, in the ox from the pudendoepigastric vein and in the small ruminants either from the latter or from the femoral vein. In the goat it can also branch from the external iliac vein. In carnivores it runs first medially over the internal oblique abdominis muscle and then between this and the transverse abdominis in a cranial direction. In the dog laterally directed branches reach as far as the external oblique abdominis. In small ruminants the caudal abdominal vein supplies only the internal oblique abdominis muscle but in the ox it also drains the transverse abdominis muscle. Anastomoses of this vessel with the caudal epigastric vein have been

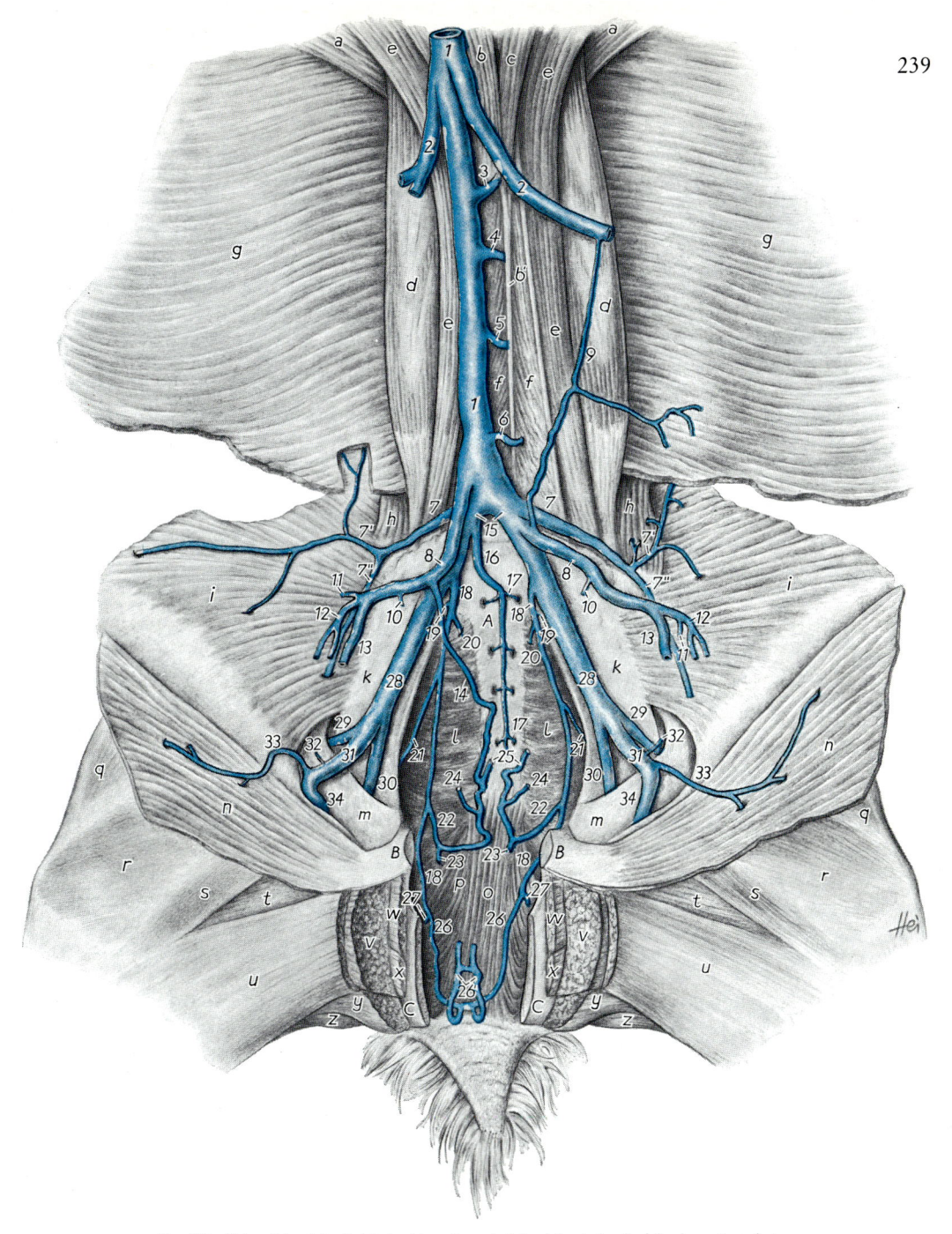

Fig. 189. Veins of the abdominal and pelvic cavity and of the abdominal wall of the sheep. Ventral view.
(After Rauhut, 1962, Diss., Hanover.)

A os sacrum; *B* ramus caudalis ossis pubis; *C* tabula ossis ischii

a m. retractor costae; *b, b', c* diaphragma, pars lumbalis: *b, b'* crus dextrum, *c* crus sinistrum; *d* m. quadratus lumborum; *e* m. psoas major; *f* m. psoas minor; *g* m. transversus abdominis; *h* m. iliocostalis lumborum; *i* m. obliquus internus abdominis; *k* fascia iliaca; *l* lig. sacrotuberale latum; *m* pelvic tendon of the m. obliquus externus abdominis; *n* m. rectus abdominis; *o* m. sacrocaudalis ventralis medialis; *p* m. sacrocaudalis ventralis lateralis; *q* m. tensor fasciae latae; *r* m. quadriceps femoris; *s* m. sartorius; *t* m. pectineus; *u* m. gracilis; *v* m. adductor; *w* mm. gemelli; *x* m. quadratus femoris; *y* m. semimembranosus; *z* m. semitendinosus

1 v. cava caudalis; *2* v. renalis; *3* common vessel of origin of the vv. lumbales I and II of the right and left side with the termination of the v. azygos sinistra; *4–6* common vessels of origin for the vv. lumbales III–V of both sides; *7* v. circumflexa ilium profunda, *7'* r. cranialis, *7"* r. caudalis; *8* v. ovarica; *9* r. anastomoticus between v. renalis sinistra and v. ovarica sinistra; *10* v. vesicalis cranialis; *11* r. tubarius, *12* terminal branches to the ovary; *13* r. uterinus of *8*; *14* r. anastomoticus between *8* and v. uterina caudalis dextra; *15* v. iliaca communis; *16* v. sacralis mediana; *17* rr. sacrales; *18* v. iliaca interna; *19* v. iliolumbalis; *20* v. glutaea cranialis; *21* v. obturatoria; *22* v. vaginalis; *23* v. rectalis media; *24* v. vesicalis caudalis; *25* r. uterinus; *26* v. pudenda interna; *26'* v. labialis dorsalis et mammaria; *27* v. glutea caudalis; *28* v. iliaca externa; *29* v. femoralis; *30* v. profunda femoris; *31* v. pudendoepigastrica; *32* v. abdominalis caudalis; *33* v. epigastrica caudalis; *34* v. pudenda externa

described in the cat, with the cranial abdominal vein in the dog and with the deep circumflex iliac vein in both the cat and the dog.

V. epigastrica caudalis
(Comparative: 149–152/*58*; 190–193/*15*; cat: 194/*16*; pig: 188/*28*; sheep: 189/*33*; 195/*12"*; horse: 197/*8*)

The **v. epigastrica caudalis** branches, while still within the abdominal cavity, from the pudendoepigastric vein. In the cat it sometimes arises from the external iliac vein. In company with the homonymous artery the caudal epigastric vein runs in a cranial direction along the dorsal surface of the rectus abdominis. It enters this muscle and in the dog, ox and horse, rarely in the pig, it unites with the cranial epigastric vein in the region of the umbilicus. In the ox and carnivores there are other anastomoses with the neighbouring veins of the body wall. The caudal epigastric vein of ruminants gives off the *v. cremasterica* which, like the artery of that name, follows the external cremaster muscle into the sheaths of the testis. In the dog this latter vein frequently originates from the pudendoepigastric vein.

V. pudenda externa
(Comparative: 149–152/*59*; 190–193/*16*; cat: 194/*13*; pig: 188/*29*; sheep: 189/*34*; 195/*12'*; horse: 197/*11*)

The **v. pudenda externa,** the second terminal branch of the pudendoepigastric vein, leaves the abdominal cavity through the inguinal canal. In the cat only, it gives off the *v. vesicalis media* to the ventral aspect of the bladder before leaving the abdomen. In male horses this vein, which passes through the inguinal canal in company with the external pudendal artery, is only slender. A thicker, additional vein arises independently from the deep femoral and passes, without arterial accompaniment, caudal to the pectineus muscle along the cranial part of the gracilis muscle to form a net-like distribution between the thighs. Like the artery, the external pudendal vein divides into the superficial caudal epigastric and the ventral scrotal veins or, in females, the ventral labial veins. In the horse it also gives rise to the cranial vein of the penis.

The *v. epigastrica caudalis superficialis* runs in a cranial direction along the superficial aspect of the ventral abdominal wall and joins with the superficial cranial epigastric vein. In the dog and ox there are also anastomoses with the superficial ramus of the deep circumflex iliac vein. The branches of the superficial caudal epigastric vein are distributed in the skin of the ventral abdominal wall and in males, as the *rr. preputiales,* in the prepuce. In females the *rr. mammaria* are distributed in the inguinal and abdominal mammary complexes. In the female of ruminants and horses this vein represents the *v. mammaria cranialis,* known as the milk vein, and it, together with the cranial superficial epigastric vein, transports a large proportion of the blood from the udder vessels to the cranial vena cava (see p. 195). Like the homonymous arterial branches, the *v. scrotalis ventralis* and *v. labialis ventralis* are distributed on the cranial and caudal surfaces of the scrotum or the labia of the vulva. There are certain modifications in distribution in the different species. In the female of ruminants and horses the ventral labial vein also forms the *v. mammaria caudalis.* In female ruminants this vein links up with the *v. labialis dorsalis et mammaria,* a branch of the ventral perineal vein, in the space between the thighs.

The *v. penis cranialis* of the horse is the stoutest vessel contributing to the formation of the *v. dorsalis penis.*

Veins of the pelvic limb

The v. profunda femoris has already been described as a branch of the v. iliaca externa (see p. 238).

V. circumflexa femoris medialis
(Comparative: 149–152/*56*; 190–193/*18*; pig: 111/*10*; sheep: 195/*13*; ox: 196/*17*; horse: 197/*10*)

The **v. circumflexa femoris medialis** is a branch of the deep femoral vein. It ramifies in the adductor and rotator muscles ventral to the pelvic floor and the hip joint down to the long ischiatic muscles. It gives rise to the *r. obturatorius* which passes cranially through the obturator foramen to those parts of the obturator muscles which lie in the pelvic cavity. In pigs and ruminants it anastomoses with the obturator vein. Thereafter the medial circumflex femoral vein gives off the acetabular, deep, ascending and the transverse (descending) branches in a sequence which varies with the species. The *r. acetabularis* goes to the hip joint and the rotator muscles. The current nomenclature of the other branches corresponds to that of man. The structural continuation of the medial circumflex femoral vein is the *r. profundus* which runs between the external obturator and the quadratus femoris muscles and anastomoses with the lateral circumflex femoral vein. The *r. ascendens* courses towards the ischiatic tuberosity and so supplies the adductors and the long muscles of the ischium. In the domestic mammals the largest branch of the medial circumflex femoral vein and, in fact, its functional continuation is known at present as the *r. transversus* but it would be more appropriately termed the *r. descendens*. It runs between the long ischiatic muscles towards the flexor aspect of the knee but its length varies with the species. Its branches are disseminated in the long ischiatic muscles and are most widespread in pigs and ruminants; in the dog the caudal branches of the deep femoral and in the horse the obturator vein are more involved in the supply of the long ischiatic muscles. The direct continuation of the transverse ramus in the pig and ruminant is the lateral saphenous vein (see. p. 248). In carnivores and horses the latter vein is a branch of the distal caudal femoral vein. In carnivores and ruminants the transverse ramus also anastomoses with the distal caudal femoral vein and in the horse this ramus is already linked to the obturator vein, ventral to the pelvic floor, and with the distal caudal femoral vein in the flexor aspect of the knee joint.

V. femoralis

(Comparative: 149–152/*62*; 190–193/*19*; cat: 194/*17*; pig: 111/*12*; sheep: 189/*29*; 195/*15*; ox: 196/*38*; horse: 104/*16*; 197/*12*)

The **v. femoralis** is the continuation of the external iliac and it runs distad in the femoral canal. In so doing it passes in a cranial direction along the pectineus muscle caudal to the femoral artery and medial to the saphenous nerve. At the distal half of the femur it crosses to the caudal surface of that bone and passes through the adductor magnus and brevis muscle into the hollow of the knee. Here it becomes the *v. poplitea*. In the dog the femoral vein gives off the superficial circumflex iliac vein and in all domestic mammals it gives off, still in the first part of the femoral canal, the lateral circumflex femoral vein. Then, as it crosses over to the caudal aspect of the femur, it gives rise in a caudodistal direction to the medial saphenous vein and craniodistally to the genus descendens vein. Several caudal femoral veins leave the v. femoralis in a caudal direction, and in all domestic mammals the last branch of the femoral vein is the distal caudal femoral vein which leaves the parent vein in the hollow of the knee.

V. circumflexa ilium superficialis

(dog: 190/*20*)

The **v. circumflexa ilium superficialis** occurs only in carnivores. In the cat it arises from the lateral circumflex femoral vein, but in the dog, although it may have a similar origin, it is more common for this vein to leave the femoral vein immediately proximal to the lateral circumflex femoral vein. The superficial circumflex iliac vein runs craniodorsally over the medial surface of the rectus femoris muscle to extend between the tensor fasciae latae and the caudal mass of the sartorius muscle. These muscles are supplied by several branches and another branch, which takes a superficial course towards the cranial ventral spine of the ilium, goes to the cranial mass of the sartorius muscle.

V. circumflexa femoris lateralis

(Comparative: 190–193/*21*; cat: 194/*19*; pig: 111/*13*; ox: 196/*39*; horse: 104/*17*; 197/*13*)

The **v. circumflexa femoris lateralis** arises in the proximal part of the femoral canal and, except in the horse, it divides into ascending, descending and transverse rami. The *r. ascendens* gives off branches to the hip joint and then continues to the gluteus profundus and gluteus medius muscles. The pig and ox do not possess a superficial circumflex iliac vein and as a result a secondary branch of the ascending ramus, or of the lateral circumflex femoral, goes to the tensor fasciae latae and anastomoses with the deep

Fig. 190.

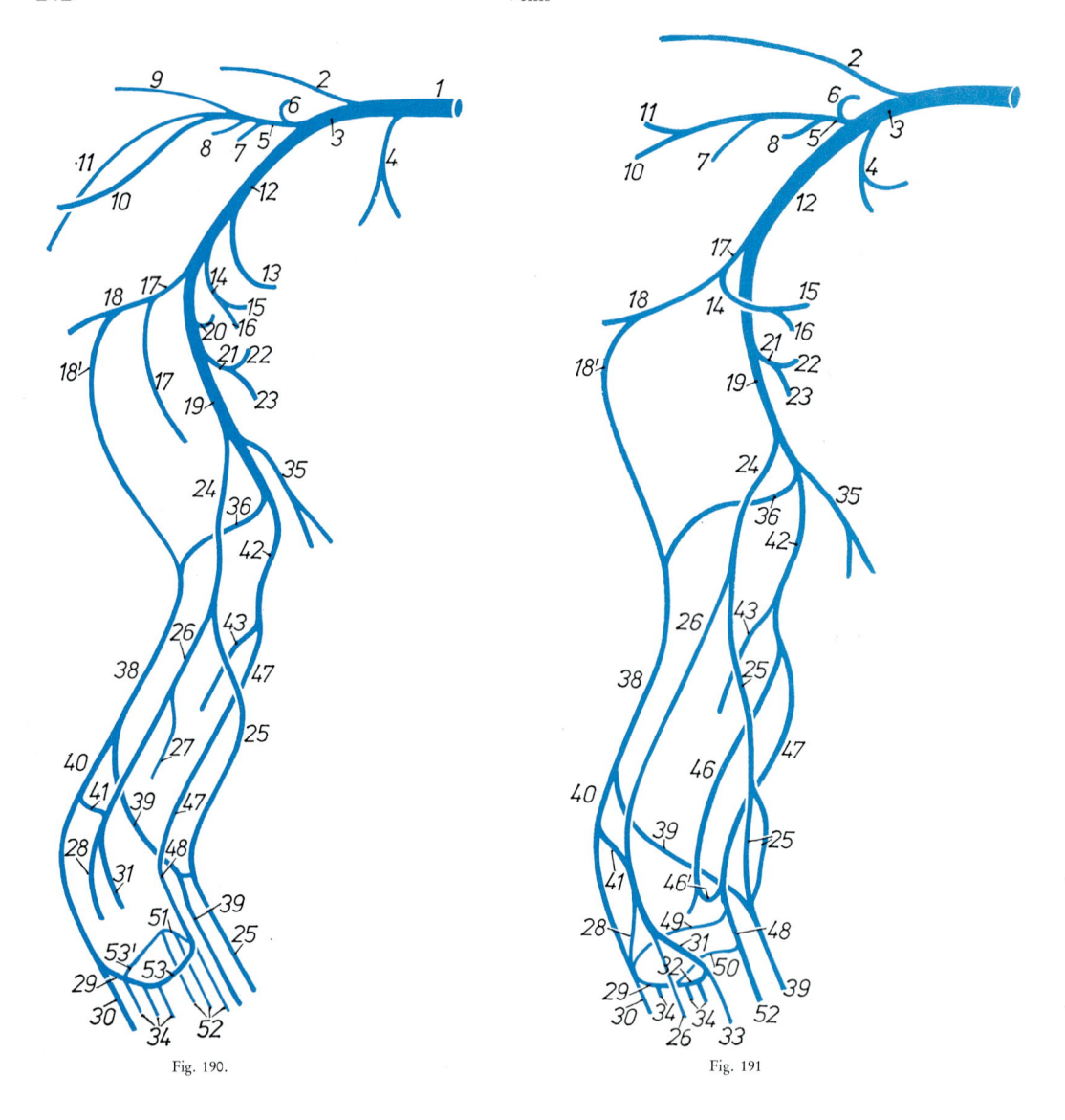

Fig. 191.

Figs 190, 191, 192, 193. Veins of the left pelvic limb down to the tarsal region of the dog, pig, ox and horse. Diagrammatic. Medial view. (After Badawi, Münster and Wilkens, in preparation, work carried out at the Institute of Veterinary Anatomy, Hanover.)

1 v. cava caudalis; *2* v. sacralis mediana; *3* v. iliaca communis; *4* v. circumflexa ilium profunda; *5* v. iliaca interna; *6* v. iliolumbalis; *7* v. obturatoria; *8* v. glutea cranialis; *9* v. caudalis lateralis superficialis; *10* v. pudenda interna; *11* v. glutaea caudalis; *12* v. iliaca externa; *13* v. abdominalis caudalis; *14* v. pudendoepigastrica; *15* v. epigastrica caudalis; *16* v. pudenda externa; *17* v. profunda femoris; *18* v. circumflexa femoris medialis, *18'* r. descendens; *19* v. femoralis; *20* v. circumflexa ilium superficialis; *21* v. circumflexa femoris lateralis, 22 r. ascendens; *22'* v. iliacofemoralis (horse); *23* r. descendens of *21*; *24* v. saphena medialis, *25* r. cranialis, *26* r. caudalis; *27* branch of *26*, not yet named; *28* v. plantaris lateralis, *29* r. profundus, *30* r. superficialis; *31* v. plantaris medialis, *32* r. profundus, *33* r. superficialis; *29* and *32* arcus plantaris profundus; *34* v. metatarseae plantares; *35* v. genus descendens; *36* v. caudalis femoris distalis; *37* v. comitans n. tibialis; *38* v. saphena lateralis, *39* r. cranialis, *40* r. caudalis, *41* r. anastomoticus cum v. saphena mediali; *42* v. poplitea; *43* v. tibialis caudalis; *44* r. anastomoticus cum v. saphena; *45* v. malleolaris caudalis lateralis; *46* v. interossea cruris; *46'* r. interosseus s. perforans; *47* v. tibialis cranialis; *48* v. dorsalis pedis; *49* v. tarsea perforans proximalis; *50* v. tarsea perforans distalis; *51* arcus dorsalis profundus; *52* vv. metatarseae dorsales; *53* r. perforans proximalis II; *53'* r. perforans proximalis IV

circumflex iliac vein. The *r. descendens* is the stoutest branch and it mainly ramifies in the quadriceps femoris muscle. The *r. transversus* is but a narrow vessel and forms the true continuation of the vein. Being laterally directed, it courses between the rectus femoris and medial vastus muscles, giving off branches to the intermediate and lateral vastus muscles. In the proximal part of the thigh it anastomoses with the medial circumflex femoris vein. In the horse the proximal area drained in other animals by the

Fig. 192.

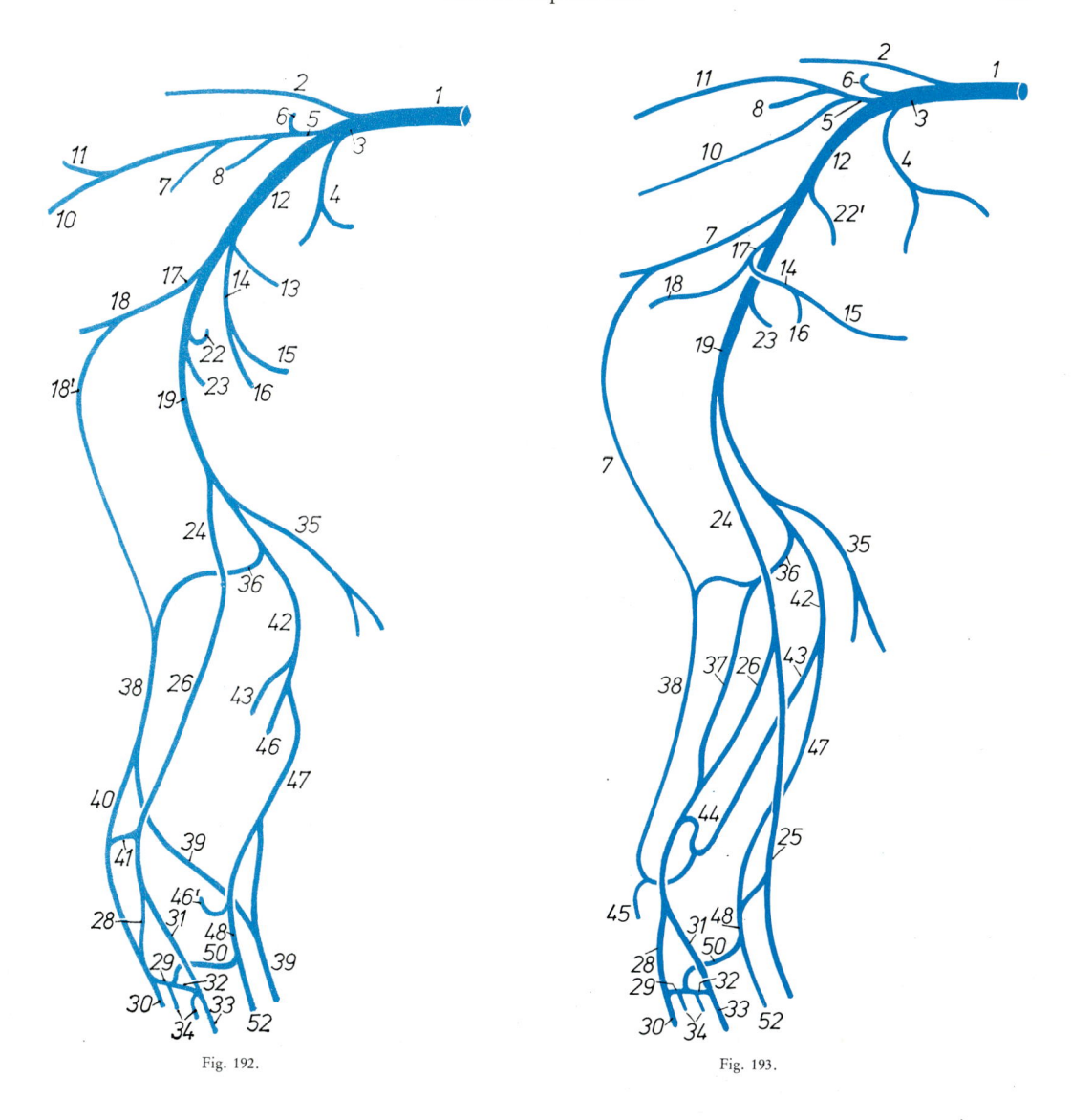

Fig. 193.

lateral circumflex femoris vein is served by the iliacofemoral vein (see p. 238) and the lateral circumflex femoral vein consists of only the descending ramus which drains a corresponding area.

V. saphena medialis (magna)

(Comparative: 190–193/*24*; 198–201/*11*; cat: 194/*26*; dog: 92/*c'*; 202/*4*; pig: 111/*14*; 188/*30*; 203/*4*; sheep: 195/*16*; ox: 196/*42*; horse: 123/*1, 19*; 197/*18*; 205/*4*)

The **v. saphena medialis** arises from the femoral vein at the distal end of the femoral canal. It accompanies the saphenous artery and nerve along its course. A little distal to the knee, near the insertion of the semitendinosus, the medial saphenous vein divides into a caudal and a cranial ramus, except in ruminants in which only the caudal ramus is developed. All the way along its course the large medial saphenous vein gives off muscular branches to such neighbouring muscles as the gracilis and the deep digital flexor.

The *r. cranialis*, which in the pig divides further into a *r. lateralis* and a *r. medialis*, runs superficially along the cranial part of the shank to the flexor aspect of the hock joint. Here the cranial ramus in the dog anastomoses with the cranial ramus of the lateral saphenous vein and these two venous branches can remain joined for a short distance. Subsequently the cranial ramus participates in the formation of the dorsal common digital vein. In the cat the cranial ramus is continued directly as the *v. digitalis dorsalis communis II*. In the dog the *v. tarsea medialis* joins the cranial ramus (p. 250). The initial part of the medial tarsal vein is superficial in position and it gives rise to the superficial plantar ramus which contributes to the formation of the superficial plantar arch. In the pig the lateral ramus, which has become reunited with the medial ramus, anastomoses with the cranial ramus of the lateral saphenous vein in the hollow of the hock joint and thus contributes to the formation of the dorsal common digital vein.

Together with the corresponding artery, the *r. caudalis* crosses the flexor digitalis pedis longus muscle medially and in a caudodistal direction. In carnivores the first part of the caudal ramus sends forth a vein which runs parallel to the artery as it passes between the tibia and parts of the deep digital flexors in a laterodistal direction to reach the distal end of the tibia. In the cat at this stage it becomes the *r. interosseus s. perforans* which, through the interosseous membrane, unites the cranial tibial vein to the caudal veins of the shank. Like the corresponding artery (p. 144) this vein has not yet been named. Proximal to the tarsal joint and craniomedial to the achilles tendon, the caudal ramus reaches the tibial nerve in company with which it passes over the sustentaculum tali. Still proximal to the hock there is, except in the horse, a stout *r. anastomoticus* to the caudal ramus of the lateral saphenous vein. As it reaches the hock joint the caudal ramus divides into the *v. plantaris medialis* and the *v. plantaris lateralis*. These medial and lateral plantar veins each give off a *r. profundus* which, together with the caudal ramus of the lateral saphenous vein, form the deep plantar arch. This arch in turn is the source of the *vv. metatarseae plantares* and, via the *r. superficialis*, the source of the *vv. digitales plantares*. Species differences to this arrangement occur in carnivores and pigs. In the cat only the medial plantar vein is present. Both plantar veins are small vessels in the dog and they end at the extensor aspect of the tarsal joint. The medial plantar vein of the dog is linked to the medial tarsal vein. In the pig the caudal ramus gives off first the slender lateral plantar vein and subsequently the medial plantar vein which latter continues as the superficial middle vessel to the superficial plantar arch.

V. genus descendens

(Comparative: 190–193/*35*; cat: 194/*21–25*; sheep: 195/*19*; ox: 196/*82*; horse: 197/*15*)

The **v. genus descendens** arises from the femoral vein after the medial saphenous has been given off and before the femoral vein reaches the caudal surface of the femur. It courses along the caudal border of the medial vastus muscle to the knee and gives off two or three branches. These supply the medial vastus, contribute (with species differences) in the vascularization of the remaining parts of the quadriceps muscle and supply branches to the adductor magnus and brevis and the semimembranosus muscles. In the cat the vein also supplies the sartorius. It finally supplies the medial region of the knee joint, the patellar joint and the infrapatellar adipose body.

Vv. caudales femoris

(Comparative: 190–193/*36*; cat: 194/*20*; pig: 111/*15*; sheep: 195/*20, 20'*; ox: 196/*40, 85, 86*; horse: 197/*16*)

Apart from the smaller muscular branches, the femoral vein gives off in a caudal direction two or three stout muscular branches known as the **vv. caudales femoris proximalis, media** and **distalis.** The first of these leaves the femoral vein proximal to the medial saphenous vein. The third and largest is present in all the domestic mammals and arises proximal to the heads of the gastrocnemius muscle; it is the last branch of the femoral vein.

The distal caudal femoral vein divides into two branches. The first is caudally directed and lies between the long ischiatic muscles and the second runs caudodistally over the lateral head of the gastrocnemius. However, in the pig and ruminants this second branch joins immediately at its origin, the lateral saphenous vein which in these species arises far proximal from the medial circumflex femoris vein. In carnivores and horses the distal caudal femoral vein gives off the lateral saphenous vein instead of the distally-directed branch. In the horse this lateral saphenous vein is very slender. In this species

Veins of the pelvic limb   245

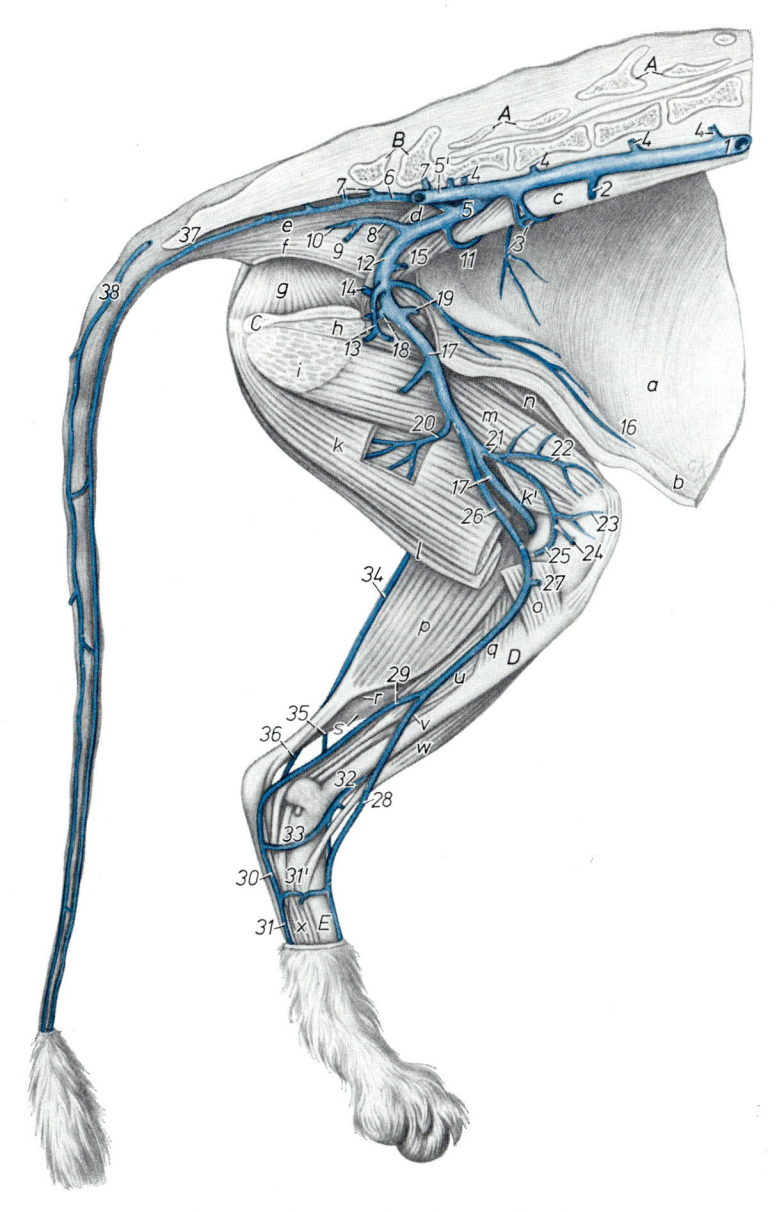

Fig. 194. Veins of the left pelvic limb of the cat. Medial view.
(After Biel, 1966, Diss., Hanover.)

A vertebrae lumbales; *B* vertebrae sacrales; *C* symphysis pelvina; *D* tibia; *E* os metatarsale II

a m. transversus abdominis; *b* m. rectus abdominis; *c* m. psoas minor; *d* m. iliopsoas; *e* m. sacrocaudalis ventralis lateralis; *f* m. coccygeus; *g* m. obturatorius internus; *h* m. adductor longus and m. pectineus; *i* m. adductor; *k, k'* m. semimembranosus; *l* m. semitendinosus; *m* m. vastus medialis; *n* m. rectus femoris; *o* insertion of the caudal mass of the m. sartorius; *p* m. gastrocnemius, caput mediale; *q* m. popliteus; *r* m. flexor digitalis superficialis; *s* m. gastrocnemius, caput laterale; *t* m. flexor hallucis longus; *u* flexor digitalis longus; *v* m. tibialis caudalis; *w* m. tibialis cranialis; *x* mm. interossei

1 v. cava caudalis; *2* v. renalis; *3* v. circumflexa ilium profunda; *4* vv. lumbales IV–VII; *5* v. iliaca communis sinistra; *5'* v. iliaca communis dextra; *6* v. sacralis mediana; *7* rr. sacrales; *8* v. iliaca interna; *9* v. pudenda interna; *10* v. glutaea caudalis; *11* r. anastomoticus with the v. circumflexa ilium profunda; *12* v. iliaca externa; *13* v. pudenda externa; *14* v. vesicalis media; *15* v. abdominalis caudalis; *16* v. epigastrica caudalis; *17* v. femoralis; *18* v. profunda femoris; *19* v. circumflexa femoris lateralis; *20* v. caudalis femoris; *21–25* v. genus descendens; *26* v. saphena medialis; *27* r. cutaneus; *28* r. cranialis; *29* r. caudalis; *30* v. plantaris medialis; *31* r. superficialis; *31'* r. profundus; *32* transition of the v. tibialis cranialis into the v. dorsalis pedis; *33* r. tarsea medialis; *34* v. saphena lateralis, *35* r. cranialis; *36* r. caudalis; *37* v. caudalis mediana; *38* v. caudalis lateralis superficialis dextra

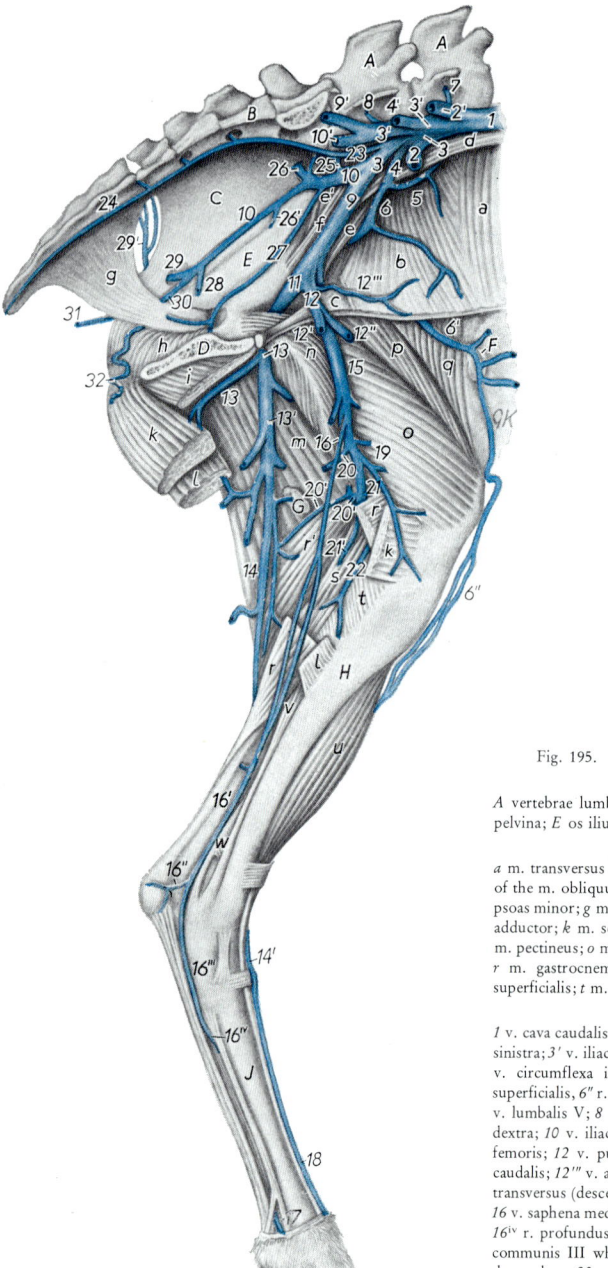

Fig. 195. Veins of the left pelvic limb of the sheep. Medial view. (After Freytag, 1962, Diss., Hanover.)

A vertebrae lumbales; *B* os sacrum; *C* lig. sacrotuberale latum; *D* symphysis pelvina; *E* os ilium; *F* ln. subiliacus; *G* ln. popliteus; *H* tibia; *J* os metatarsale III + IV

a m. transversus abdominis; *b* m. obliquus internus abdominis; *c* pelvic tendon of the m. obliquus externus abdominis; *d* m. psoas major; *e, e'* m. iliacus; *f* m. psoas minor; *g* m. coccygeus; *h* m. obturatorius externus, pars intrapelvina; *i* m. adductor; *k* m. semimembranosus; *l* m. semitendinosus; *m* m. glutaeobiceps; *n* m. pectineus; *o* m. vastus medialis; *p* m. rectus femoris; *q* m. tensor fasciae latae; *r* m. gastrocnemius, caput mediale, *r'* caput laterale; *s* m. flexor digitalis superficialis; *t* m. popliteus; *u* m. fibularis tertius; *v* m. flexor digitalis longus; *w* m. tibialis caudalis

1 v. cava caudalis; *2* v. ovarica sinistra; *2'* v. ovarica dextra; *3* v. iliaca communis sinistra; *3'* v. iliaca communis dextra; *4* v. circumflexa ilium profunda sinistra; *4'* v. circumflexa ilium profunda dextra, *5* r. cranialis, *6* r. caudalis, *6'* r. superficialis, *6"* r. anastomoticus with the r. cranialis of the v. saphena lateralis; *7* v. lumbalis V; *8* v. lumbalis IV; *9* v. iliaca externa sinistra; *9'* v. iliaca externa dextra; *10* v. iliaca interna sinistra; *10'* v. iliaca interna dextra; *11* v. profunda femoris; *12* v. pudendoepigastrica; *12'* v. pudenda externa; *12"* v. epigastrica caudalis; *12'''* v. abdominalis caudalis; *13* v. circumflexa femoris medialis, *13'* r. transversus (descendens); *14* v. saphena lateralis, *14'* r. cranialis; *15* v. femoralis; *16* v. saphena medialis, *16'* r. caudalis, *16"* rr. calcanei; *16'''* v. plantaris medialis; *16ⁱᵛ* r. profundus; *17* v. digitalis plantaris communis II; *18* v. digitalis dorsalis communis III which is the continuation of the v. dorsalis pedis; *19* v. genus descendens; *20* v. caudalis femoris media; *20'* v. caudalis femoris distalis; *21* v. poplitea; *21'* v. suralis; *22* v. tibialis caudalis; *23* v. sacralis mediana with rr. sacrales; *24* v. caudalis mediana; *25* v. iliolumbalis; *26* v. glutaea cranialis, *26'* r. muscularis; *27* v. obturatoria; *28* v. vaginalis; *29* v. glutaea caudalis, *29'* r. muscularis; *30* v. pudenda interna; *31* v. perinealis ventralis; *32* v. labialis dorsalis et mammaria

also the *v. comitans n. tibialis,* lying parallel to the artery, is given off the distal caudal femoral vein and anastomoses with the caudal ramus of the medial saphenous vein proximal to the hock joint.

The caudal femoral veins and their smaller muscular branches participate in draining the adductors and the long ischiatic muscles. They are assisted in this drainage by branches of the deep femoral vein in the dog, of the medial circumflex femoral vein in the cat, pig and ruminant and of the obturator vein in the horse. These veins form anastomoses between one another. The drainage area of the distal caudal femoral vein extends as far as the caudal part of the shank.

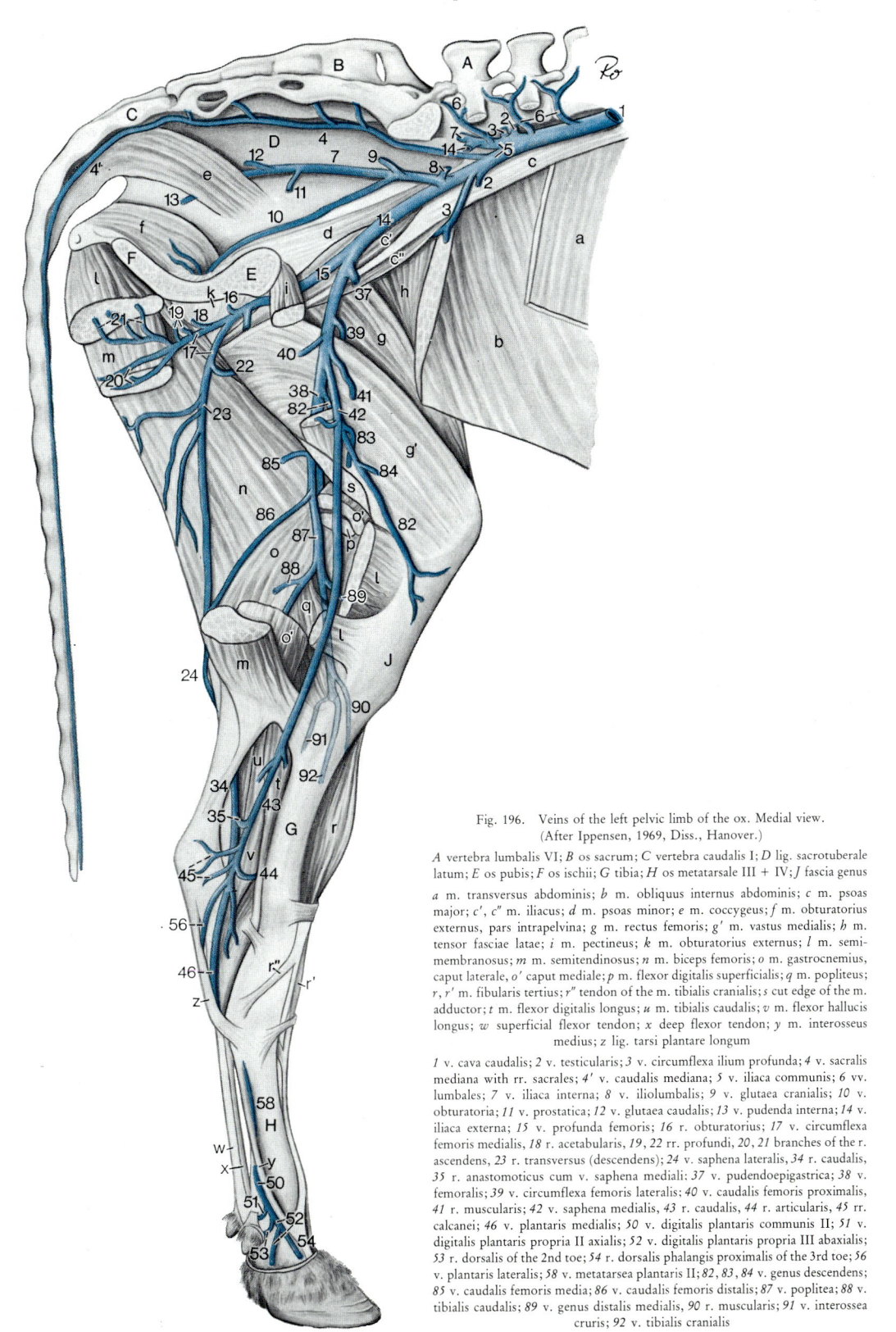

Veins of the pelvic limb

Fig. 196. Veins of the left pelvic limb of the ox. Medial view. (After Ippensen, 1969, Diss., Hanover.)

A vertebra lumbalis VI; *B* os sacrum; *C* vertebra caudalis I; *D* lig. sacrotuberale latum; *E* os pubis; *F* os ischii; *G* tibia; *H* os metatarsale III + IV; *J* fascia genus

a m. transversus abdominis; *b* m. obliquus internus abdominis; *c* m. psoas major; *c'*, *c''* m. iliacus; *d* m. psoas minor; *e* m. coccygeus; *f* m. obturatorius externus, pars intrapelvina; *g* m. rectus femoris; *g'* m. vastus medialis; *h* m. tensor fasciae latae; *i* m. pectineus; *k* m. obturatorius externus; *l* m. semimembranosus; *m* m. semitendinosus; *n* m. biceps femoris; *o* m. gastrocnemius, caput laterale, *o'* caput mediale; *p* m. flexor digitalis superficialis; *q* m. popliteus; *r*, *r'* m. fibularis tertius; *r''* tendon of the m. tibialis cranialis; *s* cut edge of the m. adductor; *t* m. flexor digitalis longus; *u* m. tibialis caudalis; *v* m. flexor hallucis longus; *w* superficial flexor tendon; *x* deep flexor tendon; *y* m. interosseus medius; *z* lig. tarsi plantare longum

1 v. cava caudalis; *2* v. testicularis; *3* v. circumflexa ilium profunda; *4* v. sacralis mediana with rr. sacrales; *4'* v. caudalis mediana; *5* v. iliaca communis; *6* vv. lumbales; *7* v. iliaca interna; *8* v. iliolumbalis; *9* v. glutaea cranialis; *10* v. obturatoria; *11* v. prostatica; *12* v. glutaea caudalis; *13* v. pudenda interna; *14* v. iliaca externa; *15* v. profunda femoris; *16* r. obturatorius; *17* v. circumflexa femoris medialis, *18* r. acetabularis, *19*, *22* rr. profundi, *20*, *21* branches of the r. ascendens, *23* r. transversus (descendens); *24* v. saphena lateralis, *34* r. caudalis, *35* r. anastomoticus cum v. saphena mediali; *37* v. pudendoepigastrica; *38* v. femoralis; *39* v. circumflexa femoris lateralis; *40* v. caudalis femoris proximalis, *41* r. muscularis; *42* v. saphena medialis, *43* r. caudalis, *44* r. articularis, *45* rr. calcanei; *46* v. plantaris medialis; *50* v. digitalis plantaris communis II; *51* v. digitalis plantaris propria II axialis; *52* v. digitalis plantaris propria III abaxialis; *53* r. dorsalis of the 2nd toe; *54* r. dorsalis phalangis proximalis of the 3rd toe; *56* v. plantaris lateralis; *58* v. metatarsea plantaris II; *82*, *83*, *84* v. genus descendens; *85* v. caudalis femoris media; *86* v. caudalis femoris distalis; *87* v. poplitea; *88* v. tibialis caudalis; *89* v. genus distalis medialis; *90* r. muscularis; *91* v. interossea cruris; *92* v. tibialis cranialis

V. saphena lateralis
(Comparative: 190–193/*38*; 198–201/*2*; cat: 194/*34*; dog: 92/*d*; 202/*1*; pig: 111/*11*; 203/*1*; sheep: 195/*14*; ox: 196/*24*; 204/*1*; horse: 124/*23*; 197/*20*)

In carnivores and horses the **v. saphena lateralis** is the direct continuation of the distal caudal femoral vein. In pigs and ruminants it arises more proximally from the medial circumflex femoral. Between the biceps femoris and semitendinosus muscles it runs along the caudal aspect of the gastrocnemius muscle to the gastrocnemius tendon and then moves into a superficial position. It accompanies the caudal cutaneous sural nerve and, except in ruminants, the distal branch of the distal caudal femoral artery in a craniodistal direction to the calcaneus. In carnivores and ruminants it gives off muscular branches to the gastrocnemius and a superficial branch which runs laterally along the common tendon of the calcaneus and then crosses the plantar surface to lie medial to the calcaneus. The lateral saphenous vein of the horse is only small and ends here by anastomosing with the lateral caudal malleolar vein. In the other domestic mammals it divides into a cranial and a caudal ramus at the point where the superficial digital flexor tendon winds around the gastrocnemius tendon.

The *r. cranialis*, which is absent in the horse, crosses the shank laterally to reach the flexor aspect of the tarsal joint. It is a larger vessel than the cranial ramus of the medial saphenous vein. By means of the *r. anastomoticus cum v. saphena mediali* it links up with the medial saphenous vein, or in the case of the pig, with the lateral and medial ramus of this vein. In the dog the two cranial rami may unite for a short distance. In the dog the lateral tarsal vein is joined to the cranial ramus of the lateral saphenous vein (p. 250). The cranial rami of the two saphenous veins are the vessels of origin for the dorsal digital veins.

The *r. anastomoticus cum v. saphena mediali* joins the *r. caudalis* to the caudal ramus of the medial saphenous vein proximal to the hock joint and caudal to the deep digital flexor. Distally directed, the caudal ramus courses on the lateral aspect of the calcaneus and unites with the more slender lateral plantar vein distal to this bone. This is not the case in carnivores and only rarely in the small ruminants. Together with the medial plantar vein this vascular link, or in the dog and usually also the small ruminants the caudal ramus itself, forms the deep plantar arch. Further distally they form the superficial plantar arch which is the source of the plantar metatarsal or digital metatarsal veins.

V. poplitea
(Comparative: 190–193/*42*; pig: 111/*16*; sheep: 195/*21*; ox: 196/*87*; horse: 197/*17*)

In analogy with the homonymous artery, the **v. poplitea** could be considered as the continuation of the femoral vein after the origin of the distal caudal femoral vein. It passes between the heads of the gastrocnemius muscle and over the popliteal fascia where it is covered by the popliteus muscle. Here, or in the cat on the proximal border of this muscle, it gives off the *v. tibialis caudalis*. Shortly thereafter it may give rise to the *v. interossea cruris*. In the proximal part of the crural interosseous space it becomes the *v. tibialis cranialis*. This latter vein, therefore, represents the true continuation of the popliteal vein, while the branches running caudal to the tibia are of little significance for the vascularization of the foot and only serve as muscular branches. This is the reason why there is no uniform nomenclature for the vessels situated on the caudal part of the shank. Up to this division the popliteal vein gives off firstly the *vv. surales*, which are muscle branches draining mainly the gastrocnemius and the long digital flexors, and secondly the *vv. genus*. The development of the latter varies with the species but there are paired medial and lateral *vv. genus proximales* and *distales* and a single *v. genus media*. They are cranially directed and lie lateral, medial and caudal to the knee joint. Not all five vv. genus are present in all the domestic mammals and, in addition, some of these vessels may originate from veins which neighbour on the popliteal vein.

V. tibialis caudalis
(Comparative: 190–193/*43*; sheep: 195/*22*; ox: 196/*88*; horse: 123/*24*; 197/*19*; 201/*32*)

The **v. tibialis caudalis** arises from the popliteal vein on the proximal part of the caudal surface of the tibia, between this bone and the popliteus muscle. Whereas it runs cranial to the popliteus muscle in the pig and horse, in carnivores and ruminants it crosses the caudal surface of this muscle and supplies the

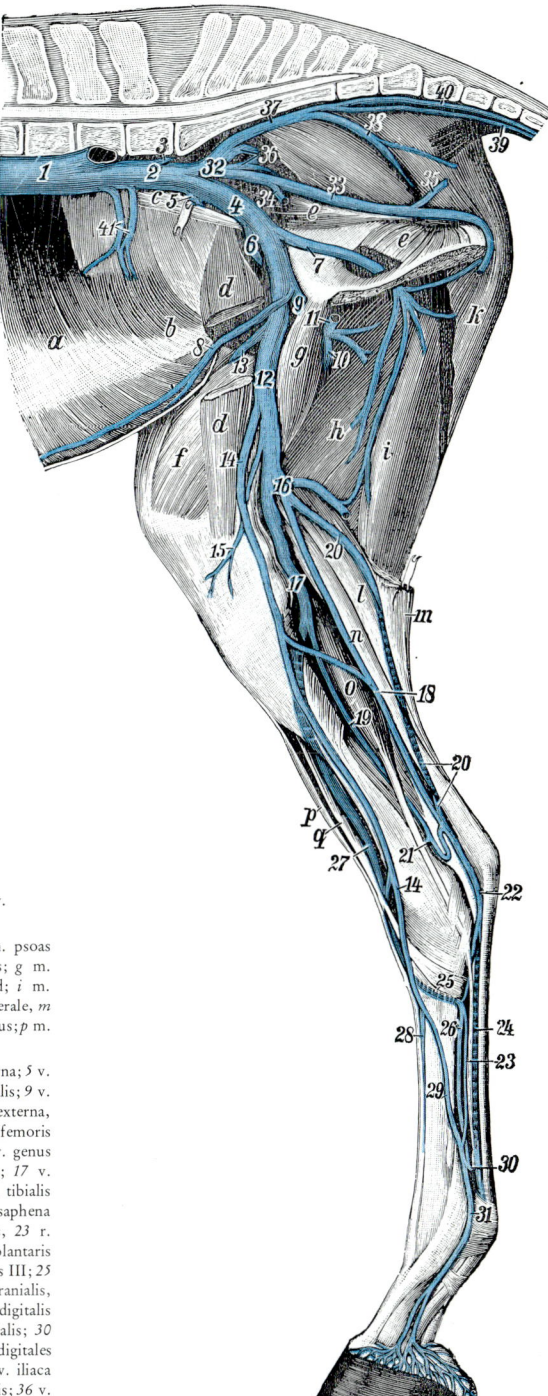

Fig. 197. Veins of the right pelvic limb of a horse. Medial view. (After Ellenberger and Baum, 1932.)

a m. transversus abdominis; *b* m. obliquus internus abdominis; *c* m. psoas minor; *d* m. sartorius; *e* m. obturatorius internus; *f* m. quadriceps; *g* m. pectineus; *h* m. biceps femoris, medial side, m. adductor removed; *i* m. semitendinosus; *k* m. semimembranosus; *l* m. gastrocnemius, caput laterale, *m* caput mediale; *n* m. flexor digitalis superficialis; *o* m. flexor digitalis longus; *p* m. extensor digitalis longus; *q* m. fibularis tertius

1 v. cava caudalis; *2* v. iliaca communis; *3* v. lumbalis VI; *4* v. iliaca externa; *5* v. iliolumbalis; *6* v. iliacofemoralis; *7* v. obturatoria; *8* v. epigastrica caudalis; *9* v. profunda femoris; *10* v. circumflexa femoris medialis; *11* v. pudenda externa, vessel not parallel to the artery; *12* v. femoralis; *13* v. circumflexa femoris lateralis, r. descendens; *14* v. saphena medialis, distal r. cranialis; *15* v. genus descendens; *16* v. caudalis femoris distalis, rr. musculares (cut off); *17* v. poplitea; *18* v. saphena medialis, r. caudalis receives the v. comitans n. tibialis from the v. caudalis femoris distalis; *19* v. tibialis caudalis; *20* v. saphena lateralis; *21* v. malleolaris caudalis lateralis; *22* v. plantaris medialis, *23* r. superficialis, continuing as v. digitalis plantaris communis II; *24* v. plantaris lateralis, r. superficialis, continuing as the v. digitalis plantaris communis III; *25* v. tarsea perforans distalis; *26* v. metatarsea plantaris II; *27* v. tibialis cranialis, continuing as the v. dorsalis pedis; *28* v. metatarsea dorsalis II; *29* v. digitalis dorsalis communis II from the r. cranialis of the v. saphena medialis; *30* anastomosis of the arcus plantaris profundus distalis with the vv. digitales plantares communes; *31* v. digitalis plantaris propria III medialis; *32* v. iliaca interna; *33* v. pudenda interna; *34* v. prostatica; *35* v. perinealis ventralis; *36* v. glutaea cranialis; *37*, *38* v. glutaea caudalis; *39* v. caudalis mediana; *40* v. caudalis ventrolateralis; *41* v. circumflexa ilium profunda

extensors of the tarsal joint and the flexors of the toe joints. In pigs and horses a connection has been described between the caudal ramus of the medial saphenous and the caudal tibial vein at the level of the calcaneus. In the horse this connection gives rise to the *v. malleolaris caudalis lateralis* which ramifies in the lateral area of the joint and anastomoses with the caudal ramus of the lateral saphenous vein.

V. interossea cruris
(pig: 191/46; ox: 192/46; 196/91)

The **v. interossea cruris** arises from the popliteal vein after the caudal tibial vein has been given off but while the popliteal is still located between the tibia and the popliteus muscle. In the pig and ox this vein supplies the deep parts of the deep digital flexors. Only in the pig does it extend further distad where it is connected to the cranial tibial vein by the *r. interosseus.*

V. tibialis cranialis
(Comparative: 190–193/47; 198–201/35; cat: 194/32; ox: 196/92; horse: 124/28; 197/27; 206/1)

At the distal border of the popliteus muscle of domestic mammals the **v. tibialis cranialis** leaves the popliteal vein and, in fact, forms its main continuation. It passes through the proximal part of the crural interosseous space and then continuing distally, usually as a double vein, it runs along the craniolateral part of the tibia under cover of the cranial tibialis muscle. Thereby it supplies the flexors of the tarsal joints and the extensors of the toe joints. In the ox one of these muscular branches perforates the crural interosseous membrane independent of the cranial tibial vein. The *r. superficialis,* which lies parallel to the vein, arises from the cranial tibial vein, in the cat in the proximal and in the ox in the distal half of the shank. This ramus passes through the fascia and gains a superficial position where it connects with the cranial ramus of the lateral tibial vein. In the cat this union occurs in the distal third of the shank and in the ox at the level of the malleolar bone. Proximally to the tarsal joint, the cranial tibial vein gives off the *r. interosseus s. perforans* but this branch has been recorded only in the cat, pig and ox. It passes through the crural interosseous membrane to the caudal aspect of the tibia; in the pig it unites here with the crural interosseous vein. It is only in the pig that this latter vessel extends so far distally. In the ox the interosseous or perforating ramus runs dorsally towards the crural interosseous vein and in the cat and pig the ramus, running more caudally, forms a link with an articular branch of the caudal ramus of the lateral saphenous vein. In all the domestic mammals the cranial tibial vein becomes the *v. dorsalis pedis* at the tarsal joint.

V. dorsalis pedis
(Comparative: 190–193/48; 198–201/36; cat: 194/32; sheep: 195/18; ox: 196/95; horse: 124/29; 197/27;206/2)

The **v. dorsalis pedis** is a paired, deeply situated vessel. It is the continuation of the cranial tibial vein and runs dorsally over the tarsus. In the cat and the pig and also occasionally in the ox, it gives off the *v. tarsea medialis* and the *v. tarsea lateralis.* These veins, which in the dog arise from the cranial ramus of the medial or lateral saphenous vein (see p. 243) and which are not present as independent vessels in the horse, run in either a medial or lateral direction to the appropriate side of the tarsal joint, giving off branches along their course. In the pig and occasionally the ox the lateral tarsal vein gives rise to the *v. tarsea perforans proximalis* which passes between the talus and calcaneus to the planta to anastomose with the lateral plantar vein. Subsequently the dorsal pedal vein gives off the *v. tarsea perforans distalis* which passes through the tarsal canal and also reaches the planta where it terminates in the deep plantar arch. Thereafter the dorsal pedal vein becomes the source of the dorsal metatarsal veins.

Veins of the hindfoot of carnivores

Plantar veins
(cat: 194/29–31'; dog: 190; 198)

In the cat the caudal ramus of the medial saphenous vein, unlike its arterial counterpart, continues only as the *v. plantaris medialis*. In the dog there is yet another division of this ramus into the *vv. plantares medialis* and *lateralis* but these terminate as rudimentary vessels in the tarsal region. The medial plantar vein of the dog unites with the medial tarsal vein. The medial plantar vein of the cat divides into a *r. profundus* and a *r. superficialis*. The second caudal vein to the plantar vascular system of the foot in the cat is the caudal ramus of the lateral saphenous vein. In the dog this is the only caudal vein of that system. Passing laterally over the calcaneus, this caudal ramus reaches the planta where it divides into the deep and the superficial rami. In the dog this bifurcation takes place at the proximal part of the metatarsus and in the cat more distally, about half way down this bone. The *arcus plantaris profundus* is formed in both dog and cat by the deep ramus of the lateral saphenous vein and the proximal perforating ramus II and additionally in the cat the medial plantar vein contributes to the arch. In the dog this deep plantar arch is also connected through the *r. perforans proximalis IV* with the deep dorsal arch. The deep plantar arch of both cat and dog gives rise to the *vv. metatarseae plantares II–IV* although the second of these veins may be incomplete in the dog. These plantar metatarsal veins are linked to the dorsal metatarsal veins by the *rr. perforantes distales* and they do not terminate directly in the plantar common digital veins but in the superficial plantar arch.

In the cat the superficial ramus of the medial plantar vein and the superficial ramus of the caudal ramus of the lateral saphenous vein form, in the middle third of the metatarsus, the *arcus plantaris superficialis*. This arch carries large connecting branches; medially they join with the cranial ramus of the medial saphenous vein and laterally with the cranial ramus of the lateral saphenous vein. In the dog the superficial plantar arch is formed by the superficial ramus of the caudal ramus of the lateral saphenous vein and the superficial plantar ramus of the medial tarsal vein which curves medially round the middle of the second metatarsal bone to reach the planta superficially. In both cat and dog the superficial plantar arch receives the plantar metatarsal veins and gives off the *vv. digitales plantares communes II–IV*. In the cat it also gives rise to the *vv. digitales plantares II abaxialis* and *V abaxialis*. The common digital plantar vein III is rudimentary in the cat and consists only of the *r. tori metatarsei*. The remaining common plantar digital veins divide into the *vv. digitales plantares propriae* whereby the proper plantar digital veins III axial and IV abaxial of the cat are linked, mainly through the *rr. plantares phalangium proximalium*. Certain axial and abaxial segments of the proper plantar veins of the third and fourth digits may be missing in the dog. The *vv. interdigitales II* and *IV* are joined to the plantar proper abaxial veins of the third and fourth toes respectively. In the dog there may also be a *v. interdigitalis III* which is then connected to the plantar proper axial vein of the third or fourth toes.

Dorsal veins
(cat: 194/32, 33, 35; dog: 190; 202)

The **v. dorsalis pedis** gives off the *vv. tarseae medialis* and *lateralis* at the level of the talus and it anastomoses, in both the cat and dog, with the medial saphenous vein about half way down the tarsal joint. This forms a single vessel in the dog which extends down to the deep dorsal arch. The *arcus dorsalis profundus* is imcomplete in both domestic carnivores. It originates at the proximal part of the metatarsus from a transverse branch of the dorsal pedal vein. This branch is parallel to the arcuate artery and connects, in the dog only with the deep plantar arch through the proximal perforating ramus IV. From this deep dorsal arch arise the *vv. metatarsea II–IV*. The third dorsal metatarsal vein is usually absent in the cat and in both the cat and the dog the second dorsal metatarsal vein is rudimentary subsequent to the origin of the proximal perforating ramus II. In the cat the fourth dorsal metatarsal vein is also rudimentary. The *r. perforans proximalis II* is the stout connecting link between the dorsal and plantar venous systems of the foot of the cat and dog. But only in the latter species do the dorsal metatarsal veins, after combining with the plantar metatarsal veins through the distal perforating rami, terminate in the common dorsal digital veins.

252 Veins

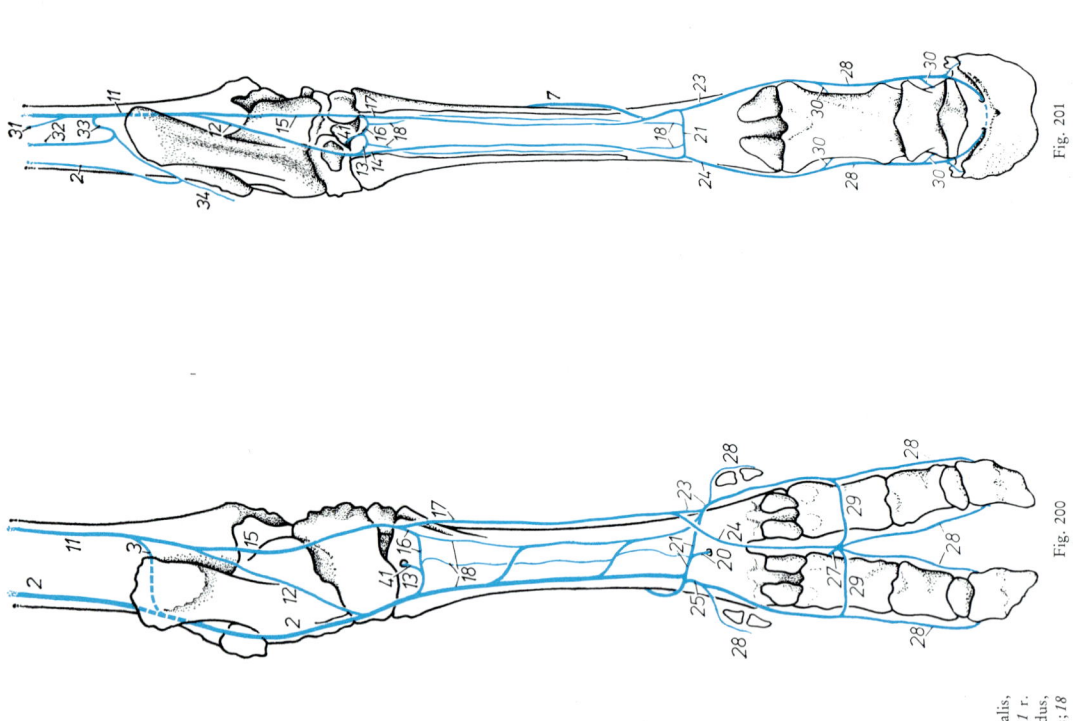

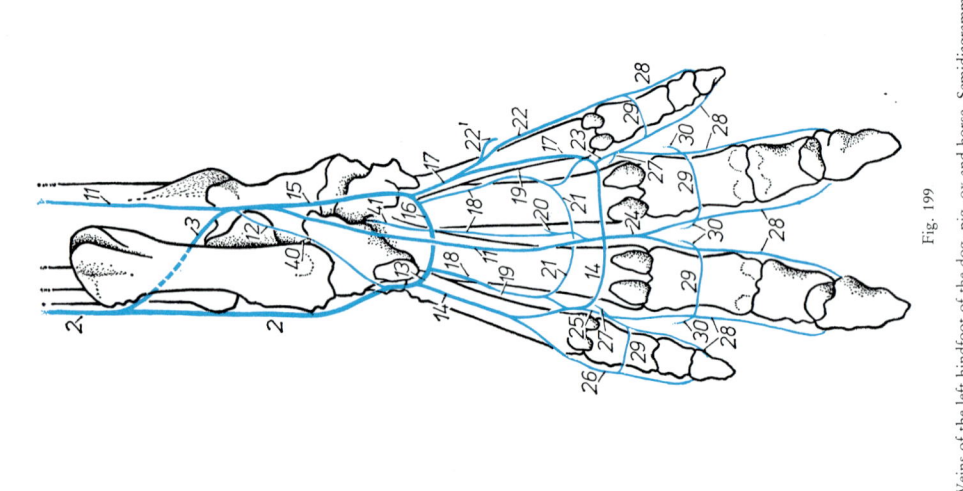

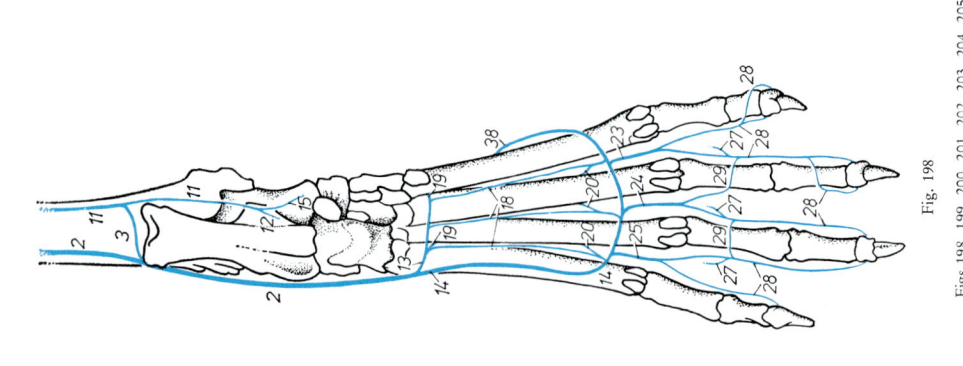

Figs 198, 199, 200, 201, 202, 203, 204, 205. Veins of the left hindfoot of the dog, pig, ox and horse. Semidiagrammatic. (After Munster, Badawi and Wilkens, in preparation, work performed at the Institute of Veterinary Anatomy, Hanover.)

Figs 198–201: plantar view, Figs 202–205: dorsal view.

1 r. cranialis, *2* r. caudalis of the v. saphena lateralis; *3* r. cranialis of the v. saphena medialis; *4* r. caudalis of the v. saphena medialis, *4'* r. medialis, *4''* r. lateralis; *5* arcus dorsalis superficialis; *6–9* vv. digitales communes I–IV; *10* vv. digitales propriae; *11* r. caudalis of the v. saphena medialis; *12* v. plantaris lateralis, *13* r. profundus, *14* r. superficialis; *15* v. plantaris medialis, *16* r. profundus, *17* r. superficialis; *13* and *16*, in the dog only *13*, arcus plantaris profundus; *14* and *17*, in the dog only *14*, arcus plantaris superficialis; *18*

Veins of the hindfoot

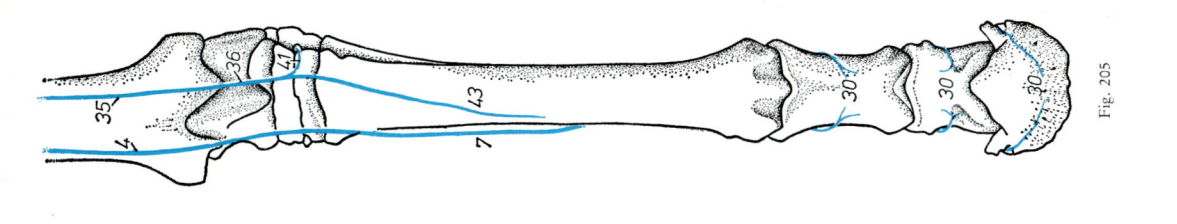

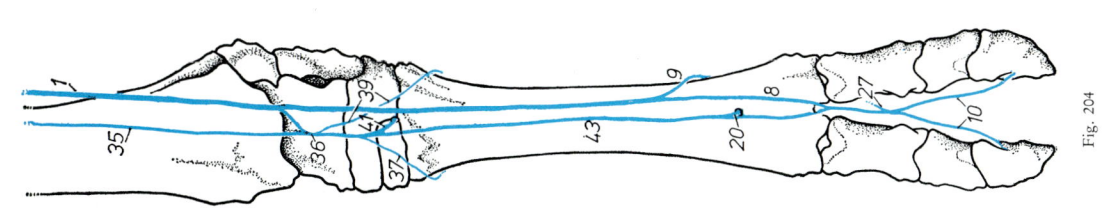

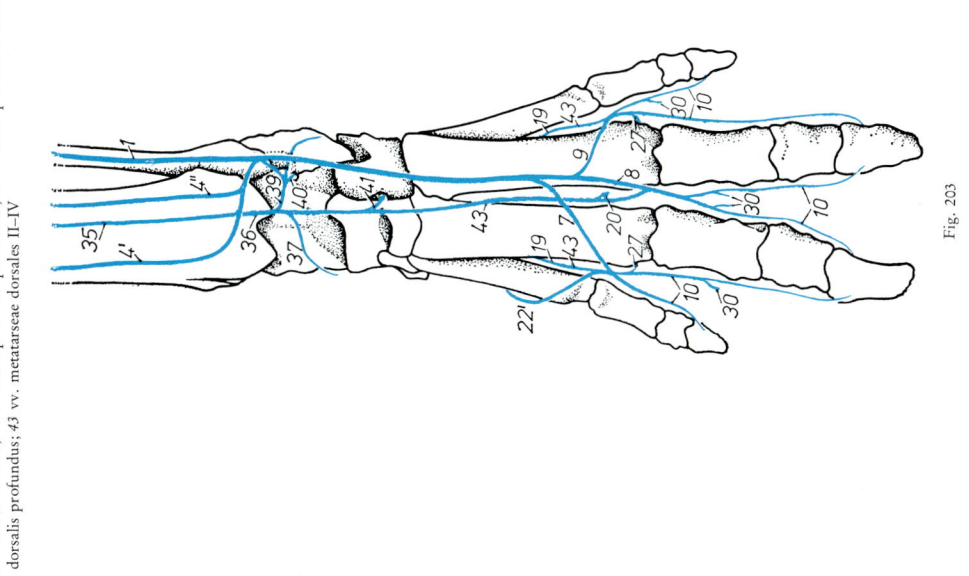

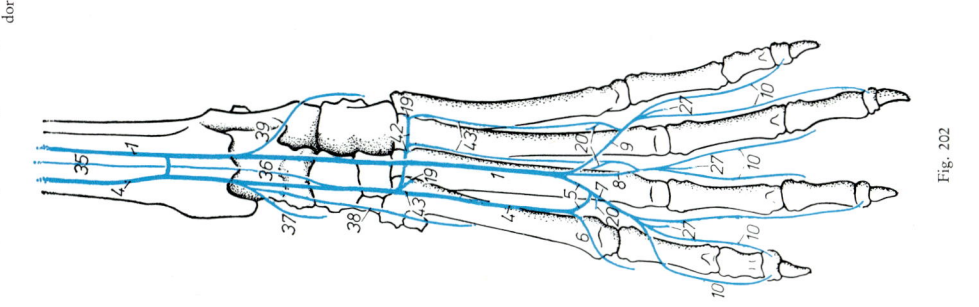

vv. metatarseae plantares II–IV; *19* rr. perforantes proximales II and IV; *20* rr. perforantes distales; *21* arcus plantaris profundus distalis; *22–25* vv. digitales plantares communes I–IV; *22'* anastomosis to the v. digitalis dorsalis communis II; *26* v. digitalis plantaris V abaxialis; *27* v. interdigitalis; *28* vv. digitales plantares propriae; *29* rr. plantares phalangium proximalium; *30* rr. dorsales phalangium proximalium or, in the horse, phalangium proximalis, mediae and distalis; *31* v. comitans n. tibialis; *32* v. tibialis caudalis; *33* r. anastomoticus cum v. saphena mediali; *34* v. malleolaris caudalis lateralis; *35* v. tibialis cranialis; *36* v. dorsalis pedis; *37* v. tarsea medialis; *38* r. plantaris superficialis; *39* v. tarsea lateralis; *40* v. tarsea perforans proximalis; *41* v. tarsea perforans distalis; *42* arcus dorsalis profundus; *43* vv. metatarseae dorsales II–IV

Fig. 205

Fig. 204

Fig. 203

Fig. 202

In the distal third of the feline metatarsus the cranial ramus of the medial saphenous vein gives rise to the medial connecting branch to the superficial plantar arch. The cranial ramus continues thereafter as the *v. digitalis dorsalis communis II*. The cranial ramus of the lateral saphenous vein sends the lateral connecting branch to the superficial plantar arch half way down the metatarsus and somewhat more distally it then forks into the *vv. digitales dorsales communes II* and *III*.

In the dog the cranial ramus of the medial saphenous vein gives off the *v. tarsea medialis* on the flexor aspect of the tarsus; in turn this vessel immediately gives rise to the *r. plantaris superficialis*. At about the same level the cranial ramus of the lateral saphenous vein gives rise to the *v. tarsea lateralis*. The cranial rami of both the medial and the lateral saphenous veins unite at the level of the distal part of the metatarsus and form the *arcus dorsalis superficialis*. From this arch arise the *vv. digitales dorsales communes I–IV*. Since the first toe is usually missing, the common dorsal digital vein I only gives off the *v. digitalis dorsalis propria II abaxialis*. The common dorsal digital veins unite with the dorsal metatarsal veins only in the dog and, in the region of their division into the *vv. digitales dorsales propriae*, they also unite with the *vv. interdigitales*. The third interdigital vein of the cat does not participate in the latter union.

Veins of the hindfoot of the pig

Plantar veins
(pig: 111/*14'*, *19, 20*; 191; 199)

The caudal ramus of the medial saphenous vein increases in diameter distal to the junction with the anastomotic ramus to the lateral saphenous vein and, at the level of the sustentaculum tali, this caudal ramus gives off the slender **v. plantaris lateralis.** It then continues superficial to the planta as a more slender vessel although it is usually still paired. The **v. plantaris medialis** divides at the level of the tarsometatarsal articulation into a more robust *r. profundus* and a more delicate *r. superficialis*. The lateral plantar vein unites with the stout caudal ramus of the lateral saphenous vein, receives the proximal perforating tarsal vein and then divides at the same level as the medial vein into a thicker deep and a thinner superficial ramus. The two deep rami form the *arcus plantaris profundus* to which the distal perforating tarsal vein also contributes. From this arch arise the *vv. metatarseae plantares II–IV*. The second and fourth plantar metatarsal veins give off respectively the *r. perforans proximalis II* and *IV* from which issue the dorsal metatarsal veins of the same number. Only the third plantar metatarsal vein unites with the corresponding dorsal metatarsal vein through the *r. perforans distalis III*. The plantar metatarsal vein II and IV join the superficial plantar arch but they also unite with the plantar metatarsal vein III to form the *arcus plantaris profundus distalis*. Through the plantar metatarsal vein III this arch joins the superficial or caudal ramus of the medial saphenous vein which itself joins the superficial arch.

Together with the caudal ramus of the medial saphenous vein, the superficial rami of both the medial and the lateral plantar veins form the *arcus plantaris superficialis* in the region of the distal part of the metatarsus. From this arch arise the *vv. digitales plantares communes I–IV* and the *v. digitalis plantaris V abaxialis*. The common plantar digital veins divide into the *vv. digitales plantares propriae*. Only the first common plantar digital vein gives off the *v. digitalis plantaris propria II abaxialis*, prior to which a stout anastomosis to the common dorsal digital vein is given off. The *vv. interdigitales II* and *IV* join with the dorsal proper digital veins.

Dorsal veins
(pig: 111/*14"*, *18*; 191; 203)

At the proximal part of the tarsus the **v. dorsalis pedis** gives off the *vv. tarseae medialis* and *lateralis* and more distally the *v. tarsea perforans distalis*, which is usually duplicated, to the deep plantar arch. As it crosses over to the metatarsus, the dorsal pedal vein becomes the *v. metatarsea dorsalis III*. This vein in turn joins the corresponding plantar metatarsal vein by means of the *r. perforans distalis III* and terminates in the third dorsal common digital vein. The *vv. metatarseae dorsales II* and *IV* originate via the *rr. perforantes proximales II* and *IV* respectively from the plantar veins of the same number and they terminate in the second and fourth dorsal common digital vein respectively. Shortly before its termination this second vein receives an anastomosis from the *v. digitalis plantaris communis I.*

At the talocrural joint the medial and lateral rami of the cranial ramus of the medial saphenous vein unite in an arch. Before this union, however, the medial ramus gives off two veins which generally course to the medial plantar vein. The united medial and lateral rami terminate in the cranial ramus of the lateral saphenous vein. This cranial ramus anastomoses at the same level with the lateral tarsal vein. At the distal third of the metatarsus the cranial ramus of the lateral saphenous vein gives rise to the *vv. digitales dorsales communes II–IV.* After receiving the dorsal metatarsal vein of the corresponding number, each of the latter divides into the *vv. digitales dorsales propriae.* The *vv. interdigitales II* and *IV* form stout connections with the plantar digital veins.

Veins of the hindfoot of ruminants

Plantar veins
(sheep: 195/*16'–17*; ox: 192; 196/*34, 35, 43–46, 50–54, 56, 58*; 200)

The caudal ramus of the medial saphenous vein divides into the **v. plantaris medialis** and the **v. plantaris lateralis.** However, the latter is frequently absent in the small ruminants. The slender lateral plantar vein unites distal to the tarsus with the stout caudal ramus of the lateral saphenous vein. Both plantar veins (or in the absence of the lateral one, the caudal ramus of the lateral saphenous vein) form, in the proximal part of the metatarsus, the *arcus plantaris profundus* by means of their respective deep rami. The distal perforating tarsal vein terminates in this arch and from the arch issue the *vv. metatarseae plantares II–IV.* In the small ruminants, especially in the proximal part of the metatarsus, these are represented by a single vessel. In the ox the third plantar metatarsal vein is the smallest and the fourth and second are of about equal calibre and freely anastomose with one another distally. In the distal part of the metatarsus the plantar metatarsal veins unite to form the *arcus plantaris profundus distalis.* This latter arch receives laterally the dorsal common digital vein IV and anastomoses, via the *r. perforans distalis III,* with the dorsal metatarsal vein of the same number.

The distal deep plantar arch is linked medially with the superficial ramus of the medial plantar vein which latter is absent in the small ruminants. The stout *v. digitalis plantaris communis II* arises from this union in the ox but in the small ruminants it stems directly from the arch. The superficial ramus of the lateral plantar vein occurs exclusively, and even then infrequently, in the ox and it joins the arch laterally. At this junction or, as the case may be, directly from the arch, arises the stout *v. digitalis plantaris communis IV.* The *v. digitalis plantaris communis III* is a vessel of smaller calibre in small ruminants and arises from the distal deep plantar arch. In the ox it is particularly slender and stems either from the superficial ramus of the medial plantar vein, from the lateral plantar vein or from the plantar common digital vein IV. The plantar common digital veins divide into the *vv. digitales plantares propriae.* Before this division, however, the slender third plantar common digital vein receives a stout connection from the third dorsal common digital vein by way of the interdigital vein III.

Dorsal veins
(sheep: 195/*14', 18*; ox: 192; 204)

The **v. dorsalis pedis,** which is usually paired, anastomoses at the proximal part of the tarsus with the cranial ramus of the lateral saphenous vein and shortly thereafter it gives off the medial and lateral tarsal veins. After having given off the distal perforating tarsal vein the dorsal pedal vein becomes the slender, and also usually double, *v. metatarsea dorsalis III.* Through the *r. perforans distalis III* this vein is linked to the distal deep plantar arch and it terminates in the dorsal common digital vein III.

The cranial ramus of the lateral saphenous vein divides at the distal half of the metatarsus into the *vv. digitales communes III* and *IV.* The dorsal common digital vein IV does not proceed further towards the toe but runs parallel to the corresponding nerve across the lateral surface to the origin of the plantar common digital vein IV. The dorsal common digital vein III receives the dorsal metatarsal vein III, gives off the *v. interdigitalis III* and then divides into the *vv. digitales dorsales propriae III axialis* and *IV axialis.* The *vv. digitales dorsales propriae III abaxialis* and *IV abaxialis* are formed via the *r. dorsalis phalangis proximalis* of the appropriate proper digital vein.

Veins of the hindfoot of the horse

Plantar veins
(horse: 123; 124; 193; 197/*18, 21–24, 26, 30, 31*; 201)

The caudal ramus of the medial saphenous vein divides at the level of the sustentaculum tali into the **v. plantaris medialis** and the **v. plantaris lateralis**. Each of these veins then divides again at the proximal part of the metatarsus into the *r. profundus* and *r. superficialis*. Together the deep rami form the *arcus plantaris profundus* to which the distal perforating tarsal vein also contributes. The *vv. metatarseae plantares II* and *III* arise from the arch and on the distal part of the metatarsus they unite to form the *arcus plantaris profundus distalis*.

The superficial ramus of the medial plantar vein becomes the *v. digitalis plantaris communis II*. This receives the dorsal common digital vein II and unites a little further distally with the distal deep plantar arch. The distal continuation of this vein is the *v. digitalis plantaris (propria III) medialis*. The superficial ramus of the lateral plantar vein becomes the *v. digitalis plantaris communis III* and this in turn connects with the distal deep plantar arch laterally and then continues as the *v. digitalis plantaris (propria III) lateralis*.

Dorsal veins
(horse: 123; 124; 193; 197/*25, 27–29*; 205; 206/*2–9*)

The **v. dorsalis pedis** receives a sturdy anastomosis from the cranial ramus of the medial saphenous vein. It then gives off the distal perforating tarsal vein to the deep plantar arch and continues as the *v. metatarsea dorsalis II*. This is only a slender vessel which accompanies the homonymous nerve over the medial surface of the third metatarsal bone but does not extend as far as the groove between this bone and the second metatarsus.

The cranial ramus of the medial saphenous vein swings medially on the proximal part of the metatarsus and becomes the *v. digitalis dorsalis communis II*. The latter vessel does not extend to the dorsal surface of the toe but anastomoses medially beyond the distal end of the second metatarsus with the plantar common digital vein II. The ramification area of the dorsal proper digital vein is supplied by the *rr. dorsales phalangium proximalis mediae* and *distalis* of the plantar proper digital veins.

Veins of the pelvic and tail regions

V. iliaca interna
(Comparative: 149–152/*63*; 187; 190–193/*5*; 212–215/*12*; cat: 194/*8*; pig: 111/*21*; 188/*18*; sheep: 189/*18*; 195/*10*; ox: 196/*7*; horse: 104/*19*; 197/*32*)

The **v. iliaca interna** is the medial branch of the division of the common iliac vein; it is directed caudally into the pelvic cavity. It divides into the *v. glutaea caudalis* and the *v. pudenda interna*. In the horse this division occurs at the level of the body of the ilium and in carnivores it occurs dorsal to the ischiatic spine and therefore further caudal than the corresponding artery. In pigs and ruminants the division is found at the level of the lesser ischiatic notch. In carnivores, pigs and small ruminants the internal iliac vein gives off first the iliolumbar vein while in the ox the slender uterine vein arises before this. The branch vessels from the internal iliac vein and the order in which they arise vary considerably from species to species, as shown in the table. Only in the dog is the superficial lateral caudal vein a branch of the internal iliac. In the horse, since the latter vein bifurcates after only a short course, the prostatic or, in the female, the vaginal vein arises as a branch of the internal pudendal and the cranial gluteal vein stems from the caudal gluteal. In this species also the iliolumbar vein springs from the common iliac and the obturator vein from the external iliac.

External iliac veins

V. iliaca interna

carnivore	pig	ruminant	horse
		v. uterina (ox)	
v. iliolumbalis	v. iliolumbalis	v. iliolumbalis	
v. prostatica or v. vaginalis			
v. glutaea cranialis	v. glutaea cranialis	v. glutaea cranialis	
	v. prostatica or v. vaginalis		
	v. obturatoria	v. obturatoria	
v. caudalis lateralis superficialis (dog)		v. prostatica or v. vaginalis	
v. glutaea caudalis	v. glutaea caudalis	v. glutaea caudalis	v. glutaea caudalis
v. pudenda interna	v. pudenda interna	v. pudenda interna	v. pudenda interna

Fig. 206. Veins and arteries at the tarsal joint of the horse. Dorsal view. (After Schmaltz, 1939.)

A malleolus medialis; *B* malleolus lateralis tibiae; *C* trochlea tali; *D* os metatarsale III
a terminal tendon of the m. fibularis tertius; *b* terminal tendon of the m. tibialis cranialis; *c* tendon of the m. extensor digitalis longus; *d* tendon of the m. extensor digitalis lateralis; *e* retinaculum extensorum medium; *f* retinaculum extensorum distale

1 a. and v. tibialis cranialis with n. fibularis profundus; *2* a. and v. dorsalis pedis, *3* rr. articulares; *4* a. and v. tarsea perforans distalis; *5* a. metatarsea dorsalis III with n. metatarseus dorsalis III; *6* v. metatarsea dorsalis II with n. metatarseus dorsalis II; *7* r. cranialis of the v. saphena lateralis; *8* r. anastomoticus; *9* v. digitalis dorsalis communis II

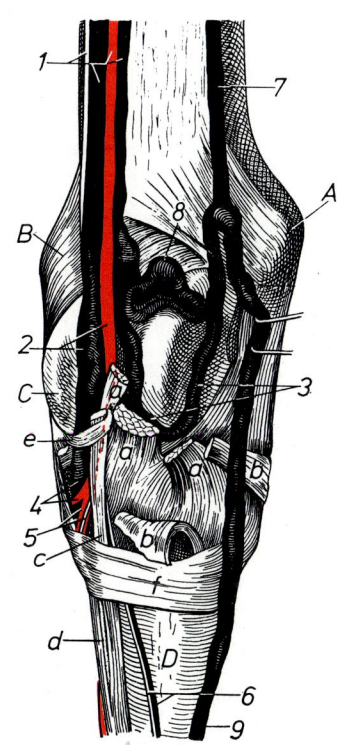

V. iliolumbalis
(Comparative: 149–152/*64*; 190–193/*6*; 212–215/*14*; sheep: 189/*19*; 195/*25*; ox: 196/*8*; horse: 197/*5*)

In carnivores, pigs and small ruminants the **v. iliolumbalis** arises ventrally to the sacroiliac joint as the first branch of the internal iliac vein. In the ox the uterine vein is given off the external iliac beforehand

and in the horse the iliolumbar vein has already branched from the common iliac ventral to the promontory. The iliolumbar vein accompanies the corresponding artery into its supply area which varies between species.

V. obturatoria
(Comparative: 149–152/67; 190–193/7; 212–215/6; pig: 111/24; sheep: 189/21; 195/27; ox: 196/10; horse: 197/7)

The **v. obturatoria** of carnivores is a branch of either the external or internal iliac vein and in pigs and ruminants it originates from the internal iliac vein. Without arterial accompaniment but with the obturator nerve, it courses medially over the body of the ilium to the obturator foramen. Whereas in carnivores it is said to terminate in the obturatorius internus muscle, in pigs and ruminants it anastomoses with the obturator ramus of the medial circumflex femoral vein.

The obturator vein of the horse arises from the external iliac and is accompanied by the homonymous artery which, however, originates from the cranial gluteal artery. The vein, like the artery, is very well developed and it runs with the artery through the obturator foramen and then gives off the medial vein of the penis or the clitoris. The *v. penis media* participates, together with the stout *v. penis cranialis*, in the formation of the *v. dorsalis penis*. The latter actually originates from the *v. penis* but its vessel of origin is only very slender. These vessels result in the formation of an extensive venous network on the dorsum of the penis. The *v. clitoridis media* is the largest vessel participating in the formation of the *v. dorsalis clitoridis*. After the medial vein of the penis or clitoris has been given off, the obturator vein is usually double and accompanies the corresponding artery. The vessels ramify in the long muscles of the ischium and anastomose with the distal caudal femoral vein in the hollow of the knee near the popliteal lymph node.

V. glutaea cranialis
(Comparative: 149–152/69; 190–193/8; 212–215/15; pig: 111/26; sheep: 189/20; 195/26; ox: 196/9; horse: 197/36)

In carnivores, pigs and ruminants the **v. glutaea cranialis** arises from the internal iliac and in the horse it originates from the caudal gluteal vein. It courses with the corresponding artery through the greater ischiatic notch and together they ramify in the gluteal musculature.

V. caudalis lateralis superficialis
(dog: 149/66; 190/9)

The **v. caudalis lateralis superficialis** occurs only in carnivores. In the dog it arises from the internal iliac vein shortly before that vessel bifurcates. In the cat it originates from the first part of the caudal gluteal vein, medial to the tendon of origin of the abductor cruris cranialis muscle. In both these animals it is a stouter vessel than the homonymous artery which it accompanies along the lateral superficial part of the tail. The two veins run along either side of the tail of the cat where they are linked by several dorsal anastomoses from which arises the unpaired *v. caudalis dorsalis*.

V. glutaea caudalis
(Comparative: 149–152/65; 190–193/11; 212–215/20; cat: 194/10; pig: 111/29; sheep: 195/29; ox: 196/12; horse: 197/37, 38)

In all the domestic mammals the **v. glutaea caudalis** and the internal pudendal vein are the two terminal branches of the internal iliac vein. In the horse the caudal gluteal vein arises immediately after the origin of the internal iliac itself and it then courses lateral to the corresponding artery in a caudal direction along the dorsal part of the pelvic cavity. The terminal bifurcation of the internal iliac, and therefore the origin of the caudal gluteal artery, lies dorsal to the ischiatic spine in carnivores; in the pig and ruminant it is at the level of the lesser ischiatic notch. In the horse the caudal gluteal vein gives off the cranial gluteal vein, the sacral rami, the median caudal vein and the ventrolateral caudal vein with the caudal rami and the dorsolateral caudal vein. These veins are described later together with those of the other domestic mammals (p. 260). In all the domestic species the caudal gluteal vein runs laterally at the level of the lesser ischiatic notch in company with the corresponding artery. The two vessels subdivide similarly. In the cat there is a stout distally directed branch which gives off the superficial lateral caudal vein and then anastomoses with the lateral saphenous vein at the level of the popliteal lymph nodes. The caudal gluteal vein of carnivores and pigs also gives rise to the *v. perinealis dorsalis* which in turn gives issue to the *v. rectalis caudalis* in the pig.

V. pudenda interna
(Comparative: 149–152/*70*; 190–193/*10*; 212–215/*22*; cat: 194/*9*; pig: 111/*27*; 188/*20*; sheep: 189/*26*; 195/*30*; ox: 196/*13*; horse: 104/*20*; 197/*33*)

The **v. pudenda interna** follows the *v. glutaea caudalis* as the second terminal branch of the internal iliac vein. Only in the horse is there a venous "long pudendal type" since in this animal the vein arises at the commencement of the internal iliac. In carnivores the internal pudendal vein arises from the internal iliac vein dorsal to the ischiatic spine and in the pig and ruminants it is given off this vessel at the level of the lesser ischiatic notch. In the horse its initial course follows that of the internal iliac and then, as in all domestic mammals, it runs caudad with the internal pudendal artery as a continuation of the internal iliac vein. Together the artery and vein pass, in the region of the lesser ischiatic notch, through the broad sacrotuberal ligament, or in the dog through the levator ani muscle, to re-enter the pelvic cavity. Medial to the broad sacrotuberal ligament the internal pudendal vein of the horse has a parallel vein. The internal pudendal vein reaches the pelvic exit and unites with the vein of the other side to form the *arcus ischiaticus*. In horses the internal pudendal gives rise to the prostatic or vaginal vein cranial to the ischiatic spine. In carnivores the *v. urethralis* and in the ox the *v. vestibularis* are branches of the internal pudendal vein. In all the domestic mammals the internal pudendal vein divides at the pelvic exit into the ventral perineal vein and the vein of the penis or clitoris. However, before this division the internal pudendal gives rise to the dorsal vein of the penis or clitoris in carnivores and to the *v. rectalis caudalis* in sheep and male cattle.

V. perinealis ventralis
(Comparative: 149–152/*74*; 212–215/*24*; pig: 111/*28*; 188/*21*; sheep: 195/*31*; horse: 197/*35*)

The **v. perinealis ventralis** is one of the two terminal branches of the internal pudendal vein. In carnivores and horses it gives off the *v. rectalis caudalis,* in male carnivores and male pigs the *v. scrotalis dorsalis* and in all domestic mammals the *v. labialis dorsalis* or, in ruminants, the *v. labialis dorsalis et mammaria*. These veins are distributed in a similar manner to their corresponding arteries. Special mention should be made of the v. labialis dorsalis et mammaria which links with the caudal mammary vein arising from the external pudendal, because the valves of the first vein show individual variations in their alignment. Therefore this vein has different functional significance in relation to the udder.

V. penis
(Comparative: 149–152/*75*; 212–215/*25*)

The **v. penis** is the second terminal branch of the internal pudendal in males and it gives rise to the *v. bulbi penis,* the *v. profunda penis* and, except in carnivores, the *v. dorsalis penis*. In carnivores the latter has already been given off independently by the internal pudendal vein before its terminal division. The above veins are distributed along with the corresponding arteries. The dorsal vein of the penis participates, especially in the horse, in the formation of the superficially-situated venous plexus at the dorsum of the penis.

V. clitoridis
(Comparative: 149–152/75; 212–215/25; pig: 188/22, 23)

The **v. clitoridis** is the second terminal branch of the internal pudendal vein of females. It gives off the *v. bulbi vestibuli*, the *v. profunda clitoridis* and, except in carnivores, the *v. dorsalis clitoridis*. In carnivores the latter arises independently from the internal pudendal prior to its terminal division. These veins branch in unison with their corresponding arteries. This also applies to the horse in which, unlike the arteries, the deep and dorsal veins of the clitoridis are also branches of the v. clitoris.

The visceral branches of the internal iliac and internal pudendal veins are described together with those of the caudal vena cava (see below).

V. sacralis mediana and V. caudalis mediana
(Comparative: 149–152/45, 47; 190–193, 212–215/2; cat: 194/6, 37; pig: 111/30, 32; 188/17, 32; sheep: 189/16; 195/23, 24; ox: 196/4, 4'; horse: 197/39)

The **v. sacralis mediana**, which is absent or only weakly developed in the horse, arises from the angle of division of the caudal vena cava or from one of the two common iliac veins. It courses ventromedially along the sacrum. Except in horses, the medial sacral vein gives issue to the *rr. sacrales*, which behave like all the other segmental vessels and terminate in the *v. caudalis mediana*. This latter vessel gives rise to the *rr. caudales* which only supply branches to the musculature of the tail; they link ventral to the rudimentary transverse processes to form the *v. caudalis ventrolateralis* and dorsal to them to form the *v. caudalis dorsolateralis*.

In the horse, even when the medial sacral vein is present, the sacral rami arise from the ipselateral caudal gluteal vein. The median caudal vein also stems from one of the caudal gluteal veins, but it is slender and may be absent. The caudal rami arise from the ventrolateral caudal vein which also originates from the ipselateral caudal gluteal vein. But in the horse, as in the preceding animals, the anastomoses lying dorsal to the rudimentary transverse processes form the dorsolateral caudal vein.

Visceral veins of the v. cava caudalis

Vv. hepaticae
(Comparative: 149–152/42; pig: 188/7; horse: 211/9)

In the sulcus venae hepatis the caudal vena cava supplies numerous **vv. hepaticae** of varying calibre directly to the liver and these vessels ramify interlobularly. The hepatic veins thus differ not only topographically from the branches of the hepatic artery which are destined for the liver; through the hepatic capillary system they link the portal vein with the caudal vena cava.

V. portae
(Comparative: 207–210/1; horse: 211/11)

While the arteries to the spleen, stomach, pancreas, small intestine and the major part of the large intestine originate from the abdominal aorta via three primary trunks, namely the coeliac, cranial mesenteric and caudal mesenteric arteries, the corresponding veins are not joined directly to the caudal vena cava. On the contrary, they are united to a single vessel, the **v. portae**, which is then connected through the hepatic capillary system and the hepatic veins to the caudal vena cava. It is thus obvious that the hepatic veins differ both in their course and function from the hepatic artery because they carry into the caudal vena cava not only the "nutritive" blood from the hepatic artery but also the "functional" blood from the portal vein. The portal vein can therefore be characterized as a vein which is followed by a capillary network, namely the sinusoids of the liver. Nevertheless, the course and branches of the portal vein will be described in a retograde manner as were the other veins.

The portal vein leaves the porta of the liver by an *r. dexter* and *r. sinister*. In the left ramus we differentiate a *pars umbilicalis* and a *pars transversa*. In the foetus the umbilical part is continued as the *v. umbilicalis* to the foetal placenta and this latter vein is connected in carnivores and ruminants through the *ductus venosus* directly to the caudal vena cava. In post-foetal life the umbilical vein persists in an obliterated state as the lig. theres hepatis in the falciform ligament of the liver. While still within the hepatic porta the portal vein gives rise, except in the horse, to the *vv. cysticae*. Then from the hepatic porta the portal vein runs in the edge of the hepatoduodenal ligament caudodorsally to reach the body of the pancreas. In so doing it forms the ventral limit of the epiploic foramen. In carnivores and ruminants it passes through the inc. pancreatis, which in the pig and horse is the anulus pancreatis. Before this it gives off the *v. gastrica dextra* in the pig and in the horse the *v. gastrica sinistra parietalis*, which latter continues from the left side of the lesser curvature to the parietal surface of the stomach. Also in the horse the portal vein gives rise to the *rr. pancreatici*. Thereafter, in all domestic mammals, the portal vein gives rise in the pancreatic region to the *v. gastroduodenalis* and the *v. lienalis*. Caudal to the pancreas and to the right of the cranial mesenteric artery the portal vein divides into a prominent *v. mesenterica cranialis* and a more slender *v. mesenterica caudalis*.

V. gastroduodenalis
(Comparative: 207–210/4; horse: 211/*12*)

The **v. gastroduodenalis** arises from the portal vein near the pancreas. In carnivores, ruminants and horses, the v. gastroduodenalis gives off the *v. gastrica dextra* which reaches the lesser curvature of the stomach from the right. In the pig it follows this lesser curvature and reaches the greater curvature on the left. In the horse it is confined to the pyloric region. Thereafter the gastroduodenal vein gives rise to the *v. gastroepiploica dextra* in all domestic mammals and this runs from the right side to the greater curvature of the stomach supplying branches to the stomach(s) and the greater omentum. Another branch of the gastroduodenal vein is the *v. pancreaticoduodenalis cranialis* which courses in company with the homonymous artery along the duodenum where it links with the caudal pancreaticoduodenal vein. In the dog there is an additional anastomosis with the caudal pancreaticoduodenal vein through the pancreatic branch of the cranial pancreaticoduodenal vein.

V. lienalis
(Comparative: 207–210/8)

Near the body of the pancreas the portal vein gives off the large **v. lienalis** (splenic vein) which is directed to the left. This gives rise in turn to the *vv. pancreaticae* and then, in carnivores, pigs and ruminants, the *v. gastrica sinistra* followed by the *vv. diverticuli* in the pig and in ruminants the *v. gastroepiploica sinistra*. In the horse the splenic vein gives issue to the *v. gastrica sinistra visceralis* with more *rr. pancreatici*. Then, except in ruminants, the splenic vein supplies the *vv. gastricae breves* to the left side of the greater curvature of the stomach and the *v. gastroepiploica sinistra*. In ruminants there is a special *r. epiploicus*, then the *v. ruminalis dextra* with the *r. collateralis*, the *v. reticularis* and the *v. ruminalis sinistra* with the *v. oesophagea caudalis*. All these veins of the ruminant, except the collateral ramus running ventral to the insula ruminis, are accompanied by the corresponding arteries.

V. mesenterica cranialis
(Comparative: 207–210/*16*; horse: 211/*13*)

The **v. mesenterica cranialis**, the stoutest of the terminal branches of the portal vein, is generally disseminated in company with the cranial mesenteric artery and its branches. However, there are individual and species differences in the sequential origin of the various veins from the cranial mesenteric.

The cranial mesenteric vein gives off the *v. pancreaticoduodenalis caudalis*, the *vv. jejunales*, the *vv. ilei* and the *v. ileocolica*. In the ox the *r. collateralis* accompanies that part of the cranial mesenteric vein which extends between the points of origin of the jejunal veins. The ileocolic vein sends a branch, the *r.*

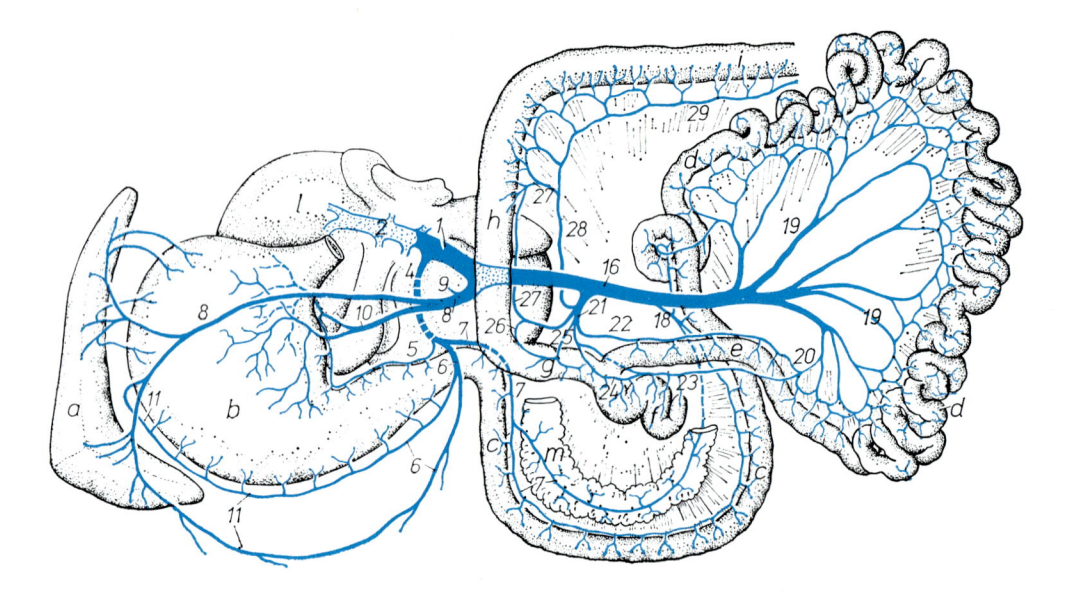

Fig. 207

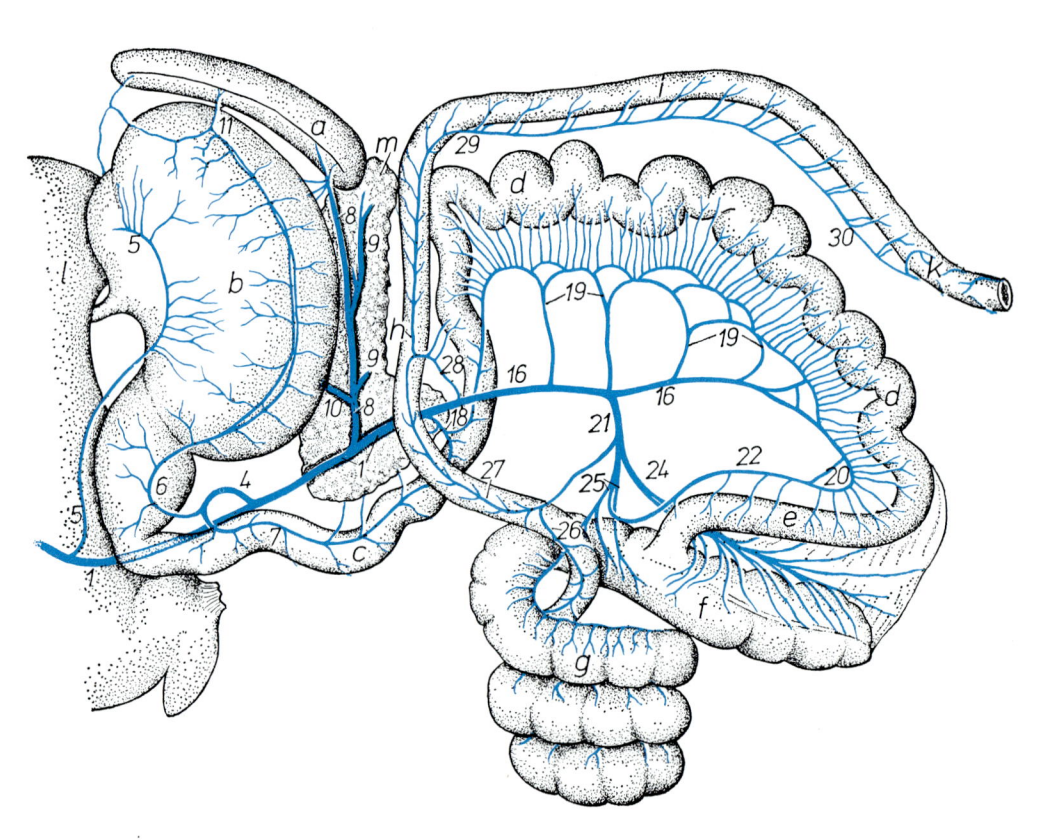

Fig. 208

Caudal vena cava 263

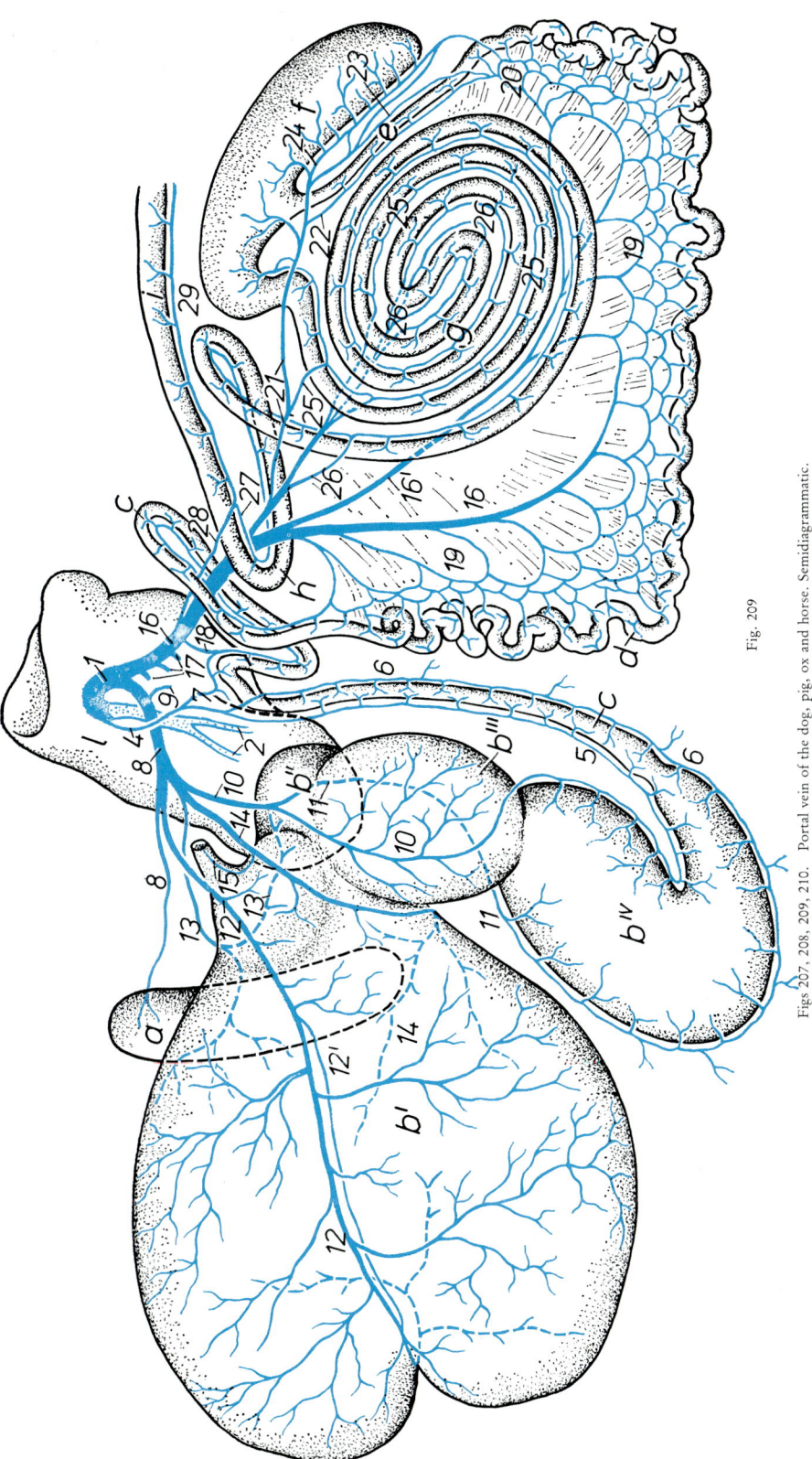

Fig. 209

Figs 207, 208, 209, 210. Portal vein of the dog, pig, ox and horse. Semidiagrammatic.
(After Schmitz, 1910, Diss., Leipzig; after Hapke, 1957, Diss., Hanover.)

a lien; *b* ventriculus; *b'* rumen; *b''* reticulum; *b'''* omasum; *b''''* abomasum; *c* duodenum; *d* jejunum; *e* ileum; *f* caecum; *g* colon ascendens; *h* colon transversum; *i* colon descendens; *k* rectum (illustrated only in the pig and horse); *l* hepar; *m* pancreas (only shown in the dog and pig)

1 v. portae, *2* rr. hepatici, *3* r. pancreatici (horse); *4* v. gastroduodenalis; *5* v. gastrica dextra; *6* v. gastroepiploica dextra with rr. gastrici and rr. epiploici; *7* v. pancreaticoduodenalis cranialis with rr. pancreatici and rr. duodenales; *8* v. lienalis with rr. lienales and vv. gastricae breves; *9* vv. pancreaticae; *10* v. gastrica sinistra; *10'* v. gastrica sinistra parietalis, *10''* v. gastrica sinistra visceralis (horse); *11* f. gastroepiploica sinistra with rr. gastrici and rr. epiploici; *12* v. ruminalis dextra; *12'* r. collateralis; *13* v. reticularis; *14* v. ruminalis sinistra; *15* v. oesophagea caudalis (ox); *16* v. mesenterica cranialis, *16'* r. collateralis (ox); *17* rr. pancreatici (ox); *18* v. pancreaticoduodenalis caudalis; *19* vv. jejunales; *20* vv. ilei; *21* v. ileocolica; *22* r. ilei mesenterialis; *23* r. ilei antimesenterialis; *24* v. caecalis; *24'* v. caecalis medialis, *24''* v. caecalis lateralis (horse); *25* r. colicus (dog, pig, horse), rr. colici (ox); *26* v. colica dextra (dog, pig, horse), vv. colicae dextrae (ox); *27* v. colica media; *28* v. mesenterica caudalis; *29* v. colica sinistra; *30* v. rectalis cranialis (shown only in the pig and horse)

Fig. 210

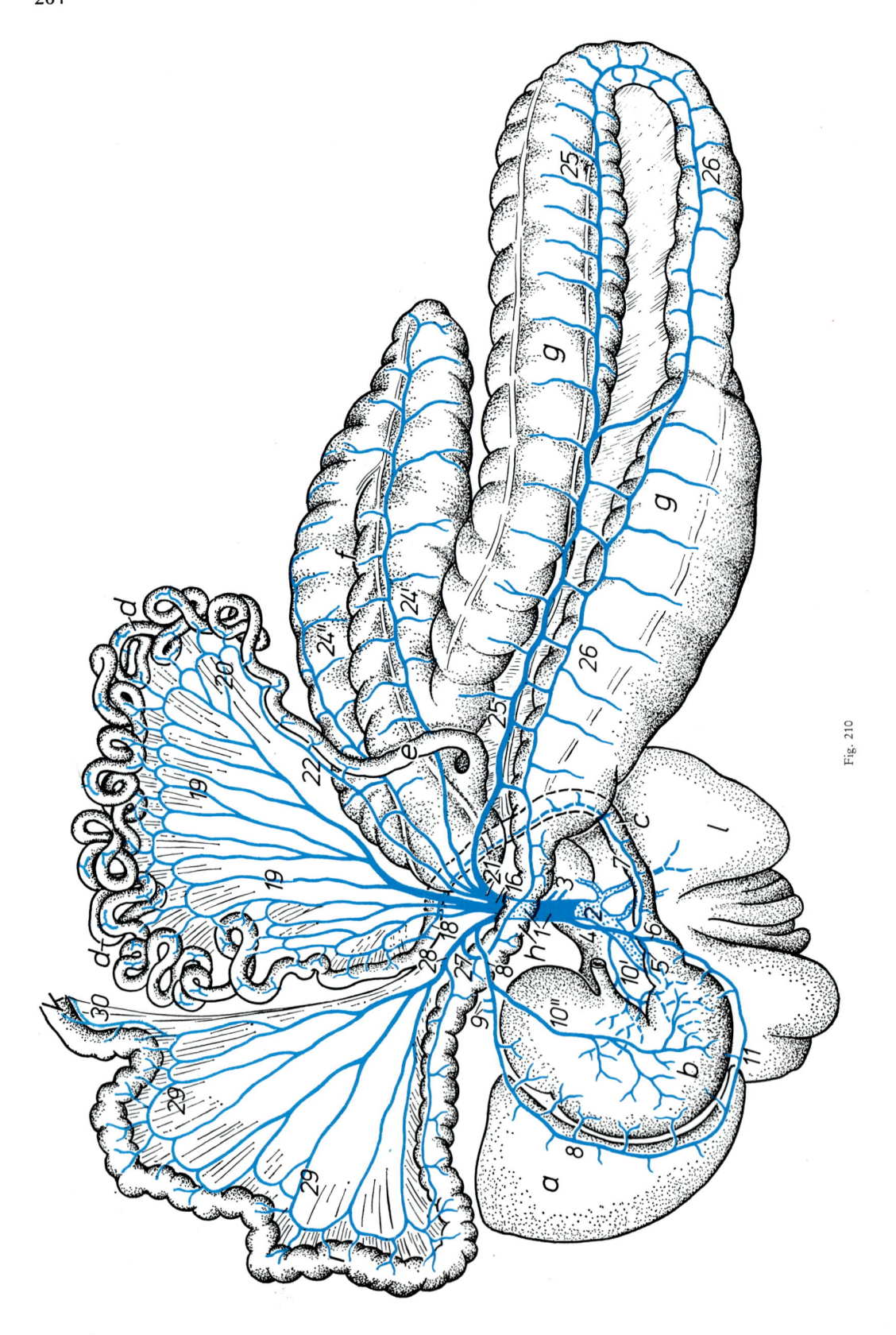

ilei mesenterialis to the ileum. The proximal half of the ascending colon is supplied by the ileocolic vein through the *r. colicus* or, in ruminants, the *rr. colici*. The same parent vessel supplies the caecum with the *v. caecalis* which is augmented in carnivores, pigs and ruminants by the *r. ilei antimesenterialis* and in the horse by the *vv. caecales mediales* and *laterales*. Furthermore, the ileocolic vein gives off the *v. colica dextra* and *v. colica media* (which have a common stem in carnivores and pigs), the *v. colica dextra* in the horse and the *vv. colicae dextrae* of the ruminant. The latter share a common stem of origin with the colic rami.

V. mesenterica caudalis
(Comparative: 207–210/*28*; horse: 211/*15*)

The **v. mesenterica caudalis** is the weaker terminal branch of the portal vein. Its origin is situated in the cranial mesentery and is thus more cranial than the artery of the same name to which, in fact, it bears no topographical relationship. In ruminants and horses it at once gives off the *v. colica media* and then continues immediately, as in all the other domestic mammals, as the *v. colica sinistra*. This caudally directed vein runs along the descending colon giving off along its course the *vv. sigmoideae* until it reaches the rectum when it becomes the *v. rectalis cranialis*. This cranial rectal vein anastomoses with the *v. rectalis media* or *v. rectalis caudalis*. These two latter veins (pp. 259, 268) are developed bilaterally and linked through the veins of the pelvic cavity directly to the caudal vena cava. It is thus possible that drugs administered per rectum can reach the systemic circulation directly by by-passing the portal vein and the liver.

V. renalis
(Comparative: 149–152/*43*; 187; cat: 194/*2*; pig: 188/*10, 11*; sheep: 189/*2*; ox: 144/*1*; horse: 104/*11*)

The **vv. renales dextra** and **sinistra** arise from the caudal vena cava between the first and fourth lumbar vertebrae depending on the species; in the cat they originate at the level of the 3rd–4th lumbar vertebrae, in the dog the 2nd–3rd, in the pig the 1st–2nd, in the ox the 2nd and in the sheep and horse at

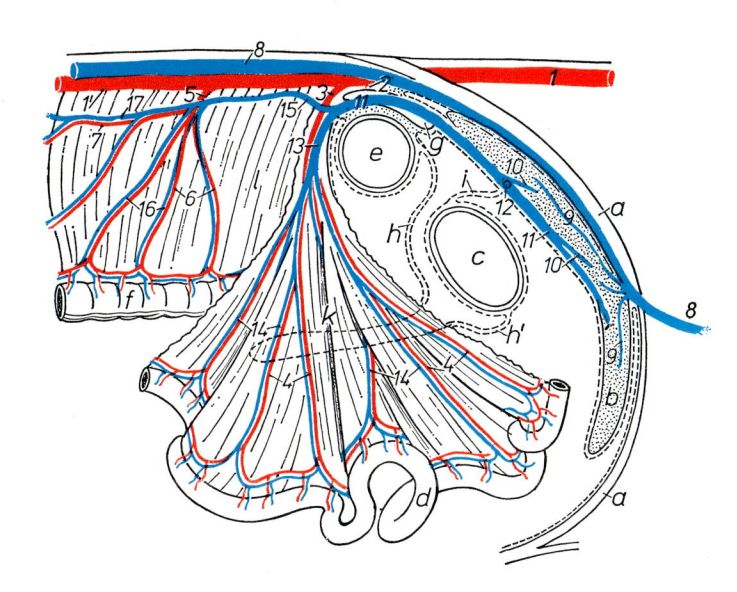

Fig. 211. Portal vein of the horse. Diagrammatic. Right lateral view.
(After Zietzschmann, 1943.)

a diaphragma; *b* hepar; *c* ventriculus; *d* jejunum; *e* colon transversum; *f* colon descendens; *g* pancreas; *h, h'* omentum majus: *h* visceral, *h'* parietal leaf; *i* omentum minus; *k* mesenterium craniale; *l* mesenterium caudale

1 aorta thoracica; *1'* aorta abdominalis; *2* a. coeliaca; *3* a. mesenterica cranialis; *4* aa. jejunales; *5* a. mesenterica caudalis; *6* a. colica sinistra; *7* a. rectalis cranialis; *8* v. cava caudalis; *9* vv. hepaticae; *10* rr. hepatici of *11* v. portae; *12* gastroduodenalis; *13* v. mesenterica cranialis; *14* vv. jejunales; *15* v. mesenterica caudalis; *16* v. colica sinistra; *17* v. rectalis cranialis

the 1st lumbar vertebra. The vein of each side goes to the corresponding renal hilus and the left renal vein, which in the pig gives off the *v. abdominalis cranialis*, crosses the aorta ventrally. In ruminants and horses the *r. suprarenalis caudalis* issues from each renal vein. Only in carnivores does the left renal vein give rise to *v. testicularis sinistra* or *v. ovarica sinistra*.

In the ox the *vv. suprarenales* arise, caudal to the renal vein, directly from the caudal vena cava.

V. testicularis or v. ovarica
(Comparative: 149–152/*44*; 187; pig: 188/*14*; sheep: 189/*8*; 195/*2*; ox: 144/*4*; 196/*2*; horse: 104/*12*)

The **vv. testiculares** or **vv. ovaricae dextra** and **sinistra** show considerable species variation in both the vessel of their origin and the level at which they arise. These differences are shown in figure 187.

The **v. testicularis** runs, together with the testicular artery, in the proximal mesorchium of the plica vasculosa to the internal inguinal ring and thence continues in the company of the artery along the spermatic cord to the testis. In so doing it forms round the artery the *plexus pampiniformis*. The testicular vein drains the epididymes by the *rr. epididymales* which, together with the *rr. ductus deferentis*, participate in the vascularization of the ductus deferens.

The **v. ovarica** is several times the calibre of the corresponding artery, in the company of which it courses in the mesovarium to the ovary. In the pig the *v. uterina* is usually the first vessel it gives off. The ovarian vein gives rise to the *r. tubarius* to the oviduct and its largest branch, the *r. uterinus*, to the uterine horn, and there the ovarian vein anastomoses with the uterine vein. The uterine vein is not present in the small ruminants. Thus the ovarian vein is one of the major veins of the uterus and during pregnancy it surpasses the uterine vein in size.

Without going into details, it should be mentioned that in ruminants the testicular or ovarian vein can sometimes give rise to the *v. vesicalis cranialis*.

Visceral veins of the v. iliaca interna and the v. pudenda interna

V. uterina
(dog: 212/*17*; pig: 213/*13*; ox: 144/*11*; 151/*71*; 214/*13*; horse: 215/*13*)

Only in the ox does the **v. uterina** arise from the internal iliac. It may be missing altogether but if present it is a delicate vessel. This vein has not been described in the small ruminants. In carnivores too this vein, like the corresponding arterial vessel to the uterus, is really absent, being replaced by the uterine ramus of the vaginal vein which in effect becomes the uterine vein. In the pig the uterine vein arises from the ovarian vein, in most cases before the origin of the stout *r. uterinus* and, having given off a *r. uretericus*, it reaches the uterine artery. Only in the horse does the uterine vein arise, at the same level as its artery, from the external iliac vein.

In the ox and the horse the uterine vein is functionally less important than the uterine artery which it accompanies because the uterine rami of both the ovarian and the vaginal veins, and also the accessory vaginal vein in the ox, form the main venous supply to the uterus. In the pig the uterine vein gives off the *v. vesicalis cranialis*; the drainage area of this latter vessel is taken over by the *v. vesicalis caudalis* in the other domestic mammals.

V. prostatica
(Comparative: 149–152/*73*; 212–215/*16*; ox: 196/*11*; horse: 197/*34*)

In carnivores, pigs and ruminants the **v. prostatica** arises from the internal iliac vein whereas in the horse it stems from the internal pudendal vein. The site of origin of this vein lies in the region of the pelvic inlet. In carnivores and ruminants it gives off the *v. ductus deferentis* and in the horse the *r. ductus deferentis*. From this vein, except in the pig in which it arises directly from the prostatic vein, springs the *v. vesicalis caudalis* and this accompanies the corresponding artery to the bladder. In carnivores, ruminants and horses its supply area extends to the apex of the bladder because these animals do not

Internal iliac vein

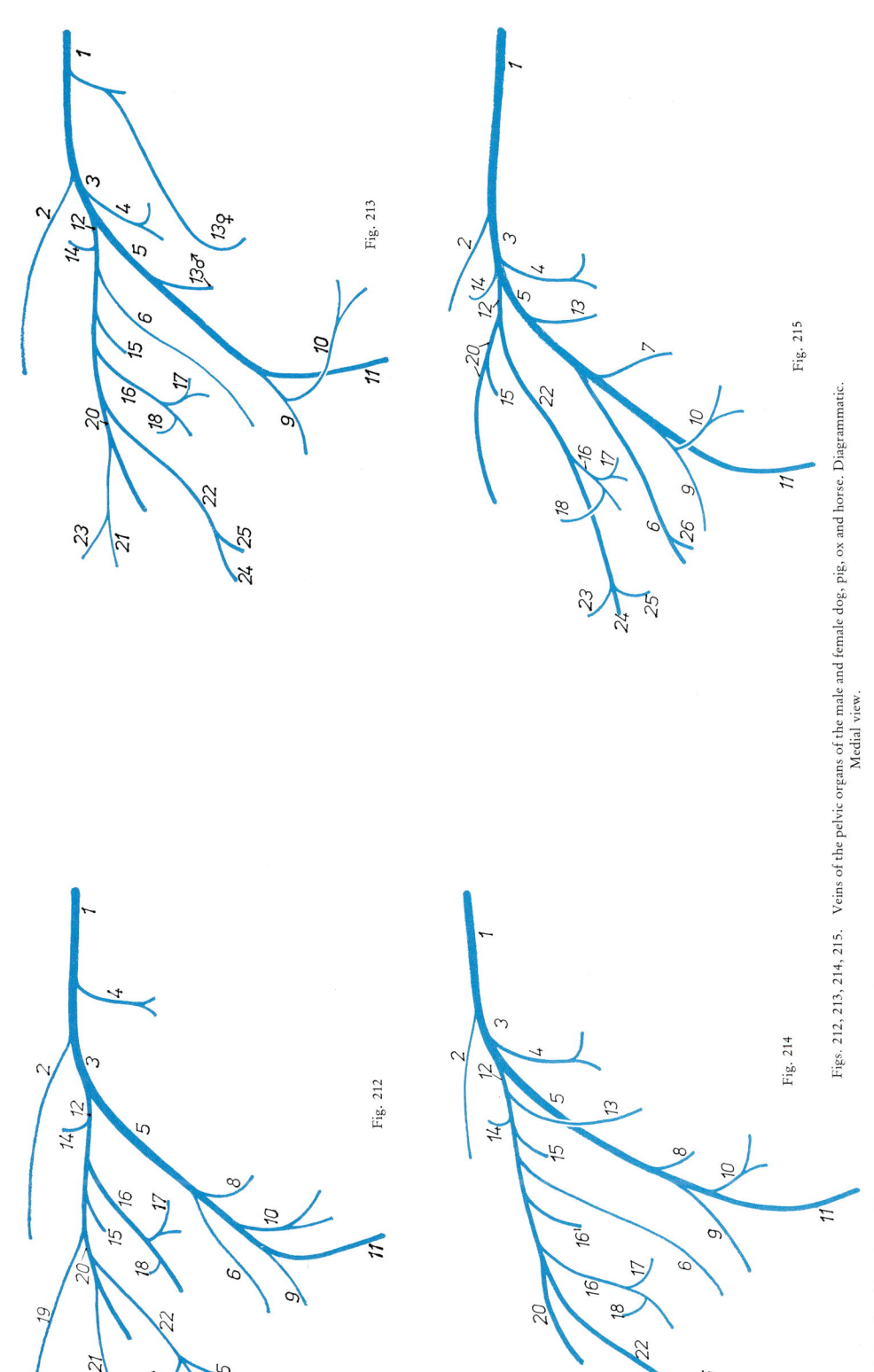

Figs. 212, 213, 214, 215. Veins of the pelvic organs of the male and female dog, pig, ox and horse. Diagrammatic. Medial view.

The names before the oblique line indicate structures in the male and those after the oblique line those of the female. *v. iliolumbalis; 15 v. glutea cranialis; 16 v. prostatica/v. vaginalis; 16′ v. vaginalis accessoria; 17 r. ductus deferentis, 1 v. cava caudalis; 2 v. sacralis mediana; 3 v. iliaca communis; 4 v. circumflexa ilium profunda; 5 v. iliaca externa; 6* in the dog and ox v. ductus deferentis/r. uterinus, in the dog v. uterina with v. vesicalis caudalis; *18 v. rectalis media; v. obturatoria; 7 v. iliacofemoralis; 8 v. abdominalis caudalis; 9 v. profunda femoris; 10 v. pudendoepigastrica; 11 v. 19 v. caudalis lateralis superficialis; 20 v. glutea caudalis; 21 v. perinealis dorsalis; 22 v. pudenda interna; 23 v. femoralis; 12 v. iliaca interna; 13 v. ductus deferentis (pig, horse)/v. uterina (pig from the v. ovarica; ox, horse); 14* rectalis caudalis; *24 v. perinealis ventralis; 25 v. penis/v. clitoridis; 26 v. penis media/v. clitoridis media*

have a cranial vesical vein. The prostatic vein of carnivores and horses gives rise to the *v. rectalis media* to the rectum.

V. ductus deferentis
(dog: 212/*17*; pig: 213/*13*; ox: 214/*17*; horse: 215/*13*)

In carnivores and ruminants the **v. ductus deferentis** arises from the prostatic vein, as does the *r. ductus deferentis* of the horse. In the pig and horse the vein of the ductus deferens stems from the external iliac vein. It thus becomes clear why it is the ductus deferens ramus in the pig and horse, and not the vein of that name, which provides the venous vascularization of the ductus deferens. The origin of the vein of the ductus deferens from the external iliac in the pig and horse is not at the same level as the artery and this is analogous to the origin of the uterine vein in the female pig and of the uterine artery and vein in the horse. Thus the area drained by the vein of the ductus deferens is supplied by various arteries. In the pig the v. ductus deferentis gives off the *v. vesicalis cranialis*, which is absent from the other domestic mammals. In carnivores and ruminants the vein, and in the horse the ramus, of the ductus deferens, gives rise to the *v. vesicalis caudalis* which in these animals takes over the drainage of the area of the cranial bladder vein.

V. vaginalis
(Comparative: 149–152/*73*; 212–215/*16*; dog: 212/*17*; pig: 111/*23*; 188/*19*; sheep: 189/*22*; 195/*28*; ox: 144/*17*; 151/*72*; 214/*16'*)

At the pelvic inlet the **v. vaginalis** leaves the internal iliac vein in carnivores, pigs and ruminants and the internal pudendal vein in the horse. The vaginal vein gives off the *r. uterinus* in the pig, ruminant and horse; this functions as the caudal uterine vein and runs parallel to the artery (p. 183). In carnivores this branch is the uterine vein. In the ox this ramus is supplemented particularly by the *v. vaginalis accessoria*, which arises from the internal iliac about half way between the uterine and vaginal veins and caudal to the cranial gluteal. There is no artery corresponding to the accessory vaginal vein. The *v. vesicalis caudalis* arises from the uterine ramus or vein and, in the pig, directly from the vaginal vein. In carnivores and ruminants the vaginal vein gives off the *v. rectalis media*; in the horse this stems from the caudal vesical vein and goes to the rectum. Other branches of the vaginal vein in ruminants are the *v. perinealis dorsalis* and in the goat and ox the *v. rectalis caudalis*.

V. urethralis
(ox: 144/*19*)

The **v. urethralis** occurs in carnivores and the ox. It is the first branch-vessel to arise from the internal pudendal vein and it is distributed in the company of the corresponding artery. It forms a prominent network in the ox.

V. vestibularis
(ox: 144/22)

Only the ox has a **v. vestibularis** and its parent vein is the internal pudendal. Together with the vestibular artery it courses toward the vestibule of the vagina.

Lymphatic system (Systema lymphaticum)

Introduction

Our knowledge of the structure and function of the organs of the lymphatic system has substantially increased during recent decades. This is equally true of those aspects of the system which are of practical application in veterinary medicine. It is thus desirable to precede the anatomical description of the lymphatic system by an account of its function and it is hoped that this will lead to an understanding of basic disciplines such as immunology, pathology and oncology and also of applied subjects such as clinical diagnosis and meat inspection.

From the anatomical viewpoint the lymphatic system can be divided into (1) the *cellular component*, that is, the *lymphoreticular* or *lymphatic tissue* of which all lymphatic organs are composed and (2) the *vascular component*, the actual *lymphatic vessel system*.

The function of the **lymphatic tissue** is defense. Its *fixed cells*, the *reticulum cells*, are found in the lymph nodes, the spleen, Peyer's patches, the tonsils and the thymus. These star-shaped cells are interconnected and form a three-dimensional meshwork which makes close contact with the permeating fluids and corpuscular elements and, because of its phagocytic property, selectively extracts substance foreign to the body. The *mobile elements* of the lymphatic tissue are represented by *lymphocytes, plasma cells* and *macrophages*. They circulate between the blood, the tissue spaces and the lymph stream. Their significance in the recognition of foreign substances and the dissemination of immune reactions is discussed in the subsequent section on the immune system. Thus both the fixed and the motile cells of the lymphatic tissue are part of the defense mechanism against infection.

The **lymphatic vessel system** includes *lymph capillares, lymph vessels* and *lymph collecting ducts* and it has a supporting function for the venous side of the blood circulation. The relationship between these two transport systems can even be recognised from their ontogenesis and phylogenesis. It is maintained in the *lymphovenous anastomoses*. On the other hand, the lymph vessel system has some characteristics which differ from the venous system; these include the special resorption property of its terminal parts and its innate motor ability.

Lymphatic organs

The term lymphatic organs encompasses those independent organs and organoid formations which are built up of lymphoreticular tissue.

The lymphatic organs are defense organs. Their reticulum cells have phagocytic ability and lymphocytes are formed by them (*lymphopoiesis*). Since immune reactions take place in the lymphopoietic centres, the lymphatic organs are also termed immune organs.

Phylogenesis of lymphatic organs

Immune reactions have so far been demonstrated only in vertebrates. Invertebrates do not show this; their defense reaction is restricted to *phagocytosis*.

In the slimefish, a forerunner of fish which belongs to the Agnatha, there is a primitive spleen and a primitive haemopoietic organ in the pronephros. On the other hand thymus, lymph nodes and lymphoepithelial structures of the digestive tract are all lacking. There are no plasma cells in the connective tissue and the blood has no lymphocytes. Only primitive granulocytes are present which, in the case of injury, infiltrate the local inflammatory lesion together with "macrophage derivatives". Various experiments with antigen injections have demonstrated that this primitive vertebrate species is unable to form antibodies and it is therefore incapable of a specific immune response.

The *higher agnatha*, such as the Lampreys (Petromyzon) possess a primitive epithelial thymus with sparse lymphocytic deposits. Both blood and spleen contain lymphocytes. No plasma cells are present in the tissues and lymph nodes are lacking. Experiments with the lamprey have clearly shown that it can mobilize its mononuclear cells against certain antigens. They react to tuberculin with a so-called delayed hypersensitivity. These animals will accept autotransplants but they gradually reject homotransplants. This would appear to demonstrate a still incomplete immune mechanism. One may perhaps assume that the evolutionary step to the capability of an immune response must have occurred in a lower vertebrate descended from the higher agnatha.

In *fish*, diffusely distributed lymphatic tissue is present in the parenchyma of the viscera and especially in the pronephros. The thymus is encountered as a defined organ on the inner surface of the gill cavity in the form of a raised white patch in the modified epithelium. Histologically one can differentiate a cortex tightly packed with lymphocytes and a less cellular medulla. In cartilaginous fish the spleen has no follicles but in bony fish these are present. The plasma cells form antibodies of the first order (class IgM). Thus, in addition to a cellular immune reaction, we now have the first humoral antibody production.

In *amphibia* the lymphatic tissue is evenly distributed in the wall of the lymph sinuses where these communicate with the veins. It possesses filtration and possibly also immune functions. It is interesting to note that some amphibian species also have lymphatic tissue which is organised, that is to say, it is surrounded by a delicate connective tissue capsule. Although it is still difficult to make definite comparisons, these structures are interpreted as forerunners of such lymphatic organs as thymus, spleen and lymph nodes. The plasma cells produce immunoglobulins of primary and secondary response (IgM and IgG).

Although the lymphatic tissue of *reptiles* is fairly sparse almost all the components of the mammalian immune response have been described in this class. Lymphatic tissue is found not only in the spleen and thymus but also in a diffuse form around the smaller and larger lymph vessels, the postcapillary veins and the precapillary arteries. Thus it occurs in those parts of the vessel where there is intense exchange activity. Reaction centres are present and the plasma cells produce antibodies of the classes IgM and IgG.

In *birds* lymphatic tissue is amply developed. As well as lymphoreticular structures in the mucous membrane of the digestive tract (caecal tonsil) and of the respiratory tract, there are lymph nodes (present particularly in the goose and duck), the spleen and especially the thymus and bursa of Fabricius all of which belong to the immunocompetent lymphatic cell system. Experiments with bursectomised, thymectomised and irradiated chicks have stimulated new lines of thought in the investigation of the immune system of mammals. We know today that the immune apparatus of the fowl is regulated by two systems: the thymus-dependent or T-cell system and the bursa-dependent or B-cell system. The *T-cell system* includes the thymus and the T-lymphocytes of the peripheral lymphatic organs. It is responsible for cell-transmitted immunity (rejection of transplants, graft-versus-host reaction, allergies of the delayed type). The *B-cell system* consists of the bursa Fabricii and the B-lymphocytes and plasma cells which occur mainly in the reaction centres of the peripheral lymphatic organs. The antibody producing plasma cells mature and differentiate in this system and these cells are responsible for the humoral immune reactions.

In *mammals* the lymphatic system participates in immune reactions by means of the numerous lymph nodes, the rich supply of lymphatic structures in the mucous membranes, the thymus, the spleen and the bone marrow. Only the bursa of Fabricius is lacking. It is assumed that its function is taken over by the bone marrow, so that the mammal, too, has immunologically active T-cell and B-cell systems, the latter deriving from the bone marrow.

Immune system

The immune system is, in fact, a molecular activity aimed at the recognition and elimination of substances foreign to the body. It thus provides the organism with *specific defense reactions*. Foreign substances can enter or be introduced into the body in the form of infective agents or their metabolic products (toxins), or as foreign tissues. On the other hand they may arise in the body itself (tumor cells).

Phylogenesis of the immune organs

animal class	central lymphatic organs – Thymus	central lymphatic organs – Bursa Fabricii	peripheral lymphatic organs – spleen	peripheral lymphatic organs – lymph nodes	peripheral lymphatic organs – aggregate lymphatic organs like tonsils or Peyer's patches	peripheral lymphatic organs – germinal centres	free immuno-competent cells – circulating lymphocytes	free immuno-competent cells – plasma cells	capacity for adaptive immune reaction
AGNATHA MYXINOIDEA	–	–	primitive	–	–	–	–	–	no, only round cell infiltration and non-specific macrophage resistence
PETROMYZO-NOIDEA	primitive	–	+	–	–	–	+	–	primitive cellular immune reaction; antibody formation against some antigens
PISCES CHONDRICH-THYES	+	–	+	–	+	–	+	+	formation of immuno-globulins (IgM)
OSTEICHTHYES	+	–	+	–	+	(splenic follicles)	+	+	formation of immuno-globulins (IgM)
AMPHIBIA	+	–	+	lymphocyte deposition in the walls of the lymph sacs	+	–	+	+	formation of immuno-globulins (IgM and IgG)
REPTILIA	+	–	+	–	+	+	+	+	formation of immuno-globulins (IgM and IgG)
AVES	+	+	+	lymph nodes in water birds and waders	+	+	+	+	full immunobiologic capacity; immunoglobulins IgM, IgG and IgA
MAMMALIA	+	bone marrow as a source of B cells	+	+	+	+	+	+	full immunologic capacity; immunoglobulins IgM, IgG, IgA and IgE

IgM = immunoglobulin of primary response; *IgG* = immunoglobulin of secondary response; *IgA* = also locally produced immunoglobulin; *IgE* = allergy antibody

In order to develop an immunity there must be a confrontation between the organism and the foreign substance. It is the *antigen*, that is to say the foreign substance of plant, animal or synthetic origin, which stimulates the body to produce *antibodies*[*].

[*] Antibody, also immune body, is an immunoglobulin molecule of type IgM, IgG, IgA or IgE; see also footnote to the table on Phylogenesis of the immune organs.

Antigen and antibody undergo a chemical reaction with one another which is very specific. Each antigen requires its complementary antibody. The adaptation of the body to the environment antigenicity is known as *active* immunization and results in *adaptive* immunity. Antibody production can, on the other hand, be undertaken by the B-cell system immediately antigen appears. The plasma cells of the germinal centres can discharge circulating antibodies into the blood stream and so initiate the humoral immune reaction. The plasma cells localised in the peripheral connective tissue can produce *in situ* antibodies of IgA type and so set up the local immune reaction. On the other hand the T-cell system is responsible for cellular immunity. The rejection of transplated or degraded (neoplastic) tissues is such a cell-mediated immune reaction: it is due primarily to the immediate reaction of the T-lymphocytes with the specific tissue antigen. In exactly the same way that an antibody reacts with its specific antigen in the humoral immune reaction, so the specifically sensitized lymphocytes find the complementary tissue antigen by means of their surface receptors. A successful cell-mediated immune reaction results in the destruction and discharge of the foreign cell complex. (In order to prevent such undesirable immune reactions in therapeutic organ transplantations, immunosuppressives such as antilymphocytic sera are used).

The antigen may enter the body by natural infection but it can also be introduced intentionally by inoculation of, for instance, an attenuated organism (vaccine). The ability to produce these specific antibodies may be retained for several months, years or throughout the life of the animal.

The described immunological processes are dependent on the availability of *immunocompetent cells*[*], the distribution and function of which will be further discussed on page 273.

Passive immunity is achieved by passively transferring certain antibodies from a specifically resistant to a non-resistant individual. The uptake of colostrum by the neonate is comparable to passive immunisation. This transmits an immediate, though transient, protection against certain antigens.

Lastly it is possible to transfer immunocompetent cells from one individual to another so that these introduced, adopted cells bring about an *adoptive immunity* in the recipient.

Structure and function of lymphatic organs

The lymphatic organs include lymph nodes, spleen, tonsils and thymus. Furthermore almost all mucous membranes contain circircumscribed areas of lymphoreticular tissue such as the *folliculi lymphatici solitarii* (solitary follicles) and *folliculi lymphatici aggregati* (aggregated follicles). These also belong to the lymphatic system.

Before discussing the structure and function of the individual lymphatic organs we might summarize the morphological and functional characteristics they have in common:

Fixed cells of the lymphatic organs

The first common morphological element is the reticular connective tissue (216). This presents as a sponge-like, three-dimensional meshwork of star-shaped *reticular cells* (/R) which are interconnected by desmosome-like contacts between their cell processes. Unlike the mesenchyme or embryonic connective tissue, the cell processes here are supported by argyrophil connective tissue fibres (*reticular fibres*) (/Rf). The reticular cells have *fibrillogenetic* function and they *monitor* the physico-chemical properties of the *ground substance*. Furthermore they are capable of *phagocytosis* and *storage*. As part of the defense mechanism of the body, the foreign substances adhere to the surface of the phagocytic cells, then they are surrounded by the plasmalemma of the protruding pseudopodia and taken into the cell as *phagosomes*. Phagocytosed material can either be broken down by lysosomal enzymes, in which case undigested parts often remain in vacuoles, or it can be stored unaltered in the cell for prolonged periods. Finally, the reticular cells are able to further differentiate into certain free cells, which will be discussed later, and into the *littoral cells*. These littoral cells are endothelial-like, flattened reticular cells which are insinuated in, and morphologically assimilated by, the endothelial complex of neighbouring blood and

---

[*] Immunocompetent cells are cells which are capable of specific recognition and response to antigen.

lymph vessels but they differ from true endothelial cells because they have retained their phagocytic and storage capacity. Because of their common properties Ludwig Aschoff grouped them together with their stem cells, the reticular cells, into the *reticulo-endothelial system* (**RES**).

Recently it has been considered more appropriate to expand the original concept of the RES to include the histiocytes and monocytes which are capable of phagocytosis, storage and the transmission of immunological information. It is now referred to as the *reticulo-histiocytic system* (**RHS**).

The medical significance of this activity is that not only blood cells and cell debris but also tumour cells, microorganisms and therapeutically administered colloid particles may be phagocytosed.

Free cells of the lymphatic organs

The second common factor in lymphatic organs is the rich content of *lymphocytes* (216/L). Besides these there are other free cells such as *plasma cells* (/P), *macrophages* (/M) (*histiocytes* and *monocytes*) and also *granulocytes* and *mast cells*.

The **lymphocytes** (216/L; 217) of all the lymphatic organs with the exception of the thymus, are not diffusely distributed but are arranged in spherical accumulations known as *lymph follicles* or *lymph nodules*. This accumulation of lymphocytes in follicles is probably due to the fact that mainly B-lymphocytes carrying special complement receptors on their surfaces are deposited in the peripheral lymphatic organs.

Lymphocytes occur in various forms. It is only recently that some of the interrelationships between the form and function of these cells have been understood. It appears certain, however, that the small lymphocyte holds a key position in immune processes because it has the ability to initiate an *"immune memory"*. It is therefore able to recognize foreign proteins. The small lymphocyte can then pass on this information and so set in motion a cell-dependent immune reaction. From the morphological viewpoint it is interesting to know that the preadapted, differentiated small lymphocyte can revert and dedifferentiate to the lymphoblast which is then able to divide. Subsequent mitotic division produces

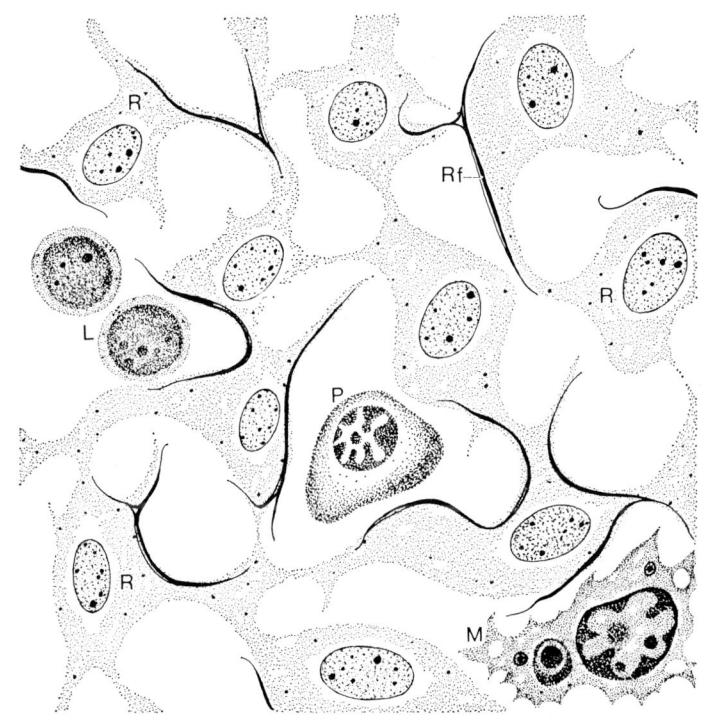

Fig. 216. Diagrammatic representation of the lymphoreticular tissues.
Star-shaped reticulum cells (*R*) form a three-dimensional network, which is traversed by reticulum fibres (*Rf*). In the meshes there are numerous lymphocytes (*L*), some plasma cells (*P*) and isolated macrophages (*M*).

not only small lymphocytes which are carriers of the immunological memory, so-called *memory cells*, but probably also *plasma cells* which form the specific humoral antibodies (γ-globulins, immune globulins).

Plasma cells (216/P) appear in the reaction centres about 2–3 days after the introduction of an antigen into the body. They are probably formed by the lymphoblasts which stem from dedifferentiated B-lymphocytes, although it has been suggested that they may arise from undifferentiated reticular cells.

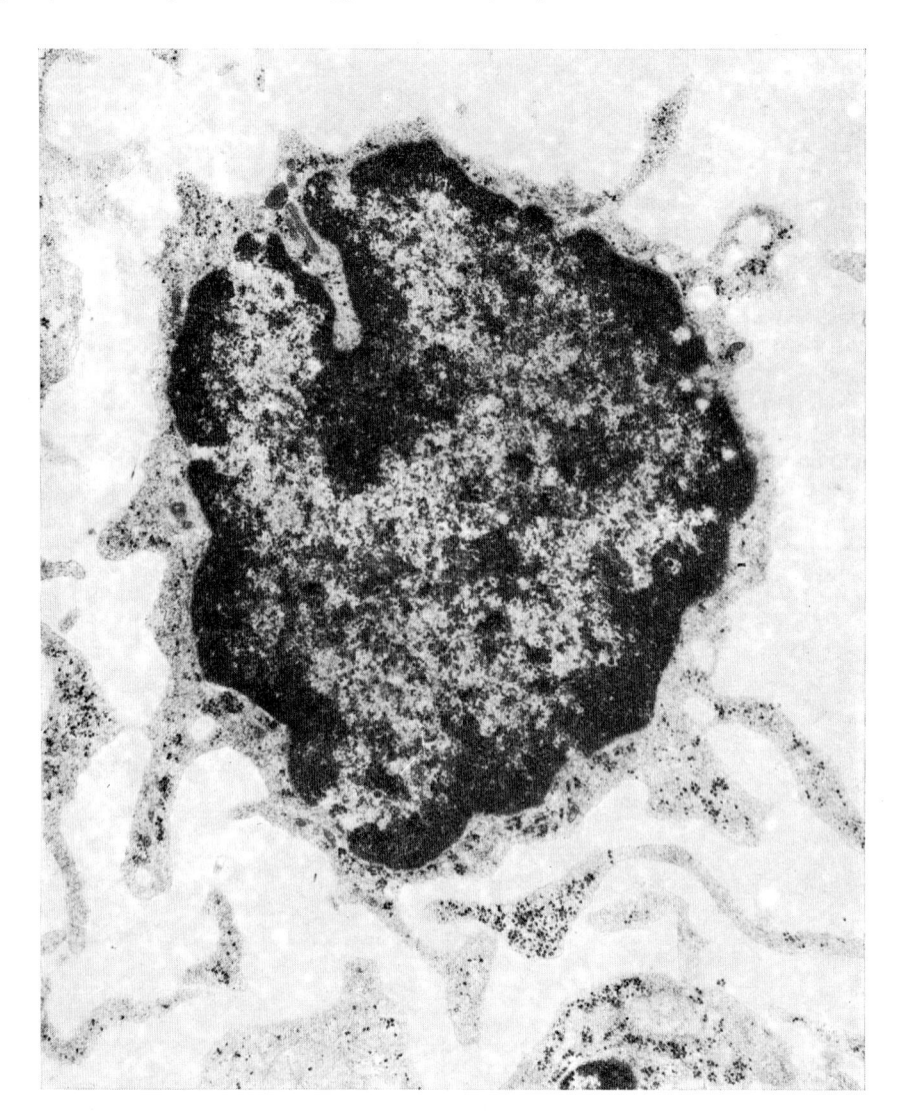

Fig. 217. Electron micrograph of a T-lymphocyte from the medulla of the cervical lymph node of an ox. (Preparation by Prof. Dr. P. Walter; Magnification approx. 24,000 x.)

The plasma cells are the producers of antibodies and in consequence are also called the *immunocytes*. They have a life span of about 10–30 days and they occur in all lymphatic organs and, following emigration, in connective tissue. Usually they are present in small, interconnected groups.

Macrophages (216/M) play a role in the immune process as mediator cells. As *histiocytes* (resting wandering cells) they probably derive directly from the reticular cells. They are usually situated in the neighbourhood of vessels and they migrate immediately to the locus of an infection. Following phagocytosis of foreign substances they transmit the antigenic information to immunologically competent lymphocytes, transforming the latter into memory cells. The *monocytes* are macrophages which have derived from the myeloid series in the bone marrow. They also possess phagocytic properties and, in times of need, when the number of histiocytes normally available is insufficient, they can quickly be carried by the blood to a focus of inflammation. The monocytes thus form the great majority of inflammatory macrophages. After phagocytosis of foreign substances the monocytes also secrete immunological information. Further details can be obtained from textbooks on immunology.

Classification of organs of the immune system

Because of their very specialized duties the cells of the immune system are grouped in various lymphatic organs. From a purely descriptive point of view one could speak of *central* and *peripheral lymphatic organs*. The **central organs** include, firstly, the *thymus* and, secondly, the *bursa Fabricii* of birds or the *bone marrow* of mammals. The two subpopulations of the small lymphocytes, **T**–*lymphocytes* (*thymus dependent*) and **B**-*lymphocytes* (*bone marrow* or *bursa dependent*), are produced in these two organs. After involution of the thymus, and also the bursa in birds, the ability to differentiate into the two types of lymphocytes (T- and B-cells) is passed on to the **peripheral lymphatic organs,** namely the lymph nodes, spleen, tonsils and Peyer's patches.

However, since cells of both systems are present in all the lymphatic organs a classification by function is more appropriate. One specific function is the *"recognition"* of antigens and the second specific function lies in the *production of antibodies*.

From these facts the following scheme of the immune reaction has now been developed:
1. Bacteria or viruses enter the body through mucous membranes, rarely through the skin.
2. The antigen is seized and phagocytosed by the macrophages. The macrophages "mediate" and "explicate" by breaking down and rearranging the antigenic information, probably by means of m-RNA (hence mediator cells).
3. T- and B-lymphocytes and possibly also reticular cells of the regional lymph nodes, take up the information.
4. T- and B-lymphocytes "recognise" the antigen as foreign to the body.
5. a) After transformation into the blast stage the T-lymphocytes become carriers with cell bound antibodies (mainly in virus infections).
    b) The B-lymphocytes become differentiated to lymphoblasts in the germinal centres. They divide into memory cells and plasma cells. The latter produce humoral antibodies (mainly in bacterial infections).
6. Then follows the fusion of the antigens to the specific antibody. Active immunity is now established and is maintained, sometimes throughout life, by the memory cells of both cell systems.
7. The body is protected against excessive amounts of antigen-antibody complexes resulting from the current and subsequent infections by eosinophil granulocytes which probably phagocytose these complexes and break them down enzymically.

From the above it becomes obvious that a local infection first causes a reaction at the infection site but that its effects are very quickly passed via lymph vessels to the nearest "regional" lymph node. Before pursuing this process further, the characteristics of the structure and function of the individual lymphatic organs will be described.

Peripheral lymphatic organs

Lymphatic tissue

Under normal physiological conditions *lymphocyte accumulations* occur in all the mucous membranes of the digestive, respiratory and urogenital tracts. These lymphocytic infiltrations are part of the local immunological defense mechanism.

In its simplest form the infiltration appears as diffuse lymphoid tissue in the propria of the mucosa. Similar accumulations are seen as "milk spots" in the greater omentum or as *"arachnoid cell accumulations"* in the pia mater.

The formation of spherical lymphoid colonies brings about the *primary follicles* (218/A). Here the uniformly differentiated small lymphocytes are situated diffusely in the meshes of the reticular tissue, so that little of the latter remains visible. Such primary follicles are encountered mainly in newborn and SPF-animals (specific pathogen free, that is to say, experimental animals reared in an environment free from certain pathogens). But soon after the first interaction between the youngster and its environment, the picture changes and *secondary follicles* develop (218/B, C). The latter are characterized as spherical structures in the centres of which, known as *reaction centres,* occur light cells with ample cytoplasm and variable differentiation. These are surrounded by a rim of darkly staining lymphocytes with sparse cytoplasm (/B). Where such secondary nodules occur in a subepithelial position, the eccentrically placed reaction centre is not surrounded by a continuous rim but a "bell" or cap of small lymphocytes, directed towards the epithelium (/C). Reactive changes, such as growth and cell division, occur continuously in the reaction centres and there is multiplication of DNA and RNA as an expression of the local immune reaction. The *lymphoblasts* and the short-lived *plasma cells* develop here. Some secondary follicles lying in the lamina propria mucosae and extending into the submucosa are known as solitary follicles *(folliculi lymphatici solitarii)*. Their occurrence in the mucosa of the gut, the respiratory and urogenital tracts has already been discussed in volume II. They also occur in the conjunctiva and in the mucous membranes of all natural body orifices where they are of practical significance in clinical diagnosis (inspection of the visible mucous membranes).

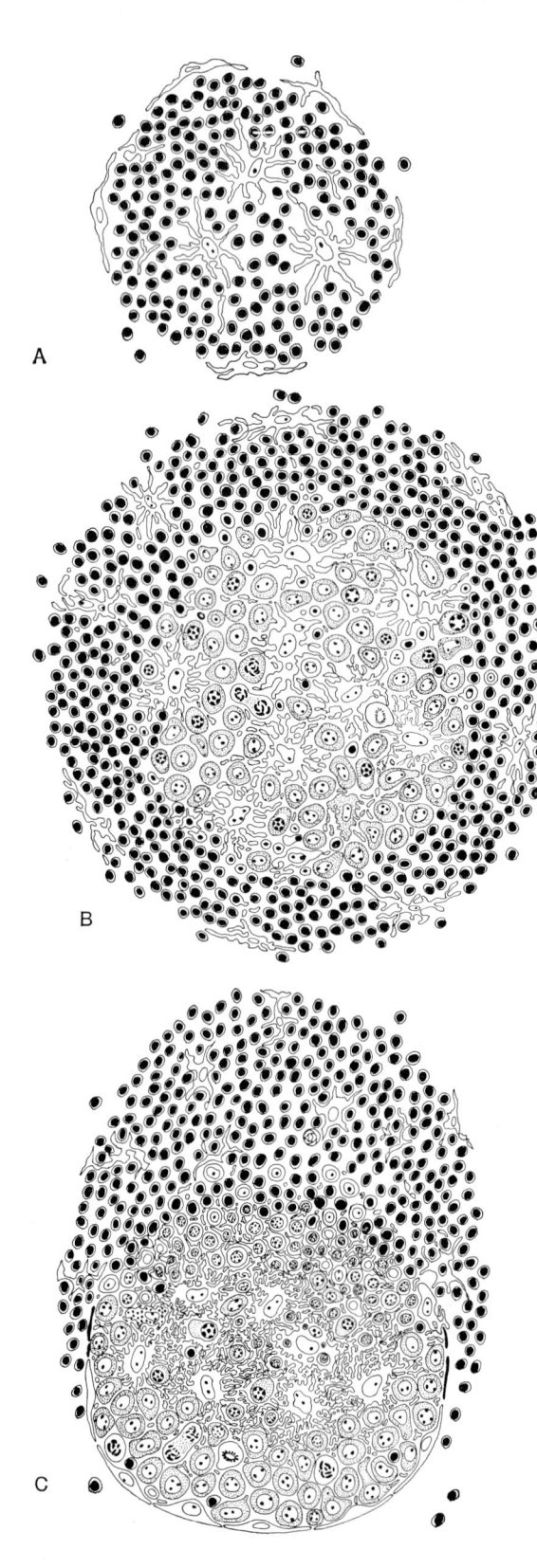

Fig. 218. Diagrammatic representation of the structure of a lymph nodule or follicle.

A primary follicle; *B* secondary follicle with centrally situated reaction centre and rim of lymphocytes; *C* secondary follicle with excentrically situated reaction centre and cap of lymphocytes pointing towards the epithelium.
(The diagrammatic representation of the reaction centres closely follows the investigations of Gorgollon and Krsuldvic, 1973)

Secondary follicles also occur as large, connected accumulations and they are then spoken of as *folliculi lymphatici aggregati*, Peyer's patches. They are well illustrated in the antimesenteric surface of the gut, especially the small intestine of domestic animals. They vary in length from a few centimetres to several metres (see volume II). Their form and number is dependent on exogenous factors such as diet and intestinal flora and on endogenous factors such as age, species and the intestinal segment. Their variable reaction in different intestinal infections exerts a significant influence on the course of the disease. It is known that in man an excessive reaction of such follicles in the vermiform process can lead to appendicitis.

In the following lymphatic organs the lymph follicles have developed into discrete organs; tonsils, lymph nodes, spleen, haemolymph nodes.

Tonsils

The lymphatic tissue of the tonsils (219) is in close functional relationship with its covering epithelium, which is either non-keratinized squamous or respiratory epithelium, lining the pharyngeal cavity. The general topographical arrangement of the tonsils and their specific peculiarities are extensively dealt with in volume II.

Fig. 219. Diagram of the microscopic structure of a tonsil.

A overall view of a non-follicular tonsil with crypts. The numerous secondary follicles are characterized by lymphocyte caps directed towards the epithelia. Below the tonsil are the tonsillar glands. B Reticulating zone of the tonsillar epithelium (enlarged)

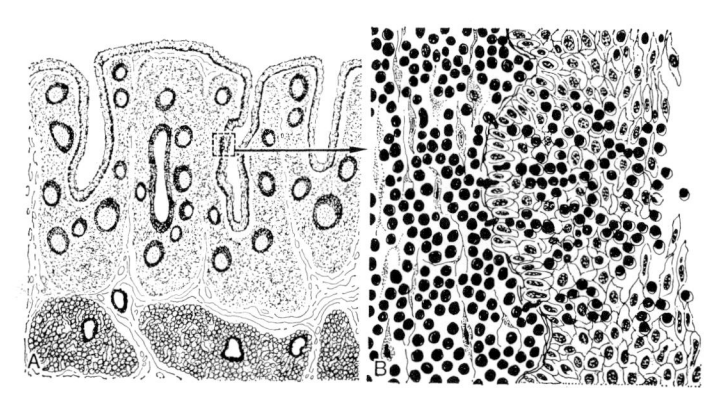

The **ontogenesis** of the lymphatic organs of the pharynx (also known as the lymphatic pharyngeal ring) have been studied in some detail in the ox. The *palatine tonsil* develops from a two-chambered *tonsillar sinus* which incorporates the remnants of the second gill pouch. The entodermal epithelium lining the sinus drives solid buds into the mesenchyme and these buds later become canalized thus forming the *tonsillar crypts* into which the *tonsillar glands* empty. The epithelium overlying the pharyngeal tonsil shows similar budding and this leads to the formation of the lingual tonsils. The glands of the palatine and lingual tonsils develop in the third month of gestation and those of the pharyngeal tonsil develop in the fourth month. Typical lymphatic tissue with a vascularized reticular cell complex and migrated lymphocytes can be seen in the mesenchymal blastema below the epithelial component of the tonsils in the pharyngeal tonsils during the third month and in the palatine tonsils during the fourth month but in the lingual tonsil not until the seventh month. It has been convincingly demonstrated that these first lymphocytes migrated from the thymus, the pacemaker of lymphopoiesis.

The five main tonsils – the *tonsillae palatina, lingualis, veli palatini, pharyngica* and *tubaria* – form a ring at the entrance to oesophagus and larynx. It is their function to make primary and continued contact with pathogenic organisms conveyed by the alimentary or aerogenic routes. For this reason the texture of the epithelium overlying the tonsil has been transformed into a spongy mass of cells. This epithelial zone is called the reticulating zone (219/B).

This is an important prerequisite for the movement of the lymphocytes between the lymphoreticular network and the tonsillar epithelium; by this means the lymphocytes reach the free surface of the tonsil where they can make contact with antigen and carry immunological information back to the tonsillar matrix. The macrophages as mediator cells and the reaction centres ensure that (1) the information is made available to the whole body via the memory cells and (2) that the information is responded to by the formation of antibodies.

This function of the tonsil is aided by other morphological peculiarities:
1. The structure of the tonsillar secondary nodule is eccentrically orientated towards the epithelial surface and therefore, unlike the secondary nodules of other lymphatic organs, it does not have a rim. Instead there is a *cap of lymphocytes* because the majority of the lymphocytes migrate from the epithelium.
2. The presence of *tonsillar crypts* increases the contact surface between lymphoreticular tissue and epithelium.

Desquamated epithelial cells mixed with lymphocytes and ubiquitous, and perhaps also pathogenic, organisms form *detritus* which lies in the crypts. In some cases this can result in constant irritation and inflammation which leads to an exaggerated reaction by the tonsil causing a worsening of the general condition of the patient. This plug of detritus can be expressed, or, if the tonsil is circumscribed and surrounded by a well defined capsule, the whole tonsil can be removed surgically. Tonsillectomies are performed on the palatine tonsil of carnivores.

Lymph nodes (nodi lymphatici, lymphonodi)

The *ontogenesis* of lymph nodes is discussed on p. 294 in the context of the development of lymph vessels.

The special function of the lymph nodes is to monitor the lymph. They are complex encapsulated organs which are placed along the course of the lymph vessels (220). Their colour is greyish-yellow to brown-red. In ruminants and carnivores they are bean-shaped, compressed or even flattened solitary nodes. In pigs they are irregular structures lying singly or in groups. The horse has small spherical lymph nodes which are often aggregated into large groups. They lie, surrounded by loose connective tissue, more or less hidden in fat tissue.

The connective tissue *capsule* (220, 221/*1*) can contain smooth muscle fibres. It sends trabeculae (220/*2*) into the substance of the node. This coarse scaffolding is spanned by the delicate meshwork of reticular cells and, especially in the *cortical region* (/*4*), there are meshes occupied by lymphocytes. In some areas of the cortex the lymphocytes collect in dense groups which measure about 1 mm in diameter and are referred to as *lymph nodules*. The parenchyma of the cortex continues in columns towards the hilus; these are known as *medullary cords* (/*5*), and they contain numerous lymphocytes but no primary nodules. Several lymph vessels enter the concave side of the lymph node (*vasa afferentia*) (220 A/*3*). Thus the lymph passes through the capsule and into a sinus (220/*6*) which lies immediately under the capsule (*marginal* or *terminal sinus*), and thence into the radially directed *intermediate sinuses* (/*7*) which traverse the cortex and dilate in the medulla into the *medullary sinus* (/*8*). One or two out-going lymph vessels (*vasa efferentia* (220 A/*9*)) issue from the hilus. It is the function of the marginal sinus to distribute the incoming lymph to several intermediary sinuses. An indirect, longer, much narrower and therefore less important route along the marginal sinus to the medullary sinus is also possible. The direct route through the intermediate sinus is thus preferred and the lymph node is divided into functional sectors which represent preferential routes and filtration zones for individual afferent lymph vessels. This is important in interpreting lymphographic pictures.

It is noteworthy that in the lymph nodes of pigs the lymph flows in the opposite direction (220 B). That is to say the vasa afferentia (220/*3*) enter at the hilus and the efferent vessels (/*9*) leave the lymph node at the convex side. In consequence the cortical and medullary areas have been rearranged (220 B/*4'*, *5'*).

The lumina of all the sinuses (221) are strengthened by reticular fibres and their walls are lined by endothelium-like reticular cells (littoral cells) (/*a*). The lumen is furthermore spanned by branching reticular cells or macrophages (/*b*) and this explains the close contact between the lymph and the reticular cells which are thus capable of a degree of phagocytosis amounting to filtration. Since the lining cells of the sinus can apparently fluctuate between a closed and a fenestrated state, the reticular cells of the cortex and the medullary cords are also involved in the uptake and retention of substances. In all the reaction centres there are, as well as lymphocytes, lymphoblasts and, in their neighbourhood, plasma cells, macrophages and granulocytes. It is normal for granulopoiesis to take place in the lymph nodes of the dog.

Appreciation of the structure of the lymph node will facilitate understanding of its function. It is composed of cells the function of which is to protect the body against pathogenic organisms and other

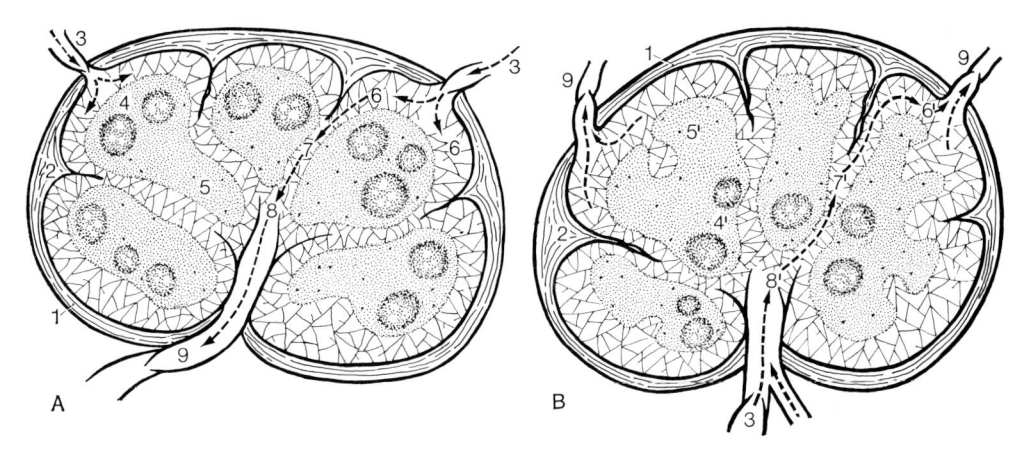

Fig. 220. Diagrammatic representation of the structure of a lymph node of A the dog and B the pig.

1 capsule, *2* trabecula, *3* vas efferens entering through the capsule in the dog and the hilus in the pig, *4* cortical parenchyma with lymph nodules and *5* medullary region, in the pig (*4'*, *5'*) these structures are interchanged; *6*, *7*, *8* passage of lymph through the marginal sinus (*6*), the intermediate sinus (*7*) and the medullary sinus (*8*); in the pig the sinus *8'* receiving the lymph is situated near the hilus. It passes the lymph to the intermediate sinuses (*7'*) and thence to the marginal sinus (*6'*) which collects the lymph and passes it on to the efferent vessels, *9* vasa efferentia, in the dog at the hilus, in the pig at the convex surface of the node

injurious substances. These cells always appear outwith the lymphatic organs when an inflammatory reaction occurs. For this reason some pathologists compare the lymph node to an organ of inflammation. When bacteria or other noxious substances appear in the lymph node drainage area, they stimulate a hyperplasia of the littoral, reticular cells and macrophages which increase in size and number. Secondary nodules develop with lymphoblasts in their centre. Plasma cells appear and the lymphocytes increase in number. Overall the lymph nodes enlarge, their capsules are stretched due to the increased internal pressure and so the lymph nodes become painful. Enlargement, increased sensitivity or pain and perhaps also increased temperature can be established in palpable lymph nodes so that they are an important clinical indication about the site and type of illness.

The substances which have been phagocytosed in the lymph node are deposited in the reticular cells. Some of these float away as macrophages but many remain for an extended period in the lymph nodes and this may result in alteration in the consistency and colour of the sectioned node. This phenomenon is utilized during meat inspection.

It is of considerable medical importance that *tumour cells* carried away in the lymph may be trapped in the regional lymph nodes where they initiate *metastases*. Subsequently, they may involve other, more distant nodes.

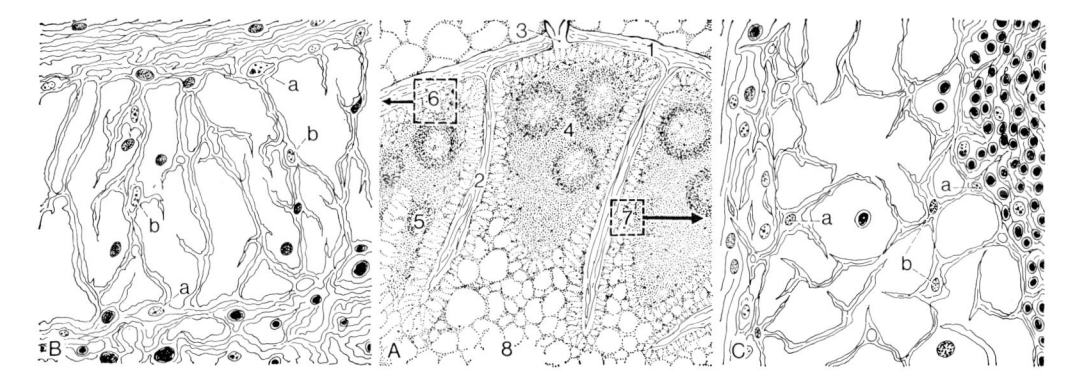

Fig. 221. Diagram of the microscopic structure of a lymph node.

A portion of lymph node with capsule (*1*) and trabeculae (*2*), entering afferent vessel (*3*), cortical parenchyma with lymph nodules (*4*), medullary cord (*5*), marginal sinus (*6*), intermediate sinus (*7*), medullary sinus (*8*); *B* marginal or terminal sinus; *C* intermediate sinus, both these enlarged areas show litoral cells (*a*) and reticular cells (*b*)

In this context it is important to recall that the lymph flow is directed towards the blood stream. The mechanism of the lymph flow will be considered later. But, like tumour cells, other particulate elements can be phagocytosed during their passage through the RES of the lymph node while antigens also can be bound to antibodies at these locations. However, the effectiveness of the lymph filter is dependent on the composition of the noxious substances, their amount and the period during which they continue to be presented to the node. As a general rule one may state that smaller amounts of corpuscular elements will be almost completely extracted whereas soluble, proteinaceous substances will pass through. As more and more corpuscular elements are presented, the probability is increased that some of them will escape phagocytosis or binding. This is not uncommon in natural infections when large numbers of microorganisms are liberated from a focus of infection. If they reach the blood stream they cause a bacteraemia or viraemia. This, of course, is the reason why complex problems result when surgical procedures involve the gut where there are enormous numbers of microorganisms. Movement of infected limbs stimulates the flow of lymph and may thus exhaust the filtration capacity of the nodes. In cases where tumour cells have escaped the filter of the lymph nodes and gained access to the blood stream, haematogenous metastases occur and successful local treatment can no longer be expected.

Haemolymph nodes (lymphonodi haemales)
Haemal nodes (nodi haemales)

In various mammals, particularly some rodents and ruminants including the domestic ruminants, reddish *haemolymph nodes* are intercalated in the vascular system between arterioles and venules. Although some questions pertaining to their development and function still remain unanswered, it seems probable that these structures have some of the functions of the spleen and bone marrow. Their external structure is reminiscent of lymph nodes, but there are neither afferent nor efferent lymph vessels and their sinuses are filled with blood.

With regard to their *structure,* they lie somewhere between lymph nodes and the spleen. For this reason they have also been referred to as *lymphoid* or *splenoid haemal nodes.* In sheep especially, the *capsule* and *trabeculae* contain collagen, elastic fibres and also smooth muscle cells. In the ox the capsule is thin, but in the small ruminants it is thick and composed of two distinct layers. The outer layer is fibrous and the inner layer is characterized by a dense network of blood capillaries. The parenchyma is made up of a three-dimensional *reticular meshwork*. In the sheep, but not the goat, a *cortex* and a *medulla* can be differentiated. Secondary nodules occur in the sheep in the cortical substance only while in the diffuse lymphoreticular tissue of the medulla, erythrocytes, erythroblasts and giant cells are encountered. In the haemolymph nodes of the goat secondary nodules are more evenly distributed in the parenchyma. Thus in some cases they resemble lymph nodes in structure, whereas in other cases they are more like the spleen. Between the capsule and the cortex there is a *marginal sinus* which is broad in the sheep but narrower in the other ruminants. The marginal sinus gives rise to *intermediary sinuses* which radiate centripetally into the medullary substance. In the neighbourhood of the hilus the *medullary sinus* is situated around a collecting venule into which congregate the capillaries of the nodule. Blood flows through the sinuses. Numerous erythrocytes and other blood cells are present in the reticular meshes, especially those of the medulla.

The reticular cells of haemal nodes are capable of *phagocytosis* and *storage* with the result that deposits of pigment can cause them to appear brown.

From the functional viewpoint the haemolymph nodes are related to the spleen, because they undertake blood filtration, and to the bone marrow because erythropoiesis and myelopoiesis (Erencin) takes place in them. Antibodies are said to be produced in haemal nodes and thus they clearly belong to the lymphatic system.

Haemolymph nodes are found mainly in the region of the head, neck, nucha, shoulder, the large blood vessels of the thoracic, abdominal and pelvic cavities and quite generally in the immediate neighbourhood of certain lymph nodes (222). They are easily distinguished from the latter by their reddish-brown colour. Haemal nodes are found in the immediate neighbourhood of the following lymph nodes:

Head region: nl. parotideus, nl. mandibularis, nl. retropharyngeus lateralis;

Cervical region: nl. cervicalis superficialis accessorius, nll. cervicales profundi craniales, medii et caudales;

Shoulder and axillary region: nl. costocervicalis, nl. infraspinatus, nl. axillaris primae costae;
Thoracic region: nll. thoracici aortici, nll. intercostales, nll. mediastinales craniales, nl. phrenicus, nll. sternales caudales, nll. bifurcationis, nll. pulmonales;
Lumbar region: nl. renalis, nll. lumbales aortici, nl. iliacus internus;
Abdominal wall: nl. fossae paralumbalis, nl. coxalis accessorius;
Pelvic region: nll. sacrales, nll. anorectales;
Pelvic limb: nll. poplitei, occasionally nl. inguinalis superficialis.

The size of the nodes varies between 1 and 20 mm. In small ruminants they rarely exceed 5 mm; in cattle they are rarely more than 10 mm. They are ellipsoidal or roundish and flattened in shape, and they feel firm and full on palpation. The fluid content of the nodes can be expressed but this requires

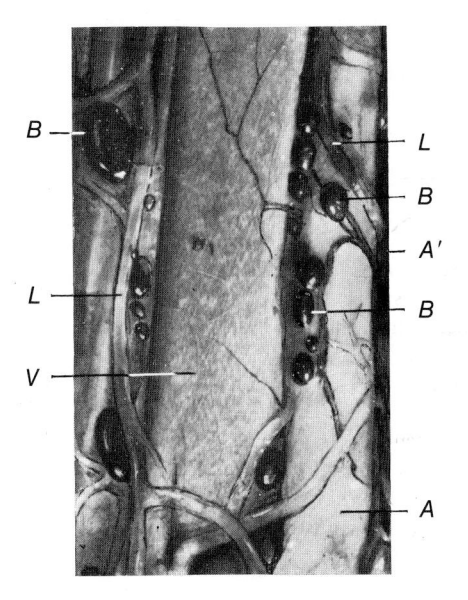

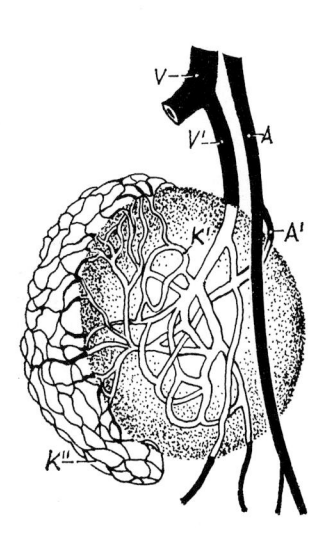

Fig. 222. Haemolymph nodes of the sheep.
left: topography of the haemolymph nodes on the abdominal aorta and the caudal vena cava
(after Grau, 1960 from Krölling and Grau.)
A abdominal aorta, *A'* smaller blood vessel whose branches supply a group of haemolymph nodes, *B, B* the haemolymph nodes, *L, L* trunci lymphatici lumbales without connection to the haemolymph nodes, *V* v. cava caudalis;

right: vascularization of the haemolymph node of a four-month-old lamb, after vascular injection
(redrawn after von Schumacher, 1913.)
A artery, whose branch *A'* supplies the haemolymph node, *K'* capillary network in the haemolymph node, *K"* capillaries of the surrounding adipose tissue, *V* vein, *V'* efferent venule

considerable pressure. In colour they are bluish-red, shining red, dark red, pink to brownish and, in the rat, even ochre. The amount of blood and pigment present in the node significantly effects its color. It is not exactly known how many nodes are present but the sheep is supposed to have between 30 and and 300.

Haemolymph nodes should not be confused with lymph nodes which have taken up erythrocytes in their vasa afferentia after a haemorrhage in their drainage area. They become reddish for a time, but a reliable differentiating characteristic is that the true lymph nodes have afferent and efferent lymph vessels linking them to the lymph vessel system whereas such vessels are absent from haemal nodes.

Spleen (lien, spleen)

The spleen has been extensively dealt with in a special chapter of volume II, so that now we have only to deal with its significance as part of the lymphatic system.

In domestic mammals the ontogenesis of the spleen commences in the third or fourth embryonic week with the appearance of a mesenchymal thickening in the dorsal gastric mesentery. The structure of the spleen is determined by the developing vascularization. The mesenchymal cells differentiate either to reticular cells which form the framework of the splenic pulp or to basophil round cells which lie in the mechwork of the reticulum as free cells. These round cells develop into erythrocytes, megakaryocytes, granulocytes and lymphocytes. As foetal development advances lymphocyte differentiation dominates but under pathological conditions granulopoiesis and erythropoiesis may recommence.

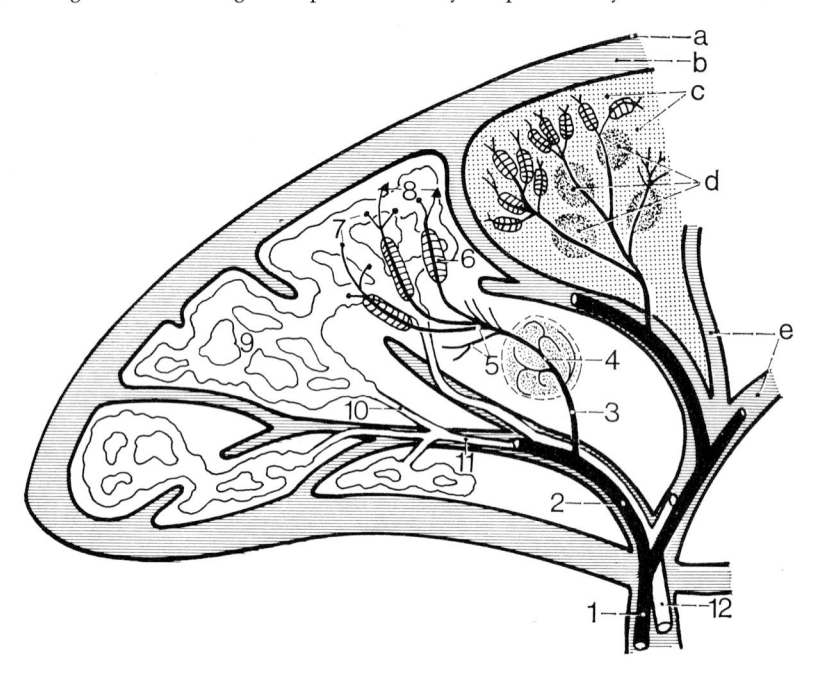

Fig. 223. Structure of the spleen (diagrammatic).

a peritoneal covering, *b* splenic capsule, *c* red pulp, *d* splenic follicle, white pulp, *e* splenic trabecula

1 splenic artery, *2* trabecular artery, *3* pulp artery, *4* follicular artery, *5* penicillate artery, *6* ellipsoid or sheath capillaries, *7, 8* endocapillaries terminating in (*7*) the splenic sinus and (*8*) the perisinusal pulp reticulum, *9* splenic sinus, *10* pulp vein, *11* trabecular vein, *12* splenic vein

The external form and topography of the spleen, which explains its function as a controlling organ of the blood, has been discussed in volume II. The a. lienalis (223/1) (or its branches) perforates the capsule and enters the spleen at the *hilus*. Numerous *trabecular arteries* (/2) follow the large trabeculae between which lies the splenic parenchyma or *red* and *white* pulp. The *pulp arteries* (/3) leave the trabeculae and so enter the substance of the spleen. The white pulp is disseminated in the form of splenic nodules (/d) (Malpighian corpuscles, *folliculi lymphatici*), through which the *follicular arteries* (/4) usually follow an eccentric course. In the ox and pig such splenic nodules are just visible to the naked eye. The delicate meshes of their reticular connective tissue contain white blood cells, mainly lymphocytes, macrophages and plasma cells. Up to 50 penicillate arteries (*penicilli*) (/5) are given off one follicular artery; they extend beyond the limit of the follicle into the red pulp, where they divide further and become capillaries. The capillaries are surrounded for a short distance by a spindle-shaped *sheath* (ellipsoid or Schweiger-Seidel's sheath) (/6). The sheaths consist of densely packed reticular cells which form a specialized RES structure having phagocytic capabilities. The terminal capillaries arise from the sheath capillaries and they take the blood by two routes to the *splenic sinuses* (/9) situated in the red pulp.

1. Either the blood flows directly (/7) into the splenic sinus in which case the blood vessel suddenly enlarges. The wall of the sinus is formed by the net-like endothelium and is thus permeable. These endothelial cells have the character of littoral cells, that is to say, reticular cells which occur in the endothelium and possess phagocytic function. Apart from these cells, the sinus is also supported by circular reticular fibres, the *ring fibres*.

2. The indirect route for the blood is through the pulp reticulum bordering on the sinus (/8) and this forms a mantle-like network around the sinus.

From the splenic sinus the blood enters the *pulpa vein* (/10), and then traverses the *trabecular veins* (/11) to the *v. lienalis* (/12) which leaves the spleen at the hilus.

The **functions of the spleen** can be summarized as follows:

1. The blood entering the splenic sinus and the perisinual pulp is monitored and the aged erythrocytes and thrombocytes are bound and phagocytosed by the littoral cells and reticular cells (RES). The blood pigment liberated during this screening is broken down into the iron-free component bilirubin, which is taken to the liver via the portal vein, and the iron-containing components ferritin and haemosiderin. Ferritin is transported to the bone marrow for erythropoiesis while haemosiderin is stored in the reticular cells of the spleen. If there is an excessive amount of iron then this storage produces a brown colouration of the spleen which can be recognised with the naked eye.

2. The Malpighian corpuscles of the spleen participate in lymphopoiesis and therefore generally contain reaction centres. If infection occurs plasma cells and macrophages also develop and this is considered to be part of the immune response. In *leukaemia* (lymphatic leucosis) of cattle swelling of the spleen results from excessive lymphopoiesis. If there is an insufficiency of bone marrow the spleen may also produce cells of the myeloid series which, of course, were produced by the spleen during the foetal period (see above). Thus the spleen is also involved in granulopoiesis in *myeloid leukaemia* (myelosis), although this serious condition of man occurs less often in animals.

3. The RE cells of the spleen are able to engulf and store abnormal metabolites, such as lipids, which can develop during disease. Bacteria and tumour cells can also be removed from the blood. Fully laden littoral cells can leave the cell complex and be carried in the blood as *splenic macrophages*. Certain *storage diseases* are also associated with splenic enlargement.

4. Another function of the spleen, especially in carnivores, is the storage of blood. Up to 16% of the circulating blood volume can be held in the spleen of dogs, thus relieving the general circulation. Contraction of the capsule, which contains much smooth muscle tissue, discharges this stored blood.

Thymus

Ontogenesis

The thymus develops from the ventral diverticulum of the paired third pharyngeal pouch and it is therefore, except in the pig, of purely entodermal origin. Early in development (in the ox embryo at a length of 15 mm) an epithelial bud on either side grows into a tube-like structure with a narrow lumen which extends cranially towards the neck and contacts the pericardium caudally. In some species (carnivores and horses) the connection with the pharynx is largely lost whereas in others (ruminants and pigs) the original part remains more or less fixed in the pharyngeal region and gives rise to the cranial part of the thymus. The longitudinal growth of the thymus coincides with the migration of the heart so that the thymus extends to the anterior part of the thoracic cavity. In the lower third of the neck and in the precardial part of the thorax, the right and left thymic anlagen come into contact due to the constriction of the thoracic aperture. Finally these parts of the organ more or less completely fuse (224). The narrow lumen becomes obliterated and the original epithelial structure assumes a sponge-like meshwork (*epitheliogenous reticular cells*). This is presumably followed by a migration of mesenchymal cells (of *mesodermal* origin) into the cortical regions of the organ which stimulates the formation of *thymocytes* (lymphocytes of *epithelial genesis*). The possibility that the stem cells of thymocytes may be situated in the bone marrow is still debated. Later the thymocytes are deposited in ever increasing numbers in the periphery, so that the organ is clearly divided into a medulla and a cortex. The medulla develops centrally by cell proliferation and it is devoid of lymphocytes. At the cortical periphery the epitheliogenous lymphocytes enter the blood and lymph streams to become localized in other lymphatic organs.

Microscopic structure and function

As stated earlier, the thymus is a central site of formation of T-lymphocytes. It is recognised as the pace-maker of lymphopoiesis, that is to say, if it should fail prematurely then the immune system cannot be established.

Lymphatic system

The thymus is a paired organ which lies in the cervical region and in the precardiac mediastinum. It regresses completely with advancing age but in the neonate it is fully developed and is the largest and most important lymphatic organ. In the course of the first years of life to about the time of sexual maturity (see species differences) involution occurs whereby true thymic tissue is replaced by connective and adipose tissue. But even these thymic adipose bodies of adult animals may contain isolated active parenchymal foci and this is especially the case in the dog and ox. The juvenile thymus is characterized by lobulation (225/A). A chord-like linked and branching medulla is surrounded by a dark mantle of cortex which contains masses of cells with prominent nuclei.

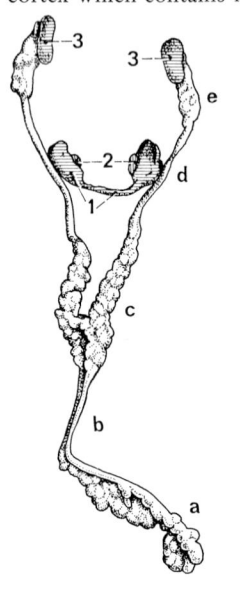

Fig. 224. Thymus anlage of a 3.7 cm bovine embryo.
(Redrawn after Hagström, 1921.)
By the 7th week the development is so advanced that the definitive form can be recognised

a pars thoracalis thymi, *b* isthmus cervicothoracalis thymi, *c* pars cervicalis thymi, *d* isthmus craniocervicalis thymi, *e* pars cranialis thymi

1 thyroid; *2* parathyreoidea IV; *3* parathyreoidea III

Fig. 225. Microscopic structure of the thymus (diagrammatic).
A overall view of the lobular structure of the juvenile thymus. *B* medulla with epithelioid reticulum cells and sparse lymphocyte population and a Hassal's corpuscle; *B'* cortex with large-meshed reticulum network and numerous lymphocytes. *C* Hassal's corpuscle (corpusculum thymi), higher magnification

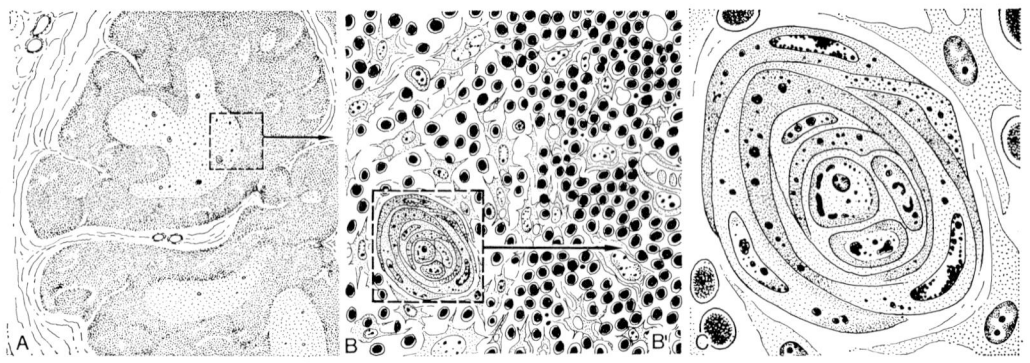

The vascular connective tissue of the central part of the medulla (/B) supplies the lobules and chords. In the outer part of the medulla the cells of the reticular connective tissue become densely aggregated and this occasionally gives them an epithelial appearance. Lymphocytes and macrophages are only rarely seen. *Hassall's corpuscles (corpusculi thymi)* (/C) are characteristic structures of this organ. These are spherical bodies just too small to be seen by naked eye. They consist of layers of modified reticulum cells of the RES arranged around centrally situated cell particles. The corpuscles are short-lived structures which are frequently replaced; a reticulum cell becomes rounded and enlarged (single-celled Hassall's corpuscle) and is then surrounded by neighbouring medullary cells. In acute infections their number may increase to more than a million and this indicates their participation in the stimulated defense mechanism.

The cortex (/B') consists of coarsely-meshed reticular connective tissue which is compact towards the surface and borders of the lobules. All the meshes of the network are filled with small lymphocytes which are therefore diffusely distributed and, unlike the other lymphatic organs, do not form follicles.

According to the latest theory, the small lymphocytes (*thymocytes*) of the cortex arise at this site from epithelial (entodermal) thymus elements under the inductive influence of immigrating mesenchyme, but one cannot exclude the possibility that they derived from the bone marrow. At any rate, in the cortex of the thymus they differentiatie into *immuno-competent T-lymphocytes*. These lymphocytes then spread from the thymus to populate the other lymphatic organs. If the thymus becomes diseased, or is experimentally excised, at the time of this lymphocyte migration, the body is unable to establish an immune system, and the individual dies after a few weeks. Thus at birth the thymus is the most significant and the largest lymphatic organ and it has a *pace-maker function* but later in life the

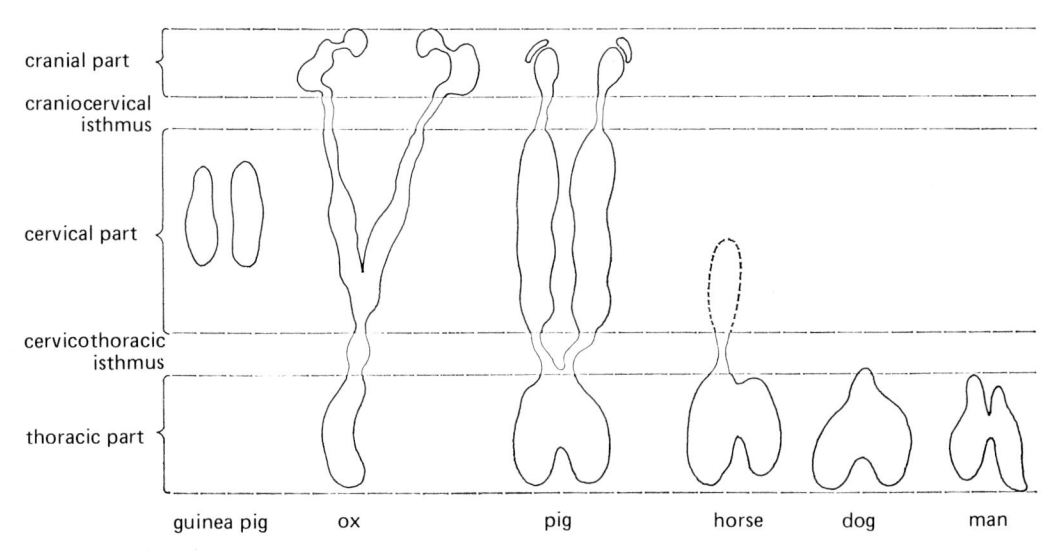

Fig. 226. Diagram showing the position and nomenclature of the fully developed thymus of some mammalian species.

multiplication of T-lymphocytes can take place in other lymphatic organs so that the effects of thymectomy are less pronounced.

It is a normal physiological process for the thymus to gradually involute at about the time of sexual maturitiy. The reticular cells collect in epithelioid groups, Hassall's corpuscles calcify and the number of lymphocytes diminishes. The parenchyma is replaced by connective tissue and especially by fat tissue. Rapid involution has been described in man under conditions of stress.

Unlike other lymphatic organs, the walls of the thymic blood vessels are impervious to antigens (*blood-thymus barrier*) and this is of considerable functional significance.

For a long time it was suspected that the thymus had some endocrine function but this is no longer considered likely. On the other hand it has recently been suggested that the thymus may produce an acellular factor of immunological significance. The possible relationship between the thymus and the gonads, especially in respect of oestrogen secretion, is controversial. It has been demonstrated experimentally that folliculin has a strong involuting effect on the thymus.

Macroscopic description of the thymus

The thymus is of variable external appearance; it shows not only variations in morphology in the different species but goes through a gradual evolution until the onset of sexual maturity and then succumbs to a progressive involution which ultimately affects the entire organ. The following description of the thymus in the different species refers to the completely developed organ (226).

It has already been mentioned that the thymus develops from the pharyngeal pouch and grows in length so that, except in guinea pigs, moles and some marsupials, it extends into the thoracic cavity. This craniocaudal-directed growth is also followed during the involution of the organ so that in all domestic animals the most caudally situated part of the thymus persists the longest. In some mammals such as dog, man, horse and cat, only the thoracic part is developed. It is therefore understandable that in comparative macroscopic descriptions the thoracic part (*pars thoracalis thymi*) receives the greatest attention since this is present in all the domestic animals. The cervical part (*pars cervicalis thymi*) is prominent in ruminants and pigs but even in the horse and cat there may sometimes be suggestions of a cervical part. In ruminants the caudal third of the organ is unpaired. The thoracic and cervical parts are linked by a parenchymal bridge which is constricted by the thoracic inlet. This thoraco-cervical connection, which is usually unpaired (except in pigs), is termed the *isthmus cervicothoracalis thymi*. A cranial part (*pars cranialis thymi*) is present in the ox and pig only to the end of intrauterine development. The narrow link between the cervical and cranial parts of either side must logically be termed *isthmus craniocervicalis thymi*.

Thymus of carnivores

In the fresh state the **thymus of the dog** (227) is pink and distinctly lobulated. It is represented by the *thoracic part* only and this is incompletely divided into a larger right and a smaller left lobe (*lobus dexter et sinister*). The thymus lies in the ventral part of the precardiac mediastinum. At the time of birth it is relatively large but it continues to grow during the following weeks. From the 4th week its relative weight drops and a few weeks later the absolute weight also gradually decreases. American authors have given maximum measurements for the thymus of the beagle: length 12cm, height 6 cm, thickness 3 cm; weight 50 g. The onset of involution coincides with the time of appearance of the second teeth. However, the involution of the canine thymus is incomplete so that even in older dogs some lymphatic regions can be demonstrated in the thymic fat body.

Size of the thymus in puppies (after Schneebeli, 1958)

	small breeds		large breeds	
	length	breadth	length	breadth
Shortly before birth	1.02—2.22 cm	0.66—1.09 cm	1.40—2.23 cm	0.66—1.20 cm
1st and 2nd week of life	1.32—2.73 cm	0.41—1.32 cm	1.53—3.68 cm	0.78—1.99 cm
3rd to 8th week of life	no data		4.53—6.00 cm	1.85—2.60 cm

Position: when its development is maximal the thymus lies against the sternum. Its cranial pole lies under the trachea and extends beyond the 1st pair of ribs by some 5 mm. This protrusion cannot be interpreted as a cervical part. Its caudal limit extends to about the 5th or 6th costal cartilage. Its caudal part is applied closely to the pericardium which distinctly separates the right and left lobes. The bulk of the larger right lobe extends dorsally along the cranial surface of the pericardium while the greater proportion of the smaller left lobe lies, with a broad base, against the sternum. When opening the thoracic cavity ventrally the left lobe appears to be the larger (227). The cranial parts of both lobes are fused medially by connective tissue. The trachea is related dorsally, the vena cava and phrenic nerve ventrally. The lateral sufaces carry shallow depressions where the apical lobes of the lungs impinge. Ventrally the internal thoracic artery and vein cut into the tissue of the thymus.

The **thymus of the cat** is an elongated, lobulated structure of pink or slightly greyish colour. Its *thoracic part* is situated against the sternum in the mediastinum and is covered by the apical lobes of the lungs. Its caudal end is closely applied to the pericardium and is divided into a shorter right and a longer left lobe. When completely developed, its cranial end, which is the short cervical part, protrudes some 1–2 cm from the thoracic cavity and in exceptional cases it may be cleft into two limbs.

Thymus of the pig

Unlike that of the other domestic animals, the thymus of the pig is not of purely entodermal origin because the blind end-piece of the ectodermal part of the ductus praecervicalis also makes a small contribution to the initial development of the cranial thymus. Furthermore, the pig is supposed to have an independent additional *"thymus superficialis"* which derives solely from the precervical duct and is therefore entirely of ectodermal origin. The microscopic structure of this superficial thymus corresponds to that of the "true" thymus.

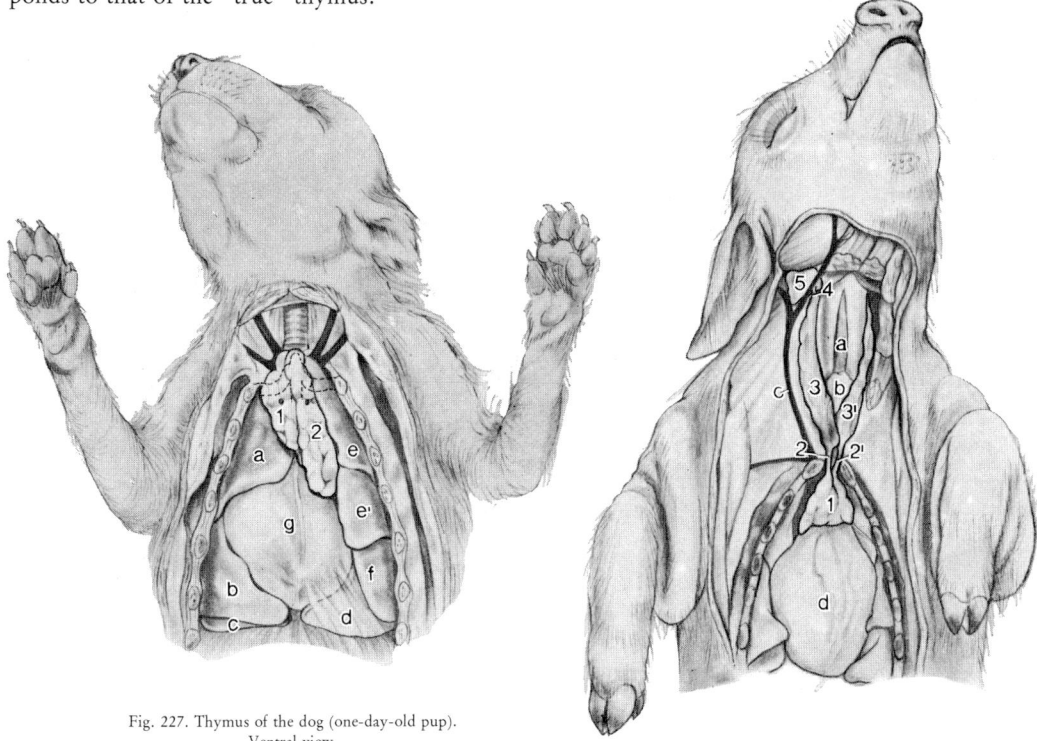

Fig. 227. Thymus of the dog (one-day-old pup). Ventral view.

1, 2 thymus, *1* right lobe, *2* left lobe

a–f lung, *a* lobus cranialis pulmonis dextri, *b* lobus medius pulm. dext., *c* lobus caudalis pulm. dext., *d* lobus accessorius pulm. dext., *e* pars cranialis and *e'* pars caudalis lobi cranialis pulmonis sinistri, *f* lobus caudalis pulm. sin., presternum and cartilage of the 1st pair of ribs shown in dotted lines.

Fig. 228. Thymus of the pig (7-day-old piglet) Ventral view.

1–5 thymus with *1* pars thoracalis thymi, *2, 2'* isthmus cervicothoracalis thymi, *3, 3'* pars cervicalis thymi, *4* isthmus craniocervicalis thymi and *5* pars cranialis thymi (the left cranial part is not shown)

a larynx, *b* thyroid, *c* v. jugularis externa, *d* pericardium

Weights of the pig's thymus

	Absolute weight	Relative weight
foetus, 40 days	no data	0,09 %
foetus, 84 days	—	0.5 %
foetus, 116 days	—	0.2 %
5 months	47—168 g	0.076%—0.157%
10 months	39—119 g	0.02 %—0.114%
21—24 months	24— 91 g	0.01 %—0.07 %
more than 24 months	20— 59 g	0.004%—0.05 %
2—3 years	average 33 g	—

Position: The *thoracic* part makes extensive contact with both the pericardium and the sternum. A caudal notch indicates the subdivision into a *left* and a *right* lobe. The flat thoracic part measures 0.5 cm in thickness and 10 cm in length and each lobe is 3.5 cm wide.

The thoracic part gives rise to the thread-like, paired *isthmus cervicothoracalis*, each 1.5 cm in length, which are followed by the paired *cervical part*. The cervical part is about 20 cm long and 3–4 cm in both thickness and width, and it accounts for about 70% of total thymic tissue. The cervical part is related to the trachea, lying initially ventral and then lateral to it, in the anterior part of the neck. Dorsolaterally it borders on the external jugular vein while the common carotid artery and the internal jugular vein lie against its dorsomedial surface. Thus the cervical part extends to the level of the larynx.

In both the calf and piglet there is a thymic lobe which extends to below the base of the skull and is separated from the cervical part by a bridge of parenchyma. This lobe also incorporates the already-mentioned superficial thymus. Thus in the full-term foetus one should differentiate a *cranial part* and a *craniocervical isthmus*. The frequently notched and divided cranial part is in contact with the jugular process of the occipital bone; it is situated on the mandibular gland and below the medial retropharyngeal lymph node.

The blood and nerve supply have not been studied to date but are probably similar to the ox.

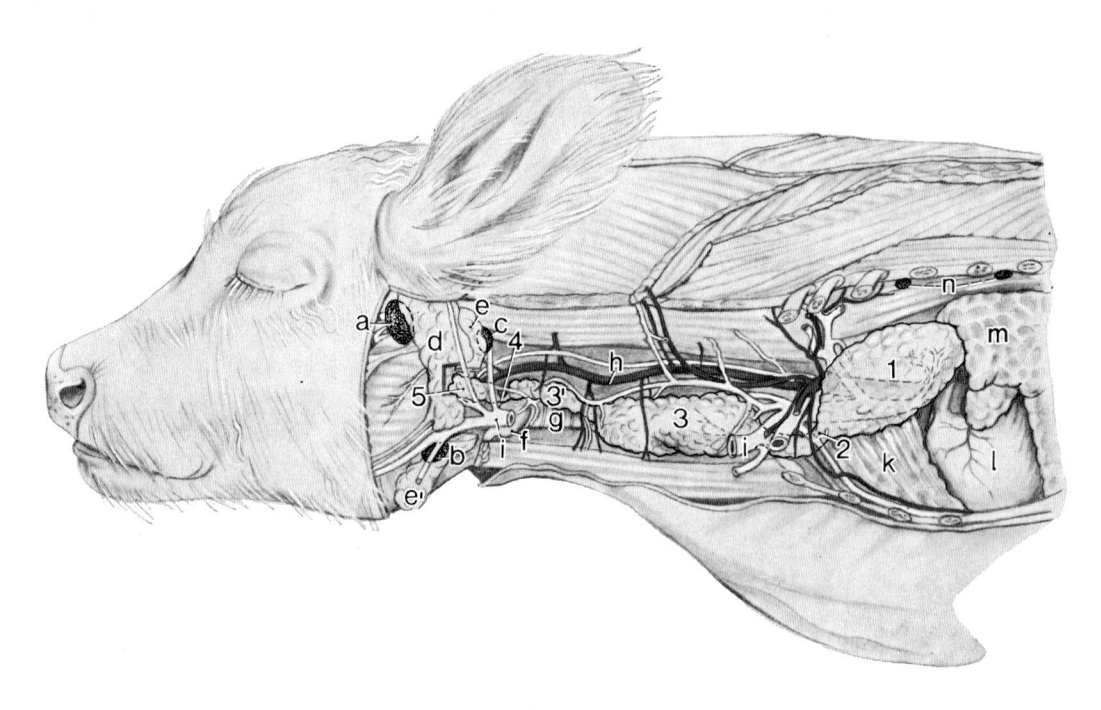

Fig. 229. Thymus of the calf. Left lateral view.

1–5 thymus with *1* pars thoracalis thymi, *2* isthmus cervicothoracalis thymi, *3* body and *3'* left limb of the pars cervicalis thymi, *4* isthmus craniocervicalis sinister thymi, *5* pars cranialis sinistra thymi

a nl. parotideus, *b* nl. mandibularis, *c* nl. retropharyngeus lateralis, *d* parotid gland, partly removed to show the cranial part of the thymus, *e, e'* glandula mandibularis, its middle part removed, *f* thyroid gland, *g* trachea, *h* a. carotis communis sinistra, *i, i* v. jugularis externa sinistra, its middle part removed, *k* lobus apicalis of the right lung, visible through the mediastinum, *l* heart in the pericardium, *m* lobus apicalis pulmonis sinister, *n* nll. intercostales

Thymus of ruminants

The **thymus of the calf** (224, 229, 230) is strikingly lobulated. The single *thoracic part* (229/1) lies asymmetrically on the left side of the dorsal half of the precardiac mediastinum. Dorsally it is related to the vertebral column and the thoracic part of the longus colli muscle, caudally to the pericardium and ventrally to the brachiocephalic trunk and its branches, the cranial vena cava and the apical lobe of the right lung. Its right surface lies against the trachea and oesophagus and is therefore invisible from the right pleural cavity. Its left surface is partly covered by pleura.

Thymus

The thoracic part of the thymus is connected to the unpaired cervical part by the single *cervicothoracic isthmus* (/2). The latter is a strip of parenchyma running along the left of the trachea from caudodorsal to cranioventral.

In the *cervical part* (/3, 3') we can differentiate a caudally situated unpaired *body* (/3) and two *limbs* (/3') lying cranially to it. The cervical part is the longest part of the calf's thymus and it is roughly in the form of a "V", with the point directed towards the thorax. The body lies against the dorsal surface of the trachea and is flanked by the two jugular veins, while the limbs lie against the lateral surfaces of the

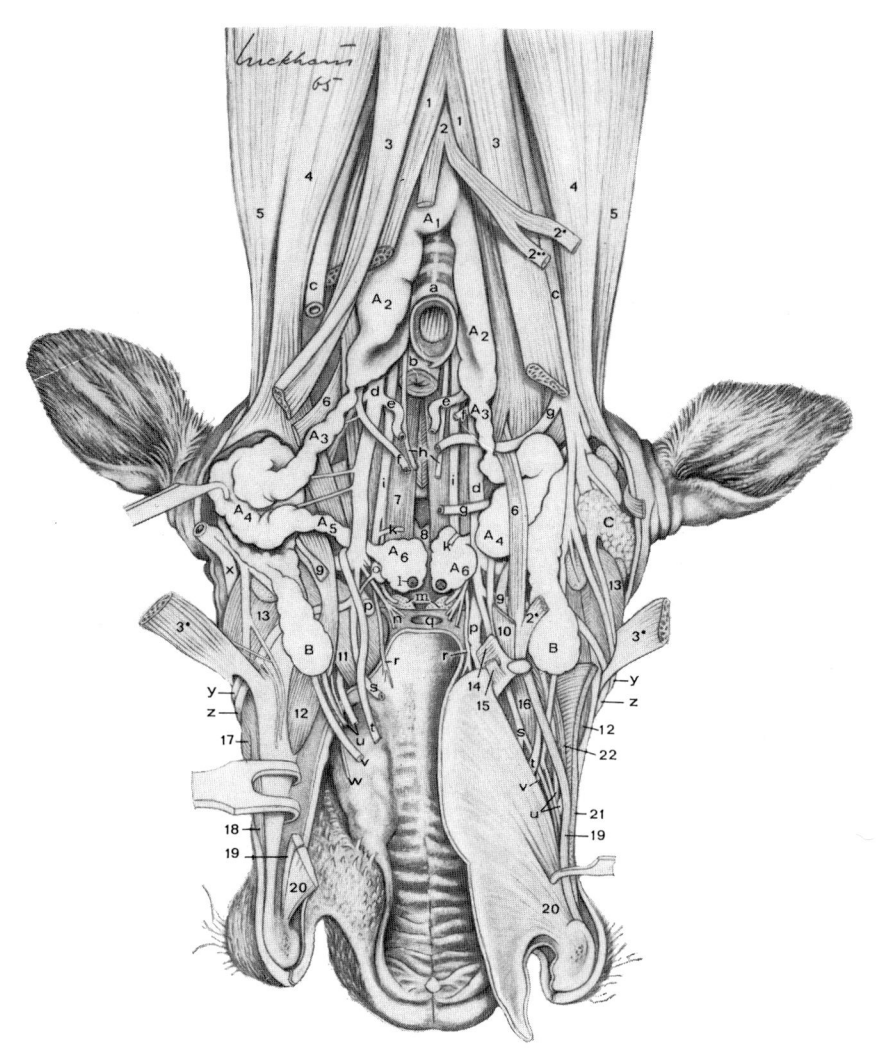

Fig. 230. Cranial part of the thymus of a male bovine foetus.
(After Luckhaus, 1966.)

Tongue split down the middle; left half of the tongue, soft palate, part of the pharynx, larynx, first parts of the oesophagus and trachea have been removed.

A_1 body of the cervical thymus; A_2 limb of the cervical thymus; A_3 craniocervical isthmus; A_{4-6} cranial part with A_4 retroglandular and A_6 subbasilar portions

a trachea, *b* oesophagus, *c* v. jugularis externa, *d* a. carotis communis (displaced somewhat laterally), *e* a. thyroidea cranialis, *f* v. jugularis interna, *g* v. thyroidea cranialis, *h* nn. lanryngei recurrentes, *i* truncus vagosympathicus, *k* n. laryngeus cranialis (the left cranial laryngeal nerve is slightly lifted off the caudal surface of the subbasilar segment of the cranial part, *l* left parathyreiodea III, *m* lnn. retropharyngei mediales, rr. pharyngei, *n* diagramatic presentation of branches of the a. palatina ascendens entering the lateral wall of the pharynx, *p* stylohyoid, *q* choanal orifice, *r* n. glossopharyngicus, *s* a. lingualis, *t* n. hypoglossus, *u* n. lingualis and ductus mandibularis, *v* v. lingualis, *w* left n. mylohyoideus, *x* left v. maxillaris interna, *y* v. facialis, *z* a. facialis

1 m. sternomastoideus, *2, 2', 2''* mm. sternothyroidei et -hyoidei, *2* common muscle trunk, *2'* proximal and distal stumps of the right sternohyoid muscle, *2''* proximal stump of the right sternothyroid muscle, *3, 3'* m. sternomandibularis, *4* m. cleidomastoideus, *5* m. cleidooccipitalis, *6* m. omohyoideus, *7* left m. longus capitis, *8* incisura intercondylica ossis occipitalis, *9* m. stylohyoideus, *10* right m. thyrohyoideus, *11* left m. pterygoideus medialis, *12* m. digastricus, venter rostralis, *13* m. masseter, *14* right m. ceratohyoideus, *15* right m. hyoepiglotticus, *16* right m. hyoglossus, *17* left m. buccinator, pars buccalis, *18* left m. depressor labii mandibularis, *19* m. geniohyoideus, *20* m. genioglossus, *21* right half of the mylohyoid muscle, *22* right m. styloglossus

trachea. Cranially they extend to the thyroid gland. The cervical part is covered laterally and ventrally by the sternocleidomastoideus muscle and the ventral muscles of the hyoid.

On each side the limbs of the cervical part are followed by a meandering *craniocervical isthmus* (/4; 230/A_3).

Recent investigations of bovine foetuses have shown that the *cranial part* (229/5; 230/A_4, A_5, A_6) is present right up to birth. The right and left cranial parts each consist of a *retroglandular portion* (230/A_4), lying immediately behind the mandibular gland, and a *sub-basilar portion* (/A_6). The latter extends to the medial retropharyngeal lymph nodes and contains the parathyroid III. Both portions are connected by a fine cord of parenchyma.

Occasionally one encounters *accessory* thymic bodies and various authors consider them to be derived from the 2nd or 4th pharyngeal pouches.

Involution commences in the ox after the 8th week of post-natal life. The cranial part regresses first followed by the isthmi. Then the limbs and body of the cervical part separate so that at that time four independent regions of thymus may be present: a right and a left anterior cervical part, an unpaired posterior cervical part and an unpaired thoracic part. When the cervical parts have disappeared the thoracic part remains as the thymic adipose body which may persist for 6 years and sometimes much longer.

Recent studies have elucidated in detail the blood supply of the bovine thymus.

The thoracic thymus is supplied by a stout vessel from the brachiocephalic trunk and by a more slender branch of the left internal thoracic artery. Sometimes there is an additional supply from the vertebral artery of the costocervical trunk. The cervicothoracic isthmus receives its arterial blood from a branch of the right or left internal thoracic artery and a branch of the superficial cervical artery. The cervical part of the thymus receives 2–6 arteries, depending on the development of the organ, on both the right and left sides. These arise as offshoots from arterial branches destined for the trachea, oesophagus and the ventral muscles of the neck which have arisen from the right and left common carotid. The craniocervical isthmus and the retroglandular portion of the cranial thymus receive direct and indirect branches from the common carotid and, additionally, also from the cranial thyroid artery. Exceptionally a branch of the external carotid or the occipital artery may also be involved. The sub-basilar part of the cranial thymus always receives its blood supply from the ascending palatine artery.

The venous drainage of the thoracic thymus is mainly achieved by a vessel which crosses the brachiocephalic trunk and terminates in the cranial vena cava. Smaller additional veins join the pericardial, vertebral or costocervical veins and the left internal thoracic veins.

The venous blood from the cervicothoracic isthmus passes through tributaries of the left internal jugular and the left and right internal thoracic veins.

The blood leaving the cervical and cranial thymus and the isthmus joining them enters the internal jugular vein, occasionally the external jugular vein or sometimes both vessels. The thyroid, laryngeal and occipital veins receive branches that drain the cranial part.

The fine blood vessels of the thymus (231) stem from the above-mentioned arteries and their branches follow the connective tissue which binds the lobules into lobes. These lobules are only just visible. Thus one *a. thymica* gives rise to several *aa. lobares*, these in turn give off several *aa. interlobares* and finally several *aa. lobulares* are produced.

Each thymic lobule is supplied by 1–4 such lobular arteries. Every lobular artery divides into a slender superficial and a stout deep branch. The former supplies the border region of apposed neighbouring lobules while the deep branch forms an incomplete arterial circle at the border between cortex and medulla. Retrograde vessels to the cortex arise from this circle which also supplies the medulla, although more sparsely. Each thymic lobule is drained by a superficial and a deep venous system. The superficial system is better developed, so that the blood flow is mainly centrifugal through the cortex. The efferent veins follow the course of the arteries and they are given corresponding names.

The vagus, sympathetic and, possibly, the hypoglossal nerves are involved in the innervation of the bovine thymus.

The lymph vessels of the thymus drain to the mediastinal, cervical and retropharyngeal lymph nodes.

The **thymus of the small ruminants** is similar in form to that of the ox. The *thoracic part* lies more to the left in the dorsal part of the precardiac mediastinum. Its left surface is in contact with the trachea, oesophagus and the large blood vessels. On the left it can be insinuated between the thoracic wall and the pericardium. Ventrally it is surrounded by the apical lobe of the right lung.

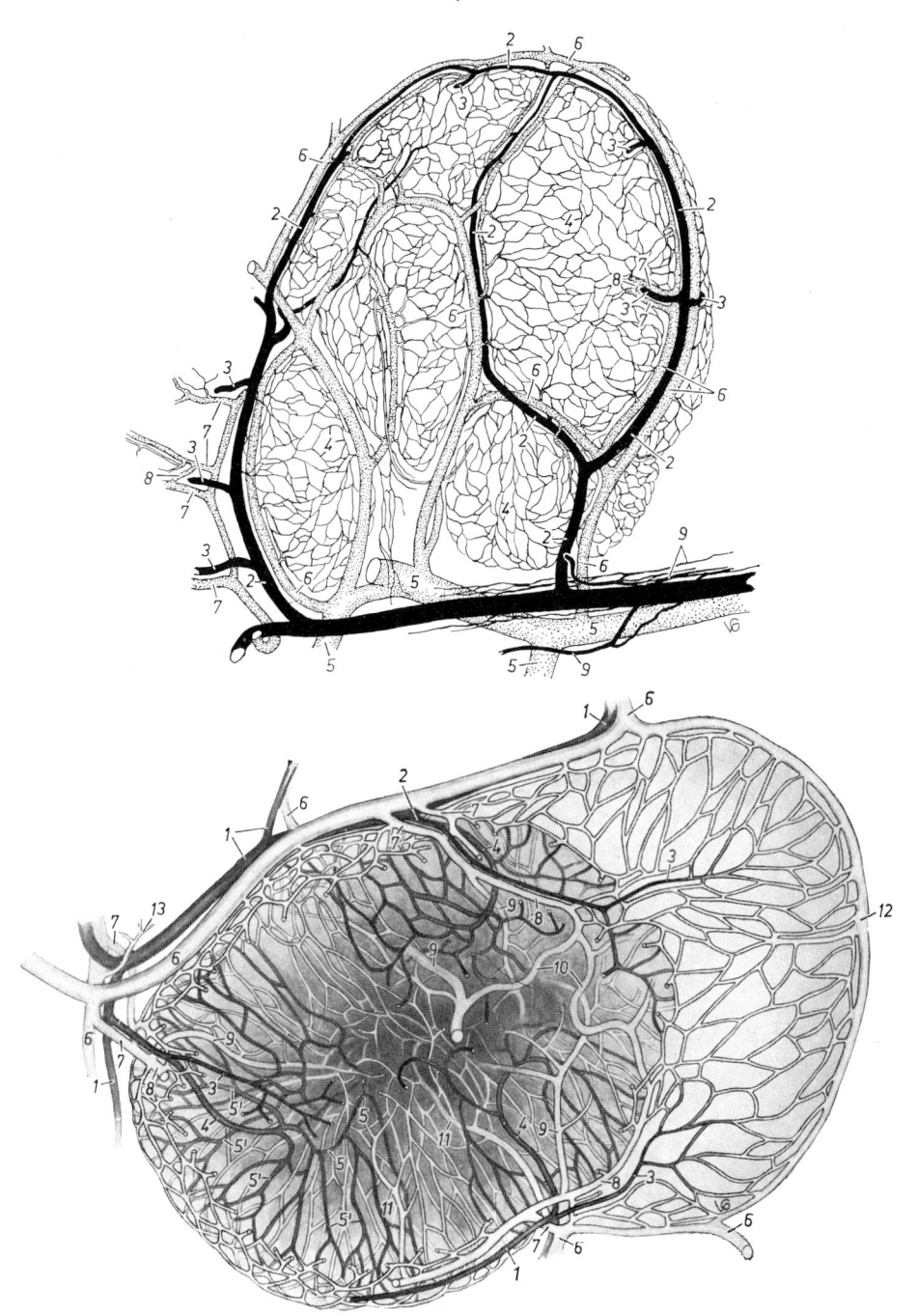

Fig. 231. Details of the blood supply to a thymus lobule of a bovine foetus.
(After Deniz, work performed at the Institute of Anatomy, Giessen, 1964.)

Above: A. the superficial blood supply of a thymus lobule

1 a. interlobaris; *2* a. interlobularis; *3* a. lobularis; *4* superficial capillary network of the isolated lobule; *5* v. interlobaris; *6* v. interlobularis; *7* vv. lobulares; *8* bridge-like anastomosis between the two lobular veins; *9* arteries to the interlobular connective tissue

Below: B. interior blood vessels of a thymus lobule

1 a. interlobularis; *2* a. lobularis; *3* superficial, *4* deep arteriole of the a. lobularis; *5* arterial arch in the cortico-medullary junction, *5'* precapillary arterioles arising from the arterial arch and supplying the cortex; *6* vv. interlobulares; *7* vv. lobulares; *8* superficial, *9* deep venule of the v. lobularis; *10* anastomosis between the superficial and deep systems; *11* radial venous connection between the superficial and deep systems; *12* superficial venous bridge between the two vv. interlobulares; *13* vein entering the interstitial connective tissue

The *cervical part* is unpaired in the lower third of the neck where it is linked by the *isthmus cervicothoracalis* with the thoracic part. The two limbs of the cervical part extend over the upper two thirds of the neck to the larynx.

In the lamb a *cranial part* (also termed the "parotid terminal piece") has been described. The cranial part of the thymus of the kid has not been investigated, nor has the blood supply to the thymus in these species. The thymus of the lamb continues to grow after birth until at least the onset of sexual maturity (6th–8th month). It amounts to about 0.1% of the body weight.

In the sheep involution is complete in two years but in the goat considerable amounts of thymic tissue are present in the thorax even at five years.

Thymus of the horse

In general the thymus of the horse consists only of a thoracic part although occasionally an unpaired cervical part may be present.

The *thoracic part* is situated against the sternum in the lower part of the precardiac mediastinum, closely applied to the pericardium. The left lobe is usually the larger; it extends from the thoracic inlet to the 4th or 5th ribs and, dorsally, to the brachiocephalic trunk. Mediodorsally it lies under the cranial lobe of the left lung. The right lobe of the thoracic thymus extends only from the 1st or 2nd to the 4th rib. Dorsally it may reach the cranial vena cava and because it lies under the cranial lobe of the right lung, it loses contact with the chest wall in older individuals. The following measurements give an indication of the size of the thoracic thymus:

	length	height	breadth
12 month old foal:	15 cm	10–12 cm	2–3 cm
Newborn foal:	16.5 cm	8 cm	6.5 cm

When a *cervical part* is present it is usually unpaired and is situated to the left of the trachea. Most frequently connected to the thoracic part by a distinct isthmus, it extends some 15 cm towards the head. Occasionally the cervical part is no more than a 3–4 cm long protrusion which lies between the two external jugular veins at about their termination.

Branches of the common carotid and internal thoracic arteries supply blood to the thymus. Venous drainage is through the external jugular, cranial vena cava and internal thoracic veins. The thymus is innervated via autonomic plexuses.

Lymphatic vessel system
General considerations

The *lymphatic vessels* (*vasa lymphatica*) pervade the entire body, forming a second tubular system in addition to the blood vessels. They contain *lymph*, a fluid of very varying composition. Thus during digestion the lymph vessels of the gut carry absorbed fats with the result that the lymph appears as a cloudy, milky emulsion termed *chyle*. On the other hand, the content of the lymphatic vessels of the extremities has a certain resemblance to blood plasma although it contains more water and less protein. Stated simply, the tissues may be said to be continually permeated by a stream of fluid originating from the blood vessels, drained in part by the lypmh vessels and ultimately returned to the blood. Larger molecules and cellular elements are carried in this stream. Thus the lymph vessel system has a function supplementary to the venous side of the blood circulation. The relationship between lymph vessels and veins is most clearly illustrated during embryonic development for the veins give rise to parts of the lymph vessels and the lymphovenous anastomoses remain as evidence of this. After their development, however, each system assumes a different function. It is of considerable clinical interest that the veins and lymph vessels take up and transport substances of different molecular size. Pathogenic organisms, toxins and cancer cells are among those disseminated by lymph routes. They can become lodged in the lymph nodes which are situated along the lymph vessels and act as a sort of filter. After passing through the nodes the lymph is not only "cleansed" but numerous lymphocytes are added to it. Before passing through the node the lymph is practically cell-free; it contains only 200–2000 lymphocytes per cu mm. On the other hand, the central lymph leaving the lymph node is said to contain between 1700 and 152 000 cells per cu mm. The lymph vessels are therefore important in the circulation of lymphocytes.

Phylogenesis of lymphatic vessels

In all *vertebrates* except agnatha and cartilaginous fishes, there is a lymph vessel system which supports the venous system in carrying fluid from the tissues back to the heart.

In *bony fishes* complete separation of the blood and lymphatic systems is encountered for the first time. There are four superficial lymph vessels which run parallel to the axis of the body from the origin of the tail fin to the base of the head. The vertebral canal harbours another lymph vessel and there is a paired longitudinal vessel under the vertebral column which is interpreted as the precursor of the thoracic duct of higher vertebrates. These are all lymph vessels of large calibre and they empty behind the head into the lymph sacs. These lymph sacs also receive vessels directly from the head. Small vessels from the viscera enter the subvertebral longitudinal vessels.

The lymph vessel system is completely developed in *amphibia*. These animals have *lymph hearts* which are specialized structures of the lymph vessel system. The lymph hearts, containing cross striated musculature, are contractile structures situated at the segmental junction between lymph vessels and the venous system. They also contain sphincters or valves. The function of the lymph hearts is to regulate the lymph flow rather than to provide the driving force for it; the latter is supplied by the movement of the body itself. However, they are also supposed to aid the flow of blood in the venous system.

The number of lymph hearts varies between the three orders of amphibia. The Gymnophiona can have more than 100 pairs. In the Urodela they number between 14 and 20 while in the Anura they are reduced to only two pairs. The lymph vessels themselves do not have valves with the result that lymph often dams back into the lymph sacs; the sacs can suddenly empty when the body makes the appropriate movement. Frogs have very large lymph sacs.

In *reptiles* there is a pair of lymph hearts at the side of the cloaca. Apart from lymph sacs and reticulated lymph spaces this is the first class of animal to have regularly-arranged tubular lymph vessels. The thoracic duct is still duplicated in the thoracic region but it becomes single caudally and develops a lymph cistern which collects lymph from the gut and the pelvic region. The most important, if not the only, connection between lymph and blood systems are the jugular lymph sacs of the cervical region.

Birds generally have lymph hearts only during their embryonic development. Lymph nodes occur for the first time in waders and water birds. Further details are given in volume V.

The lymph vessel system of *mammals* is characterized by the occurrence of a large number of lymph nodes which are situated both along the major collecting routes and also at the periphery where they are responsible for the filtration of the lymph from a circumscribed drainage area.

With the exception of certain monkeys and the kangaroo, in which lymph vessels also empty into the caudal vena cava, the lymphovenous connections of mammals are confined to the link between the thoracic duct and the jugular vein. No lymph hearts are present. Lymph valves are very frequent and the lymph stream, directed by these valves, is maintained by the movement of the lymph vessels themselves, by tissue pressure, by the movement of the body, its organs, its musculature and, above all, by respiratory movements and the suction in the venous angle. Even in mammals therefore, the function of the lymph vessel system to carry fluid from the tissues is safeguarded, despite the absence of lymph hearts. It has already been mentioned that by virtue of the numerous lymph nodes situated along the lymph stream, the lymph vessel system participates, along with the other lymphatic organs, in the immune processes of the body.

Ontogenesis of lymph vessels and lymph nodes

Two processes are important in the development of lymph vessels: *Firstly*, endothelial buds appear on certain parts of the venous system (e. g. jugular and iliac veins) and these generally lose their connections with their parent vessel. It seems very probable that the funnel-shaped, valve-bearing terminal section of the so-called jugular lymph sac is venous in origin. A connection also remains for some time between the lumbar lymph sac and the iliac veins. *Secondly*, the lymph vascular system can develop from endothelium-lined perivenous mesenchymal clefts which at first consist of individual lacunae which later coalesce and form a secondary link with the venous system.

By this means a primitive lymphovascular system develops in mammals which consists of the following sections, as illustrated in figure 232:

1. *Saccus lymphaticus jugularis* (232/1a, 1b) is situated in the neck region and extends from the arm

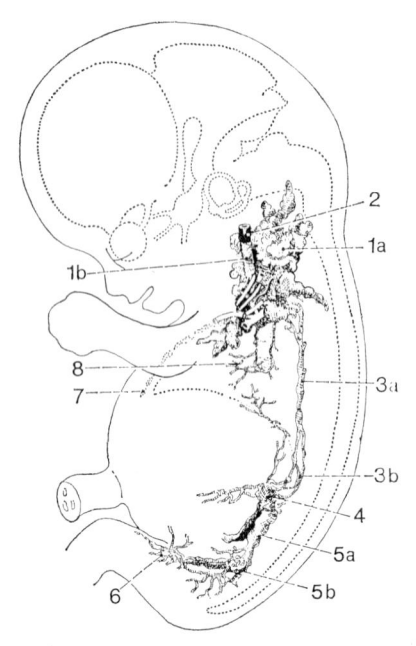

Fig. 232. Primitive lymphatic system of a 30 mm human embryo. (After Töndury and Kubik, 1972).
1 saccus lymphaticus jugularis, *1a* its superficial, *1b* its deep part; *2* v. jugularis interna; *3a* ductus thoracicus, *3b* anlage of the cysterna chyli; *4* saccus retroperitonaealis; *5* saccus lymphaticus caudalis, *5a* its pars lumbalis, *5b* its pars iliaca; *6* saccus or plexus lymphaticus inguinalis; *7* anlage of the sternal lymphatic route; *8* pulmonary lymph vessels

buds to the base of the skull. It is joined to the venous system at the level of the junction of the internal jugular, external jugular and subclavian veins, the so-called "venous angle". This lymph sac grows, not by budding, but by the fusion of new, separately-formed mesenchymal clefts.

2. *Saccus lymphaticus caudalis* (/5a, 5b) lies in the lumbar region and consists of two parts; a paired *lumbar part* with a wide lumen and a reticulate *iliac part* which has many lacunae. It is linked with the left iliac vein. This sac gives rise to the lymph vessels and node chains of the lumbar and iliac regions.

3. *Saccus lymphaticus inguinalis* (/6) splits into a network that goes to the inguinal region and the hind limb bud. It gives rise to the inguinal lymph nodes.

4. *Saccus lymphaticus retroperitonealis* (/4) is unpaired and situated in the mesentery. It later forms the junction between the lumbar lymph sac and cisterna chyli and gives rise to the lymph nodes of the gut.

5. *Cisterna chyli* (/3b) and *ductus thoracicus* (/3a). At first the former is a complex network at the level of the kidney anlage. The thoracic duct arises from a venous plexus. Its dilated terminal part, known as the *pars ampullaris*, meets the left jugular sac and its anterior, arched part is unpaired and runs on the left between the oesophagus and vertebral column. Its posterior part is paired and accompanies the right and left azygos veins. The right limb becomes the main stem and, curving to the left, it joins the unpaired anterior part.

Lymph nodes arise in association with the lymph sacs in two ways. Firstly, at the edges of the lymph sacs there are circumscribed areas to which are joined large numbers of endothelium-lined lacunae which form a vascular network with small meshes. This is traversed by numerous connective tissue septa and blood vessels. Intensive capillary formation causes the accumulation of lymphoblasts. The entire anlage is surrounded by a capsule and has a superficial lymph capillary sinus (subsequently becoming the marginal sinus). Gradually the larger lymph node anlage at the edge of the lymph sacs divide into different regions and give rise to the lymph node chains of the cervical, thoracic, lumbar and pelvic regions. Secondly, lymph nodes can also develop from lymph vessels as cell groups protruding into the lumen. This form of development is most common in the gastro-intestinal lymph nodes and those of the limbs. There is also a third form of lymph node formation, the so-called *micro-lymph nodes*, which show histological peculiarities and are of clinical significance because they can enlarge rapidly under certain pathological conditions.

Structure and function of lymphatic vessels

The lymphatic vessels can perform the function of continual drainage of the tissues and the return of large molecular plasma proteins and lipids because they consist of consecutive segments of different structure:

1. The lymph passages start as delicate tubules, the *lymph capillaries*, which are closed at one end. Because of their specialized make up they permit the trans- and inter-endothelial transfer of fluids and other substances from the tissue spaces to the lumen of the vessel.

The lymph capillaries unite to form complex capillary networks.

2. The lymph next reaches the *lymph vessels* which have a larger lumen and contain numerous bicuspid valves. They carry the lymph towards the blood stream. For this reason we term this first part of the lymph vessels the *"conducting vessels"*. Segmentally arranged muscle fibres appear in the walls of the second part of the vessels. This muscle layer is particularly well developed between two valves and, by contraction, it can propel the lymph in a centripetal direction. This second part is termed the *"transport vessel"*.

3. Before their termination in the venous system the lymph vessels unite into large *lymph collecting ducts* (lymph trunks) (233). The largest of these is the *ductus thoracicus* which, commencing behind the diaphragm as the dilated, usually ampulla-like *cisterna chyli*, carries the lymph from the posterior two-thirds of the body to the left venous angle. Shortly before its termination the thoracic duct receives the *truncus jugularis sinister*, carrying lymph from the left anterior third of the body.

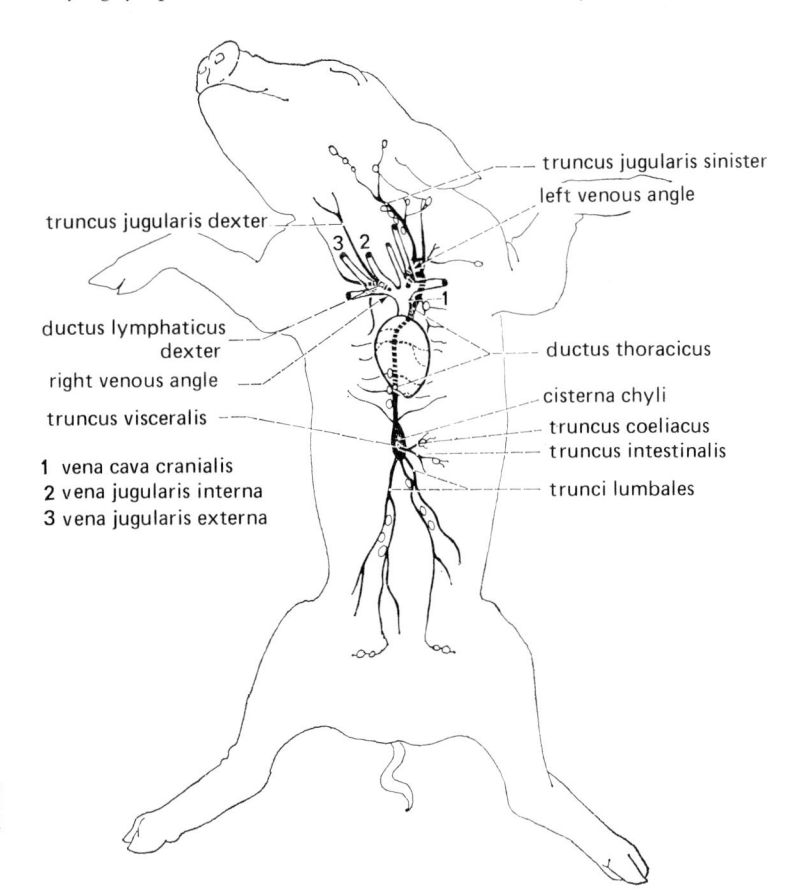

Fig. 233. Diagrammatic representation of the large lymph collecting ducts and the junction between the lymphatic and venous system

The lymph from the right anterior third of the body flows through the *truncus jugularis dexter*, the dilated terminal part of which is consequently called the *ductus lymphaticus dexter*, and it enters the right venous angle independently.

The following chapters provide detailed information about the structure and function of the different parts of the lymph passages.

Lymph capillaries

The microscopic structure of the first part of the lymph passage, the *lymph capillary* (234), depends on its drainage function. The single layer of *endothelium* is between 0.1 and 0.2 μm thick. The cell boundaries are irregularly notched (/1). In some areas the cell membranes form circumscribed contact complexes (cell junctions like zonulae occludentes, zonulae and maculae adherentes). The width of the

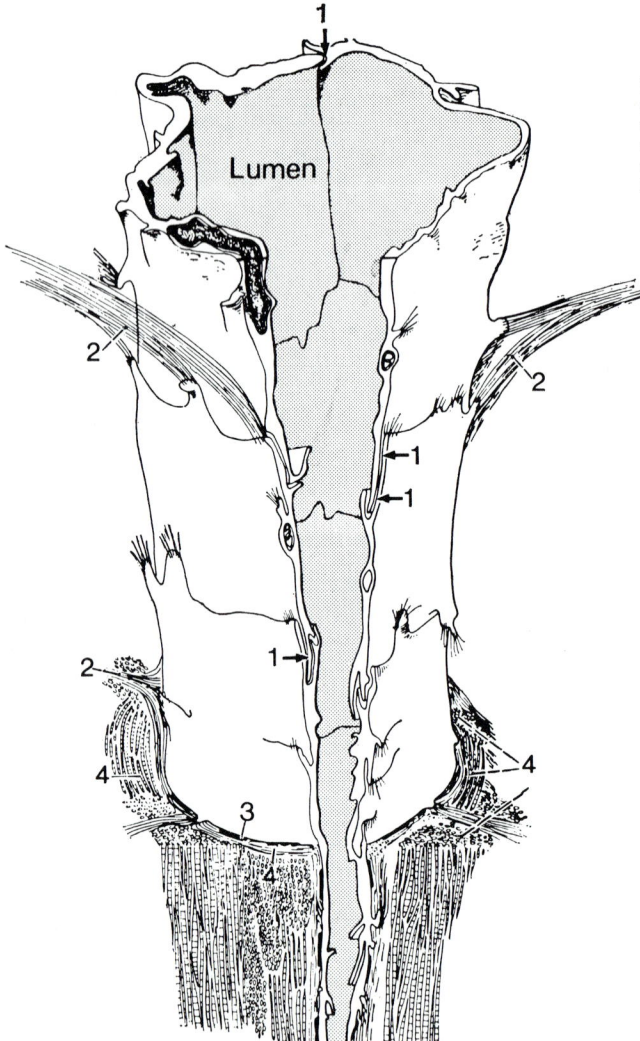

Fig. 234. Structure of a lymph capillary (diagrammatic). (Simplified from Leak and Burke, 1968.)

The vessel has been opened in transverse and longitudinal directions, so that the interdigitations of the edges of the endothelial cells (*1*) can be seen. Reticulum fibres (*2*) form the connection between the endothelial cell borders and the neighbouring connective tissue. The basal membrane (*3*) is incomplete and borders on the collagen fibres (*4*) of the interstitium

intercellular space is said to be 90 Å normally and 150–200 Å in the chyle capillaries of the intestinal villi. This permits the passage of macromolecules up to a molecular weight of 40,000. Unlike the endothelial cells of blood capillaries, those of lymph capillaries are not fenestrated although like them they contain numerous vesicles of both small (rhopheosomes) and large (symphosomes) size. These facilitate the transcellular transport of molecules of between 2,000 and 5,000 molecular weight. In contrast to blood capillaries, the basal membranes of lymph capillaries are either poorly developed or incomplete (/3). Delicate, undulated reticulum fibres bind the capillary wall to the surrounding connective tissue; pericytes are lacking. The delicate walls of the capillaries are very distensible when full and collapse completely when empty so that they are invisible in ordinary histological preparations.

The diameter of the lymph capillaries varies depending on whether they are full or empty. It is of clinical interest that, with increasing tissue pressure such as occurs in oedema during inflammation, the lymph capillaries are forced to dilate. This is because the reticular fibres which fix the capillary wall to the tissues are tensed and pull upon the lymphatic walls and then maintain the open lumen against the increased tissue pressure.

Lymph capillaries form into closed networks (235) from which spring blind processes, the true roots of the lymph circulation. Unlike the blood capillaries, the first segments of the lymph passages are of variable structure; narrow tube-like regions alternate with dilated portions (/*A*, *B*). According to Grau's theory such lymph capillary networks are only seen where collagenous connective tissue occurs, that is to say, in the subepithelial connective tissue of the "external and internal body surfaces" and in the interstitial connective tissue of parenchymatous organs. There are no lymph capillaries in epithelium, cartilage, the cornea and lens of the eye, in the purely epithelial parenchyma of certain glands, in the central nervous system and in the placenta.

Extravascular circulation

The biological significance of the double drainage of the body tissues by blood and lymph capillaries can only be appreciated by understanding the movement of water and its solutes within tissue spaces, so-called extravascular circulation. The fluid lying in the tissue spaces, such as that between the fibres of the connective tissue, is known as tissue fluid. It can fluctuate considerably in quantity and this increase may be pathological. At one time the tissue spaces were erroneously referred to as "lymph spaces" or "lymph sheaths" because they were assumed to be extensive exchange areas between the tissues and the beginning of the lymph capillaries. It was also believed that the composition of tissue fluid was identical with that of lymph but this is not always the case. On the contrary, we must imagine the tissues in these regions as comprising several spaces separated by semipermeable membranes between which occurs a more or less intensive exchange. Cells and tissues must be sufficiently supplied for their maintenance and function. The blood vessels take substances to the tissues (235A/1) whereas both blood and lymph vessels remove others (/2, 3).

The extravascular circulation relies on two groups of substances; those with a relatively low molecular weight and high diffusion rate (236/A) and those with high molecular weight and low exchange rate (/B, C).

It appears that the behavior of the macromolecules influences the structure of the blood and lymph capillaries and the osmotic forces which act on the tissues and are of importance in the formation of lymph.

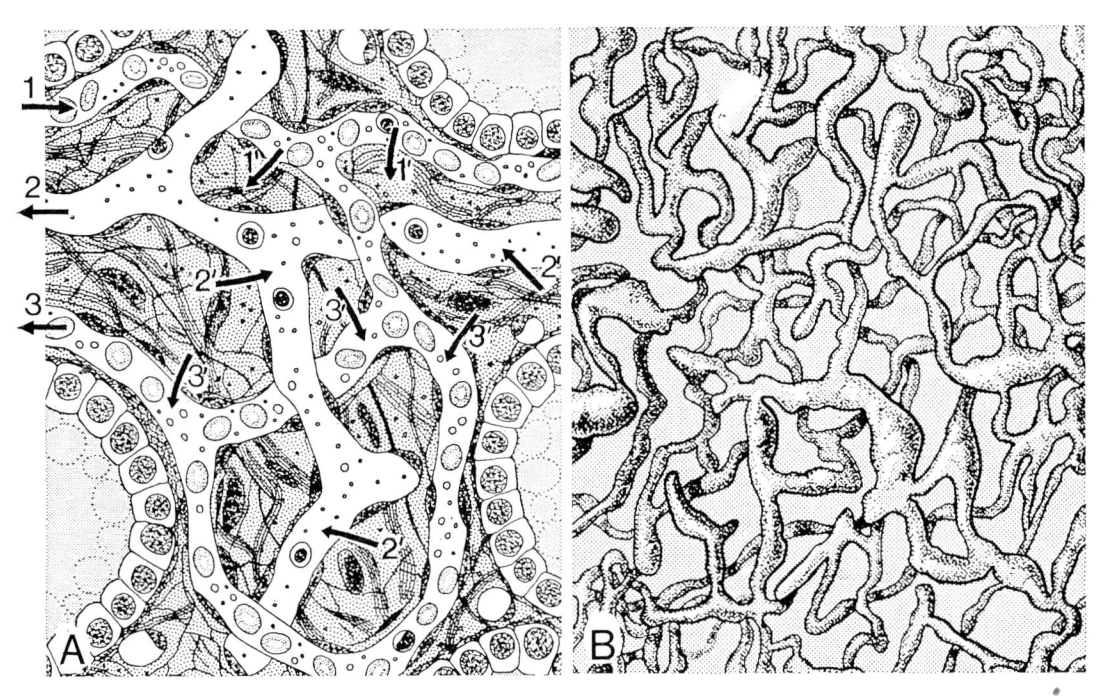

Fig. 235. Organization of the lymph capillaries and capillary networks.

A (after Kampmeier from Wenzel, 1972.)

1 arteriole, *2* lymph capillary, *3* venule

The arrows in the diagram indicate, on the one hand, the direction of diffusion from the arterial side of the blood capillary into the interstitium (1') and on the other hand, from the interstitium into the lymph capillary (2') or the venous side of the blood capillary (3').

B (after Sushko from Wenzel, 1972.)

Net-like arrangement of the lymph capillary with blind terminal saccules and variable width of the vascular lumina

Extravascular circulation of macromolecules

Each day between 50% and 100% of the quantity of circulating plasma proteins are permitted to pass from the blood capillaries into the tissues (236/B). These proteins are of importance not only to the protein metabolism of the body but by acting as vehicles for such bound substances as iron, cholesterol, lactoflavin and carotene and by their function as antibodies. Their absorption and removal from the tissues is performed almost exclusively by the lymph passages. If this route should be blocked in any way, then a lymphostatic oedema develops because the protein leaving the blood capillaries remains in the tissues and exerts an osmotic tension effect with consequent water retention.

The lymph capillaries of the intestinal *lacteals* are of primary importance to lipid absorption (/C). Long chain fatty acids can only be taken up and transported by the lymph passages and after a meal of high fat content the flow rapidly increases in the lacteals. Indeed this phenomenon led Asellius in 1622 to discover lymph vessels (237). Fatty acids of short or medium chain length can also be removed by the veins of the hepatic system.

However, lipids bound to protein can leave the blood capillaries and so participate in the extravascular circulation. Such substances have considerable molecular weight (up to 130,000) and fat droplets (chylomicrons with a diameter of 1.3 microns) can also occur in lymph.

Extravascular circulation of corpuscular elements

The blood capillaries regularly release leucocytes, including lymophocytes, into the tissues. They are carried back to the blood stream by the lymph passages. It must be remembered, however, that the majority of lymphocytes occurring in the lymph passages stem from the lymph nodes. Other corpuscular elements are also taken up by the lymph capillaries and carried through the lymph vessels to the lymph nodes where they are filtered out. These include micro-organisms which enter the interstitium either by way of the blood capillaries or directly through the skin or mucous membranes.

Lymph formation

Lymph is sometimes known as the "pale sister" of the blood. It is only recently that the morphologist Casley-Smith (1967) discovered by electronmicroscopical studies the mechanism of lymph production and his theory has become generally accepted today. The starting point in his description (238/15) is the collapsed, closed lymph capillary which terminates in the tissue space (intercellular space, interstitium). The production of small molecular, osmotically-active metabolites by cellular functions (/3, 4, 5) leads to hyperaemia and increased permeability of the blood capillaries (/2). There consequently follows a rise in water content of the tissues. Other processes, too, such as increased capillary blood pressure or a drop in the effective colloidal osmotic pressure of the blood, can cause increased filtration of water into the tissues and swelling of the latter (/6, 11).

Under these circumstances the reticulum fibres, which anchor the walls of the lymph capillaries to the surrounding connective tissue, are tensed by the swelling and so pull the endothelial cells apart and open the lymph capillaries (/10). Because of the gradient between the blood capillary pressure or the interstitial pressure on the one hand, and the intralymphatic pressure on the other, the interstitial fluid, including corpuscular elements, streams into the lumen of the lymph capillaries (/12). The corpuscles can hold the interendothelial spaces open for a short time and even provide mechanical support. The movement of tissues may also play a part in the absorption phase. In addition, the lymph capillaries have a greater permeability potential than blood capillaries because the former have an incomplete or absent basal membrane. At this time of absorption the first valve of the efferent lymph conducting vessel is still closed (/13). But almost at once some of the water again returns to the interstitium whereas protein and corpuscular elements are retained with the result that the lymph becomes concentrated and thus differs in composition from tissue fluid. This can be seen in histological preparations in which lymph is stained more intensively. If the lymph capillaries are tightly filled by this process then, due to increased tissue pressure following muscle contraction, the interendothelial clefts are closed (/15) and the lymph is propelled into the conducting vessels and the fist lymph valve opens passively (/16). The process of lymph formation can proceed afresh in the now empty lymph capillary.

Fig. 236. (p. 299) Diagrams showing where the main constituents of lymph originate.
(After Courtice, 1972.)

Above: The metabolic processes of the cells alter the effective colloidal osmotic pressure within the interstitium and are therefore involved in the movement of small molecules in the extravascular circulation.

Centre: The proteins move only in one direction in the interstitium, towards the lymph capillaries.

Below: Fat droplets (chylomicrons) and lipids of very low density are formed in the intestinal mucosa and they enter the chyle capillaries (lymph vessels of the villi). Lipids of high and low density derive mainly from the blood plasma. Lipids of all densities are transported via the thoracic duct to the blood circulation

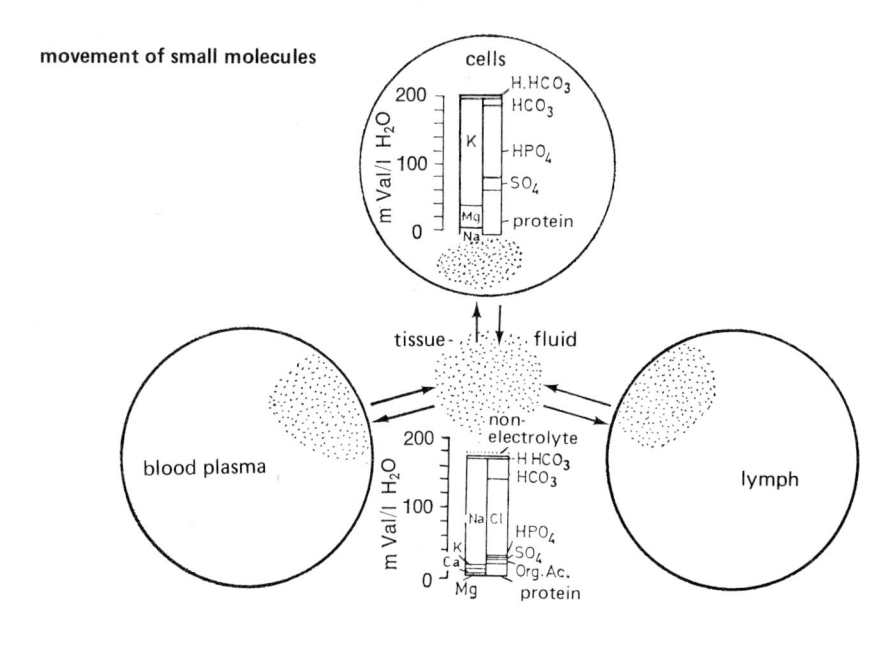

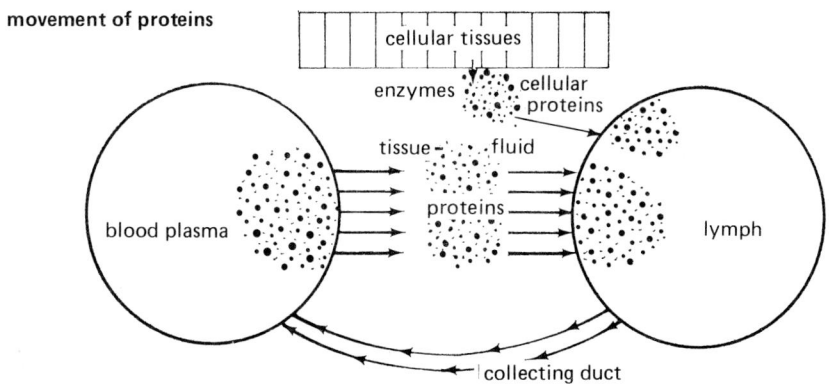

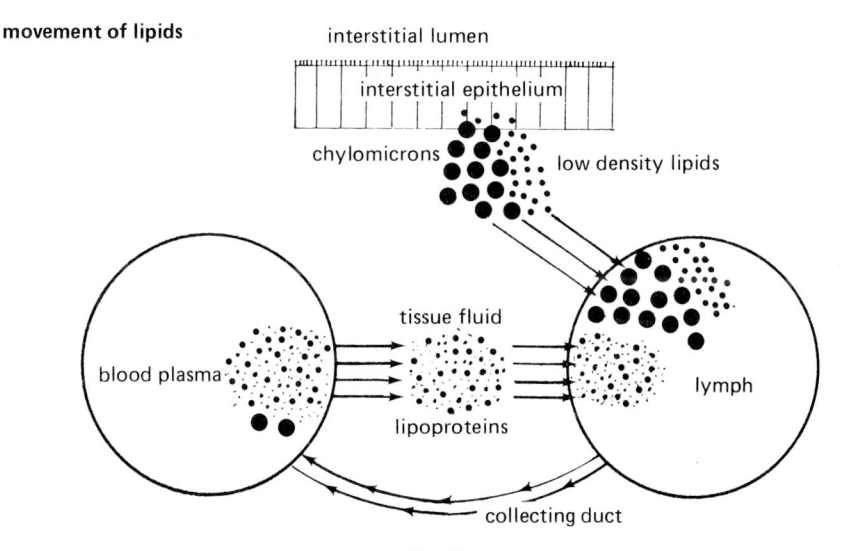

Fig. 236

The study of lymph formation in the lymph capillaries of the villi of the small intestine (239) is particularly impressive. If a few ml of oil are introduced into the small intestine of an experimental animal, within 21 minutes some of it is absorbed and present in the form of fine droplets in the lymph capillaries of the connective tissue stroma of the villi.

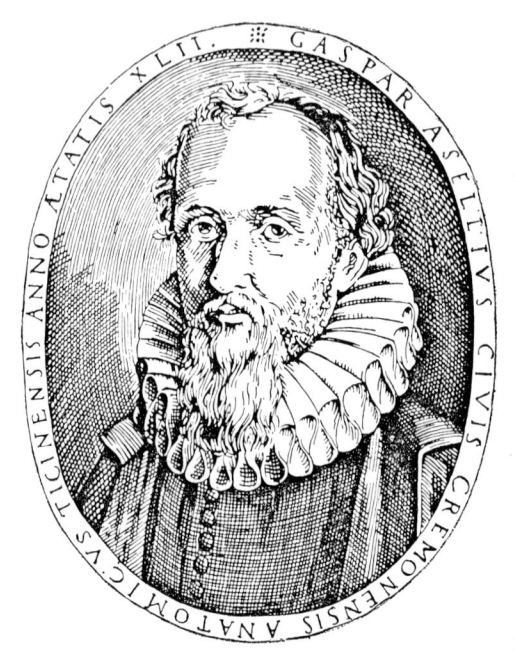

Fig. 237. Milestones in the discovery of the lymphatic system.

Above left: Gaspare, known as Asellius (1581–1626), anatomist at Pavia. In 1622, during the vivisection of a dog which had been fed a fat-rich diet, he discovered the lymphatic vessels of the intestinal mesentery, which he interpreted as "milk veins". He also saw the jejunal lymph nodes which he believed to be a type of pancreas (pancreas aselli).

Below from left to right:

Paul Ehrlich (1854–1915) developed histological and bacteriological staining methods based on the affinity of cells and bacteria to certain dyes. Results of his outstanding research activities are the differentiation of the free connective tissue cells (Ehrlich's mast cells), the establishment of the "Ehrlich side-chain theory" and fundamental studies on chemotherapy (development of the antisyphilitic agent Salvarsan).

Ludwig Aschoff (1866–1942), pathologist in Freiburg/Breisgau, introduced the concept of the reticuloendothelial system (RES). This widely disseminated system of mesenchymal elements phagocytoses and stores various substances from the body's tissue fluids. It is involved in the formation of antibodies.

Frank Macfarlane Burnet (born 1899) showed that the immunological phenomenon is the ability of the body to differentiate, by means of its immunocompetent cells, between the body's own and foreign tissues. This ability is not inherited but is acquired by the cells of the thymus (thymocytes or T-lymphocytes) during their ontogenesis.

Jaques F. A. P. Miller (born 1931) was able to demonstrate by experiment that the thymus possesses a "pacemaker" function in the immunological capacity of the organism.

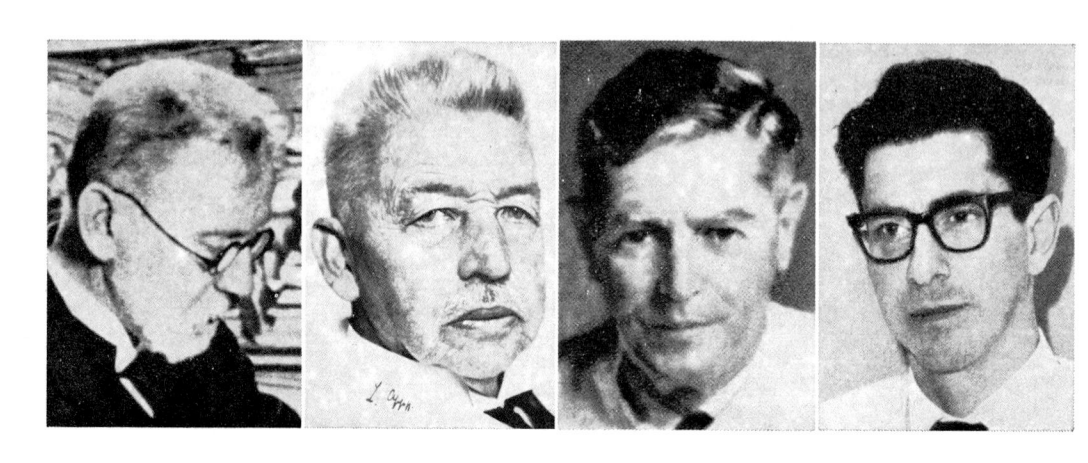

The membranes of neighbouring endothelial cells are disengaged by fluid and fat droplets which enter the spaces between them. Apart from areas of adhesion, the cell membranes are so widely separated that fluid can easily pass. These observations have finally answered the controversial question of whether the lymph capillaries are open or closed: *the degree of opening depends on swelling of the interstitium and the tension exerted on the reticulum fibres attached to their cell borders.* Additionally, small amounts of fluid can be transported through the endothelial cells by small vesicles during cytopempsis. The lymph of the intestinal villus is emptied into the conducting vessel by contraction of muscle fibres situated along the axis of every villus.

Lymph vessels

It has already been pointed out that the lymph capillary is followed by the lymph vessel (240 A, B) which has a wider lumen. It is the function of this vessel to carry the lymph from the lymph capillary to the lymph node and finally to the blood stream. Since the first lymph valves are situated in this region, the direction of flow is centripetal and we therefore call these vessels *"conducting vessels"*. Like the capillary network, these conducting vessels have numerous branches which are interconnected into a reticulation. They do not differ from the capillaries in the structure of their walls but they are of greater calibre and bear a large number of cusped valves. The forces which drive the lymph centripetally along these vessels are exerted from outside. In the conducting vessels of the skin such forces can result from the tension of the vessels during movement. In the conducting vessels of the locomotor apparatus the forces are due to the contraction of neighbouring muscle bundles. Conducting vessels are situated along the intestines running from the mucous membrane to the peritoneum and passing between the bundles of intestinal muscles and they are therefore expressed during peristaltic movement.

On the other hand the more distally situated sections of lymph vessels have muscle fibres in their own walls and are themselves capable of movement. For this reason we refer to them as the *"transport vessels"*. They also have numerous, regularly-distributed valves and these divide the transport vessel into a chain of valved segments. Each *valve segment*, also known as a *lymphangion*, therefore consists of a pair of valves and the following length of vessel, which has a lining endothelium and a *cuff of muscle tissue*. Depending on the size of this vessel, the cuff consists of one or more layers of muscle fibres arranged in a complex pattern. It is interesting to note that the walls of small transport vessels are free from muscle fibres at the point of insertion of the valves. Thus the muscular cuffs of the individual lymphangion are separated from one another and can function independently. If lymph flows from the periphery towards a valve segment then it distends between the valves, because the muscular cuff relaxes and the vessel can be stretched. When the segment is filled, muscle contraction follows with the result that the lymph in the valve segment is put under pressure. The entry valve now closes and the lymph is released centripetally through the passively opened exit valve into the next lymphangion. In this latter lymphangion the muscular cuff is again stretched and the process repeated. This theoretically-satisfactory modus operandi may be demonstrated by experimentation.

If the vessels are filled with contrast medium, their consecutive dilation and collapse *in vivo* gives an appearance like a string of pearls (240 B).

The lymph transport vessels often run parallel to one another and have lateral intercommunications. They link the *drainage* area with the regional lymph nodes. This arrangement provides a safety measure against prolonged occlusion of a single vessel and it ensures the full use of the extravascular forces of lymph transport. Besides their own contractability, the transport vessels are also able to utilise external factors for the propulsion of lymph. These include physico-chemical forces, the movement of muscles and organs, the pulsation of arteries and veins and the effect of respiration and circulation.

On the other hand, we generally do not find a confluence of several small vessels forming a larger lymph vessel, as is the rule in veins. Several lymph vessels, the *vasa afferentia*, enter one lymph node; only one or two *vasa efferentia* issue from it. Thus the number of lymph vessels is substantially reduced along the chain of lymph nodes.

In this context it should be stressed that a node lying in the course of the lymph passage presents considerable resistance to the lymph flow and this resistance must be overcome by the lymphangions situated both before and after the node.

The lymph vessel wall is permeable to substances of small molecular weight to a limited degree. This is important in the nourishment of the lymph vessels themselves because they are only sparsely furnished with *vasa vasorum*. It also ensures further concentration of the lymph when it travels a long distance from a peripheral region to the blood vessel.

The clinical significance of perfectly functioning lymphangions is not a series of distinctly interrupted stages as each segment fills and empties, but it is a wave-like motion of considerable propulsive force running along the vessel. The extent to which the vessel is filled thus gradually increases centripetally. Between 10 and 12 rhythmic waves per minute can be observed in the lacteals following a diet rich in fat. Experiments on isolated lymphangions have shown that reaction can be elicited by natural stimuli such as pressure, stretching and temperature, and also by various chemical substances and drugs. This suggests the possibility of therapy in cases of failure of the lymph transport vessels.

The preceding observations explain why retrograde injections of lymph vessels fail. Experimentation

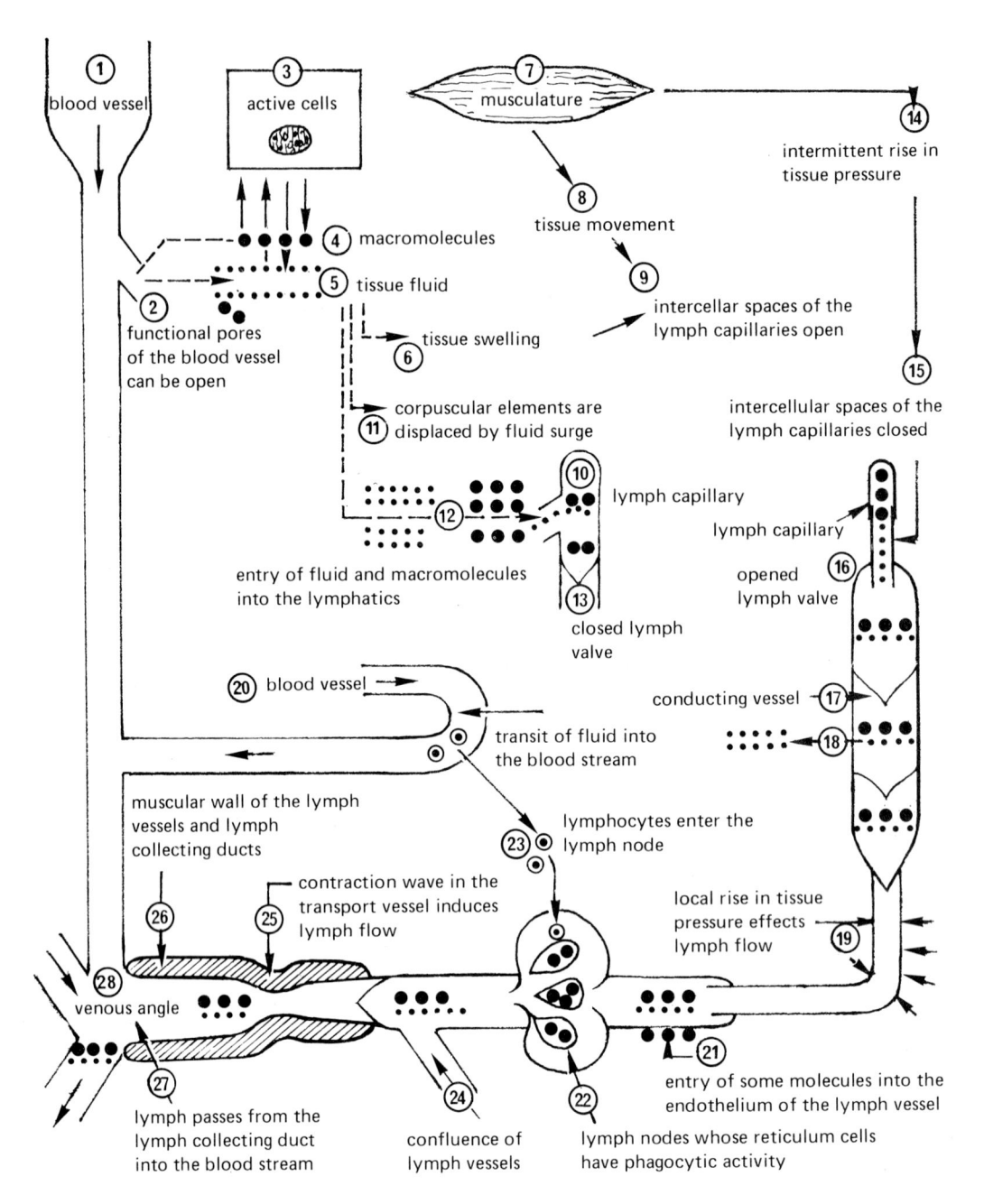

Fig. 238. Diagrammatic representation of lymph formation and lymph flow. (After Casley-Smith, 1967.)

has also demonstrated that the valves of healthy lymph vessels close completely, that is to say, they are *sufficient*. We know, on the other hand, that the valves in veins are not infrequently insufficient and so do not close completely. Infections can never be carried against the flow in lymph vessels. Extreme back-pressure of lymph can occur in exceptional circumstances when unusual conditions, including mechanical blockage of the vessels, occur. These structural peculiarities of the transport vessels are of inportance because they are the longest parts of the lymph tracts and sometimes cover considerable distances. They are placed in loose connective tissue which allows them autonomous movement. They

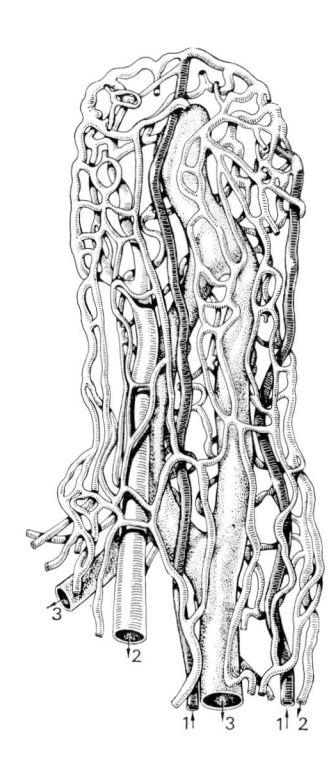

Fig. 239 (left). Diagrammatic representation of the vascularization of a villus of the small intestine.
(After Horstmann, 1968, monochrome reproduction.)
1 arteriole, *2* venule, *3* lymph capillary in the centre of the stroma of the villus (chyle capillary)

Fig. 240. Pearl-string-like appearance of the lymph vessels.

Below: visible when the lymphatics of the mesometrium of a pig are filled with lymph (After Baum and Grau, 1938.)

Right: lymphogram of the hind limb of a horse after direct lymphography
(from Auer, Diss. med. vet., Zurich, 1974.)

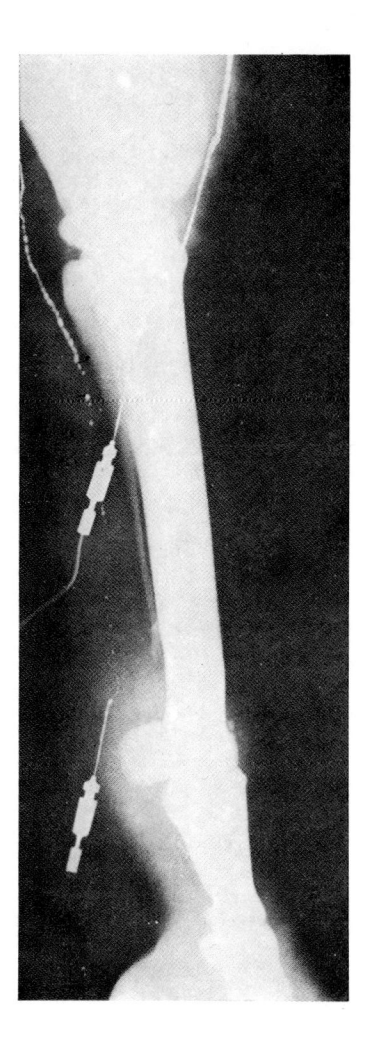

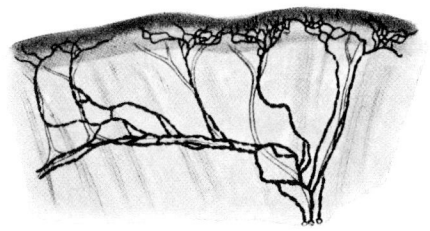

can only be identified when full in which state the chain-like arrangement of numerous lymphangions resembles a string of pearls (240 A). In the patient one can recognize the well filled or congested lymph vessels lying under the skin where they form an important pointer to the site of disease. Lymphography show that lymph flow cannot be overstressed because retention of lymph is in effect similar to the accumulation of proteins and metabolites which turn the tissues into a quagmire. Oedema develops as a result of retained tissue fluids and leads to deformation and painful swelling of certain parts of the body, the sequelae to which are the severest functional disturbances. A modern therapeutic method tried especially in human medicine consists in careful, patient massage directed by an exact consideration of the topography of the lymph tracts.

Special arrangement of lymph capillaries and lymph vessels in various organs

The pattern of distribution of the lymph capillaries and lymph vessels is largely determined by the function of the organ. The following summary will illustrate this point.

Occurrence and distribution pattern in the organs

1. *Locomotor apparatus*:

Skeleton: Sparse networks of lymph capillaries are present in the periosteum and endosteum. The lymph capillaries within compact bone follow the pattern of the Haversian canals. No lymph capillaries are present in bone marrow and cartilage.

Musculature: Small lymph capillaries are present in the endomysium between individual muscle fibres. The origin of the initial lymph capillaries follows the perimysium internum. A network is found in the external perimysium, also below the muscle fascia. Lymph vessels passing obliquely through the epimysium are linked to the efferent lymph tracts.

Tendons: Longitudinally directed networks, running between the tendon fibres, can unite into a capillary plexus below the peritenonium externum. Plexuses are also found subsynovially in tendon sheaths and synovial bursae. The efferent lymph vessels of associated muscles and tendons can either lead to the same or, as in the case of muscles with long tendons, to different lymph nodes.

Joints: Here there is the first subsynovially-situated capillary plexus which also participates in the reabsorption of synovial fluid. Occasionally a second plexus in the joint capsule is linked to the efferent lymph vessels.

2. *Serous membranes*:

In the serous membranes of the large body cavities there are two networks of different densities. One is superficial, immediately below the mesothelial lining, and the other is deep, in the subserosa. They participate in the reabsorption of serous fluid from the cavities. Apparently there are some circumscribed areas where this fluid transfer is especially intense and possibly the only method of fluid reabsorption. At such sites the subserosa is differentiated into a spongy meshwork-like reticular connective tissue. Kihara terms these regions *"maculae cribriformes"*. In the more dense surrounding collagenous connective tissue the lymph and blood capillary networks form much smaller meshes. Such specialized regions have been identified in the peritoneal surface of the diaphragm and on the costal and mediastinal pleura. The "milk spots" on the greater omentum differ in that the venous capillary limb alone takes over the absorption, while lymph capillaries and lymph vessels are only sparsely present.

3. *Digestive organs*:

There are differences in the arrangement of the lymph capillaries in the different intestinal segments but they all have in common a subserous and a submucous plexus. Both these plexuses are connected by intermuscular lymph networks which are so arranged that a plexus is stretched between each muscular layer. The reason for this is that lymph passages coming from the mucosa have a purely ducting purpose unless there is an increased amount of lymph, when they also assume a storage and propellant function. The actual mucosal plexuses are particularly adapted to the individual segments of the digestive tract. In the gastric mucosa the networks follow the glandular structures. In the small intestine the central lymph capillary of the villus lacteal is remarkable. Recently it has been suggested that this central lymph capillary of the villus is preceded by very fine lymph capillaries. Chyle capillaries of neighbouring villi anastomose at the base of the villi. Thence the capillaries go to the muscularis mucosae where they form plexuses and then continue on into the extensive network of the submucosa. The mucous membranes of both the *small* and the *large intestine* are richly supplied with solitary lymph nodules and Peyer's patches. The lymph capillaries surround the lymph follicles in a net-like manner, but they do not enter the follicles as do the blood capillaries. For details of the lymph vessels and lymph capillaries of the rumen see Schnorr et al.

The deep initial lymph capillaries of the *liver* and *pancreas* lie in the interstitial connective tissue, that is to say in a perilobular or periacinar location. They arise neither in the liver lobule nor in the acini of the pancreas nor are they in open communication with the spaces of Disse. Along with the large blood vessels the lymph passages attain the surface of the glands where they unite with extensive superficial lymph plexuses of the capsule. The distribution of the lymph capillaries of the salivary glands is similar to that of the deep lymph passages of the liver and pancreas.

4. *Respiratory system*:

The alveoli of the lungs do not have any lymph capillaries. The peribronchial and perivascular connective tissue carries a deep plexus and subpleurally there is a superficial plexus; these two anastomose. The respiratory mucosa of the air passages contains a submucous network and there is a second, deeper net in certain segments.

5. *Urogenital system*:

There are no lymph passages in the parenchyma of the renal cortex or medulla. The roots of the lymph capillaries lie in the perivascular connective tissue of the interlobular arteries. Around the subcortical and interlobular arteries there are lymph plexuses from which valve-bearing conducting vessels pass to the hilus of the kidney. The extent to which the subcapsular lymph plexus is developed varies between species but it anastomoses at the hilus with the deep lymph passages which also carry lymph from the renal sinus. The ureter has lymph vessels in its adventitia but opinions vary about the arrangement of the lymph plexuses of the urinary bladder. Some authors believe that only an intermuscular network is present while others contend that there are additional submucous and subserous networks.

In the *testis* the lymph capillaries commence in the septula testis. Some proceed thence to the rete testis and others to the tunica albuginea, where several plexuses may be superimposed upon one another. No lymph passages are present between the seminiferous tubules. At the border between the testis and epididymis the lymph tracts of the epididymis meet the subcapsular plexuses of the testis and then continue by common efferent routes along the spermatic cord. Between the convolutions of the epididymis and between the efferent ductuli there are numerous lymph capillaries draining towards the capsule of the organ.

The lymph passages of the *ovary* are subject to continual change in accordance with the cyclical changes in that organ. The lymph capillaries arise below the tunica albuginea. They enter the stratum parenchymatosum and surround both primary and secondary follicles and eventually groups of the interstitial cells. Maturing and atretic follicles as well as corpora lutea are surrounded by many layered capillary networks. The lymph capillaries enter the centre of the florid corpus luteum with the connective tissue. There are no lymph capillaries between the lutein cells.

All lymph passages of the stratum parenchymatosum go to the stratum vasculosum where they form into stout lymph plexuses. It is believed that by maximal filling this plexus participates in the process of ovulation.

Oviduct and *uterus* have both mucosal and subserous lymph plexuses which are linked by networks of lymph capillaries lying in the muscularis. The ampulla carries more lymph vessels than any other segment of the oviduct and the congestion of the lymph vessels associated with the ovarian cycle is of significance. The lymph capillaries of the uterine mucosa are reorganised during pregnancy. The *placenta* has no lymph capillaries.

6. *Circulatory and defense system*:

Heart: The lymph capillaries start in a subendocardial position. Forming into networks they continue into the interstitial connective tissue of the myocardium. The efferent subepicardial lymph vessels pass towards the coronary grooves and there they are joined by a finely meshed supbepicardial lymph capillary network.

Blood vessels: In the larger blood vessels (aorta, pulmonary artery, portal and caval veins) the lymph capillaries enter from without and proceed as far as the internal elastic lamina. The intima is free of lymph capillaries. Depending on its thickness the media has one or several lymph plexuses and they drain into the perivascularly-situated lymph passages.

Spleen: Lymph capillaries and lymph vessels are present in the capsule and trabeculae. They sometimes become confluent at the hilus. The splenic pulp does not have lymph passages.

Thymus: The capsule and interlobular connective tissue are supplied with lymph capillaries and the blood vessels supplying the thymus are accompanied by rope ladder-like lymph vessels. Hassall's corpuscles are supposed to be surrounded by lymph capillaries and this would be in keeping with their continual remodelling. It is not certain as yet whether lymph capillaries are present in the medulla and the cortex. On the other hand it has been conclusively demonstrated that large numbers of lymphocytes (12 million have been calculated in the guinea pig) leave the thymus via the lymph tract each day.

7. *Skin*:

The epidermis has no lymph capillaries. In the corium there is a superficial network containing ampulla-like dilated areas and a deeper layer of capillaries of varying calibre which constitute the start of the efferent route. The density of the lymph capillary network varies from area to area but in regions which are exposed to greater mechanical stress the network has very small meshes.

8. *Central nervous system*:

The tissues of the central nervous system and its meninges do not have lymph vessels. It is of interest, however, that lymph vessels have been demonstrated in the extradural fat tissue, in the intervertebral foramina and in the connective tissue surrounding the large blood vessels of the central nervous system. It is particularly important to stress the functional significance of drainage of the cerebrospinal fluid via the lymph passages which accompany the olfactory nerves to the nasal cavity. The "lymphogenous fluid circulation" of the brain involves the lymph capillaries outwith the dural sheaths, namely those of the cranial and spinal nerves and of the perineural and perivascular connective tissue.

9. *Endocrine system*:

Thyroid: The roots of the lymph capillaries lie perifollicularly, between the thyroid follicles. The lymph reaches the double-layered capsular plexus by following the trabeculae. The capsular plexus also has lymph capillaries dilated into sinus-like structures. The arrangement of the efferent lymph passages as they follow the blood vessels resembles a rope ladder.

Adrenal: The net-like lymph capillaries of the capsule and the perivascular plexuses, especially those around the central vein, link to form two or three efferent lymph vessels.

Lymph collecting vessels and lymphovenous anastomoses

Before terminating in the so-called "venous angle" the lymph vessels fuse into larger *lymph collecting* trunks and ducts. Particularly in the thoracic duct, but to some extent in the other collecting trunks also, the histological differentiation into tunica intima, tunica media and tunica adventitia can clearly be recognised. These three layers are least well developed in carnivores in which the lymph trunks have little muscle tissue. There are marked differences in the proportion of muscular, elastic and collagenous tissue in the thoracic duct, not only in the different species but in members of the same species and in different segments of the same duct.

The lymph collecting ducts carry many valves. At the base of the valves the muscle fibres of the vessel wall are arranged mainly in longitudinal direction. It is likely, therefore, that they exhibit autonomous movement, as in lymphangions. Of considerable importance in the movement of the lymph in these ducts is the intrathoracic inspiratory suction force and the pull produced by the large veins near the heart.

Normally the lymph vessel system joins the venous system in the "venous angle" (233, 241). This is the point of confluence of the external and internal jugular veins or, if only one of these veins is present, its junction with the ipselateral subclavian vein. We thus recognise a *left venous angle (angulus venosus sinister)* and a *right venous angle (angulus venosus dexter)*. The *ductus thoracicus* and the *truncus jugularis sinister* terminate in the *left* venous angle either separately or as one ampulla-like dilated vessel with one or more branches. The *right* venous angle receives the *truncus jugularis dexter,* the terminal 1–4 cm of which constitute the *ductus lymphaticus dexter.* This is greatly dilated since numerous efferent vessels from neighbouring lymph nodes in the right part of the neck and thoracic inlet terminate in it. There are other ways in which the collecting ducts near the venous angles can terminate in the various veins of the neck and axilla or in the cranial vena cava and this is brought about by the close developmental interrelationship between the venous and lymph vascular systems.

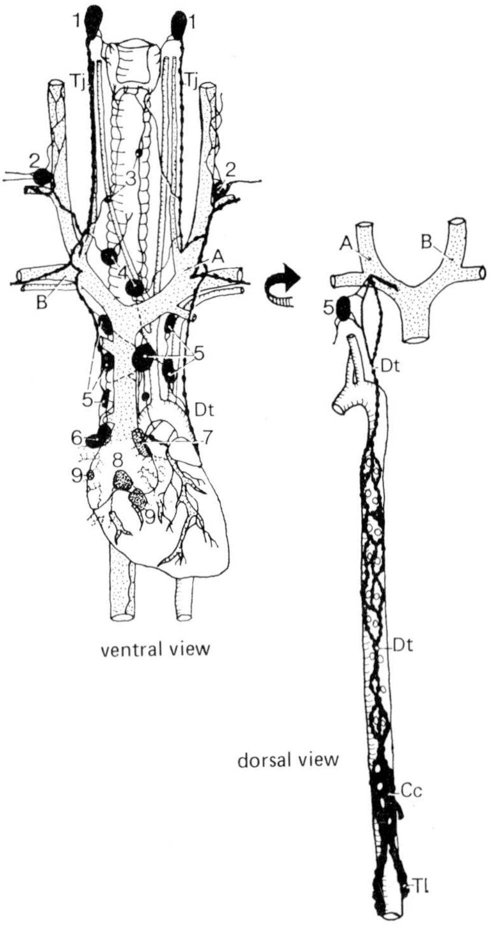

Other lymphovenous anastomoses in excess of normality have become of practical importance in medicine. The occurrence in animals of such additional lymphovenous junctions as the lymphovenous termination in the iliac, deep circumflex iliac, sacral and cephalic veins and the anastomosis between the thoracic duct and the azygos veins, have initiated a search for similar structures in man but without conclusive results. However, there are anastomoses of congenital or pathological origin which should be considered in lymphography. Lymphovenous anastomoses can be established experimentally and such procedures have indicated the feasability of producing these surgically in the treatment of such conditions as lymph stasis and lymph oedema.

It should be mentioned at this stage that the thoracic duct takes its origin from a more or less distinct lymph cistern which is situated dorsal to the aorta between the crura of the diaphragm. This is known as the *cisterna chyli.* Later, on pages 325, 326, 330 and 331, we shall record the lymph trunks emptying into this lumbar cisterna; these are the *trunci lumbales, truncus visceralis, truncus coeliacus, truncus intestinalis, truncus colicus, truncus jejunalis, truncus gastricus* and *truncus hepaticus.*

Fig. 241. Lymph collecting ducts of the cat and their termination in the venous system (diagrammatic). *Left* in the cervical and thoracic regions (ventral view), *right* in the thoracic and part of the abdominal regions (dorsal view).
(Redrawn and amplified after Sugimura, Kudo and Takahata, 1959.)
A, A angulus venosus sinister, left venous angle; *B, B* angulus venosus dexter, right venous angle; *Dt* ductus thoracicus, *Cc* cisterna chyli, *Tj* truncus jugularis, *Tl* truncus lumbalis

1, 1 nll. retropharyngei mediales, *2, 2* nll. cervicales superficiales ventrales, *3* nll. cervicales profundi medii, *4* nll. cervicales profundi caudales, *5, 5* nll. mediastinales craniales, *6* nl. bifurcationis dexter, *7* nl. bifurcationis sinister, *8* nl. bifurcationis medius, *9, 9* nll. pulmonales

Systematics and topography of lymph vessels and lymph nodes

General considerations

In the preceding chapters it has been shown that the lymph vascular system is both a transport and a defense system. Although in subsequent pages the accent will be placed on a morphological description of lymph vessels and lymph nodes, it will become evident that an exact topographical knowledge of the lymph vascular system is necessary to make a correct diagnostic interpretation.

Before commencing it is important do define certain terms (242): The term *"regional lymph nodes"* (242/a–f) will be used repeatedly. This refers to a lymph filtration point which receives and controls the *"primary lymph"* of an organ or body region. Disease involvement of such a regional lymph node indicates that the preceding organ is diseased.

Fig. 242. Diagram of lymph flow.
(In continuation of a comparable figure by Kubik, 1973.)
A–F lymph drainage areas (tributary regions) of the left (*A–C*) and the right (*D–F*) halves of the body
a–f regional lymph nodes for the drainage areas designated with the same capital letters, *g* lymph node without its own tributary region.
1–10 lymph vessels: *1* carrying primary lymph to the primary stage node, *2* secondary lymph being carried to the secondary or tertiary stage nodes, *3* carrying primary lymph past the regional node to a more distally situated lymph node (*b*), *4* primary lymph being carried to a lymph node (*f*) past two nodes of the chain, *5* transverse anastomosis to the opposite half of the body, *6* oblique anastomosis to the opposite side of the body, *7* recurrent oblique anastomosis, *8* an efferent vessel leading back to the same lymph node, *9* lymph vessel forming longitudinal meshes, *10* lymph collecting vessel

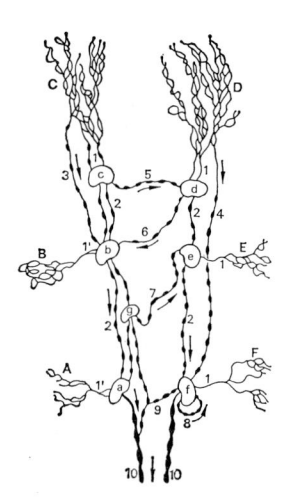

Conversely the *"drainage area"* (242/A–F) of such a regional lymph node is the tributary region from which it receives its *"primary lymph"*. This lymph flows from the lymph capillary region via the lymph vessels to reach the lymph nodes in *afferent vessels* (vasa afferentia) (/1). Two to four *efferent vessels* (vasa efferentia) (/2) leave the lymph node, carrying lymph which is filtered and enriched with lymphocytes. In contrast to the primary lymph we refer to this as the *"secondary lymph"*.

Lymph nodes are placed in chains mainly around the large blood vessel trunks. For this reason a lymph node which is not situated at the extreme periphery, can receive both primary lymph from its own drainage area and secondary lymph from a preceding lymph node (/a, b, e, f). Thus the lymph node is both the *"primary stage"* for the primary lymph and the *"secondary stage"* for the secondary lymph.

Sometimes the afferent vessels (/3, 4) by-pass the nearest lymph node and enter the node next to it. Thus they link directly a more distant lymph node with a drainage area that is actually related to another node. Furthermore there are interconnections between nodes of a group lying at the same level (/5, 6, 7). This means, of course, that the lymph nodes are linked not only in chains one behind the other but also in parallel to one another. Under certain circumstances this increases the number of filtration points through which the lymph has to pass and this increases not only the defense capacity but also the spread of disease processes along the lymphatic route. In view of this lateral connection, one can describe the organisation of the regional lymph nodes and their drainage areas only with certain reservations.

The nomenclature of the lymph nodes is based on their location. This is surprisingly constant in the different species, so that comparisons are possible, although one should remember that in dogs and ruminants there are usually only one or two lymph nodes at each site whereas the pig and horse have a group of many small nodes. It is therefore appropriate to use the term "lympho-centre" for functionally analogous groups.

A difficult diagnostic problem is the question of the "normal size" of a lymph node, because there is practically no absolute norm. In any one area the number and size of the nodes are usually in inverse proportion to one another. The total amount of lymphatic tissue available for the drainage of each region of the body has not yet been determined exactly. There can be considerable size variation between individual nodes. Increasing age is said to cause involution of the medulla rather than the cortex and its follicles.

There is, in fact, such great variation in the number and size of lymph nodes, not only between species but also from animal to animal, that even in the same individual differences occur between one side of the body and the other. This fact must be borne in mind when examining lymph nodes clinically by palpation or in the lymphogram (240 B), during meat inspection or at autopsy. Interpretation of the examination often depends on the personal experience of the examiner. However, allowing for the limitations of the method, the findings in the lymphatic system can be important, or even decisive, in the final diagnosis.

This is the reason, of course, why our knowledge of the topography of the lymph vascular system has been very good for many years. The veterinary anatomist Hermann Baum (243) has produced numerous papers and excellent atlases on the lymph vascular system of the domestic animals and many of his illustrations are reproduced in the comparative part of this chapter.

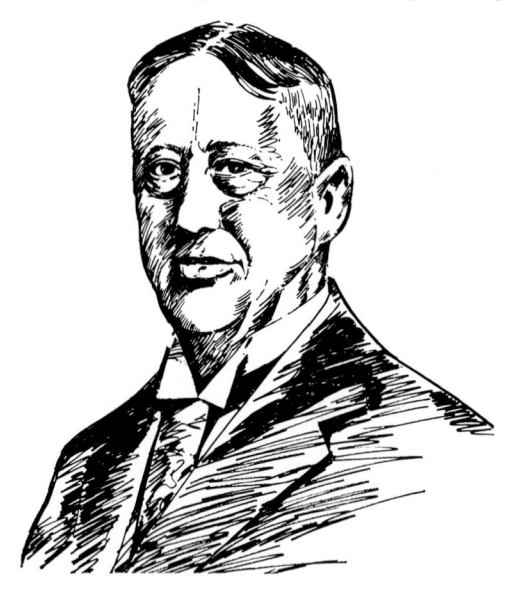

Fig. 243. Hermann Baum, Prof. Dr. phil., Dr. med vet. h. c., Dr. med. h. c. (1864–1932), veterinary anatomist at Dresden and Leipzig. From 1911 he studied systematically the lymph vascular system of the domestic animals devoting 5 comprehensive monographs and more than 50 papers to this subject alone.

Comparative description of the lymph vessel system

In the following chapter the terms lymph centre and lympho-nodes will be abbreviated to **lc.** (*lymphocentrum*) and **nl.** (*nodus lymphaticus*) or **nll.** (*nodi lymphatici*) respectively.

Lymph vessel system of the head

We differentiate three lymphocentres in the heads of domestic mammals: 1. the *lc. parotideum* which receives lymph from the superficial regions of the upper part of the head (except the anterior parts of the nose), 2. the *lc. mandibulare*, which is responsible for the superficial and deep regions of the lower jaw including the oral cavity and also the anterior parts of the nose and 3. the *lc. retropharyngeum* which collects lymph from the deeper parts of the head such as the base of the nose, the paranasal sinuses, the pharynx and larynx.

Lymphocentrum parotideum
(244/*1, 1'*; 245/*P*)

The **nll. parotidei** (parotid lymph nodes) lie ventral to the mandibular joint below the aural end of the parotid gland. Nodes may sometimes be embedded in the parotid glandular tissue itself. In the dog and ox they are palpable. In the pig, ox and horse they are regularly examined in meat inspection but in the small ruminants only in special circumstances is it necessary to inspect them.

Drainage area: the parotid lymph nodes collect primary lymph from the skin of the frontal, parietal, ocular, aural, masseter and parotid regions, from the external ocular and masticatory muscles, from the frontal, zygomatic, temporal and parietal bones, from the mandible and mandibular joint, the eyelids and lacrimal apparatus, the external ear and the parotid gland. The parotid lymph nodes are exclusively primary stage nodes.

Outflow: their transit lymph is passed on to the medial and lateral retropharyngeal lymph nodes.

Lymphocentrum parotideum	dog	cat	pig	ox	sheep	goat	horse
Nll. parotidei	337	354	364	383	405	405	420

The numbers refer to the pages where these are described in detail.

Lymphocentrum mandibulare
(244/3, 3'; 245/M, Ma)

In dogs, ruminants and horses this centre consists of one group of lymph nodes, the **nll. mandibulares**, but in the cat and pig there is a second group, the **nll. mandibulares accessorii**. The mandibular lymph nodes are situated in the posterior part of the intermandibular space, near the angle of the jaw and in the dog and ox they are readily palpable. In the horse they can be found at the level of the

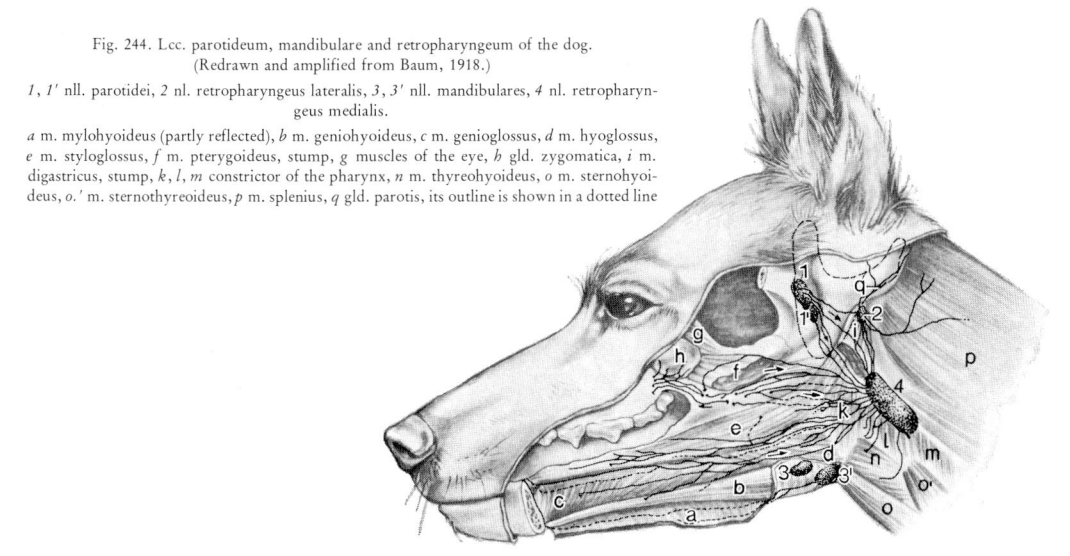

Fig. 244. Lcc. parotideum, mandibulare and retropharyngeum of the dog. (Redrawn and amplified from Baum, 1918.)
1, 1' nll. parotidei, *2* nl. retropharyngeus lateralis, *3, 3'* nll. mandibulares, *4* nl. retropharyngeus medialis.
a m. mylohyoideus (partly reflected), *b* m. geniohyoideus, *c* m. genioglossus, *d* m. hyoglossus, *e* m. styloglossus, *f* m. pterygoideus, stump, *g* muscles of the eye, *h* gld. zygomatica, *i* m. digastricus, stump, *k, l, m* constrictor of the pharynx, *n* m. thyreohyoideus, *o* m. sternohyoideus, *o.'* m. sternothyreoideus, *p* m. splenius, *q* gld. parotis, its outline is shown in a dotted line

notch for the facial vessels and the groups from the two sides join into a V-shaped structure which is palpable. This structure is characteristically involved in strangles. In meat inspection they are always examined in the pig, ox and horse but in small ruminants they are inspected only to confirm previously suspected conditions.

Drainage area: primary lymph is collected from the skin of the nose, the nares, lips, cheeks and the regions of the masseter, eyes and intermandibular space, almost all facial muscles, the muscles of mastication and those of the intermandibular space, also certain bones such as the maxilla, incisive bone, lacrimal, nasal, frontal, zygomatic bones and mandible. The teeth, gums, the tongue and its muscles, the hard palate, the mucosa of the cheeks, the anterior part of the nasal cavity and all the glands of the head fall into the drainage area of this node.

Outflow: the vasa efferentia go to the accessory mandibular lymph nodes (cat and pig), to the medial retropharyngeal and especially the cranial deep cervical lymph nodes.

In the ox the **nl. pterygoideus** (245C/Pt) can, in some instances, precede the mandibular lymph node. It receives and filters the primary lymph from the palate and passes it to the mandibular lymph node.

The mandibular lymph nodes are therefore the primary stage for large areas of the head and sometimes (in the ox) the secondary stage for lymph from the palate.

The accessory mandibular lymph nodes (cat and pig) are mainly secondary stage.

Lymphocentrum mandibulare	dog	cat	pig	ox	sheep	goat	horse
nll. mandibulares	337	354	365	383	405	405	420
nll. mandibulares accessorii	—	*354*	366	—	—	—	—
nl. pterygoideus	—	—	—	383	—	—	—

The numbers refer to the pages where these are described in detail; **bold** type indicates that they are always present, *italics* that they are inconstant in occurrence.

Lymphocentrum retropharyngeum
(244/2, 4; 245/Rl, Rm)

In all the domestic mammals this lymphocentre consists of two groups of lymph nodes, the lateral and the medial retropharyngeal lymph nodes.

The **nll. retropharyngei laterales** (244/2) lie in the retromandibular fossa near the atlantal fossa. They are palpable in the ox and, when present, in the dog. In the horse they are related to the lateral wall of the guttural pouch (guttural lymph node). The **nll. retropharyngei mediales** (/4) lie against the pharynx. Both groups of retropharyngeal lymph nodes are regularly examined at meat inspection in the pig, ox and horse but in small ruminants only for confirmation.

Drainage area: skin of the parotid region, the intermandibular muscles, the inner muscles of mastication, the muscles of the hyoid bone, the muscles of the cranial part of the neck and of the nape, the occipital, the sphenoid, temporal, palatine, frontal and maxillary bones as well as the mandible, the glands of the head, the tongue, lingual muscles, hard and soft palate, the lymphatic pharyngeal ring, the gums, maxillary teeth, floor of the nose, paranasal sinuses, guttural pouch (horse), pharynx, larynx, thyroid gland and external ear.

The retropharyngeal lymph nodes also receive transit lymph from the parotid lymphocentre in all domestic mammals and also from the mandibular lymphocentre in carnivores and bovines.

In the ox the inconstant **nl. hyoideus rostralis** and the **nl. hyoideus caudalis**, which filter lymph from the tongue and the glands of the head and then pass it on to the lateral retropharyngeal nodes, are also present.

Lymphocentrum retropharyngeum	dog	cat	pig	ox	sheep	goat	horse
nll. retropharyngei mediales	340	355	366	384	406	406	422
nll. retropharyngei laterales	*341*	355	368	384	406	406	422
nl. hyoideus rostralis	—	—	—	*385*	—	—	—
nl. hyoideus caudalis	—	—	—	*385*	—	—	—

The numbers refer to the pages on which these are described in detail: **bold** type indicates that they are constant in occurrence, *italics* that they are inconstant.

Lymph drainage from the head varies considerably between the species. The following is a general picture which does not take into account individual variation and small secondary routes.

In the **dog** (245A) the parotid node, mandibular nodes and the inconstant lateral retropharyngeal node pass their lymph mainly to the medial retropharyngeal lymph node where the jugular trunk commences.

In the **cat** the jugular trunk also commences at the medial retropharyngeal node. The interconnection between the individual lymph nodes of the head is more or less a combination of the situation in the other domestic mammals and it is described in the special section on the cat's lymphatic system.

Two main drainage routes are recognised in the **pig** (245B). 1. The parotid nodes and the lateral pharyngeal nodes send their lymph to the medial retropharyngeal nodes where the truncus jugularis

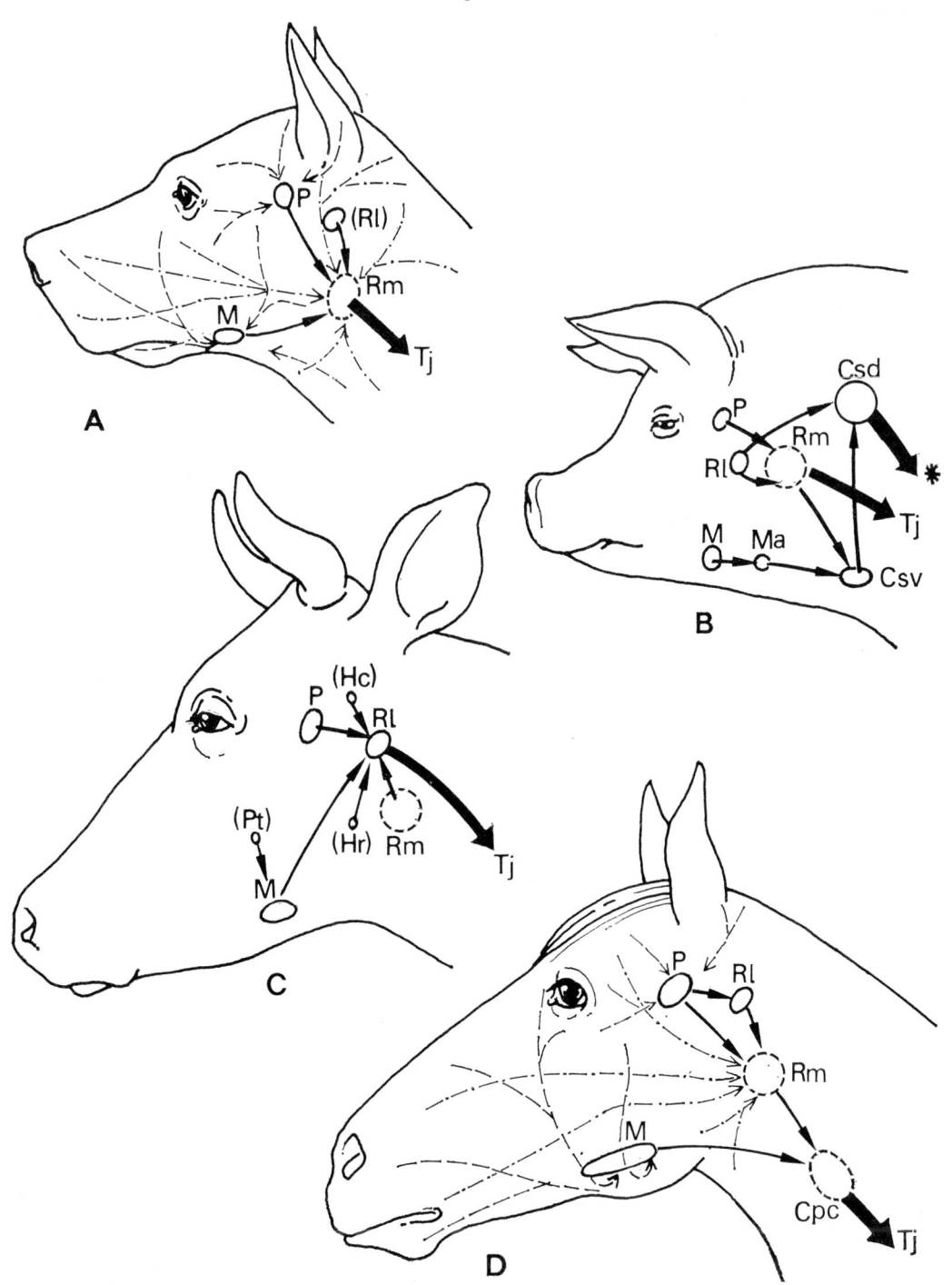

Fig. 245. Diagrams of lymph drainage from the head; only the principal routes are shown.
A dog, B pig, C ox, D horse.

The lymph nodes are shown as single units even when they occur as several nodes or in groups. The superficially situated nodes are drawn in solid lines, the deep nodes in broken lines. Lymph nodes of inconstant occurrence are in brackets.

Lymph nodes of the head: P nll. parotidei, M nll. mandibulares, Ma nll. mandibulares accessorii (pig), Rl nll. retropharyngei laterales, Rm nll. retropharyngei mediales, Hr nl. hyoideus rostralis (ox), Hc nl. hyoideus caudalis (ox), Pt nl. pterygoideus (ox).

Lymph nodes of the neck (in as far as they are involved in the filtration of lymph from the head): Csd nll. cervicales supff. dorss. (pig), Csv nll. cervicales supff. ventrr. (pig), Cpc nll. cervicalis proff. crann. (horse).

Lymphatic routes: Tj truncus jugularis, *Lymph drainage via the superficial cervical node (pig). The vasa afferentia are shown as interrupted lines only in the dog and horse.

commences. This trunk passes on a small amount of the lymph from the head. 2. The mandibular lymph nodes pass their lymph to the accessory mandibular nodes which in turn connect with the ventral superficial cervical nodes. The latter also receive a contribution from the medial retropharyngeal nodes which they pass on to the dorsal superficial cervical nodes. Since these dorsal superficial cervical nodes also collect lymph directly from the lateral retropharyngeal nodes, they receive the bulk of the lymphatic drainage of the head.

In the **ox** (245C) lymph from the parotid node, the mandibular node and the medial retropharyngeal node goes to the lateral retropharyngeal nodes. The jugular trunk arises from the latter nodes. It carries all the lymph from the head.

In **small ruminants** drainage of lymph from the head is similar to the ox although in the goat the jugular trunk arises from two roots originating in the efferent vessels of the lateral and medial retropharyngeal nodes respectively.

In **horses** (245D) lymph passes from the parotid nodes and the lateral retropharyngeal nodes to the medial retropharyngeal nodes. In turn the latter, and the mandibular nodes, drain into the cranial deep cervical nodes, the efferent branches of which give rise to the jugular trunk.

In the dog, ruminants and horse the lymph from the head is thus drained exclusively by the jugular trunk whereas in the pig, although the trunk also carries some efferent lymph, the bulk drains via the dorsal superficial cervical nodes.

Lymph vessel system of the neck

We differentiate two lymphocentres in the neck of domestic mammals: 1. the superficial lymph vessels collect in the superficial cervical lymphocentre, the drainage area of which also includes some parts of the head, forelimb and trunk. 2. the deep lymph vessels meet in the deep cervical lymphocentre, which may consist of a chain of cranial, middle and caudal lymph nodes situated along the trachea. Its drainage area also extends to the head, shoulder and upper arm.

Lymphocentrum cervicale superficiale
(246/i; 247/Cs, Csa, Csd, Csm, Csv)

The **nll. cervicales superficiales** is the largest of the superficial lymph nodes of the neck. This node, or group, is situated cranial to the shoulder joint under the brachiocephalicus muscle and sometimes also under the omotransversarius. In the horse this group can be palpated in front of the prescapular part of the deep pectoral muscle but in the dog and ox the single node is accessible at the cervical border of the supraspinatus muscle. Only in the cat are there other superficial cervical lymph nodes, apart from that situated at the shoulder joint. The cat has two groups, namely the *nll. cervicales superficiales dorsales et ventrales*, and the pig has three groups, the *nll. cervicales superficiales dorsales, medii et ventrales*. The dorsal group corresponds to the shoulder lymph nodes of the other domestic mammals. It may be examined in meat inspection in special circumstances.

The *drainage area* is not confined to the neck, its skin and superficial muscles. It extends on the one hand to the head, especially the parietal, aural, masseter and parotid regions, and on the other hand it encompasses the dorsal, lateral and ventral wall of the thorax and in the horse even the lateral and ventral wall of the abdomen. Furthermore considerable regions of the pectoral limb, their skin, some of the muscles of the shoulder girdle, extensors and flexors of the toe, shoulder, carpal and toe joints and almost all the bones of the forelimb contribute lymph to these glands.

It must be stressed that in the pig the ventral group of the superficial cervical nodes also receives lymph vessels from the anterior portions of the mammary gland and for this reason they must be examined if breeding sows are slaughtered. Furthermore, it should be remembered that in this species the dorsal group has not only its own drainage area but it also acts as a secondary and even tertiary stage for all three lymphocentres of the head and for the middle and ventral group of superficial cervical nodes.

In the ox and sheep there are *nll. cervicales superficiales accessorii* (247/Csa) which are in anteposition to the superficial cervical node and act as a primary stage for the lymph from the back of the neck.

In the dog the efferent lymph vessels of the superficial cervical nodes (247) enter the terminal section of the jugular trunk or the terminal part of the thoracic duct, sometimes even passing directly into the external jugular vein. In the pig the three groups are linked together by means of the efferent vessels. The ventral group passes its lymph to the middle or dorsal group. The efferent vessels of the middle group generally flow directly to the venous angle while those of the dorsal group pass to the jugular trunk or to the middle group. In the ox the efferent vessels of the superficial cervical lymph nodes empty directly into the jugular trunk or the thoracic duct. In the horse the efferent vessels of the superficial nodes go to the caudal deep cervical lymph nodes or sometimes, on the right, they run directly to the right lymphatic duct.

Fig. 246. Lcc. parotideum, retropharyngeum, cervicale superficiale, cervicale profundum, mediastinale and axillare of the horse. (After Baum, 1928.)

a, a nll. cervicales profundi craniales, *b, b', b''* nll. cervicales profundi medii, *c, c'* nll. cervicales profundi caudales, *d* nll. parotidei, *e* nll. retropharyngei laterales, *e'* nll. retropharyngei mediales, *f* nl. nuchalis, *g* nll. mediastinales craniales, *h* nll. axillares proprii, *i* nll. cervicales superficiales, *k, k* truncus jugularis

1 thyroid, *2* trachea, *3* oesophagus, *4* a. carotis communis, *5* first rib, *6* axillary vessels, *7* a. cervicalis superficialis sinistra, ramus ascendens, *8* a. cervicalis profunda, *9* part of the m. omohyoideus

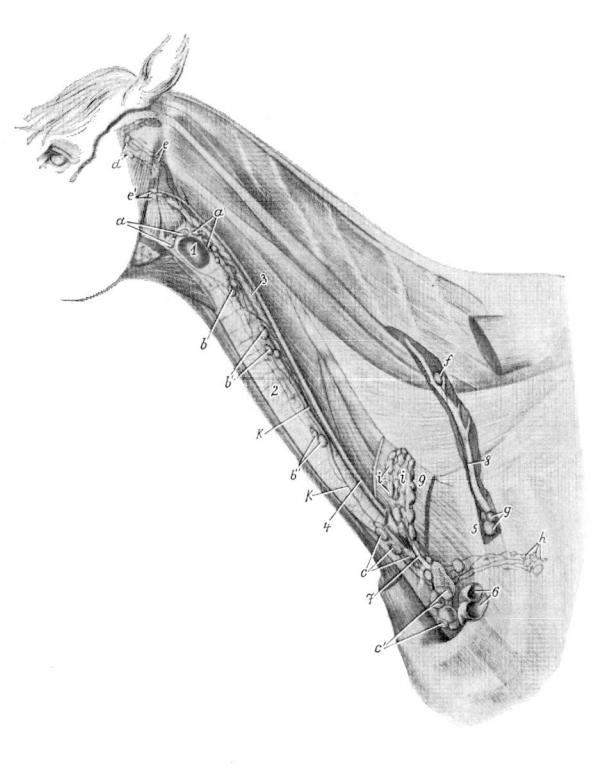

Lymphocentrum cervicale superficiale	dog	cat	pig	ox	sheep	goat	horse
nll. cervicales superficiales	341	—	—	386	407	407	422
nll. cervicales superficiales (dorsales)	—	355	368	—	—	—	—
nll. cervicales superficiales medii	—	—	369	—	—	—	—
nll. cervicales superficiales ventrales	—	355	369	—	—	—	—
nll. cervicales superficiales accessorii	—	—	—	386	*407*	—	—

The numbers refer to the pages where these are described in detail; **bold** type indicates that they are constant, *italics* that they are inconstant in occurrence.

Lymphocentrum cervicale profundum
(246/*a, b, b', b'', c*; 247/*Cpc, Cpm, Cpca*)

The deep lymph nodes of the neck are related to the cervical part of the trachea and the deep blood vessels. They can be subdivided into three groups, namely the **nll. cervicales profundi craniales, medii et caudales**. The cranial and middle groups are smaller and can be absent altogether (dog, cat, pig, small ruminants), the caudal group is constant and, apart from the dog, it is particularly large. The caudal deep cervical nodes of the pig, ruminants and horse and the costocervical node of ruminants (see below) are sometimes examined in meat inspection.

The *drainage area* includes the deeper regions of the neck, such as cervical vertebrae, cervical musculature, larynx, trachea, oesophagus, thyroid gland and thymus. The cranial deep cervical lymph nodes also receive lymph from the head, especially the parotid, masseter and nape regions. The ramifications of the caudal group extend to the regions of the shoulder and upper arm, including the musculature of the shoulder girdle and of the shoulder and elbow joints, the shoulder blade and the shoulder joint itself.

In the ox, sheep and goat the caudal group of deep cervical lymph nodes is preceded by a *nl. costocervicalis* (247/Cc; 250, 251/2) which lies below the ventral scalenus muscle. Furthermore the ox also has an inconstant *nl. subrhomboideus* (247/Sr) which lies under the cervical part of the rhomboideus muscle. The latter may itself precede the costocervical lymph node, or pass lymph to the cranial mediastinal node.

The *efferent vessels* of the deep cervical nodes go directly or indirectly to the jugular trunk. In the pig only they go to the nll. axillares primae costae or to the cranial vena cava.

It is noteworthy that the caudal deep cervical lymph nodes of the ox also act as a secondary stage for lymph from the axillary lymphocentre.

Lymphocentrum cervicale profundum	dog	cat	pig	ox	sheep	goat	horse
nll. cervicales profundi craniales	*342*	—	*369*	*387*	*407*	*407*	*423*
nll. cervicales profundi medii	*342*	*356*	*370*	*387*	*407*	*407*	*424*
nll. cervicales profundi caudales	*342*	*356*	*370*	**387**	**408**	**408**	**424**
nl. costocervicalis	—	—	—	**388**	*408*	*408*	—
nl. subrhomboideus	—	—	—	*388*	—	—	—

The numbers refer to the pages where these are described in detail; **bold** type indicates that they are constant, *italics* that they are inconstant in occurrence.

Truncus jugularis
(247/Tj)

There is one jugular trunk, the large collecting vessel of the neck, on each side. The *trunci jugulares dexter et sinister* receive the vasa efferentia of the lymphocentres of the head and neck and pass their lymph directly to the venous angle.

The **truncus jugularis dexter** is related in its entire length to the cervical part of the trachea and for this reason it is sometimes referred to as *truncus trachealis dexter*. Also related to the right jugular trunk are the common carotid artery, the recurrent nerve and, when present (except in small ruminants), the internal jugular vein. At the cranial thoracic aperture the trunk either unites with the axillary lymph vessels and the efferent vessels of the deep cervical and of the cranial mediastinal lymph nodes to form the *ductus lymphaticus dexter*, or the right jugular trunk empties independently in the venous angle. In the latter case the thickened terminal part is known as the *ductus lymphaticus dexter*.

The **truncus jugularis (trachealis) sinister** lies against the oesophagus in the upper third of the neck, then it progresses alongside the trachea to reach the terminal part of the thoracic duct at the thoracic aperture. Alternatively it can also empty into the venous angle independently. Both jugular trunks may be duplicated. Species peculiarities will be discussed in a separate chapter, special attention being given to the intercalation in its course of the caudal deep cervical lymph nodes in the horse and the two roots of origin and single termination which occur in small ruminants.

Lymph vessel system of the forelimb

In the main the superficial lymph vessels of the pectoral limb drain into the already-mentioned superficial cervical lymphocentre. A separate lymphocentre, the *lc. axillare* is responsible for receiving the deep lymph vessels of the forelimb. This latter lymphocentre also drains the lateral thoracic wall and, in the dog, the mammary gland.

Lymphocentrum axillare
(248/e, e'; 249/Ap, Apc, Aa)

This lymphocentre includes:

The **nll. axillares proprii**. These are situated caudal to the shoulder joint in the bifurcation of the axillary and subscapular arteries; they are absent in the pig.

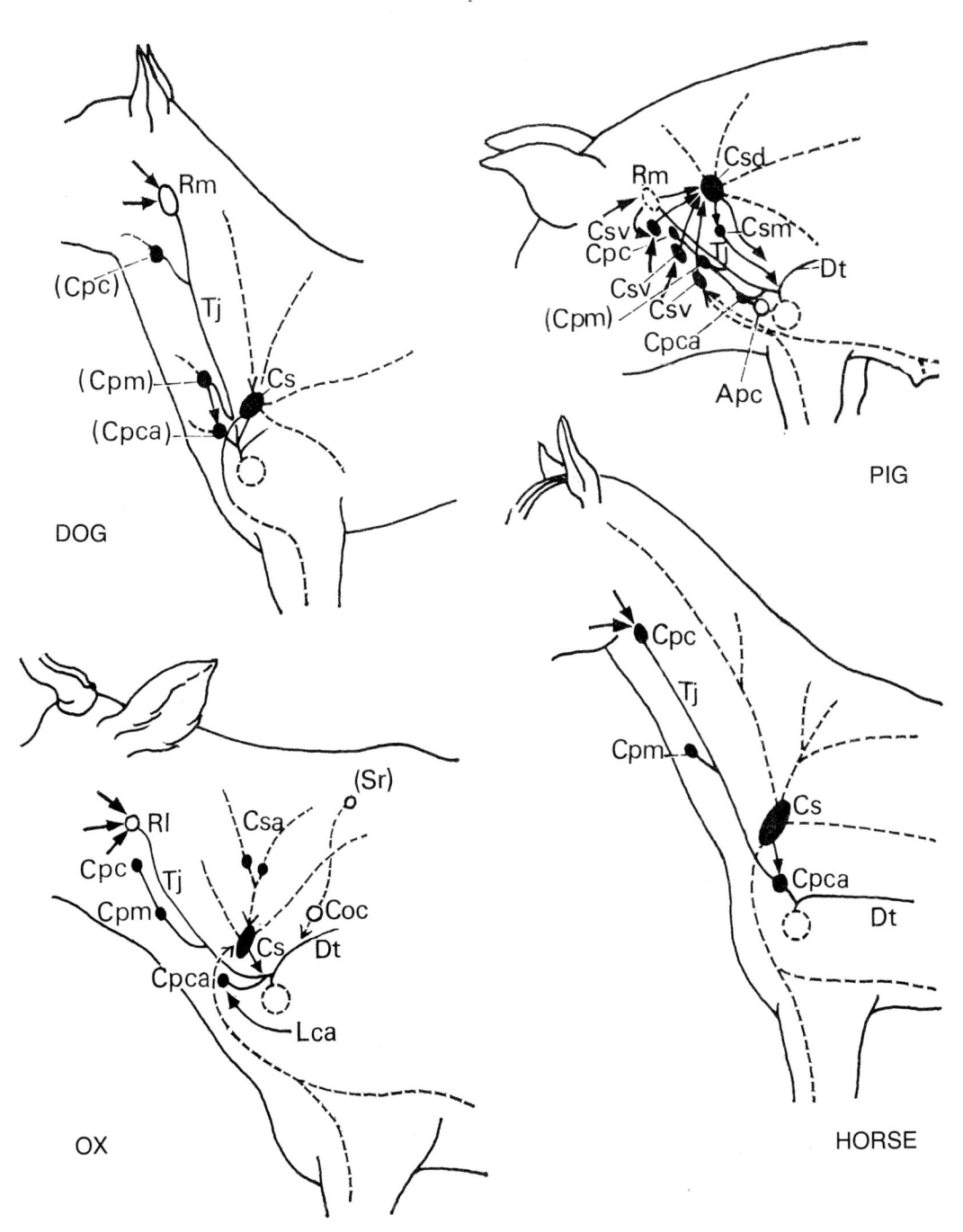

Fig. 247. Diagram of the lymph drainage from the neck; only the principal routes are shown. The lymph nodes of the superficial and deep cervical lymphocentres are shown solid; inconstantly occurring nodes are in brackets.

Lymph nodes of the lc. cervicale superficiale: Cs nll. cervicales superficiales (dog, ox, horse), Csa nll. cervicales superficiales accessorii (ox), Csd nll. cervicales superficiales dorsales (pig), Csm nll. cervicales superficiales medii (pig), Csv nll. cervicales superficiales ventrales (pig);

Lymph nodes of the lc. cervicale profundum: Cpc nll. cervicales profundi craniales, Cpm nll. cervicales profundi medii, Cpca nll. cervicales profundi caudales;

Lymph nodes which are not part of the cervical centres: Rm nll. retropharyngei mediales where the truncus jugularis begins in the dog and pig, Rl nl. retropharyngeus lateralis, where the truncus jugularis begins in the ox, Coc nl. costocervicalis (ox) and Sr nl. subrhomboideus (ox) the lymph node of the cervicothoracic transition; Apc nl. axillares primae costae (pig), a secondary stage for the lymph from the neck.

Lymph collecting ducts: Dt ductus thoracicus, Tj truncus jugularis, Lca lymph vessel from lymphocentrum axillare (ox); venous angle is shown as interrupted circle

The **nll. axillares primae costae**. These lie lateral to the first rib at the level of the axillary artery; they are absent in the dog and the horse.

The **nll. axillares accessorii** are found in dogs and cats and sometimes in bovines and sheep against the 3rd or 4th ribs at the level of the lateral thoracic vein.

Clinically the above-mentioned lymph nodes are collectively referred to as the axillary lymph nodes.

The **nll. cubitales** (249/*Cu*) lie medial to the elbow joint. They are found regularly only in the horse although they may occur inconstantly in the sheep.

The inconstant **nl. infraspinatus** (249/*I*) is to be found only in the ox. It is situated in the upper third of the caudal border of the infraspinatus muscle.

Of all these lymph nodes only the axillaries of the dog and the cubital lymph nodes of thin horses are palpable. In all meat animals the axillary nodes are examined at meat inspection under certain circumstances.

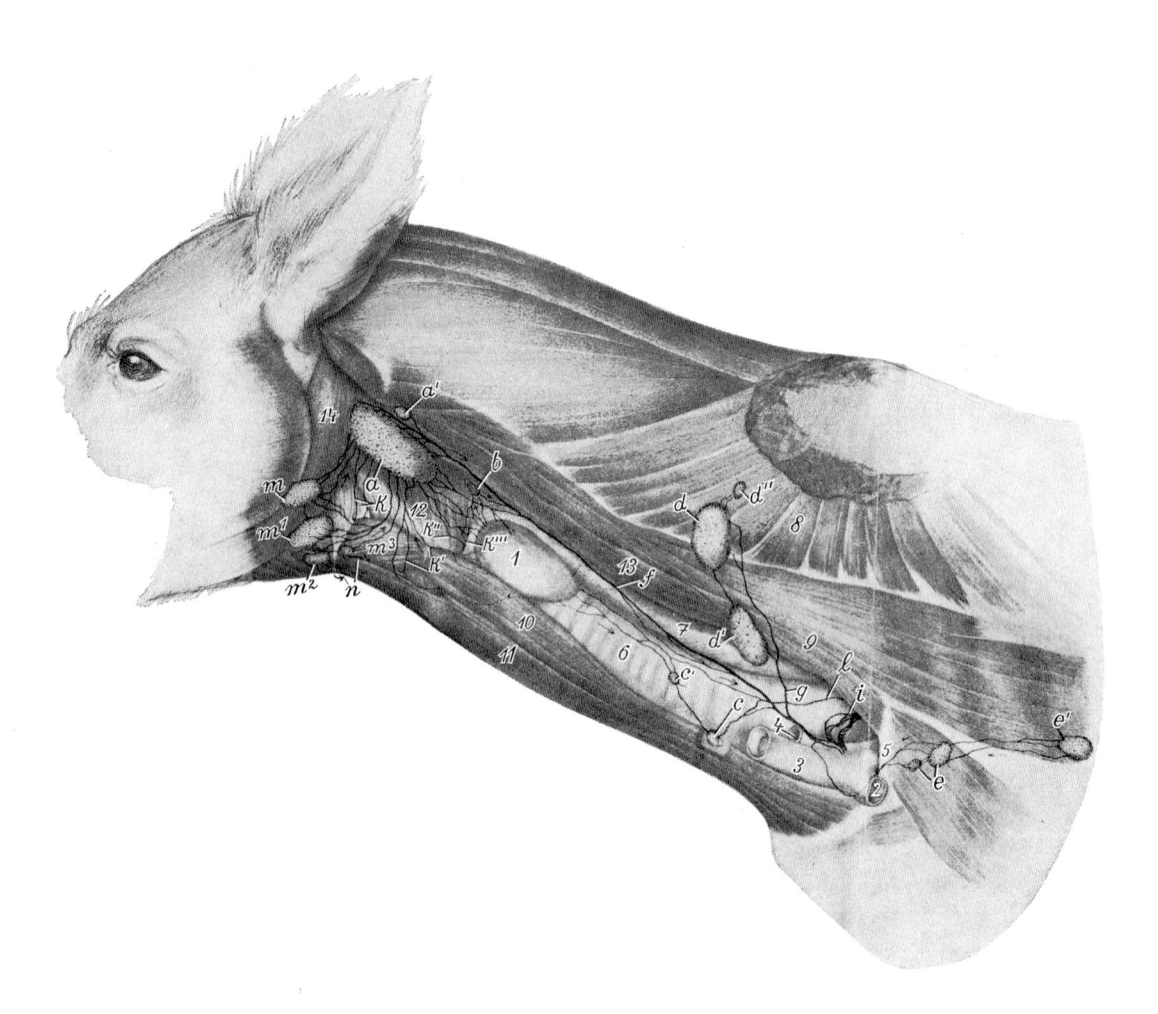

Fig. 248. Lcc. mandibulare, retropharyngeum, cervicale superficiale, cervicale profundum and axillare of the dog. (Amplified from Baum, 1918.)

a, a' nll. retropharyngei mediales, *b* nl. cervicalis profundus cranialis, *c, c'* nll. cervicales profundi caudales, *d, d', d''* nll. cervicales superficiales, *e* nl. axillaris proprius, *e'* nl. axillaris accessorius, *f* truncus jugularis sinister, *g* vas efferens of the nll. cervicales superficiales, *i* ductus thoracicus with its terminal part, *k, k', k'', k'''* lymph vessels from the larynx, *l* lymph vessel which ends in one of the cranial mediastinal nodes, *m, m¹, m², m³* nll. mandibulares, *n* vasa efferentia of the nll. mandibulares which go to the nll. retropharyngei mediales of the other side.

1 thyroid, *2* v. axillaris, *3* v. jugularis externa, *4* v. jugularis interna, *5* first rib, *6* trachea, *7* oesophagus, *8* m. serratus ventralis, *9* m. scalenus, *10* m. sternothyreoideus, *11* m. sternohyoideus, *12* pharyngeal musculature, *13* m. longus capitis, *14* m. digastricus

The *drainage area* of the axillary lymphocentre includes the deeper parts of the entire forelimb and superficial regions, the extent of which varies according to the species. The superficial regions include the anterior and ventral parts of the chest, in the pig also the ventral part of the neck, in the horse the lateral chest wall, in the dog the dorsal wall of the thorax, the ventral abdominal wall and the thoracic and anterior abdominal mammary complexes.

Lymphocentrum axillare	dog	cat	pig	ox	sheep	goat	horse
nll. axillares proprii	**342**	**356**	—	**388**	**408**	**408**	**424**
nll. axillares primae costae	—	*357*	**370**	**389**	**409**	**409**	—
nl. axillaris accessorius	*342*	*357*	—	*389*	*409*	—	—
nll. cubitales	—	—	—	—	**410**	—	**424**
nl. infraspinatus	—	—	—	*389*	—	—	—

The numbers refer to the pages where these are described in detail; **bold** type indicates that they are constant, *italics* that they are inconstant in occurrence.

Lymph drainage from the axillary lymphocentre
(249)

When the axillary lymph nodes are present in three groups, as in cats and perhaps oxen and sheep, or in two groups as in dogs and ruminants, they form a lymph node chain with a flow direction from caudal to cranial. From either the axillary lymph nodes of the first rib or the proper axillary lymph nodes (in the cat from both), the efferent vessels go directly (in the cat), indirectly (in the ox and horse) or by both routes (in the dog and pig), to the venous angle. In the dog the indirect route is via the jugular trunk or the terminal section of the thoracic duct. In the pig the indirect route goes to the ventral superficial cervical nodes and the jugular trunk. In the ox this indirect route goes via the thoracic duct and the cervical lymph nodes and in the horse it goes through the caudal deep cervical nodes. The cubital lymph nodes pass their lymph to the proper axillary nodes (horse and sheep) and the axillary nodes of the first rib (sheep).

Thus the majority of the deep lymph vessels of the forelimb drain into the axillary lymphocentre. In the dog lymph from the mammae is also drained by these nodes which are clinically palpable in this species. The superficial lymph vessels of the pectoral limb, and in some species also the efferent vessels of the axillary lymphocentre, flow to the superficial and deep cervical lymph nodes. They collect in the dorsal and ventral superficial cervical ones in the pig. But, except in the horse, the axillary lymphocentre also passes its lymph directly to either the venous angle or the lymph collecting ducts at the thoracic entrance.

Lymph vessel system of the chest wall and thoracic organs
(250, 251, 252)

There are four lymphocentres in the thoracic cavity. Two are mainly concerned with drainage of the chest wall; these are the dorsal thoracic lymphocentre and the ventral thoracic lymphocentre. The third receives lymph from the mediastinum and its organs and it is therefore known as the mediastinal lymphocentre. The fourth, known as the lc. bronchale, drains the heart and lungs.

Lymphocentrum thoracicum dorsale
(250/7, 8, 8'; 251/8, 9, 9')

Two groups of lymph nodes belong to this lymphocentre. They both extend below the thoracic vertebral column and are separated from one another by the sympathetic trunk. They are the thoracic aortic lymph nodes and the intercostal lymph nodes.

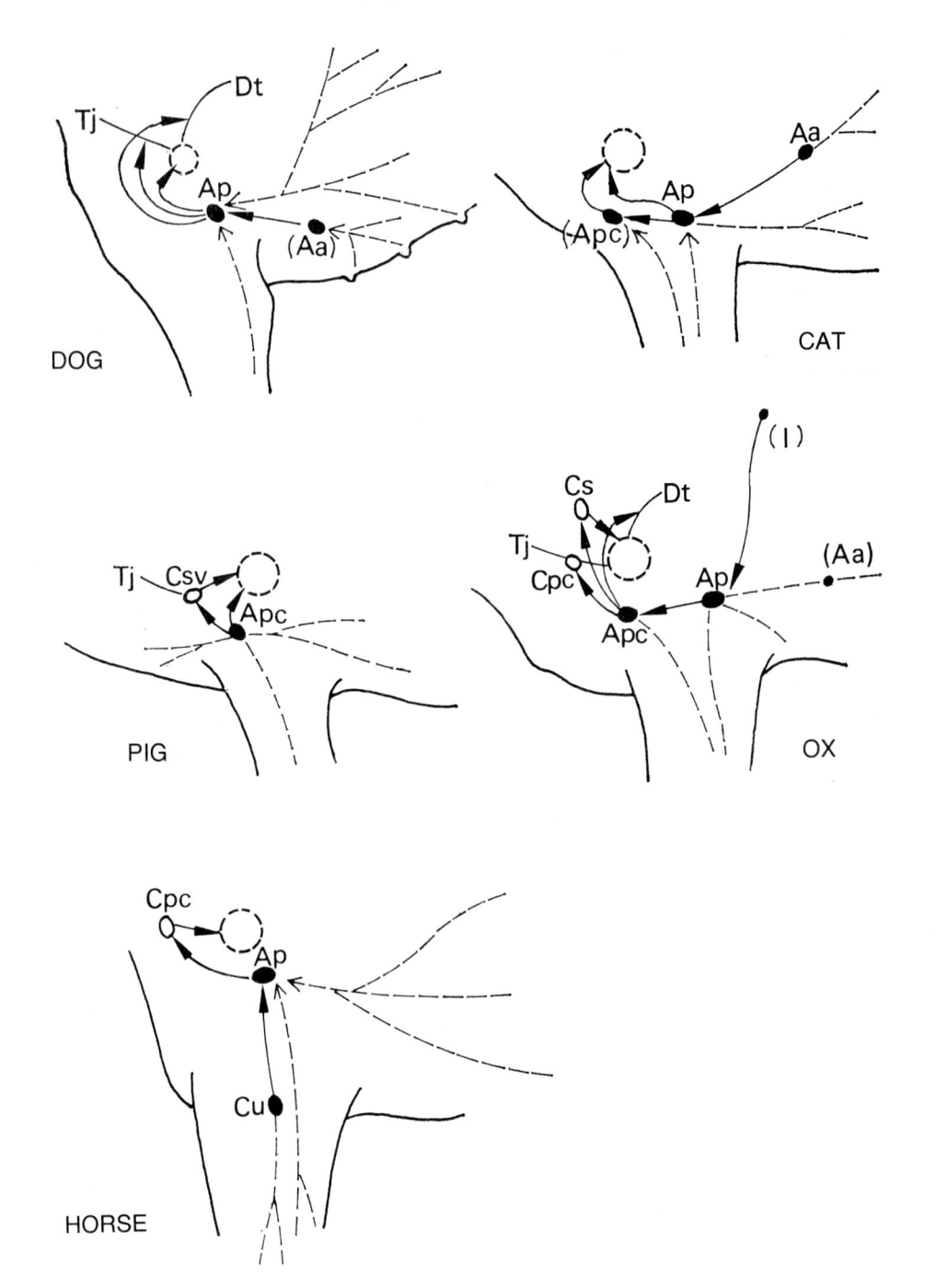

Fig. 249. Diagram of the lymph drainage from the lc. axillare; only the principal routes are shown.
Lymph nodes of the lc. axillare, shown solid: *Ap* nll. axillares proprii (except pig), *Apc* nll. axillares primae costae (cat, pig, ox), *Aa* nl. axillaris accessorius (carnivores, ox), *Cu* nll. cubitales (horse), *I* nl. infraspinatus (ox, inconstant)
Cervical lymph nodes which act as secondary stage nodes: *Cs* nll. cervicales supff. (ox), *Csv* nll. cervicales supff. ventrr. (pig), *Cpc* nll. cervicales proff. caudd. (ox, horse)
Lymph collecting ducts which are involved: *Tj* truncus jugularis, *Dt* ductus thoracicus
Venous angle is shown as an interrupted circle

The **nll. thoracici aortici** (250/7; 251/8) are situated below the pleura immediately next to the thoracic aorta. They are absent in the dog. The **nll. intercostales** (250/8, 8'; 251/9, 9') lie in the intercostal spaces near the rib heads under cover of the pleura and endothoracic fascia. The two groups of lymphocentres converge in the caudal region of the thoracic vertebrae but they can always be differentiated by the position of the sympathetic trunk. In the dog there is generally only one intercostal lymph node on each side in the 5th or 6th intercostal space and in the cat also the intercostal lymph nodes are inconstant. They are absent in the pig. The thoracic aortic nodes are examined in meat inspection in the pig, ruminant and horse, and under special circumstances they, and the intercostal nodes, are removed in ruminants and horses.

Drainage area of the dorsal thoracic lymphocentre consists of the dorsal and lateral chest wall including the shoulder girdle, partly also the abdominal wall immediately next to it, the diaphragm, pleura and mediastinum. In the ox and horse it receives efferent vessels from the spleen or liver.

Efferent lymph vessels of the intercostal lymph nodes go to the thoracic aortic nodes, except for the cranial intercostal nodes which have a variable drainage to the cranial mediastinal nodes or, in the ox, to the left costovertebral or thoracic aortic nodes situated at the aortic arch. The cranial intercostal nodes of the horse form a chain one behind the other. The thoracic aortic nodes of this species pass their efferent vessels directly to the thoracic duct or to the mediastinal lymph nodes.

Lymphocentrum thoracicum dorsale	dog	cat	pig	ox	sheep	goat	horse
nll. thoracici aortici	—	*357*	370	389	410	410	425
nll. intercostales	*344*	*358*	—	389	410	410	425

The numbers refer to the pages where these are described in detail; **bold** type indicates that they are constant, *italics* that they are inconstant in occurrence.

Lymphocentrum thoracicum ventrale
(250/3, 9; 251/3, 16)

Lying against the sternum, these lymph nodes can be divided into a discrete cranial and a diffuse caudal group.

The **nll. sternales craniales** are present in all the domestic mammals. They are situated in the presternum in the adipose tissue of the precardiac mediastinum or in the spaces between the first costal cartilages. Under certain circumstances they may be removed in meat inspection in the pig, ruminant and horse; in breeding sows they are regularly examined.

The **nll. sternales caudales** occur regularly only in ruminants but inconstantly also in the cat and horse. They are irregularly distributed along the internal thoracic artery and vein, above or below the transverse thoracic muscle. In the cat the **nl. epigastricus cranialis** occurs inconstantly in the abdominal wall and the sternal lymph nodes drain into it because its afferent vessels flow to the ventral thoracic lymphocentre.

The *drainage area* of the ventral thoracic lymphocentre comprises the lateral and ventral chest wall including the pectoral girdle, part of the ventral abdominal wall, the diaphragm, pleura and mediastinum. In the horse it also includes the superficial lymphatic vessels of the liver and in carnivores and pigs the mammae. It is for this reason that the gland should be inspected in slaughtered breeding sows.

The *efferent vessels* go to the cranial mediastinal lymph nodes in carnivores and to the terminal part of the thoracic duct or the axillary nodes of the first rib in the pig. In the ox and sheep the caudal sternal lymph nodes drain into the cranial nodes and thence to the thoracic duct or the right jugular trunk, or, as is invariably the case in the horse, to the cranial mediastinal nodes.

Lymphocentrum thoracicum ventrale	dog	cat	pig	ox	sheep	goat	horse
nll. sternales craniales	344	358	372	390	410	410	*426*
nll. sternales caudales	—	*358*	—	390	*410*	—	*426*
nl. epigastricus cranilis	—	*358*	—	—	—	—	—

The numbers refer to the pages where these are described in detail; **bold** type indicates that they are constant, *italics* that they are inconstant in occurrence.

Lymphocentrum mediastinale
(250/4, 4', 4'', 6, 6'; 251/4, 4', 4'', 6, 7, 7')

Three groups of lymph nodes are situated in the mediastinum: the cranial, middle and caudal mediastinal nodes. They are not always clearly separated from one another or from the lymph nodes of other centres.

The **nll. mediastinales craniales** are situated in the cranial mediastinum near the thoracic inlet. It is difficult to separate them from the caudal deep cervical nodes and from the cranial nodes of the ventral and dorsal thoracic and bronchial lymphocentres. All these nodes are partly connected to the cranial mediastinal nodes by their afferent vessels. Furthermore, they also receive efferent vessels from the heart and neighbouring mediastinal organs. They are present in all the domestic mammals. In carnivores they can be demonstrated by x-ray, especially if they are enlarged. In the horse this group of lymph nodes is frequently preceded by the **nl. nuchalis** which lies against the deep cervical artery medial to the longissimus cervicis muscle at the projected level of the first intercostal space.

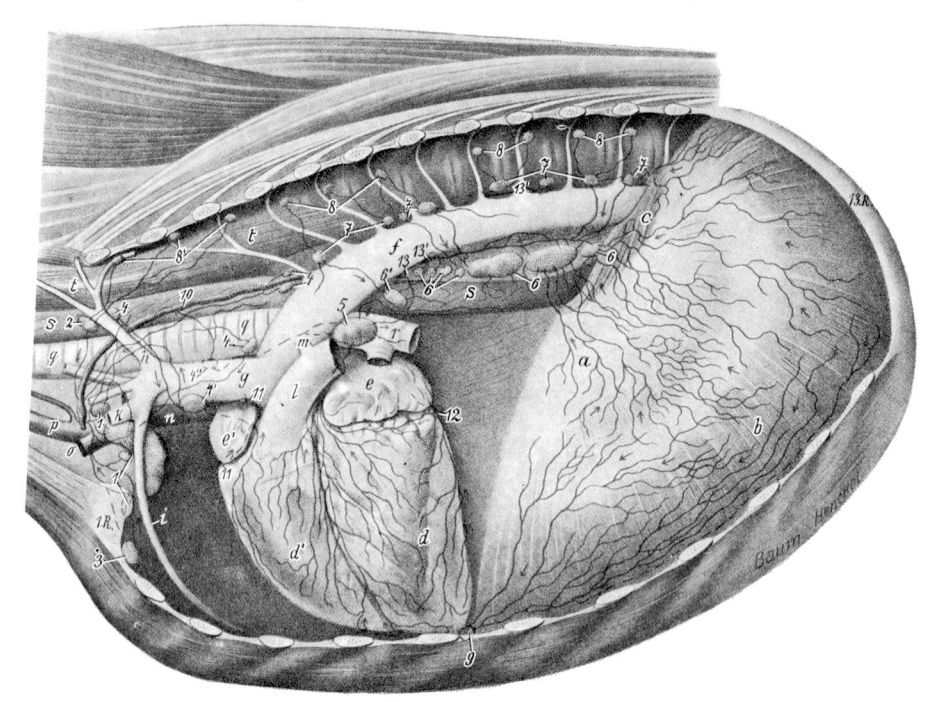

Fig. 250. Lcc. thoracicum dorsale, thoracicum ventrale, mediastinale and bronchale of the ox, viewed from the left side.
(After Baum, 1912.)
The left thoracic wall and left lung have been removed. The arrows indicate the direction of lymph flow.

1, 1' nll. cervicales profundi caudales, *2* nl. costocervicalis, *3* nl. sternalis cranialis, *4, 4', 4''* nll. mediastinales craniales sinistri, *5* nl. bifurcationis sinister, *6, 6, 6'* nll. mediastinales caudales, *7, 7, 7* nll. thoracici aortici, *8, 8, 8'* nll. intercostales, *9* nl. sternalis caudalis, *10* ductus thoracicus, *11, 11* lymph vessel which stems from the right part of the sulcus coronarius and which is labelled *14* in fig. 251, *12* lymph vessel which curves round from the right and is labelled *13* in fig. 252, *13, 13', 13''* lymph vessels which cross over from the left to the right side

a centrum tendineum, *b* pars costalis and *c* pars lumbalis of the diaphragm, *d* left and *d'* right ventricle, *e* left and *e'* right atrium, *f* aorta thoracica, *g* truncus brachiocephalicus, *h* truncus costocervicalis, *i* a. thoracica interna, *k* end of the a. subclavia, *l* truncus pulmonalis, *m* lig. arteriosum, *n* v. cava cranialis, *o* v. axillaris, *p* v. jugularis externa, *q, q* trachea, *r* bronchus principalis sinister (cut off), *s, s* oesophagus, *t, t* m. longus colli, *1.R.* and *13.R.* 1st and 13th ribs respectively

Nll. mediastinales medii are lacking in carnivores and pigs. In ruminants and horses they are situated over the base of the heart to the right of the aortic arch and usually to the right of the trachea and oesophagus.

There is no **nl. mediastinalis caudalis** in carnivores but in all the other domestic mammals it lies in the caudal mediastinum, immediately next to the oesophagus. It comprises an inconstantly-occurring group in the horse but in ruminants this caudal mediastinal node is very large. If it is pathologically enlarged it can cause stenosis of the oesophagus and this can be recognised by the sudden resistance encountered on passing the probang. All the mediastinal nodes are regularly examined in meat inspection. In the ox and cat **nl. phrenicus** (251/10) is sometimes present and is situated on the tendinous centre of the diaphragm.

The *drainage area* of the mediastinal lymphocentre includes the bones of the chest and partly those of the neck and shoulder, of the inner thoracic musculature, the diaphragm and some deep muscles of the neck, the pleura, pericardium, heart, the thoracic parts of the thymus and oesophagus, the trachea and, directly or indirectly via the bronchial lymphocentre, the lungs. In the ox and horse even the spleen and liver drain into the mediastinal lymphocentre because lymphatic vessels from these organs pass through the diaphragm and link up with the caudal mediastinal lymph nodes.

The *efferent vessels* terminate in the large lymph collecting ducts in dogs. In pigs the vasa efferentia of the caudal mediastinal nodes go to the bronchial lymphocentre, thence to the cranial mediastinal nodes and, after receiving tributaries from the neighbouring lymphocentres, they go to either the thoracic duct or the right lymphatic duct. In the ox and horse the lymph flows directly into the thoracic duct.

Lymphocentrum mediastinale	dog	cat	pig	ox	sheep	goat	horse
nll. mediastinales craniales	**344**	**359**	**372**	**390**	**410**	**410**	**427**
nl. nuchalis	—	—	—	—	—	—	*428*
nll. mediastinales medii	—	—	—	**391**	**411**	**411**	**428**
nll. mediastinales caudales	—	—	**372**	**391**	**411**	**411**	**428**
nll. phrenici	—	*359*	—	*391*	—	—	—

The numbers refer to the pages where these are described in detail; **bold** type indicates that they are constant, *italics* that they are inconstant in occurrence.

Lymphocentrum bronchale

(250/5; 251/5, 20)

At the hilus of the lung there are three groups of lymph nodes, the **nll. bifurcationis seu tracheobronchales dextri, sinistri et medii**. The right and middle tracheobronchial nodes are always absent in the sheep but they are inconstantly present in the ox and goat. In ruminants and pigs there are the additional **nll. tracheobronchales craniales** (251/5) which lie against the bronchus trachealis of artiodactylic animals. Finally there are, in carnivores, ox, goat and horse, small and inconstant **nll. pulmonales** lying against the principal and lobar bronchi within the lung, and these are a preceding stage to the nll. bifurcationis. The tracheobronchial lymph nodes are always examined in meat inspection.

The *drainage area* of the bronchial lymphocentre includes the lung, the terminal part of the trachea, the heart and pericardium and the cranial part of the thoracic oesophagus and the neighbouring mediastinum. Efferent vessels from the caudal and middle mediastinal nodes can join the bronchial lymphocentre.

Efferent vessels of the bronchial lymphocentre are linked to the cranial or middle mediastinal nodes and sometimes run directly to the thoracic duct.

Lymphocentre bronchale	dog	cat	pig	ox	sheep	goat	horse
nll. bifurcationis seu tracheobronchales sinistri	**345**	**359**	**372**	**391**	**411**	**411**	**428**
nll. bifircationis seu tracheobronchales dextri	**345**	**359**	**372**	*391*	—	*412*	**428**
nll. bifurcationis seu tracheobronchales medii	**345**	**359**	**372**	*392*	—	—	—
nll. tracheobronchales craniales	—	—	**373**	**392**	**412**	*412*	—
nll. pulmonales	**346**	*359*	—	**392**	—	*412*	**428**

The numbers refer to the pages where these are described in detail; **bold** type indicates that they are constant; *italics* that they are inconstant in occurrence.

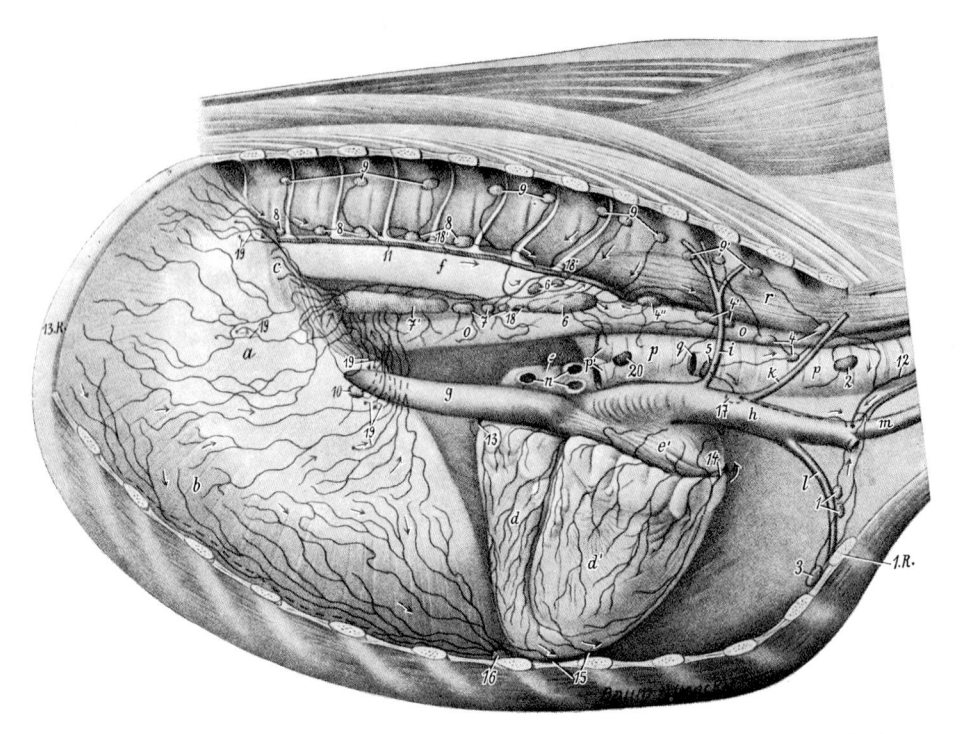

Fig. 251. Lcc. thoracicum dorsale, thoracicum ventrale, mediastinale and bronchale of the ox, viewed from the right side.
(After Baum, 1912.)

The right thoracic wall and the right lung have been removed, the former up to the 13th rib. The arrows indicate the direction of lymph flow

1 nll. cervicales profundi caudales, *2* nl. costocervicalis, *3* nl. sternalis cranialis, *4*, *4'*, *4"*, nll. mediastinales craniales, *5* nl. tracheobronchialis cranialis, *6* nll. mediastinales medii, *7*, *7'*, nll. mediastinales caudales, *8*, *8* nll. thoracici aortici, *9*, *9'* nll. intercostales, *10* nl. phrenicus, *11* ductus thoracicus, *12* truncus jugularis and ductus lymphaticus dexter, *13* lymph vessel which curves to the left and into the sulcus coronarius, *14* lymph vessel which curves to the left and reappears again designated *11* in fig. 250, *15* lymph vessels which curve towards the sulcus interventricularis paraconalis, *16* nl. sternalis, *17* nl. mediastinalis cranialis which lies deep, between the trachea, cranial vena cava and brachiocephalic trunk, *18*, *18'* lymph vessels which curve round from the left, *19* lymph vessels of the liver which perforate the diaphragm, *20* nl. bifurcationis seu tracheobronchialis dexter

a centrum tendineum, *b* pars costalis and *c* pars lumbalis of the diaphragm, *d* left and *d'* right ventricle, *e* left and *e'* right atrium, *f* aorta thoracica, *g* v. cava caudalis, *i* v. azygos dextra, *k* v. costocervicalis, *l* v. thoracica interna, *m* v. jugularis externa, *n* transected pulmonary veins, *o*, *o* oesophagus, *p*, *p* trachea, *p'* both bronchi principales (cut off), *q* bronchus trachealis (cut off) *r* m. longus colli, *1.R.*, *13.R.* 1st and 13th ribs respectively

Ductus thoracicus
(250/*10*; 251/*11*; 252)

The thoracic duct conveys lymph from the cisterna chyli to the venous angle. It also receives efferent vessels from neighbouring lymphocentres. It will be described under the following sections: 1. Origin from the cisterna chyli, 2. its diaphragmatic transit, 3. the right segment lying in the postcardiac region of the thorax, 4. the left segment of the precardiac region of the thorax, 5. its termination in the venous angle and 6. its valve system.

1. The thoracic duct always arises from the cisterna chyli as a single trunk in ruminants and pigs but in the dog and horse it is double and in the dog there are sometimes even three trunks of origin.
2. In horses, carnivores and pigs it always passes through the aortic hiatus of the diaphragm in company with the aorta. In ruminants it passes into the thoracic cavity through a gap in the musculature of the lumbar portion of the diaphragm.
3. The right or post-cardiac segment of the thoracic duct is generally situated to the right and dorsal to the thoracic aorta and ventral to the right azygos vein. Even when there is only a single trunk of origin, the thoracic duct may subsequently divide and the second vessel then passes dorsal and to the left of the aorta. Olique and cross linking anastomoses between these two vessels can produce a "rope ladder" pattern. Most of these variations are to be found in the dog.
4. Transition of the thoracic duct from right to left into the left or precardiac segment usually occurs in the horse at the level of the 6th thoracic vertebra and in the other domestic mammals at the 5th thoracic vertebra. During its subsequent course the duct dips, at first gradually and then increasingly

steeply, ventrad. In so doing it crosses in a medial direction the large blood vessels at the thoracic inlet and this is invariably the case in the ox. Collateral ducts develop in the precardiac segment, especially in the dog.

5. The thoracic duct ends in the venous angle. Its termination is usually at the distal end of the cranial vena cava near the point of origin of the left (common, external, internal) jugular vein or of the left subclavian vein or immediately caudal thereto. Occasionally one may find two, rarely several, terminal branches which then show considerable variation in the way they link to the veins. However, the termination of the thoracic duct is always at the level of the 1st rib or immediately (up to 2 cm) cranial to it. Generally in the dog and horse, and often in the ox, the terminal part dilates into an ampulla. At its termination the orifice of the thoracic duct is closed by a pair of valves, by a single valve or simply by a reduction in the size of its lumen. Despite the presence of a pair of valves the closure is incomplete in the horse, so that *post mortem* there is always a retrograde flow of venous blood into the precardiac part of the duct. Numerous papers have dealt with the important variations of the terminal region and surgical techniques for introducing catheters to collect lymph from the thoracic duct of experimental animals.

6. In the thoracic duct of all the domestic mammals there are about 10–15 lymph valves. The distance between them is less at the terminal end than at the origin although generally, except in the horse, the portion nearest the cisterna chyli is free from valves.

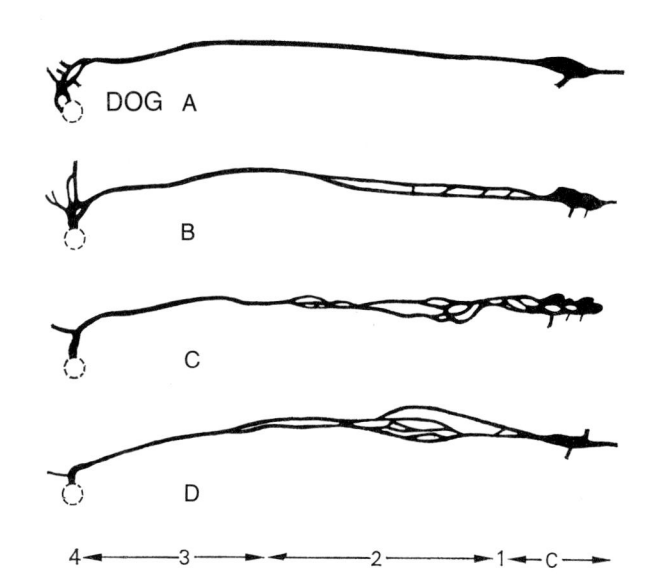

Fig. 252. Diagrammatic representation of the ductus thoracicus of the dog. Some variations are illustrated. (According to a study by Huber, 1909.)

1–4 ductus thoracicus, *1* its origin from *C* the cisterna chyli, *2* its postcardiac or right part, *3* its precardiac or left part and *4* its termination in the venous angle

Lymph vessel system of the dorsal abdominal wall and the abdominal viscera

Four lymphocentres drain the dorsal abdominal wall, the organs arising in the lumbar regions and the abdominal viscera. The lumbar lymphocentre is responsible for the lumbar region. The coeliac, cranial mesenteric and caudal mesenteric lymphocentres serve those regions which are supplied by the homonymous arteries and their branches.

Lymphocentrum lumbale
(253/*a*; 258/2, 2', 2")

The lumbar aortic lymph nodes occur in a long chain in the lumbar region of the domestic mammals and they are responsible for the deep layers of the dorsal abdominal wall. One or more of them have the additional duty of filtering lymph from the kidney and these are known as the renal lymph nodes. There are special lymph nodes in the ox, horse and pig which are classed with the lumbar lymphocentre. This centre deals with lymph drainage not only from the dorsal abdominal wall but also from the lumbar part of the diaphragm and all the organs which have arisen in the lumbar region. The nodes are also partly responsible for drainage of the lateral abdominal wall (dog, pig and ox) and areas of the pleura (dog and horse).

The **nll. lumbales aortici** lie, in a chain-like manner, below the lumbar vertebral column along the abdominal aorta or the abdominal part of the caudal vena cava. In meat inspection they are of significance in special circumstances in pigs, ruminants and horses. They are removed in diseases of the peritoneum.

Isolated small **nll. lumbales proprii** precede the lumbar aortic nodes of the ox. They are situated between the last rib and the transverse process of the first lumbar vertebra or occasionally between the transverse processes of the 1st and 2nd, the 4th and 5th and the 5th and 6th lumbar vertebrae. Their relationship to the lumbar aortic nodes is comparable to that between the intercostal and thoracic aortic nodes.

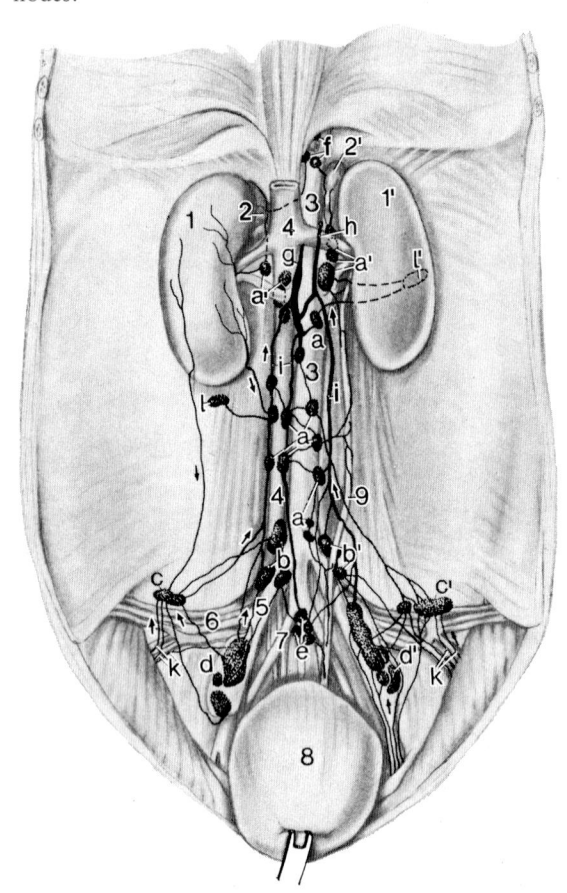

Fig. 253. Lymphocentrum lumbale, iliosacrale and inguinale profundum of the pig.
(Redrawn after Baum und Grau, 1938.)

a, a, a nll. lumbales aortici, a', a' nll. renales, b, b' nll. iliaci mediales, c, c' nll. iliaci laterales, d, d' nll. iliofemorales, e nll. sacrales, f nll. coeliaci, g first part of the cisterna chyli (pulled a little forward), h truncus visceralis, i trunci lumbales, k vasa efferentia of the nll. subiliaci, l right, l' left nl. phrenicoabdominalis (l' is shown in interrupted lines because it is overlaid by the kidney.)

1 right and 1' left kidney, 2, 2' adrenals, 3, 3 aorta abdominalis, 4, 4 v. cava caudalis, 5 a. and v. iliaca externa, 6 a. and v. circumflexa ilium profunda, 7 a. and v. iliaca interna, 8 urinary bladder (reflected), 9 left ureter.

The first part of the a. renalis can lie either on the v. cava caudalis (as shown) or below it

One or two lymph nodes of the lumbar aortic chain must be discussed in more detail. These include the **nll. renales** (253/a'; 258/3, $3'$) which lie near the renal hilus and receive lymph from the kidney. They are regularly examined at meat inspection in the pig, ruminants and horse. It is noteworthy, however, that some lymph vessels from the kidney can go to other neighbouring lymph nodes, as occurs in the dog where the renal lymph nodes are absent. In the latter species the lymph from the kidneys goes to all the lumbar aortic nodes but especially to those situated more cranially. Since the latter also receive efferent vessels from the lumbar region, they cannot be termed renal lymph nodes.

It is not uncommon for lymph nodes of the lumbar centre of the pig and horse to migrate into the suspensory ligament of the gonads. They are then termed **nll. ovarici** (horse) when they lie in the ovarian suspensory ligament or **nl. testicularis** (pig) when they are in the membrane of the internal spermatic artery and vein. Finally, in the majority of pigs there is a **nl. phrenicoabdominalis** below the mesentery, at the lateral border of the iliopsoas muscle and caudal to the cranial abdominal artery and vein (253/1, $1'$).

The *drainage area* of the lumbar lymphocentre includes the last thoracic and the lumbar vertebrae, the pelvic bones, the lumbar musculature including the long extensors of the back, the lumbodorsal fascia, the transverse fascia and the peritoneum of the lumbar region. In the dog and horse this lymphocentre also drains the costal pleura, the kidneys, ureter, urinary bladder, the urethra in females, the adrenals and large blood vessels of the lumbar region, the testis, epididymis, spermatic cord, ovary and oviduct. The lymph nodes of the lumbar lymphocentre also receive efferent vessels from the iliosacral lymphocentre.

From the lumbar lymphocentre the lymph drains via the lumbar trunks, which also transport lymph from the pelvis and the pelvic limb, to the cisterna chyli. In the dog efferent vessels from some lumbar lymph nodes can link directly with the cisterna chyli.

Lymphocentrum lumbale	dog	cat	pig	ox	sheep	goat	horse
nll. lumbales aortici	346	360	373	393	412	412	429
nll. lumbales proprii	—	—	*393*	—	—	—	—
nll. renales	—	—	373	393	412	412	429
nl. ovaricus	—	—	—	—	—	—	429
nl. testicularis	—	—	*373*	—	—	—	—
nl. phrenicoabdominalis	—	—	*373*	—	—	—	—

The numbers relate to the pages where these are described in detail; **bold** type indicates that they are constant, *italics* that they are inconstant in occurrence.

Lymphocentrum coeliacum
(254, 255, 256)

Those organs which are situated in the intrathoracic part of the abdominal cavity send tributaries to the coeliac lymphocentre. The lymphatic routes and the chain of lymph nodes generally follow the course of the branches of the coeliac artery. Thus the nomenclature of the lymph nodes corresponds to that of the associated arterial tree. One can differentiate: the **nll. coeliaci** which are situated (except in carnivores) at the origin of the coeliac artery. In ruminants the coeliac lymph nodes are united with the cranial mesenteric nodes to comprise one group. Along the branches of the left gastric artery and especially along the lesser curvature of the stomach, we find, except in ruminants, the **nll. gastrici**. Along the hepatic artery, near the porta of the liver, the **nll. hepatici seu portales** are situated. In the ox we also recognise the **nll. hepatici accessorii** lying near the impression of the vena cava. The **nll. pancreaticoduodenales** can be found alongside the pancreaticoduodenal artery. The splenic artery is associated with the **nll. lienales**. In ruminants the superordinate position of this lymph node in the filtration of the lymph from the stomach is indicated by the name **nll. lienales seu atriales**. Finally mention should be made of the **nll. omentales**, situated in the greater omentum of the horse. There is further differentiation of the gastric lymph nodes in ruminants because of the special development of their stomach. We differentiate **nll. ruminales dextrei, ruminales sinistri** (ox), **ruminales craniales, reticulares, omasiales, ruminoabomasiales** (ox, sheep), **reticuloabomasiales, abomasiales dorsales** and **abomasiales ventrales**. The disposition of these nodes in relation to the stomach is shown diagramatically in figure 254. A more detailed description follows on pages 394 to 396 and 413 to 414.

Of all these preceding lymph nodes only a few are important in meat inspection. The hepatic nodes are regularly examined in the pig, ruminants and horse, the gastric nodes in the pig and horse and in ruminants the splenic nodes. The latter were at one time known only as the nll. atriales, the lymph nodes of the atrium of the rumen.

The *drainage area* of the individual lymph nodes generally corresponds to the organs after which they are named – the stomach, liver, spleen, pancreas and duodenum. However, the coeliac lymphocentre also receives lymph from the diaphragm and, in the dog, pig and horse, from the thoracic cavity.

The *outflow* is achieved in the dog by many efferent vessels which collect into a lymph vessel network which ultimately gives rise to the truncus visceralis. Lymph from the intrathoracic abdominal organs of the pig and horse is collected by the truncus coeliacus which terminates in the pig in the visceral trunk and in the horse directly in the lumbar cistern. There is no coeliac trunk in the ox where the truncus gastricus, the truncus hepaticus and the truncus intestinalis all join to form the truncus visceralis.

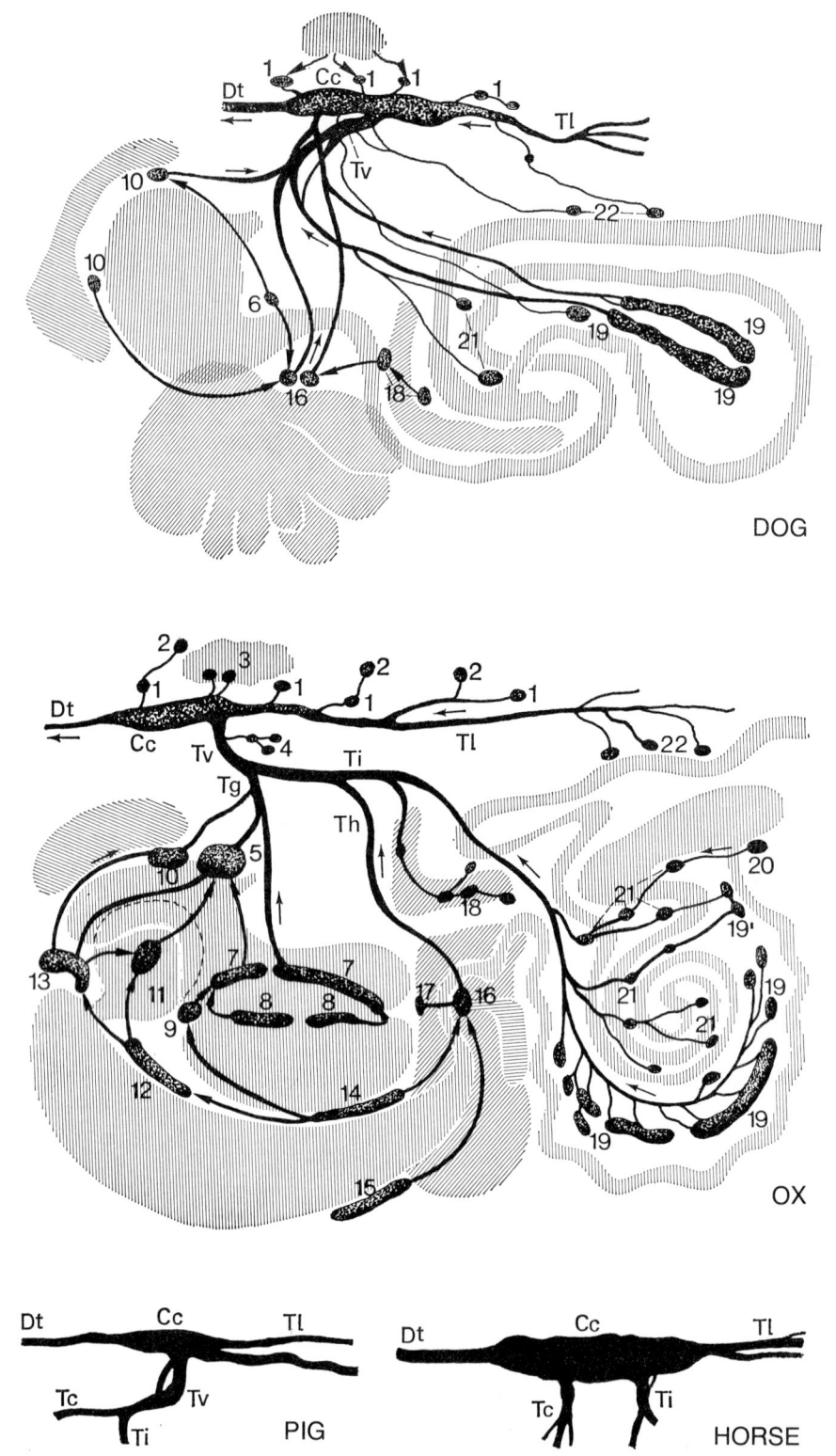

Fig. 254. Lymph drainage from the abdominal viscera in the dog and ox. The specific arrangement of the cisterna chyli of the pig and horse is shown diagrammatically.

1 nll. lumbales aortici, *2* nll. lumbales proprii (ox), *3* nll. renales (ox), *4* nll. coeliaci et mesenterici craniales (ox), *5* nll.lienales (dog), or lienales seu atriales (ox), *6* nll. gastrici (dog), *7* nll. ruminales dextri (ox), *8* nll. ruminales sinistri (ox), *9* nll. ruminales craniales (ox), *10* nll. reticulares (ox), *11* nll. omasiales (ox), *12* nll. ruminoabomasiales (ox), *13* nll. reticuloabomasiales (ox), *14* nll. abomasiales dorsales (ox), *15* nll. abomasiales ventrales (ox), *16* nll. hepatici, *17* nll. hepatici accessorii (ox) *18* nll. pancreaticoduodenales, *19* nll. jejunales, *19'* similar nodes in the mesoileum (ox), *20* nl. caecalis (ox), *21* nll. colici, *22* nll. mesenterici caudales

Dt ductus thoracicus, *Cc* cisterna chyli, *Tl* truncus lumbalis, *Tv* truncus visceralis (excluding horse), *Tc* truncus coeliacus (pig and horse), *Tg* truncus gastricus (ox), *Th* truncus hepaticus (ox), *Ti* truncus intestinales

Lymphocentrum coeliacum		dog	cat	pig	ox	sheep	goat	horse
nll. coeliaci et mesenterici craniales	(ruminants)	—	—	—	393	412	412	—
nll. coeliaci	(excl. ruminants)	—	—	374	—	—	—	430
nll. lienales	(excl. ruminants)	346	360	374				430
nll. lienales seu atriales	(ruminants)	—	—	—	393	413	413	—
nll. gastrici	(excl. ruminants)	347	360	374	—	—	—	430
nll. ruminales dextri	(ruminants)				394	413	413	
nll. ruminales sinistri	(ruminants)				394	414	414	
nll. ruminales craniales	(ruminants)				395	414	414	
nll. reticulares	(ruminants)				395	414	414	
nll. omasiales	(ruminants)				395	414	414	
nll. ruminoabomasiales	(ruminants)				395	414	—	
nll. reticuloabomasiales	(runimants)				395	414	414	
nll. abomasiales dorsales	(ruminants)				395	414	414	
nll. abomasiales ventrales	(ruminants)				396	414	414	
nll. hepatici seu portales		347	360	375	396	414	414	431
nll. hepatici accessorii		—	—	—	396	—	—	—
nll. pancreaticoduodenales		347	360	375	397	414	414	431
nll. omentales		—	—	—	—	—	—	431

The numbers relate to the pages where these nodes are described in detail; **bold** type indicates that they are constant, *italics* that they are inconstant in occurrence.

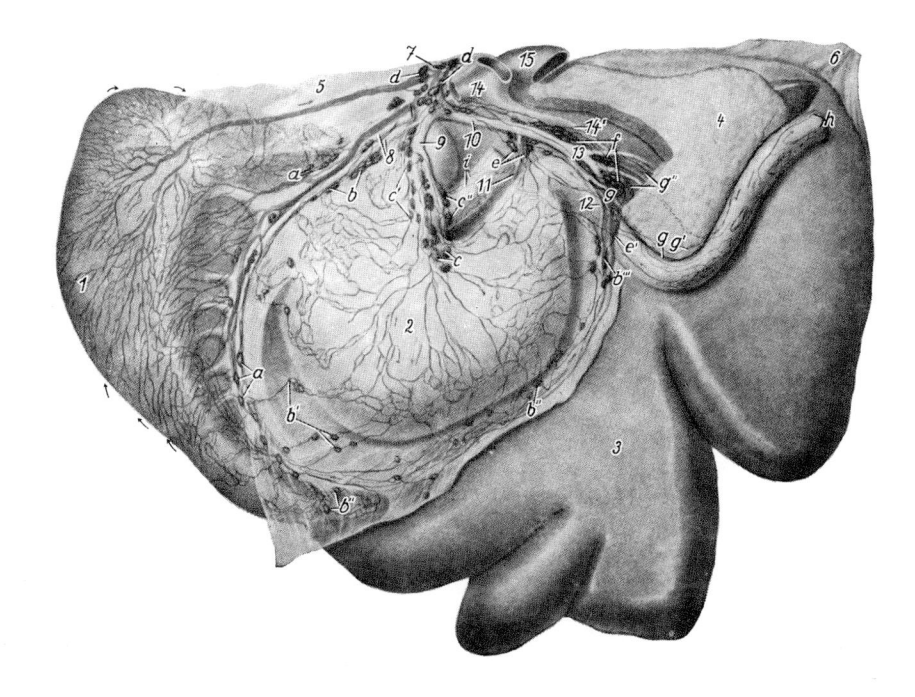

Fig. 255. Lc. coeliacum of the horse.
(After Baum, 1928.)

a, a nll. lienales, *b, b′, b″, b‴* nll. omentales, *c, c′, c″* nll. gastrici, *d, d* nll. coeliaci, *e, e′* nll. pancreaticoduodenales, *f* nll. hepatici, *g, g′, g″, g‴* lymph vessels of the pancreas, *h* lymph vessels of the duodenum which go to the caecal nodes, *i* lymph vessels of the oesophagus

1 spleen, *2* stomach, *3* liver, *4* pancreas (partly excised), *5* lig. phrenicolienale, *6* lig. triangulare dextrum, *7* a. coeliaca, *8* a. and v. lienalis, *9* a. gastrica sinistra, *10* a. hepatica, *11* a. gastrica dextra, *12* a. gastroepiploica dextra, *13* a. hepatica and its terminal branches, *14, 14′* v. portae (cut off), *15* v. cava caudalis (cut off)

Lymphocentrum mesentericum craniale
(254, 256, 257)

The *drainage area* of the cranial mesenteric lymphocentre includes the entire gut except for the proximal part of the duodenum, the descending colon and the rectum. There are differences in arrangement of the lymph nodes according to the differences in the course of the gut in the different species. We differentiate the following groups:

The **nll. mesenterici craniales** are situated at the origin of the cranial mesenteric artery. These nodes are absent in carnivores and in ruminants they are combined with the coeliac lymph nodes.

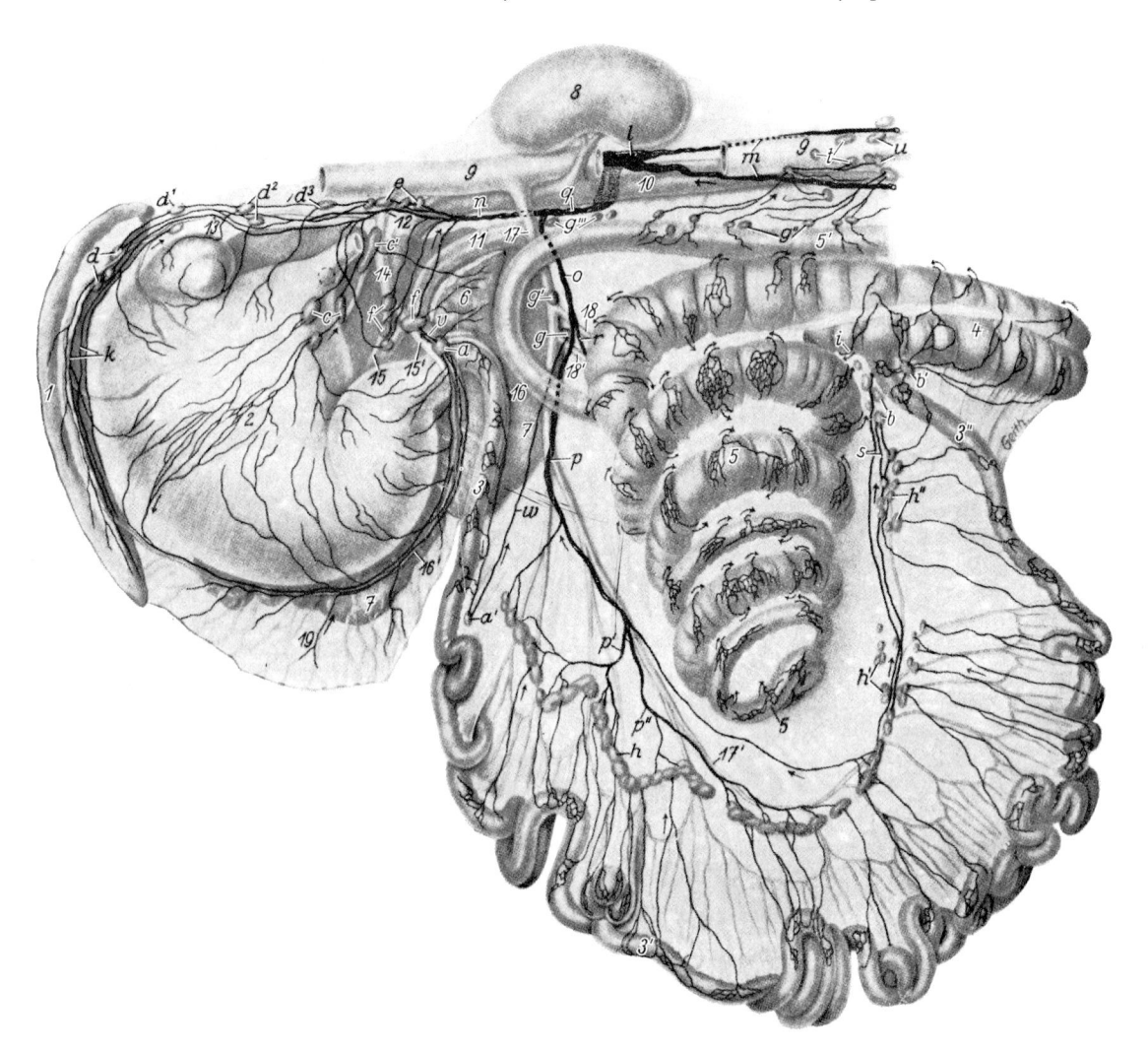

Fig. 256. Lcc. coeliacum, mesentericum craniale and mesentericum caudale of the pig, semidiagrammatic.
(After Baum and Grau, 1938.)

(The spleen has been displaced a considerable distance to the left in order to show the lymph nodes and vessels related to it. The pancreas (6) has been largely removed. The jejunal loops are placed around the cone of colon spirals which themselves are shown in reduced size)

a, a' nll. pancreaticoduodenales, b, b' nll. ileocolici, c, c' nll. gastrici, d, d^1, d^2, d^3 nll. lienales, e nll. coeliaci, f, f nll. hepatici, g, g' nll. colici, g'' nll. mesenterici caudales, g''' nll. mesenterici craniales, h, h', h'' nll. jejunales, i lymph vessel at the junction between the caecum and colon which enters the colic nodes, k lymph vessels of the spleen which have joined a gastric lymph vessel, l cisterna chyli, m trunci lumbales, n truncus coeliacus, o truncus intestinalis, p truncus jejunalis, p', p'' its first branches, q truncus visceralis, r truncus colicus, s vasa efferentia of the nll. jejunales, which go to the ileocolic nodes, t nll. lumbales aortici, u nll. iliaci mediales, v vas efferens of the nl. pancreaticoduodenalis (proximalis), w vas efferens of the nl. pancreaticoduodenalis (distalis)

1 spleen, *2* stomach, *3* duodenum, *3'* jejunum, *3"* ileum, *4* caecum, *5, 5* colon ascendens, *5'* colon descendens, *6* pancreas, *7, 7* liver, *8* left kidney (reflected), *9, 9* aorta (with a portion excised), *10* v. cava caudalis, *11* portal vein, *12* a. coeliaca, *13* a. lienalis, *14, 15* a. hepatica, *15'* a. gastroduodenalis, *16* a. pancreaticoduodenalis cranialis, *16'* a. gastroepiploica dextra, *17* a. mesenterica cranialis, *17'* a. jejunalis, *18, 18'* aa. colicae, *19* greater omentum

The **nll. jejunales** are situated in the mesentery of the jejunum. In carnivores their distribution in the middle of the mesentery is somewhat gland-like and for this reason Asellius thought that they represented a special kind of pancreas (*pancreas Aselli*) in the dog. In the pig and ruminant they form a chain of lymph nodes along the jejunal vessels. In the pig they lie on both sides of the mesojejunum, in the ox between the jejunal and colonic spiral and in the small ruminants between the last centrifugal and the first centripetal coil of the ascending colon. In the horse they are numerous (35–90); they lie at the origin of the jejunal arteries or in the middle of the mesojejunum. The jejunal lymph nodes of all the domestic mammals are of great importance in the progress of alimentary infections and they are therefore always examined at meat inspection (in pigs on both sides of the mesentery).

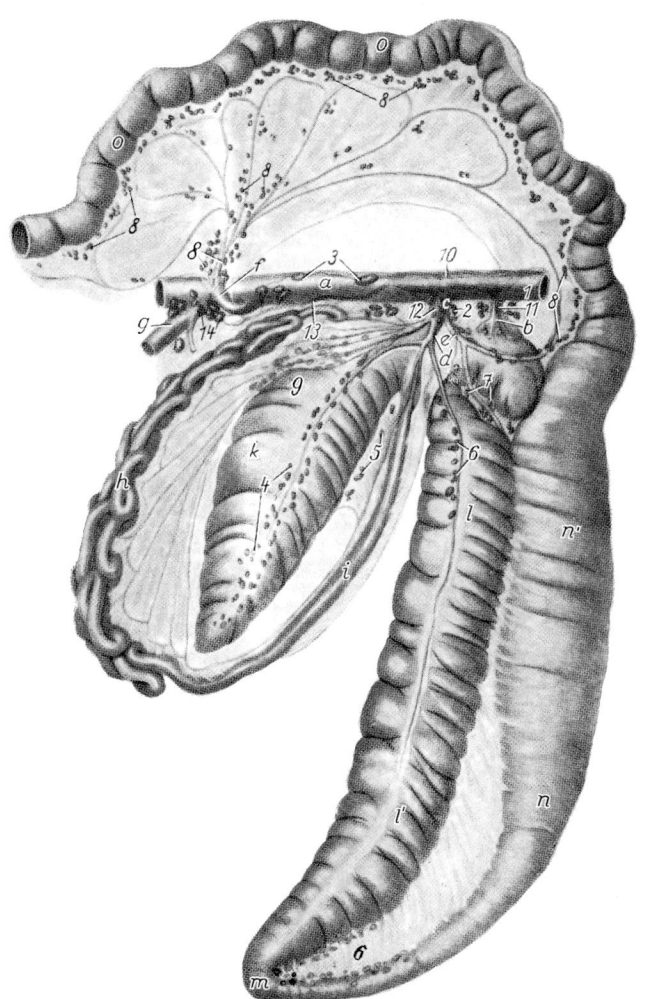

Fig. 257. Lymphocentrum mesentericum craniale and lymphocentrum mesentericum caudale and cisterna chyli of the horse, diagrammatic.
(Expanded from Baum, 1928.)

1 nll. coeliaci, *2* nll. mesenterici craniales, *3* nll. lumbales aortici, *4*, *5* nll. caecales, *6*, *7* nll. colici, *8* nll. mesenterici caudales, *9* nll. jejunales, *10* cisterna chyli, *11* truncus coeliacus, *12* truncus intestinalis, *14* nll. iliaci mediales

a aorta, *b* a. coeliaca, *c* a. mesenterica cranialis, *d* a. ileocolica, *e* common stem of the middle and right colic artery, *f* a. mesenterica caudalis, *g* a. iliaca externa, *h* jejunum, *i* ileum, *k* caecum, *l* right and *l'* left ventral colon, *m* pelvic flexure, *n* left and *n'* right dorsal colon, *o* descending colon

The **nll. colici** occur in all the domestic mammals but in the herbivores with their voluminous large intestine, they are divided into subgroups. In the horse they number between 2,000 and 4,000. They lie next to vessels in the mesentery of the ascending and transverse colon and in the dog of some vessels of the descending colon. Examination during meat inspection is confined to a few of the more prominent nodes.

The arrangement of the lymph nodes at the transition of the small to the large intestine varies according to the species. In the dog there are no special nodes at that location. In the pig and goat this group lies at the level of the ileal orifice, receiving lymph vessels from the ileum, caecum and colon and being known as the **nll. ileocolici**.

In the ox, sheep and cat the **nl. caecalis** lies in the ileocaecal fold. In the horse there are numerous

(500–700) lymph nodes along the medial, lateral and dorsal bands of the caecum and they filter lymph derived mainly from the caecum but to some extent from the ileum and duodenum. They are sometimes referred to as the **nll. caecales**. In meat inspection of pigs and goats the iliocaecal nodes are regularly inspected and in the ox, sheep and horse the caecal nodes are examined.

In carnivores the *outflow* of lymph from the intestine into the lumbar cistern is by way of the visceral trunk. In the other species the jejunal and colic trunks carry lymph from the homonymous nodes and then join to form the intestinal trunk. In the horse this goes directly to the lumbar cistern but in pigs and ruminants it first links with the efferent vessels from the coeliac lymphocentre to form the visceral trunk and then empties into the cistern.

Lymphocentrum mesentericum craniale	dog	cat	pig	ox	sheep	goat	horse
nll. mesenterici craniales	—	—	*357*	—	—	—	432
nll. jejunales	348	361	376	397	415	415	432
nll. caecales	—	362	—	398	415	—	433
nll. ileocolici	—	—	376	—	—	415	—
nll. colici	349	362	376	398	415	415	433

The numbers relate to the pages where these nodes are described in detail; **bold** type indicates that they are constant, *italics* that they are inconstant in occurrence.

Lymphocentrum mesentericum caudale
(254; 257/8, 9)

Those parts of the gut which are supplied by the caudal mesenteric artery, namely the descending colon and first part of the rectum, send their lymph to the **nll. mesenterici caudales.** In the horse these nodes are very numerous and they lie at the intestinal reflection of the mesentery and also half way up the mesentery and near its origin. In pigs and ruminants they are few in numbers and in the small ruminants they occur inconstantly. They are regularly examined at slaughter in all meat animals.

The caudal mesenteric lymph nodes of the dog discharge their lymph partly into the visceral trunk and partly, as in the other domestic mammals, to the middle iliac nodes of the lumbar trunk. In the horse the former nodes are sometimes preceded by the **nl. vesicalis** which lies in the lateral ligament of the urinary bladder.

Lymphocentrum mesentericum caudale	dog	cat	pig	ox	sheep	goat	horse
nll. mesenterici caudales	358	362	377	398	*415*	*415*	433
nl. vesicalis	—	—	—	—	—	—	*434*

The numbers relate to the pages where these nodes are described in detail; **bold** type indicates that they are constant, *italics* that they are inconstant in occurrence.

Cisterna chyli
(254; 257/10; 258/15)

Generally the cisterna chyli of domestic mammals lies on the right of and dorsal to the aorta, between the origin of the two crura of the diaphragm. It extends from the 2nd lumbar to the last thoracic vertebra. In the dog there is occasionally also a dilatation which extends to the left and partly on to the ventral aspect of the aorta. The shape of the cisterna is subject to considerable individual variation. The following main types are differentiated in the different species: in the pig and horse it is elongated oval or spindle shaped, in the dog it has a relatively larger lumen and has been described as sack-shaped. It is very pleiomorphic in ruminants; in some cases it is present in the form of elongated loops arising from the lumbar trunks and collecting into the thoracic duct whereas in others one or two barely-thickened, elongated lymph trunks occur which correspond to the cisterna chyli of other animals.

It can be taken as a general rule, however, that the cisterna chyli receives the lumbar trunks at its posterior end and gives off the thoracic trunk at its cranial end. Other lymph collecting ducts like the truncus visceralis (carnivores, pigs and ruminants) or truncus intestinalis and truncus coeliacus (horse), drain the abdominal viscera and enter the cisterna from ventral and the right. Since the cisterna chyli lies against the dorsal wall of the aorta, it is often perforated by dorsal branches of this vessel (dorsal and lumbar intercostal arteries). Furthermore, in its position between the crura of the diaphragm, the rhythmic contraction of the diaphragm is said to aid the lymph flow. With the exception of the horse, there are no valves in the cisterna so that the valves in the afferent and efferent lymph trunks must control the direction of flow of the lymph.

Lymph vessel system of the lateral and ventral abdominal wall, the pelvis, the pelvic viscera and the pelvic limb (258, 259, 260)

There are five lymphocentres in the region of the pelvic inlet, the pelvic cavity and the hind limb.

The iliosacral lymphocentre includes all the nodes at the aortic bifurcation and below the pelvic surface of the sacrum. It is responsible for drainage of the pelvic region and is a secondary stage for all subsequent lymphocentres.

The deep inguinal or iliofemoral lymphocentre includes lymph nodes which are situated on the external iliac artery or its continuation, the femoral artery, in front of the body of the ilium or on the medial aspect of the thigh. Its drainage area includes the superficial and deep regions of the thigh and it also receives efferents from the popliteal lymphocentre.

The superficial inguinal or inguinofemoral lymphocentre includes lymph nodes of the groin and stifle fold. Its afferent lymphatics derive from the ventral abdominal and pelvic walls, the mammary gland and the external genitalia, including the scrotum, the dorsal and lateral abdominal wall and the superficial layer of the thigh region.

The ischiatic lymphocentre consists of lymph nodes which lie on the broad pelvic ligament in the gluteal region and at the pelvic outlet. They are responsible for draining the pelvic wall.

The popliteal lymphocentre is situated in the hollow of the knee and drains the distal parts of the hind limb.

Lymphocentrum iliosacrale
(258; 260/1, 1^i, 1^{ii}, 1^{iii}, 1^{iv}, 1^v)

The **nll. iliaci mediales** are located at the bifurcation of the aorta. They are present in all the domestic mammals and, depending on the species, they are the largest and most numerous lymph nodes of the pelvis. Their extensive *drainage area* includes the wall and organs of the pelvis as well as the proximal parts of the hind limb. Besides this, they receive secondary lymph from the other lymph nodes of this lymphocentre and the four lymphocentres to be described directly. These lymph nodes therefore occupy a superordinate position. On rectal examination (horse and ox) they can be identified only if they are enlarged. In meat inspection of pigs, ruminants and horses they are subjected to careful examination under special circumstances.

The *lymph outflow* is variable; generally it is indirect via the lumbar trunks or the aortic lumbar nodes, sometimes it is also direct to the cisterna chyli.

The **nll. iliaci laterales** are situated at the bifurcation of the deep circumflex iliac artery, that is, lateral to the foregoing lymph nodes. They are absent in carnivores and goats. They receive lymph from the hip region and efferent vessels from the superficial inguinal lymphocentre. In special cases they are examined during meat inspection of pigs, sheep and horses.

The **nll. sacrales** can be found behind the aortic bifurcation, around the middle sacral artery or medial to the iliac arteries. Their sub-classification into *nll. sacrales* and *nll. hypogastrici* is still subject to discussion. We include all lymph nodes lying under the sacrum and on the inner surface of the broad pelvic ligaments in the term *nll. sacrales*. They *drain* the deep musculature of the pelvic wall, the tail, anal region and perineum. The *outflowing* lymph goes to the medial iliac nodes.

The **nll. anorectales** lie against the lateral aspect of the rectum. Carnivores do not have these nodes. They *drain* the rectum, anus and tissues in the region of the pelvic outlet; their *efferent* vessels go to the medial iliac and sacral lymph nodes.

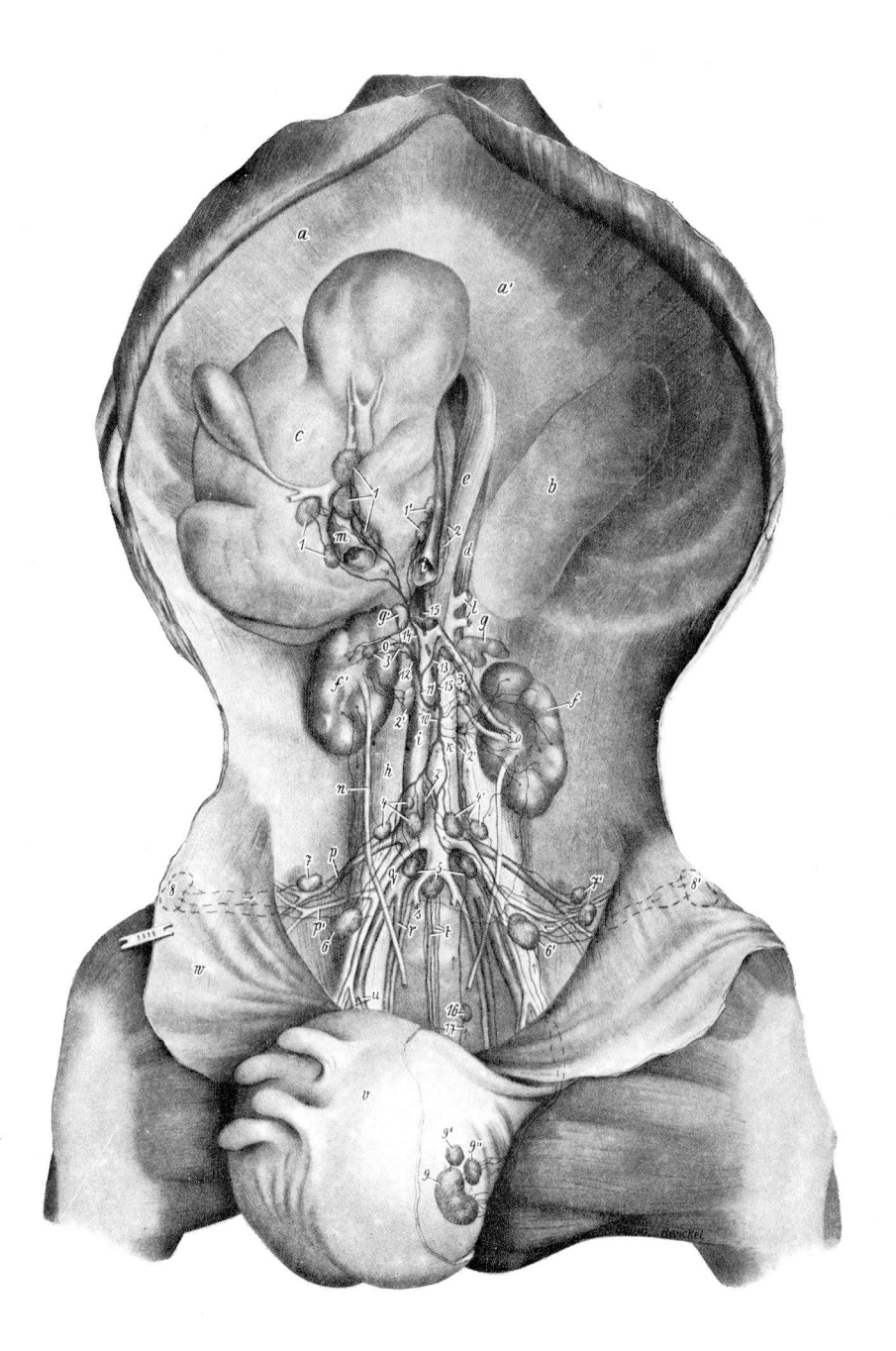

Fig. 258. Lcc. lumbale, iliosacrale, inguinale profundum and inguinale superficiale of the ox.
(After Baum, 1912.)
Ventral wall of the abdomen and stomach and intestines have been removed.

1, 1 nll. hepatici, *1'* nll. hepatici accessorii, *2, 2', 2"* nll. lumbales aortici, *3, 3'* nll. renales, *4, 4'* nll. iliaci mediales, *5* nll. sacrales, *6, 6'* nll. iliofemorales, *7, 7'* nll. iliaci laterales, *8, 8'* nll. subiliaci, *9, 9', 9"* nll. mammarii (inguinales superficiales), *10* truncus lumbalis, *11* truncus visceralis, *12* truncus intestinalis (cut off), *13* truncus gastricus (cut off), *14* truncus hepaticus, *15, 15* cisterna chyli, (the part overlaid by the vena cava is drawn in broken lines), *16* nll. sacrales, *17* lymph vessels from the tail muscles

a, a' diaphragm, *b* spleen, *c* liver, *d* left and *e* right crus of the diaphragm, *f* left and *f'* right kidney, *g* left and *g'* right adrenal, *h* inner lumbar musculature, *i, i* v. cava caudalis (partly excised), *k* aorta abdominalis, *l* a. coeliaca and a. mesenterica cranialis, *m* portal vein, *n* right ureter (cut off in the removal of the bladder), *o, o* a. and v. renalis, *p* v. and *p'* a. circumflexa ilium profunda, *q* a. and v. iliaca externa, *r* a. and v. iliaca interna, *s* a. umbilicalis (cut off), *t* a. and v. sacralis mediana, *u* a. and v. profunda femoris, *v* udder, *w* abdominal wall (reflected)

Nll. uterini are lymph nodes which may or may not be present in the broad ligament of the uterus in horses and pigs and which drain the uterus. Finally, the horse sometimes has a small **nl. obturatorius** lying next to the obturator artery.

Lymphocentrum iliosacrale	dog	cat	pig	ox	sheep	goat	horse
nll. iliaci mediales	350	362	377	399	415	415	435
nll. iliaci laterales	—	—	377	399	*416*	*416*	435
nll. sacrales	350	362	377	399	416	416	435
nll. anorectales	—	—	377	400	416	416	435
nll. uterini	—	—	*378*	—	—	—	*435*
nl. obturatorius	—	—	—	—	—	—	*436*

The numbers relate to the pages where these nodes are described in detail; **bold** type indicates that they are constant, *italics* that thay are inconstant in occurrence.

Lymphocentrum inguinale profundum seu iliofemorale
(258; 260/2, 2', 2'', 2''')

The lymph nodes of this centre lie against the external iliac artery or its direct continuation, the femoral artery. The level of their position determines their name. If they lie within the body cavity in front of the body of the ilium they are termed the **nll. iliofemorales** (carnivores, pigs, ox, sheep). If they are situated at the entrance to the femoral canal they are called **nll. inguinales profundi** (goat and horse). If they lie deeper within the interfemoral space they are known as the **nll. femorales** (carnivores). In the dog and the cat the iliofemoral and femoral lymph nodes respectively are very inconstant in occurrence. The iliofemoral node of the ox is palpable rectally and in this species it is preceded by a **nl. epigastricus** which drains the ventral abdominal wall. In pigs, cattle and horses and also, if present, in the small ruminants, the iliofemoral or deep inguinal nodes are examined in special circumstances at meat inspection.

The *drainage area* of the deep iliac lymphocentre includes the superficial and deep parts of the thigh. It also receives the efferent vessels of the popliteal centre. The *outflow* is to the iliosacral lymphocentre.

Lymphocentrum inguinale profundum seu iliofemorale	dog	cat	pig	ox	sheep	goat	horse
nll. iliofemorales	*350*	*363*	*379*	400	*417*	—	—
nll. inguinales profundi	—	—	—	—	—	417	436
nl. femoralis	*351*	*363*	—	—	—	—	—
nl. epigastricus	—	—	—	400	—	—	—

The numbers relate to the pages where these nodes are described in detail; **bold** type indicates that they are constant, *italics* that they are inconstant in occurrence.

Lymphocentrum inguinale superficiale seu inguinofemorale
(258; 259; 260/3; 3^i, 3^{ii}, 3^{iii}, 3^{iv})

The two important lymph node groups of this centre are the superficial inguinal nodes situated in the groin and the subiliac nodes lying in the stifle fold. The drainage area of both groups is the skin and superficial layers of the thigh and the abdominal wall. The drainage area of the **nll. inguinales superficiales,** in males also known as *nll. scrotales*, is the scrotum and copulatory organ; in the female these nodes, which are known as the *nll. mammarii*, drain the udder (ruminants, horses) or the inguinal (dog, pig) and parts of the abdominal (carnivores, pig) mammary complexes. The **nl. epigastricus caudalis** occurs in the cat and can be considered as a preceding node. It is noteworthy that in the dog, ruminant and horse the superficial inguinal nodes are palpable and that in pigs, ruminants and horses they are thoroughly examined at meat inspection amd may be excised.

The **nll. subiliaci** (259/*1*, *1'*) are always absent in dogs and rarely present in cats. In ruminants they are single but they occur as conglomerates about 8 cm long in the horse and they are palpable in both species at the cranial border of the tensor fasciae latae muscle about half way between the ischiatic tuberosity and the knee cap. In special circumstances they are examined at meat inspection in pigs, ruminants and horses.

The **nl. coxalis** (259/*2*) can be considered a primary-stage node which is usually present in the ox but seldom in horses and sheep. It lies immediately below the ischiatic tuberosity, covered by the tensor fasciae latae muscle. Occasionally one can find in the ox, lateral to this muscle, a **nl. coxalis accessorius** (259/*7*) and more rarely in the paralumbar fossa a subcutaneous **nl. fossae paralumbalis** (259/*5*).

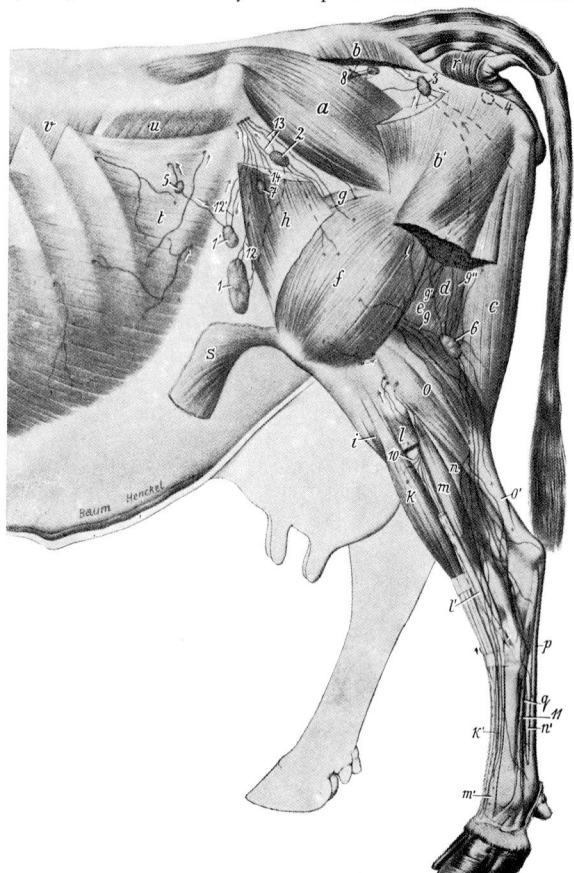

The *outflow* of lymph from the nodes of the superficial inguinal lymphocentre is usually direct to the iliosacral lymphocentre, sometimes indirect by way of the interposed deep inguinal lymphocentre.

Fig. 259. Lcc. inguinale superficiale, ischiadicum and popliteum of the ox.
(After Baum, 1912.)
Part of the superficial muscle has been removed

The small crosses (+ + +) indicate the approximate position where the corresponding lymph vessels were injected

1, 1' nll. subiliaci, *2* nl. coxalis, *3* nl. ischiadicus, *4* nl. tuberalis, *5* nl. fossae paralumbalis, *6* nl. popliteus profundus, *7* nl. coxalis accessorius, *8* nl. glutaeus, *9, 9', 9''* vasa efferentia of the lc. popliteum, *10* lymph vessels from the m. tibialis cranialis, *11* lymph vessel coming through from the medial side, *12, 12'* vasa efferentia of the nll. subiliaci, *13* vasa efferentia of the nl. coxalis, *14* lymph vessels of the m. tensor fasciae latae

a m. glutaeus medius, *b, b'* m. glutaeobiceps, large parts of which have been excised, *c* m. semitendinosus, *d* m. semimembranosus, *e* m. adductor, *f* m. vastus lateralis, *g* m. rectus femoris *h* m. tensor fasciae latae, the proximal part of which has been removed, *i* m. tibialis cranialis, *k* m. peronaeus tertius and m. extensor digitorum communis, *l* m. peronaeus longus, a large part of which has been excised, *l'* its tendon, *m* m. extensor digitorum lateralis, *m'* its tendon, *n* m. flexor digitorum profundus, *n'* its tendon, *o* m. gastrocnemius, caput laterale, *o'* Achilles tendon, *p* superficial flexor tendon, *q* m. interosseus medius, *r* m. coccygeus, *s* terminal part of the m. cutaneus trunci, *t* m. obliquus externus abdominis, *u* m. obliquus internus abdominis, *v* m. serratus dorsalis caudalis

Lymphocentrum inguinale superficiale seu inguinofemorale	dog	cat	pig	ox	sheep	goat	horse
nll. inguinales superficiales (nll. scrotales, mammarii)	351	363	380	**401**	**417**	**417**	**436**
nl. epigastricus caudalis	—	*363*	—	—	—	—	—
nll. subiliace	—	*363*	*380*	**401**	**417**	**417**	**436**
nl. coxalis	—	—	—	**401**	*417*	—	*437*
nl. coxalis accessorius	—	—	—	*401*	—	—	—
nl. fossae parlumbalis	—	—	—	*402*	—	—	—

The numbers relate to the pages where these nodes are described in detail; **bold** type indicates that they are constant, *italics* that they are inconstant in occurrence.

Lymphocentrum ischiadicum

(259/3, *4*, *8*; 260/4; *4'*, *4"*)

This centre is absent in the dog but in the other animals the lymph nodes lie externally on the broad pelvic ligament. The most cranial is the **nl. glutaeus** (pig, occasionally ox) which is situated at the level of the greater ischiatic notch beside the transition point of the ischiatic nerve and cranial gluteal artery. At about the level of the lesser ischiatic notch, near the caudal border of the broad pelvic ligament and the perforation point of the caudal gluteal artery, lie the **nll. ischiadici** (cat, pig, ruminants, horse). Both these groups of lymph nodes are covered laterally by the gluteal and biceps muscles. In special cases in the meat inspection of pigs, ruminants and horses, these nodes have to be exposed from the medial side and carefully examined.

Medial to the dorsal angle of the ischiatic tuberosity we find in ruminants the inconstant **nl. tuberalis**.

The *drainage* area of the ischiatic lymphocentre includes the skin at the pelvic exit, the root of the tail and the powerful pelvic musculature. The *efferent* route is to the iliosacral lymphocentre.

Lymphocentrum ischiadicum	dog	cat	pig	ox	sheep	goat	horse
nll. ischiadici	—	363	**380**	**402**	**417**	*417*	**437**
nl. glutaeus	—	—	**380**	*403*	—	—	—
nl. tuberalis	—	—	—	*403*	*418*	*418*	—

The numbers relate to the pages where these nodes are described in detail; **bold** type indicates that they are constant, *italics* that they are inconstant in occurrence.

Lymphocentrum popliteum

(259/6; 260/5, *5'*)

These lymph nodes, lying in the hollow of the knee, occur in all domestic mammals and we can sometimes differentiate both superficial and deep groups.

In carnivores there are only **nll. poplitei superficiales** which lie in the groove between the biceps femoris and semitendinosus muscles. They are palpable subcutaneously.

Ruminants and horses have only the **nll. poplitei profundi**. They lie deep between the above named muscles, on the popliteal artery and the belly of the gastrocnemius.

The pig has both the superficial and the deep popliteal nodes; the former in 80% of individuals and the latter in 40%. One can assume that in this species about 30% of individuals have both groups, while 10% have neither.

In meat inspection of pigs, ruminants and horses, the popliteal lymph nodes are examined in special cases.

The *drainage* area comprises the distal part of the hind limb. The *efferents* go directly, or via the deep inguinal lymphocentre (dog, pig, ruminants, horse) or the ischiatic centre (pig), to the iliosacral lymphocentre.

Lymphocentrum popliteum	dog	cat	pig	ox	sheep	goat	horse
nll. poplitei profundi	—	—	*381*	**403**	**419**	**419**	**438**
nll. poplitei superficiales	**352**	**364**	*381*	—	—	—	—

The numbers relate to the pages where these nodes are described in detail; **bold** type indicates that they are constant, *italics* that they are inconstant in occurrence.

Outflow of lymph from the pelvis and pelvic limb

There is great variation in individuals and species in the pattern by which the superficial lymphatic vessels flow to the superficial inguinal lymph nodes and the popliteal lymph nodes. The deep lymphatic vessels of the hind limb go to the popliteal nodes in all domestic mammals, to the ileofemoral nodes in the dog, pig and ox and to the deep inguinal lymph nodes in the horse. Subsequent transport is by the following routes (260): from the superficial inguinal nodes (260/3) the efferent vessels pass through the inguinal canal to the medial inguinal nodes (dog, pig) and the lateral iliac nodes (pig) and through the femoral canal to the iliofemoral nodes (pig, dog, ox) or the deep inguinal nodes (horse). From the popliteal lymphocentre (250/5, 5') the vasa efferentia can take two routes. They may accompany the tibial and ischiatic nerves to the sacral lymph nodes, possibly via the ischiatic (pig, ox), and from the sacral nodes proceed to the iliosacral centre at the aortic bifurcation. In the alternative route secondary

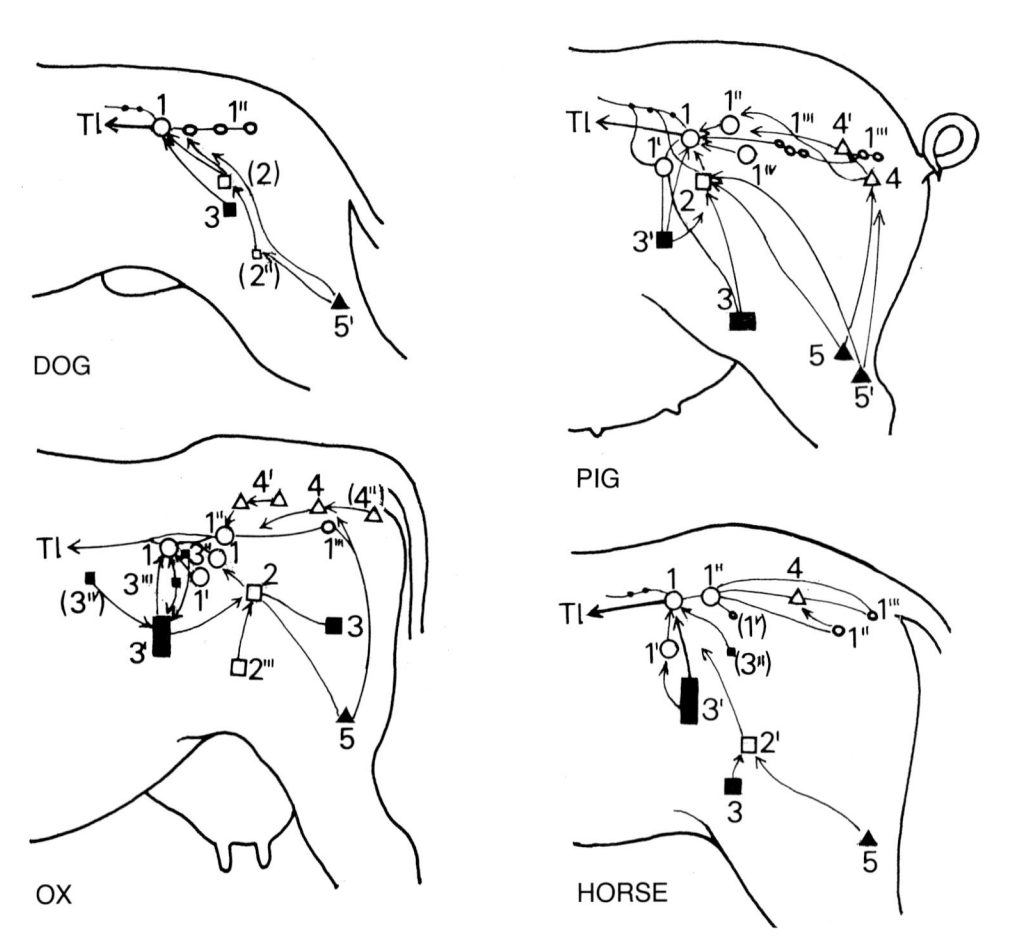

Fig. 260. Principal drainage routes from the pelvis and the pelvic limb (diagrammatic).
Tl = truncus lumbalis

1–1^v lymphocentrum iliosacrale, represented by circles: *1* nll. iliaci mediales, *1'* nll. iliaci laterales (excluding dog), *1"* nll. sacrales, *1'''* nll. anorectales (excluding dog), *1^{iv}* nll. uterini (pig), *1^v* nl. obturatorius (horse); *2–2'''* lymphocentrum inguinale profundum, represented by open squares; *2* nll. iliofemorales (excluding horse), *2'* nll. inguinales profundi (horse), *2"* nl. femoralis (dog) *2'''* nl. epigastricus (ox); *3–3^{iv}* lymphocentrum inguinale superficiale, represented by black squares: *3* nll. inguinales superficiales, *3'* nll. subiliaci (excluding dog), *3"* nl. coxalis (ox, horse), *3'''* nl. coxalis accessorius (ox), *3^{iv}* nl. fossae paralumbalis (ox); *4–4"* lymphocentrum ischiadicum (excluding dog), represented by open triangles; *4* nll. ischiadici, *4'* nl. glutaeus (ox, pig), *4"* nl. tuberalis (ox); *5, 5'* lymphocentrum popliteum, represented by black triangles: *5* nll. poplitei profundi (except dog), *5'* nll. poplitei superficiales (dog, pig)

lymph from the popliteal nodes passes between the adductor muscles to the femoral canal reaching, perhaps after the interposition of the nodes of the deep inguinal centre, the medial iliac nodes in all domestic mammals and the lateral iliac nodes in the pig and ox. The subiliac lymph nodes (260/3') are linked in the pig and horse through their efferent vessels to the lateral iliacs and to the medial iliacs in the pig, horse and ox. In the latter species they sometimes first pass through the coxal node. The lymph nodes at the aortic bifurcation, namely the medial (260/1) and lateral (/1') iliac nodes and the sacral nodes (/1″), receive not only the already-mentioned efferent vessels but also their own afferent contribution from the deep lymphatics of the pelvic limb and pelvic cavity.

The nodes of the iliosacral and to some extent also those of the deep inguinal lymphocentre, give off stout efferent vessels which lead to the formation of the truncus lumbalis. The latter may also occur as several parallel vessels or a network of vessels. The lumbar trunk joins the nodes of the lumbar lymphocentre or their efferent vessels before it empties into the cisterna chyli.

Concluding remarks on comparative aspects

In the preceding chapter an attempt was made to present the lymph vascular system of the domestic mammals in a comparative form and to provide an introductory overall view of the subject. However, when this information is applied practically it will soon become obvious that the finer details are very different in the various species. Further details are therefore recorded in the following chapter which may be consulted as required.

Lymph nodes and lymph collecting ducts of the dog

The lymph vascular system is of considerable importance in the clinical examination of the dog because the superficial nodes are readily palpable while the deep nodes can occasionally be demonstrated in radiograms. In both cases assessment of their condition will aid clinical diagnosis. For these reasons detailed information is provided about their position, size, drainage areas and efferent routes. Baum (1918) collected authentic data to this end.

Lymphocentrum parotideum
nl. parotideus of the dog
(244/1, 1′; 254 A/P; 261/1; 262/1; 263/1)

This large node lies caudal to the mandibular joint. It measures 1.0–2.5 cm in length, 0.5–1.5 cm in breadth and 0.4–1.0 cm in thickness. Its posterior part is covered by the parotid gland while its anterior portion lies against the edge of the mandible and the masseter muscle. It is palpable in this location.

Drainage area: nasal, frontal, parietal, zygomatic and temporal bones; mandible, mandibular joint; zygomatic, temporal and masseter muscles; muscles of the ear and facial skin; external nares, external ear, eyelids, lacrimal apparatus, parotid gland; skin covering the posterior part of the dorsum of the nose, the frontal region, the anterior half of the parietal region, the zygomatic and masseter regions and the skin of the eyelids and external ear.

Efferent routes: medial and also, when present, the lateral retropharyngeal lymph node.

Lymphocentrum mandibulare
nll. mandibulares of the dog
(244/3, 3′; 245 A/M; 261/2; 262/3, 3′, 3″, 3‴; 263/2, 2′, 2″)

Two to five individual nodes, each varying in length from 1.0 to 5.5 cm, are situated caudolateral to the angular process of the mandible. They are palpable. The pattern of grouping above and below the facial vein is not constant.

Drainage area: incisive, nasal, zygomatic, palatine and mandibular bones; mandibular joint; masseter, temporal and digastric muscles, muscles of the lips, cheeks, intermandibular space and the skin muscles of the face and neck; upper and lower lips, apex of the tongue, gums, cheeks, soft and hard palate, floor of the oral cavity; sublingual and zygomatic glands; external nares, eyelids and lacrimal apparatus; skin covering the external nares, the anterior part of the dorsum of the nose, lips, lateral part of the nose, cheeks, intermandibular space, the masseter, frontal, zygomatic and parotid regions, skin of the eyelids and the cranial half of cranial third of the front of the neck.

Efferent routes: the medial, possibly also the lateral, retropharyngeal lymph node. A proportion of the efferent vessels cross to the mandibular nodes of the other side.

Summary of the lymph nodes of the domestic mammals

Consideration is given to their importance from a clinical and meat inspection* view point.

Key to symbols:

- ● = lymph nodes which can be palpated under physiological conditions,
- ○ = inconstant node, palpable when present,
- ▲ = lymph node regularly to be examined at meat inspection,
- △ = inconstant node, to be examined at meat inspection if present,
- ■ = lymph node which is to be examined at meat inspection and if necessary removed in doubtful cases,
- □ = inconstant node, to be examined at meat inspection if present,
- ◆ = only in breeding sows, regularly examined at meat inspection (regional lymph node for the mammary gland),
- ● = lymph node constantly present but without special clinical significance,
- ○ = inconstantly present lymph node, present in the majority of cases,
- · = inconstantly present node, present in less than half the cases.

Lymphocentrum parotideum
  nll. parotidei

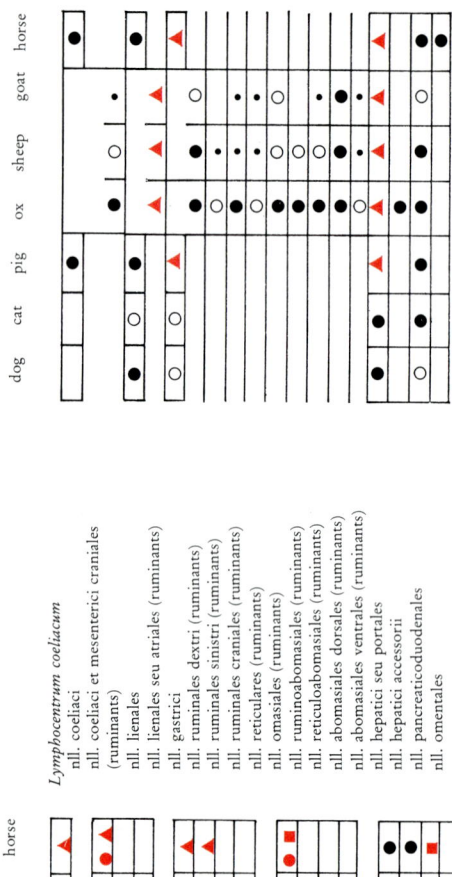

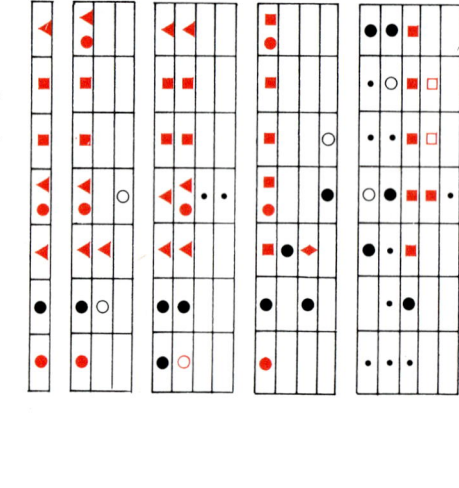

Lymphocentrum mandibulare
  nll. mandibulares
  nll. mandibulares accessorii
  nl. pterygoideus

Lymphocentrum retropharyngeum
  nll. retropharyngei mediales
  nll. retropharyngei laterales
  nl. hyoideus rostralis
  nl. hyoideus caudalis

Lymphocentrum cervicale superficiale
  nll. cervicales superficiales (dorsales)
  nll. cervicales superficiales medii
  nll. cervicales superficiales ventrales
  nll. cervicales superficiales accessorii

Lymphocentrum cervicale profundum
  nll. cervicales profundi craniales
  nll. cervicales profundi medii
  nll. cervicales profundi caudales
  nl. costocervicalis
  nl. subrhomboideus

Lymphocentrum coeliacum
  nll. coeliaci
  nll. coeliaci et mesenterici craniales (ruminants)
  nll. lienales
  nll. lienales seu atriales (ruminants)
  nll. gastrici
  nll. ruminales dextri (ruminants)
  nll. ruminales sinistri (ruminants)
  nll. ruminales craniales (ruminants)
  nll. reticulares (ruminants)
  nll. omasiales (ruminants)
  nll. ruminoabomasiales (ruminants)
  nll. reticuloabomasiales (ruminants)
  nll. abomasiales dorsales (ruminants)
  nll. abomasiales ventrales (ruminants)
  nll. hepatici seu portales
  nll. hepatici accessorii
  nll. pancreaticoduodenales
  nll. omentales

Tabular Summary

	dog	cat	pig	ox	sheep	goat	horse
Lymphocentrum axillare							
nll. axillares proprii	●		·				■
nll. axillares primae costae	○	·	■	■	■	■	●
nll. axillaris accessorius		●		·	·		
nll. cubitales							
nll. infraspinatus							
Lymphocentrum thoracicum dorsale							
nll. thoracici aortici	·	·	◀	◀	■	■	◀
nll. intercostales		·	■	■	■	■	
Lymphocentrum thoracicum ventrale							
nll. sternales craniales	●	·	◀	■	■	■	■
nll. sternales caudales	●	·	◆	◀	◀	◀	◀
nll. epigastricus cranialis	·	·					
Lymphocentrum mediastinale							
nll. mediastinales craniales	●		◀	◀	◀	◀	◀
nl. nuchalis							
nll. mediastinales medii							○
nll. mediastinales caudales				○		□	△
nll. phrenici							
Lymphocentrum bronchale							
nll. bifurcationis seu tracheobronchales sinistri	●	●	◀	◀	◀	◀	◀
nll. bifurcationis seu tracheobronchales dextri	●	●	◀	◀	◀	◀	◀
nll. bifurcationis seu tracheobronchales medii				△	△	△	
nll. tracheobronchales craniales	●	·	◀	○	○	·	○
nll. pulmonales							
Lymphocentrum lumbale							
nll. lumbales aortici	●	●	◀	■	■	■	■
nll. lumbales proprii	●	●	◀	◀	◀	◀	◀
nl. renales				○			
nl. ovaricus							·
nl. testicularis			·				
nl. phrenicoabdominalis			○				

	dog	cat	pig	ox	sheep	goat	horse
Lymphocentrum mesentericum craniale							
nll. mesenterici craniales (excluding ruminants)	●	·	◀	◀	◀	◀	●
nll. jejunales	●	●	◀	◀	◀	◀	◀
nll. caecales							◀
nll. ileocolici			◀	◀	△	△	·
nll. colici							
Lymphocentrum mesentericum caudale							
nll. mesenterici caudales	●	●	■	■	■	■	■
nl. vesicalis	●	●	◀	◀	◀	◀	●
Lymphocentrum iliosacrale							
nll. iliaci mediales							●
nll. iliaci laterales				□	□	□	·
nll. sacrales			○	·	·	·	
nll. anorectales	·		○				
nll. uterini	·						
nl. obturatorius							
Lymphocentrum inguinale profundum seu iliofemorale							
nll. iliofemorales	·		■	■	■	■	■
nll. inguinales profundi						□	
nl. femoralis				○			
nl. epigastricus							
Lymphocentrum inguinale superficiale seu inguinofemorale							
nll. inguinales superficiales (nll. scrotales, mammarii)	●	·	■◀	■◀	■◀◀◀◀●	■◀◀◀◀●	■◀◀◀◀▲
nl. epigastricus caudalis	●		◀	■	■	■	●
nl. subiliaci			■	■	●	●	●
nl. coxalis	·			·	·	·	·
nl. coxalis accessorius	●		●	○			■
nl. fossae paralumbalis	●			○			■
Lymphocentrum ischiadicum							
nll. ischiadici	●	·	□	○	□	□	■
nl. glutaeus	●		□	○			
nl. tuberalis							·
Lymphocentrum popliteum							
nll. poplitei profundi							■
nll. poplitei superficiales	●	●	●				

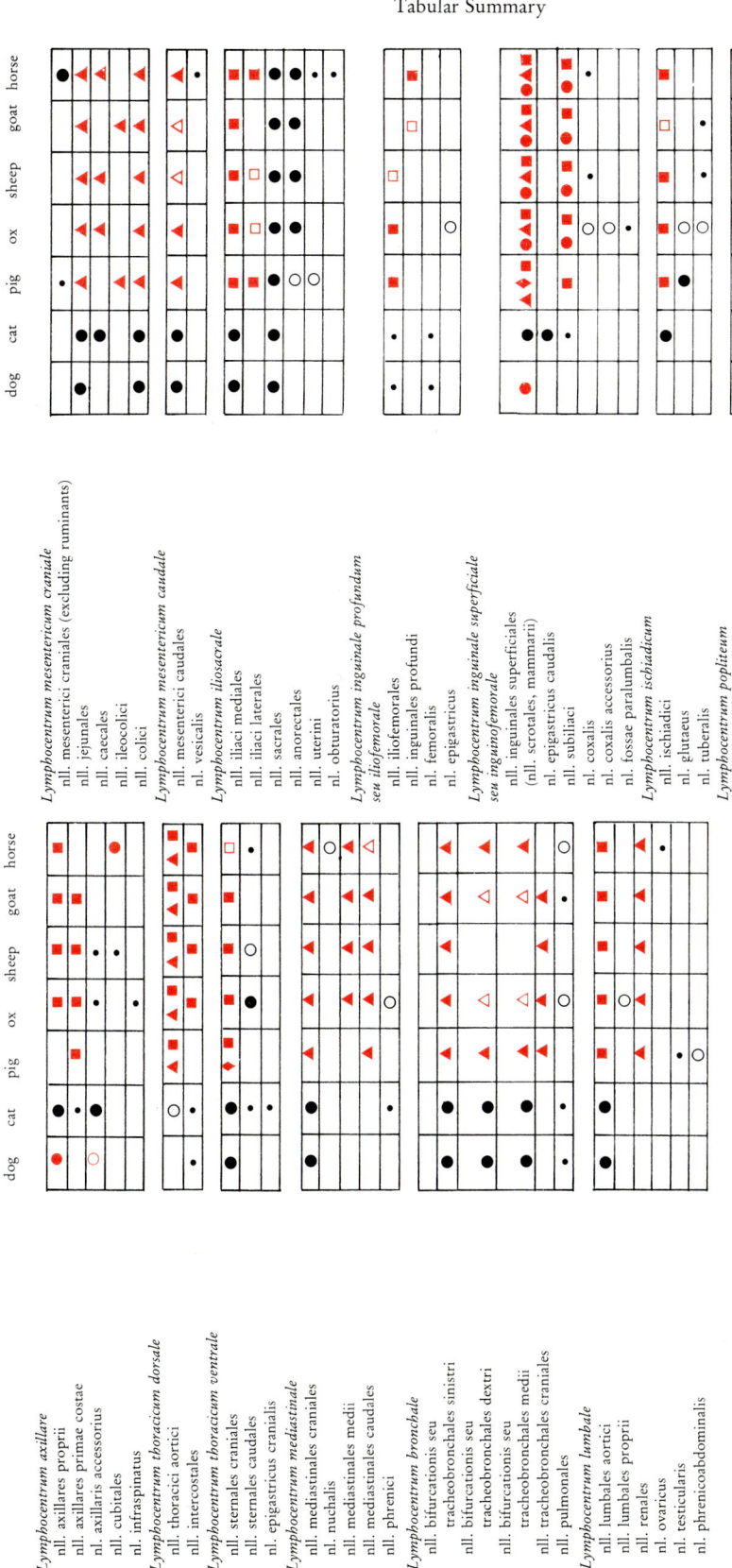

* Meat inspection regulations do not always make use of unequivocal, scientifically-founded nomenclature for lymph nodes and they are therefore prone to variable interpretation. In respect of the pig, ox and horse the above summary largely follows the wide interpretation of Hadlok (1974). In my opinion meat inspection regulations for the small ruminants are inadequate and they correspond to those of the ox and consequently the same applies to this summary.

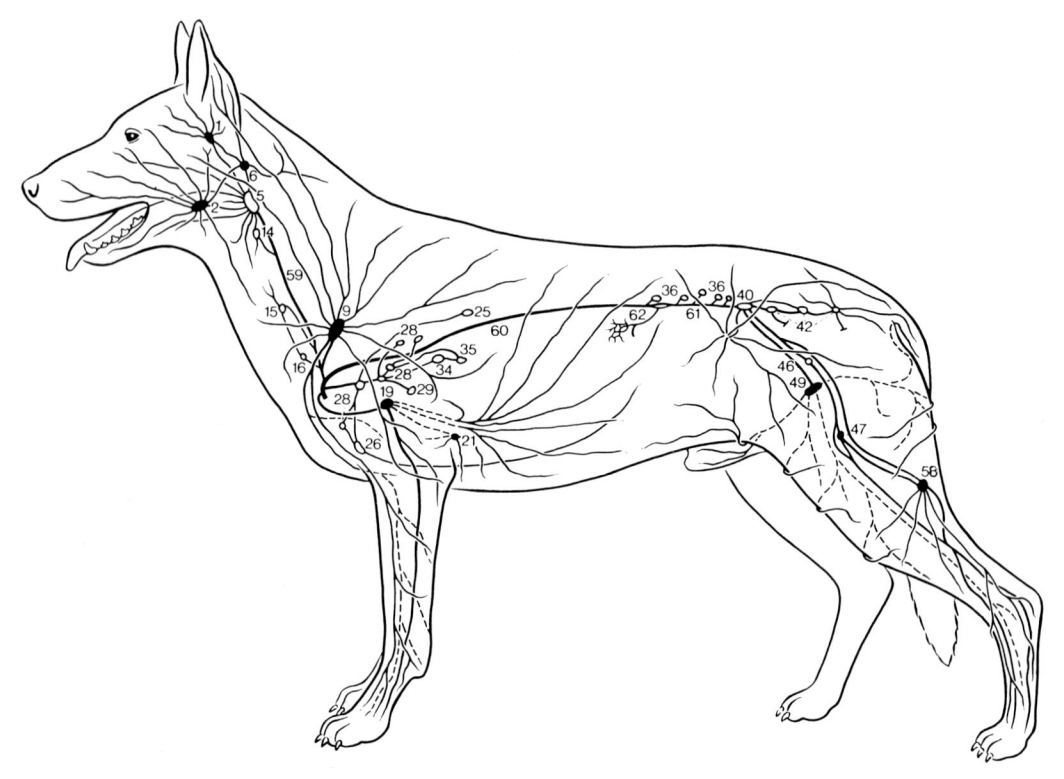

Fig. 261. Diagrammatic representation of the lymph nodes of the dog.
(After Wilkens and Münster, 1972.) The lymph nodes of the abdominal viscera are not depicted.

Lc. parotideum: *2* nll. parotidei; lc. mandibulare: *1* nll. mandibulares; lc. retropharyngeum: *5* nll. retropharyngei mediales, *6* nll. retropharyngei laterales (inconstant); lc. cervicale superficiale: *9* nll. cervicales superficiales: lc. cervicale profundum: *14* nll. cervicales profundi craniales (inconstant), *15* nll. cervicales profundi medii (inconstant), *16* nll. cervicales profundi caudales (inconstant); lc. axillare: *19* nll. axillares proprii, *21* nl. axillaris accessorius (inconstant); lc. thoracicum dorsale: *25* nll. intercostales (inconstant); lc. thoracicum ventrale: *26* nll. sternales craniales; lc. mediastinale: *28* nll. mediastinales craniales, *29* nll. mediastinales which are situated on the pericardium; lc. bronchale: *34* nll. tracheobronchales (bifurcationis) sinistri, *35* nll. tracheobronchales (bifurcationis) medii; lc. lumbale: *36* nll. lumbales aortici; lc. iliosacrale: *40* nll. iliaci mediales, *42* nll. sacrales; lc. iliofemorale (inguinale profundum): *46* nll. iliofemorales, *47* nl. femoralis (inconstant); lc. inguinofemorale (inguinale superficiale): *49* nll. inguinales superficiales (nll. scrotales ♂), nll. mammarii (♀); lc. ischiadicum: absent in the dog; lc. popliteum: *58* nl. popliteus superficialis, *59* truncus jugularis, *60* ductus thoracicus, *61* truncus lumbalis, *62* truncus visceralis

Lymphocentrum retropharyngeum

nl. retropharyngeus medialis of the dog
(244/4; 245 A/Rm; 261/5; 262/4)

There is usually one, seldom two, flat and elongated nodes measuring 1.5 to 8 cm in length, situated dorsolaterally on the pharynx, caudal to the digastric muscle and ventromedial to the wing of the atlas. Aborally it extends to the caudal end of the constrictor muscle of the pharynx. Laterally it is covered by the maxillary gland, the sterno- and cleido-mastoideus muscles and the ventral ramus of the accessory nerve. Medially it is related to the m. longus capitis, the musculature of the pharynx and the large vessels lying upon the latter as well as the vagus, hypoglossus and sympathetic nerves.

Drainage area: parietal, occipital, temporal, sphenoid, palatine and mandibular bones, 1st and 2nd cervical vertebrae; mandibular joint; muscles of mastication, the tongue and hyoid bone, cervical region of the muscles of the pectoral girdle, superficial and deep muscles of the neck; tongue, gums, soft and hard palate, floor of the mouth pharyngeal ring, external ear, lymph vessels of the nervous system in the cranial region. It is also a secondary node receiving afferent vessels from the parotid, mandibular and possibly also the lateral retropharyngeal lymph nodes.

Efferent routes: the delicate vasa efferentia unite to form 3 to 5 stouter ducts which in turn form the left and right jugular trunk. If a cranial deep cervical lymph node is present then one or two of the efferent vessels go to it.

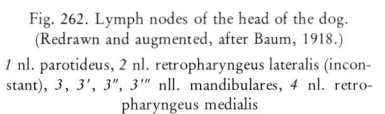

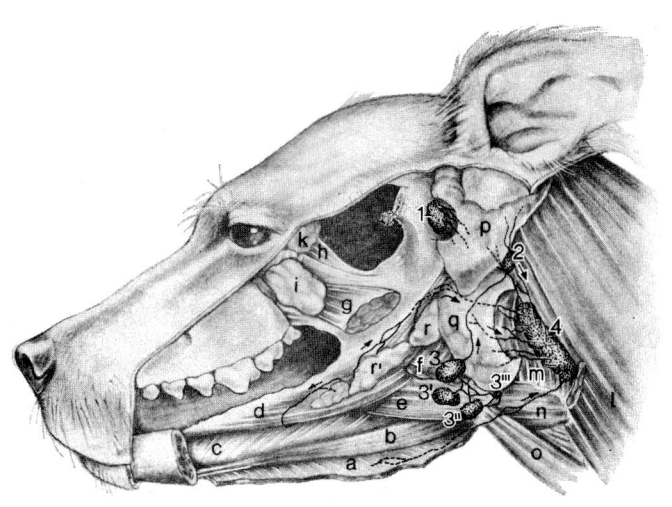

Fig. 262. Lymph nodes of the head of the dog. (Redrawn and augmented, after Baum, 1918.)

1 nl. parotideus, *2* nl. retropharyngeus lateralis (inconstant), *3, 3', 3", 3'''* nll. mandibulares, *4* nl. retropharyngeus medialis

a m. mylohyoideus (reflected), *b* m. geniohyoideus, *c* m. genioglossus, *d* m. styloglossus, *e* m. hyoglossus, *f* stump of the m. digastricus, *g* stump of the m. pterygoideus, *h* eye muscles, *i* glandula zygomatica, *k* lacrimal gland, *l* m. sternomastoideus and m. cleidomastoideus from both of which a portion has been excised so as to expose the ml. retropharyngeus medialis, *m* constrictors of the pharynx, *n* m. thyreohyoideus, *o* m. sternohyoideus, *p* gland, parotis, *q* gland, mandibularis, *r* gland. sublingualis monostomatica, *r'* gland. sublingualis polystomatica

Nl. retropharyngeus lateralis of the dog
(244/2; 245A/*Rl*; 261/6; 262/2)

This lymph node is inconstant, being present in only one in three dogs. When present, there is usually only one, but sometimes two or three, nodes of 0.5 to 0.75 cm diameter. It is palpable. It is situated near the cartilaginous acoustic meatus at the dorsal border of the maxillary gland on the tendon of the sternomastoideus muscle or on the origin of the diagastricus muscle. It is partly covered by the parotid gland, projecting beyond its caudal border.

Drainage area: muscles lying over the 1st and 2nd cervical vertebrae; cutaneous muscles of the neck, posterior aural muscle and external ear. There are no cutaneous lymphatic vessels.

It also receives the efferent vessels of the parotid and mandibular lymph nodes.

Efferent routes: 1 or 2 efferent vessels go to the medial retropharyngeal node.

Lymphocentrum cervicale superficiale
nll. cervicales superficiales of the dog
(247/*Cs*; 248/*d, d', d"*; 261/9; 263/3, 3')

In the majority of cases this group consists of two oval, flat nodes; less often there may be only one or sometimes three or four nodes. They are of considerable size, up to 7.4 cm in length, 3.4 cm in breadth and 2.1 cm in thickness. They lie cranial to the supraspinatus muscle on the lateral surface of the neck, covered by skin and fascia and by the cutaneous muscle of the neck and the trapezius, omotransversarius and brachiocephalicus muscles. Thus they are very superficial in position and may be palpated.

Drainage area: skin of the parietal, ear, nape and parotid regions, of the caudal half of the front of the neck, of the lower arm and foot, large parts of the lateral shoulder and upper arm region and of the medial upper arm regions and cranial part of the chest and cranial part of the sternal region; muscles of the pectoral girdle and shoulder joint; all bones of the forelimb and all joints of the foot.

Efferent routes: these are extremely variable. Usually 6–8 efferent vessels from each node unite to form 2–3 ducts which empty into either the jugular trunk or the terminal part of the thoracic duct, or both, or pass directly into the venous angle. On the right side, the confluence of the jugular trunk and the efferent vessels can produce a short ductus lymphaticus dexter.

Lymphocentrum cervicale profundum

The lymph nodes of this centre lie close to the cervical part of the trachea and are but poorly developed in the dog; sometimes they may be absent altogether. However, three groups can sometimes be differentiated.

Nl. cervicalis profundus cranialis of the dog
(247/*Cpc*; 248/*b*; 261/*14*)

This is inconstant, being present in only one dog in three. The single node is situated at the craniodorsal or dorsomedial border of the thyroid gland. It is of similar size to the parathyroid gland and can thus be confused with it.

Drainage area: larynx, thyroid gland, upper portion of the cervical part of the trachea and oesophagus.

Efferent route: it links directly to the jugular trunk.

Nl. cervicalis profundus medius of the dog
(247/*Cpm*; 261/*15*)

Only in one tenth of dogs is this small, round node present and it lies behind the thyroid gland in the middle third of the cervical trachea.

Drainage area: some lymph vessels of the thyroid gland, trachea and oesophagus.

Efferent routes: to the caudal deep cervical node, the jugular trunk, the thoracic duct or right lymphatic duct or one of the cranial mediastinal nodes.

Nl. cervicalis profundus caudalis of the dog
(247/*Cpca*; 248/*c, c'*; 261/*16*)

This single node is present in only about one dog in three and may be present on only one side. It measures 1.5 to 2.5 cm in diameter and lies immediately cranial to the first rib against the trachea and it is covered by the sternohyoideus, sternothyreoideus and brachiocephalicus muscles.

Drainage area: isolated lymph vessels from the splenius, sternohyoideus, sternothyreoideus, longus colli, longus capitis muscles; the last 5–6 cervical vertebrae, thyroid gland, trachea and oseophagus.

Efferent route: it drains into one of the lymph collecting ducts near the thoracic inlet or, after forming a lymph network, into one of the cranial mediastinal nodes.

Lymphocentrum axillare

Nl. axillaris proprius of the dog
(248/*e*; 249/*Ap*; 261/*19*)

This spherical node occurs almost always singly and measures between 0.3 and 0.5 cm in length. When the limb is advanced the node can be palpated at the level of the shoulder joint on the transversus costarum or pectoralis profundus muscles over the 1st intercostal space or the 2nd rib. The teres major muscle overlies the node laterally.

Drainage area: the skin of the thorax and abdomen to the level of the last rib; the skin covering the shoulder and the upper arm; thoracic part of the musculature of the shoulder girdle; the first three of the five mammary complexes; bones and joints of the forelimb with the exception of the toes. It may also receive secondary lymph from the inconstantly-occurring accessory axillary node.

Efferent routes: on the left it drains into the left jugular trunk or the thoracic duct or directly into the venous angle. On the right side into the right jugular trunk, the right lymphatic duct or directly into the venous angle.

Nl. axillaris accessorius of the dog
(248/*e'*; 249/*Aa*; 261/*21*; 263/*4*)

Only one dog in four has this relatively small lymph node. When present it is situated vertically above the olecranon on the dorsal border of the deep pectoral muscle or on the ventral border of the latissimus dorsi in the angle formed by these two muscles. It is covered only by skin and cutaneous muscle. When present it is therefore palpable.

Drainage area: the skin of the surrounding area, abdominal cutaneous muscle, deep pectoral muscle and the mammary gland.

Efferent route: proper axillary node.

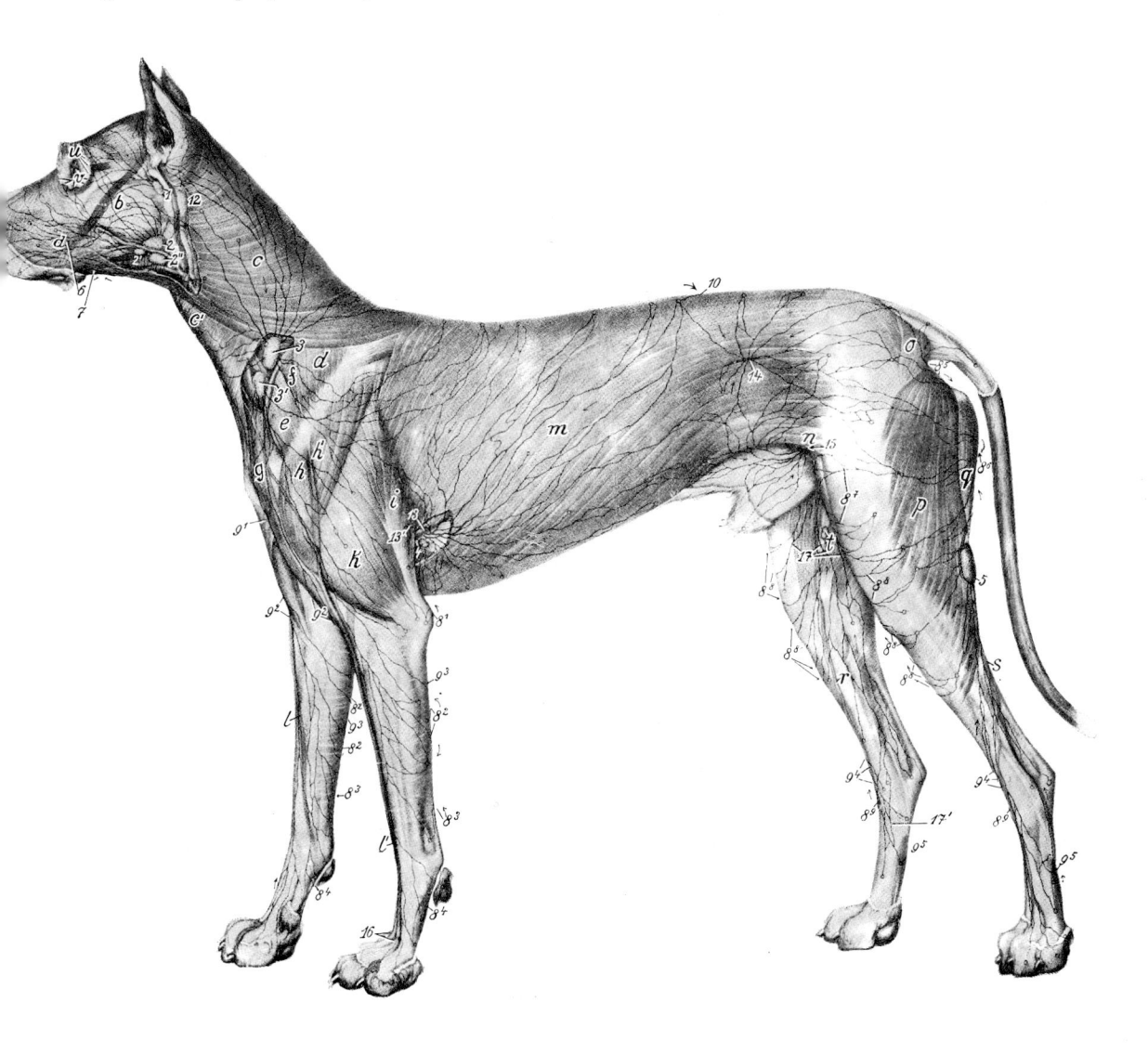

Fig. 263. Lymph vessels of the skin and palpable nodes of the dog.
(After Baum, 1918.)

1 nl. parotideus, *2, 2', 2"* nll. mandibulares, *3, 3'* nll. cervicales superficiales, *4* ln. axillaris accessorius, *5* nl. popliteus superficialis, *6* lymph vessels from the gums on the buccal side of the maxillary teeth, *7* lymph vessels from the gums on the buccal side of the mandibular teeth, 8^1–8^9 lymph vessels which curve to the medial side of the lower arm or lower shank; nodes marked 8^5–8^8 go to the nll. inguinales superficiales 9^1 lymph vessels from the skin of the ventral aspect of the chest, 9^2–9^5 lymph vessels which are reflected to the lateral surface of the upper and lower arm or shank, *10* lymph vessels which extend beyond the midline of the back, *11* lymph vessels of the external surface of the nose, *12* lymph vessels which go deep to the nl. retropharyngeus medialis, *13, 13'* lymph vessels going to the nl. axillaris proprius, *14* lymph vessels to the nll. iliaci mediales, *15* lymph vessels ending in the nll. inguinales superficiales, *16* lymph vessels passing from the palmar aspect to the dorsal surface of the paw, *17, 17'* lymph vessels going to the nll. inguinales superficiales

a cheek muscles, *b* m. masseter, *c, c'* cutaneous muscles of the neck, *d* m. trapezius, pars cervicalis, *e* m. omotransversarius, *f* m. supraspinatus, *g* m. brachiocephalicus, *h, h'* m. deltoideus, *i* caput longum and *k* caput laterale of the m. triceps brachii, *l* v. cephalica, *l'* v. cephalica accessoria, *m* cutaneous muscles of the abdomen, *n* stifle fold, *o* m. gluteus superficialis, *p* m. biceps femoris, *q* m. semitendinosus, *r* v. saphena medialis, *s* v. saphena lateralis, *t* nl. femoralis, *u* upper and *v* lower eyelids

Lymphocentrum thoracicum dorsale
Nl. intercostalis of the dog
(261/25; 264/g; 265/9)

Only one dog in four has this single node. It is about 2–7 cm in length and is located in the 5th or 6th intercostal space at the level of the rib-head articulation or at the 6th rib-head joint.

Drainage area: lymph vessels which pass through the 6th to 8th intercostal spaces carry primary lymph from the back, shoulder, chest and abdominal musculature; thoracic vertebrae, spinal meninges, aorta, pleura.

Efferent route: cranial mediastinal lymph nodes.

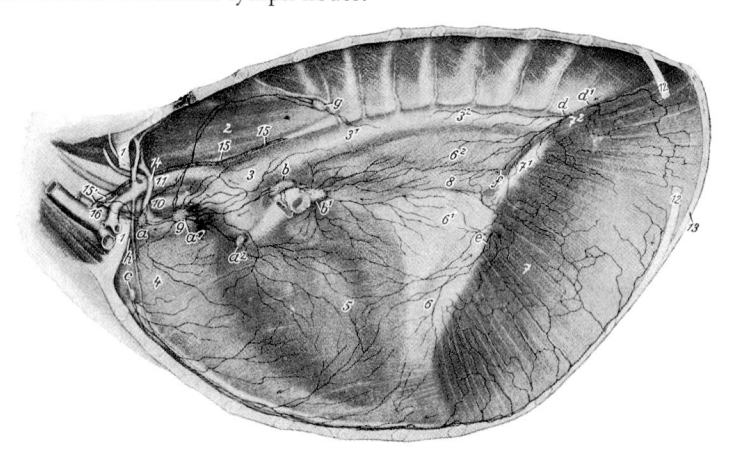

Fig. 264. Lymph nodes and lymph vessels of the thoracic cavity of the dog. Left lateral view. The left lung, left thoracic wall and the m. transversus thoracic have been removed.
(After Baum, 1918).

a, a^1, a^2 nll. mediastinales craniales, b nl. bifurcationis (tracheobronchalis) sinister, b^1 nl. bifurcationis (tracheobronchalis) medius, c nl. sternalis cranialis, d, d^1 lymph vessels going to the nll. lumbales aortici, e lymph vessels which pass through the diaphragm into the abdominal cavity to terminate in the nll. lienales, nll. gastrici, nll. hepatici or the nll. lumbales aortici, f lymph vessels passing with the oesophagus into the abdominal cavity, g nll. intercostales, h an efferent vessel which passes to the right side and reappears as 10 in fig. 265.

1, 1 first rib from which a piece has been removed, *2* m. longus colli, *3, 3¹, 3²* aorta, *4* precardiac mediastinum, *5* pericardium and cardiac mediastinum, *6, 6¹, 6²* post cardiac mediastimum, *7, 7¹, 7²* diaphragm, *8* oesophagus, *9* v. cava cranialis, *10* truncus brachiocephalicus, *11* a. subclavia sinistra, *12, 12* twelfth rib from which a piece has been removed, *13* thirteenth rib, *14* v. costocervicalis, *15* ductus thoracicus *15'* termination of the ductus thoracicus, shown here with a secondary branch, *16* venous angle, point of bifurcation of the subclavian vein into the axillary and jugular veins

Lymphocentrum thoracicum ventrale
Nl. sternalis cranialis of the dog
(261/26; 264/c; 265/6)

As a rule this is a single node 3–20 mm in length situated on each, or only one, side, medial to the 2nd costal cartilage or 2nd intercostal space. It is absent only exceptionally.

Drainage area: neighbouring shoulder, chest and abdominal musculature, ribs, sternum, diaphragm, mediastinum, pleura, parts of the peritoneum, thymus and certain lymph vessels which pass through the ventral chest wall from the cranial half of the mammary complex.

Efferent route: cranial mesenteric lymph nodes.

Lymphocentrum mediastinale
Nll. mediastinales craniales of the dog
(261/28; 264/a, a^1, a^2; 265/3, 3^1, 3^2, 3^3, 3^4, 3^5; 266/8, 8^1)

The number, size and position of these lymph nodes varies considerably but on each side of the body there are 1–6 individual nodes ranging in size from 0.3 to 3 cm in length. One very constant node is that which is situated in the 1st intercostal space immediately in front of the costocervical vein. The remainder follow on up to the aortic arch or even onto the pericardium. If a single node is present on one side only, then it lies in the first position recorded above. In young animals these nodes may be partially embedded in the thymus. Otherwise they lie between the vessels and organs of the precardiac mediastinum.

Drainage area: subscapular muscle and muscles of the shoulder girdle, chest and abdomen, ventral muscles of the neck, flexor muscles of the neck and extensors of the back; scapula, cervical vertebrae (excluding atlas), thoracic vertebrae, ribs; trachea, oesophagus, thyroid gland, thymus, mediastinum, costal pleura, heart, aorta, spinal meninges. They also receive secondary lymph from the intercostal, cranial sternal, middle and caudal deep cervical, tracheobronchial and pulmonary lymph nodes.

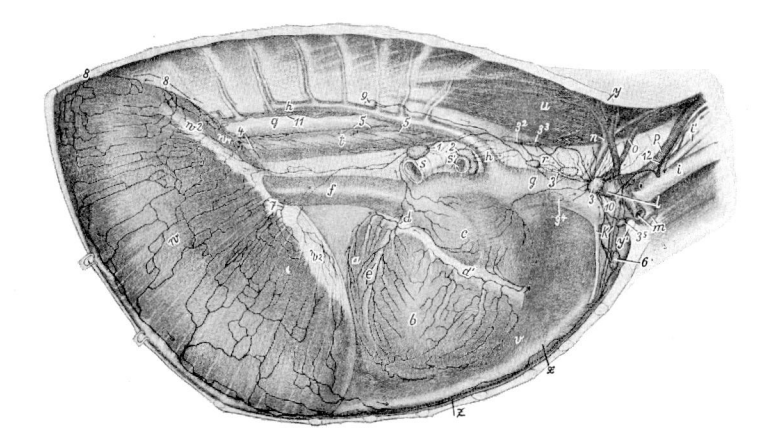

Fig. 265. Lymph nodes and lymph vessels of the thoracic cavity of the dog. Right lateral view. The right thoracic wall and right lung have been removed. (After Baum, 1918.)

1 nl. bifurcationis medius, *2* nl. bifurcationis dexter, *3, $3^1, 3^2, 3^3, 3^4, 3^5$* nll. mediastinales craniales, *4* lymph vessels of the oesophagus entering the thoracic cavity, *5, 5* oesophageal lymph nodes curving towards the dorsal border of the oesophagus and thence to the left, to terminate in the left tracheobronchial node, *6* nl. sternalis cranialis, *7* lymph vessels which terminate in the nl. gastricus, nll. lienales, nll. hepatici or nll. lumbales aortici, *8, 8* lymph vessels going to the nll. lumbales aortici, *9* nl. intercostalis, *10* vas efferens of a nl. mediastinalis cranialis, *11* ductus thoracicus, *12* ductus lymphaticus dexter
a left ventricle, *b* right ventricle, *c* right atrium, *d, d'* sulcus coronarius, *e* sulcus interventricularis subsinuosus, *f* v. cava caudalis, *g* v. cava cranialis, *h* v. azygos dextra, *i* v. jugularis externa, *i'* v. jugularis interna, *k* a. and v. thoracica interna, *l* a. subclavia dextra, *m* a. and v. axillaris dextra, *n* v. costocervicalis dextra, *o* a. vertebralis dextra, *p* a. carotis communis dextra, *q* aorta, *r* trachea, *s* right bronchus principalis, *s'* right bronchus lobaris cranialis, *t* oesophagus, *u* m. longus colli, *v* left m. transversus thoracis, *w* pars costalis, *w^1* pars lumbalis and *w^2* centrum tendineum of the diaphragm, *x* sternum, *y, y'* dorsal and ventral part of the 1st rib, *z* right m. transversus thoracis (cut off)

Efferent routes: on the left side these go to the terminal part of the thoracic duct and possibly also to the left jugular trunk. On the right side they convey the lymph to the right jugular trunk and the right lymphatic duct.

Lymphocentrum bronchale
Nll. bifurcationis dexter, sinister et medius of the dog
(261/34, 35; 264/b, b^1; 265/1, 2; 266/1, 2, 3)

One lymph node is found respectively on the right, left and dorsum of the trachea at the point of its bifurcation into the main bronchi. Each is 0.6 to 3.2 cm in diameter but the dorsally situated node is always the largest. The nodes are always prominent because of their black colour which results from the deposition of dust particles.

Drainage area: thoracic parts of the oesophagus and trachea, bronchial tree and lungs, mediastinum, diaphragm, heart and aorta. They also receive secondary lymph from the inconstant pulmonary nodes.

Efferent routes: the tracheobronchial lymph nodes are interlinked through their efferent vessels. Thus the right and left tracheobronchial nodes pass some of their secondary lymph to the middle tracheobronchial node. The latter sends some of its secondary lymph to the left tracheobronchial node, and efferent vessels from all three tracheobronchial nodes go to the cranial mediastinal lymph nodes.

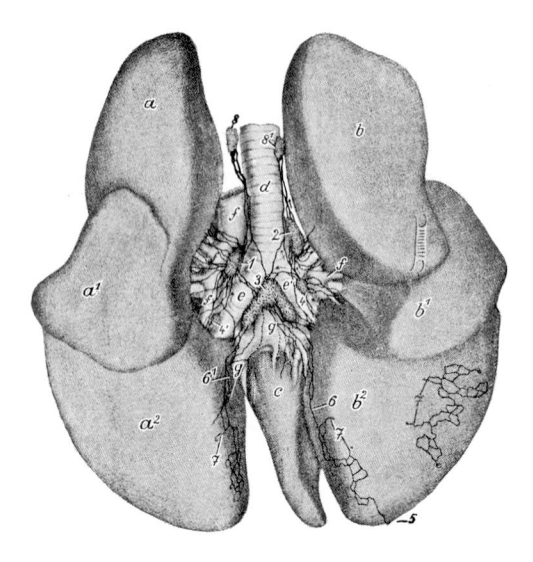

Fig. 266. Lymph nodes and lymph vessel of the lungs of the dog. Dorsal view.
(After Baum, 1918.)

1 nl. bifurcationis sinister, *2* nl. bifurcationis dexter, *3* nl. bifurcationis medius, *4, 4'* lnn. pulmonales, *5* subserous lymph vessel which passes round the margo acutus onto the diaphragmatic surface and thence into the deeper tissues, *6, 6'* subserous lymph vessels which run in the insertion of the ligamentum pulmonale, *7, 7, 7* subserous lymph vessels which dip into the deeper tissues, *8, 8'* nll. mediastinales craniales

a, a¹ lobus cranialis sinister, pars cranialis and pars caudalis, *a²* lobus caudalis sinister, *b* lobus cranialis dexter, *b¹* lobus medius, *b²* lobus caudalis dexter, *c* lobus accessorius, *d* trachea, *e* bronchus principalis sinister, *e'* bronchus principalis dexter, *f* a. pulmonalis and its branches, *g, g* vv. pulmonales

Nll. pulmonales of the dog
(266/4, 4')

These small nodes are inconstant, occurring in but a third of all dogs. They are blackish structures, 4–10 mm in diameter, and they lie on the extrapulmonary part of the right or left primary bronchi.
Drainage area: lungs.
Efferent routes: to one or both of the tracheobronchial or cranial mediastinal lymph nodes.

Lymphocentrum lumbale
Nll. lumbales aortici of the dog
(261/36; 267/3, 3'; 268/5; 269/h; 270/1, 1', 2, 3, 3'; 271/2, 2'; 272/2, 3)

The lumbar aortic nodes are usually very small, measuring no more than 1–2 mm in diameter, and they lie in an irregular manner dorsal, ventral and lateral to the abdominal aorta or caudal vena cava. They extend from the diaphragm to the origin of the deep circumflex iliac arteries. Their number is very variable. The cranial pair of nodes is almost constant and its individual nodes, measuring 1–2 cm in diameter, are much larger than the rest. Subsequent nodes may be completely lacking or there may be as many as 17 of them.
Drainage area: ribs, last thoracic and all lumbar vertebrae; lumbar and abdominal musculature, extensors of the back; mediastinum, pleura, peritoneum, diaphragm, liver, kidneys, adrenals, ureter, ovary, uterine tubes, uterus or testes, epididymis, spermatic cord, vaginal process and cremaster muscle; aorta and spinal meninges. Secondary lymph also comes from the caudal mesenteric and iliosacral lymphocentres.
Efferent routes: lymph is either passed directly into the cisterna chyli or the efferent vessels participate in the formation of the lumbar trunks.

Lymphocentrum coeliacum
Nll. lienales of the dog
(267/8, 8'; 268/3, 3'; 269/d, d')

This is a group of between 1 and 5 nodes located near the splenic artery and vein and their terminal branches. Their size varies between 0.5 and 4 cm in diameter.
Drainage area: oesophagus, stomach, pancreas, spleen, liver, diaphragm, mediastinum, omentum; secondary lymph from the gastric lymph node.
Efferent route: to the visceral trunk.

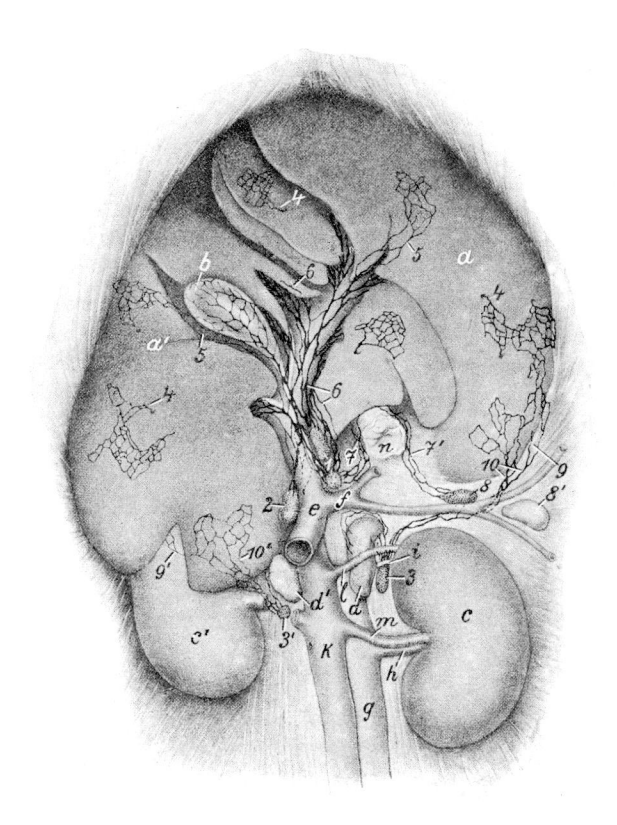

Fig. 267. Lymph nodes and lymph vessels of the liver of the dog, in situ. (After Baum, 1918.)

1, 2 nll. hepatici, *3, 3'* nll. lumbales aortici, *4, 4, 4* subserous lymph vessels which go deep into the tissues, *5, 5* subserous lymph vessels which can be traced in subserous position to the nll. hepatici, *6, 6* deep lymph vessels of the liver, *7, 7'* lymph vessels which follow the end of the oesophagus, *8, 8'* nll. lienales, *9, 9'* subserous lymph vessels which originate from the parietal surface of the liver and *10, 10'* subserous lymph vessels from the visceral surface of the liver, which go to the nll. lumbales aortici (*3, 3'*)

a, a' liver, *b* gall bladder, *c* left and *c'* right kidney, *d, d'* adrenals, *e* v. portae, *f* v. lienalis, *g* aorta, *h* a. renalis, *i* a. abdominalis cranialis, *k* v. cava caudalis, *l* v. abdominalis cranialis, *m* v. renalis, *n* stump of the oesophagus

Nl. gastricus of the dog
(269/*o*)

This is usually a small node of between 5 and 25 mm diameter. It lies on the small curvature of the stomach near the pylorus. Sometimes it is absent but occasionally it is duplicated.
Drainage area: oesophagus, stomach, liver, diaphragm, mesentery, peritoneum.
Efferent route: hepatic or splenic lymph nodes.

Nll. hepatici seu portales of the dog
(267/1, 2; 268/1, 2; 269/*b, c*)

These nodes lie to the right and left of the portal vein. The left node is usually moderately elongated and slightly flattened, measuring 1–6 cm in length. It extends to the beginning of the duodenum. Rarely there are 2 or 3 nodes. On the right side there is a group of 1–5 flat nodes, each of which ranges in size from 1 to 5 cm.
Drainage area: mainly the liver, including the gall bladder, stomach, pancreas and duodenum. However, it also receives tributaries from the oesophagus, diaphragm, mediastinum and peritoneum. Secondary lymph is contributed from the gastric and pancreaticoduodenal nodes.
Efferent route: the visceral trunk.

Nll. pancreaticoduodenales of the dog
(269/*a*)

This small node is almost always present and is located at the cranial flexure between the duodenum and the right lobe of the pancreas. In about fifty per cent of dogs there is a second node, and sometimes

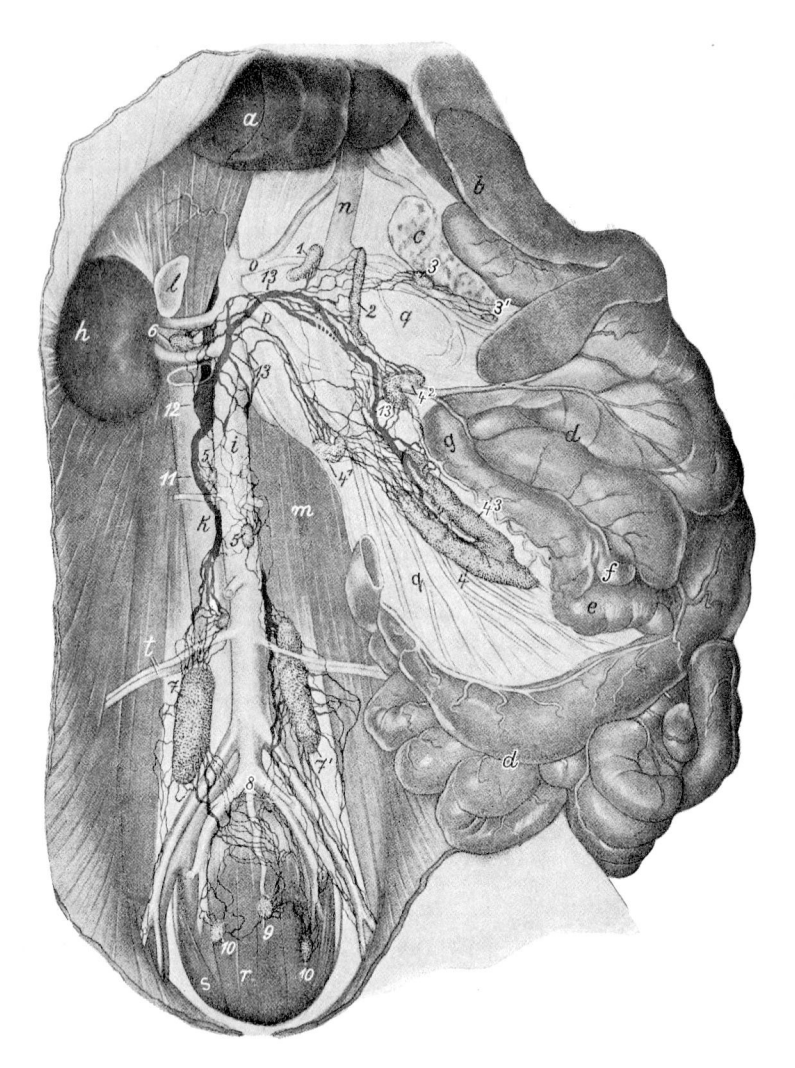

Fig. 268. Lymph nodes and lymph vessels of the abdominal cavity of the dog. The abdomen has been opened and most of the viscera lifted out of the cavity.
(After Baum, 1918.)

1, 2 nll. hepatici, *3, 3'* nll. lienales, *4, 4¹, 4², 4³* nll. jejunales, *5, 6* nll. lumbales aortici, *7, 7'* nll. iliaci mediales, *8, 9, 10* nll. sacrales, *11* truncus lumbalis, *12* cisterna chyli, *13, 13, 13* truncus visceralis

a liver, *b* spleen *c* pancreas, *d* jejunum, *e* ileum, *f* caecum, *g* colon, *h* right kidney, *i* aorta, *k* caudal vena cava, *l* right adrenal, *m* lumbar musculature, *n* v. portae, *o* a. coeliaca, *p* a. mesenterica cranialis, *q* mesentery with blood vessels, *r* depressor muscle of the tail, *s* lateral flexor of the tail, *t* a. and v. circumflexa ilium profunda

two or even three nodes, in the visceral layer of the greater omentum about 2–5 cm distant from the duodenum. The latter measures approximately 4–10 mm.

Drainage area: greater omentum, duodenum, pancreas, stomach.
Efferent route: to the hepatic lymph nodes.

Lymphocentrum mesentericum craniale

Nll. jejunales of the dog
(268/4, 4¹, 4², 4³)

Usually these consist of two elongated, flattened main nodes which are tapered at the ends and measure 0.5–20 cm in length, 0.4–2 cm in breadth and 0.3–1 cm in thickness. Some smaller nodes are occasionally also associated with them. The jejunal nodes are grouped around the jejunal arteries and veins and they extend from the root of the mesentery into the mesojejunum up to the point where the blood vessels undergo terminal division.

Drainage area: jejunum, ileum, pancreas.
Efferent route: the efferent vessels form a network which, together with those of the coeliac lymphocentre forms the visceral trunk.

Nll. colici of the dog
(269/e, f)

In the short mesentery of the ascending colon and 5–7 cm from the transverse colon there are 1 to 2 nodes, each measuring between 0.3 and 2.5 cm in length.

Drainage area: ileum, caecum, colon and secondary lymph from the caudal mesenteric lymph nodes.
Efferent route: visceral trunk.

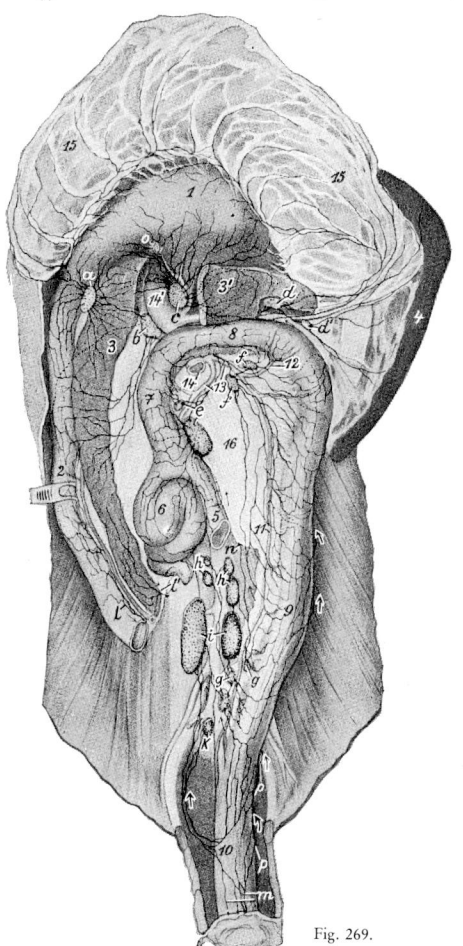

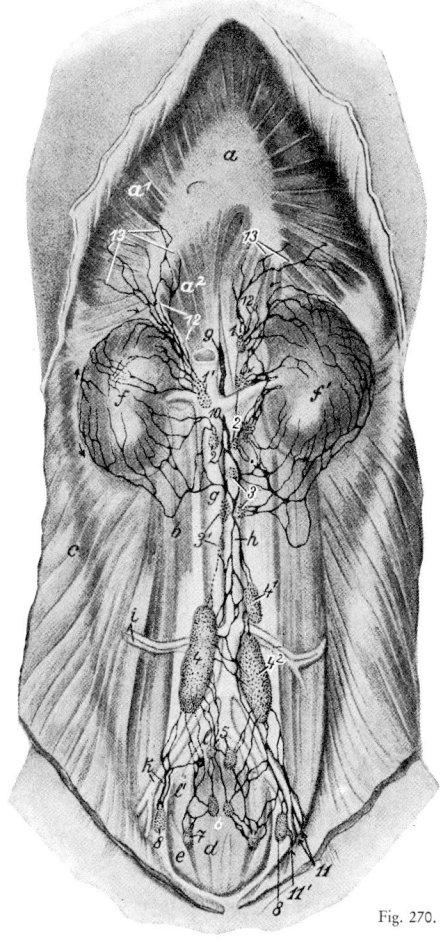

Fig. 269.

Fig. 270.

Fig. 269. Lymph nodes and lymph vessels of the stomach, spleen, pancreas, duodenum and large intestine of the dog. The small intestine, except the first part of the duodenum and the end of the ileum, has been removed.
(After Baum, 1918.)

a nl. pancreaticoduodenalis, *b*, *c* nll. hepatici, *d*, *d'* nll.lienales (part of the pancreas has been removed to expose *c* and *d*), *e*, *f*, *f* nll. colici, *g*, *g* nll. mesenterici caudales, *h*, *h* nll. lumbales aortici, *i* nll. iliaci mediales (part of the mesocolon has been excised to expose the groups *h* and *i*), *k* nll. sacrales, *l* lymph vessels of the duodenum and *l'* lymph vessels of the pancreas which go to the nll. jejunales and have therefore been removed, *m* lymph vessels of the anus and rectum, *n* lymph vessel which runs directly to the cisterna chyli, *o* nl. gastricus, *p*, *p* lymph vessels to the rectum which cross over the dorsal surface of the rectum and go to the nll. sacrales and iliaci mediales

1 stomach, *2* duodenum (ascending part), *3*, *3'* pancreas, *4* spleen (deflected to one side), *5* ileum (cut off), *6* caecum, *7*, *8*, *9* colon, *10* rectum, *11* v. colica sinistra, *12* v. colica media, *13* v. iliocolica, *14*, *14'* v. portae, *15*, *15* ventral wall of the omental bursa, reflected, *16* mesocolon

Fig. 270. Lymph nodes of the lumbar region of the dog.
The abdominal viscera, except the kidneys, have been removed and the right kidney (f) has been pushed posteriorly so that the diaphragmatic lymph vessels could be shown.
(After Baum, 1918.)

1, *1'*, *2*, *3*, *3'* nll. lumbales aortici, *4*, *4¹*, *4²* nll. iliaci mediales, *5*, *6*, *7* nll. sacrales, *8*, *8* nl. iliofemoralis, *9* cisterna chyli, *10* truncus lumbalis, *11* vasa efferentia of the nll. inguinales superficiales and the nl. femoralis (some of these [*11'*]) enter the nl. iliofemoralis [*8*]), *12* lymph vessels which pass with the n. sympathicus and n. splanchnicus major from the thoracic to the abdominal cavity, *13* lymph vessels of the diaphragm

a, *a¹*, *a²* diaphragm, *b* lumbar muscularure, *c* lateral abdominal wall, *d* depressor and *e* lateral flexor muscle of the tail, *f*, *f'* kidneys, *g* v. cava caudalis, *h* aorta abdominalis, *i* a. and v. circumflexa ilium profunda, *k* a. and v. iliaca externa, *l*, *l'* a. and v. iliaca interna

Lymphocentrum mesentericum caudale
Nll. mesenterici caudales of the dog
(269/g)

Two to five nodes each of 0.3–1.5 cm diameter lie in the mesentery of the descending colon.
Drainage area: colon, rectum.
Efferent routes: lymph drains partly to the colic nodes or directly to the visceral trunk and partly to the lumbar aortic nodes.

Lymphocentrum iliosacrale
Nll. iliaci mediales of the dog
(261/40; 268/7, 7'; 269/i; 270/4, 4¹, 4²; 271/1; 272/1)

Below the 5th and 6th lumbar vertebrae, to the left of the aorta and to the right of the caudal vena cava, there is usually one lymph node which extends from the origin of the deep circumflex iliac artery to that of the external iliac. In large dogs it can measure up to 6 cm in length. Occasionally there may be two or even three nodes on one or both sides.
Drainage area: lymph is drawn from the skin which covers the dorsal abdominal wall caudal to the last rib; from the skin in the region of the pelvis, tail root, cranial part of the lateral aspect of the thigh and the knee joint; abdominal musculature, muscles and bones of the pelvic limb, pelvic and lumbar musculature; colon, rectum, anus, vagina, vulva or testes, epididymis, spermatic cord, vaginal process and cremaster muscle, prostate gland; in both males and females the ureter, bladder and urethra; aorta, spinal meninges and finally secondary lymph from all the lymphocentres to be described below.
Efferent routes: the efferent vessels go partly to the lumbar aortic node and partly to form the lumbar trunks.

Nll. sacrales of the dog
(261/42; 268/8, 9, 10; 269/12; 270/5, 6, 7; 271/3; 272/4, 7)

Below the 7th, but sometimes under the 6th, lumbar vertebra in the angle between right and left internal iliac arteries there are one, two or occasionally even more nodes, each measuring up to 2.5 cm in length. In half the population of dogs these are joined by smaller nodes of 3–15 mm diameter, which lie against the roof or dorsolateral wall of the pelvis.
Drainage area: inner lumbar and gluteal and posterior thigh musculature, the deep muscles of the thigh and the muscles of the tail; lumbar vertebrae, sacrum, coccygeal vertebrae, pelvic bones, femur; colon, rectum, anus, uterus, vagina, vulva or, in males, prostate and penis; bladder, ureter, urethra; spinal meninges. They also receive secondary lymph from the deep inguinal lymphocentre.
Efferent route: medial iliac lymph nodes.

Lymphocentrum inguinale profundum (seu iliofemorale)
Nl. iliofemoralis of the dog
(261/46; 270/8)

This is a small, inconstantly-occurring node of 2–11 mm diameter, which is present in only one dog out of three. When present, it is situated at the insertion point of the tendon of the psoas minor muscle on the iliopectineal crest.
Drainage area: some of the lymphatic vessels of the femoral canal are filtered by this node. If the node is absent they continue to the iliosacral lymphocentre.
Efferent routes: to the medial iliac and sacral nodes.

Nl. femoralis of the dog
(261/47; 236/t)

This is usually absent but if present it is situated at the distal end of the femoral canal. In large dogs it is barely 1 cm in length, in small dogs only 2–3 mm.

Drainage area: skin lying medially over the knee joint, shank and foot; knee and hock joints; patella, bones of the shank and foot; Achilles tendon and tendons of the short digital extensors, interosseous muscles. It also receives secondary lymph from the popliteal node.

Efferent routes: the lymph from the femoral lymph node may pass to the iliofemoral or the medial iliac and sacral nodes.

Lymphocentrum inguinale superficiale (seu inguinofemorale)
Nll. inguinales superficiales of the dog
(nll. scrotales 261/49; 271/4)
(nll. mammarii 272/5; 273/1, 1')

In the male there are one to three, but usually two, nodes which measure 0.5–6.8 cm in length. They form a group which is palpable on the dorsolateral border of the penis in the subcutaneous connective tissue $\frac{1}{2}$ to 1 cm in front of the spermatic cord. In the bitch there is usually one, although not infrequently two, nodes of 1–2 cm length which are palpable dorsolateral to the mamma about 2–4 cm in front of the pecten of the pubis.

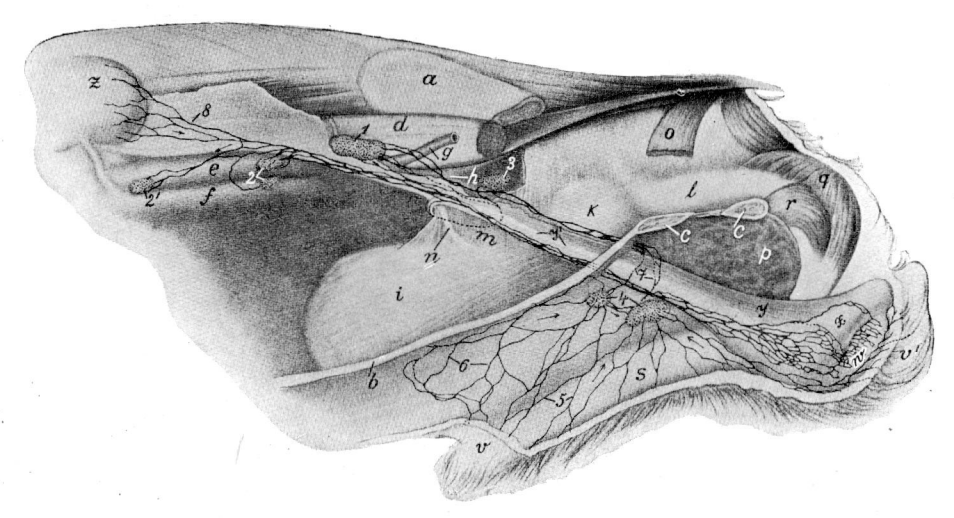

Fig. 271. Lymph nodes and lymph vessels of the urinary and male sex organs of the dog, in situ.
(After Baum, 1918.)
(The left abdominal and pelvic walls and the intestine have been removed)

1 nll. iliaci mediales, *2, 2'* nll. lumbales aortici, *3* nll. sacrales, *4* nll. inguinales superficiales (scrotales), *5, 6* lymph vessels of the prepuce, *7* vasa efferentia of the nll. inguinales superficiales, *8* lymph vessels of the renal capsule which, like the lymph vessels of the testis, go to the nll. lumbales aortici

a ilium (cut off), *b* ventral wall of the abdomen, *c, c* pelvic floor, *d* lumbar musculature, *e* aorta, *f* caudal v. cava, *g* left a. iliaca externa, *h* right a. iliaca interna, *i* urinary bladder, *k* prostate, *l* urethra, *m* lateral wall of the bladder, *n* ureter, *o* m. coccygeus (cut off), *p* cut surface of the m. adductor, *q* m. bulbospongiosus, *r* m. ischiocavernosus, *s* penis, *v* prepuce, *v'* skin of the scrotum, *w* testis, *x* epididymis, *y* spermatic cord, *y'* ductus deferens, *z* left kidney

Drainage area: the skin of the ventral abdomen from the costal arch onwards, skin of the prepuce and scrotum or, in the bitch, the posterior half of the mamma, skin of the pelvic outlet, tail, thigh, shank and foot; cutaneous musculature of the abdomen; vulva, clitoris and the caudal three of the five glands of the mammary complexes or, in the male, the scrotum, prepuce, penis, glans and urethra.

Efferent route: medial iliac lymph nodes.

Lymphocentrum popliteum
Nl. popliteus superficialis of the dog
(261/57; 263/5)

This is almost invariably only a single large node, up to 5 cm in length, lying in the flexor aspect of the knee between the biceps femoris and the semitendinosus muscles. As a rule it is situated immediately under the skin and fascia and it is therefore easily palpable.

Drainage area: skin plantar to the knee joint and shank, skin of the foot; bones of the shank and foot; distal parts of the posterior thigh muscles and the quadriceps femoris and all the short muscles as well as the tendons of the foot.

Efferent routes: lymph drains directly to the medial iliac nodes and to the femoral node if it is present.

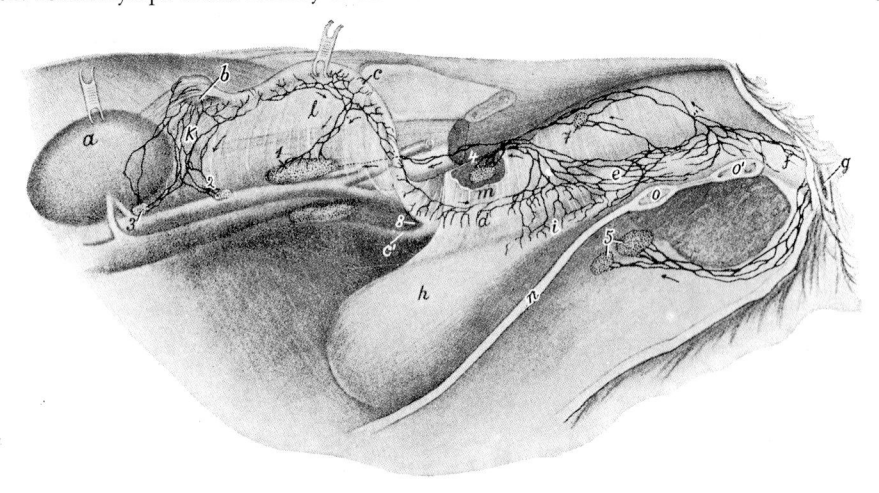

Fig. 272. Lymph nodes and lymph vessels of the female genital organs of the bitch.
(After Baum, 1918.)

1 nll. iliaci mediales, *2, 3* nll. lumbales aortici, *4, 7* nll. sacrales, *5* nll. inguinales superficiales (mammarici), *8* lymph vessel curving onto the dorsomedial surface of the uterine horn

a left kidney (reflected), *b* left ovary within the bursa ovarica (seen from the medial surface), *c* left uterine horn (lifted up), *c'* right horn of the uterus, *d* body of the uterus, *e* vagina, *f* vestibulum vaginae, *g* vulva, *h* urinary bladder, *i* urethra, *k* ligamentum suspensorium ovarii, *l* ligamentum latum uteri, *m* ligamentum vesicae laterale, *n* ventral wall of the abdomen, *o, o'* floor of the pelvis

Lymph collecting ducts
Ductus thoracicus of the dog
(252; 261/60; 264/15, 15'; 265/11)

The thoracic duct arises from cisterna chyli by one, two or even three roots. Initially it lies to the right of and dorsal to the thoracic aorta and it passes through the diaphragm at the aortic hiatus. It runs ventral to the right azygos vein as far as the 5th or 6th thoracic vertebra, passes dorsally over the aorta to the left side and continues on the left of the oesophagus to the thoracic inlet. When there is only one trunk the lumen is uniformly 3–4 mm in diameter. However, a double thoracic duct is not uncommon in the dog (see fig. 252), and the second duct then lies to the left and dorsal to the aorta and is linked to the right duct by cross anastomoses. The intercostal arteries pass through the meshes of these anastomoses. The left part can form into a coarse network; it lies between the costocervical and vertebral arteries and veins laterally, and the left common carotid artery medially. Its terminal part has an ampulla-like dilatation but, immediately before it enters the venous angle, it reduces so much in diameter that in a large dog the actual termination is not more than 1 mm wide.

The thoracic duct empties into the left common jugular vein, usually from a dorsal direction but sometimes from lateral or ventral. In large dogs this junction is situated 1–3 cm cranial to the 1st rib. In the majority of cases the terminal piece divides into two, or sometimes three or four, branches which are interconnected by a very variable arrangement of cross anastomoses. The thoracic duct has valves at intervals of about 1–3 cm as far as the 11th or 12th thoracic vertebra, caudal to which none are found. The valves close the lumen completely even in dead animals.

Fig. 273. Lymph nodes and lymph vessels of the mammary glands of the bitch. (After Baum, 1918.)

1 nll. inguinalis superficialis seu mammaricus (retracted somewhat from beneath the mammary gland), *1'* nl. inguinalis superficialis (covered by the mamma), *2* nl. axillaris accessorius, *3, 3* glandular tissue, *4, 4* teasts, *5* m. obliquus externus abdominis

a, a parenchymal lymph vessels rising onto the surface, *b, b* lymph vessels protruding from the base of the mammary complex, *c, c* cutaneous lymph vessels going deep into the tissues (the remaining lymph vessels are skin and teat lymph vessels), *d* lymph vessels going to the nl. axillaris propius, *e, e', e"* lymph vessels going deep and to the nl. sternalis cranialis

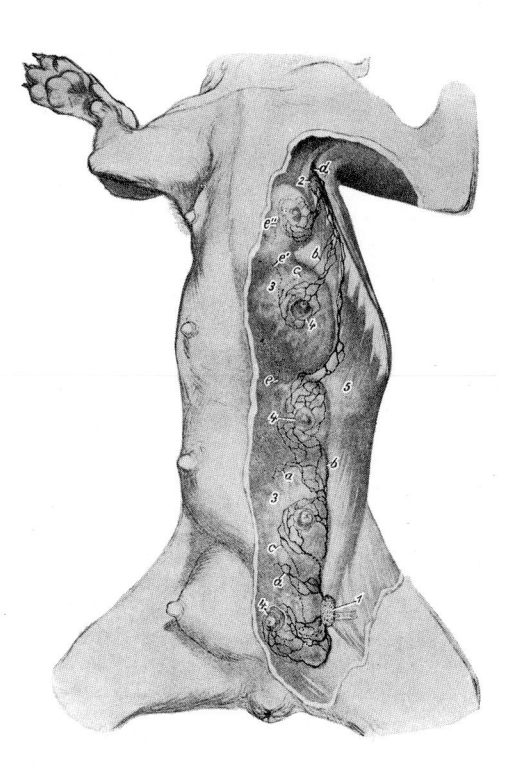

Cisterna chyli of the dog
(254/*Cc*; 268/*12*; 270/*9*)

The cisterna chyli extends from the 4th to the 1st lumbar vertebrae. Its shape is subject to considerable variation. It is generally a sack-like structure which usually lies dorsal and to the right of the abdominal aorta between the crura of the diaphragm and the lumbar musculature. It is often perforated by the lumbar arteries. Sometimes the sack also extends to the lateral and ventral surfaces of the aorta. The lumbar trunk, which is usually double or net-like, terminates at the caudal end and the visceral trunk empties by one or more branches into the cisterna chyli from ventral. The cranial end merges into the thoracic duct. The cisterna is free of valves.

Truncus visceralis of the dog
(254/*Tv*; 261/*62*; 268/*13*)

The stout visceral trunk is very variable in shape and it arises from a network which is formed by the efferent vessels of the lymph nodes of the coeliac and cranial mesenteric lymphocentres. The confluence of the network is variable and it ends in two or three stout, or a number of smaller, branches which enter at about the middle of the cisterna chyli. Sometimes a distinct truncus is not developed at all and the efferent vessels then weave about on the right and left of the aorta and enter the cisterna chyli dorsal to the aorta.

Truncus lumbales of the dog
(260/*Tl*; 261/*61*; 268/*11*; 270/*10*)

As a rule there are two net-like interconnected ducts of which the larger runs along the left dorsal border of the aorta whereas the more slender one runs along its right ventral border. The left dorsal duct may sometimes be absent. Both originate from the medial iliac lymph nodes.

Truncus jugularis of the dog
(248/f; 249/Tj; 261/59; 265)

The left and right tracheal trunks (*truncus jugularis; truncus trachealis*) of the dog arise from the efferent vessels of the medial retropharyngeal lymph node of the appropriate side. When full they measure 2.5–4 mm in diameter. The ductus jugularis sinister follows the trachea and oesophagus on the left side, while the ductus jugularis dexter lies to the right of the trachea. Both ducts go towards the thorax in company with the common carotid artery and the internal jugular vein. It is not unusual for the main trunk to be double for part of, or almost its entire, length. Towards its termination the left duct is joined by the efferent vessels of the superficial cervical lymph nodes and sometimes also those of the axillary nodes. It empties in a very variable pattern into the thoracic duct. After receiving the lymphatic vessels from the right superficial nodes, the right duct terminates by becoming the right lymphatic duct.

Ductus lymphaticus dexter of the dog
(265/12)

This duct measures some 1.5 cm in length and 4–6 mm in diameter; it terminates in the right subclavian vein. Alternatively it can divide and terminate in the venous angle. Usually the right lymphatic duct also receives efferent vessels from the right axillary nodes, from the cranial mediastinal nodes and from the cranial sternal node.

Lymph nodes and lymph collecting ducts of the cat

The lymph nodes of the cat have not hitherto been of great importance in clinical diagnosis because insufficient information has been available about their occurrence, position and size. However, the investigations of Sugimura, Kudo and Takahata (1955–1960) have provided us with reliable data which has been included in this textbook after some revision of nomenclature. It must be pointed out that the occurrence and arrangement of the lymph nodes of the cat sometimes differ substantially from those of the dog.

Lymphocentrum parotideum
Nl. parotideus of the cat
(274/1)

As a rule there is a single parotid lymph node but very rarely there are two or more and rarely it is absent altogether. Most frequently it is flat and disc-like with a maximum diameter of between 0.1 and 0.8 cm. It lies against the superficial temporal vein at the cranial border of the parotid gland or hidden in the glandular tissue.

Drainage area: the upper, and parts of the lower, eyelid, the parotid gland and other parts of the upper half of the head.

Efferent route: to the lateral retropharyngeal nodes.

Lymphocentrum mandibulare
Nll. mandibulares et nll. mandibulares accessorii of the cat
(274/3, 3')

There are usually two large mandibular nodes lying medial and lateral to the facial vein under cover of the cutaneous muscle. Less commonly 1–4 smaller accessory mandibular nodes lie behind the caudal pole of the larger ones. The larger lateral nodes are 0.4 to 1.9 cm in length and the medial ones are 0.25–2.4 cm in length. The smaller nodes are 0.05–0.35 cm in length.

Drainage area: the upper and lower lips, chin region, mouth cavity, cheek glands, eyelids. Sometimes also secondary lymph from the parotid and lateral retropharyngeal nodes.

Efferent routes: the mandibular and accessory mandibular nodes are linked by their efferent vessels in a variable pattern. The mandibular lymphocentre passes its lymph partly to the medial retropharyngeal and partly to the ventral superficial cervical nodes or, if the latter are absent, to the dorsal superficial cervical nodes.

Lymphocentrum retropharyngeum
Nl. retropharyngeus medialis of the cat
(274/4)

This kidney-shaped node has a maximum diameter of 0.15–2.25 cm and is regularly present on each side of the body. It lies against the pharynx and is flanked by the internal jugular vein.

Drainage area: the oral cavity including the tongue; proximal part of the cervical sections of the oesophagus and trachea; thyroid and mandibular glands and part of the parotid gland. It also receives secondary lymph from all the cranial nodes.

Efferent routes: its efferent vessels form the jugular trunk (274/7). Some efferent vessels appear, however, to join with both groups of superficial cervical nodes.

Nll. retropharyngei laterales of the cat
(274/2)

There may be from 1 to 7 of these nodes although the average number is 3 to 4, and they are of very variable shape. Most frequently they are club-shaped but spherical nodes are also seen. The diameter of the individual nodes varies between 0.05 and 3.1 cm. They are embedded in the adipose tissue which occurs behind the parotid gland where they lie along the caudal auricular vein.

Drainage area: region of the ear and parotid gland; in some cases lips and eyelids, surface of the platysma and other areas of the upper half of the head and nape.

Efferent routes: it drains mainly into the medial retropharyngeal lymph node but to some extent also into the mandibular lymphocentre and the superficial cervical nodes.

Lymphocentrum cervicale superficiale
Nll. cervicales superficiales dorsales of the cat
(274/5; 275B/2)

One to three, but usually two, flat elliptical nodes with a maximum diameter of 0.1–3.2 cm are situated in the adipose tissue in front of and below the cervical part of the trapezius muscle and under the omotransversarius muscle.

Drainage area: dorsal area of the neck and the forelimb. It also receives secondary lymph from the ventral superficial node and in some cases from the medial retropharyngeal and lateral pharyngeal nodes. If, in exceptional cases, the ventral superficial cervical node is absent, then the lymphatic vessels from the areas usually drained by it, and especially the efferent vessels of the mandibular nodes, go directly to this dorsal superficial cervical node.

Efferent routes: to the terminal part of the jugular trunk or directly into the venous angle.

Nl. cervicalis superficialis ventralis of the cat
(274/5; 275A/1; 275B/1; 241/2)

There is usually one (seldom two) oval node with a maximum diameter of 0.1–1.5 cm situated on the external jugular vein close to the point of origin of the superficial cervical vein. This node is nearly always present.

Drainage area: ventral part of the neck, thoracic inlet and secondary lymph from the mandibular lymphocentre and from the lateral, sometimes also the medial, retropharyngeal nodes.

Efferent routes: terminal part of the jugular trunk or the venous angle.

Lymphocentrum cervicale profundum
Nl. cervicalis profundus medius of the cat
(274/6; 241/3)

This small round node is present in less than one cat in four and it occurs only unilaterally. It measures 0.1–0.45 cm in diameter. This inconstant node is placed against the cervical part of the trachea and the internal jugular vein at about halfway up the neck.

Drainage area: the thyroid gland and cervical parts of the trachea and oesophagus. Secondary lymph from the medial retropharyngeal node.

Efferent route: to the jugular trunk.

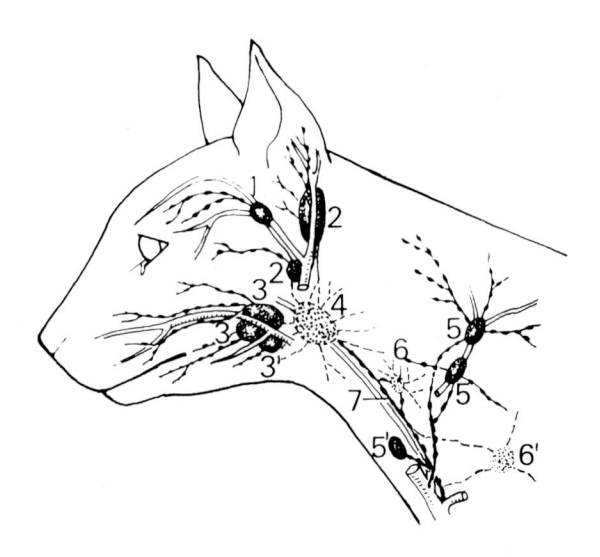

Fig. 274. Lymph nodes and lymph vessels of the head and neck of the cat.
(Diagrammatic, redrawn after Sugimura, Kudo and Takahata, 1955.)

1 nl. parotideus, *2* nll. retropharyngei laterales, *3* nll. mandibulares, *3'* nll. mandibulares accessorii, *4* nl. retropharyngeus medialis, *5* nll. cervicalis superficiales dorsales, *5'* nl. cervicalis superficialis ventralis, *6* nl. cervicalis profundus medius, *6'* nll. cervicales profundi caudales, *7* truncus jugularis

Nll. cervicales profundi caudales of the cat
(274/6; 241/4)

One to six (usually two to four) flat, roundish or elliptical nodes of 0.1–1.3 cm diameter are found regularly on the ventral surface of the trachea near the thoracic inlet, at the bifurcation of the brachiocephalic veins.

Drainage area: trachea, oesophagus, thyroid gland. Secondary lymph from nodes of the mediastinal, bronchial and ventral thoracic lymphocentres and from the middle deep cervical node. Secondary branches of the terminal part of the jugular trunk also enter these nodes.

Efferent routes: venous angle, terminal part of the lymph collecting ducts.

Lymphocentre axillare
Nl. axillaris proprius of the cat
(249/Ap; 275A/4)

At the fork between the lateral thoracic and the axillary veins one can regularly find one or two flat, elliptical nodes of 0.1–2 cm diameter.

Drainage area: skin and subcutaneous region of the medial aspect of the upper and lower arm, the lateral thoracic wall and occasionally also the palmar aspect of the forelimb. Secondary lymph from the accessory axillary nodes.

Efferent routes: from this node lymph goes partly to the inconstantly-present axillary node of the first rib and partly to the venous angle.

Nl. axillaris primae costae of the cat
(249/Apc; 275A/3)

This small, inconstant, slightly flattened and rounded node, measuring about 1–4.5 mm in diameter, lies against the axillary vein.

Drainage area: lateral wall of the thorax; skin of the upper and lower arm. Secondary lymph is received from the proper axillary node; occasionally it may receive a secondary branch of the jugular trunk.

Efferent route: venous angle.

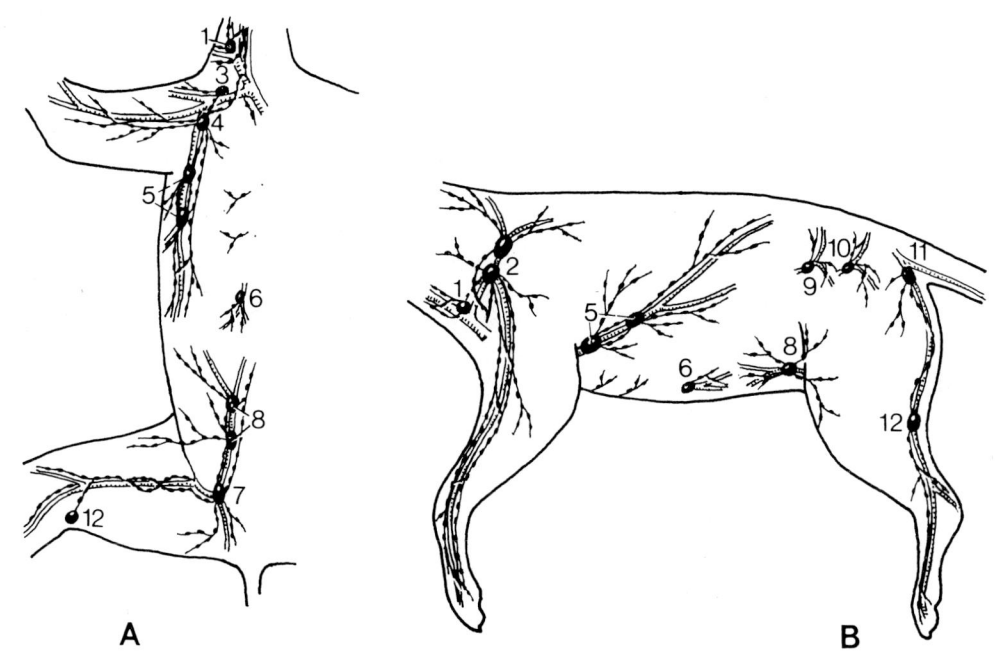

Fig. 275. Diagrammatic representation of the superficial lymph nodes and lymph vessels of the trunk and limbs of the cat. A ventral view, B left lateral view. (Redrawn after Sugimura, Kudo and Takahata, 1956.)
1 nl. cervicalis superficialis ventralis, *2* nll. cervicales superficiales dorsales (only in Fig. B), *3* nl. axillaris primae costae (A), *4* nl. axillaris proprius (A), *5* nll. axillares accessorii, *6* nl. epigastricus cranialis, *7* nl. inguinalis superficialis (A), *8* nll. epigastrici caudales, *9* nl. subiliacus, *10* nl. femoralis (B), *11* nl. ischiadicus (B), *12* nl. popliteus superficialis

Nll. axillares accessorii of the cat
(249/Aa; 275A/5; 275B/5)

Along the lateral thoracic vein from the level of the 3rd to 6th intercostal spaces there are as many as 7, but usually 3 to 5, ellipsoidal nodes.

Drainage area: skin of the inside of the upper and lower forelimbs, the lumbar region and the lateral and dorsal chest wall; lymph vessels from the mamma.

Efferent route: to the proper axillary node.

Lymphocentrum thoracicum dorsale
Nll. thoracici aortici of the cat
(276/1)

One to five round nodes occur in barely more than half of all cats. They are usually present on only one side, on the ventral surface of the thoracic vertebrae, particularly the more distal thoracic vertebrae. Their diameter varies from 0.5–5 mm.

Drainage area: peritoneum; they may also receive secondary lymph from the inconstant intercostal node.
Efferent route: to the thoracic duct.

Nl. intercostalis of the cat
(276/2)

Very infrequently there is one round node of 0.8–2 mm diameter at the dorsal end of the intercostal space. In quite exceptional cases two nodes may occur.
Drainage area: the pleura.
Efferent route: to the thoracic duct.

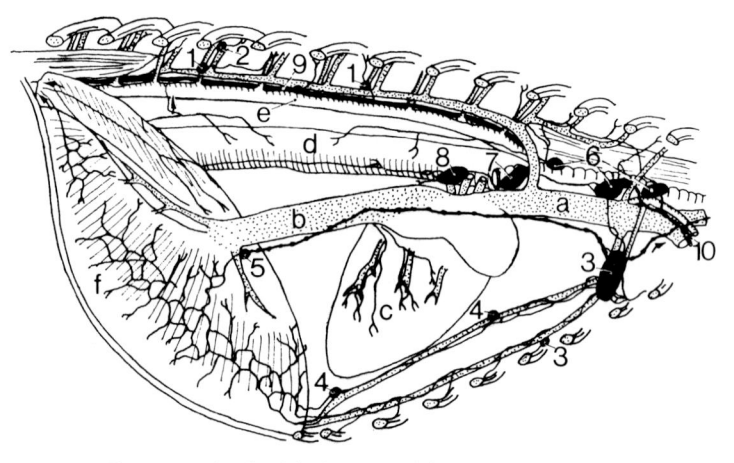

Fig. 276. Lymph nodes of the thoracic cavity of the cat. Right lateral view.
(Redrawn after Sugimura, Kudo and Takahata, 1959.)
1 nll. thoracici aortici, *2* nl. intercostalis, *3* nll. sternales craniales, *4* nll. sternales caudales, *5* nl. phrenicus, *6* nll. mediastinales craniales, *7* nl. bifurcationis dexter, *8* nl. bifurcationis medius, *9* ductus thoracicus, *10* ductus lymphaticus dexter

a cranial v. cava, *b* caudal v. cava, *c* heart, *d* oesophagus, *e* aorta thoracica, *f* diaphragm

Lymphocentrum thoracicum ventrale
Nl. sternalis cranialis of the cat
(276/3)

Lying along the internal thoracic artery and vein at the level of the 2nd, somtimes even up to the 4th, intercostal space there is regularly one node of 0.1–1.5 cm diameter. Occasionally as many as 5 nodes may be present.
Drainage area: ventral thoracic and abdominal wall, diaphragm and pericardium. Secondary lymph is received from the inconstant caudal sternal and phrenic nodes and also from the cranial mediastinal and caudal deep cervical nodes.
Efferent routes: this gland drains into the terminal part of the thoracic duct or the right lymphatic duct. It may also empty directly into the venous angle or indirectly to the cranial mediastinal nodes. There appears to be an anastomosis with the lumbar aortic nodes via the diaphragmatic lymphatic vessels.

Nl. sternalis caudalis of the cat
(276/4)

In about one cat out of four there is one round node of 1–3.5 mm diameter on the sternum, near the apex or the cranial surface of the pericardium. Two nodes may be infrequently observed.
Drainage area: pleura, pericardium, diaphragm.
Efferent route: to the cranial sternal node.

Nl. epigastricus cranialis of the cat
(275A/6; 275B/6)

This small node is found only in very exceptional cases. It lies behind the xyphoid cartilage over the rectus abdominis muscle.

Lymphocentrum mediastinale
Nll. mediastinales craniales of the cat
(241/5; 276/6)

At the level of the first and second ribs there are between 2 and 8 nodes, each of 0.1–2 cm diameter, and this large group of thoracic lymph nodes is constantly present in the precardiac mediastinum. Regularly occurring on the right side as far as the termination of the right azygos vein, there are another 1–3 nodes which measure 0.1–1 cm in diameter. This second group is inconstant on the left side.

Drainage area: heart, trachea, thymus, oesophagus, pleura, pericardium. Secondary lymph is received from the cranial sternal node, the bronchial and dorsal thoracic lymphocentres and the thoracic duct can occasionally give off a secondary branch to it.

Efferent routes: its outflowing vessels terminate independently in the venous angle or in the terminal part of the large lymph collecting ducts.

Nl. phrenicus of the cat
(276/5)

Beneath the diaphragmatic pleura, near the foramen venae cavae, is an inconstant and usually single node which measures 1.5–8.5 mm in diameter. It is present in about 25% of all cats.

Drainage area: diaphragm.
Efferent route: to the cranial sternal node.

Lymphocentrum bronchale
Nl. bifurcationis seu tracheobronchalis dexter of the cat
(276/7; 241/6)

Nl. bifurcationis seu tracheobronchalis sinister of the cat
(241/7)

Nl. bifurcationis seu tracheobronchalis medius of the cat
(276/8; 241/8)

There is a node lying respectively right, left and caudal to the point of division of the trachea into its primary bronchi. They are between 0.15 and 1.4 cm diameter. Sometimes two nodes occur at each location.

Drainage area: mainly the lung, but also the heart, pericardium, mediastinum and diapragm.

Efferent routes: to the cranial mediastinal nodes, sometimes directly to the thoracic duct or the venous angle.

Nl. pulmonalis of the cat
(241/9)

This node is only present in one cat in three in which it lies on the primary bronchus. It measures 2–6 mm in diameter. It is sometimes paired.

Drainage area: lungs.
Efferent route: tracheobronchial nodes.

Lymphocentrum lumbale
Nll. lumbales aortici of the cat
(278/1, 1')

Several lymph nodes are to be found in rows on either side of the abdominal aorta. The group situated cranial to the renal artery is always present and consists of 2–5, sometimes up to 7, nodes. Caudal to the renal artery there are usually 3–7 nodes, although up to 10 may occur and even 19 nodes have been recorded in an exceptional case. However, this caudal group may occasionally be entirely lacking. The individual nodes are rounded or elongated and measure 0.1–1.8 cm.

Drainage area: diaphragm, kidneys, adrenals, dorsal abdominal wall, ovary, oviduct and uterus or testes. Secondary lymph is received from the iliofemoral lymphocentre and through some vessels from the coeliac, cranial mesenteric and caudal mesenteric lymphocentres.

Efferent routes: lymph flows to the cisterna chyli and the lumbar trunks. However, there is also a connection with the cranial sternal lymph node via the diaphragmatic lymphatic vessels.

Lymphocentrum coeliacum
Nll. lienales of the cat
(277/1)

There are one to three roundish nodes lying along the splenic vein in the majority of cats and they vary between 0.2 and 2.2 cm in diameter.

Drainage area: spleen, greater curvature of the stomach and left lobe of the pancreas.

Efferent route: visceral trunk and hepatic nodes.

Nll. gastrici of the cat
(277/2)

There are almost always 1–4 roundish or elliptical nodes, 0.1–2.0 cm in length, situated on the lesser curvature of the stomach between the cardia and pylorus.

Drainage area: stomach, liver and oesophagus.

Efferent routes: lymph passes to the visceral trunk and the hepatic lymph nodes. There is apparently also a link with the cranial sternal node via the diaphragm.

Nll. hepatici (seu portales) of the cat
(277/3)

Two to four, although sometimes even as many as eight, roundish or elliptical nodes which are between 0.2 and 3 cm in diameter are generally grouped around the portal, splenic and gastroduodenal veins close to their junction.

Drainage area: liver, greater curvature of the stomach, oesophagus, diaphragm, body and left lobe of the pancreas and cranial part of the duodenum. It also receives secondary lymph from all peripheral nodes of the coeliac lymphocentre.

Efferent route: to the visceral trunk.

Nl. pancreaticoduodenalis of the cat
(277/4)

This elongated node is always present on the cranial pancreaticoduodenal vein. It is 0.3–1.5 cm in diameter. Sometimes two nodes are present.

Drainage area: pylorus, duodenum, body and right lobe of the pancreas.

Efferent routes: hepatic lymph nodes and via the diaphragmatic lymphatic vessels to the cranial sternal node.

Lymphocentrum mesentericum craniale
Nll. jejunales of the cat
(277/5, 5')

A large group of nodes (277/5) consisting of 2–5, sometimes even as many as 20, individual nodes, extends from the root of the mesentery on both sides of the jejunal arteries and veins far into the mesojejunum in all cats. This group is always present. Individual nodes may attain a length of up to 8 cm. In 50 per cent of cats there are smaller nodes (277/5') of 1–9 mm length located in the distal mesentery near the jejunum and, especially, near the ileum.

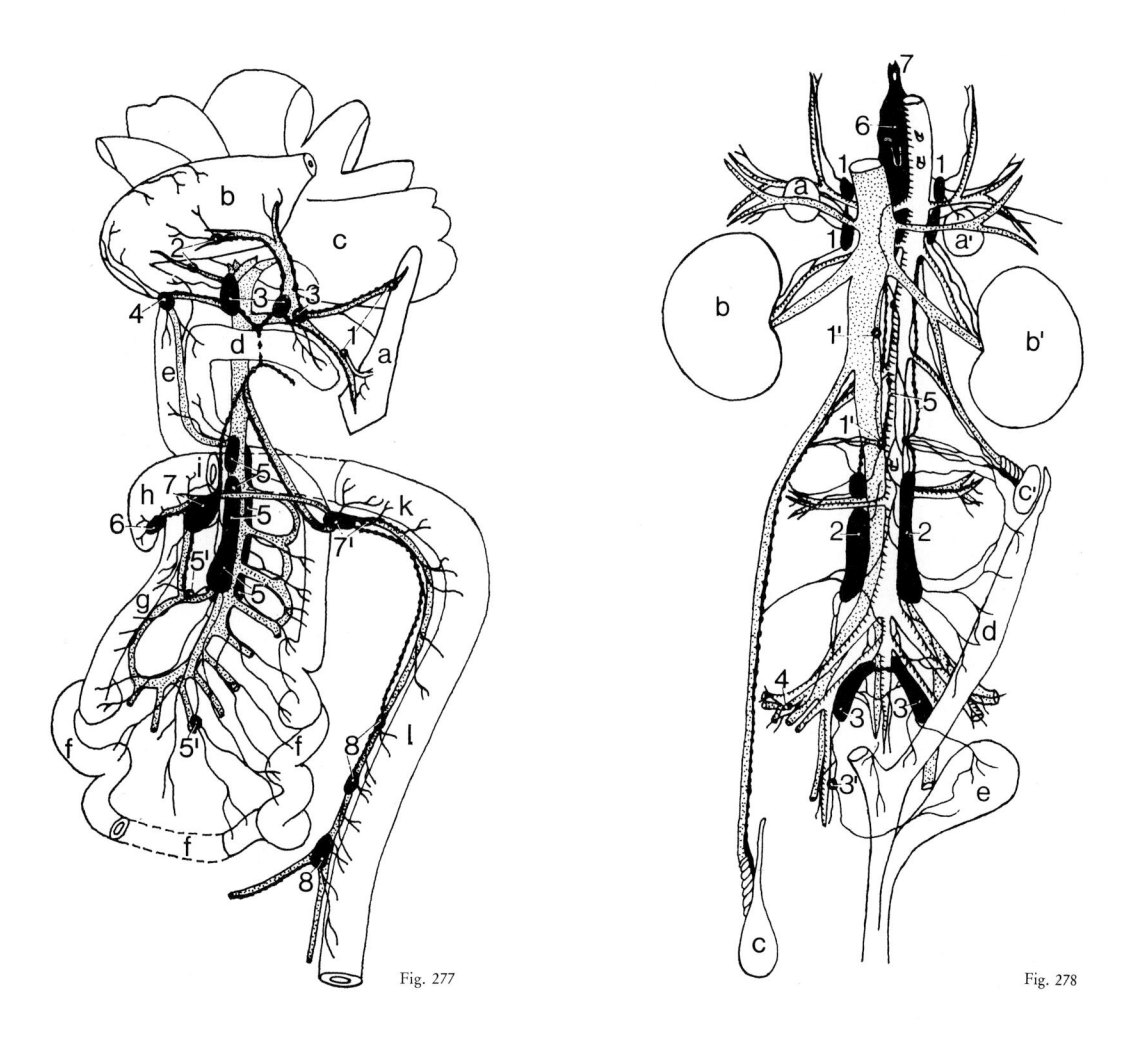

Fig. 277

Fig. 278

Fig. 277. Lymph nodes of the stomach and gut of the cat. Ventral view.
(Redrawn after Sugimura, Kudo and Takahata, 1958.)
1 nll. lienales, *2* nll. gastrici, *3* nll. hepatici, *4* nl. pancreaticoduodenalis, *5, 5'* nll. jejunales, *6* nll. caecales, *7, 7'* nll. colici, *8* nll. mesenterici caudales.
a spleen, *b* stomach, *c* liver, *d* pancreas, *e* duodenum, *f* jejunum, *g* ileum, *h* caecum, *i* colon ascendens, *k* colon transversum, *l* colon descendens; branches of the portal vein stipped

Fig. 278. Lymph nodes of the urogenital apparatus and lymph vessels of the lumbar and sacral regions of the cat. Ventral view.
(Redrawn after Sugimura, Kudo and Takahata, 1958.)
(This diagram shows the genital organs of the male on one side and those of the female on the other)
1 nll. lumbales aortici (constant), *1'* more nll. lumbales aortici (inconstant), *2* nll. iliaci mediales, *3* nll. sacrales (constant), *3'* more nll. sacrales (inconstant), *4* nl. iliofemoralis, *5* truncus lumbalis, *6* cisterna chyli, *7* ductus thoracicus
a right and *a'* left adrenals, *b* right and *b'* left kidneys, *c* testis, *c'* ovary, *d* uterus, *e* urinary bladder

Drainage area: entire small intestine and the body of the pancreas. It receives secondary lymph from the caudal mesenteric nodes.
Efferent route: to the visceral trunk.

Nll. caecales of the cat
(277/6)

On both sides of the caecum we generally find two (1–3) nodes which are 0.3–1.4 cm in length.
Drainage area: caecum, ileum; secondary lymph from the neighbouring colic nodes.
Efferent routes: jejunal nodes and lumbar trunks.

Nll. colici of the cat
(277/7, 7')

In the mesentery of the ascending and transverse colon there are regularly 3–9, sometimes even more, nodes which are 0.3 to 3.0 cm in diameter.
Drainage area: ileum, ascending and transverse colon, parts of the descending colon and the caecum. Secondary lymph is received from the caudal mesenteric and jejunal nodes.
Efferent route: lumbar trunks.

Lymphocentrum mesentericum caudale
Nll. mesenterici caudales of the cat
(277/8)

In the mesentery of the descending colon, near the division of the caudal mesenteric artery, there are always 1–3, and sometimes up to 5, elongated nodes of 0.5–1.5 cm diameter.
Drainage area: descending colon and rectum.
Efferent routes: colic nodes and lumbar trunks as well as lumbar aortic lymph nodes.

Lymphocentrum iliosacrale
Nll. iliaci mediales of the cat
(278/2)

On both sides of the abdominal aorta, between the origin of the deep circumflex iliac arteries and the aortic bifurcation, there are regularly 2–4 ribbon-like nodes with individual lengths of between 0.1 and 2.8 cm. Infrequently, more than 4 nodes may be found.
Drainage area: pelvic wall, pelvic limb; uterus and sometimes oviduct or testes; urinary bladder. Secondary lymph enters these nodes from all lymphocentres to be described below.
Efferent routes: the outgoing vessels form mainly the lumbar trunks but some of them go to the lumbar aortic nodes.

Nll. sacrales of the cat
(278/3, 3')

1–3, but even up to 6, nodes are arranged in a horse-shoe manner around the aorta immediately after the origin of the internal iliac arteries. Each of these nodes is between 0.1 and 2.8 cm long. Besides these one cat in three has smaller, roundish nodes of 0.1 to 0.5 cm diameter, lying along the further course of the internal iliac artery on the roof and lateral wall of the pelvis.
Drainage area: rectum, uterus, vagina, urinary bladder, ureter, wall of the pelvis, pelvic outlet, tail and hind limbs. Secondary lymph is also drawn from the inconstantly-present iliofemoral node.
Efferent route: to the medial iliac nodes.

Lymphocentrum inguinale profundum (seu iliofemorale)
Nl. iliofemoralis of the cat
(278/4)

This small, roundish node, 0.1 to 0.5 cm in diameter, is rarely present near the entrance to the femoral canal.
Drainage area: parts of the neighbouring ventral abdominal wall and some lymph vessels from the hind limb. Secondary lymph also drains from the superficial inguinal and popliteal lymph nodes.
Efferent routes: to the medial iliac and sacral nodes.

Nl. femoralis of the cat
(275B/10)

This node, measuring only 1–3 mm in diameter, is rare. When present, it occurs on the lateral circumflex femoral artery and vein between the tensor fasciae latae and sartorius muscles.
Drainage area: gluteal region and thigh.
Efferent route: to the iliosacral lymphocentre.

Lymphocentrum inguinale superficiale (seu inguinofemorale)
Nl. inguinalis superficialis of the cat
(275A/7)

This is a constant node which is related to the external pudendal artery and vein in the femoral canal. Occasionally it is duplicated. Its shape is elongated.
Drainage area: lymph vessels of the inguinal and gluteal regions; in females also the posterior half of the mamma.
Efferent route: iliosacral lymphocentre.

Nll. epigastrici caudales of the cat
(275A, 275B/8)

These 1–3, or sometimes up to 5, nodes occur almost constantly on the ventral abdominal wall alongside the caudal epigastric artery and vein. They are ellipsoidal and 0.1 to 2.5 cm in length.
Drainage area: caudal part of the ventral abdominal wall and subcutis of the thigh.
Efferent routes: superficial inguinal node and the ventral thoracic lymphocentre.

Nl. subiliacus of the cat
(275B/9)

This node, 1–5 mm in length, is only occasionally found. If present it is situated on the posterior branch of the deep circumflex iliac artery and vein.

Lymphocentrum ischiadicum
Nl. ischiadicus of the cat
(275B/11)

This node is situated on the caudal gluteal artery and vein and is 0.1 to 1 cm in diameter. It is almost constantly present.
Drainage area: skin, subcutis and fasciae of the thigh; lymphatic vessels of the anal region; deeper lymphatics of the hind limb; secondary lymph from the popliteal node.
Efferent route: iliosacral lymphocentre.

Lymphocentrum popliteum
Nl. popliteus superficialis of the cat
(275A, 275B/*12*)

This constant, rounded node, 0.1 to 1.2 cm in diameter, lies subcutaneously in the flexor region of the knee.
Drainage area: hind foot, skin, subcutis of the shank.
Efferent routes: iliofemoral lymphocentre and ischiatic node.

Lymph collecting ducts
Ductus thoracicus of the cat
(241/*Dt*; 276/*9*; 278/*7*)

The thoracic duct arises between the crura of the diaphragm from the cisterna chyli. Above the dorsal surface of the thoracic aorta it forms a rope-ladder-like system through the meshes of which pass the intercostal arteries. A single trunk is formed as it passes over to the left side of the aortic arch. However, this trunk may again split into individual branches before it enters the venous angle.

Cisterna chyli of the cat
(241/*Cc*; 278/*6*)

The cisterna chyli is 0.7–3 cm long, sack-like and lies between the renal vessels and the crura of the diaphragm on the dorsal surface of the abdominal aorta.
The other lymph collecting ducts behave substantially like those of the dog.

Lymph nodes and lymph collecting ducts of the pig

The lymph vascular system of the pig is of considerable practical importance in meat inspection. In Germany at any rate, the pig is numerically the most important slaughter animal.

Attention has already been drawn to the morphological peculiarity of the lymph nodes of this species in which the course of the afferent and efferent lymph vessels has resulted in "inversion" of cortex and medulla. The lymph nodes of pigs also differ from those of other domestic mammals in number, form and size. In respect of the number per group they take up an intermediate position between the dog and ox in which there is usually only one large node, and the horse in which numerous small nodes are present. In young pigs most of the groups consist of a large number of small nodes but in older pigs the number of individual nodes is reduced, presumably as a result of fusion. This would explain the distinctly lobulated form of the large nodes in older pigs and the considerable variation in the number and size of the individual nodes of comparable groups.

The comprehensive monograph of Baum and Grau (1938) and various papers by Egehoj (1935 to 1937) and other workers, contain detailed information which forms the basis of the following account.

Lymphocentrum parotideum
Nll. parotidei of the pig
(245B/*P*; 279/*1*; 280/*c, c'*; 282/*5*)

This usually comprises one or two nodes but infrequently even six nodes have been found. Depending on the age of the animal, they measure from 0.5 to 5.5 cm or more in length. They are situated ventral to the mandibular joint behind the ramus of the mandible on the maxillary artery. At meat inspection this node should always be examined.
Drainage area: skin over the parietal, frontal, parotid and masseter regions, over the cheek, upper lip and external nares; most of the facial muscles, the masticatory and cutaneous muscles of the face;

numerous skull bones; mandibular joint; hard palate, gums, nasal cavity, eyelids and external ear; parotid, mandibular and lacrimal glands.

Efferent routes: the lymph drains mainly to the medial retropharyngeal nodes; also to the lateral retropharyngeal nodes and occasionally directly to the ventral superficial cervical nodes.

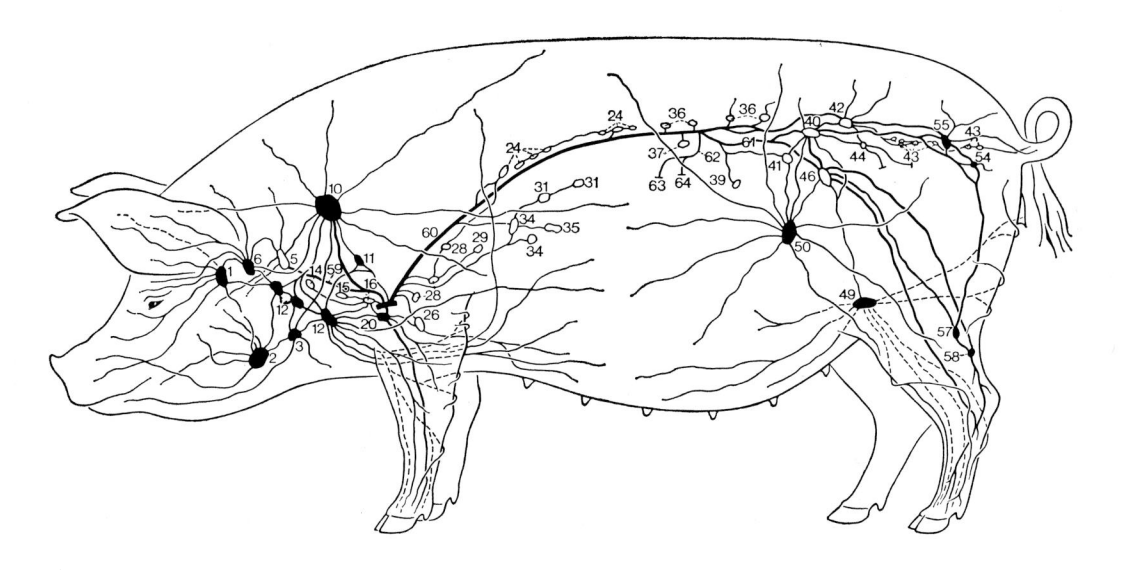

Fig. 279. Diagrammatic outline of the lymph nodes of the pig.
(After Wilkens and Münster, 1972.)
The nodes of the abdominal viscera are excluded.

lc. parotideum: *1* nll. parotidei; lc. mandibulare: *2* nll. mandibulares, *3* nll. mandibulares accessorii; lc. retropharyngeum: *5* nl. retropharyngeus medialis, *6* nll. retropharyngei laterales; lc. cervicale superficiale: *10* nll. cervicales superficiales dorsales, *11* nll. cervicales superficiales medii, *12* nll. cervicales superficiales ventrales; lc. cervicale profundum: *14* nll. cervicales profundi craniales, *15* nll. cervicales profundi medii (inconstant), *16* nll. cervicales profundi caudales; lc. axillare: *20* nll. axillares primae costae; lc. thoracicum dorsale: *24* nll. thoracici aortici; lc. thoracicum ventrale: *26* nll. sternales craniales; lc. mediastinale: *28* nll. mediastinales craniales, *29* nll. mediastinales which are situated on the pericardium, *31* nll. mediastinales caudales; lc. bronchale: nll. tracheobronchales (bifurcationis) sinistri, *35* nll. tracheobronchales (bifurcationis) medii; lc. lumbale: *36* nll. lumbales aortici, *37* nll. renales; lc. iliosacrale: *40* nll. iliaci mediales, *41* nll. iliaci laterales, *42* nll. sacrales, *43* nll. anorectales (inconstant), *44* nl. urogenitalis; lc. iliofemorale (inguinale profundum): *46* nll. iliofemorales; lc. inguinofemorale (inguinale superficiale): *49* nll. inguinales superficiales (nll. scrotales [♂], nll. mammarii [♀]), *50* nll. subiliaci; lc. ischiadicum: *54* nll. ischiadici, *55* nl. glutaeus; lc. popliteum: *57* nll. poplitei profundi (inconstant), *58* nll. poplitei superficiales (not entirely constant), *59* truncus jugularis, *60* ductus thoracicus, *61* truncus lumbalis, *62* truncus visceralis, *63* truncus coeliacus, *64* truncus intestinalis

Lymphocentrum mandibulare
Nll. mandibulares of the pig
(245B/*M*; 279/2; 280/*a*; 281/*a*; 282/*I*)

This flat group is formed by 2–6 nodes lying close together. According to the age of the animal, the individual nodes vary from 0.75–5 cm in length. The measurements of the whole group are 4–6 cm in length and 2–3 cm in breadth and thickness.

Laterally the group of lymph nodes is covered by the ventral border of the parotid gland. It lies under and medial to the linguofacial vein on the sternohyoideus muscle at the level of the mandibular angle. The mandibular gland can be found immediately behind and partially under this group of lymph nodes. The nodes should always be examined during meat inspection.

Drainage area: skin of the intermandibular space, the nasal, lip, cheek and masseter regions; the facialis muscles of the lip and cheek regions; muscles of mastication and those of the intermandibular region; muscles of the tongue and hyoid bone; numerous skull bones; external nares and snout; lips, cheeks and their glands, tongue, oral mucosa and gums, soft and hard palate, pharyngeal lymphatic ring; nasal cavity, larynx; parotid, sublingual and mandibular glands.

Efferent routes: after uniting into 1–6 ducts, the efferent vessels run to the accessory mandibular nodes; some may go directly to the ventral superficial cervical nodes and rarely to the lateral retropharyngeal nodes.

Nll. mandibulares accessorii of the pig
(245B/Ma; 279/3; 280/b; 281/b; 282/2)

This comprises 2–4 nodes which individually are 0.3–2 cm long. The group lies on the sternohyoideus muscle at the level of the bifurcation of the external jugular vein and the initial part of the external maxillary vein, below the cervical angle of the parotid gland. It is routinely examined at meat inspection.

Drainage area: skin of the throat, the parotid region and the cranial half of the ventral part of the neck; cutaneous muscles of the face; parotid gland. It receives secondary lymph from the mandibular nodes.

Efferent routes: the main outflow is to the ventral superficial cervical nodes; occasionally directly to the dorsal superficial cervical or lateral retropharyngeal nodes.

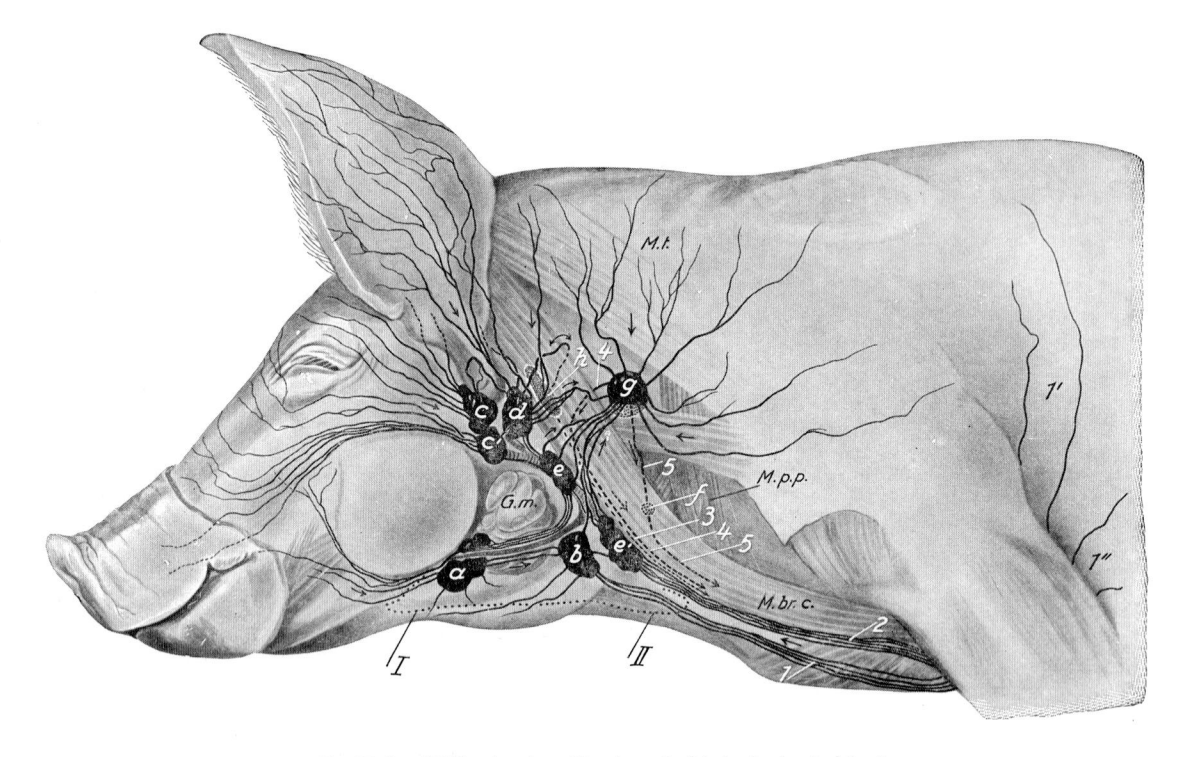

Fig. 280. Superficial lymph nodes and lymph vessels of the head and neck of the pig.
(After Zietzschmann, from Schönberg-Zietzschmann, 1958.)

The parotid gland has been removed, its cervical part (*I*, *II*) is dotted in outline; *I* mandibular angle, *II* cervical angle of the parotid

a nll. mandibulares; *b* nll. mandibulares accessorii; *c*, *c'* nll. parotidei; *d* nll. retropharyngei laterales; *e*, *e'* nll. cervicales superficiales ventrales (only two groups are seen here), *f* nl. cervicalis medius, lying below the m. brachiocephalicus; *g* nll. cervicales superficiales dorsales, partly below the m. omotransversarius; *h* nl. retropharyngeus medialis, situated below the m. brachiocephalicus

1 lymph vessels running from the sternal region to the nl. mandibulares accessorii; *1'*, *1"* lymph vessels from the lateral wall of the thorax: *2* superficial lymph nodes of the pectoral limb going to the nll. cervicales superficiales ventrales; *3* truncus jugularis arising from the medial retropharyngeal node; *4*, *5* vasa efferentia to the nll. cervicales superficiales dorsales, a second drainage route for the lymph from the head but it also drains other regions

G m gland. mandibularis; *M. br. c.* m. brachiocephalicus; *M. p. p.* prescapular part of the m. pectoralis profundus; *M. t.* m. trapezius

Lymphocentrum retropharyngeum
Nl. retropharyngeus medialis of the pig
(245 B/Rm; 297/5; 280/h; 281/h)

This is a very lobulated node, 1.5–4 cm in length. In about one pig in three there is a second, smaller node on one side. The main node is situated on the dorsolateral wall of the pharynx on a transverse plane through the free ends of the jugular processes. It also projects onto the longus capitis muscle. Below the node are found large vessels and nerves such as the occipital and internal carotid arteries, internal jugular veins, vagus, sympathetic and hypoglossus nerves. The accessory nerve curves around the ventral border of the lymph node to the lateral side and then runs towards the neck. This lymph node is examined routinely at meat inspection, when it can best be seen on the split head from medially, immediately behind the soft palate on the pharynx and directly under the first occipital joint.

Drainage area: masticatory muscles, muscles which run between the head and neck, certain cranial bones; pharynx, hard and soft palate, tonsils, nasal cavity, larynx, thymus, auditory tube. Secondary lymph is received from the parotid and lateral retropharyngeal nodes.

Efferent routes: its efferent vessels give rise to the jugular trunk and some go to the superficial cervical lymphocentre.

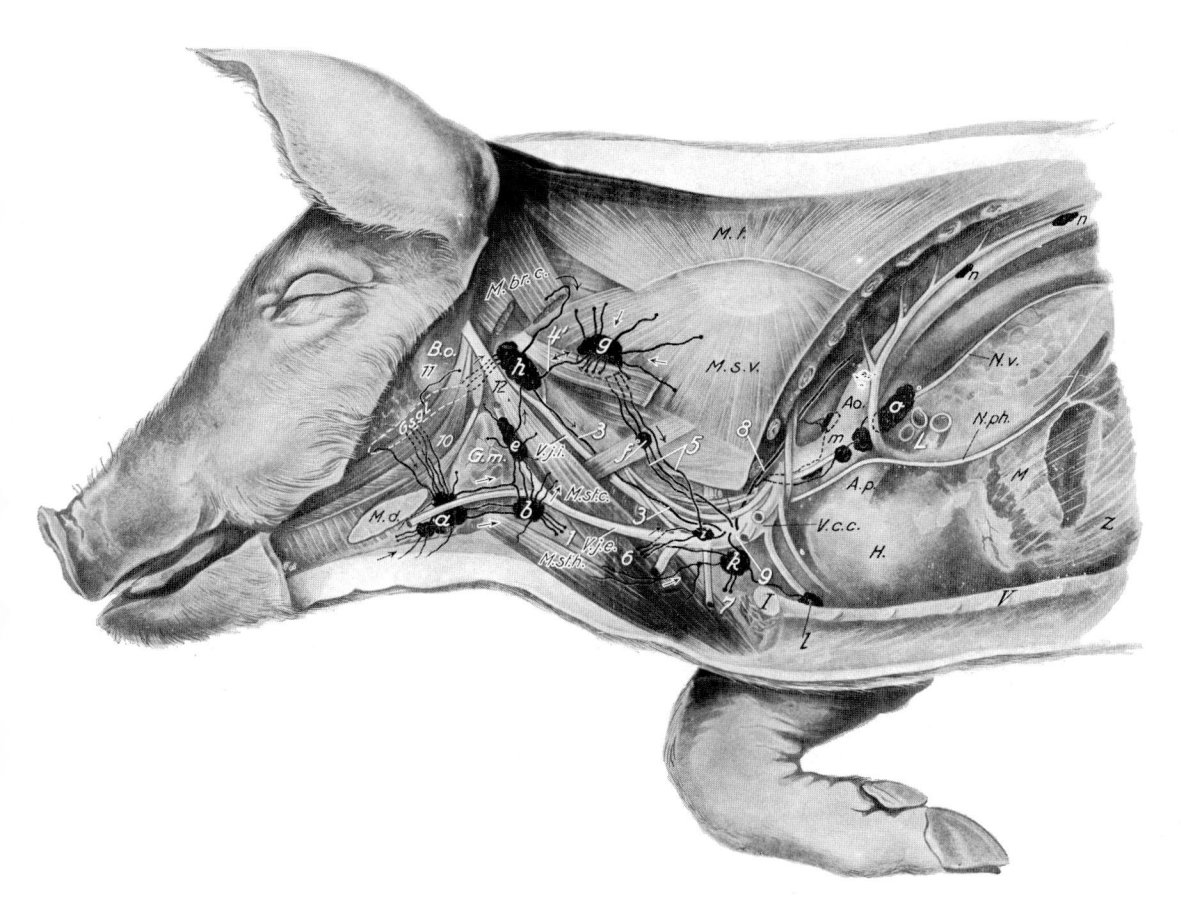

Fig. 281. Deep lymph nodes and lymph vessels of the head and neck and within the thoracic cavity of the pig.
(After Zietzschmann, from Schönberg-Zietzschmann, 1958.)
The thoracic cavity has been opened, after removal of the pectoral limb.

a nll. mandibulares; *b* nll. mandibulares accessorii; *e* one of the nll. cervicales superficiales ventrales (the more caudally situated nodes of this group have been removed with the brachiocephalic muscle); *f* nl. cervicalis superficialis medius, lying on the omohyoideus muscle; *g* nll. cervicales superficiales dorsales, partly under the omotransversarius muscle; *h* nll. retropharyngeus medialis; *i* nl. cervicalis profundus caudalis; *k* nll. axillares primae costae; *l* nll. sternales craniales; *m* nll. mediastinales craniales; *n* nll. thoracici aortici; *o* nll. bifurcationis sinistri

1 stumps of lymph vessels which run from the sternal region to the accessory mandibular nodes; *3* truncus jugularis arising from the medial retropharyngeal node; *4'* vessel in which the lymph can flow in either direction between nodes *g* and *h*; *5* three efferent vessels of the dorsal superficial cervical nodes on the course of some of which the nl. cervicalis superficialis medius may be inserted; *6* vasa efferentia from the caudal groups of the ventral superficial cervical nodes going to the axillary nodes of the first rib and the caudal deep cervical node; *7* deep lymph vessels of the pectoral limb; *8* ductus thoracicus; *9* termination of the lymph collecting ducts in the left venous angle; *10, 11, 12* lymph vessels of the soft palate which go (*10*) to the mandibular nodes, (*11*) to the lateral pharyngeal nodes and (*12*) to the medial retropharyngeal node

Ao. aorta thoracica; *A.p.* a. pulmonalis; *B.o.* Bulla tympanica; *Gsgl.* soft palate: *H.* pericardium and heart; *M.* mediastinum with accessory lobe visible through; *M. br.c.* m. brachiocephalicus; *M.d.* m. digastricus; *M.st.c.* m. sternocephalicus; *M. st.h.* m. sternohyoideus; *M.s.v.* m. serratus ventralis; *M.t.* m. trapezius; *N.ph.* n. phrenicus; *N.v.* n. vagus; *V.c.c.* v. cava cranialis; *V.j.e.*, *V.j.i.* v. jugularis externa or interna; *Z* diaphragm; *I, V* cartilage of the first and fifth ribs respectively

Nll. retropharyngei laterales of the pig
(245 B/*Rl*; 279/6; 280/*m*; 282/6)

There are usually two nodes although occasionally only one or rarely, three, are present. They each measure 0.7–3.8 cm in length. They are situated on the cleidocephalicus muscle at the posterior border of the parotid on the caudal auricular vein. They are routinely examined at meat inspection.

Drainage area: skin of the head (masseter, frontal, parietal and parotid regions), parietal and temporal bones; temporalis, digastricus, brachiocephalicus, longissimus capitis muscles; larynx, pharynx, external ear; occasionally it also receives secondary lymph from the parotid and mandibular lymphocentres.

Efferent routes: both to the medial retropharyngeal node and thus to the jugular trunk and also to the dorsal superficial cervical nodes, that is to say, the second efferent route for lymph from the head.

Lymphocentrum cervicale superficiale
Nll. cervicales superficiales dorsales of the pig
(247/*Csd*; 279/10; 280/*g*; 281/*g*; 282/7; 285/*f*)

This node corresponds to the superficial cervical nodes of the other domestic mammals. Generally there is a flat, lobulated node 3.6–4.8 cm long which is occasionally accompanied by one or two smaller nodes. It is situated on the ventral serratus muscle proximal to the shoulder joint and dorsal to the brachiocephalicus muscle in the angle between the cervical part of the trapezius and omotransversarius muscles and the pectoralis profundus muscle. This node is sometimes examined at meat inspection.

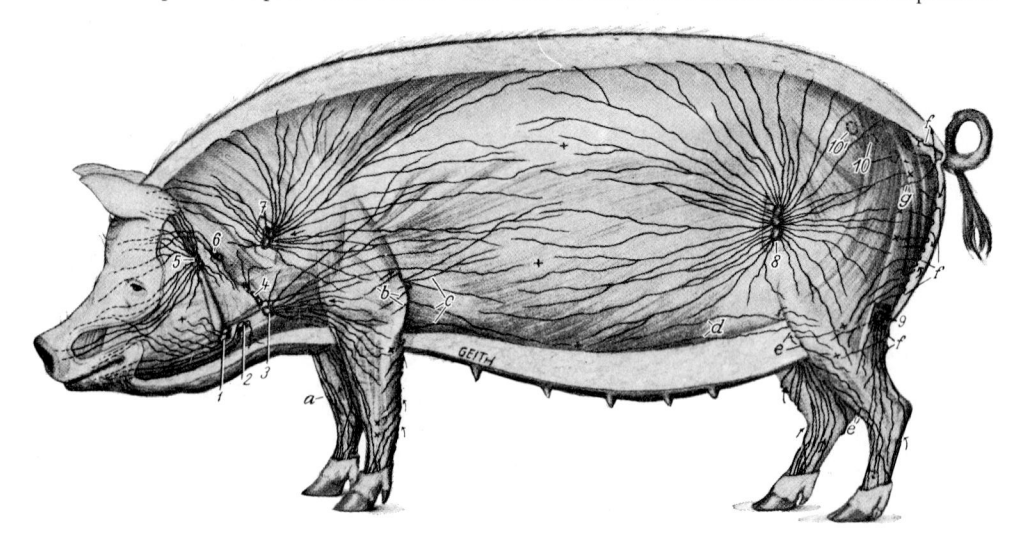

Fig. 282. Lymph nodes and lymph vessels of the skin of the pig.
(Slightly simplified after Baum and Grau, 1938.)

1 nll. mandibulares, *2* nll. mandibulares accessorii, *3*, *4* nll. cervicales superficiales ventrales, *5* nll. parotidei, *6* nll. retropharyngei laterales, *7* nll. cervicales superficiales dorsales, *8* nll. subiliaci (with part of the overlying cutaneous muscle removed), *9* nl. popliteus superficialis, *10* nll. ischiadici, *10'* nl. glutaeus

a, *b*, *c* lymph vessels going to the ventral superficial cervical nodes; *d*, *e*, *f* lymph vessels to the superficial inguinal nodes; *g* cutaneous lymph vessels which go deep to one of the ischiatic nodes; all the other cutaneous lymph nodes illustrated, can be followed to their respective regional lymph nodes. The small crosses (+) mark the points of injection whence the lymphatic routes can be filled in two directions (rather analogous to a watershed)

Drainage area: skin of the parietal and nape regions, external ear, shoulder, lateral surface of the upper arm and the lateral wall of the chest; parts of the musculature of the shoulder girdle, scapula, and supraspinatus muscle. It is important to note that this node receives the bulk of the secondary lymph from the head and from the ventral superficial cervical nodes (245B/*Csd*).

Efferent routes: terminal parts of the lymph collecting ducts (thoracic duct, jugular trunk, right lymphatic duct) or directly into the venous angle.

Nll. cervicales superficiales medii of the pig
(247/Csm; 279/11; 280/f; 281/f; 285/g)

This small group consists of one or two, rarely up to four, nodes which are to be found on the external jugular vein under the cleidocephalicus muscle.

Drainage area: skin of the ventral part of the neck; parts of the musculature of the shoulder girdle, long hyoid muscles; axis; secondary lymph from the two neighbouring groups of the superficial cervical nodes.

Efferent routes: there is considerable variation in the pattern by which they empty into the neighbouring lymph collecting ducts, the venous angle or possibly into the caudal deep cervical nodes.

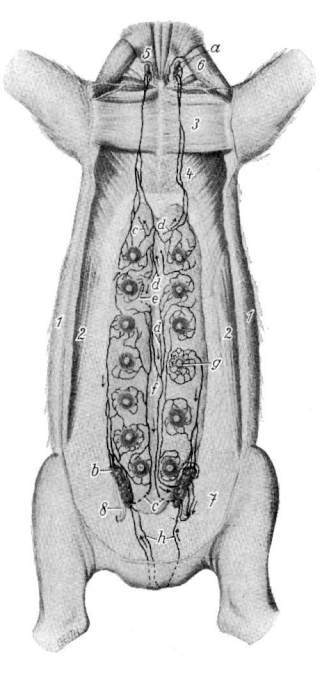

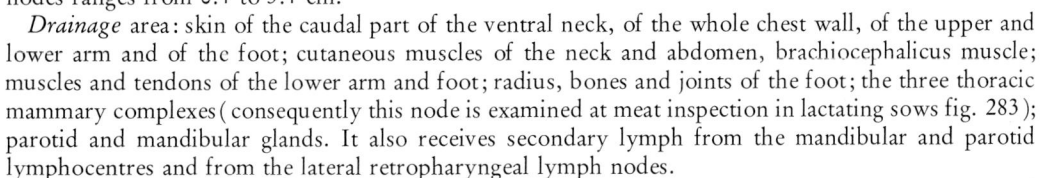

Fig. 283. Lymph nodes and lymph vessels of the mammary glands of the pig.
(After Baum and Grau, 1938.)

a nll. cervicales superficiales ventrales, *b* nll. inguinales superficiales seu mammarii, *c* lymph vessels going deep; *d* lymph vessel coming to the surface from the parenchyma of the gland, *f* lymph vessel which crosses the median plane of the body, *g* teat from which the skin has been dissected to show the garland of lymph vessels

1 outer skin, *2* m. abdominis obliquus, *3* m. pectoralis superficialis, *4* m. pectoralis profundus, *5* cutaneous muscle of the neck, *6* m. brachiocephalicus, *7* subcutaneous adipose tissue, *8* a. and v. pudenda externa

Nll. cervicales superficiales ventrales of the pig
(247/Csv; 279/12, 280/e, e'; 281/e; 282/3; 4; 283/a)

This group rarely consists of less than six to nine nodes which form a row in front of the shoulder joint between the cleido-occipitalis muscle and the caudal border of the parotid gland. The most caudally situated node (282/3) is the largest but the size of the nodes ranges from 0.4 to 3.4 cm.

Drainage area: skin of the caudal part of the ventral neck, of the whole chest wall, of the upper and lower arm and of the foot; cutaneous muscles of the neck and abdomen, brachiocephalicus muscle; muscles and tendons of the lower arm and foot; radius, bones and joints of the foot; the three thoracic mammary complexes (consequently this node is examined at meat inspection in lactating sows fig. 283); parotid and mandibular glands. It also receives secondary lymph from the mandibular and parotid lymphocentres and from the lateral retropharyngeal lymph nodes.

Efferent routes: the nodes of this group are interconnected. The outflowing lymph goes to the dorsal superficial cervical and the middle superficial cervical nodes.

Lymphocentrum cervicale profundum
Nll. cervicales profundi craniales of the pig
(247/Cpc; 279/14)

1–5 nodes of 0.2–1.5 cm diameter are situated between the pharynx, larynx and first part of the trachea. Accessory thyroids, not infrequently found in front of the thyroid gland, can easily be confused with the nodes of this group.

Drainage area: pharynx, larynx, cervical parts of the trachea, oesophagus thymus, thyroid, longus colli muscle.

Efferent routes: its lymph flows to the inconstantly present middle deep cervical nodes or to the caudal deep cervical nodes.

Nll. cervicales profundi medii of the pig
(247/*Cpm*; 279/15)

These are 2–7 inconstant nodes; in the majority of pigs they are absent. When present they lie against the trachea and are between 2–10 mm in diameter.

Drainage area: neighbouring musculature, larynx, cervical parts of the trachea and oesophagus, thymus, thyroid. Secondary lymph from the cranial deep cervical nodes.

Efferent route: to the caudal deep cervical nodes.

Nll. cervicales profundi caudales of the pig
(247/*Cpca*; 279/16; 281/*i*; 284/1''; 285/*h'*)

This is an unpaired group consisting of 1–14 nodes which lie close against the trachea immediately before the thoracic inlet. The size of the individual nodes varies from 1–10 mm. In meat inspection they are examined in special cases.

Drainage area: long hyoid muscle, longus colli muscle, 3rd to 7th cervical vertebrae, cervical parts of the trachea and oesophagus, thymus and thyroid glands. It also receives secondary lymph from the cranial and middle deep cervical and cranial mediastinal lymph nodes.

Efferent routes: its efferent vessels open into the terminal part of the thoracic duct, the axillary lymph nodes of the first rib or the right lymphatic duct.

Lymphocentrum axillare
Nll. axillares primae costae of the pig
(249/*Apc*; 279/20; 281/*k*; 284/1; 285/*h*)

Lying laterally against the trachea in front of the thoracic inlet and in close contact with the first rib on each side of the body, there is a group of nodes which includes a large one, 3–4 cm in length, and up to 4 other smaller nodes. They are examined at meat inspection in certain conditions because they are so important in the lymphatic drainage of the pectoral limb.

Drainage area: ventral musculature of the neck, cutaneous muscle of the abdomen, musculature of the shoulder girdle; 3rd to 7th cervical vertebrae, sternum, thyroid, thymus; *all* muscles, bones and joints of the pectoral limb; skin of the toes. Secondary lymph from the cranial mediastinal and cranial sternal nodes and from the deep cervical lymphocentre.

Efferent routes: terminal part of the thoracic duct or right lymphatic duct.

Lymphocentrum thoracicum dorsale
Nll. thoracici aortici of the pig
(297/24; 281/*n*; 284/4, 4', 4'', 4'''; 285/1, 1', 1'')

This consists of 2–10 unpaired nodes lying between the thoracic aorta and the 6th–14th thoracic vertebrae. The nodes are overlaid by the right or left azygos vein and thus not immediately seen when the thorax is opened. In front and to the right of the left azygos vein there is a constant node (284/4) which is readily visible, and on the dorsolateral aspect of the thoracic aorta there are other isolated nodes (284/4'', 4''') which are also easily identified. These are subpleural in position and are more common on the left than on the right; they measure 0.5–4 cm in length. These nodes are examined as a routine during meat inspection and they are removed in certain conditions.

Drainage area: dorsal and lateral chest wall including the musculature of the shoulder girdle but excluding the skin; diaphragm, pleura, mediastinum. Secondary lymph from the caudal mediastinal lymph nodes.

Efferent routes: these nodes are interconnected by their efferent vessels. They drain into the thoracic duct or the cranial mediastinal lymph nodes.

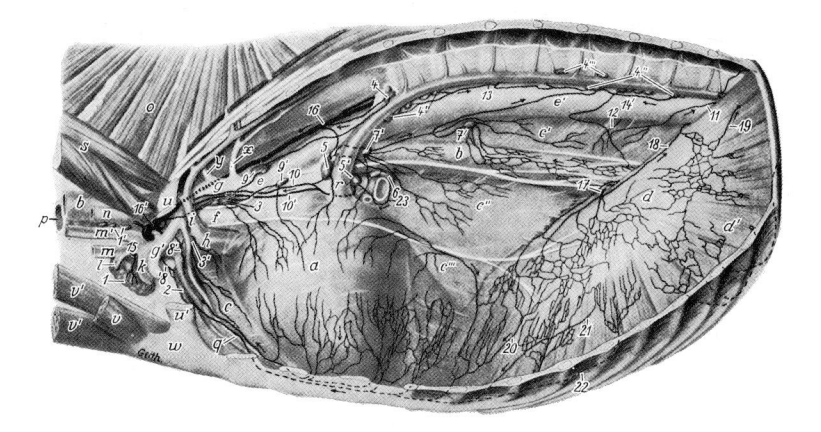

Fig. 284. Lymph nodes and lymph vessels of the thoracic cavity of the pig. Left lateral view.
(After Baum and Grau, 1938.)
(The left chest wall and left lung have been removed)

1 nll. axillares primae costae, *1'* nll. cervicales profundi caudales, *2* nll. sternales craniales, *3, 3', 9, 9'* nll. mediastinales craniales, *4, 4', 4", 4'''* nll. thoracici aortici, *5, 5'* nll. bifurcationis sinistri, *6* nll. bifurcationis medii, *7, 7'* nll. mediastinales caudales, *8, 8'* vasa efferentia of the nll. sternales craniales, *10, 10'* vasa efferentia of the nll. bifurcationis sinistri, *11* lymph vessel from the caudal mediastinum which goes to the coeliac node or terminates in the cisterna chyli, *12* lymph vessel from the caudal mediastinum which crosses over to the right side and enters the aortic thoracic node, *13* vas efferens from the aortic thoracic nodes marked *4'*, *14* efferent vessel from the aortic thoracic nodes marked *4"*, *15* vas efferens of the axillary nodes of the first rib which crosses over to the right side and appears at *b* in fig. 285, *16* ductus thoracicus, *16'* its ampulla, *17* lymph vessels of the diaphragm which pass through the oesophageal hiatus to the gastric nodes, *18* lymph vessels of the diaphragm, passing through the aortic hiatus to the coeliac node, *19* lymph vessels of the diaphragm, perforating the crus, *20, 21, 22* lymph vessels of the diaphragm which accompany the internal thoracic artery and vein to the sternal nodes, *23* efferent vessel of the middle tracheobronchial nodes

a heart and pericardium, *b, b* oesophagus, *c* mediastinum craniale, *c', c", c'''* caudal mediastinum, with the accessory lobe of the right lung discernible through at *c"*, *d* tendinous part, *d'* muscular part of the diaphragm, *e* arcus aortae, *e'* aorta thoracica, *f* truncus brachiocephalicus, *g* a. subclavia sinistra, *g'* a. axillaris, *h* v. cava cranialis, *i* v. costocervicalis, *k* v. axillaris, *l* v. cephalica, *m* v. jugularis externa, *m'* v. jugularis interna, *n* a. carotis communis, *o* m. serratus ventralis, *p* trachea, *q* a. and v. thoracica interna, *r* v. azygos sinistra, *s* m. scalenus, *t* stump of the left principal bronchus, *u, u'* first rib from which a large part has been removed, *v* m. sternomastoideus, *v'* m. sternothyreoideus und m. sternohyoideus, *w* sternum, *x* truncus costocervicalis, *y* a. cervicalis profunda

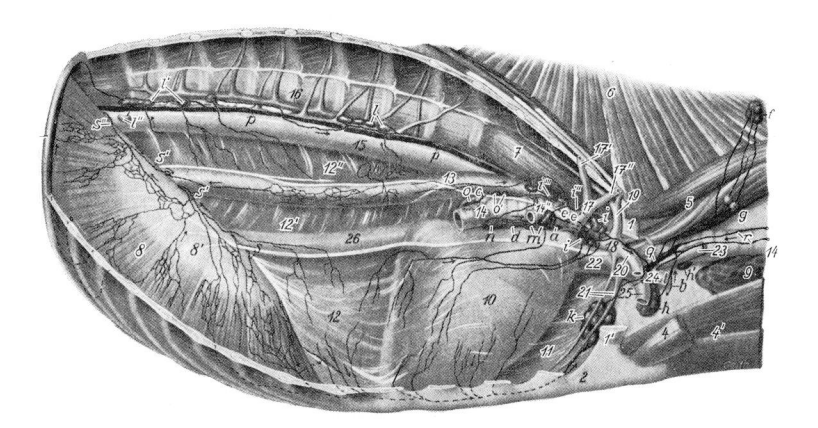

Fig. 285. Lymph nodes and lymph vessels of the thoracic cavity of the pig. Right lateral view.
(After Baum und Grau, 1938.)
(The right chest wall and right lung have been removed)

a vas efferens of the nll. bifurcationis sinistri, *b* vas efferens of the left nll. axillares primae costae, *c* efferent vessel of the middle tracheobronchial node which enters a left tracheobronchial node, *d* efferent vessel of the right tracheobronchial node going to the left tracheobronchial node, *e, e'* vasa efferentia of the nll. tracheobronchales craniales, *f* nll. cervicales superficiales dorsales, *g* nll. cervicales superficiales medii, *h* axillares primae costae, *h'* nll. cervicales profundi caudales, *i, i', i", i'''* nll. mediastinales craniales, *k* nll. sternales craniales, *l, l', l"* nll. thoracici aortici, *m* nll. tracheobronchales craniales, *n* nll. bifurcationis dextri, *o* nll. bifurcationis medii, *p* ductus thoracicus, *q* ductus lymphaticus dexter, *r* double truncus jugularis dexter, *s* lymph vessels of the diaphragm passing into the abdominal cavity through the caval orifice, *s"* lymph vessels passing through the aortic cleft into the abdominal cavity

1, 1' first rib, *2* sternum, *3* last rib, *4* m. sternomastoideus, *4'* m. sternohyoideus and m. sternothyroideus, *5* m. scalenus, *6* m. serratus ventralis, *7* m. longus colli, *8, 8'* diaphragm, *9* thyroid, *10* heart and pericardium, *11* mediastinum craniale, *12, 12', 12"* mediastinum caudale, *13* oesophagus, *14, 14'* trachea, *14'* tracheal bronchus (cut off), *15* aorta, *16* v. azygos dextra, *17, 17'* v. costocervicalis, *17"* v. cervicalis profunda, *18* a. subclavia dextra, *19* a. costocervicalis, *20* a. axillaris, *21* a. and v. thoracica interna, *22* v. cava cranialis, *23* v. jugularis interna, *24* v. jugularis externa, *25* v. axillaris, *26* v. cava caudalis

Lymphocentrum thoracicum ventrale
Nll. sternales craniales of the pig
(279/26; 281/1; 284/2; 285/k)

An unpaired group of 1–4 nodes, each 0.3–5 cm long, is situated on the presternum between the internal thoracic artery and vein of each side. The group as a whole is 4–5 cm in thickness and 2–2.5 cm broad. At meat inspection they should be examined in breeding sows but in other pigs only in special circumstances.

Drainage area: ventral chest wall, pleura, mediastinum, suspending membrane of the vena cava, diaphragm, peritoneum and anterior half of the mamma – hence the necessity for examination of these nodes in slaughtered breeding sows at meat inspection.

Efferent routes: terminal part of the thoracic duct or right lymphatic duct or, alternatively, directly into the venous system. Sometimes the efferent vessels may go to the caudal deep cervical nodes.

Lymphocentrum mediastinale
Nll. mediastinales craniales of the pig
(279/28, 29; 281/m; 284/3, 3', 9, 9'; 285/i, i', i", i''')

This group is variably arranged in the precardiac mediastinum. It is separated into a left and a right group but the left group is often absent. In total there are between 1 and 8 nodes, each of 0.2–3 cm diameter. Occasionally a node may be implanted in the pericardium on the left side (279/29; 284/9, 9'). This group should be examined as a routine during meat inspection.

Drainage area: bones and muscles of the cranial part of the chest wall and the lower part of the neck; trachea, thymus, oesophagus, pleura, mediastinum, suspensory membrane of the vena cava, pericardium; secondary lymph from the dorsal thoracic and bronchial lymphocentres.

Efferent routes: terminal part of the thoracic duct or the right lymphatic duct.

Nll. mediastinales caudales of the pig
(279/31; 284/7, 7')

There are 1–3 constant nodes situated against the oesophagus immediately behind the aortic arch. Another node may sometimes be found dorsal or ventral to the oesophagus, halfway to the oesophageal hiatus. These nodes are 0.4–2 cm in diameter and they should always be examined at meat inspection.

Drainaige area: postcardiac part of the oesophagus, mediastinum and pericardium.

Efferent routes: bronchial lymphocentre but the posterior node may drain to one of the thoracic aortic nodes.

Lymphocentrum bronchale
Nll. bifurcationis (seu tracheobronchales) dextri of the pig
(285/n; 286/10)
Nll. bifurcationis (seu tracheobronchales) sinistri of the pig
(279/34; 281/0; 284/5, 5'; 286/8)
Nll. bifurcationis (seu tracheobronchales) medii of the pig
(279/35; 284/6; 285/0; 286/9)

There are 1–3 right and 2–7 left tracheobronchial lymph nodes, which are more or less hidden, at the origin of the primary bronchi. The 2–5 middle nodes are situated dorsally to the bifurcation of the trachea. Their size varies from 0.2–6.5 cm. They should be regularly examined at meat inspection.

Drainage area: thoracic part of the trachea, lung; the left and middle nodes also receive lymph vessels from the mediastinum, heart and pericardium and the left node from the oesophagus. Secondary lymph is received from the caudal mediastinal nodes.

Efferent routes: to the cranial mediastinal nodes or the terminal or even precardiac parts of the thoracic duct.

Nll. tracheobronchales craniales of the pig
(285/*m* ; 286/*11*)

As a rule there are 2–5 nodes located at the angle of origin of the tracheal bronchus but often there is only a solitary large node. These nodes may be situated caudoventrally to the bronchus or, alternatively, ventral to the trachea and extending craniad to the level of the costocervical vein. They are 0.3–3.5 cm in size. They should be examined as a routine at meat inspection.
Drainage area: lung, pericardium, heart; there is an interchange of efferent vessels with the other tracheobronchial nodes.
Efferent routes: lymph goes to the cranial mediastinal nodes.

Lymphocentrum lumbale
Nll. lumbales aortici of the pig
(253/*a* ; 256/*t* ; 279/*36* ; 288/*16* ; 290/*2* ; 291/*4*)

8 to 20 nodes, each 0.2–2.5 cm long, are situated ventral and lateral, partly also dorsal, to the abdominal aorta and caudal vena cava. The chain extends from the aortic hiatus to the deep circumflex iliac artery. In certain conditions they should be examined during meat inspection.
Drainage area: dorsal and lateral abdominal wall, peritoneum, renal capsule, kidney, adrenal, ureter, testes, epididymis or ovary and oviduct; secondary lymph from the iliosacral and caudal mesenteric lymphocentres and also from preceding nodes such as the phrenicoabdominal and testicular.
Efferent routes: the nodes of this group are interconnected but finally their efferent vessels form the lumbar trunks which in turn lead into the cisterna chyli.

Nl. renales of the pig
(253/*a'* ; 279/*37*)

On the renal artery and vein near the hilus one can identify 2–4 small lymph nodes. Alternatively they may also lie on the dorsal side of the vena cava. They are examined routinely during meat inspection.
Drainage area: mainly kidney and capsule, but also adrenal, ureter and circumscribed areas of the dorsal abdominal wall. Secondary lymph is received from the neighbouring lumbar aortic and phrenicoabdominal nodes.
Efferent routes: to the lumbar trunks or directly into the cisterna chyli.

Nl. phrenicoabdominalis of the pig
(253/*1, 1'*)

Although present in the majority of pigs, this small node is inconstant and sometimes confined to one side of the body. It is situated at the caudal surface of the cranial abdominal artery and vein or somewhat further towards the pelvis at the level of the lateral border of the iliopsoas muscle.
Drainage area: dorsal wall of the abdomen, diaphragm.
Efferent route: aortic lumbar or renal nodes.

Nl. testicularis of the pig
(290/*2'*)

This node is inconstant but if present it is situated on the testicular artery and vein. It is a small node, up to 10 mm in size, lying subserously.
Drainage area: testes, epididymis.
Efferent route: lumbar aortic nodes.

Lymphocentrum coeliacum
Nll. coeliaci of the pig
(253/f; 256/e)

There are 2-4 coeliac lymph nodes of 0.3-4 cm in length, situated in the vicinity of the coeliac artery and its division.

Drainage area: lung, mediastinum, diaphragm, spleen, liver, adrenal. Secondary lymph is received from all the nodes of the coeliac lymphocentre to be described below.

Efferent routes: efferent vessels unite to form the coeliac trunk.

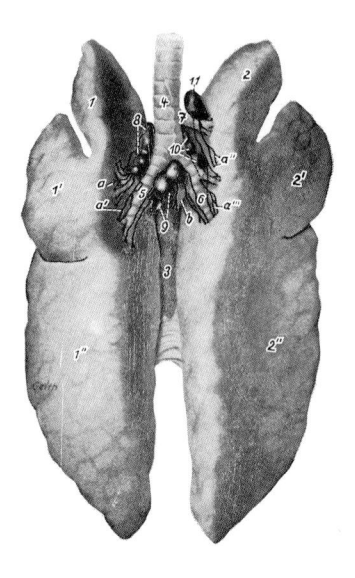

Fig. 286. Lymph nodes and deep vessels of the lung of the pig. (After Baum and Grau, 1938.)

1, 1' lobus cranialis sinister with *1* pars cranialis and *1'* pars caudalis, *1''* lobus caudalis sinister, *2* lobus cranialis dexter, *2'* lobus medius, *2''* lobus caudalis dexter, *3* lobus accessorius, *4* end of the trachea, *5* left and *6* right principal bronchus, *7* bronchus trachealis, *8* nll. bifurcationis sinistri, *9* nll. bifurcationis medii, *10* nll. bifurcationis dextri, *11* nll. tracheobronchales craniales

a, a', a'', a''', b deep lymph vessels of the lung

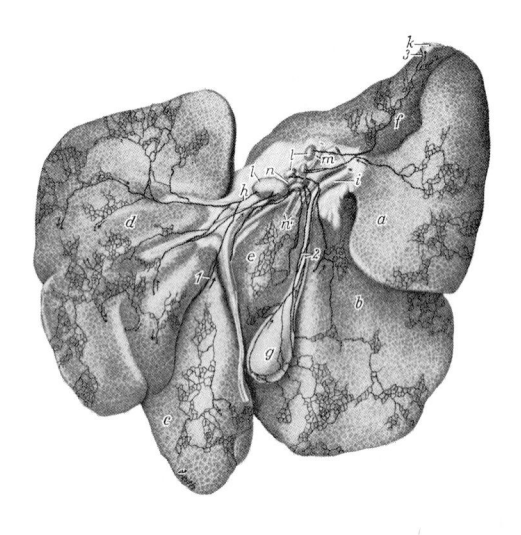

Fig. 287. Lymph nodes and lymph vessels of the liver of the pig. (After Baum and Grau, 1938.)

a lobus hepatis dexter lateralis, *b* lobus hepatis dexter medialis, *c* lobus hepatis sinister medialis, *d* lobus hepatis sinister lateralis, *e* lobus quadratus, *f* lobus caudatus, *g* gall bladder, *h* portal vein, *i* ductus choledochus, *k* vena cava caudalis (cut off where it meets the dorsal border of the liver), *l* nll. hepatici, *m, n, n'* a. hepatica and branches

1 lymph vessel which stems from the parietal surface of the liver, *2* lymph vessels of the gall bladder, *3* lymph vessel entering the ligamentum triangulare dextrum

Nll. lienales of the pig
($256/d, d^1, d^2, d^3$)

1-10 nodes, 0.2-2.5 cm in size, are strung along the splenic artery and vein. They are found either in the dorsal quarter of the splenic hilus or along the vessels running in the mesentery. They must always be examined at meat inspection.

Drainage area: stomach, omentum, pancreas, spleen.

Efferent routes: either to the coeliac nodes or directly to the coeliac trunk.

Nll. gastrici of the pig
(256/c, c')

These consist of 1-5 nodes, 0.3-6 cm long, which are situated either subserously on the cardia of the stomach or along the left gastric artery which runs in the mesentery. These nodes must be examined at meat inspection.

Drainage area: thoracic part of the oesophagus, mediastinum, suspending membrane of the vena cava, diaphragm, stomach, abdominal part of the oesophagus, pancreas.

Efferent routes: coeliac nodes or directly to the coeliac trunk.

Nll. hepatici (seu portales) of the pig
(256/*f*; 287/*1*; 288/*1*)

2–7 nodes, which measure 0.7 to 8.8 cm in length, are situated at the porta of the liver or on the trunk of the portal vein. These nodes should be examined routinely during meat inspection.

Drainage area: liver, gallbladder, pancreas. Secondary lymph from the pancreaticoduodenal nodes.

Efferent routes: coeliac trunk or coeliac lymph nodes.

Fig. 288. Lymph nodes, lymph vessels and lymph collecting ducts of the abdominal cavity of the pig in situ. Right lateral view.
(After Baum and Grau, 1938.)

The liver is reflected so as to show its visceral surface.

1 nll. hepatici, *2, 2', 2'', 2''', 2''''* external conglomerate of nll. jejunales, *3, 3', 3'', 3'''* nll. ileocolici, *4, 5, 6* nll. pancreaticoduodenales, *7* lymph vessels which curve round the dorsal border from the left to the right side of the caecum, *8* truncus intestinalis, *8', 8'', 8'''* truncus jejunalis and branches, *9* vasa efferentia which go from the first jejunal nodes to the intestinal trunk, *10* efferent vessels going from the distal jejunal nodes to the ileocolic nodes, *11* vas efferens of the nll. ileocolici, *12* cisterna chyli, *13* trunci lumbales, *14* truncus visceralis, *15* truncus coeliacus, *16* nll. lumbales aortici, *17* nll. mesenterici caudales, *18* vas efferens from a pancreaticoduodenal node (6)

a, a', a'', a''' liver, *b* stomach, *c, c* duodenum, *d, d* jejunum, *e* ileum, *f* jejunal mesentery, *g* caecum, *h* plica ileocaecalis, *i* colon ascendens, *k* colon descendens, *l* pancreas, *m* right kidney, *n* v. cava caudalis, *o* v. portae, *p, p'* a. mesenterica cranialis, *q* aorta, *r* gall bladder

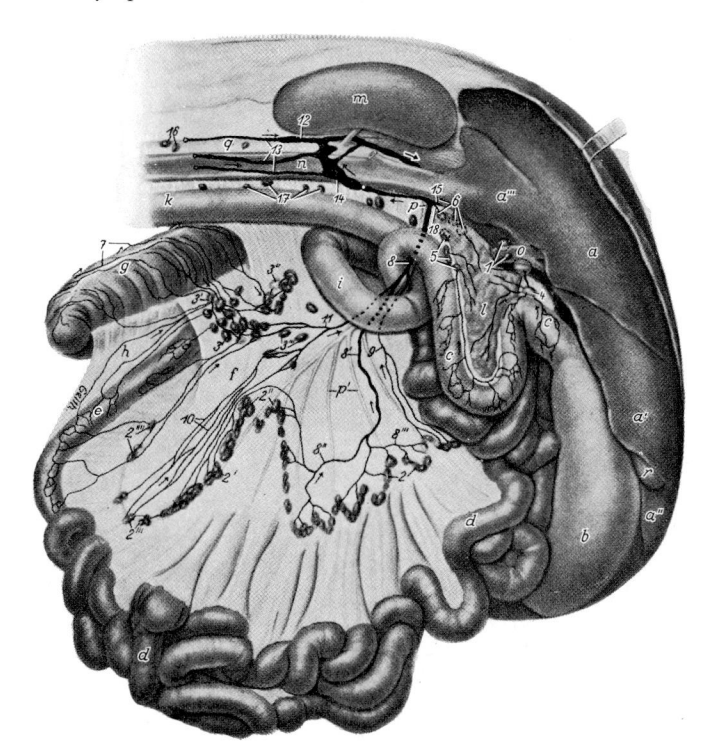

Nll. pancreaticoduodenales of the pig
(256/*a, a'*; 288/*4, 5, 6*)

These 4–9 nodes are situated on the duodenum or embedded in the pancreas. They are found near the site where the cranial pancreaticoduodenal artery arises from the gastroduodenal artery. They also extend on the left to the end of the descending duodenum and towards the right as far as the end of the right lobe of the pancreas. At the pancreas they are situated near the cranial mesenteric artery.

Drainage area: pancreas, duodenum, stomach and omentum.

Efferent routes: from these nodes the lymph passes partly to the coeliac trunk and partly to the colic nodes.

Lymphocentrum mesentericum craniale

Nl. mesentericus cranialis of the pig
(256/*g'''*; 288/ at *p*)

On the main trunk of the cranial mesenteric artery one occasionally finds one or more nodes. It is uncertain whether these actually form an independent group.

Nll. jejunales of the pig
(266/h, h′, h″; 288/2, 2′, 2″, 2‴, 2⁗; 289/b, b′)

These important and numerous nodes are accommodated in the mesentery of the small intestine in two long rows. One of these groups lies under the outer serous lamella furthest from the colonic cone, while the other group is situated below the inner lamella which faces the cone of colonic coils. Thus the two groups are separated from one another by the blood vessels, connective- and adipose-tissue of the central layer of the mesentery. Each chain of lymph nodes follows the convolutions of the small intestine for a distance of about 60 cm from the duodenum to the ileum. Both chains consist of 4–40 individual nodes, each 0.4–6 cm long, and so closely packed together that each chain almost resembles a single long node. Towards the ileum individual nodes are more widely separated. However, instead of chains, there are sometimes only a few nodes scattered through the mesentery. Both these rows of jejunal nodes, the outer and the inner, should always be examined in meat inspection because of their importance in assessing the significance of alimentary diseases.

Drainage area: jejunum, ileum, last part of duodenum.

Efferent routes: with the exception of the first and last nodes of each row, the efferent vessels of the majority of the jejunal nodes form the jejunal trunk. This trunk joins the colic and intestinal trunks at the root of the mesentery. The lymph from the last, distally situated, nodes passes to the ileocolic nodes; efferent vessels from the first, proximally situated, nodes go directly to the intestinal trunk.

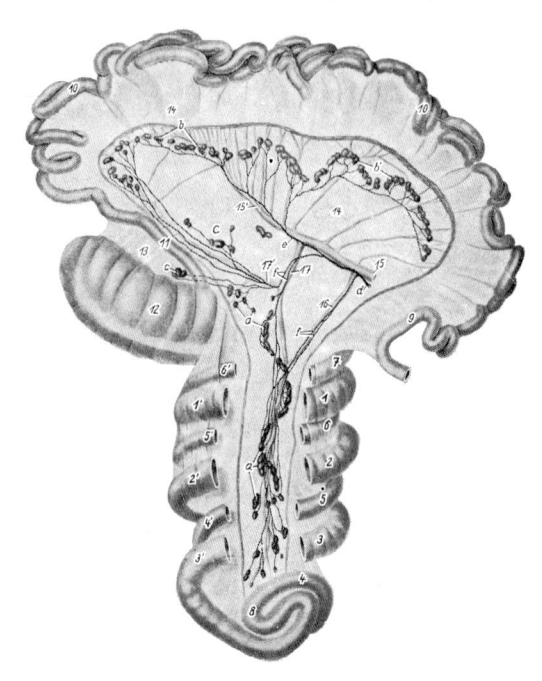

Fig. 289. Lymph nodes and lymph vessels of the gut of the pig. (After Baum and Grau, 1938.)

For the sake of clarity this is presented in semidiagrammatic form. The loops of the colonic cone have been cut through and slightly separated. The jejunum is reflected.

a, a nll. colici, *b, b′* nll. jejunales, *c* nll. ileocolici, *d* truncus intestinalis, *e* truncus jejunalis, *f* vasa efferentia of the nll. colici

1, 1′, 2, 2′, 3, 3′ centripetal layers of colon, *4, 4′, 5, 5′, 6, 6′* centrifugal layers of colon, *7* terminal loop of colon, *8* apex of colonic cone, *9* duodenum, *10* jejunum, *11* ileum, *12* caecum, *13* ileocaecalis

Nll. ileocolici of the pig
(256/b, b′; 288/3, 3′, 3″, 3‴; 289/c)

This is a group of 5–9 nodes, each 0.6 to 3.2 cm long, which is situated near the ileal orifice in the mesoileum and in the plica ileocaecalis. It should always be examined at meat inspection.

Drainage area: caecum, ileum, terminal part of the jejunum.

Efferent routes: coeliac and intestinal trunks.

Nll. colici of the pig
(256/g, g′; 289/a)

On the axis of the cone of the colon, that is to say, lying against the right colic artery and the colic ramus of the ileocolic artery, one can identify up to 50 nodes, each measuring 0.2–9 cm. At meat inspection examination must be restricted to those lying near the ileocolic nodes.

Drainage area: the ascending, transverse and first part of the descending colon; caecum.

Efferent routes: the majority of efferent vessels form the colic trunk while others lead directly to the intestinal trunk. The latter develops from the confluence of the colic and jejunal trunks.

Lymphocentrum mesentericum caudale
Nll. mesenterici caudales of the pig
(256/g; 288/17)

In the mesentery of the descending colon there are 7–12 nodes, each 2–12 mm in diameter. They must be examined and their condition assessed at meat inspection.
Drainage area: descending colon and pancreas.
Efferent routes: lumbar aortic and medial iliac nodes.

Lymphocentrum iliosacrale
Nll. iliaci mediales of the pig
(253/b, b'; 256/u; 260/1; 279/40; 290/3; 291/3; 292/c)

On each side of the terminal part of the abdominal aorta and then accompanying each external iliac artery as far as the origin of the deep circumflex iliac artery, are 2–6 nodes. Each node is 0.3–2.5 cm in diameter. This is an important group of lymph nodes which should be examined during meat inspection under certain circumstances.
Drainage area: extensor muscles of the back, lumbar musculature, gluteal musculature and the muscles at the back of the thigh, adductors: lumbar vertebrae, sacrum, patella; peritoneum, ureter, bladder and urethra; male and female sex organs; secondary lymph from all the lymphocentres described below and from the caudal mesenteric nodes.
Efferent routes: the efferent vessels partly empty into the lumbar aortic nodes and partly are involved in forming the lumbar trunks.

Nll. iliaci laterales of the pig
(253/c, c'; 260/1'; 279/41; 292/e)

At the bifurcation of the deep circumflex iliac artery and at its cranial terminal branch, there are 1 or 2, sometimes even up to 7, nodes. They are 0.3–2.6 cm long. They are examined in special conditions at meat inspection.
Drainage area: inner lumbar musculature, abdominal muscles, lumbodorsal fascia and fascia lata; quadriceps femoris; pelvic bones, bladder, kidney and renal capsule, peritoneum; secondary lymph from subiliac, iliofemoral and superficial inguinal lymph nodes.
Efferent routes: medial iliac and lumbar aortic nodes.

Nll. sacrales of the pig
(253/e; 260/1''; 279/42; 290/4, 4'; 291/5)

2–5 nodes, each 0.7–2 cm in diameter, are present at the angle of bifurcation of the internal iliac arteries. Rarely there are a further 1 or 2 smaller nodes along the course of these vessels in the pelvic cavity. In females one sometimes encounters another, occasionally unpaired node, in the posterior part of the broad ligament of the uterus. This could be given the name *nl. urogenitalis* (279/44; 291/9) but it is part of the sacral group.
Drainage area: deep gluteal muscles, gracilis muscle, musculature of the tail, pelvic bones, sacrum, coccygeal vertebrae; ureter, bladder, urethra; in males the accessory sex glands and the bulbocavernosus muscle; in females the vagina and vulva; secondary lymph from the anorectal and gluteal nodes.
Efferent routes: medial iliac nodes.

Nll. anorectales of the pig
(260/1'''; 279/43; 290/5)

This group consists of 6–10 nodes, each 0.2–2.2 cm in diameter. They are situated at the dorsolateral border of the rectum. Sometimes they are absent.

378   Lymph vessel system

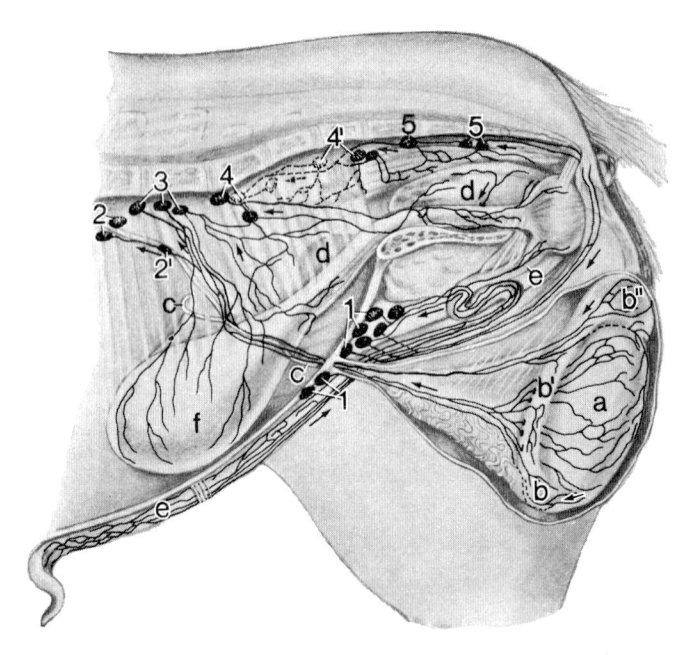

Fig. 290. Lymph nodes and lymph vessels of the male genital organs of the pig, in situ.
(After Baum and Grau, 1938).

1, 1 nll. inguinales superficiales seu scrotales, *2* nll. lumbales aortici, *2'* nl. testicularis, *3* nll. iliaci mediales, *4, 4'* nll. sacrales, *5, 5* nll. anorectales

a left testis, *b, b', b"* head, body and tail of the epididymis, *c, c* ductus deferens, *d, d* accessory sex glands lying over the pelvic portion of the urethra, *e, e* penis, *f* urinary bladder

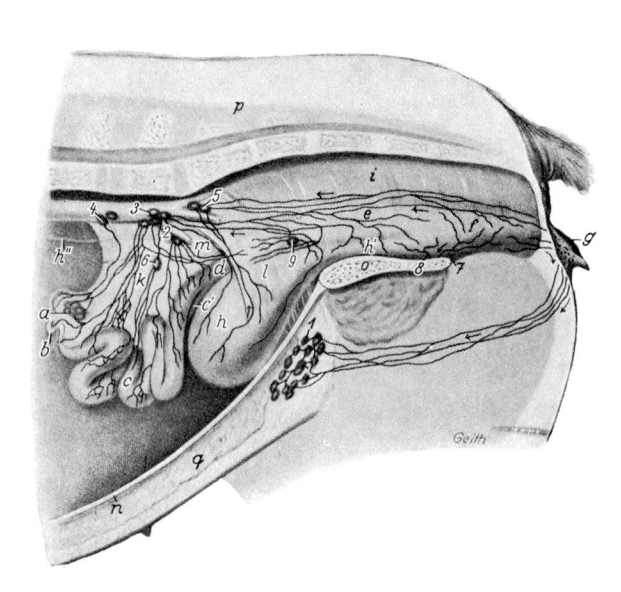

Fig. 291. Lymph nodes and lymph vessels of the female genital organs of the pig in situ.
(After Baum and Grau, 1938)

1 nll. inguinales superficiales seu mammarii, *2* nll. iliofemorales, *3* nll. iliaci mediales, *4* nll. lumbales aortici, *5* nll. sacrales, *6* nl. uterinus, *7* lymph vessel from the vaginal vestibule and *8* lymph vessel from the urethra, both of which run to the ischiatic nodes, *9* nl. urogenitalis

a left ovary, *b* left uterine tube, *c* left, *c'* right horn of the uterus, *d* body of uterus, *e* vagina, *f* vestibulum vaginae, *g* vulva, *h* urinary bladder, *h'* urethra, *h"* ureter, *i* rectum, *k* ligamentum suspensorium ovarii and ligamentum latum uteri, *l* ligamentum vesicae laterale, *m* ligamentum latum uteri, *n* ventral wall of the abdomen, *o* floor of the pelvis, *p* dorsal wall of the abdomen and pelvis, *q* udder

Drainage area: rectum, anus, tail muscles.
Efferent routes: sacral and medial iliac nodes.

Nll. uterini of the pig
(291/6)

Some smaller lymph nodes situated in the anterior part of the broad ligament of the uterus can be considered to precede the medial iliac nodes. They are 1.2–1.8 cm in diameter. They may be lacking.
Drainage area: ovary, oviduct, uterus.
Efferent routes: medial iliac, lumbar aortic nodes or lumbar trunks.

Lymphocentrum inguinale profundum (seu iliofemorale)
Nll. iliofemorales of the pig
(253/d, d'; 260/2; 279/46; 291/2; 292/d)

This group usually consists of 2–3 nodes distributed against the external iliac artery and vein between the origins of the deep circumflex iliac on the one hand and the deep femoral artery on the other. Less frequently there may be only 1 node or as many as 6 and their size varies. A solitary node is generally large (3–5.5 cm) but if several are present each is smaller (0.2–3.5 cm). Because of the way they are grouped together they have the overall appearance of a single node. They are of importance in meat inspection and have to be examined in certain circumstances.

Drainage area: all muscles, bones and joints of the pelvic limb, abdominal muscles, peritoneum; vaginal process and cremaster muscle or, in the female, the uterus; bladder; secondary lymph from the superficial inguinal and subiliac nodes and from the popliteal lymphocentre.

Efferent routes: medial iliac and aortic lumbar nodes and lumbar trunks.

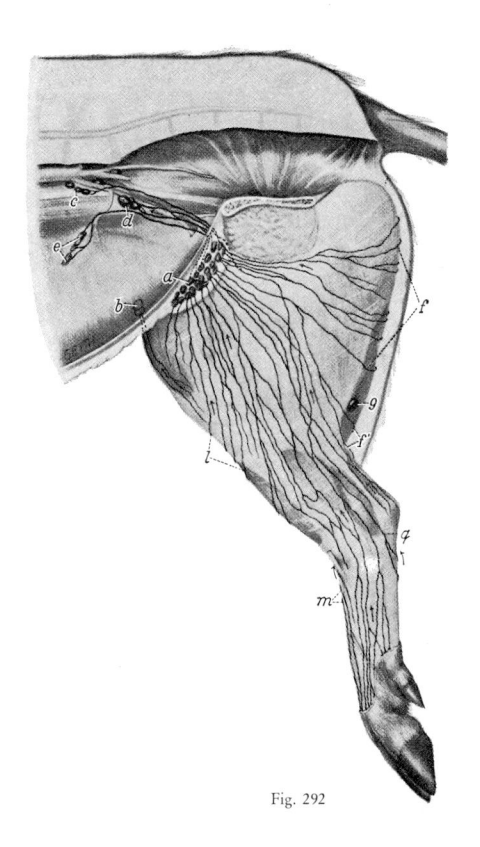

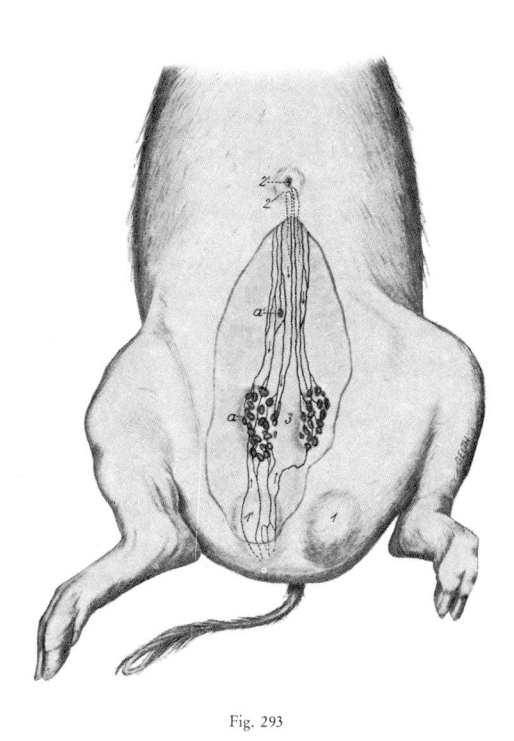

Fig. 292

Fig. 293

Fig. 292. Lymph nodes and superficial lymph vessels of the pelvic limb of the pig. Medial view.
(After Baum and Grau, 1938).

a nll. inguinales superficiales, *b* nll. subiliaci, *c* nll. iliaci mediales, *d* nll. iliofemorales, *e* nll. iliaci laterales, *f, f'* lymph vessels from the lateral surfaces of the knee and thigh curving round to the medial side (in fig. 282 these vessels are marked *f*), *g* nl. popliteus superficialis, *l* lymph vessels from the lateral surface of the shank running onto the medial side, *m* lymph vessels from the medial side of the foot crossing over dorsal and lateral to the popliteal nodes, *q* lymph vessels going from the lateral to the medial side of the foot

Fig. 293. Lymph nodes and lymph vessels of the male genital organs and scrotum of the pig, in situ
(After Baum and Grau, 1938.)

a nll. inguinales superficiales seu scrotales, *a'* accessory lymph nodes of this group

1, 1' scrotum, at *1'* its skin has been lifted off to show the lymph vessels; *2* praeputium, *2'* ostium praeputiale; *3* location of penis

Lymphocentrum inguinale superficiale (seu inguinofemorale)
Nll. inguinales superficiales of the pig
(Nll. scrotales 290/1; 293/a)
(Nll. mammarii 260/3; 279/49; 283/b; 291/1)

The nodes of this group form a complex measuring 5–8 cm in length which lies in the pubic region, between the skin and the outer layer of the rectus sheath. In the male the nodes are close to the penis and in the female they lie against the mamma. In both sexes the complex consists of 2–6 nodes; infrequently there is only one node. The nodes should be examined routinely at meat inspection. In some cases, such as with breeding sows, they should be inspected with particular care.

Drainage area: skin of the ventral and lateral abdominal wall, inner surface of the thigh, posterior part of the outer surface of the thigh including the skin over the ischiatic tuberosity, skin covering the shank, foot and tail; abdominal cutaneous muscle and abdominal musculature; gracilis, pectineus, glutaeobiceps, quadriceps femoris muscles; bones, joints and tendons of the foot; in males the scrotum, penis, prepuce, urethra, ischiocavernosus and bulbocavernosus muscles; in females the vaginal vestibule, vulva, abdominal and inguinal part of the mamma up to the 2nd mammary complex (therefore careful examination during meat inspection of breeding sows); anus.

Efferent routes: iliofemoral and possibly also medial and lateral iliac nodes.

Nll. subiliaci of the pig
(260/3'; 279/50; 282/8; 292/b; 294/8)

This is a complex of 1–6 closely packed nodes which measures 3.5–5.5 cm in length. The complex is situated in the stifle fold almost in the centre of a line connecting the tuber coxae with the patella. The posterior branch of the deep circumflex iliac artery is immediately related to it. It is examined at meat inspection under special circumstances.

Drainage area: the skin a hand's breadth in front of and above the costal arch, the skin of the dorsal and lateral abdominal wall and of the front and middle parts of the pelvis, of the lateral region of the thigh and of the anterior part of the medial thigh region, over the area of the knee and over the proximal half of the shank; cutaneous musculature of the abdomen, tensor fasciae latae and glutaeobiceps muscles; coxal tuber.

Efferent routes: lateral iliac nodes, also iliofemoral and medial iliac nodes.

Lymphocentrum ischiadicum
Nll. ischiadici of the pig
(260/4; 279/54; 282/10; 294/7)

At the border of the broad sacrotuberal ligament one invariably finds 1–2 nodes, each 0.4–2.5 cm in length. Sometimes this group is joined by another node which is pushed between the ischium and the glutaeobiceps muscle. In special cases this is examined during meat inspection; generally it is exposed by incision behind the broad sacrotuberal ligament.

Drainage area: skin covering the pelvic outlet, superficial gluteal and posterior thigh muscles, internal obturator muscle, pelvic bones, sacrum, coccygeal vertebrae; anus, vagina, vaginal vestibule, urethra, bulbourethral gland. Secondary lymph from the popliteal lymphocentre.

Efferent routes: gluteal, sacral and medial iliac nodes.

Nl. glutaeus of the pig
(260/4'; 279/55; 282/10'; 294/7')

One or two nodes up to 2.5 cm long are situated on the outer surface of the broad sacrotuberal ligament at the level of the greater ischiatic notch. The node is related to the ischiatic nerve and the cranial gluteal artery and vein.

Drainage area: see ischiatic nodes.

Efferent route: lymphocentrum iliosacrale

Lymphocentrum popliteum
Nl. popliteus profundus of the pig
(260/5; 279/57; 294/9')

This lymph node occurs in 40% of pigs. It is hidden between the biceps and semitendinosus muscles and lies 3–6 cm down on the gastrocnemius.

It may be duplicated and sometimes there may be three or even four nodes. It is 0.3–2.5 cm in diameter. Small nodes are not easily found in the adipose tissue.

Drainage area and *efferent* routes – see below.

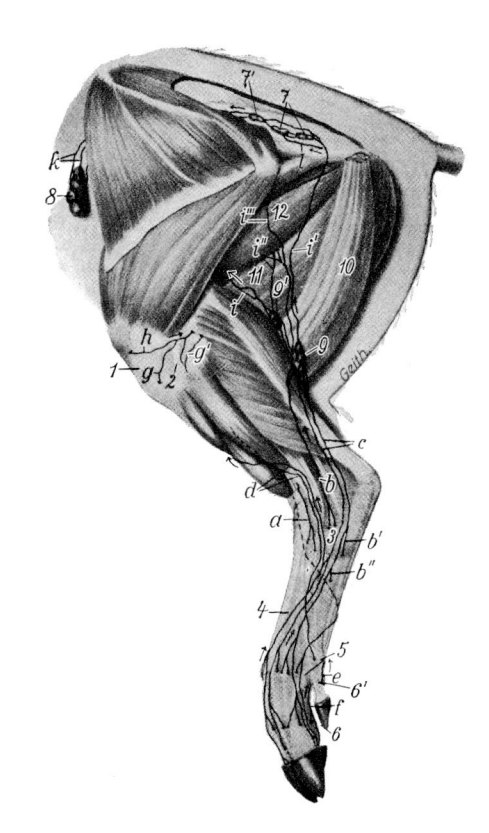

Fig. 294. Lymph nodes of the pelvic limb and lymph vessels of the joints of the pig. Lateral view.
(After Baum and Grau, 1938.)

1 capsule of the femoropatellar joint, *2* lateral collateral ligament of the femorotibial joint, *3* tarsus, *4* metatarsus, *5* metatarsophalangeal joints, *6* 2nd interphalangeal joint of the 4th toe, *6'* 1st interphalangeal joint of the 5th toe, *7* nll. ischiadici, *7'* nl. glutaeus, *8* nll. subiliaci, *9* nl. popliteus superficialis, *9'* nl. popliteus profundus, *10* m. semitendinosus, *11* m. semimembranosus, *12* m. adductor

a, *b*, *b'*, *b"* lymph vessels of the tarsal joint, *c* lymph vessels which rise from the dorsal surface of the metatarsus to the lymphocentrum popliteum, *d* lymph vessels which run from the dorsal surface of the metatarsus round the anterior aspect of the shank to the medial surface of the thigh and to the superficial inguinal or the iliofemoral lymph nodes. *e* lymph vessel which emerges on the posterior surface of the 2nd interphalangeal joint of the 5th digit, *f* lymph vessel which emerges on the caudal surface of the 2nd and 3rd interphalangeal joints of the 4th digit, *g*, *g'* lymph vessels of the femorotibial joint, *h* lymph vessels from the femoropatellar joint, *i*, *i'*, *i"*, *i'''* vasa efferentia of the lymphocentrum popliteum, *k* vasa efferentia of the nll. subiliaci

Nl. popliteus superficialis of the pig
(260/5'; 279/58; 282/9; 292/g; 294/9)

80% of pigs have a superficial popliteal node. It lies subcutaneously between the biceps and semitendinosus muscles, generally where they diverge in their distal course.

In the majority of cases only one of these nodes, either the superficial or the deep, is present; in about one pig in three both are represented. On the other hand, neither of them can be found in about 10% of cases. Nevertheless, meat inspection regulations rightly require that one of the two nodes be examined in certain circumstances because their drainage area is important in assessing the disease status of the hind limb.

Drainage area of the lc. popliteum: skin of the caudal part of the shank and foot; musculature of the shank and foot; fibula, bones and joints of the foot.

Efferent routes of the popliteal lymphocentre: if both popliteal nodes are present then they are interconnected and the efferent vessels go partly to the ischiatic and partly to the iliofemoral nodes.

Lymph collecting ducts

Ductus thoracicus of the pig
(252; 279/60; 284/16, 16'; 285/p)

The thoracic duct originates from the cisterna chyli, without a sharp line of division, at the level of the last thoracic vertebra or sometimes at the transition to the first lumbar vertebra. Up to the 9th thoracic vertebra it remains under the right azygos vein to the right of and dorsal to the aorta. For short distances it may divide into two vessels. From the 9th to the 5th thoracic vertebrae it lies laterally between the aorta and vertebral column turning left at the level of the 5th, rarely the 4th or 6th, thoracic vertebrae. It now lies between the laterally situated blood vessels (left subclavian artery and its branches) and the oesophagus and trachea which are situated medially. A short distance before its termination, the thoracic duct bends ventrad to end 2–15 mm in front of the 1st rib in the venous angle. Its diameter is 2–4 mm throughout its course. In its postcardiac part it has 3–4 bicuspid valves; in the precardiac part 2–4 such valves. At the point where it enters the vein there is also a valve, usually with two cusps, rarely with only one. These terminal valves may occasionally be absent. The thoracic duct receives the efferent vessels of the following lymph nodes: thoracic aortic, cranial mediastinal, cranial sternal, left tracheobronchial, caudal deep cervical and axillary nodes of the first rib. A short distance before its termination it receives the left jugular trunk. The ampulla ductus thoracici is not well developed and may be absent.

Cisterna chyli of the pig
(253/g; 254/Cc; 256/1; 288/12)

The cisterna chyli extends from the 2nd or 3rd lumbar to the last thoracic vertebra and lies against the right dorsal surface of the aorta. Its form is that of an elongated spindle but it can also be subdivided into several branches. At its widest part it measures 5–10 mm in diameter. The cisterna itself is without valves and the visceral trunks which empty into it are said to have no terminal valves.

Truncus visceralis of the pig
(253/h; 254/Tv; 256/n, o, q; 279/62, 63, 64; 288/14, 15, 8)

The origin of the visceral trunk from the coeliac and intestinal trunks is illustrated in figures 254; 256/n, o, q. The truncus visceralis is about 4–5 cm long and 6–9 mm in diameter and it arises behind the cranial mesenteric artery towards the aorta and caudal vena cava. Here it first curves caudally over the ventral border of the left renal vein to reach either the left or right side of the posterior vena cava. Again it changes direction, this time craniad, to receive 1 or 2 pelvic trunks and then enter the posterior pole of the cisterna chyli.

Trunci lumbales of the pig
(253/h, i; 256/m; 260/Tl; 279/61; 288/13)

An extraordinary variable network of longitudinal meshes is formed by the efferent vessels of the iliosacral and deep inguinal lymphocentres and efferent vessels of the lumbar aortic nodes. Gradually the numerous longitudinal branches unite to form fewer, stouter trunks which either empty into the visceral trunk or the cisterna chyli. Alternatively, they may directly form the cisterna by confluence with the visceral trunk.

Truncus jugularis of the pig
(247/Tj; 279/59; 285/r, q)

The efferent vessels of the right and left medial retropharyngeal lymph nodes form the right and left jugular trunks. These are 1–3 mm in diameter. The course and position of these correspond to the description given in the comparative section. The left jugular trunk empties either into the first part of the thoracic duct or independently into the venous angle. About 2 cm before its termination into the right venous angle, the right jugular trunk dilates to 5–6 mm diameter. This dilated terminal part (285/*q*) corresponds to the *right lymphatic duct* of the other domestic mammals.

Finally, it should again be stressed that in the pig only a small proportion of the lymph from the head passes into the jugular trunks, while the bulk goes through an efferent system in which the superficial cervical nodes are an important transit point. This system is lacking in all the other domestic mammals (cf. fig. 245).

Lymph nodes and lymph collecting ducts of the ox

The lymph vascular system of the ox is of considerable practical importance. As in the dog and horse careful attention must be paid to it in clinical and pathological examinations while, additionally, cattle are the most important of the meat animals. Both aspects of the practical application of our knowledge of the lymphatic system of the ox are therefore equally important and should be given equal consideration, as Baum (1912) has done in his monograph and Egehoj (1934, 1935) has done in various papers.

Lymphocentrum parotideum
Nl. parotideus of the ox
(245/*p*; 295/1; 296/1; 298/1)

This is a flat, oval node, 6–9 cm long, which lies immediately ventral to the mandibular joint and is half covered by the parotid gland. It is palpable on the edge of the jaw and the surface of the masseter muscle. At slaughter it remains connected to the tissue of the parotid gland. It must be regularly examined at meat inspection.

Drainage area: skin of the head; mandible, incisive, nasal, frontal and zygomatic bones; mandibular joint; facial and masticatory muscles; parotid gland, external ear, lacrimal apparatus, apical half of the nasal cavity and wall, upper and lower lip, hard palate and parts of the gums, dental pad, chin.

Efferent route: lymph drains exclusively to the lateral retropharyngeal node.

Lymphocentrum mandibulare
Nl. mandibularis of the ox
(245/*M*; 295/2; 296/2; 297/1; 298/2; 299/12)

This node is 3–4.5 cm in length and of elongated oval shape. It is situated a few centimetres behind the vascular notch on the ventral border of the mandible but not in the depth of the intermandibular space. Its nodular shape is palpable and it must not be confused with the oval end of the mandibular gland. Occasionally a second, smaller node is present. The mandibular node must be examined at meat inspection.

Drainage area: skin of the head; facial and masticatory muscles; apical half of the wall of the nasal cavity, lips, cheeks, oral and nasal mucosa, parts of the hard and soft palate, tonsils, gums of the lower jaw and in part of the upper, tip of the tongue, larynx, pharynx, paranasal sinuses, salivary glands. Secondary lymph from the pterygoid node.

Efferent route: lateral retropharyngeal node.

Nl. pterygoideus of the ox
(245/*Pt*; 295/4; 297/4; 299/6)

This is an inconstant node, 0.75–1.5 cm long, situated on the medial surface of the pterygoid muscle, close to the oral border of the mandible.

Drainage area: mandibular node.
Efferent route: mandibular node.

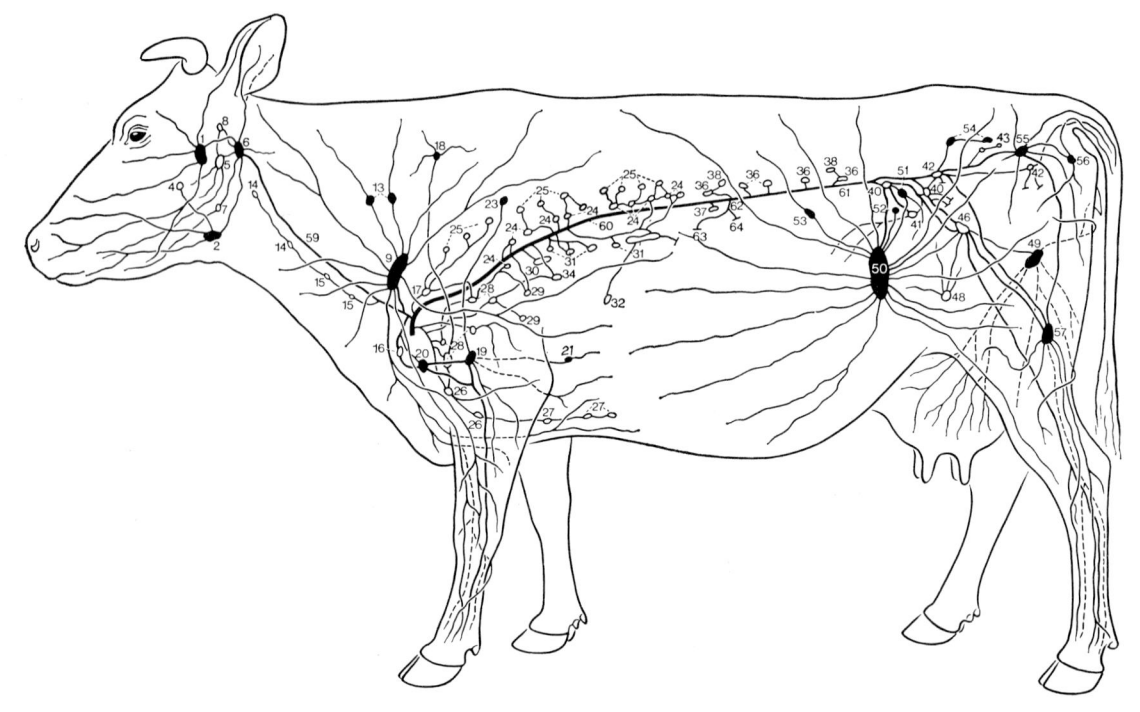

Fig. 295. Survey diagram of the lymph nodes of the ox.
(After Wilkens and Münster, 1972.)

lc. parotideum: *1* nl. parotideus ; lc. mandibulare: *2* nl. mandibularis, *4* nl. pterygoideus (inconstant); lc. retropharyngeum: *5* nl. retropharyngeus medialis, *6* nl. retropharyngeus lateralis, *7* nl. hyoideus rostralis (inconstant), *8* nl. hyoideus caudalis (inconstant); lc. cervicale superficiale: *9* nl. cervicalis superficialis, *13* nll. cervicales superficiales accessorii; lc. cervicale profundum: *14* nll. cervicales profundi craniales, *15* nll. cervicales profundi medii, *16* nll. cervicales profundi caudales, *17* nl. costocervicalis, *18* nl. subrhomboideus (inconstant); lc. axillare: *19* nl. axillaris proprius, *20* nll. axillares primae costae, *21* nl. axillaris accessorius (inconstant), *23* nl. infraspinatus (inconstant); lc. thoracicum dorsale: *24* nll. thoracici aortici, *25* nll. intercostales; lc. thoracicum ventrale: *26* nl. sternalis cranialis, *27* nll. sternales caudales; lc. mediastinale: *28* nll. mediastinales craniales, *29* nll. mediastinales which lie on the pericardium, *30* nll. mediastinales medii, *31* nll. mediastinales caudales, *32* nl. phrenicus (inconstant); lc. bronchale: *34* nl. tracheobronchalis (bifurcationis) sinister, *35* nl. tracheobronchalis (bifurcationis) medius; lc. lumbale: *36* nll. lumbales aortici, *37* nll. renales, *38* nll. lumbales proprii (inconstant); lc. iliosacrale: *40* nll. iliaci mediales, *41* nl. iliacus lateralis, *42* nll. sacrales, *43* nll. anorectales; lc. iliofemorale (inguinale profundum): *46* nl. iliofemoralis, *48* nl. epigastricus; lc. inguinofemorale (inguinale superficiale): *49* nll. inguinales superficiales (nll. scrotales (♂). nll. mammarii (♀), *50* nl. subiliacus, *51* nl. coxalis (inconstant) *52* nl. coxalis accessorius (inconstant), *53* nl. fossae paralumbalis (inconstant); lc. ischiadicum: *54* nl. ischiadicus, *55* nl. glutaeus (inconstant), *56* nl. tuberalis (inconstant); lc. popliteum: *57* nl. popliteus profundus, *59* truncus jugularis, *60* ductus thoracicus, *61* truncus lumbalis, *62* truncus visceralis, *63* truncus gastricus, *64* truncus intestinalis

Lymphocentrum retropharyngeum

Nl. retropharyngeus medialis of the ox
(245/Rm; 295/5; 297/3)

This is a 3–6 cm long, oval node which lies medial to the stylohyoid bone on the pharyngeal muscles. Less commonly there are two nodes. It should be examined during meat inspection.

Drainage area: tongue, hyoid musculature, oral mucosa and gums, hard and soft palate, tonsils, pharynx, larynx, mandibular and sublingual glands, maxillary and palatine sinuses, mandible; caudal half of the nasal cavity; longus capitis muscle.

Efferent route: lateral retropharyngeal node.

Nl. retropharyngeus lateralis of the ox
(245/Rl; 295/6; 296/12; 297/2, 2'; 298/3)

This is a flat, oval node, 4–5 cm in length. In about half of the oxen which are examined another 1–3 smaller nodes, each 1–3 cm in length, will be found. It is situated under the free border of the wing of the atlas overlaid by the upper end of the mandibular gland. It can be palpated and should be examined routinely at meat inspection.

Drainage area: skin of the posterior half of the head and the first part of the neck; lips, cheeks, lower gums in the diastema; body and tip of the tongue, salivary glands, masticatory muscles, mandible, possibly cranial and cervical parts of the thymus, neighbouring neck muscles, external ear; secondary lymph from all nodes of the head.

Efferent routes: the jugular trunk is formed by the efferent vessels of this node.

Fig. 296. Superficial lymph nodes and lymph vessels of the head of the ox.
(After Baum, 1912).

The small crosses (xxx) indicate the sites where the lymph vessel has been injected.

1 nl. parotideus, *2* nl. mandibularis, *3* lymph vessels of the conjunctiva and lower eyelid, *4* lymph vessels of the conjunctiva and upper eyelid, *5* lymph vessels of the mandibular joint, *6, 6'* lymph vessels of the external ear, *7, 8, 9, 10, 11* lymph vessels of individual muscles of the head and neck, *12* nl. retropharyngeus lateralis

a m. levator nasolabialis, *b* m. levator labii maxillaris, m. caninus and m. depressor labii maxillaris, *c* m. zygomaticus, *d* m. malaris, *e* m. buccinator, *f* m. depressor labii mandibularis, *g* m. masseter, *h* m. orbicularis oculi, *i* m. frontalis, *k* m. cleidooccipitalis, *m* m. cleidomastoideus, *n* m. sternomandibularis, *o* m. omohyoideus and sternohyoideus, *p, q, r* muscles of the external ear, *s* m. frontoscutularis, *t* v. jugularis externa, *u* glandula mandibularis, *v* glandula parotis

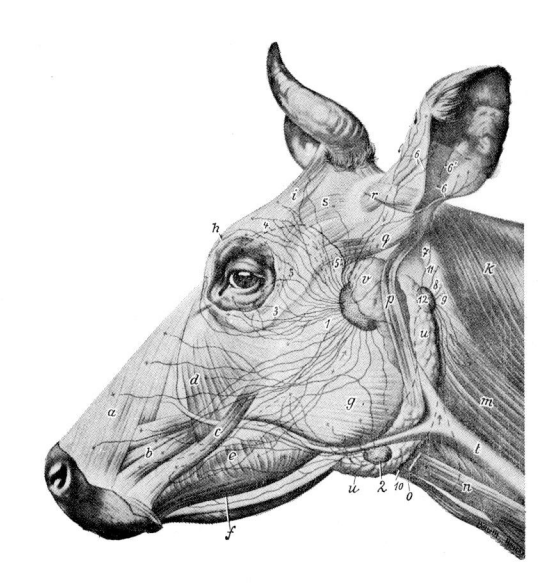

Fig. 297. Deep lymph nodes and lymph vessels of the head of the ox (the left mandible has been removed).
(After Baum, 1912).

1 nl. mandibularis, *2, 2'* nll. retropharyngei laterales, *3* nl. retropharyngeus medialis, *4* nl. pterygoideus, *5* nl. hyoideus rostralis, *6* nl. hyoideus caudalis

a, a' glandula sublingualis, *b* oral part of the glandula mandibularis (the remainder of the gland has been removed), *c* thyroid, *d* m. mylohyoideus (reflected), *e* m. geniohyoideus, *f* m. genioglossus, *g* m. styloglossus, *h* m. hyoglossus, *i* end of the m. sternohyoideus, *k* end of the m. omohyoideus, *l* m. sternothyreoideus, *m* m. thyreo- and cricopharyngeus, *n* m. pterygoideus, *o* m. temporalis, *p* m. cleidomastoideus, *q* m. longus capitis, *r* trachea

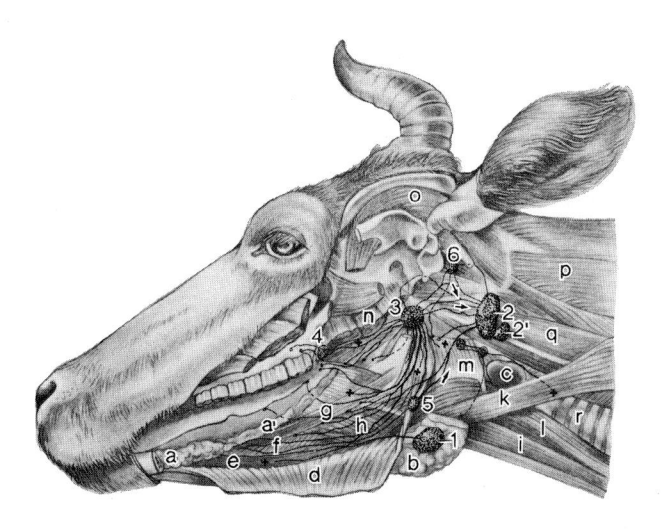

Nl. hyoideus rostralis and hyoideus caudalis of the ox
(245/Hr, Hc; 295/7, 8; 297/5, 6; 299/11)

Both these nodes are 1–1.5 cm long and very inconstant. The rostral node lies on the lateral surface of the thyreohyoid and the caudal node at the angle of the stylohyoid muscle.

Drainage area: apex of the tongue to the rostral node, mandible to the caudal node.

Efferent route: retropharyngeal lymphocentre.

Lymphocentrum cervicale superficiale
Nl. cervicalis superficialis of the ox
(247/Cs; 295/9; 298/4; 299/1)

This node, measuring 7–9 cm in length and 1–2 cm in thickness, can be palpated at the cranial border of the supraspinatus muscle where it is covered by the brachiocephalicus and omotransversarius muscles. In special cases it is examined at meat inspection.

Drainage area: skin of the neck and pectoral limb, of the dorsal, lateral and ventral thoracic walls up to about the level of the 10th–12th rib; musculature of the shoulder girdle, muscles over the scapula, fascia of the lower arm, foot, including tendons and joints; secondary lymph of the accessory superficial cervical node.

Efferent routes: on the left to the end of the thoracic duct or the left jugular trunk, and on the right to the end of the right jugular trunk.

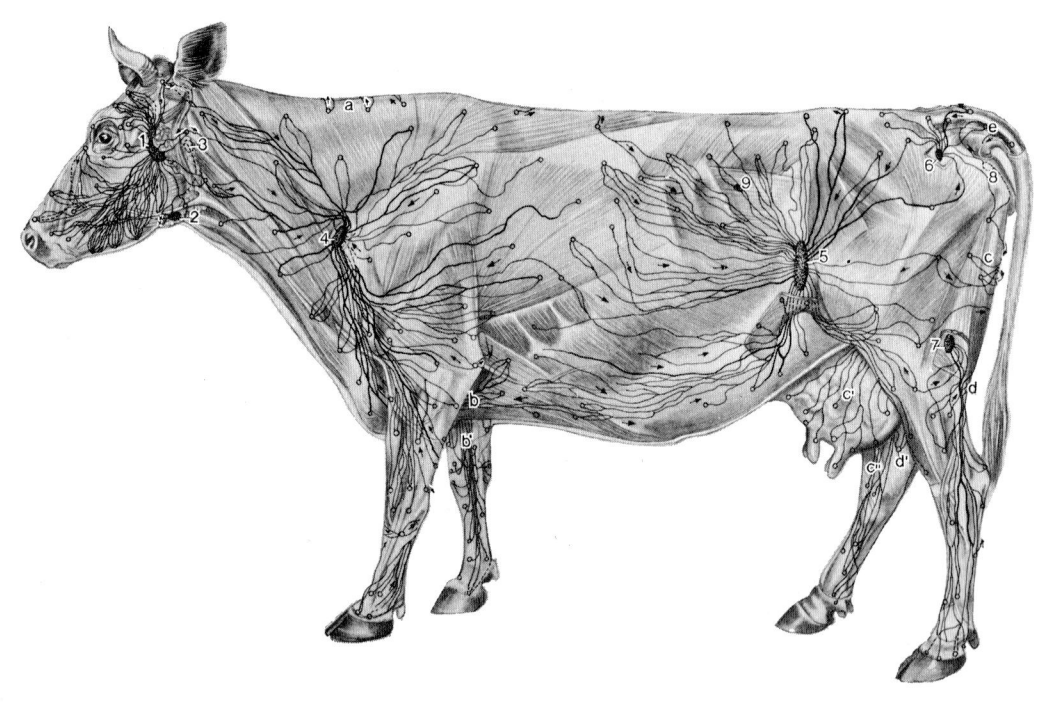

Fig. 298. Lymph nodes and lymph vessels of the skin of the ox.
(Redrawn from several illustrations of Baum, 1912).

1 nl. parotideus, *2* nl. mandibularis, *3* nl. retropharyngeus lateralis, covered by the mandibular gland, *4* nl. cervicalis superficialis, *5* nl. subiliacus, *6* nl. ischiadicus, *7* nl. popliteus profundus, *8* nl. tuberalis, *9* nl. fossae paralumbalis (inconstant)

1 nl. parotideus, *2* nl. mandibularis, *3* nl. retropharyngeus lateralis, covered by the mandibular gland, *4* nl.

a lymph vessels which cross to the superficial cervical node of the other side, *b*, *b'* lymph vessel going from the ventral chest region and the medial aspect of the leg to the superficial cervical nodes of the same side, *c*, *c'*, *c''* lymph vessels from the posterior aspect of the thigh, udder and medial surface of the hind limb going to the superficial inguinal nodes, *d*, *d'* lymph vessels to the deep popliteal node, *e* lymph vessels of the nl. tuberalis

Nll. cervicales superficiales accessorii of the ox
(247/Csa; 295/13; 299/7)

Below the trapezius and omotransversarius muscle, usually at the cranial border of the supraspinatus, there are 5–10 nodes, which are visible through the muscles because they are dark red. Some of these are haemolymph nodes whereas others are linked to the lymph vascular system and are therefore true lymph nodes, the *efferent* route of which is to the superficial cervical node.

Lymphocentrum cervicale profundum

Nll. cervicales profundi craniales of the ox
(247/*Cpc*; 295/14; 299/5, 5')

In the neighbourhood of the thyroid gland at the initial part of the trachea, there are a maximum of 4–6 nodes, each 1–2.5 cm in length. Sometimes they are absent.

Nll. cervicales profundi medii of the ox
(247/*Cpm*; 295/15; 299/4)

On each side of the middle third of the cervical part of the trachea there are 1–7 nodes, each 0.5–3 cm in length. On the right they are closely applied to the trachea but on the left they are nearer the ventral surface of the oesophagus

Nll. cervicales profundi caudales of the ox
(247/*Cpca*; 295/16; 299/3, 3', 3")

Immediately in front of the 1st rib and lying close against each side of the trachea there are 2–4 nodes. Another solitary node may also occur ventral to the trachea. In certain conditions these should be examined during meat inspection.

Drainage area of all the cervical nodes: ventral neck muscles, flexors of the neck; thyroid gland, larynx, pharynx; cervical parts of the trachea and oesophagus; cervical part of the thymus. Secondary lymph of the lateral retropharyngeal node, axillary lymphocentre, costocervical node and sometimes the superficial cervical node.

Efferent routes: on the left side their lymph is discharged into the thoracic duct, the end of the left jugular trunk or sometimes directly into the venous angle. On the right it passes into the terminal part of the right jugular trunk.

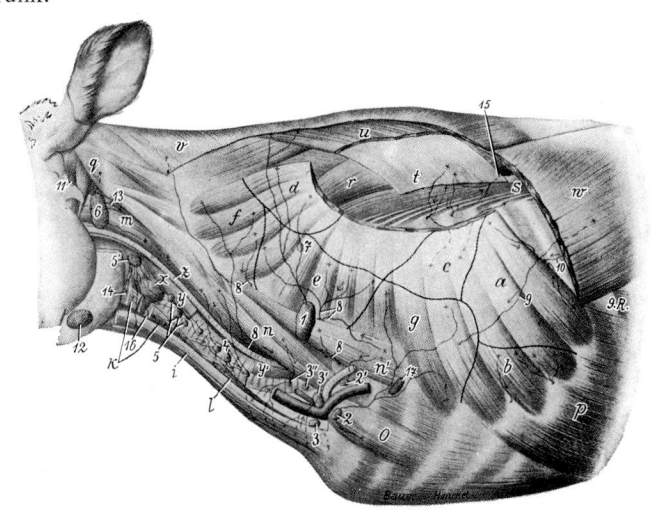

Fig. 299. Deep lymph nodes and lymph vessels of the neck of the ox.
(After Baum, 1912.)

1 nl. cervicalis superficialis, *2, 2'* nll. axillares primae costae, *3, 3', 3"* nll. cervicales profundi caudales, *4* nll. cervicales profundi medii, *5, 5'* nll. cervicales profundi craniales, *6* nl. retropharyngeus lateralis, *7* nl. cervicalis superficialis accessorius, *8, 8* lymph vessels going to the costocervical node, *9* lymph vessels from the latissimus dorsi muscle, which has been cut off, *10* lymph vessel from the latissimus dorsi muscle entering the thoracic cavity, *11* nl. hyoideus caudalis, *12* nl. mandibularis, *13* lymph vessel from the rectus capitis ventralis muscle, *14* lymph vessel from the thyreohyoideus muscle, *15* lymph vessel from the iliocostalis and serratus dorsalis muscles, this vessel enters the thoracic cavity at the medial border of the iliocostalis muscle, *16* lymph vessel from the thyroid or its isthmus; it curves round the ventral border of the trachea at the right side, *17* nl. axillaris proprius, *9 R.* = 9th rib

a, b, c individual regions of the serratus ventralis thoracic muscle, *d, e, f* individual regions of the serratus ventralis cervicis muscle, *i* m. sternomandibular muscle with a portion excised, *k* m. sternothyreoideus, *l* sternomastoideus muscle, cut off, *m* m. longus captitis, *n* m. scalenus medius, *n'* m. scalenus dorsalis, *o* m. rectus thoracis, *p* m. obliquus externus abdominis, *q* m. obliquus capitis cranialis, *r* m. longissimus dorsi, *s* m. iliocostalis thoracis, *t* m. serratus dorsalis cranialis, *u* m. rhomboideus, *v* part of the trapezius muscle, *w* initial part of the latissimus dorsi muscle, *x* thyroid, *y, y'* oesophagus with a part excised, *z* a. carotis communis

Nl. costocervicalis of the ox
(250/2; 251/2; 295/17)

At the cranial border of the arterial costocervical trunk, medial to the cranial border of the first rib, is a node which measures 1.5–3 cm in size. In special cases it should be examined at meat inspection.

Drainage area: supraspinatus and infraspinatus muscles, dorsal musculature of the shoulder girdle; extensors of the back and neck, flexor muscles of the neck, omohyoid muscle; pleura, trachea. Secondary lymph of the first intercostal, cranial mediastinal and subrhomboid nodes.

Efferent routes: on the left, generally to the thoracic duct but also, in very variable patterns, to the caudal deep cervical or cranial mediastinal nodes or directly to the venous angle. On the right the lymph flows to the right jugular trunk or the efferent vessel of the right superficial cervical node.

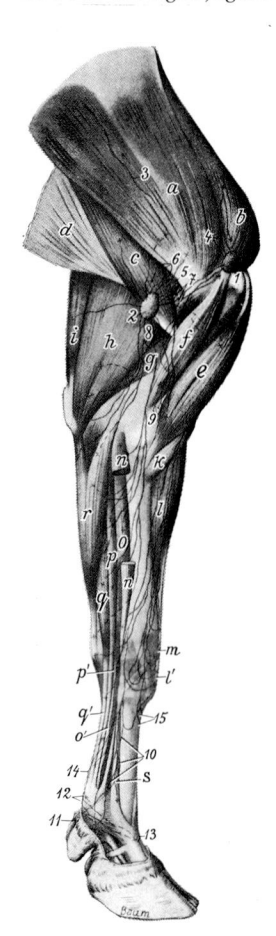

Nl. subrhomboideus of the ox
(295/18)

This node lies below the cervical part of the rhomboideus muscle, near its ventral border and close to the cranial angle of the scapula. It is very inconstant.

Drainage area: supraspinatus, rhomboideus and ventral serratus muscles.

Efferent route: costocervical node.

Fig. 300. Deep lymph nodes and lymph vessels on the medial aspect of the pectoral limb of the ox.
(After Baum, 1912.)

1 nl. axillaris primae costae, *2* nl. axillaris proprius, *3* lymph vessel from the subscapularis muscle going to an intercostal node, *4* and *5* lymph vessels from the infraspinatus muscle, *6, 7, 8, 9* lymph vessels which pass from the lateral to the medial side, *10–15* lymph vessels of the extensor and flexor tendons of the digit

a m. subscapularis, *b* m. supraspinatus *c* m. teres major, *d* m. latissimus dorsi, *e* m. biceps brachii, *f* m. coracobrachialis, *g* caput mediale and *h* caput longum of the m. triceps brachii, *i* m. tensor fasciae antebrachii, *k* m. brachialis, *l* m. extensor carpi radialis, *l'* its tendon, *m* tendon of the m. abductor digiti I longus, *n, n'* m. flexor carpi radialis with a portion excised, *o* m. digitorum profundus, *o'* its tendon, *p* deep belly of the m. flexor digitorum superficialis, *p'* its tendon, *q* superficial belly of the m. flexor digitorum superficialis, *q'* its tendon, *r* m. flexor carpi ulnaris, *s* m. interosseus medius

Lymphocentrum axillare
Nl. axillaris proprius of the ox
(249/*Ap*; 295/*19*; 299/*17*; 300/*2*)

6–10 cm caudal to the shoulder joint, in the 2nd intercostal space or over the 3rd rib on the medial surface of the teres major muscle there is a node 2.5–3.5 cm in diameter. In special cases it is examined at meat inspection.

Drainage area: nearly all the muscles of the shoulder and upper arm, some muscles of the shoulder girdle (trapezius, latissimus dorsi, pectoralis profundus), cutaneous muscle of the shoulder; bones and joints of the forelimb, excluding the metapodium and acropodium. Secondary lymph from the infraspinatus node and possibly the inconstant accessory axillary node.

Efferent routes: axillary node of the first rib, caudal deep cervical node.

Nll. axillares primae costae of the ox
(249/*Apc*; 295/20; 299/2, 2'; 300/1)

2–3 nodes, infrequently only a single node, will be found lateral to the 1st rib and in the 1st intercostal space. They are covered by the laterally situated pectoralis profundus muscle. This group is examined at meat inspection in special cases.

Drainage area: pectoral muscles, transversus costarum, serratus ventralis, and scalenus muscles; some muscles of the shoulder and fore arm; bones of the pectoral limb from the scapula to the carpus; elbow and carpal joints. Secondary lymph from the proper axillary node.

Efferent routes: caudal deep cervical nodes or thoracic duct on the left, and right jugular trunk on the right.

Nl. axillaris accessorius of the ox
(249/*Aa*; 295/21)

A very inconstant small node which can be found over the 4th rib. Its lymph is passed to the proper axillary node.

Nl. infraspinatus of the ox
(249/*J*; 295/23)

This node, 0.5–1 cm in length, is very infrequently present but can sometimes be found near the caudal border of the infraspinatus muscle at the level of the tip of the long head of the triceps brachii. Sometimes it is overlaid by the cranial border of the latissimus dorsi muscle.

Drainage area: latissimus dorsi muscle.

Efferent route: proper axillary node.

Lymphocentrum thoracicum dorsale
Nll. thoracici aortici of the ox
(250/7; 251/8; 295/24)

A variable number of nodes, of between 1 and 3.5 cm in length, is situated between the dorsal wall of the aorta and the bodies of the 5th to 13th thoracic vertebrae. On the left side most of the nodes lie ventral, although some are also dorsal, to the left azygos vein. On the right side they are situated almost exclusively along the dorsal wall of the thoracic duct. They are examined at meat inspection and removed in special cases.

Drainage area: subscapularis muscle; some muscles of the pectoral girdle, muscles of the chest wall, all extensors of the back; diaphragm, heart, occasionally the spleen; pleura, peritoneum, mediastinum; ribs. Secondary lymph of the intercostal and some cranial mediastinal nodes which are inconstantly present on the pericardium.

Efferent routes: lymph from the nodes of the right side goes to the thoracic duct. The posterior nodes of the left side are often linked to the efferent lymphatic trunk of the caudal mediastinal nodes. The outflow from the nodes lying in front of the aortic arch is very variable; it goes either to the cranial mediastinal nodes or their efferent vessels, or into the large lymph collecting ducts or directly into the venous angle.

Nll. intercostales of the ox
(250/8, 8'; 251/9, 9'; 295/25)

At the level of the joints of the rib heads there are one, exceptionally two, nodes for each intercostal space. They are located subpleurally. They are 4–20 mm in size. Numerous variations occur so that some intercostal spaces are without nodes. They are examined in speciel cases at meat inspection.

Drainage area: muscles of the lateral chest wall, extensor muscles of the back, longus colli, subscapularis, external oblique abdominis muscle; costal pleura, peritoneum; ribs and thoracic vertebrae.

Efferent routes: the efferent vessels of the nodes in the first 2–4 intercostal spaces on the right go to the cranial and middle mediastinal nodes; lymph from the nodes of the 1st, 2nd and possibly 3rd intercostal spaces on the left goes to the costocervical node. The left 3rd and 4th nodes send their efferent vessels to the cranial mediastinal nodes which are situated on the aortic arch. The lymph from all the other intercostal nodes goes to the thoracic aortic nodes situated at the same level.

Lymphocentrum thoracicum ventrale
Nl. sternalis cranialis of the ox
(250/3; 251/3; 295/26)

A pair of nodes each 1.5–2.5 cm in diameter, is present on the manubrium sterni on the ventral surface of the internal thoracic artery and vein, at the level of the first costal cartilage or first intercostal space but before these vessels enter the transversus thoracic muscle. Sometimes there is only a single node. These nodes should be examined in special circumstances during meat inspection.
Drainage area: sternum, costal cartilage; transversus thoracic muscle, thoracic musculature; pleura, pericardium. Secondary lymph from the caudal sternal nodes.
Efferent routes: cranial mediastinal nodes or jugular trunk or end of the thoracic duct.

Nll. sternales caudales of the ox
(250/9; 251/16; 295/27)

This group incluses 1–5 nodes which lie on each side of the median line under the transversus thoracic muscle in several, but not all, intercostal spaces. They are located along the internal thoracic artery and vein. It also includes 2–5 nodes which are situated on top of the transversus thoracic muscle immediately before the sternal insertion of the diaphragm.
Drainage area: diaphragm, pericardium, pleura, peritoneum; ribs, sternum; muscles of the chest wall, ventral musculature of the pectoral girdle, abdominal muscles; liver.
Efferent route: cranial sternal node.

Lymphocentrum mediastinale
Nll. mediastinales craniales of the ox
(250/1, 1', 4, 4', 4"; 251/1, 4, 4', 4"; 295/28, 29)

These lymph nodes, lying in the precardiac mediastinum, can be divided into several subgroups. Their location and appearance differ on the two sides of the body. On the left there are: 1) A group of small nodes lying cranial to the aortic arch, behind the costocervical trunk and lateral to the trachea, oesophagus and longus colli muscle. 2) Another group situated ventral to the brachiocephalic trunk or on the left of the cranial vena cava. Small nodes are sometimes insinuated between the two vessels so that they are not immediately obvious. 3) One large or several smaller nodes are found at the origin of the internal thoracic artery (referred to by Baum as the lymph nodes of the thoracic inlet). 4) A small node occasionally occurs on the pericardium behind the aortic arch and in front of the left azygos vein. On the right side there are: 1) A cranial group situated at the level of the aortic arch and dorsal to the trachea. One of these nodes, measuring between 4 and 7 cm in length, is located below the end of the right azygos vein. 1–3 nodes are found in front of and behind the azygos vein up to the costocervical trunk. 2) Another group (nodes of the thoracic inlet, see above) lies at the origin of the internal thoracic artery. 3) In exceptional cases a small node is found on the pericardium, immediately below the termination of the cranial vena cava at the right atrium. These nodes should be examined as a routine in meat inspection.
Drainage area: thoracic parts of the trachea and oesophagus, thymus, lung, pericardium, heart, pleura. Secondary lymph from the cranial intercostal nodes, the tracheobronchial nodes, on the left the thoracic aortic nodes and on the right the middle mediastinal nodes.
Efferent routes: these are very variable passing through nodes of the same group or the costocervical node or, on the left, the thoracic duct and on the right the end of the right jugular trunk.

Nll. mediastinales medii of the ox
(251/*c*; 259/*30*)

These 2–5 nodes are only visible from the right. They are situated on the dorsal and right surfaces of the oesophagus. They are regularly examined at meat inspection.
Drainage area: thoracic part of the trachea and oesophagus, lung. Secondary lymph from the first 4 intercostal and the right tracheobronchial nodes.
Efferent routes: direct to the thoracic duct, to one of the cranial mediastinal nodes of the right side or into an efferent vessel of the caudal mediastinal nodes.

Nll. mediastinales caudales of the ox
(250/*6, 6'*; 251/*7, 7'*; 295/*31*)

This group comprises several nodes situated in the postcardiac mediastinum. One node is usually very long (15–25 cm), although occasionally it may be divided into two, and it lies dorsally against the oesophagus and extends to the diaphragm. 2–3 smaller nodes (1–4 cm) are inserted in the angle between the oesophagus and aorta. Inconstantly there may also be a node immediately in front of the oesophageal hilus and 1–2 others on the left surface of the oesophagus. When enlarged due to disease, these nodes can cause partial closure of the wide but thin-walled oesophagus. Such a constricted oesophageal lumen can be diagnosed by means of a probang. At meat inspection these nodes have to be routinely examined.
Drainage area: thoracic part of the oesophagus, lung, pericardium, diaphragm, mediastinum, peritoneum; spleen and liver. Secondary lymph from the pulmonary, phrenic, left tracheobronchial and occasionally the posterior thoracic aortic lymph nodes.
Efferent routes: lymph is carried directly to the thoracic duct by a stout collecting duct. Smaller efferent vessels sometimes go to the left tracheobronchial node.

Nl. phrenicus of the ox
(251/*10*; 295/*32*)

On the thoracic surface of the diaphragm up to four nodes may be present. Most frequently, however, there is only one and it is generally situated at the foramen venae cavae near the terminal branches of the phrenic nerve.
Drainage area: diaphragm, mediastinum.
Efferent route: caudal mediastinal lymph nodes.

Lymphocentrum bronchale
Nl. bifurcationis (seu tracheobronchalis) sinister of the ox
(250/*5*; 295/*34*; 301/*1*)

This node, 2.5–3.5 cm long, lies caudal to the ligamentum arteriosum between the bifurcation of the trachea and the pulmonary trunk. It is always present and should be examined regularly in meat inspection.
Drainage area: thoracic part of the oesophagus, tracheal bifurcation, heart. Secondary lymph from the pulmonary as well as the thoracic aortic, caudal mediastinal and phrenic lymph nodes.
Efferent routes: to the lymph duct of the caudal mediastinal nodes or the thoracic duct or the caudal or cranial mediastinal nodes.

Nl. bifurcationis (seu tracheobronchalis) dexter of the ox
(251/*20*; 301/*2*)

This node, 1–3 cm in length, can be brought into view if the cranial and middle lobes of the right lung are separated, if necessary by incision of the interlobar fissure. It occurs in 75% of individuals. It should be examined at meat inspection so its obscured location must be remembered.

Drainage area: lung. Secondary lymph from the pulmonary and middle tracheobronchial nodes.
Efferent route: middle mediastinal nodes.

Nl. bifurcationis (seu tracheobronchalis) medius of the ox
(295/35; 301/3)

This node measures 0.75–1 cm in length and lies dorsal to the bifurcation of the trachea. It is lacking in 50% of cattle, but when present it must be examined at meat inspection.
Drainage area: caudal lobe of the lung.
Efferent route: right tracheobronchial node.

Nl. tracheobronchalis cranialis of the ox
(251/5; 301/6)

Cranial and ventromedial to the origin of the tracheal bronchus there is a node measuring 2–5 cm in length. Sometimes it may be accompanied by a second, smaller node. It should be examined at meat inspection.
Drainage area: lung. Secondary lymph from the pulmonary nodes of the right side.
Efferent route: cranial mediastinal nodes.

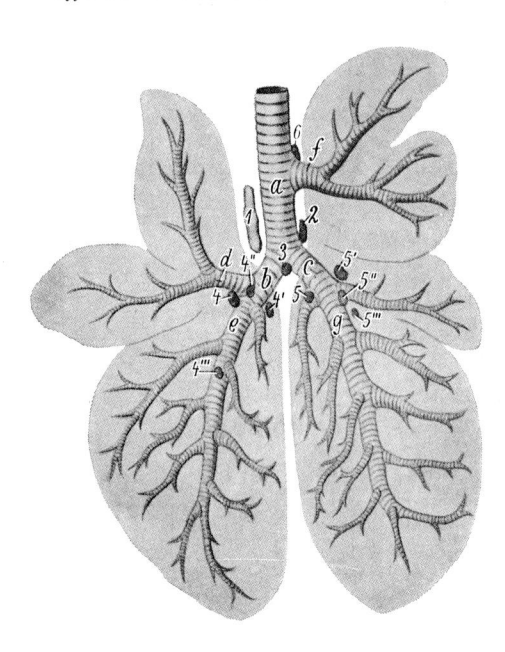

Fig. 301. Lymph nodes of the lung of the ox.
(After Baum, 1912.)

a end of the trachea, *b* left and *c* right bronchus principalis, *d* bronchus for the left cranial lobe, pars cranialis, pars caudalis, *e* bronchus for the left caudal lobe, *g* bronchus for the right caudal lobe

1 nl bifurcationis sinister, *2* nl. bifurcationis dexter, *3* nl. bifurcationis medius, *4, 4', 4", 4'''* nll. pulmonales sinistri, *5, 5', 5", 5'''* nll. pulmonales dextri, *6* nl. tracheobronchalis cranialis

Nll. pulmonales of the ox
(301/4, 4', 4", 4''', 5, 5', 5", 5''')

In at least 50% of cattle there are 1–2 nodes, each 0.5–1.5 cm diameter, located at each of the primary bronchi. They are hidden by lung tissue. At meat inspection the lung tissue is palpated to ascertain whether these nodes are excessively large.
Drainage area: all lobes of the lung with the exception of the right cranial lobe.
Efferent routes: lymph drains to the right, left and cranial tracheobronchial nodes; less often it passes to the caudal mediastinal nodes.

Lymphocentrum lumbale

Nll. Lumbales aortici of the ox
(254/1; 258/2, 2', 2"; 295/36; 309/1)

12–25 nodes are distributed along the lateral, dorsal and ventral surfaces of the abdominal aorta and caudal vena cava, between the last thoracic and the last lumbar vertebrae. They should be examined at meat inspection in special cases.

Drainage area: inner lumbar musculature, extensor muscles of the back; lumbodorsal fascia; lumbar vertebrae; kidneys, adrenals, peritoneum. Secondary lymph from the proper lumbar nodes.

Efferent route: lumbar trunk.

Nll. lumbales proprii of the ox
(254/2; 295/38)

A variable number of round nodes of 0.5 cm diameter occur unilaterally or bilaterally. Their distribution is also irregular but they generally lie near the lumbar intervertebral foramina in a position where they may be confused with sympathetic ganglia. They are most common between the last rib and the transverse process of the 1st lumbar vertebra and between the transverse processes of the 1st and 2nd, the 4th and 5th and the 5th and 6th lumbar vertebrae. The number occurring in any one animal is said not to exceed five and they may occasionally be altogether lacking.

Drainage area: extensor muscles of the back, abdominal muscles, caudal dorsal serratus muscle and lumbodorsal fascia.

Efferent route: aortic lumbar nodes.

Nll. renales of the ox
(254/3; 258/3, 3'; 295/37)

On each side of the renal vessels or in their immediate neighbourhood, there are 1–4 nodes of 0.75–5 cm length (in exceptional cases 9 cm). These are examined as a routine at meat inspection.

Drainage area: kidneys, adrenals.

Efferent routes: cisterna chyli; occasionally also the lumbar or visceral trunks.

Lymphocentrum coeliacum

Nll. coeliaci et mesenterici craniales of the ox
(254/4)

Two to five nodes are situated on the coeliac and cranial mesenteric arteries which, in the ox, arise close to one another. These nodes are not clearly differentiated from the neighbouring groups of the lumbar aortic, splenic and accessory hepatic lymph nodes.

Drainage area: spleen.

Efferent routes: gastric or visceral trunks or directly into the cisterna chyli.

Nll. lienales (seu atriales) of the ox
(254/5; 302/1, 1')

1–7 lymph nodes are insinuated between the cranial sac of the rumen and the left crus of the diaphragm. They are related to the dorsal pole and cranial border of the spleen. Another 1–3 nodes are occasionally distributed to within a short distance of the right side of the cardia. These nodes should be examined regularly at meat inspection. With incorrect evisceration of the rumen, they may adhere to the blunt border of the liver when they must be differentiated from the accessory hepatic nodes.

Drainage area: spleen, rumen including cranial sac, reticulum. Secondary lymph from all gastric nodes (infra).

Efferent routes: this is very variable. As a rule the efferent vessels form the gastric trunk.

Nll. ruminales dextri of the ox
(254/7; 302/2, 2', 3)

Along the right longitudinal groove of the rumen there are 2–8 subserously-situated nodes, each of 1–3.5 cm diameter. At the transition to the cranial groove there are a further 1–4 nodes.

Drainage area: rumen including cranial sac. Secondary lymph from the left and cranial ruminal nodes.
Efferent route: splenic nodes of gastric trunk.

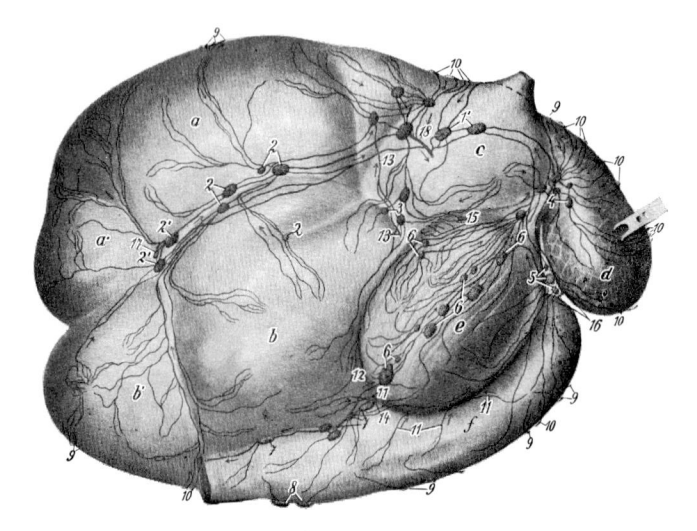

Fig. 302. Lymph vessels and lymph nodes on the right surface of the stomach of the ox.
(After Baum, 1912.)

The vasa efferentia are drawn as thicker lines to distinguish them from the others

a dorsal sac of the rumen, *a'* caudodorsal blind sac, *b* ventral sac of the rumen, *b'* caudoventral blind sac, *c* atrium of the rumen, *d* reticulum, *e* omasum, *f* abomasum

1, 1' nll. lienales seu atriales, *2, 2'* nll. ruminales dextri, *3* nll. ruminales craniales, *4* nll. reticulares, *5* nll. reticuloabomasiales, *6* nll. omasiales, *7* nll. abomasiales dorsales, *8* nll. abomasiales ventrales, *9, 9* lymph vessels curving from the right to the left side, *10, 10* lymph vessels curving from the left to the right side, *11, 11* lymph vessels going to the reticuloabomasal nodes, *12* lymph vessels going to the cranial ruminal nodes, *13* efferent vessels of the left ruminal nodes, *14* efferent vessels terminating in the ruminoabomasal nodes, *15* lymph vessels of the omasum going to the reticuloabomasal nodes, *16* efferent vessels of the ruminoabomasal nodes, *17* lymph vessels from the left side, *18* truncus gastricus.

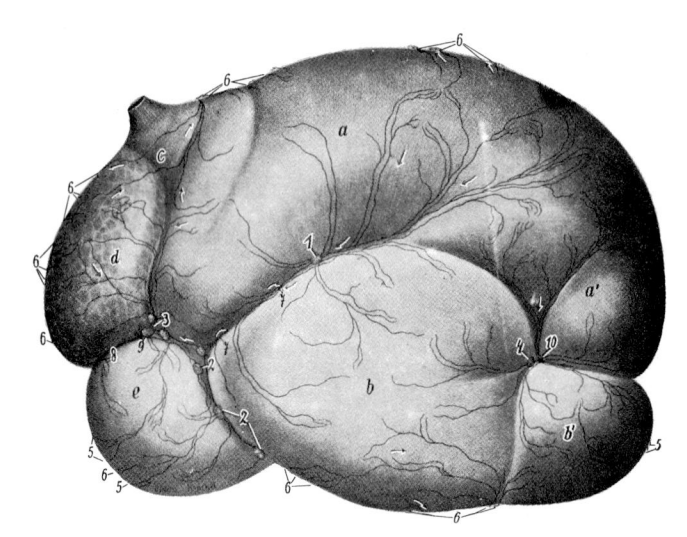

Fig. 303. Lymph vessels and lymph nodes on the left surface of the stomach of the ox.
(After Baum, 1912.)

a dorsal sac of the rumen, *a'* caudodorsal blind sac, *b* ventral sac of the rumen, *b'* caudoventral blind sac, atrium of the rumen, *d* reticulum, *e* abomasum

1 nl. ruminalis sinister, *2* nll. ruminoabomasiales, *3* nll. reticuloabomasiales, *4* inconstant node preceding the right ruminal nodes, *5* lymph vessels which curve around from the right to the left surface, *6* lymph vessels curving from the left to the right side, *7* lymph vessels running to the cranial ruminal nodes, *8, 9* lymph vessels going to the reticuloabomasal nodes, *10* lymph vessels which run in the caudal groove to the right ruminal nodes

Nll. ruminales sinistri of the ox
(254/8; 303/1, 4)

One to two inconstant nodes of 1–2 cm length are situated below the serosa of the left longitudinal groove of the rumen.

Drainage area: rumen.

Efferent routes: cranial ruminal nodes, possibly in part also via the caudal groove to one of the right ruminal nodes.

Nll. ruminales craniales of the ox
(254/9)

These are well hidden in the cranial groove of the rumen. The group comprises 2–8 nodes of 0.5–2.5 cm diameter.
Drainage area: rumen. Secondary lymph from the inconstant left ruminal nodes.
Efferent routes: right ruminal and splenic nodes.

Nll. reticulares of the ox
(254/*10*; 302/*4*)

One to seven small nodes of 0.5–1.5 cm diameter are situated on the dorsal and posterior surfaces of the reticulum at the transition to the omasum. These nodes are occasionally absent.
Drainage area: reticulum. Secondary lymph from the ruminoabomasal and reticuloabomasal nodes.
Efferent routes: splenic nodes; occasionally directly to the gastric trunk.

Nll. omasiales of the ox
(254/*11*; 302/*6*)

Near the greater curvature of the omasum on the surface facing the rumen are 6–12 nodes of 0.5–4 mm diameter.
Drainage area: omasum.
Efferent routes: these are linked one with the other along the greater curvature and they drain into the splenic nodes on the left side.

Nll. ruminoabomasiales of the ox
(254/*12*; 303/*2*)

These comprise 2–7 nodes of 0.5–4 cm diameter which lie cranial and to the left abomasal nodes. They are insinuated between the proximal half of the greater curvature of the abomasum and the rumen. They are best seen from the left.
Drainage area: rumen and cranial sac, omasum, abomasum. Secondary lymph of the cranial dorsal abomasal nodes.
Efferent routes: reticuloabomasal nodes or directly to the reticular nodes.

Nll. reticuloabomasiales of the ox
(254/*13*; 302/*5*; 303/*3*)

The cranial continuation of the preceding chain of lymph nodes is represented by 2–8 nodes of 0.5–4 cm diameter which, viewed from the left, are found to lie between the reticulum, abomasum and cranial sac of the rumen.
Drainage area: rumen, reticulum, abomasum. Secondary lymph from the ruminoabomasal nodes.
Efferent routes: reticular nodes; occasionally directly to the splenic or the omasal nodes.

Nll. abomasiales dorsales of the ox
(254/*14*; 302/*7*)

Each of these 3–6 nodes measures between 0.5 and 4 cm. They are situated along the dorsal border, that is to say, near the lesser curvature of the abomasum.
Drainage area: duodenum, omasum, abomasum.

Efferent routes: in the main the efferent vessels run towards the pylorus and in the lesser omentum to the hepatic nodes. Only the cranially situated nodes may pass their lymph to the ruminoabomasal or omasal nodes.

Nll. abomasiales ventrales of the ox
(254/15; 302/8)

These 1–4 inconstant nodes are situated on the ventral border, or near the greater curvature of the abomasum in the greater omentum. They are restricted to the pyloric part of the abomasum.
Drainage area: duodenum, abomasum.
Efferent route: hepatic nodes.

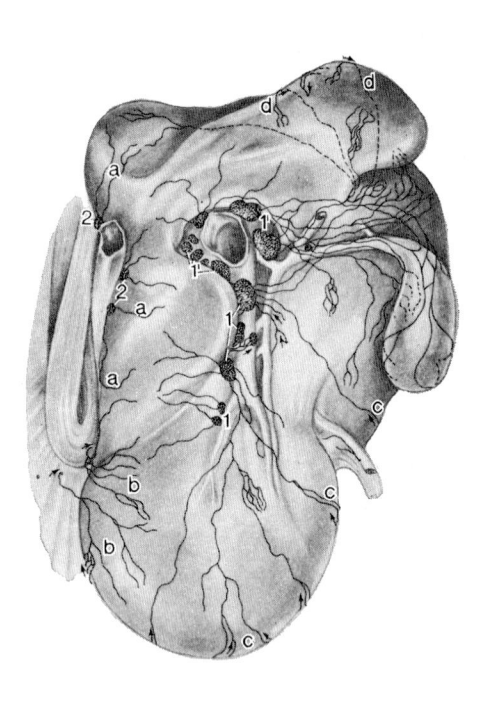

Fig. 304. Visceral surface of the liver of the ox, showing lymph nodes and lymph vessels.
(Redrawn after Baum, 1912.)

1, 1, 1', 1' nll. hepatici, surrounding the portal vein at *1', 1'*, *2, 2* nll. hepatici accessorii

The illustration shows that those superficial lymph vessels which lie near the blunt border of the liver go either to the accessory hepatic nodes (*a, a*) or through the diaphragm into the thoracic cavity (*b, b*). The remaining lymph vessels of the visceral surface of the liver go to the hepatic nodes. Note also that lymph vessels from the parietal surface of the liver curve round onto its visceral surface (*c, c, c*) and, *vice versa*, lymph vessels from the visceral surface of the caudate lobe go to its parietal surface (d, d)

Nll. hepatici (seu portales) of the ox
(254/16; 258/1; 304/1, 1')

6–15 nodes, each 1–7 cm in diameter, are grouped around the porta of the liver. They should be examined routinely at meat inspection.
Drainage area: liver, pancreas and duodenum. Secondary lymph from the dorsal and ventral abomasal nodes.
Efferent routes: the efferent vessels fuse to form the hepatic trunk.

Nll. hepatici accessorii of the ox
(254/17; 258/1'; 304/2)

At the blunt border of the liver, firmly fused to the caudal vena cava and the right crus of the diaphragm, one can detect several small nodes. [Occasionally one may see some lymph nodes loosely attached to the dorsal border of the eviscerated liver; these are splenic nodes (q. v.)].
Drainage area: liver.
Efferent route: hepatic trunk.

Nll. pancreaticoduodenales of the ox
(254/18)

Between the pancreas and duodenum on the one hand and the transverse colon on the other, there is a variable number of small nodes lying on the visceral surface of the pancreas near the point where the portal vein crosses.

Drainage area: pancreas, duodenum, neighbouring parts of the colon, particularly of the transverse colon.

Efferent route: intestinal trunk.

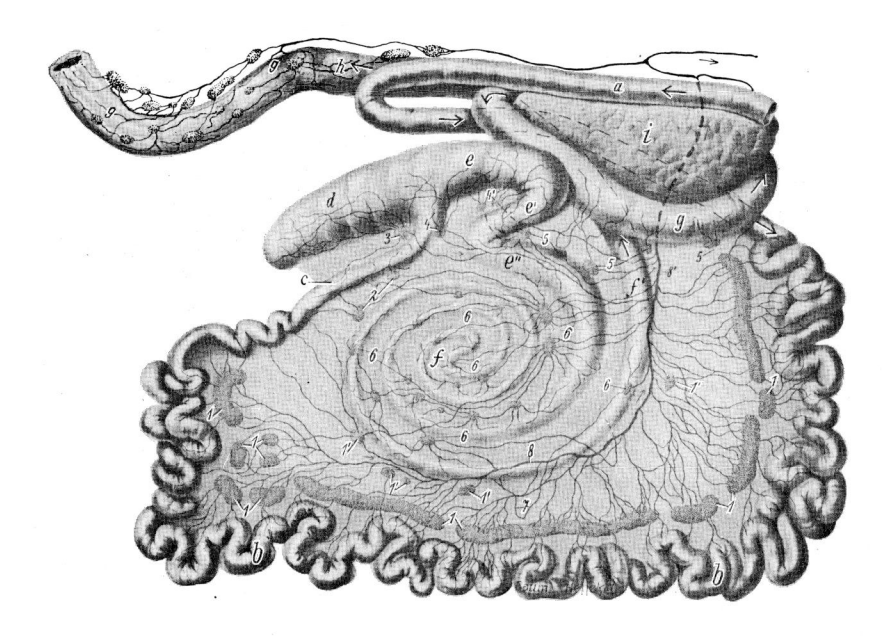

Fig. 305. Intestine of the ox (semi-diagrammatic) with lymph vessels and lymph nodes.
(Extended, after Baum, 1912.)

a duodenum, *b, b* jejunal loops (semidiagrammatic), *c* ileum, *d* caecum, *e, e', e''* first loop of colon, *f* colon labyrinth and *f'* its last loop, *g* terminal loop of colon, *h* rectum, *i* pancreas

1, 1' 2 nll. jejunales, *3* nl. caecalis, *4, 4', 5, 5, 5, 6, 6, 6* nll. colici, *7* lymph vessel of the colon forming a large loop directed towards the jejunum, *8* truncus jejunalis, *8'* truncus intestinalis, *9, 9* nll. anorectales

Lymphocentrum mesentericum craniale
Nll. mesenterici craniales of the ox

See under Nll. coeliaci et mesenterici craniales (p. 393).

Nll. jejunales of the ox
(254/19, 19'; 305/1, 1', 2)

Between the layers of serosa of the mesojejunum there is a group of lymph nodes lying near the jejunum and peripherally to the colonic disc. The number of nodes in this group varies from 10 to 50 and their length varies from 0.5 to 120 cm; there are either relatively few large nodes or a larger number of smaller ones. The group also includes up to 4 inconstant nodes situated in the mesoileum (305/2). They should be examined at meat inspection as a routine.

Drainage area: jejunum, ileum.

Efferent routes: the efferent vessels gradually unite to form the stout intestinal trunk which runs craniodorsally. The nodes lying in the mesoileum also pass their lymph to the colic nodes.

Nll. caecales of the ox
(254/20; 305/3)

One may find one to three nodes of 0.5–2 cm diameter in the ileocaecal fold. They are regularly examined at meat inspection.
Drainage area: ileum, caecum.
Efferent routes: colic nodes or directly to the intestinal trunk.

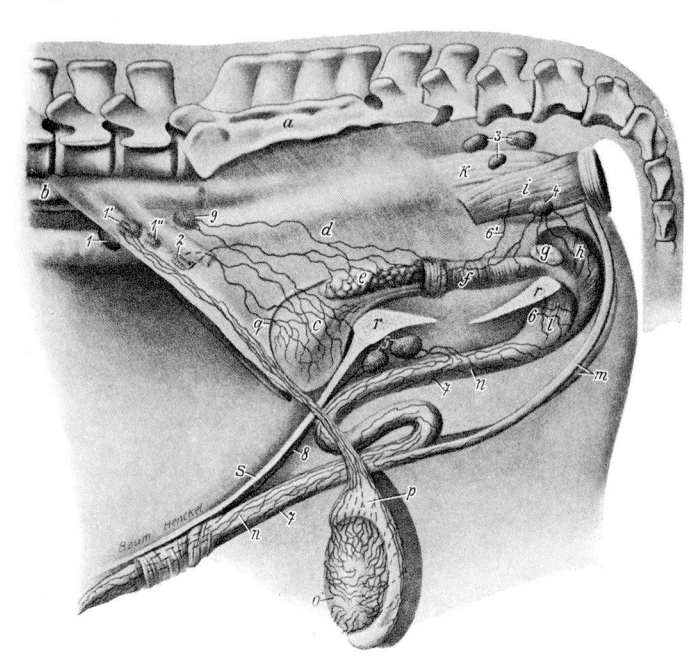

Fig. 306. Lymph vessels and lymph nodes of the male sexual organs of the ox.
(After Baum, 1912.)

1, 1' 1" nll. iliaci mediales, *2* nl. iliofemoralis, *3* nll. anorectales, *4, 9* nl. sacralis, *5* nll. scrotales (inguinales superficiales), *6, 6"* lymph vessels terminating in the left ischiatic nodes, *7* lymph vessels of the urethra, *8* lymph vessels of the visceral layer of the prepuce, *9* see *4*

a sacrum, *b* last part of the abdominal aorta, *c* urinary bladder, *d* ligamentum vesicae laterale and peritonaeum, *e* seminal vesicle, *f* m. urethralis and pelvic part of the urethra, *g* glandula bulbourethralis, *h* m. bulbospongiosus, *i* m. levator ani (cut off at its origin), *k* rectum, *l* m. ischiocavernosus, *m* retractor penis muscle, *n, n* penis *o* testis, *p* epididymis, *q* ductus deferens *r, r* ventral wall of the pelvis, *s* ventral wall of the abdomen

Nll. colici of the ox
(254/21; 305/4, 4', 5, 6)

Three subgroups of colic lymph nodes may be differentiated without difficulty: 1. On the ascending limb and between the ascending and descending limbs of the proximal loop of the colon there are 1–6 nodes (305/4, 4'). 2. Another 1–4 nodes are situated in the angle between the proximal and distal loops of the colon, cranial and dorsal to the colonic disc (305/5). 3. Finally, another 7–30 nodes, the individual size of which only rarely exceeds 0.5–4 cm, lie on the right of the spiral loop, or insinuated between the individual coils, of the colon (305/6). Only some of the nodes in subgroups 1 and 2 are accessible for examination at meat inspection.
Drainage area: ascending colon, ileum, caecum. Secondary lymph from the caecal nodes and from those jejunal nodes which are situated in the mesoileum
Efferent route: the nodes are interconnected and finally pass their lymph into the intestinal trunk.

Lymphocentrum mesentericum caudale
Nll. mesenterici caudales of the ox
(254/22)

On the lateral surface of the descending colon there are isolated lymph nodes which are only indistinctly differentiated from the lumbar aortic, medial iliac and anorectal nodes.
Drainage area: descending colon.
Efferent routes: lumbar trunk. Possibly also to the above-mentioned neighbouring nodes.

Lymphocentrum iliosacrale
Nll. iliaci mediales of the ox
(258/4, 4'; 260/1; 295/40; 306/1, 1', 1"; 307/1, 1'; 309/2)

Immediately before the aorta bifurcates into the external iliac arteries and the origin of the deep circumflex iliac arteries and their venous companion vessels there are, on each side, 1–4 nodes whose length varies between 0.5 and 5 cm. These should be examined at meat inspection in certain circumstances.

Drainage area: femur, hip joint, inner lumbar musculature, pelvic and thigh muscles; testes and spermatic cord or ovary, oviduct and uterus; urinary bladder, urethra. Secondary lymph from the other nodes of the iliosacral lymphocentre and from the deep inguinal, superficial inguinal and ischiatic lymphocentres.

Efferent route: lumbar trunk.

Fig. 307. Lymph vessels and lymph nodes of the female sexual organ of the ox.
(After Baum, 1912.)

The left uterine horn is shown in the extended position

a sacrum, *b* aorta abdominalis, *c* a. iliaca interna, *d* a. iliaca externa, *e* a. circumflexa ilium profunda, *f* rectum, *g* m. levator ani (cut off at its origin), *h* ovary, *i* uterine tube, *k* free horn of the uterus, *l* body of the uterus, *m* vagina, *n* vestibulum vaginae, *o* urinary bladder, *p* urethra, *q, q'* mesovarium and mesometrium, *r* anus, *s* vulva, *t, t'* floor of the pelvis, *u* ventral wall of the abdomen, *v* udder

1, 1' nll. iliaci mediales, *2* nl. iliofemoralis, *3, 3', 4* nll. sacrales, *5, 5* nll. mammarii inguinales superficiales, *6* lymph vessel which terminates in the ischiatic nodes (cut off)

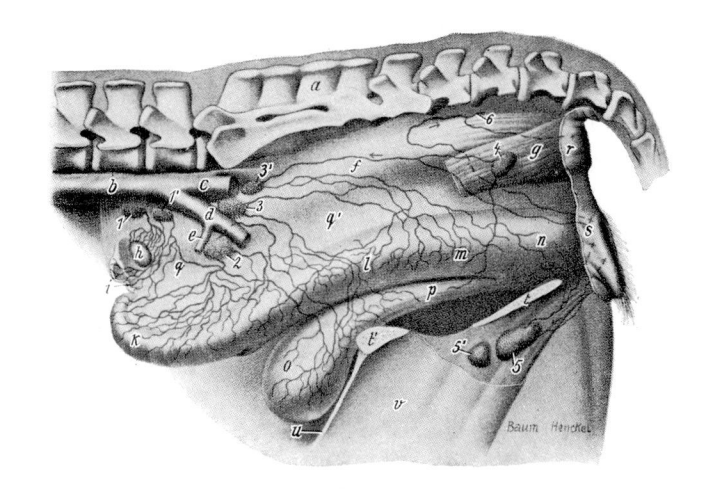

Nl. iliacus lateralis of the ox
(258/7, 7'; 260/1'; 295/41)

One, occasionally two nodes, of 1–2.5 cm in length are situated at the bifurcation of the deep circumflex iliac artery and vein. In a third of the cattle which are examined it will be found to occur only unilaterally and in 10% of cases it is absent from both sides. In special cases this should be examined at meat inspection.

Drainage area: bony pelvis; fascia lata and its extensor, abdominal muscles, deep gluteal muscle, rarely also the quadriceps femoris muscle; peritoneum. Secondary lymph from the subiliac and coxal nodes.

Efferent routes: partly to the medial iliac and partly to the iliofemoral nodes.

Nll. sacrales of the ox
(258/5, 16; 260/1"; 295/42; 306/4, 9; 307/3, 3', 4; 309/4, 5)

At the angle of origin and first part of the internal iliac arteries, and also at the end of the caudal vena cava, there are 2–8 nodes on both sides, each being 0.5–4.5 cm in length. These are accompanied by an inconstant group of smaller nodes located at the transition between the middle and posterior third of the sacrum on the inner surface of the broad sacrotuberal ligament.

Drainage area: iliopsoas, gluteus and tail muscles; ischiocavernosus, bulbospinosus and urethralis muscles; pelvic bones; uterus, vagina and vulva or prostate, seminal vesicle and root of the penis; urinary bladder and urethra. Secondary lymph from the ischiatic lymphocentre.

Efferent routes: partly to the medial iliac and partly to the iliofemoral nodes or, alternatively, directly to the lumbar trunk.

Nll. anorectales of the ox
(260/*1'''*; 295/*43*; 306/*3*)

These are as many as 12 nodes on each side of the anus and rectum and up to 17 on their dorsal surface. They are firmly implanted in the subserosa of these organs. Each is 0.5–3 cm in length.
Drainage area: descending colon, rectum, anus.
Efferent route: medial iliac nodes.

Lymphocentrum inguinale profundum (seu iliofemorale)
Nl. iliofemoralis of the ox
(258/*6, 6'*; 260/*2*; 295/*46*; 306/*2*; 307/*2*; 309/*3*)

The iliofemoral lymph node is situated on the anterior aspect of the external iliac artery before the point of origin of the deep femoral artery. It is readily palpated from the abdominal cavity. It should be examined under special circumstances in meat inspection. Its considerable size of 3.5–9 cm by 3–5.5 cm by 1–2 cm makes palpation by rectal examination possible in the living animal; in this procedure it can be located in front of the body of ilium about 8–13 cm (a hand's breadth) ventrolaterally to the sacral promontory. Another 1–2 smaller noses are occasionally found along the course of the deep femoral artery.

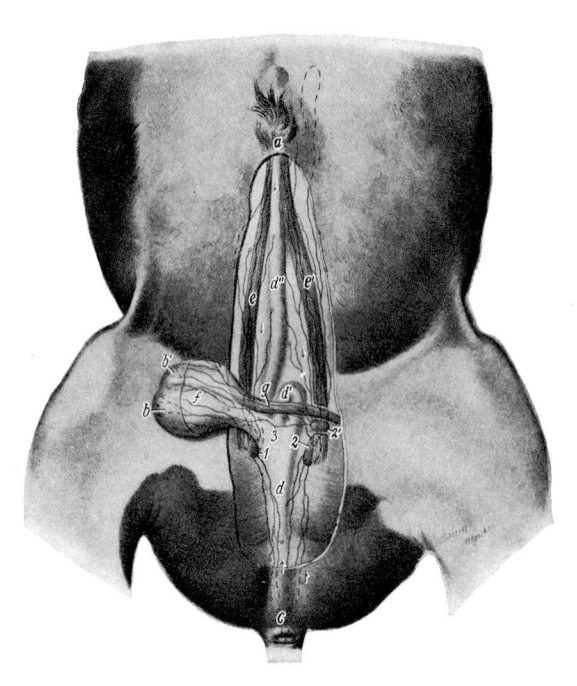

Drainage area: fasciae of the thigh and shank; most of the pelvic and thigh muscles, all leg muscles and their tendons, abdominal muscles; bones and joints of the pelvis and limb; kidneys, bladder, peritoneum; uterus and urethra in the female or, in the male, the tunica vaginalis, cremaster muscle and seminal vesicle; occasionally the skin of the shank and hock joint. Secondary lymph from the popliteal, superficial inguinal, ischiatic and epigastric lymphocentres.

Efferent routes: partly to the medial iliac nodes and in part directly to the lumbar trunk.

Fig. 308. Lymph vessels of the prepuce and scrotum of the ox. (After Baum, 1912.)

1 right, *2, 2'* left nll. scrotales (inguinales superficiales), *3* lymph vessel from the the right half of the scrotum going to a left scrotal lymph node

a prepuce, the greater part of which has been removed, *b, b'* scrotum, most of which has been removed, *c* perineum, *d, d', d''* penis, *e, e'* mm. praeputiales, *f* tunica dartos, *g* m. cremaster

Nl. epigastricus of the ox
(260/*2'''*; 295/*48*)

This is an inconstant, small node lying on the caudal epigastric artery near the pecten of the pubis on the inner surface of the rectus abdominis muscle.
Drainage area: abdominal muscles, peritoneum.
Efferent route: iliofemoral node.

Lymphocentrum inguinale superficiale (seu inguinofemorale)

Nll. inguinales superficiales of the ox
(Nl. scrotalis 306/5; 308/1, 2, 2';
Nll. mammarii 258/9, 9', 9''; 260/3; 295/49; 307/5, 5'; 309/6, 6')

In *males* there are 1, less commonly 2, 3 or 4 nodes, on each side. If only one node is present it measures 3–6 cm by 2–4 cm and lies dorsolateral to the penis at the level of the pecten of the pubis, immediately behind the spermatic cord and below the retractor penis muscle. At this point the skin of the abdominal wall and medial aspect of the thigh is reflected onto the scrotum. The node is palpable and should be regularly examined at meat inspection and removed in special cases.

Drainage area: scrotum prepuce, penis, urethra within the penis; retractor penis muscle; skin of the thigh, shank and knee.

Efferent route: through the inguinal canal to the iliofemoral node.

In *females* there are 1–3 mammary lymph nodes. They are situated relatively far caudad between the thighs and between the posterior half of the base of the udder and the ventral wall of the pelvis. By lifting the udder from behind one can palpate them in the space between the thighs. Often there is also a larger flat node 6–10 cm long, 1–4 cm wide and only 1 cm thick, and 1–2 smaller ones of about half that size. These are regularly examined at meat inspection and removed in special cases.

It is worthy of mention that Hampl found more lymph nodes in two thirds of cows at the base of the teats embedded in the udder parenchyma. These varied considerably in number and size (1–18 mm) and he termed them *nll. intramammarii*. They also occur in calves.

Drainage area: udder, vulva, vaginal vestibule, clitoris.

Efferent route: mainly to the iliofemoral node.

Nl. subiliacus of the ox
(258/8, 8'; 259/1, 1'; 260/3'; 295/50, 298/5)

This node, 6–11 cm by 1.5–2.5 cm in size, is readily palpated where it lies in front of the cranial border of the tensor fasciae latae muscle in the middle of a line between the tuber coxae and the patella. In special cases it is examined at meat inspection.

Drainage area: skin covering all of the following structures: – the ventral, lateral and dorsal walls of the abdomen, the posterior part of the thorax, the pelvis, thigh, knee and shank regions; tensor fasciae latae muscle; prepuce. Secondary lymph of the inconstant lymph node of the paralumbar fossa and the inconstant accessory coxal node.

Efferent routes: iliofemoral and medial iliac nodes. Often some of the efferent vessels pass first through the inconstant coxal node. Very rarely does the lymph flow out to the lateral iliac node.

Nl. coxalis of the ox
(259/2; 260/3''; 295/51)

In the majority of individuals a lymph node of 1.5–2 cm length occurs medial to the tensor fasciae latae muscle, about 12–15 cm in front of the hip joint.

Drainage area: fascia lata and its tensor muscle; quadriceps femoris muscle. Secondary lymph from the subiliac node.

Efferent routes: either to the lateral iliac, medial iliac or iliofemoral nodes.

Nl. coxalis accessorius of the ox
(259/7; 260/3'''; 295/52)

In about half the cases a node, measuring 0.5–1.5 cm, is found lying laterally on, or sometimes embedded in, the tensor fasciae latae muscle near its cranial border at the junction of the upper and middle thirds.

Drainage area: skin covering the pelvis.

Efferent routes: subiliac node, sometimes also the iliofemoral node.

Nl. fossae paralumbalis of the ox
(259/5; 260/3^{iv}; 295/53; 298/9)

One or two small subcutaneous nodes occur inconstantly in the middle of the flank, behind the last rib near the ends of the transverse processes of the lumbar vertebrae.

Drainage area: skin over the lumbar and flank region.

Efferent routes: to the iliofemoral and subiliac nodes.

Lymphocentrum ischiadicum
Nl. ischiadicus of the ox
(259/3; 260/4; 295/54; 298/6)

Lying on the lateral surface of the broad sacrotuberal ligament, 5 cm in front of its caudal border and 3 cm above the lesser ischiatic notch, there is a node of 2.5–3.5 cm diameter. In special circumstances this node should be examined at meat inspection in which case the pelvic ligament has either to be incised from inside at the lower border of the coccygeus muscle, or exposed from caudal.

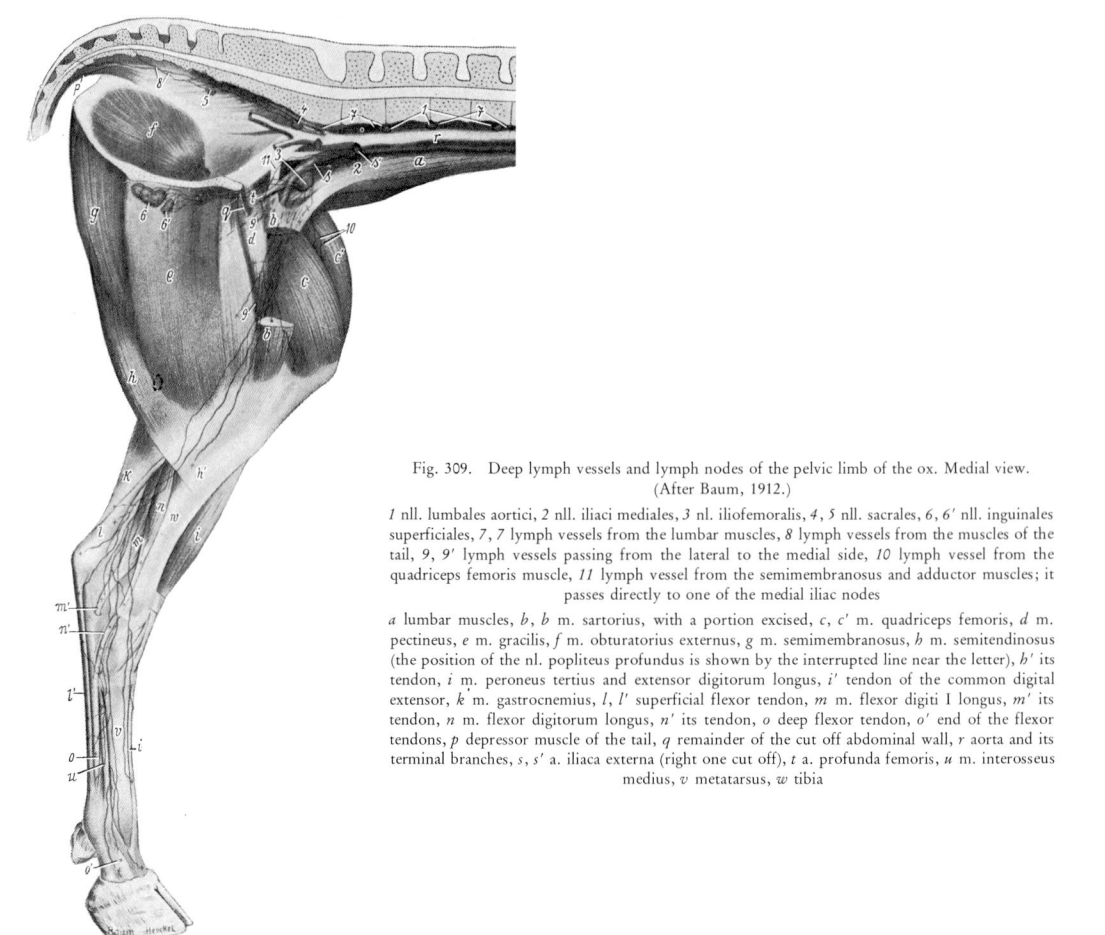

Fig. 309. Deep lymph vessels and lymph nodes of the pelvic limb of the ox. Medial view. (After Baum, 1912.)

1 nll. lumbales aortici, *2* nll. iliaci mediales, *3* nl. iliofemoralis, *4, 5* nll. sacrales, *6, 6'* nll. inguinales superficiales, *7, 7* lymph vessels from the lumbar muscles, *8* lymph vessels from the muscles of the tail, *9, 9'* lymph vessels passing from the lateral to the medial side, *10* lymph vessel from the quadriceps femoris muscle, *11* lymph vessel from the semimembranosus and adductor muscles; it passes directly to one of the medial iliac nodes

a lumbar muscles, *b, b* m. sartorius, with a portion excised, *c, c'* m. quadriceps femoris, *d* m. pectineus, *e* m. gracilis, *f* m. obturatorius externus, *g* m. semimembranosus, *h* m. semitendinosus (the position of the nl. popliteus profundus is shown by the interrupted line near the letter), *h'* its tendon, *i* m. peroneus tertius and extensor digitorum longus, *i'* tendon of the common digital extensor, *k* m. gastrocnemius, *l, l'* superficial flexor tendon, *m* m. flexor digiti I longus, *m'* its tendon, *n* m. flexor digitorum longus, *n'* its tendon, *o* deep flexor tendon, *o'* end of the flexor tendons, *p* depressor muscle of the tail, *q* remainder of the cut off abdominal wall, *r* aorta and its terminal branches, *s, s'* a. iliaca externa (right one cut off), *t* a. profunda femoris, *u* m. interosseus medius, *v* metatarsus, *w* tibia

Drainage area: skin of the pelvic and tail regions; gluteal muscles, muscles of the buttocks; internal obturator muscle; hip joint; rectum, anus, urethra; vulva or prostate, root of the penis, musculature of the pelvic outlet. Secondary lymph from the popliteal and tuberal nodes.

Efferent route: sacral nodes.

Nl. glutaeus of the ox
(259/8; 260/4'; 295/55)

This comprises two nodes. One, measuring 1 cm in diameter, is found in the majority of individuals at the greater ischiatic notch, while the other, which measures 0.5–1 cm, is inconstantly present on the broad sacrotuberal ligament where it is covered by the gluteobiceps muscle.
Drainage area: pelvic bones, hip joint; deep gluteal muscle and lumbodorsal fascia.
Efferent route: sacral nodes.

Nl. tuberalis of the ox
(259/4; 260/4"; 295/56; 298/8)

This is a very constant, 2–3 cm long, node which occurs subcutaneously immediately medial to the ischiatic tuberosity and medial to the insertion of the broad sacrotuberal ligament. It is frequently removed with the subcutaneous fat while skinning the carcase.
Drainage area: skin of the pelvic and tail regions; gluteobiceps muscle.
Efferent routes: usually to the ischiatic node, rarely to one of the sacral nodes.

Lymphocentrum popliteum
Nl. popliteus profundus of the ox
(259/6; 295/57; 298/7; 309/*h*)

This node lies on the gastrocnemius muscle in the depth of the flexor aspect of the knee. It is situated 7–9 cm from the posterior edges of the semitendinosus and gluteobiceps muscles. It is 3–4.5 cm in length. It should be examined at meat inspection in special cases.
Drainage area: skin of the foot and parts of the shank; musculature of the buttock; fasciae of the knee and shank; tendons of the shank muscles; interosseus muscle; bones of the shank and foot; hock and toe joints.
Efferent routes: mainly to the iliofemoral node but also to the sacral nodes with or without first passing through the ischiatic node.

Lymph collecting ducts
Ductus thoracicus of the ox
(250/*10*; 251/*11*; 252; 295/60)

This duct traverses the diaphragm, not at the aortic hiatus but lateral to the right crus. As a rule the thoracic duct remains single throughout its entire course but in exceptional cases the original single trunk divides within the thoracic cavity into two parallel vessels of equal calibre. The latter two vessels are linked by cross-anastomoses. The transition of the single trunk from the right to the left side, or the fusion of the two parallel trunks if duplicated, occurs at the level of the 5th, occasionally 4th, thoracic vertebra. Its diameter is 2–4 mm in calves and 6–10 mm in adult cattle. The double trunks are appropriately narrower than the single trunk. The left part of the thoracic duct runs to the left of the trachea and oesophagus and medial to the large blood vessels. It, too, may occasionally divide into several branches which, however, unite into a single vessel before the duct terminates. Only in very rare cases does one encounter double, or even three to four, terminal vessels. The duct ends a few millimetres to 2 cm anterior to the cranial border of the 1st rib. Towards the last part of the duct there may be an ampulla-like dilatation but invariably there is a constriction for the last 1–3 mm. Its terminal orifice has one or two valves and, additionally, a venous valve often lies across the opening. It is interesting to note that not infrequently there is a connecting branch from the terminal part of the thoracic duct to the right jugular trunk, running past the ventral surface of the jugular vein. The direction of flow of the lymph in this branch is unknown.

Cisterna chyli of the ox
(252; 254/Cc; 258/15)

As a rule the cisterna chyli is about twice the calibre of the thoracic duct. It extends from the 1st or 2nd lumbar to the last thoracic vertebra and lies dorsal to the caudal vena cava. The lumbar trunk and visceral trunk empty into the caudal end of the cisterna. Both these trunks are 0.75–1 cm in diameter. The cisterna continues as the thoracic duct and its cranial end can either reduce suddenly in size or become spindle-shaped. The shape of the cisterna chyli is very variable. Generally its diameter is 1.5–2 cm although occasionally it is more saccular and it can be up to 4 cm in diameter.

Truncus visceralis of the ox
(254/Tv, Th, Tg, Ti; 258/11, 12, 13, 14; 295/62, 63, 64; 305/8, 8')

The visceral trunk is 0.7–1 cm wide and arises near the origin of the cranial mesenteric artery by confluence of the gastric and intestinal trunks. It is generally a short distance thereafter that the hepatic trunk joins the visceral trunk. It is rare for all three trunks to meet at one point and thus there is no coeliac trunk.

Trunci lumbales of the ox
(258/10; 295/61)

It is not possible to describe all the many variations of this lumbar trunk. Most frequently it arises from the efferent vessels of the sacral and iliofemoral nodes which are joined by the efferents of the medial and lateral iliac nodes. The single or double trunk then receives further tributaries from the lumbar aortic and renal nodes before it joins with the visceral trunk to form the cisterna chyli.

Truncus jugularis of the ox
(247/Tj; 295/59)

The left jugular trunk arises from the efferent vessels of the lateral retropharyngeal node. It runs along the left side of the trachea and receives the lymph vessels of the superficial and deep cervical nodes and of the costocervical node. Sometimes, however, these tributaries are received by a smaller trunk running parallel to it and this unites with the jugular trunk at about the middle of the neck. The jugular trunk then terminates either in the last part of the thoracic duct or independently into the venous angle, adjacent to the opening of the thoracic duct. Alternatively it may divide into two branches before terminating, one of which then terminates in the former manner and the other in the venous angle.

The right jugular trunk behaves like the left except for the last part, because it ends as one or two branches directly in the venous angle. Along its course it receives the stout afferent vessels of the right superficial cervical, the right caudal deep cervical and the right costocervical nodes. The efferent vessels of those parts of the cranial mediastinal nodes which lie on the right at the thoracic inlet also contribute to this trunk. The duct is between 0.5 and 2 cm long and its terminal part is dilated so that, from a comparative point of view, one can refer to it as a *right lymphatic duct*.

Lymph nodes and lymph collecting ducts of the goat and sheep

In comparison with the other domestic mammals, the lymphatic vascular system of the small ruminants has not been adequately described. This means that, although there are many differences between the lymph nodes of the ox and those of the small ruminants, official national and international meat inspection regulations are mainly based on the ox. This must be rectified in the future but it seems superfluous in these circumstances to make further reference to the importance of certain lymph nodes of small ruminants in meat inspection unless the regulations expressly indicate a different procedure to that for the ox. In the case of the lymph nodes of the head of small ruminants, a different procedure is required in meat inspection.

Lymphocentrum parotideum
Nl. parotideus of the goat and sheep
(310/*1*; 318/*1, 1'*)

In the goat there is generally one node of 1.2–5.0 cm length, whereas the sheep has two to four nodes. They are situated below the mandibular joint at the posterior border of the masseter muscle, completely covered by the parotid gland. During meat inspection this node, like all the other nodes of the head, need be examined only when a disease process is suspected.

Drainage area: skin of the upper half of the head, including nostrils; mouth and nasal cavity, tongue, gums, muscles of mastication. It rarely receives secondary lymph from the mandibular node.

Efferent route: lateral retropharyngeal node.

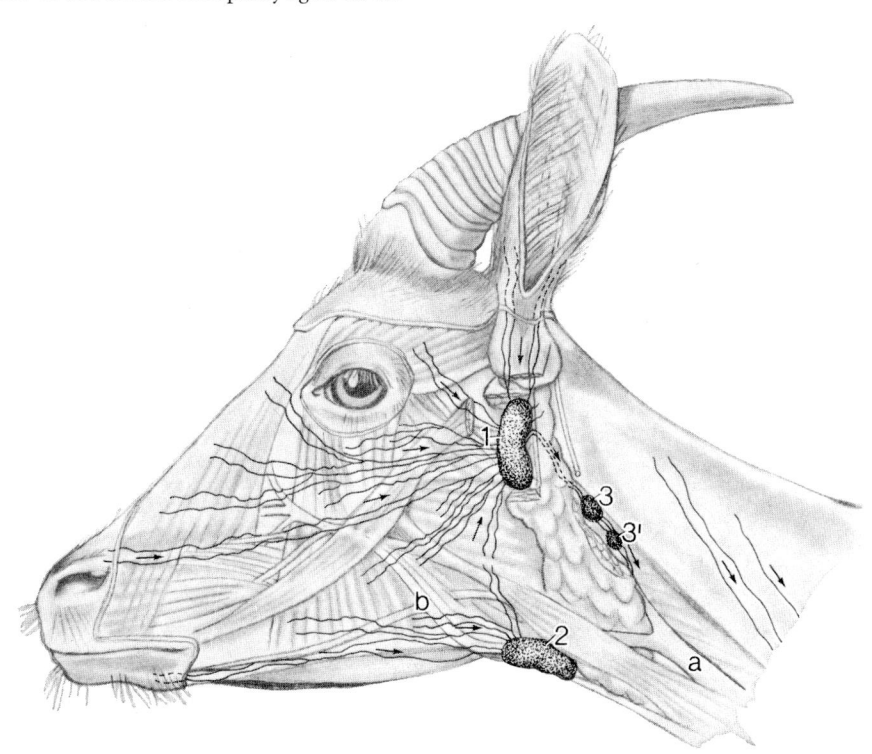

Fig. 310. Superficial lymph nodes and lymph vessels of the head of the goat.
(Redrawn after Tanudimadja and Ghoshal, 1973.)
1 nl. parotideus, *2* nl. mandibularis, *3, 3'* nll. retropharyngei laterales
a v. jugularis externa, *b* v. facialis

Lymphocentrum mandibulare
Nl. mandibularis of the goat and sheep
(310/*2*; 318/*3*)

The goat usually only has one of these nodes and it is 1.7–3.5 cm in length. In the sheep there are sometimes two and they lie at the level of, or immediately behind, the vascular notch of the mandible covered by cutaneous muscle. At meat inspection they are examined only under special circumstances.

Drainage area: skin of the lower jaw, tongue, mouth cavity, gums of the lower jaw, mandibular gland and parts of the masticatory muscles.

Efferent routes: it generally drains to the lateral retropharyngeal node or sometimes to the medial node.

Lymphocentrum retropharyngeum
Nl. retropharyngeus medialis of the goat and sheep
(312/1)

One or two triangular to oval nodes of about 2–4 cm in length are situated on the roof of the pharynx. The right and left nodes are about 0.5 cm apart. The position of the node is identical in both small ruminants. At meat inspection they are to be examined only in doubtful cases.

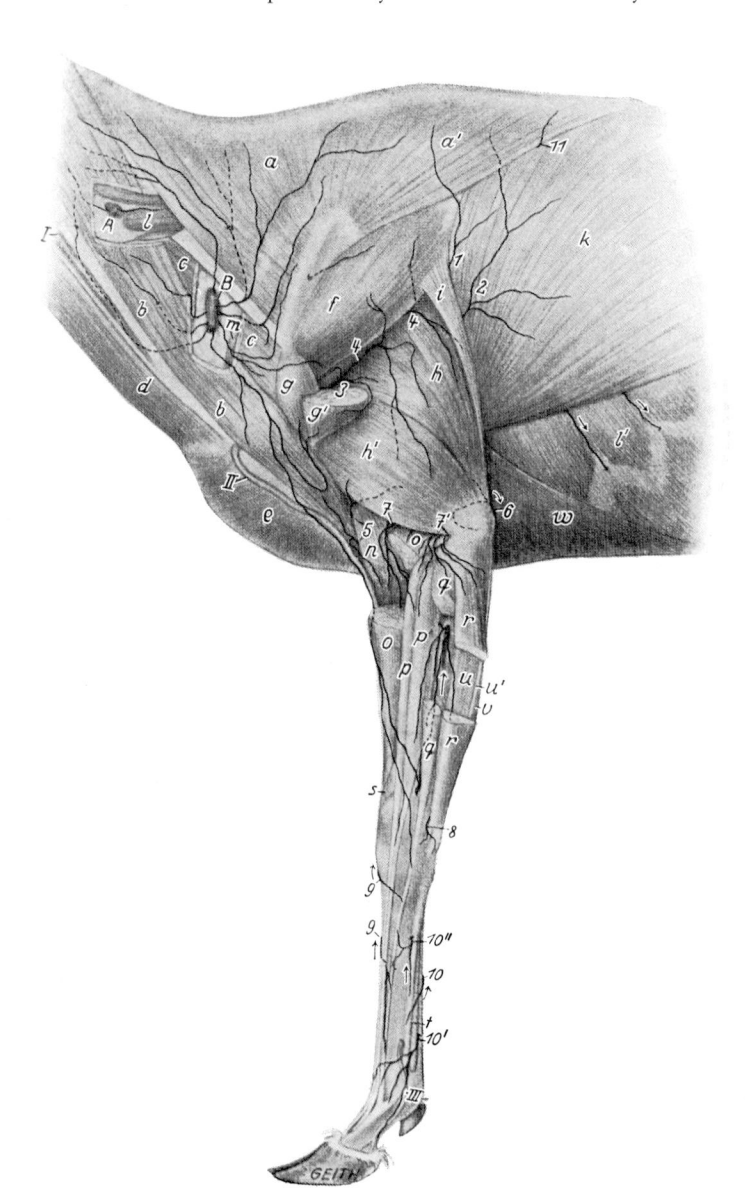

Drainage area: mouth and nasal cavity, gums, masticatory muscles, muscles of the tongue, pharynx. Sometimes secondary lymph from the mandibular node.

Efferent routes: partly to the lateral retropharyngeal node, and partly the efferent vessels are involved in the formation of the jugular trunk.

Fig. 311. Superficial cervical lymph nodes and lymph vessels of the pectoral limb musculature of the sheep.
(After Grau, 1934.)

A nl. cervicalis superficialis accessorius, *B* nl. cervicalis superficialis

1–10 lymph vessels of the musculature of the pectoral girdle and fore limb; these are tributary to the axillary lymphocentre

I v. jugularis externa, *II* v. cephalica

a–v muscles of the shoulder girdle and pectoral limb

Nl. retropharyngeus lateralis of the goat and sheep
(310/3, 3'; 312/2, 2'; 318/2)

In the sheep there is one large and up to six smaller nodes. In the goat there are two or three. They are somewhat disc-shaped and 0.7–2.8 cm in diameter. They lie below the wing of the atlas on the left border of the parotid, covered by the aponeurosis of the cleido-occipitalis muscle. Only examined at meat inspection in doubtful cases.

Drainage area: skin of the parotid region and deeper parts of the upper nape region. Secondary lymph from all the nodes of the head.

Efferent routes: they form the lateral root of the jugular trunk.

Lymphocentrum cervicale superficiale
Nl. cervicalis superficialis of the goat and sheep
(311/B; 313/A; 318/4)

At the cranial border of the supraspinatus muscle, covered by the cervical part of the trapezius, the omotransversarius and the cleido-occipitalis muscles, there is a single node of 3.4–6 cm in length in the goat. In the sheep there may be a second node.

Drainage area: skin and musculature of the neck and the dorsal and lateral wall of the thorax up to the 10th intercostal space; also a few superficial lymph vessels of the pectoral limb.

Efferent routes: the left node drains into the jugular trunk, the right directly into the venous angle.

Nll. cervicales superficiales accessorii of the sheep
(311/A)

This small node is present only in the sheep and it lies ventral to the splenius muscle between the 2nd and 3rd cervical vertebrae, under the brachiocephalicus or omotransversarius muscles. It may be absent but this is rare.

Lymphocentrum cervicale profundum
Nll. cervicales profundi craniales of the goat and sheep
(312/5)

One or two nodes, each of 0.7–1.5 cm diameter, are found dorsal to the thyroid and caudal to the constrictor muscles of the pharynx. They may be present on one or both sides. In the goat they are inconstant, being present in barely half the goats which have been examined. The incidence has not been determined in the sheep.

Drainage area: lymph vessels of the immediate neighbourhood.

Efferent route: lymph flows to the lateral root of the jugular trunk.

Fig. 312. Deep cervical lymph nodes and course of the truncus jugularis of the goat. Ventral view.
(Redrawn after Tanudimadja and Ghoshal, 1973.)

1 nl. retropharyngeus medialis, *2, 2'* nl. retropharyngeus laterales, *3* nl. cervicalis profundus medius, *4, 4* nll. cervicales profundi caudales, *5* nl. cervicalis profundus cranialis (inconstant)

a truncus bijugularis, *b* v. jugularis externa, *c* a. carotis communis, *d* thyroid, *e* medial root of the truncus jugularis, arising from the efferent vessels of the medial retropharyngeal node, *f* lymph vessels going to the lateral retropharyngeal node, *g* lateral root of the truncus jugularis formed by the efferent vessels of the lateral retropharyngeal nodes, *h* truncus jugularis sinister, *i* common duct of the two jugular trunks, which is formed by the efferent vessels of the deep caudal cervical nodes and which terminates independently in the venous angle

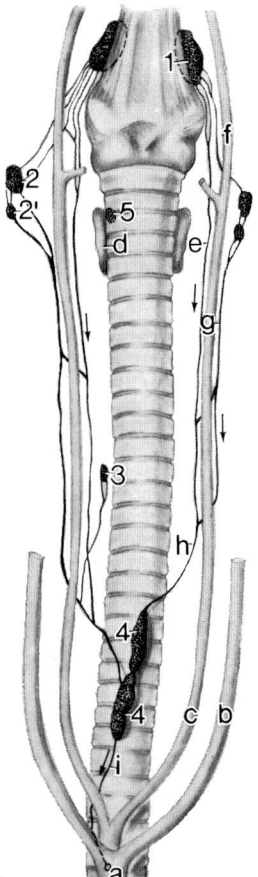

Nll. cervicales profundi medii of the goat and sheep
(312/3)

This node, which is 1–1.5 cm in diameter, is present in at least half the population. In the goat it occurs unilaterally or bilaterally but in the sheep it is unpaired. It lies ventral to the trachea.

Drainage area: trachea, oesophagus, lymph vessels of the surrounding region.

Efferent route: lateral root of the jugular trunk.

Nll. cervicales profundi caudales of the goat and sheep
(312/4)

In the goat 1–3 unpaired nodes, each 3–4 cm long, lie ventral to the trachea and 4–5 cm in front of the thoracic inlet. This group is also present in sheep.
Drainage area: surrounding musculature; trachea, oesophagus, thymus. Secondary lymph from the left and/or the right jugular trunk.
Efferent routes: venous angle (external jugular vein or bijugular trunk).

Nl. costocervicalis of the sheep and goat
(314/*1*; 315/*1*)

In both the sheep and the goat this node lies medial or immediately cranial to the first rib between the costocervical artery and vein. It is not always present.
Drainage area: muscles of the surrounding region; trachea, oesophagus.
Efferent routes: on the left, either into the thoracic duct or into the axillary nodes of the first rib. On the right, into one of the cranial mediastinal or the cranial tracheobronchial nodes.

Lymphocentrum axillare
Nl. axillaris proprius of the goat and sheep
(313/*C*)

In the sheep and goat there is one (rarely two) node on the medial surface of the teres major muscle, in the angle formed by the subscapular artery and vein and by the thoracodorsal artery and vein. In the goat it measures 1–3 cm in length.
Drainage area: lymph vessels of the carpus, of the lower and upper arm, of the medial surface of the scapula.
Efferent route: axillary nodes of the first rib.

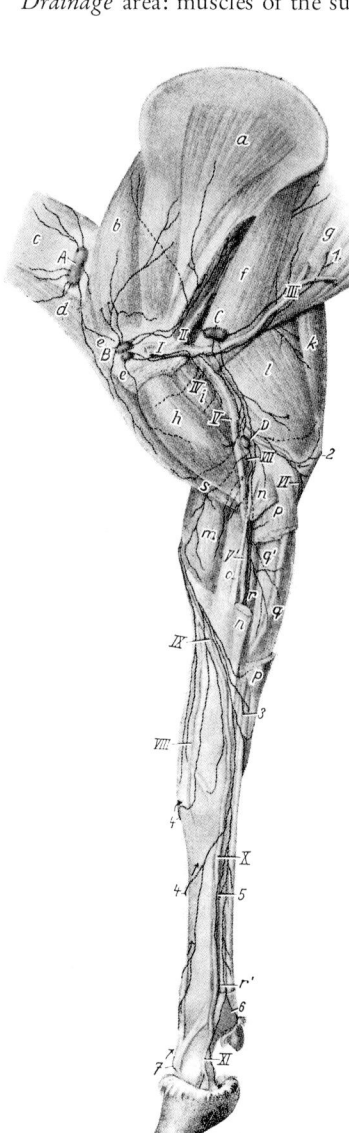

Fig. 313. Lymph nodes and deep lymph vessels of the pectoral limb of the sheep. Medial view.
(After Grau, 1934.)
A nl. cervicalis superficialis, *B* nll. axillares primae costae, *C* nl. axillaris proprius, *D* nl. cubitalis (inconstant)
1 lymph vessels of the trapezius and latissimus dorsi muscles, *2* lymph vessels of the triceps brachii muscle, *3, 4, 5, 6* lymph vessels of the flexor and extensor tendons of the foot
I to *XI* veins and *a* – *r* muscles of the pectoral limb

Nll. axillares primae costae of the goat and sheep
(313/B)

In sheep and goats there are always 2–3 nodes situated lateral to the 1st and 2nd ribs or in the 1st intercostal space at the level of the axillary artery and vein. In the goat they are 0.7–1.5 cm in length.

Drainage area: skin of the ventral and lateral walls of the thorax; serratus ventralis thoracis and pectoralis profundus muscles; parts of the abdominal musculature and the muscles of the anterior thoracic wall. Secondary lymph from the proper axillary node.

Efferent routes: on the left to the thoracic duct, the costocervical node or its efferent vessel. On the right to the efferent lymphatic vessel of the superficial cervical node.

Nl. axillaris accessorius of the sheep

This is a very small node which is only occasionally encountered in the sheep at the level of the 5th intercostal space where it is covered by the pectoralis profundus muscle. It is never present in the goat.

Fig. 314. Lymph nodes and lymph vessels of the thoracic cavity of the goat. Left lateral view.
(Redrawn after Tanudimadja and Ghoshal, 1973.)

1 nl. costocervicalis, *2 2* nll. mediastinales craniales, *3, 3* nll. intercostales, *4, 4* nll. thoracici aortici, *6, 6* nll. mediastinales caudales, *7* nl. bifurcationis sinister, *8* nl. sternalis cranialis

a lymph vessels from the left superficial cervical node, *b* ductus thoracicus

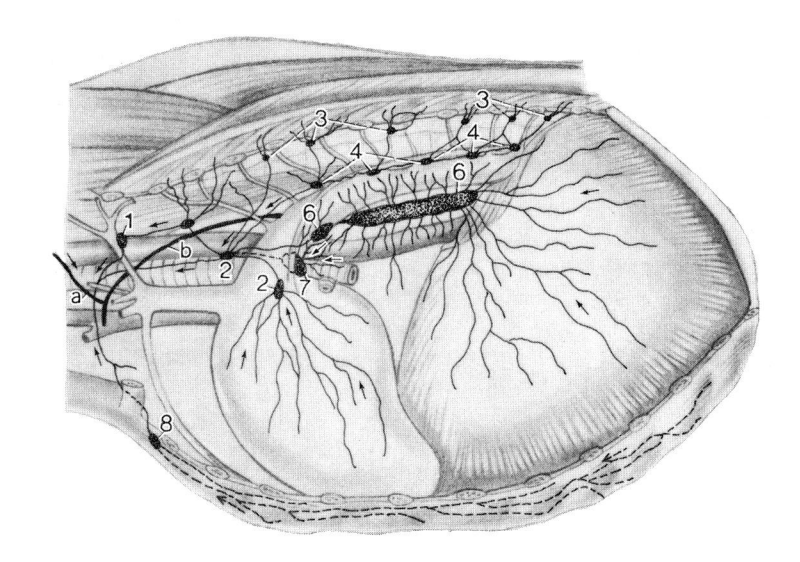

Fig. 315. Lymph nodes and lymph vessels of the thoracic cavity of the goat. Right lateral view.
(Redrawn after Tanudimadja and Ghoshal, 1973.)

1 nl. costocervicalis, *2* nll. mediastinales craniales, *3, 3* nll. intercostales, *4, 4* nll. thoracici aortici, *5* nll. mediastinales medii, *6* nl. mediastinalis caudalis, *7* nl. bifurcationis dexter, *8* nl. sternalis cranialis

a lymph vessels from the superficial cervical node, *b* lymph vessels from the deep cervical node, *c* ductus thoracicus

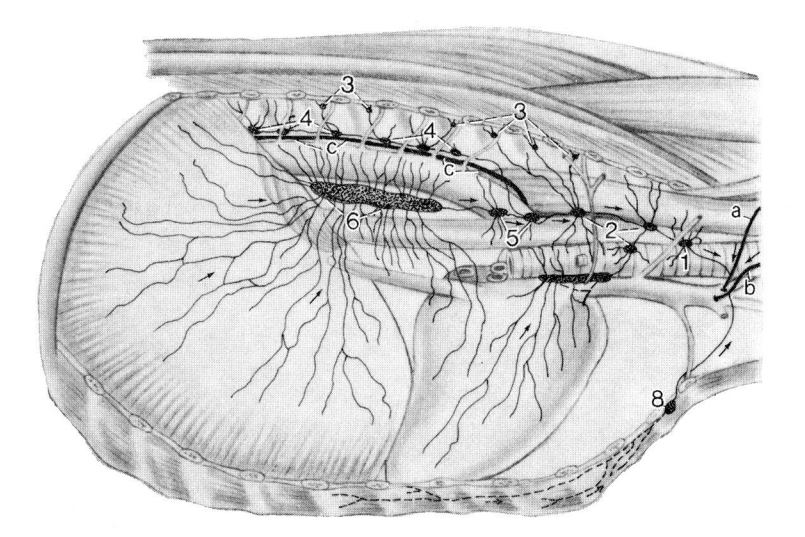

Nl. cubitalis of the sheep
(313/D)

Only occasionally will one find this small node in the sheep. It lies a little proximal to the elbow joint in the angle between the brachial and collateral ulnar veins. It has not been found in the goat.

Lymphocentrum thoracicum dorsale
Nll. thoracici aortici of the sheep and goat
(314/4; 315/4)

These nodes occur subpleurally in the sheep and goat. They lie dorsal to the thoracic aorta, immediately below the body of the thoracic vertebrae and medial to the sympathetic trunk. In the goat there are 5–6 nodes on each side measuring 0.4–1.5 cm in length.
Drainage area: oesophagus, thoracic wall. Secondary lymph from the intercostal nodes.
Efferent routes: cranial and middle mediastinal nodes.

Nll. intercostales of the goat and sheep
(314/3; 315/3)

In both goats and sheep small nodules of about 0.5 cm diameter are present below the pleura at the level of the ribhead joint or the rib angle. In the goat there are 5 or 6 on each side and in the sheep, too, the number of intercostal spaces containing a node is not constant.
Drainage area: dorsal and lateral thoracic wall.
Efferent routes: thoracic aortic or cranial mediastinal nodes.

Lymphocentrum thoracicum ventrale
Nl. sternalis cranialis of the goat and sheep
(314/8; 315/8)

In sheep and goats there is, on both sides, a node measuring 0.6–1.8 cm in length which is located on the manubrium sterni in the 1st intercostochondral space, in front of the transversus thoracic muscle.
Drainage area: transversus thoracic muscle; ventral part of the thoracic wall, pectoralis profundus muscle and parts of the abdominal musculature. In the sheep it also receives secondary lymph from the caudal sternal nodes.
Efferent routes: on the left into the efferent vessels of the superficial cervical node, on the right into the vessel of the caudal deep cervical nodes.

Nll. sternales caudales of the sheep

In the sheep there are often 1–3 nodes on the sternum under cover of the transversus thoracis muscle. Their outflowing lymph goes to the cranial sternal node. These nodes are absent in the goat.

Lymphocentrum mediastinale
Nll. mediastinales craniales of the goat and sheep
(314/2, *8*; 315/2)

In the precardiac mediastinum of both goats and sheep there are, on each side, 2–3 nodes or, less commonly, a single node. In the goat they are 0.8–1 cm in length. Occasionally one node may also be located on the left of the pericardium.

Drainage area: trachea, oesophagus, thymus; longus colli muscle. Secondary lymph of the intercostal, thoracic aortic, cranial tracheobronchial and caudal mediastinal nodes.

Efferent routes: costocervical node or its efferent vessels.

Nll. mediastinales medii of the goat and sheep
(315/5)

In the goat there are 1–2, even 3, nodes each of 0.7–3 cm in length. They are located at the base of the heart. Although these nodes also occur in the sheep, no information is available as to their number and frequency.

Drainage area: trachea, oesophagus, lung, mediastinum; longus colli muscle. Secondary lymph from the thoracic aortic and caudal mediastinal nodes.

Efferent routes: cranial mediastinal nodes.

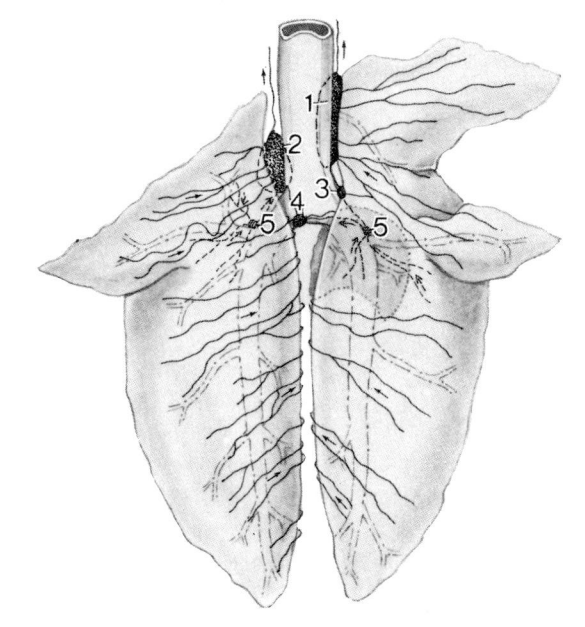

Fig. 316. Lymph nodes and lymph vessels of the lung of the goat. (Redrawn after Tanudimadja and Ghoshal, 1973.)

1 nl. tracheobronchalis cranialis, *2* nl. bifurcationis sinister, *3* nl. bifurcationis dexter, *4* nl. bifurcationis medius, *5, 5* nll. pulmonales

Nll. mediastinales caudales of the goat and sheep.
(314/5, 6; 315/6)

In both the sheep and goat there is a large and a small unpaired node lying in the postcardiac mediastinum between the thoracic aorta and the oesophagus. In the sheep, the large posterior node is 7–10 cm in length and the smaller cranial node is 1–1.5 cm in length. In the goat the corresponding measurements are 10–13 cm and 1–3 cm respectively.

Drainage area: diaphragm, oesophagus, mediastinum, pericardium, part of the dorsolateral thoracic wall between about the 6th and 13th ribs.

Efferent routes: middle mediastinal nodes.

Lymphocentrum bronchale

Nl. bifurcationis (seu tracheobronchalis) sinister of the goat and sheep.
(314/7 ; 316/2)

Anterior to the origin of the left principal bronchus there is, in both the sheep and goat, a constant large node which in the goat is 2–3.5 cm long. The left azygos vein passes over this node.

Drainage area: caudal lobe of the left lung, trachea, oesophagus, mediastinum, heart. Secondary lymph from the inconstant middle tracheobronchial node.

Efferent routes: cranial mediastinal nodes.

Nl. bifurcationis (seu tracheobronchalis) dexter of the goat.
(315/7 ; 316/3)

Nl. bifurcationis (seu tracheobronchalis) medius of the goat.
(316/4)

In the goat both these nodes are very inconstant and they appear to be entirely absent in the sheep.

The right tracheobronchial node lies to the right and dorsal to the origin of the right principal bronchus. It is 0.2 cm in length. It *drains* the middle lobe of the right lung and the heart. Its *efferent* routes go to the cranial tracheobronchial node.

The middle tracheobronchial node lies on the dorsum of the tracheal bifurcation and is 0.3 cm in length. Its *drainage* area includes both caudal lobes and the accessory lobe. Its lymph is passed to the left tracheobronchial node.

Nl. tracheobronchalis cranialis of the goat and sheep.
(316/1)

Below the tracheal bronchus there is an elongated node which is 1–7 cm in length in the goat and about 2.5 cm in length in the sheep. The right azygos vein passes over it.

Drainage area: cranial lobe of the right lung, trachea, oesophagus, pericardium. Secondary lymph from the right tracheobronchial node in the goat or, if it is lacking, the lymph vessels of the middle lobe and perhaps also of the caudal lobe.

Efferent route: cranial mediastinal nodes.

Nll. pulmonales of the goat
(316/5)

In exceptional cases one may find a large node on the right and left principal bronchus of the goat. This is 0.7–1 cm in length and is covered by lung tissue.

Lymphocentrum lumbale
Nll. lumbales aortici of the goat and sheep

In the region of the abdominal aorta and the caudal vena cava there are 14–21 subperitoneal nodes, each 0.2–1.1 cm in length, in the goat and 14–18 nodes, 0.1–4 cm in length, in the sheep. No information is available on their afferent vessels, but the outflowing lymph goes to the lumbar trunk.

Nl. renalis of the goat and sheep

Immediately behind the renal blood vessels of the goat there is one node, 2–3 cm in length, on each side. In the sheep there are reputed to be one or two nodes in this location.

Lymphocentrum coeliacum
Nll. coeliaci et mesenterici craniales of the goat and sheep
(317/1)

Two small (1 mm) nodes are found in the root of the mesentery in one goats in three. In the sheep there are said to be between 1 and 4 of these nodes. Nothing is known about their afferent vessels but they drain into the intestinal trunk.

Nll. lienales (seu atriales) of the goat and sheep
(317/2)

In the goat this group is formed by 2–4, but usually 3, nodes, each 1.5 cm in diameter. There are 2–3 nodes in the sheep. They lie on the atrium of the rumen immediately behind the cardia and they occur fairly regularly.

Drainage area: rumen. Secondary lymph from the reticular, omasal and dorsal abomasal nodes.
Efferent route: to the coeliac trunk.

Nll. ruminales dextri of the goat and sheep
(317/3)

In the cranial half of the right longitudinal groove of the rumen of the goat there are usually 2, but sometimes only 1, nodes which are about 1.5 cm in length. Occasionally these are accompanied on the right by 1–2 nodes at the transition between the longitudinal and cranial grooves. The sheep has 2–3 nodes.

Drainage area: rumen.
Efferent routes: coeliac trunk. The cranial inconstant nodes of the goat also transmit their lymph to the splenic nodes.

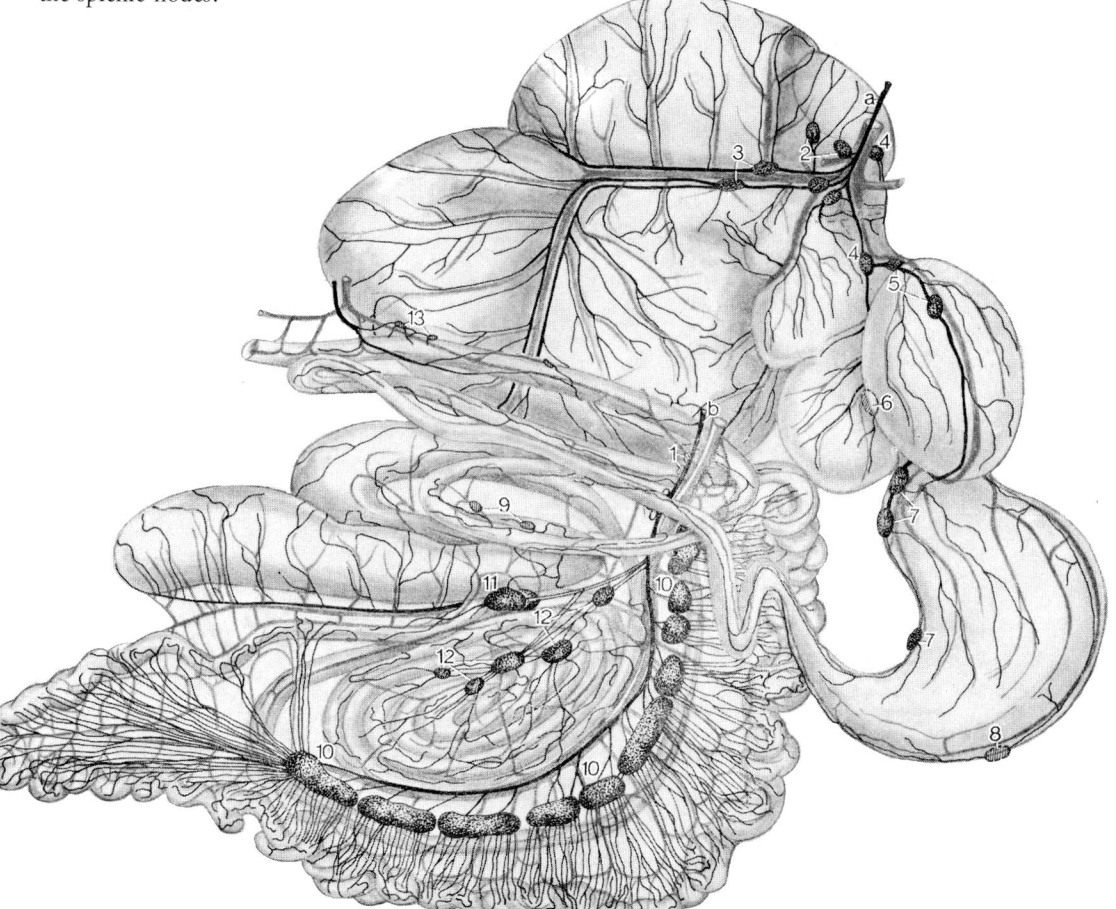

Fig. 317. Stomach and intestine of the goat showing lymph nodes and lymph vessels.
(Redrawn after von Forstner, Diss. med. vet. Munich, 1974.)

1 nll. coeliaci et mesenterici craniales (inconstant), *2* nll. lienales seu atriales, *3* nll. ruminales dextri, *4* nll. reticulares, *5* nl. omasialis, *6* nl. reticuloabomasialis (inconstant), *7, 7* nll. abomasiales dorsales, *8* nl. abomasialis ventralis (inconstant), *9* nll. pancreaticoduodenales, *10, 10* nll. jejunales, *11* nll. ileocolici, *12, 12* nll. colici, *13* nll. mesenterici caudales (inconstant);
a truncus gastricus, *b* truncus intestinalis

Nll. ruminales sinistri et craniales

These nodes are seen only occasionally in the sheep and goat.

Nll. reticulares of the goat and sheep
(317/4)

These nodes are inconstant, occurring in less than half the animals. There are up to 2 nodes on the dorsal surface of the reticulum.
Drainage area: reticulum, cranial sac of the rumen. Secondary lymph from the omasal and dorsal abomasal nodes.
Efferent route: coeliac trunk.

Nll. omasiales of the goat and sheep
(317/5)

In the majority of cases there are 1–2 nodes on the curvature of the omasum.
Drainage area: omasum. Secondary lymph from the dorsal abomasal nodes.
Efferent route: reticular nodes of coeliac trunk.

Nll. ruminoabomasiales and nll. reticuloabomasiales of the sheep (and goat)
(317/6)

These nodes are present in about every second sheep. They occur in groups of 1 to 3 nodes. In the goat the ruminoabomasal nodes are always absent and a reticuloabomasal node is only occasionally encountered.

Nll. abomasiales dorsales of the goat and sheep
(317/7)

A fairly large node (1–2 cm) occurs relatively constantly near the omasum on the lesser curvature of the abomasum. Another 1–2 nodes can extend up to the pylorus.
Drainage area: abomasum, omasum.
Efferent route: omasal nodes.

Nll. abomasiales ventrales of the goat and sheep
(317/8)

Only in one goat in five are one or two nodes present on the greater curvature of the abomasum or at the insertion of the omentum. They are also inconstant in occurrence in the sheep.
Drainage area: abomasum.
Efferent routes: proximally to the coeliac trunk and distally to the hepatic nodes.

Nll. hepatici of the goat and sheep

Around the porta of the liver there is a group of small (0.2–4 cm) nodes. Their efferent vessels form the hepatic trunk which terminates in the end of the intestinal trunk.

Nll. pancreaticoduodenales of the goat and sheep
(317/9)

In the sheep there is one group of lymph nodes in the first part of the mesoduodenum and a second group on the ventral surface of the pancreas and on the right lobe of the pancreas along the duodenum.

The goat only has the second of these groups which consists of 3 nodes and sometimes even it may be absent.

Drainage area: pancreas, duodenum and related parts of the colon.

Efferent routes: the first group (sheep) drains to the hepatic nodes; the second group (sheep and goats) goes to the intestinal trunk.

Lymphocentrum mesentericum craniale

Nll. mesenterici craniales (see nll. coeliaci et mesenterici craniales)

Nll. jejunales of the goat and sheep
(317/10)

This, the largest group of intestinal lymph nodes, is elongated and lies in the mesentery between the first centripetal and the last centrifugal coils of the spiral loop of the ascending colon. The number and size of the individual nodes varies considerably. One may observe between 2 and 25 (average about 12) nodes, each being 0.3–30 cm (average 3.5 cm) in length.

Drainage area: jejunum, ileum.

Efferent routes: The efferent vessels from the jejunal trunk which runs parallel with the cranial mesenteric artery and vein.

Nll. caecales of the sheep or Nll. ileocolici of the goat
(317/11)

In the ileocaecal fold of the sheep there are 2–3 nodes. These are always lacking in the goat. But in this latter species there are 3, less commonly only 2, nodes of 2 cm in length on the ileocolic artery near the junction of the ileum with the large gut.

Drainage area: caecum, ileum. In the goat they also drain the lymph vessels coming from the proximal loop of the colon.

Efferent routes: colic nodes or directly to the intestinal trunk.

Nll. colici of the goat and sheep
(317/12)

These nodes lie both superficially on the right side of the colonic spiral and also between the individual coils. Individual nodes can be seen in the proximal part of the mesentery. The number in the sheep varies between 7 and 11 and in the goat between 2 and 8 with an average of 5. They are between 0.2 and 5 cm in length with an average of 1.5 cm.

Drainage area: ascending colon; in the sheep they also receive lymph from the caecum and ileum.

Efferent route: intestinal trunk.

Lymphocentrum mesentericum caudale

Nll. mesenterici caudales of the goat and sheep
(317/13)

In the mesocolon descendens there are a variable number of small, inconstant nodes. These receive the lymph vessels of the descending colon and they pass their lymph to the lumbar trunk.

Lymphocentrum iliosacrale

Nll. iliaci mediales of the goat and sheep
(319B/5)

In the goat there are two, less often three, elongated nodes on the external iliac artery. The craniomedial of these attains the angle between the aorta and external iliac artery. The second, and larger, caudolateral node extends to the origin of the deep circumflex iliac artery. In the sheep there are

416   Lymph vessel system

one to three nodes in the same location, although the largest is not infrequently fused with the largest of the iliofemoral nodes.

Drainage area: skin of the tarsus and shank; foot; tarsal and knee joints; testes and epididymis or ovary. Secondary lymph from the sacral, ischiatic, superficial inguinal, subiliac nodes and partly from the popliteal and deep inguinal nodes.

Efferent routes: the efferent vessels give rise to the lumbar trunk.

Nll. iliaci laterales of the sheep and goat

Only in rare instances do these small nodes occur in sheep. They are located at the bifurcation of the deep circumflex iliac artery. In the goat they are even less common.

Nll. sacrales of the goat and sheep
(319B/3, 4)

At the bifurcation of the internal iliac arteries there is always a node. It is about 1 cm in diameter. Further small nodes occur, very inconstantly, unilaterally or bilaterally along the course of the internal iliac artery, at the level of the greater ischiatic notch of the caudal border of the broad sacrotuberal ligament.

Drainage area: vertebrae and muscles of the tail. Secondary lymph from the ischiatic node.

Efferent route: medial iliac nodes.

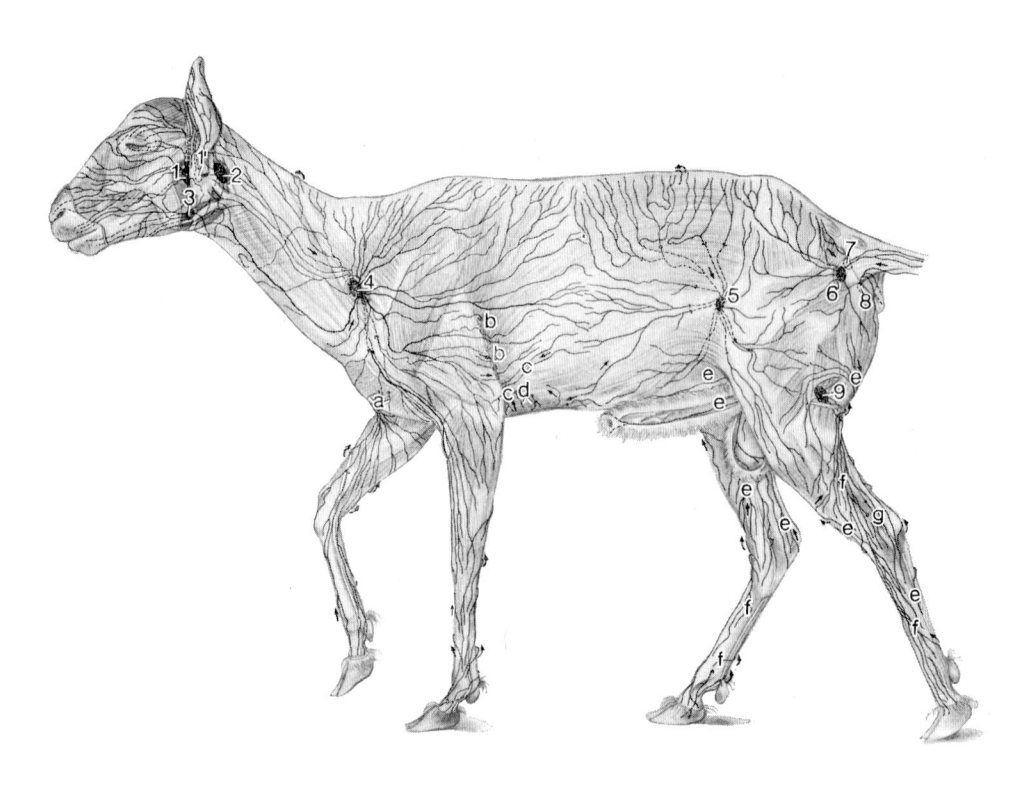

Fig. 318. Lymph vessels and lymph nodes of the skin of the sheep.
(Redrawn after Grau, 1933.)

1, 1' nll. parotidei, *2* nl. retropharyngeus lateralis, *3* nl. mandibularis, *4* nl. cervicalis superficialis, *5* nl. subiliacus, *6* nl. ischiadicus, *7* a caudal nl. sacralis, indicated by broken outline, *8* nl. tuberalis, *9* nl. popliteus profundus

a lymph vessels going to the axillary node of the first rib, *b, b* lymph vessels to the axillary lymphocentre, *c, c* lymph vessels going past the medial surface of the forelimb to the superficial cervical node, *d* lymph vessels to the ventral thoracic lymphocentre, *e, e* lymph vessels to the superficial inguinal nodes, *f* lymph vessels going to the deep popliteal node, *g* lymph vessel going to the iliofemoral node

Nll. anorectales of the goat and sheep

In front of the cranial border of the coccygeus muscle, on each of the lateral walls of the rectum, there are 2–3 nodes.
Drainage area: rectum, anus, terminal part of the descending colon.
Efferent route: medial iliac nodes.

Lymphocentrum inguinale profundum
Nll. iliofemorales of the sheep or Nl. inguinalis profundus of the goat
(319B/6)

In the sheep there are inconstantly 2–3 nodes on the external iliac artery at the entrance to the femoral canal. In the goat one occasionally finds a node of 0.4 cm diameter in the femoral canal. Nothing is known about their afferent vessels.
Efferent route: medial iliac nodes.

Lymphocentrum inguinale superficiale
Nll. inguinales superficiales of the goat and sheep.
(319B/*1*)

In *males* there is an elongated node lying dorsolaterally to the penis immediately behind the spermatic cord. In the ram there may be 2 or 3 nodes.
In *females* there are usually two bean-shaped nodes of unequal size in the immediate neighbourhood of the external pudendal artery and vein at the base of the udder. These are infrequently accompanied by a third node. They are larger in the sheep (Hampl et al.) than in the goat (Schauder).
Drainage area: in *males*: prepuce and ventral abdominal wall, penis, scrotum, anus, perineum; in *females* : lymph vessels of the udder and here there may be a cross over of the vessels from the respective sides of the body; anus, vulva. In *both sexes* : lymph vessels of the skin covering the medial surface of the thigh.
Efferent route: medial iliac nodes.

Nl. subiliacus of the goat and sheep
(318/5; 319 A/4; 319 B/2)

Usually this cylindrical node, 5 cm in length, is single and can be palpated in front of the quadriceps femoris muscle where it is covered by the cutaneus trunci muscle. It lies between tuber coxae and patella although in the goat it is nearer to the latter.
Drainage area: lateral surface of the thigh, lateral and ventral abdominal wall.
Efferent route: medial iliac nodes.

Nl. coxalis of the sheep

This very inconstant node, which is lacking altogether in the goat, lies below the tensor faciae latae muscle, immediately ventral to the tuber coxae.

Lymphocentrum ischiadicum
Nl. ischiadicus of the goat and sheep
(318/6; 319 A/2)

This is constant in the sheep although occasionally it may be present only on one side. On the other hand, the node may sometimes be duplicated. It lies against the outer surface of the broad sacrotuberal ligament near its caudal border. In the goat it is found in two thirds of cases, is 0.5 cm in length, and is occasionally divided into two or three parts.

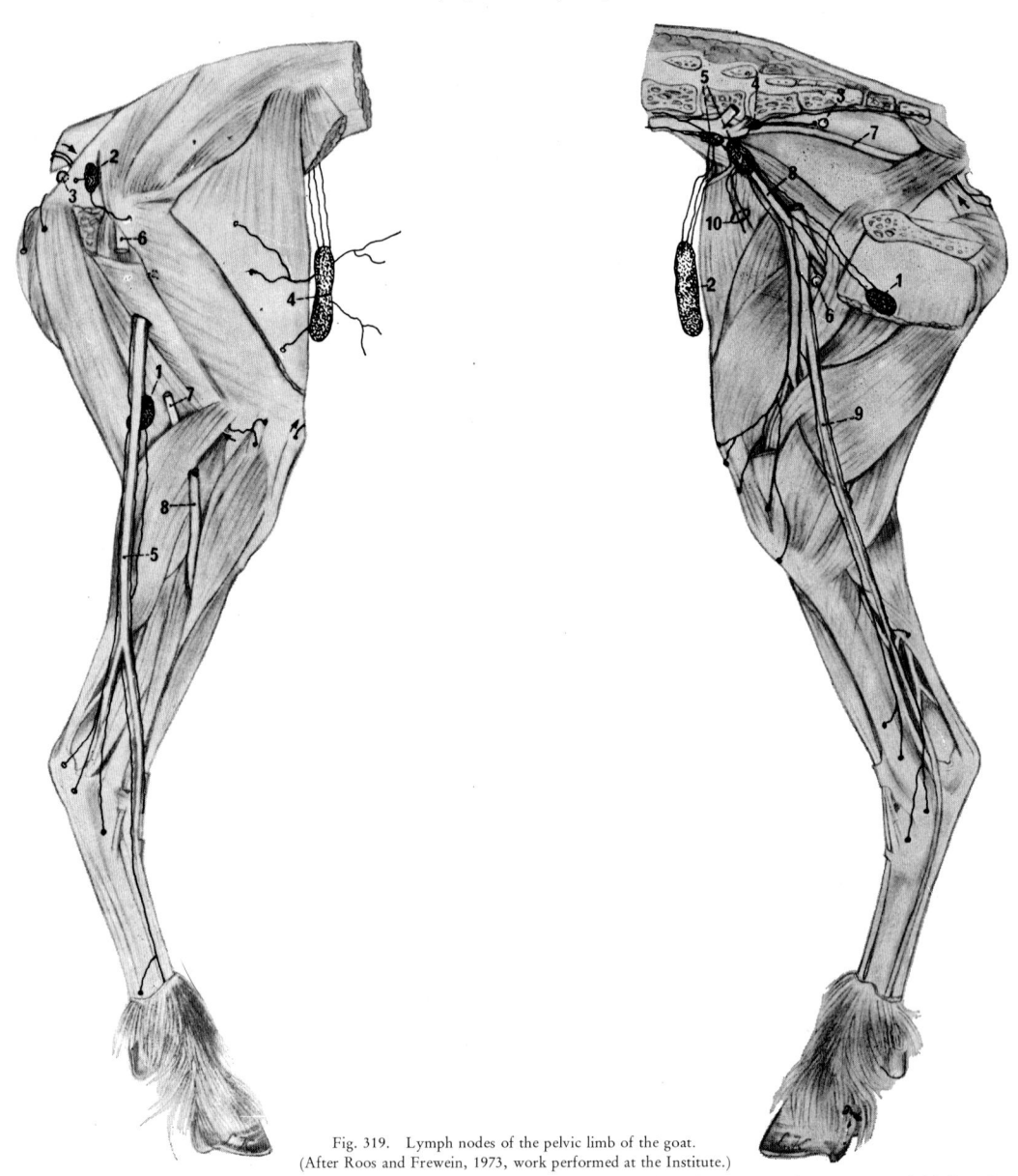

Fig. 319. Lymph nodes of the pelvic limb of the goat.
(After Roos and Frewein, 1973, work performed at the Institute.)

A (left): lateral view. *1* nl. popliteus profundus, *2* nl. ischiadicus, *3* nl. tuberalis (inconstant), *4* nl. subiliacus, *5* v. saphena parva, *6* n. ischiadicus, *7* n. tibialis, *8* n. fibularis communis;

B (right): medial view. *1* nl. inguinalis superficialis (nl. scrotalis), *2* nl. subiliacus, *3* caudal nl. sacralis (inconstant) *4* cranial nl. sacralis (constant), *5* nll. iliaci mediales, *6* nl. inguinalis profundus (inconstant), *7* a. iliaca interna, *8* a. iliaca externa, *9* v. saphena magna, *10* lymph vessels from the testis and epididymis

Drainage area: tail; ischiatic and thigh regions. Secondary lymph in some cases from the popliteal and the inconstant tuberal nodes.

Efferent route: sacral or medial iliac nodes.

Nl. tuberalis of the goat and sheep
(318/8; 319 A/3)

This is very rarely present. It is approximately 4 mm in diameter and lies about 1 cm caudodorsally to the ischiatic tuberosity on the caudodorsal border of the gluteobiceps muscle and lateral to the insertion on the tail of the coccygeus muscle. Its efferent vessels go to the ischiatic node.

Lymphocentrum popliteum
Nl. Popliteus profundus of the goat and sheep
(318/9; 319 A/*1*)

This node is 1–2.5 cm long and is usually single. It may be accompanied by a second smaller node but this is unusual. It lies hidden in the popliteal fossa, 2.5 cm deep in the space between the gluteobiceps and semitendinosus muscles.
Drainage area: foot, shank.
Efferent routes: the lymph goes in various ways either to the ischiatic node or, further towards the pelvis, to the sacral and medial iliac nodes.

Lymph collecting ducts

The arrangement of the *ductus thoracicus* of the small ruminants does not differ significantly from that mentioned in the comparative description. It should be stressed again, however, that it passes from the abdominal into the thoracic cavity through the lateral limb of the right crus of the diaphragm and *not* through the aortic hiatus.

The *cisterna chyli* resembles an extended tube and its commencement is marked by the junction between the lumbar trunk and the visceral lymph vessels.

The *truncus lumbalis* develops from the efferent vessels of the medial iliac nodes which are joined by the vessels of the inconstant lateral iliac nodes and those of the deep inguinal lymphocentre. The union of the structures from the right and left sides of the body to form the lumbar trunk occurs at different levels of the lumbar region.

Some peculiarities of the visceral lymph vessels have been reported but their general application has stil to be established. Thus in the sheep the union of the *truncus visceralis* occurs as in the ox while in the goat (317) this trunk is missing. In that species the *truncus gastricus* (–/*a*) is said to empty independently into the cisterna chyli; the *truncus intestinalis* receives the *truncus hepaticus* before it terminates.

The *truncus jugularis sinister* and *dexter* of the sheep arise from the efferent vessels of the lateral retropharyngeal node of the appropriate side of the body. The left trunk empties into the thoracic duct, the right either into the right lymphatic duct or, crossing the midline, also into the thoracic duct. In the goat (312) each jugular trunk arises by two roots of which the lateral (–/*g*) is formed from the efferent vessels of the lateral retropharyngeal node and the other, the medial, (–/*e*), by those of the medial retropharyngeal node.

The two roots of each side unite to form the right and left jugular trunks respectively. The junctions lie at different levels in the neck. It is interesting that the two lymph ducts of the neck empty into the caudal deep cervical nodes and that their efferent vessels (312/*k*) go directly to the venous angle without first linking with either the thoracic duct or the right lymphatic duct.

Lymph nodes and lymph collecting ducts of the horse

In the anatomical presentation of the lymphatic system of the horse, both clinical aspects of veterinary practice and the importance of the horse as a food animal have to be taken into account.

The lymph nodes of the horse characteristically accumulate in large groups. The individual nodes of such groups are usually between 2 and 15 mm in diameter although occasionally nodes 80 mm in diameter are seen. The number of individual nodes making up such a lymph node-group is generally 10–40; only rarely it is smaller but frequently it can be larger and several hundred or even a few (1–4) thousand nodes occur in some groups (e. g. colic nodes). This means, of course, that the total number of lymph nodes in the horse is exceptionally large and, according to Baum, amounts to 8000 on the average (compared with about 300 in the ox, 465 in man and 60 in the dog). This is impressively demonstrated in the illustrations which have been reproduced from Baum's monograph (1928).

Lymphocentrum parotideum
Nll. parotidei of the horse
(245 D/P; 246/d; 320/1; 321/1; 323/1)

This comprises a group of 6–10 small nodes, each 2–7 mm in diameter, lying ventral to the mandibular joint on the caudal border of the ramus of the mandible under cover of the parotid gland. Some of the nodes are embedded in the glandular tissue. It should be regularly examined at meat inspection.

Drainage area: skin of the frontal, parietal, masseteric, parotid and zygomatic regions; mandibular joint; zygomaticus, malaris, masseter, temporalis muscles; ocular muscles, eyelids, lacrimal apparatus, external ear, parotid gland; bones of the skull and mandible.

Efferent route: retropharyngeal lymphocentre.

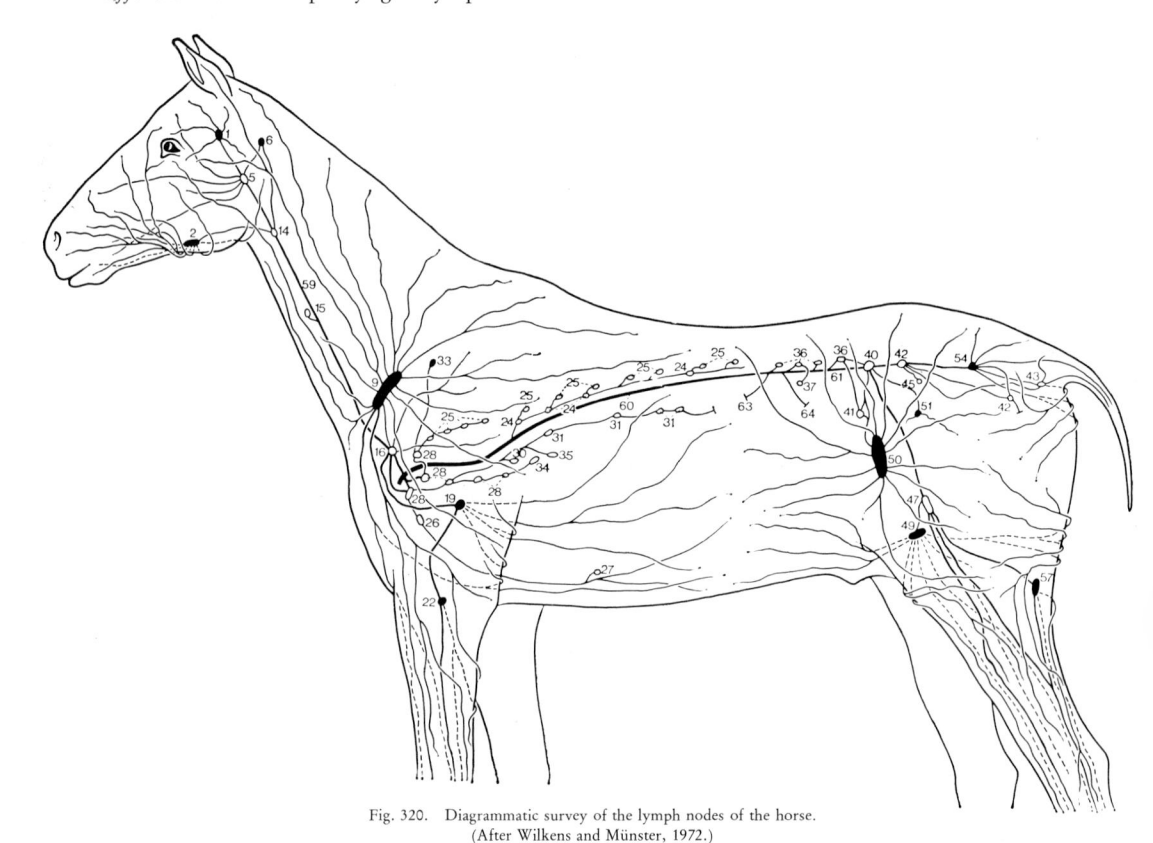

Fig. 320. Diagrammatic survey of the lymph nodes of the horse.
(After Wilkens and Münster, 1972.)

lc. parotideum: *1* nll. parotidei; lc. mandibulare: *2* nll. mandibulares; lc. retropharyngeum: *5* nll. retropharyngei mediales, *6* nll. retropharyngei laterales; lc. cervicale superficiale: *9* nll. cervicales superficiales; lc. cervicale profundum: *14* nll. cervicales profundi craniales, *15* nll. cervicales profundi medii, *16* nll. cervicales profundi caudales; lc. axillare: *19* nll. axillares proprii, *22* nll. cubitales; lc. thoracicum dorsale: *24* nll. thoracici aortici, *25* nll. intercostales; lc. thoracicum ventrale: *26* nll. sternales craniales (inconstant), *27* nl. sternalis caudalis (inconstant); lc. mediastinale: *28* nll. mediastinales craniales, *30* nll. mediastinales medii, *31* nll. mediastinales caudales (inconstant), *33* nl. nuchalis; lc. bronchale: *34* nll. tracheobronchales (bifurcationis) sinistri, *35* nll. tracheobronchales (bifurcationis) medii; lc. lumbale: *36* nll. lumbales aortici, *37* nll. renales; lc. iliosacrale: *40* nll. iliaci mediales, *41* nll. iliaci laterales, *42* nll. sacrales, *43* nll. anorectales, *45* nl. obturatorius; lc. iliofemorale (inguinale profundum): *47* nll. inguinales profundi; lc. inguinofemorale (inguinale superficiale): *49* nll. inguinales superficiales (nll. scrotales (♂), nll. mammarii (♀)), *50* nll. subiliaci, *51* nll. coxalis; lc. ischiadicum: *54* nll. ischiadici; lc. popliteum: *57* nll. poplitei profundi; *59* truncus jugularis, *60* ductus thoracicus, *61* truncus lumbalis, *63* truncus coeliacus, *64* truncus intestinalis

Lymphocentrum mandibulare
Nll. mandibulares of the horse
(245 D/M; 320/2; 322/1, 1')

This is an aggregation of lymph nodes in the intermandibular space ventral to the tongue muscles. The aggregate is 10–16 cm in length and 2–2.5 cm in breadth. It commences at the incisura vasorum or up to

Lymph nodes of the horse

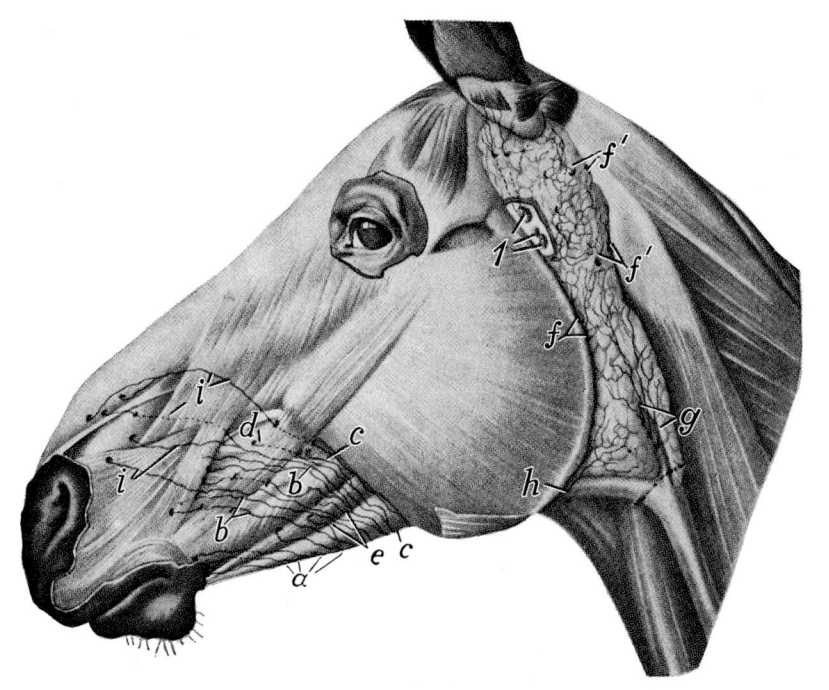

Fig. 321. Superficial lymph vessels and lymph nodes of the head of the horse.
(After Baum, 1928.)

1 nll. parotidei

a, b lymph vessels of the gums and incisor teeth, *c, c* lymph vessels of the cheek, *d* lymph vessels of the gums of the upper molars and of the hard palate, *e* lymph vessels of the gums and lower cheek teeth, *f, f'* lymph vessels going to the lateral retropharyngeal nodes, *g* lymph vessels terminating in the cranial deep cervical nodes, *h* lymph vessels going to the mandibular nodes, *i, i'* lymph vessels of the nasal cavity

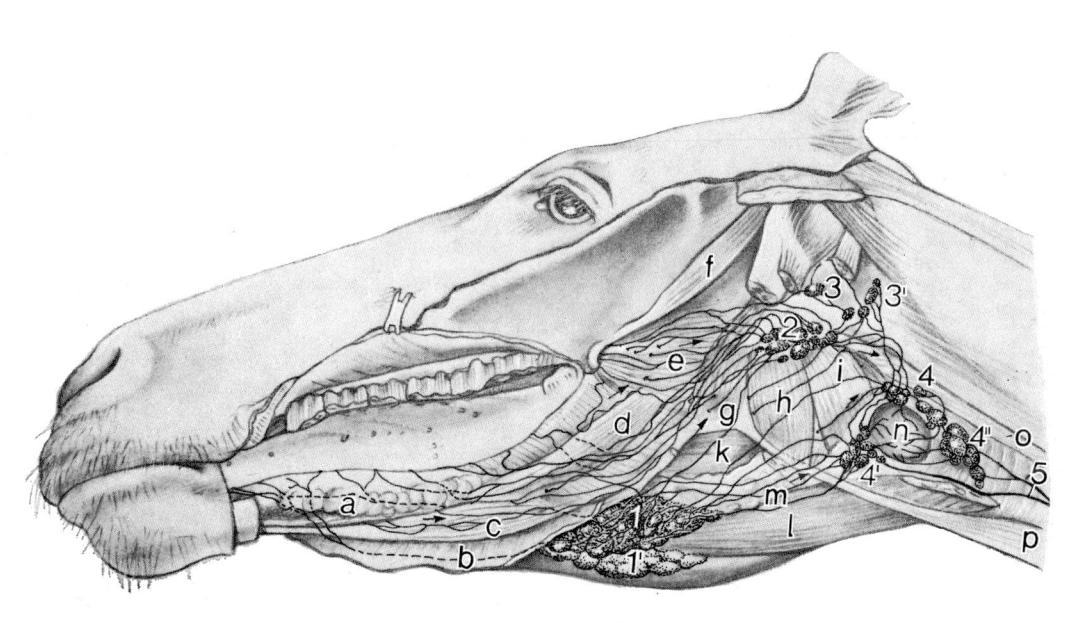

Fig. 322. Deep lymph nodes and lymph vessels of the head of the horse.
(Redrawn and expanded after Baum, 1928.)

1, 1' nll. mandibulares, *2* nll. retropharyngei mediales, *3, 3'* nll. retropharyngei laterales, *4, 4', 4"* nll. cervicales profundi craniales, *5* truncus jugularis
a glandula sublingualis, *b* m. mylohyoideus (reflected), *c* m. geniohyoideus, *d* m. styloglossus, *e* m. pterygo- and palatopharyngeus, *f* m. tensor veli palatini, *g* m. hyopharyngeus, *h* m. thyreopharyngeus, *i* m. cricopharyngeus, *k* m. thyreohyoideus, *l* end of the m. omohyoideus, *m* part of the glandula mandibularis, *n* thyroid, *o* oesophagus, *p* m. sternothyreoideus

4 cm orally to it. At this point the two aggregations from the two sides join to form a body 4–5 cm in size. Thence they diverge in an oral direction like the two limbs of an arrowhead to contact the medial pterygoid muscle and the oral belly of the digastricus. The individual nodes are between 2 and 35 mm in diameter and the entire conglomerate of both sides consists of 70–150 nodes. It is palpable and should be examined at meat inspection.

Drainage area: skin of the face; almost all the muscles of the head including those of mastication, of the intermandibular space, of the tongue and the hyoid bone; numerous cranial bones especially those of the splanchnocranium; mandibular joint; the oral two-thirds of the nasal cavity up to the orbit; eyelids; mouth and gums; all salivary glands of the head.

Efferent route: cranial deep cervical nodes.

Lymphocentrum retropharyngeum
Nll. retropharyngei mediales of the horse
(245 D/*Rm*; 246/*e'*; 320/5; 322/2)

This is a less compact group of 20–30 nodes, each measuring 3–40 mm, which is situated on the pharynx under cover of the guttural pouch and the jugulomandibular muscle. These nodes should be examined at meat inspection.

Drainage area: skin of the parotid region; all muscles around the nuchal region; numerous skull bones, especially those of the neurocranium but also the mandible, palatine bone and maxilla; atlas and axis; all the large salivary glands of the head; oral cavity, base of the nose, paranasal sinuses, pharynx, larynx, thyroid gland, external ear. Secondary lymph from the parotid and lateral retropharyngeal nodes, occasionally also the mandibular nodes.

Efferent route: cranial deep cervical nodes.

Nll. retropharyngei laterales of the horse
(245 D/*Rl*; 246/*e*; 320/6; 322/3, *3'*)

This is a group of 8–15 nodes, each measuring between 3 and 15 mm. They lie against the lateral wall of the guttural pouch and are covered by the parotid and mandibular glands and the jugulomandibular muscle. They should be examined at meat inspection.

Drainage area: this is the same as the drainage area of the medial retropharyngeal nodes. They also receive secondary lymph from parotid nodes.

Efferent route: medial retropharyngeal nodes.

Lymphocentrum cervicale superficiale
Nll. cervicales superficiales of the horse
(246/*i*; 247/*Cs*; 320/9; 322/4, *4'*, *4"*; 323/2)

This group is made up of 60–130 nodes each between 2 and 40 mm in size. The whole conglomerate measures 15–30 cm in length, 1.5–4 cm in breadth and 2 cm in thickness. Covered by the brachiocephalicus muscle, it lies immediately cranial to the shoulder joint on the cervical border of the prescapular part of the pectoralis profundus muscle. The group of lymph nodes can be palpated and its dorsal end lies up to a hand's breadth above the shoulder joint, while its ventral end reaches the beginning of the groove between the cleidobrachialis and the pectoralis descendens muscles. In surgery it is readily accessible at the lower border of the brachiocephalicus muscle. In meat inspection this conglomerate is examined under special circumstances.

Drainage area: skin of the nuchal, parietal, masseteric and parotid regions; external ear, mandibular joint; skin of the neck and pectoral limb, of the thoracic wall, of the lateral and ventral abdominal wall; some muscles of the pectoral girdle; splenius, supraspinatus and deltoideus muscles, musculature of the lower arm, cutaneous muscles of the neck and shoulder; axis, bones of the pectoral limb (except the ulna); shoulder, carpal and toe joints.

Efferent routes: on the left side the caudal deep cervical nodes; on the right side the caudal deep cervical nodes and the right lymphatic duct.

Lymphocentrum cervicale profundum
Nll. cervicales profundi craniales of the horse
(245 D/*Cpc*; 246/*a*; 247/*Cpc*; 320/*14*)

Behind the pharynx and larynx there are 30–40 nodes lying on the first part of the trachea. They are closely crowded against the thyroid gland, most frequently against its cranial and dorsomedial border but occasionally also against its caudal and ventral borders.

Drainage area: skin of the parotid region, masseter muscle, long muscle of the hyoid, brachiocephalicus, sternocephalicus, longus capitis, longissimus capitis et atlantis muscles; cervical vertebrae, occipital bone, mandible, larynx, trachea, oesophagus, thyroid and thymus glands; external ear. Secondary lymph from the mandibular and medial retropharyngeal nodes.

Efferent routes: the vasa efferentia generally form the jugular trunk. Occasionally some lymph vessels go to the middle deep cervical nodes.

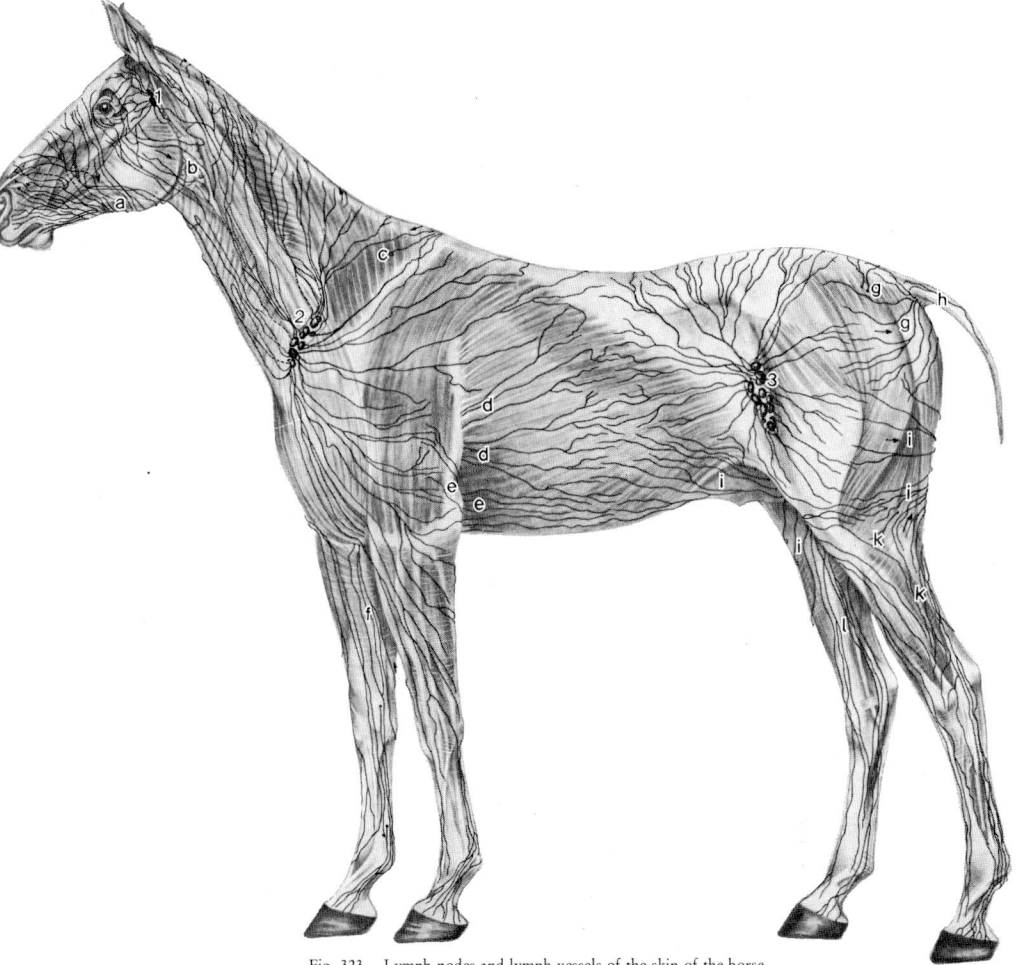

Fig. 323. Lymph nodes and lymph vessels of the skin of the horse.
(Redrawn after Baum, 1928)

1 nll. parotidei, *2* nll. cervicales superficiales, *3* nll. subiliaci

a lymph vessels going to the mandibular nodes, *b* lymph vessel which dips down behind the parotid gland and goes to the cranial deep cervical nodes, *c* lymph vessel which drains to the nuchal node or, in its absence, the mediastinal lymphocentre, *d, d* lymph vessels going to the proper axillary nodes, *e, e* lymph vessels which pass over the sternal region on their way to the superficial cervical nodes, *f* lymph vessels to the cubital nodes, *g, g* lymph vessels going partly to the ischiatic and partly to the sacral nodes, *h* lymph vessels for the anorectal nodes, *i, i, i* lymph vessels to the superficial inguinal nodes, *k, k* lymph vessel going to the deep popliteal nodes, *l* lymph vessels to the deep inguinal nodes

Nll. cervicales profundi medii of the horse
(246/*b*, *b'*, *b"*; 247/*Cpm*; 320/*15*)

Single nodes or a group of up to seven nodes lie along the trachea at about the middle of the neck in a conglomerate or a long row. They may be unilateral or bilateral.

Drainage area: sternomandibularis and scalenus muscles and the long muscles of the hyoid bone; 3rd–7th cervical vertebrae; trachea, oesophagus; thyroid and thymus glands. Secondary lymph from the cranial deep cervical nodes.

Efferent routes: jugular trunk, caudal deep cervical nodes.

Nll. cervicales profundi caudales of the horse
(246/*c*, *c'*; 247/*Cpca*; 320/*16*)

The two groups of 60–70 nodes from each side unite on the ventral surface of the trachea, flanked by the scalenus muscles and immediately in front of the first rib. This conglomerate should be examined under special circumstances at meat inspection.

Drainage area: muscles of the shoulder blade and upper arm; scalenus, longus colli, sternomandibularis, serratus ventralis muscles, long muscles of the hyoid bone, thoracic musculature and cutaneous muscles of the neck; cervical vertebrae, scapula, humerus; shoulder joint; oesophagus, thymus and thyroid glands. Secondary lymph from the superficial cervical, middle deep cervical and proper axillary nodes. *The jugular trunk also flows into this group of lymph nodes.*

Efferent routes: cranial mediastinal nodes and, on the right, to the right lymphatic duct. Also directly to the venous angle.

Lymphocentrum axillare
Nll. axillares proprii of the horse
(246/*h*; 249/*Ap*; 320/*19*; 324/*1*)

12–20 nodes are formed into a group 4–7 cm in length. This group is situated caudal to the shoulder joint and behind the angle formed by the origin of the subscapular artery from the axillary artery. In certain circumstances this group should be examined at meat inspection.

Drainage area: skin of the lateral surface of the shoulder and upper arm, of the whole of the thorax, possibly also of the lateral and ventral abdomen; all muscles situated on the shoulder and upper arm and some of those of the lower arm, cutaneous muscles of the shoulder and abdominal wall; latissimus dorsi and pectoralis profundus muscles; scapula, humerus; shoulder and elbow joints; pleura. Secondary lymph from the cubital nodes.

Efferent route: caudal deep cervical nodes.

Nll. cubitales of the horse
(249/*Cu*; 320/*22*; 324/*2*)

On the medial side of the upper arm near the elbow joint, there is a conglomerate which measures 3–4 cm by 4–5 cm in size and consists of 5–20 lymph nodes. This group can be palpated where it lies between the biceps brachii, the medial head of the triceps brachii and the tensor fasciae antebrachii muscles.

Drainage area: skin of the foot, antebrachial fascia; brachiocephalicus muscle; all muscles and tendons situated on the lower arm and foot; bones of the upper arm, lower arm and foot; elbow, carpal and toe joints.

Efferent route: proper axillary nodes.

Lymphocentrum thoracicum dorsale

Nll. thoracici aortici of the horse
(320/24; 325/f; 326/g, g')

Between the 6th and 17th thoracic vertebrae and the aorta, at about the level of each thoracic vertebra, there is usually one or sometimes as many as four nodes which may be paired or single. These nodes may be absent, especially on the right side where they are usually lacking between the 7th–15th or 9th–14th thoracic vertebrae. They should be examined routinely at meat inspection and removed under special circumstances.

Drainage area: lumbodorsal fascia; numerous muscles of the shoulder girdle and thorax; external oblique abdominis, transverse abdominis muscle; thoracic vertebrae, ribs; pleura, mediastinum, thoracic aorta; liver. Secondary lymph comes from the intercostal and caudal mediastinal nodes.

Efferent routes: these nodes are interconnected in both longitudinal and transverse directions. In the anterior region of the thorax their efferent vessels go to the cranial and middle mediastinal nodes, in the middle and posterior part the thoracic duct is preferred and in the posterior thoracic region they may extend through the aortic hiatus to the coeliac nodes.

Nll. intercostales of the horse
(320/25; 325/e; 326/f, f')

One or, less commonly, two nodes are situated subpleurally or deeper covered by the intercostal vessels in the 3rd, 4th and 5th intercostal spaces. They are located near the border of the longus colli muscle, from the 6th to 16th intercostal space at the level of the rib head joint. They may be absent from some, or even the majority, of intercostal spaces. They are always absent from the 17th, and very frequently from the 16th, intercostal space.

It is important to note that the intercostal nodes are separated from the thoracic aortic nodes by the sympathetic trunk. This is especially significant in the posterior thoracic region where these two groups are placed closely together. They are examined at meat inspection under special circumstances.

Drainage area: musculature of the pectoral girdle and thoracic wall and the extensors of the back; longus colli, psoas minor muscles; some of the abdominal muscles; thoracic and lumbar vertebrae, ribs, scapula; pleura, mediastinum, diaphragm.

Efferent routes: the nodes are often linked together longitudinally. From about the last 10 intercostal spaces the efferent vessels go to the thoracic aortic nodes or directly to the thoracic duct. From the 3rd to 5th or 6th they descend to the cranial mediastinal nodes.

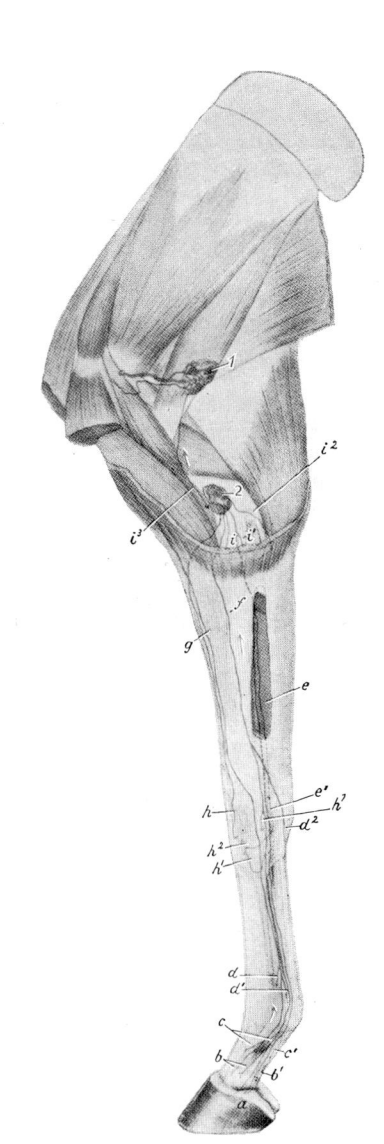

Fig. 324. Deep vessels and lymph nodes of the pectoral limb of the horse. Medial view.
(After Baum, 1928.)

1 nll. axillares proprii, *2* nll. cubitales

a lymph vessels of hoof and coffin joint, *b, b'* of pastern, *c, c'* of fetlock, *d, d', d²* lymph vessels running from lateral to medial side, *e, e'* deep, *f, g* superficial vessels to cubital nodes, *h, h', h¹, h²*, lymph vessels of carpal joint, *i, i', i², i³* elbow joint

Lymphocentrum thoracicum ventrale
Nll. sternales craniales of the horse
(320/26; 325/b; 326/a″)

This is an inconstant group of lymph nodes which lies on the manubrium of the sternum in the angle formed by the axillary artery and vein and the internal thoracic artery and vein. It may be absent altogether and is not always easy to distinguish from the cranial mediastinal nodes.

Drainage area: musculature of the thoracid wall and ventral musculature of the shoulder girdle; trachea, oesophagus, thymus; pericardium, pleura, mediastinum, suspensory ligament of the vena cava, diaphragm, liver. It sometimes receives secondary lymph from the inconstant caudal sternal node.

Nl. sternalis caudalis of the horse
(320/27; 325/a)

This is an inconstant, unpaired node of variable location. It may be found in a median position near the insertion of the diaphragm or on the right of the sternum. Alternatively, it can occur on the left in the 10th intercostal space or in the ligament of the vena cava. Baum has classed this as a diaphragmatic lymph node.

Drainage area: diaphragm, possibly also liver or pericardium.

Efferent routes: cranial sternal nodes or, if these are lacking, to the cranial mediastinal nodes.

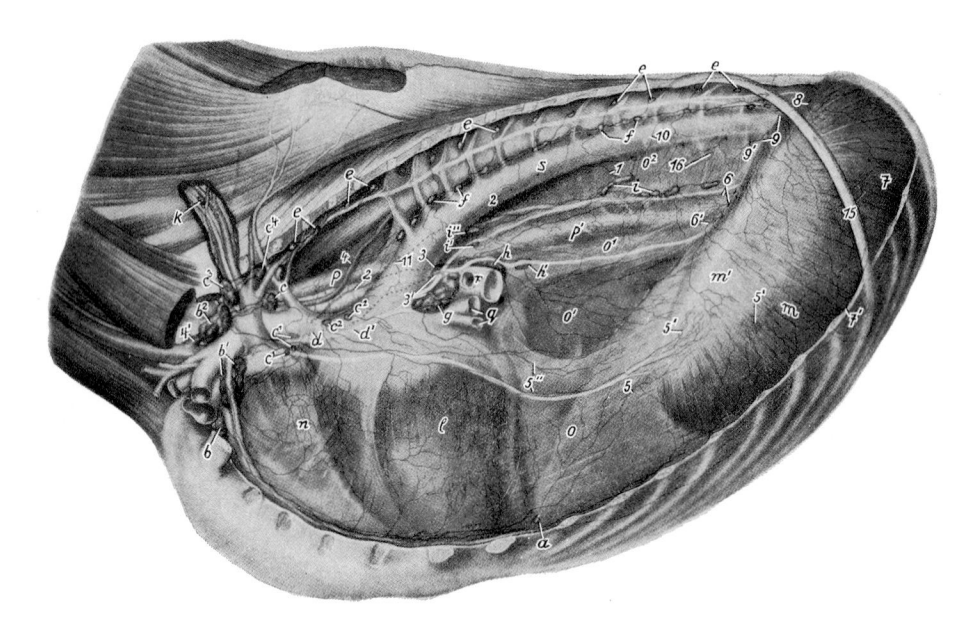

Fig. 325. Lymph vessels and lymph nodes of the thoracic cavity of the horse. Left lateral view.
(After, Baum, 1928.)

a nl. sternalis caudalis, *b* nll. sternales craniales, *b′*, *b²*, *c¹*, *c²*, *c³*, *c⁴* nll. mediastinales craniales, *d*, *d′* more cranial mediastinal nodes which are situated between the brachiocephalic trunk or the left subclavian artery and the trachea, *e*, *e*, *e* nll. intercostales, *f*, *f* nll. thoracici aortici, *g* nll. bifurcationis sinistri, *h* nll. bifurcationis medii, *h′* displaced medial tracheobronchial node, *i*, *i′*, *i″* nll. mediastinales caudales, *k* nl. nuchalis, *l* pericardium, *m*, *m′* diaphragm, *n* mediastinum craniale, *o*, *o¹*, *o²* mediastinum caudale, *p*, *p′* oesophagus, *q* branches of the pulmonary trunk, *r* bifurcation of the trachea, *s* aorta
1 efferent vessels which pass the ventral surface and right side of the aorta to reach the aortic thoracic nodes, *2, 2* efferent vessels from the caudal mediastinal nodes going to one of the cranial mediastinal nodes, *3, 3′* vasa efferentia from the left and middle tracheobronchial nodes ending in the cranial mediastinal nodes, *4, 4′* ductus thoracicus, *5, 5′, 5″, 5‴* lymph vessels of the diaphragm, *6, 6′* lymph vessels which pass through the oesophageal hiatus to go to the gastric nodes, *7, 7′* lymph vessels to the lateral iliac nodes, *8* lymph vessel of the diaphragm which passes through the crus to go to the coeliac nodes, *9, 9′* lymph vessels passing through the aortic hiatus to go to the coeliac nodes, *10* lymph vessel of the oesophagus going to an aortic thoracic node, *11* lymph vessel of the aorta which curves round to the right side and enters a middle mediastinal node, *15* 15th rib, *16* lymph vessels from the caudal mediastinum which ascend over the right side of the aorta to the aortic thoracic nodes

Lymphocentrum mediastinale
Nll. mediastinales craniales of the horse
(320/28; 325/b′, b², c, c¹, c², c³, c⁴; 326/a, a′, a″)

In the precardiac mediastinum there is a conglomerate of between 40 and 100 individual nodes divided into subgroups. Their distribution is extensive; they can be found to the left of the origin of the costocervical, deep cervical and vertebral arteries and veins, in the dorsal part of the 1st and 2nd intercostal spaces, to the left of the brachiocephalic trunk and the cranial vena cava up to the pericardium and aortic arch, ventral to the trachea between the cranial vena cava and the brachiocephalic trunk, also to the right of the cranial vena cava and finally to the right of the above mentioned vessels including the supreme intercostal artery and vein. This conglomerate extends to the level of the thoracic inlet. It should always be examined at meat inspection.

Drainage area: trapezius, rhomboideus, serratus ventralis and splenius muscles; superficial and deep muscles of the neck, supra- and infra-spinatus muscles; scapula, 2nd–7th cervical vertebrae, ribs, sternum; trachea, oesophagus, thymus, pleura, mediastinum, diaphragm, pericardium and heart; liver; thoracic aorta. Secondary lymph from the nuchal node, the caudal deep cervical, cranial and caudal sternal, caudal and middle mediastinal nodes, also from the cranial nodes of the intercostal and aortic thoracic groups.

Efferent routes: the nodes are variously interconnected. On the right side they drain to the right lymphatic duct and on the left to the terminal part of the thoracic duct.

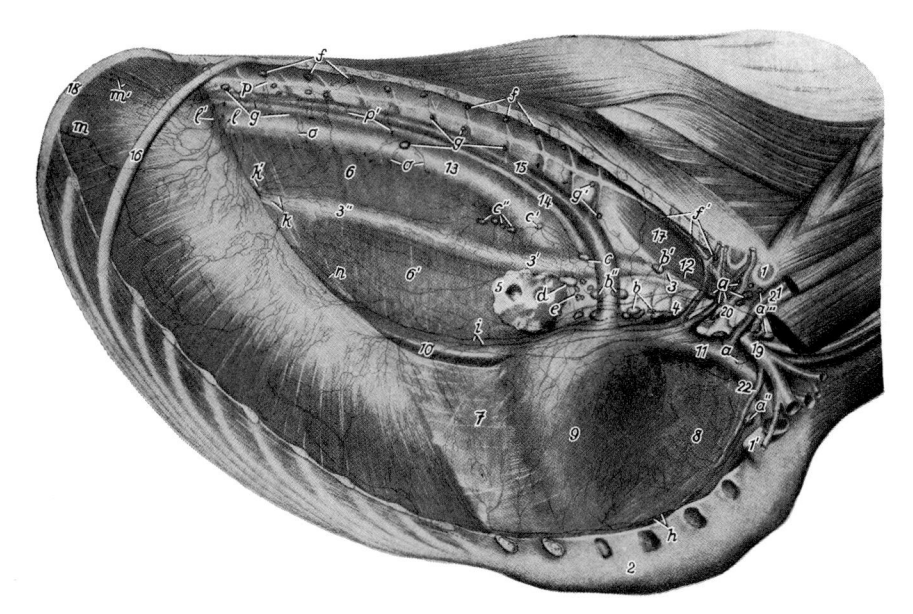

Fig. 326. Lymph vessels and lymph nodes of the thoracic cavity of the horse. Right lateral view.
(After Baum, 1928.)

a, a′, a‴, nll. mediastinales craniales, *a″* nll. sternales craniales, *b, b′, b″* nll. mediastinales medii, *c, c′, c″* nll. mediastinales caudales, *d* nll. bifurcationis medii, *e* nll. bifurcationis dextri, *f, f, f′* nll. intercostales, *g, g, g′* nll. thoracici aortici (partly obscured), *h* lymph vessels accompanying the internal thoracic artery and vein, *i* lymph vessels from the diaphragm, caudal mediastinum and caval suspensory ligament; they go to the cranial and middle mediastinal nodes, *k* lymph vessels from the diaphragm and *k′* lymph vessels of the mediastinum which pass through the diaphragm with the oesophagus and go to the gastric nodes, *l* lymph vessels passing through the aortic hiatus to go to the coeliac nodes, *l′* lymph vessel ending directly in the thoracic duct, *m, m′* lymph vessels which enter the abdominal cavity and go to the lateral iliac nodes, *n* lymph vessels of the diaphragm, passing with the vena cava into the abdominal cavity and to the gastric nodes, *o, o* lymph vessels arising from the left half of the thoracic cavity (the left mediastinum), *p, p′* lymph vessels which cross over to the left side of the thoracic cavity

1 articular surface for the 1st rib, *1′* ventral end of the 1st rib which has been largely excised, *2* sternum, *3, 3′* and *3″* oesophagus, *4* trachea, *5* remnants of the right lung, *6, 6′* mediastinum caudale, through which the left lung (*6′*) is visible, *7* caudal mediastinum, with the accessory lobe of the lung discernible, *8* cranial mediastinum, *9* pericardium and heart, *10* v. cava caudalis, *11* v. cava cranialis, *12* lymph vessel crossing over to the left side, *13* aorta, *14* ductus thoracicus, *15* v. azygos (dextra), *16* 16th rib, *17* m. longus colli, *18* 18th rib, *19* a. subclavia dextra, *20* a. costocervicalis, *21* a. and v. vertebralis, *22* a. thoracica interna

Nl. nuchalis of the horse
(320/33; 325/k)

This small node is present in about two thirds of individuals and it is situated medial to the longissimus cervicis muscle on the deep cervical artery and vein at the level of the first intercostal space.

Drainage area: the surrounding musculature of the shoulder girdle and neck; scapula, 2nd–7th cervical vertebrae.

Efferent route: cranial mediastinal nodes.

Nll. mediastinales medii of the horse
(320/30; 326/b, b', b")

This group, consisting of 4–14 nodes, lies dorsal to the base of the heart and to the right of the trachea, oesophagus and aortic arch. It should be examined regularly at meat inspection.

Drainage area: trachea and oesophagus, lung, pericardium; mediastinum; liver, thoracic aorta. Secondary lymph from the dorsal thoracic and bronchial lymphocentre and from the caudal mediastinal nodes.

Efferent routes: middle tracheobronchial and cranial mediastinal nodes.

Nll. mediastinales caudales of the horse
(320/31; 325/i, i', i"; 326/c, c', c")

The number of nodes in this group varies between 1 and 7; in exceptional cases they are absent. They lie dorsal and lateral to the oesophagus, immediately behind the aortic arch. They should be regularly examined at meat inspection.

Drainage area: lung, oesophagus, mediastinum.

Efferent routes: middle and cranial mediastinal and, possibly, aortic thoracic nodes.

Lymphocentrum bronchale

Nll. bifurcationis (seu tracheobronchales) dextri of the horse
(326/e; 327/2)

Nll. bifurcationis (seu tracheobronchales) sinistri of the horse
(320/34; 325/g; 327/3)

Nll. bifurcationis (seu tracheobronchales) medii of the horse
(320/35; 325/h; 326/d; 327/1)

These three groups are composed of 4–6, 8–10 and 9–20 nodes respectively. On the right and dorsally each conglomerate measures 4–6 cm in length, on the left even up to 10 cm. They are 2–3 cm broad. Their location at the tracheal bifurcation has been recorded in the comparative section. They should be regularly examined at meat inspection.

Drainage area: trachea, lung, heart and pericardium, oesophagus, mediastinum. Secondary lymph from the middle mediastinal and pulmonary nodes.

Efferent route: cranial mediastinal nodes.

Nll. pulmonales of the horse

These small, inconstant nodes are found in 50–60% of cases. They are situated along the principal bronchus and often on the bronchus to the apical lobe. They are covered by lung tissue but may be palpated at meat inspection if enlarged.

Drainage area: lung.

Efferent route: tracheobronchial nodes.

Lymphocentrum lumbale

Nll. lumbales aortici of the horse
(257/3; 320/36; 329/4; 332/5; 334/1)

Lying along the abdominal aorta and caudal vena cava there are 30–160 subperitoneal nodes. They are usually lateral and ventral to the abdominal aorta but in a few cases they may also be dorsal and they extend from the kidneys to the origin of the deep circumflex iliac arteries and veins. These nodes are so tightly fused to the peritoneum that when this is stripped off the nodes come away from the body wall with it. In special cases they should be examined at meat inspection.

Drainage area: inner lumbar musculature, back muscles and lumbodorsal fascia; thoracic and lumbar vertebrae, pelvic bones; pleura and peritoneum; kidneys, ureter, adrenal glands, urinary bladder; testis, epididymis or ovary, uterine tube, uterus and female urethra; abdominal aorta. Secondary lymph from the medial and lateral iliac nodes.

Efferent routes: the nodes are interconnected. The vasa efferentia terminate in, or actually form, the lumbar trunk.

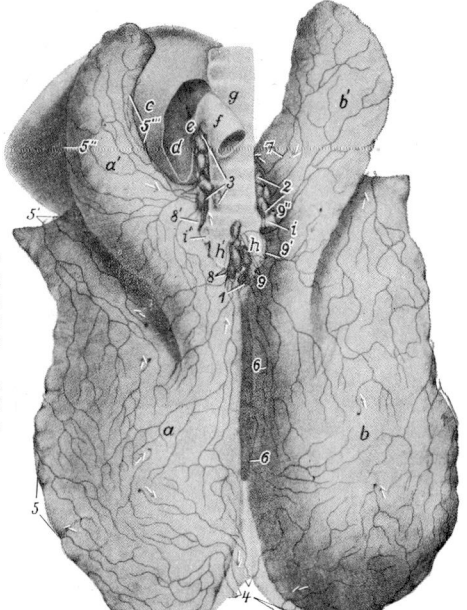

Fig. 327. Lymph nodes and lymph vessels of the lung of the horse. Dorsal view. (After Baum, 1928.)

1 nll. bifurcationis medii, *2* nll. bifurcationis dextri, *3* nll. bifurcationis sinistri, *4* lymph vessels passing through the diaphragm, *5, 5′, 5″, 5‴* lymph vessels reflected onto the diaphragmatic and mediastinal surfaces of the lung, *6, 6* lymph vessels destined for the nll. mediastinales, *7* lymph vessel which goes to the middle mediastinal nodes, *8, 8′* deep lymph vessels of the left lung, *9, 9′, 9″* deep lymph vessels of the right lung

a, a′ left lung, *b, b′* right lung, *c* pericardium with a portion of its basal part excised so as to show the aorta (*f*), pulmonary trunk (*d*) and ligamentum arteriosum (*e*), *d* truncus pulmonalis, *e* lig. arteriosum, *f* aorta, *g* trachea, *h* right and *h′* left bronchus principalis, *i* bronchus lobaris for the right and *i′* for the left cranial lobe

Nll. renales of the horse
(320/37; 332/5, 5′)

Along the course of the renal arteries and veins there are 10–18 nodes on each side of the body. These are closely associated with the aortic lumbar nodes from which they can be separated only with difficulty. They are regularly examined at meat inspection.

Drainage area: kidney, adrenal glands, ureter; liver, duodenum; testis; peritoneum and abdominal aorta.

Efferent routes: aortic lumbar nodes or directly into the cisterna chyli.

Nl. ovarius of the horse
(334/7′)

This is a small node which occurs inconstantly in the mesovarium.
Drainage area: ovary.
Efferent routes: aortic lumbar and medial iliac nodes.

Lymphocentrum coeliacum
Nll. coeliaci of the horse
(255/2; 257/1)

This is a conglomerate of 12–30 nodes which surround the coeliac artery and its main branches immediately ventral to the aorta.

Drainage area: diaphragm, lung, mediastinum; peritoneum; stomach, pancreas, liver, spleen, adrenal gland; abdominal aorta. Secondary lymph comes from all the other nodes of the coeliac lymphocentre and the caudal nodes of the dorsal thoracic lymphocentre.

Efferent routes: the efferent vessels fuse to form the coeliac trunk which in turn terminates in the anterior part of the cisterna chyli.

Nll. lienales of the horse
(255/a)

These comprise 10–30 very flattened lymph nodes located at the hilus of the spleen in the gastrosplenic ligament along the splenic artery and vein.

Drainage area: stomach, spleen. Secondary lymph from the omental nodes.

Efferent route: coeliac nodes.

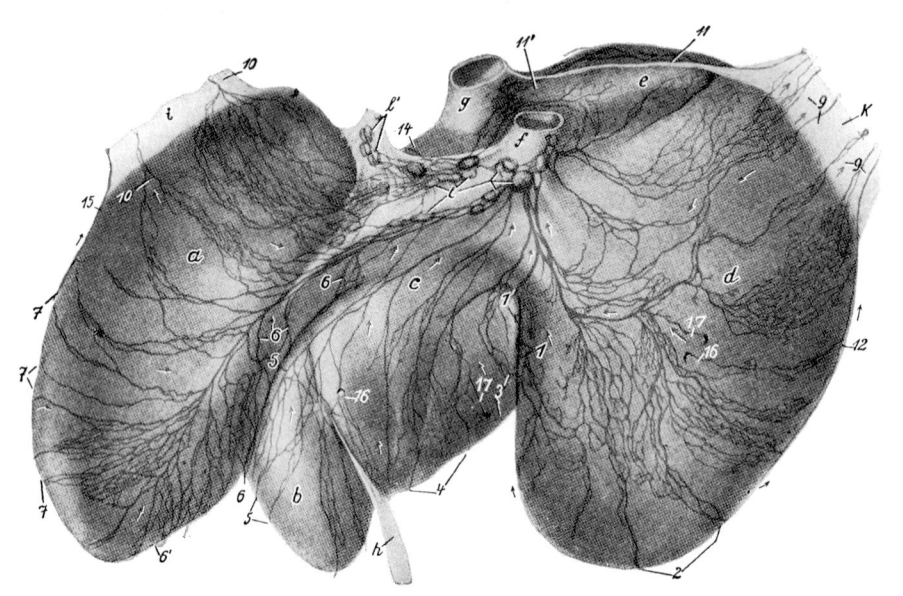

Fig. 328. Lymph vessels and lymph nodes on the visceral surface of the liver of the horse.
(After Baum, 1928.)

a lobus hepatis sinister lateralis, *b* lobus hepatis sinister medialis, *c* lobus quadratus, *d* lobus hepatis dexter, *e* lobus caudatus, *f* portal vein, *g* v. cava caudalis, *h* lig. falciforme hepatis, *i* lig. triangulare sinistrum, *k* lig. triangulare dextrum, *l* nll. hepatici which at *l'* are partly covered by the serosa of the pancreas

1–7 lymph vessels running from the parietal to the visceral surface of the liver, *9, 9'* lymph vessels which enter the right and *10, 10* the left triangular ligament, *11, 11'* lymph vessels from the visceral surface of the right hepatic lobe, *12* right marginal vessel on the lateral border of the right lobe of the liver, *14* lymph vessel from the peripheral surface entering the hepatic lymph nodes, *15* left marginal vessel, *16, 16* lymph vessels entering the substance of the liver, *17, 17* lymph vessels coming from the deeper parts of the organ

Nll. gastrici of the horse
(255/c, c', c''; 329/2)

15–35 nodes are situated along the branches of the left gastric artery on the lesser curvature of the stomach. Sometimes they are found on both surfaces of the stomach and frequently on the cardia. They should be examined regularly at meat inspection.

Drainage area: oesophagus, stomach, liver, greater omentum; also mediastinum and lung.

Efferent route: coeliac nodes.

Nll. hepatici seu portales of the horse
(255/f; 328/1, 1')

At the porta of the liver and along the blood vessels entering it, there are 4–10 nodes which are remarkably flat so that they appear almost ribbon-like. These should be regularly examined at meat inspection.

Drainage area: duodenum, liver, pancreas. Secondary lymph from the pancreaticoduodenal and omental nodes.

Efferent route: coeliac nodes.

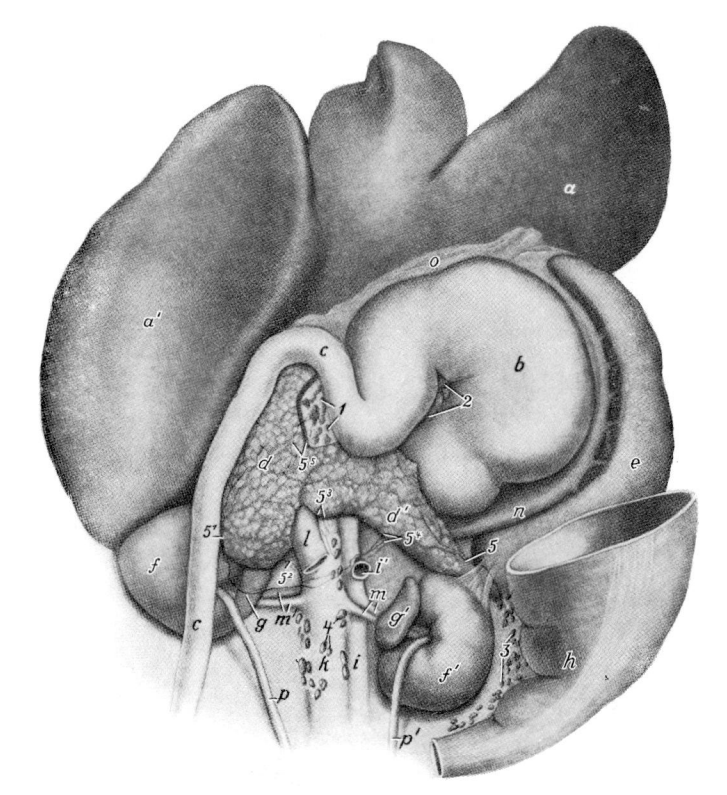

Fig. 329. Stomach, liver, spleen and pancreas in situ with lymph vessels and lymph nodes. (After Baum, 1928.)

1 nll. pancreaticoduodenales, *2* nll. gastrici, *3* nll. colici, *4* nll. lumbales aortici including nll. renales and nll. mesenterici craniales, *5, 5¹, 5², 5³, 5⁴, 5⁵* lymph vessels of the pancreas

a left and *a'* right lobe of the liver, *b* stomach, *c, c* duodenum, *d, d'* pancreas, *e* spleen, *f* right and *f'* left kidney, *g* right and *g'* left adrenal, *h* transition from the right dorsal colon to the small colon, *i* aorta, *i'* stump of the a. mesenterica cranialis, *k* v. cava caudalis, *l* v. portae, *m, m'* aa. and vv. renales, *n* blood vessels of the spleen, *o* omentum (cut off), *p, p'* ureter

Nll. pancreaticoduodenales of the horse
(255/e, e'; 329/1)

5–15 nodes are distributed in a very variable manner along the right gastric and gastroduodenal arteries and veins and their branches, and along the cranial pancreaticoduodenal and right gastroepiploic arteries and veins.

Drainage area: duodenum, pancreas, stomach, greater omentum. Secondary lymph from the omental nodes.

Efferent routes: hepatic and coeliac nodes.

Nll. omentales of the horse
(255/b, b', b'', b''')

14–20 roundish nodes comprise the omental lymph nodes. They are situated on the greater curvature of the stomach, or in its neighbourhood, in the greater omentum and the gastrosplenic ligament. It is not always possible to differentiate them from the splenic lymph nodes which are situated mainly in the dorsal part of the gastrosplenic ligament. But the latter receive lymph mainly from the spleen whereas the omental nodes drain the stomach and greater omentum.

Drainage area: stomach, omentum majus.

Efferent routes: to the left, lymph drains to the splenic and coeliac nodes; to the right it passes to the pancreaticoduodenal and hepatic nodes.

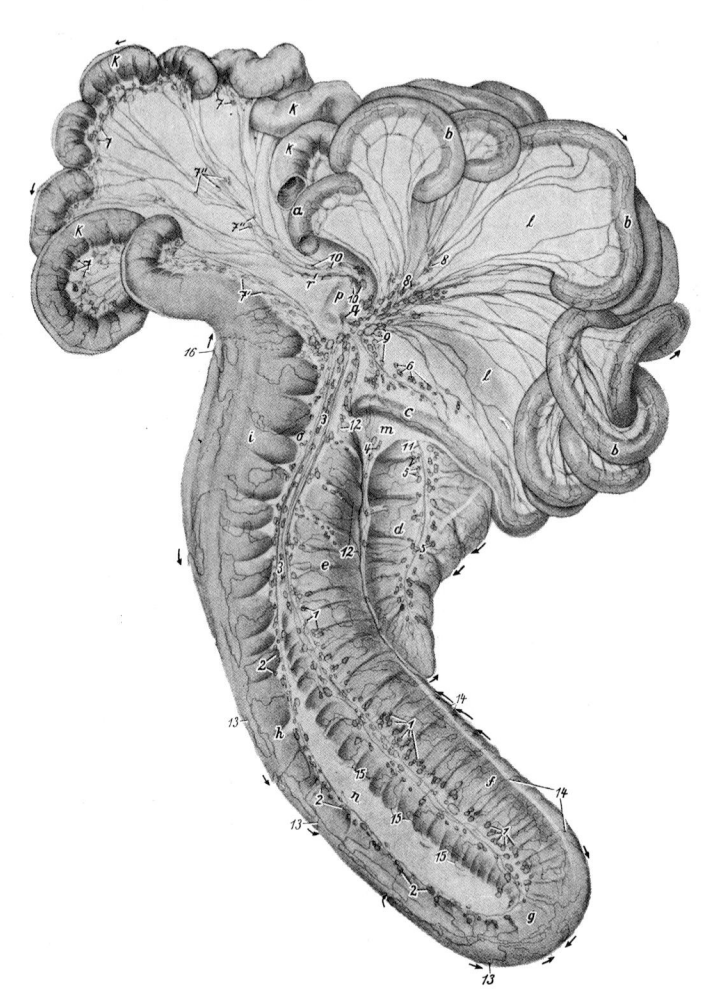

Fig. 330. Lymph vessels and lymph nodes of the intestine of the horse.
(After Baum, 1928.)

1, 1, 2, 2, 3, 3, nll. colici, *4, 5, 5* nll. caecales, *6, 8, 8* nll. jejunales, *7, 7', 7'', 10* nll. mesenterici caudales, *9* nll. mesenterici craniales, *11* lymph vessel to the cranial mesenteric lymph nodes. *12, 13, 14, 15* and *16* lymph vessels of the great colon

a duodenum (cut off), *b, b* jejunum, *c* ileum, *d* caecum, *e* right ventral and *f* left ventral colon, *g* pelvic flexure, *h* left dorsal and *i* right dorsal colon, *k, k* loops of small colon, *l* mesojejunum, *m* ileocaecal mesentery, *n* mesentery between the left limbs of the colon, *o* mesenteric fold between the dorsal and ventral right colon, *p* a piece of aorta, *q* a. mesenterica cranialis, *r* a. mesenterica caudalis

Lymphocentrum mesentericum craniale
Nll. mesenterici craniales of the horse
(257/2; 330/9)

In the cranial mesenteric root along the cranial mesenteric artey there is a group of 70–80 nodes which are not always clearly separated from the nodes of the lumbar lymphocentre, the coeliac nodes and other mesenteric nodes which will be described later.

Drainage area: duodenum, ascending colon, pancreas, adrenal; abdominal aorta. Secondary lymph from the jejunal, caecal, colic and caudal mesenteric nodes.

Efferent route: the efferent vessels join to form the intestinal trunk which terminates in the posterior part of the cisterna chyli.

Nll. jejunales of the horse
(330/8)

About 35–90 nodes are situated around the initial part of the jejunal arteries or within the mesojejunum towards the jejunal loops. A few nodes, which are mainly regional to the ileum, lie in the

supply-area of the ramus ilei mesenterialis. Their examination is obligatory at meat inspection.
Drainage area: jejunum, ileum.
Efferent route: cranial mesenteric nodes.

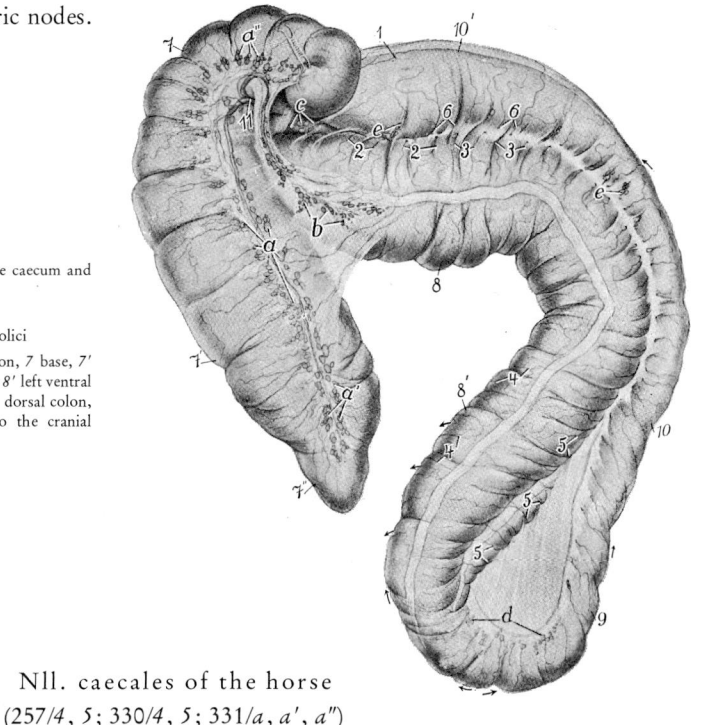

Fig. 331. Lymph vessels and lymph nodes of the caecum and large colon of the horse.
(After Baum, 1928.)

a, a', a'' nll. caecales, *b, c, d* and *e* nll. colici
1, 2, 3, 4, 5 and *6* lymph vessels of the great colon, *7* base, *7'* body and *7''* apex of the caecum, *8* right ventral and *8'* left ventral colon, *9* pelvic flexure, *10* left dorsal and *10'* right dorsal colon, *11* vasa efferentia of the caecal nodes going to the cranial mesenteric nodes

Nll. caecales of the horse
(257/4, 5; 330/4, 5; 331/a, a', a'')

500–700 individual nodes form ribbon-shaped conglomerates on the medial and lateral caecal arteries along the medial and lateral taeniae of the caecum. These conglomerates are 3–7 cm wide. Additionally, there are a further 4–18 nodes on the dorsal taenia or in the iliocaecal fold. They should be examined at meat inspection.
Drainage area: duodenum, ileum, caecum.
Efferent route: cranial mesenteric nodes.

Nll. colici of the horse
(257/6, 7; 330/1, 2, 3; 331/b, c, d, e)

Between the right longitudinal segments of the ascending colon there are laterally 100–150 individual lymph nodes. Medially, that is to say in the immediate neighbourhood of the two arteries of the great colon, there are two elongated conglomerates. Between the left longitudinal segments the lymph node conglomerates are divided into two elongated groups, a ventral and a dorsal. The total number of individual nodes in the mesocolon ascendens has been estimated at 2000–4000 and sometimes as many as 6000. These should always be examined at meat inspection.
Drainage area: ascending and transverse colon, ileum, greater omentum.
Efferent routes: the outgoing vessels of the individual nodes are linked for a considerable distance to form stout lymphatic trunks, which accompany the colic arteries. They empty into the cranial mesenteric nodes.

Lymphocentrum mesentericum caudale
Nll. mesenterici caudales of the horse
(257/8, 9; 330/7, 7', 7'', 10)

This group is situated in the mesentery of the descending colon on the caudal mesenteric artery and to some extent along its branches. The nodes are very numerous along the gut at the mesenteric reflection. 30–50 nodes have been counted at the mesenteric root and 50–100 in the mesocolon descendens while

1600–1800 individual nodes have been reported to be present at the intestinal reflection. These should be regularly examined at meat inspection.

Drainage area: descending colon, rectum, pancreas, peritoneum, greater omentum. Secondary lymph comes from the anorectal nodes.

Efferent routes: the nodes nearest the gut send their efferent vessels either to the cranial mesenteric nodes or to the nodes of their own group at the root of the mesentery. Stouter trunks take lymph to the lumbar trunk or they form vessels which run parallel to the trunk and empty into the cisterna chyli.

Nll. vesicales of the horse

In exceptional cases there are one or two small nodes in the lateral ligament of the urinary bladder which receive lymph vessels from the bladder and prostate gland.

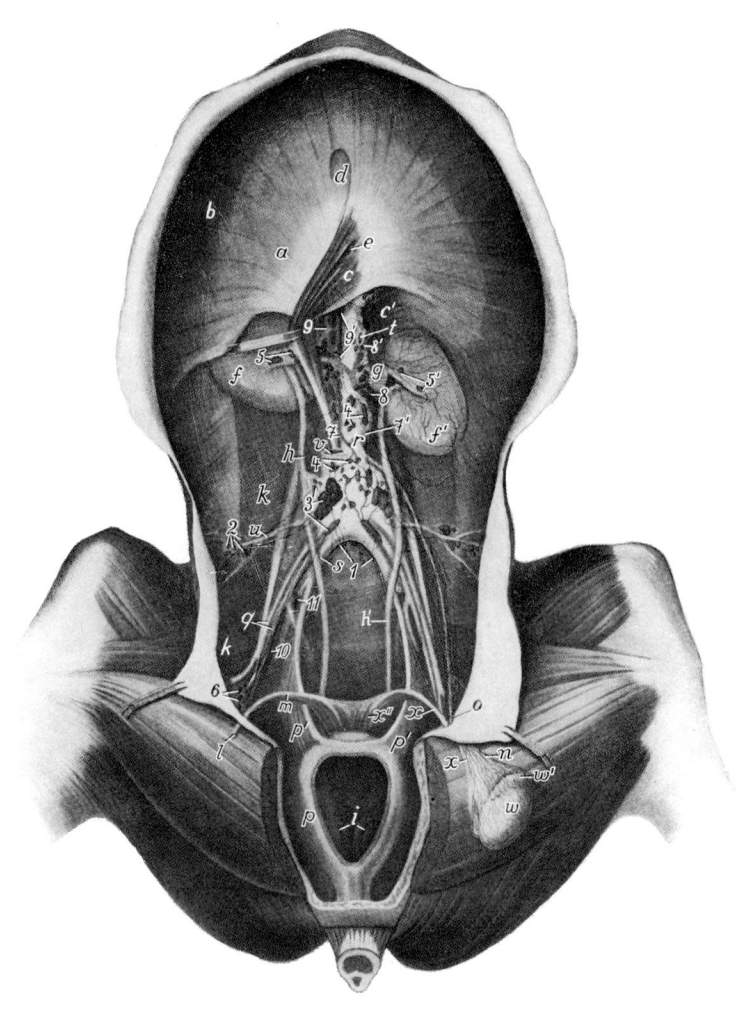

Fig. 332. Lymph nodes and lymph vessels of the dorsal wall of the abdomen of the horse. (After Baum, 1928.)

1 nll. sacrales, *2* nll. iliaci laterales, *3* nll. iliaci mediales, *4* nll. lumbales aortici, *5, 5'* nll. renales, *6* nll. inguinales profundi, *7, 7'* trunci lumbales, *8, 8'* truncus intestinalis, *9, 9'* cisterna chyli, *10* vas efferens of the nl. coxalis, *11* nl. obturatorius with vas efferens

a centrum tendineum and *b* pars costalis of the diaphragm, *c* crus of the diaphragm, *d* foramen for vena cava, *e* oesophageal hiatus, *f* right and *f'* left kidney, *g* left adrenal, *h* right and *h'* left ureter, *i* ureter openings, *k* lumbar musculature, *l* and *m* right ductus deferens, *n* left spermatic cord, *o* a. testicularis sinistra (the right counterpart is not shown), *p* bladder, *p', p''* ligg. vesicae lateralia, *q* a. and v. iliaca externa, *r* aorta, *s* a. iliaca interna dextra, *t* a. mesenterica cranialis (cut off), *u* a. and v. circumflexa ilium profunda dextra, *v* caudal vena cava (cut off), *w* left testis, *w'* left epididymis, *x, x', x''* left ductus deferens

Lymphocentrum iliosacrale

Nll. iliaci mediales of the horse
(257/14; 260/1; 320/40; 332/3; 333/3; 334/2; 335/c)

The origins of the deep circumflex iliac arteries and veins and the external iliac arteries and veins are surrounded by about 25 or more lymph nodes. Rarely there are only 3–4 of these nodes but each node is then much larger. They are situated subperitoneally but they are not so closely attached to the peritoneum as the aortic lumbar nodes with which they are in contact anteriorly. In special cases they should be examined at meat inspection.

Drainage area: inner lumbar musculature, internal oblique abdominis muscle; fascia lata and its extensor muscle; almost all the muscles of the pelvis and thigh; pelvic bones and femur; hip joint; pleura and peritoneum; ureter, urinary bladder; testis, epididymis, spermatic cord and accessory genital glands or ovary, uterine tube, uterus and female urethra; abdominal aorta. Secondary lymph comes from the lateral iliac, sacral, deep inguinal and subiliac nodes.

Efferent routes: to the aortic lumbar nodes or sometimes a few efferent vessels unite to form the lumbar trunk which goes to the cisterna chyli. The lumbar trunk may be double.

Nll. iliaci laterales of the horse
(260/1'; 320/41; 332/2; 335/f)

In the angle formed by the terminal branching of the deep circumflex iliac artery and vein there is, on each side, a small group of 4–20 nodes. This should be examined at meat inspection in special cases.

Drainage area: abdominal muscles, lumbodorsal fascia, fascia lata and its extensor muscle; ribs, pelvic bones; pleura and peritoneum; liver, kidney, diaphragm. Secondary lymph comes from the subiliac nodes.

Efferent routes: medial iliac and aortic lumbar nodes.

Nll. sacrales of the horse
(260/1''; 320/42; 332/1; 333/4, 5; 334/3, 4; 335/d)

This is a fairly constant group of lymph nodes at the angle formed by the bifurcation of the aorta into the external iliac arteries. Further individual nodes are sometimes found on the broad sacrotuberal ligament along the internal pudendal artery.

Drainage area: skin over the ischiatic tuberosity; superficial and middle glutaeus muscle, biceps femoris, semitendinosus, semimembranosus, obturator internus, quadratus lumborum, and tensor fasciae latae muscles; lumbar vertrebrae, sacrum, hip bone, femur; male urethra and accessory genital glands, ischiocavernosus muscle or uterus and vagina. Secondary lymph from the ischiatic lymphocentre and the obturator lymph node.

Efferent route: medial iliac nodes.

Nll. anorectales of the horse
(260/1'''; 320/43; 334/5)

On the dorsal border of the retroperitoneally-situated part of the rectum and in the angle between the anus and the caudal border of the buttock muscles and the tail there are about 15–45 lymph nodes.

Drainage area: descending colon, rectum, anus, skin of the pelvic outlet and tail; muscles and coccygeal vertebrae; semimembranosus muscle; urethra; vagina, vulva, clitoris, uterus.

Efferent routes: caudal mesenteric, sacral and ischiatic nodes.

Nl. uterinus of the horse
(334/7)

A small inconstant node may occur in the broad ligament of the uterus.

Drainage area: uterus.

Efferent routes: medial iliac or aortic lumbar nodes.

Nl. obturatorius of the horse
(260/1ᵛ; 320/45; 332/11; 335/e)

This is a small, very inconstantly-occurring node at the cranial border of the obturator artery and vein. It is subperitoneal in position and can usually be seen from the pelvic cavity.

Drainage area: fascia lata, iliopsoas, tensor fasciae latae, quadriceps femoris muscles and gluteal musculature; hip joint, pelvic bones.

Efferent route: sacral nodes.

Lymphocentrum inguinale profundum (seu iliofemorale)
Nll. inguinales profundi of the horse
(260/2'; 320/47; 332/6; 333/2; 335/b)

A wedge-shaped, 8–12 cm-long conglomerate consisting of 16–35 individual lymph nodes, is present in the femoral canal around the femoral artery and vein and the origin of the deep femoral artery and vein. In special cases this should be examined at meat inspection.

Drainage area: skin of the shank and foot; fasciae; almost all the muscles of the pelvis and thigh and all muscles and tendons of the shank and foot; abdominal muscles; all bones and joints of the pelvic limb; peritoneum; vaginal process and cremaster muscle, penis, ischiocavernosus muscle or uterus. Secondary lymph comes from the superficial inguinal nodes and the popliteal lymphocentre.

Efferent routes: medial iliac nodes; in exceptional cases direct to the cisterna chyli.

Lymphocentrum inguinale superficiale (seu inguinofemorale)
Nll. inguinales superficiales of the horse
(Nll. scrotales 320/49; 333/1, 1';
Nll. mammarii 260/3; 334/6, 6')

In both males and females there are 20–100 lymph nodes on each side between the ventral wall of the trunk and the prepuce and scrotum or udder. In males the laterally directed spermatic cord separates a larger cranial group, 11–13 cm long, from a smaller caudal group which measures only 4–6 cm in length. They can be readily palpated lateral to the penis. In females the conglomerate measures 10–14 cm in length and extends laterally and cranially beyond the base of the udder. Caudally it extends to the external pudendal artery and vein. A small group which lies caudally against the base of the udder may sometimes be present. The udder lymph nodes can be palpated. The nodes of both sexes should be regularly examined at meat inspection and in special cases they can be carefully removed.

Drainage area: skin of the lateral and ventral wall of the trunk, skin from the thigh down to the foot; abdominal musculature, abdominal cutaneous muscle; pubis, scrotum, prepuce, penis, ischiocavernous muscle, male urethra or vulva, clitoris and udder.

Efferent route: deep inguinal nodes.

Nll. subiliaci of the horse
(260/3'; 320/50; 323/3)

This conglomerate, measuring 6–10 cm in length, consists of 15–50 nodes and lies midway between the knee cap and the tuber coxae on the cranial or craniomedial border of the tensor fasciae latae muscle. It is palpable in this position. It should be examined under special circumstances at meat inspection.

Drainage area: skin of the dorsal and lateral wall of the trunk, of the stifle fold, over the pelvis, thigh and knee; fasciae; tensor fasciae latae muscle; cutaneous muscle of the abdomen.

Efferent routes: lateral iliac, medial iliac nodes or both.

Nl. coxalis of the horse
(260/3″; 320/51)

This node occurs in only about a quarter of horses and is situated at the flexor aspect of the hip joint on the rectus femoris muscle between the iliacus and deep or middle gluteal muscles. Sometimes, however, it is found a little more ventrolaterally on the inner surface of the tensor fasciae latae muscle related to the lateral circumflex femoris artery and vein.

Drainage area: hip joint, gluteal musculature, extensors of the knee joint, fascia lata and its extensor muscle.

Efferent route: medial iliac nodes.

Fig. 333. Lymph vessels and lymph nodes of the male genital organs of the horse.
(After Baum, 1928.)

1, 1′ nll. scrotales (inguinales superficiales), *2* nll. inguinales profundi, *3* nll. iliaci mediales, *4* and *5* nll. sacrales, *6, 7, 8* lymph vessels from the copulatory organ

a left testis and *b* left epididymis, both covered by *c* the process of the tunica vaginalis and the cremaster muscle, *d* penis, *e* glans penis, *f* praeputium, *g* m. ischiocavernosus, *h* urinary bladder, *i* urethra surrounded by the urethralis muscle, *k* seminal vesicle, *l* prostate, *m* bulbourethral gland, *n* lateral wall of the bladder, *o* rectum, *p* kidney, *q* anus, *t* ventral wall of the pelvis, *u* scrotum

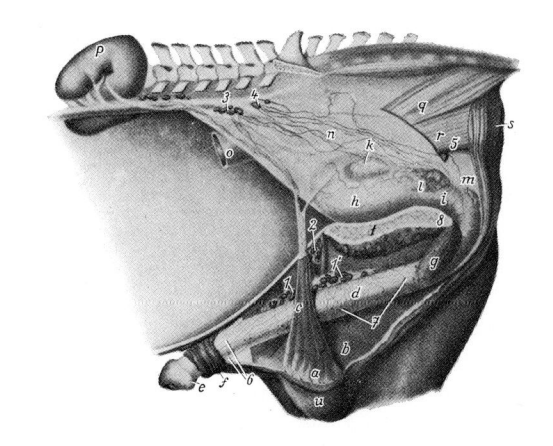

Fig. 334. Lymph nodes and lymph vessels of the female genital organs of the horse.
(After Baum, 1928.)

1 nll. lumbales aortici, *2* nll. iliaci mediales, *3* and *4* nll. sacrales, *4′* left nll. ischiadici which are situated on the outside of the broad pelvic ligament, *5* nll. anorectales, *6* and *6′* nll. mammarii, *7* nl. uterinus, *7′* nl. ovaricus, *8* vasa efferentia of the anorectal nodes which run on the lateral surface of the broad pelvic ligament to the ischiatic nodes

a ovary, *b* uterine tube, *c* left horn of the uterus, *d* body of the uterus, *e* mesovarium, *f* mesometrium, *g* urinary bladder, *h* lig. vesicae laterale (cut off), *i* urethra, *k* vagina, *l* vestibulum vaginae, *m* labium pudendi, *n* rectum, *o* anus, *p* udder, *q* ventral pelvic wall, *r* kidney, *s* ureter, *t* aorta, *u* a. iliaca ext. (cut across), *v* a. iliaca int. (cut across), *w* broad pelvic ligament (severed)

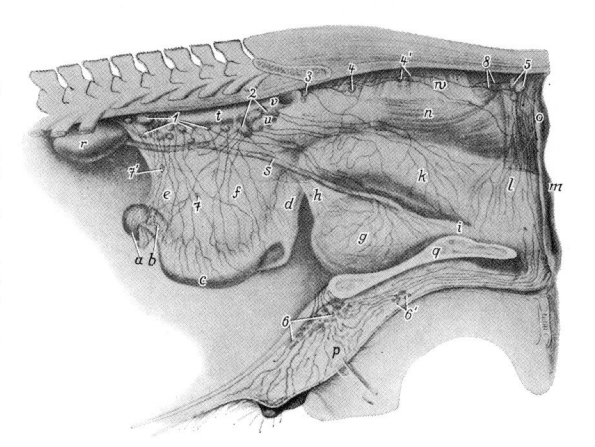

Lymphocentrum ischiadicum
Nll. ischiadici of the horse
(260/4; 320/54; 334/4′)

This group of 1–5 nodes lies on the outer surface of the broad sacrotuberal ligament, at the lateral border of the sacrum in relation to the caudal gluteal artery and vein. It is overlaid by the biceps femoris muscle. It is examined at meat inspection in special cases.

Drainage area: skin of the pelvis and tail; superficial gluteal, biceps femoris, semitendinosus and semimembranosus muscles; sacrum, hip bone, coccygeal vertebrae. Secondary lymph may be received from the posterior sacral and anorectal lymph nodes.

Efferent route: sacral nodes.

Lymphocentrum popliteum
Nll. poplitei profundi of the horse
(260/5; 320/57; 335/a)

Lying on the gastrocnemius muscle about 5 cm deep in the hollow of the knee, between the biceps femoris and semitendinosus muscles, is a group of 3–12 nodes. The conglomerate is up to 5 cm in length. In special cases it should be examined at meat inspection.

Drainage area: skin from the thigh to the toes; fascia cruris; biceps femoris, semitendinosus, semimembranosus gastrocnemius and adductor muscles; tendon of the long digital extensor and of the superficial digital flexor, tendons of the extensor muscles of the hock joint, interosseus medius muscle; all bones of the pelvic limb except the patella and fibula; all joints of the foot.

Efferent route: through the femoral canal to the deep inguinal nodes.

Lymph collecting ducts
Ductus thoracicus of the horse
(252; 320/60; 325/4, 4'; 326/14)

The course of the thoracic duct of the horse is as described in the comparative section of this text. As a rule it is single but in exceptional cases it may give off a branch either at its origin or further along its course. These two branches then run parallel to one another along the left dorsal border of the aorta. The two trunks reunite as the thoracic duct crosses from right to left at the level of the 6th thoracic vertebra. Baum records only a single case where the thoracic duct ran its entire length on the left.

In the precardiac mediastinum it is situated to the left of the oesophagus and trachea below the left subclavian artery and its branches. Occasionally it divides in its terminal segment into two, or even three, branches which reunite shortly before its termination. The thoracic duct has a diameter of 7–10 mm throughout its length; rarely occurring extremes are between 0.5 and 2 cm. The last 3–4 cm dilate into a terminal ampulla which is 13–20 mm in diameter. At the cranial border of the 1st left rib, or up to 2.5 cm cranial to it, the duct empties into either the cranial vena cava or the left external jugular vein. There are two crescentic valves at its termination but these close only incompletely, so that after death blood always enters the duct from the vein in a retrograde direction.

About 5 mm before the termination there is a second pair of valves and then further backwards in the duct there are, on average, another 10–15 valves which are partly single, partly paired. The majority of these valves are situated in the left part of the thoracic duct, while the right part carries few or none at all. After death all these valves are insufficient.

Cisterna chyli of the horse
(254; 257/10; 332/9)

The cisterna chyli is a spindle-shaped structure which extends from the 2nd lumbar to the last thoracic vertebra. It is usually about 11–12 cm in length although exceptionally it may be up to 18 cm long, and at its widest point it is 1.5–2 cm in diameter. It has 2–5 valves which are either single or paired. The lymph vessels emptying into the duct can be partially closed by valves. The lumbar trunks empty into the caudal pole and the intestinal trunk joins the caudal half of the cisterna from ventral and slightly to the right. The coeliac trunk enters the right ventral part of the cranial half. The thoracic duct arises from the cranial pole of the cisterna as a single or double trunk.

The possible variations in morphology of the cisterna are remarkable. Besides the simple, spindle-shaped dilatation there are cisterns which are only indistinctly differentiated from the lumbar trunk. On the other hand there are some individuals in which the cisterna divides into two limbs, one on each side of the aorta. Each limb carries diverticula and the limbs are interlinked by diverse cross branches so that coarse meshes span the aorta.

Truncus coeliacus and truncus intestinalis of the horse
(254/Tc, Ti; 257/11, 12; 320/63, 64; 332/8, 8')

The coeliac trunk is formed from the efferent vessels of the coeliac lymph nodes. It is only a few cm in length and 8–10 mm in diameter. It accompanies the coeliac artery on the right and penetrates between the lateral and middle limb of the right crus of the diaphragm to terminate in the cranial half of the cisterna chyli.

The intestinal trunk arises as a shorter (1–1.5 cm) but wider (7–9 mm) trunk from the union of the efferent vessels of the cranial mesenteric nodes. It ascends to the right of the cranial mesenteric artery, between the aorta and caudal vena cava, to reach the caudal end or caudal half of the cisterna chyli. This often gives the impression that the cisterna is actually formed by the confluence of the intestinal and lumbar trunks. In the majority of cases the intestinal trunk divides into two branches which then enter the cisterna independently.

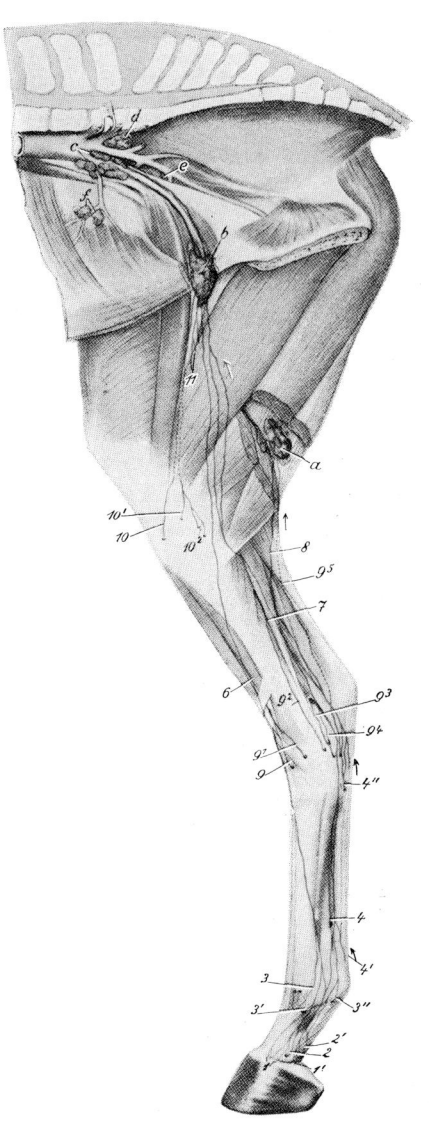

Fig. 335. Deep lymph nodes and lymph vessels of the pelvic limb of the horse. Medial view.
(After Baum, 1928.)

a nll. poplitei profundi, *b* nll. inguinales profundi, *c* nll. iliaci mediales, *d* nll. sacrales, *e* nl. obturatorius, *f* nll. iliaci laterales

1, 1' lymph vessels of the hoof and coffin joint, *2, 2'* of the pastern joint, *3, 3', 3''* of the fetlock joint; *4, 4', 4''* lymph vessels which pass from the lateral to the medial side, *6* lymph vessels lying in the neighbourhood of the saphenous vein, *7* lymph vessel running in company of the caudal tibial vein; *8* lymph vessel which terminates in the popliteal nodes, *9, 9¹, 9², 9³, 9⁴, 9⁵* lymph vessels of the tarsal joint, *10, 10¹, 10²* of the knee joint; *11* lymph vessels entering the femoral canal from the lateral side

Truncus lumbalis of the horse
(257/13; 320/61; 332/7)

The efferent vessels of the aortic lumbar lymph nodes join to form a stout trunk 1 cm in diameter. This trunk also receives the efferent vessels of the caudal mesenteric and the medial iliac nodes. It terminates in the caudal end of the cisterna chyli. The group of lymph nodes mainly responsible for the formation of the lumbar trunk is very variable. Some collecting ducts may run parallel to the lumbar trunk for a considerable distance before they terminate in it or in the cisterna chyli, and this phenomenon makes the trunk appear to be more or less duplicated.

Truncus jugularis of the horse
(246/k; 247/Tj; 320/59)

The right and left jugular trunks are 3–5 mm in diameter and they arise from the union of the efferent vessels of the cranial deep cervical nodes and terminate in the caudal deep cervical nodes. Deviations in the course of the jugular trunks along the trachea occur, particularly if the trunk is duplicated on one side.

Ductus lymphaticus dexter of the horse

The right lymphatic duct is about 4 cm long and 8–10 mm wide. It arises from the efferent vessels of the cranial mediastinal nodes on the right side. It ascends in a gentle curve, immediately in front of the first right rib, to reach the external jugular vein. In so doing it receives efferent vessels from the superficial cervical and caudal deep cervical lymph nodes. It usually terminates in the external jugular vein although occasionally it may discharge into the cranial vena cava or even the point of bifurcation of the jugular veins. The mouth of the duct carries a pair of valves. One or two further pairs of valves may be present in the right lymphatic duct despite its short course.

SKIN AND CUTANEOUS ORGANS

Common integument, integumentum commune

General and comparative considerations

The **skin** (**cutis**) is the external covering which protects the body against the environment. Even prehistoric man found that animal skin and its various formations, such as hair, were of primary importance as clothing. It soon became an object of barter so that of all an animals' organs, it was often the first known and most familiar.

Skin is the surface which separates the organism from its surroundings and as such it fulfills a number of physiological functions and contributes most significantly to the individual's survival.

The common integument not only protects the body against mechanical, chemical and physical influences and against the invasion of parasites, bacteria and viruses but serves as an *"ionic pool"* to maintain the serum electrolyte level and as an organ which regulates blood pressure. The skin is totally impermeable to water but only partially impervious to organic fats so that these are used as the basis of ointments. Certain chemical substances may thus also pass through the skin provided they are fat soluble. The intact skin prevents, to a large extent, the entry of gaseous substances. It protects the body against dessication. It is under permanent tension with the result that wound edges tend to gape.

The *sensory organs* of the skin are receptors for temperature, pressure, tension and pain and they allow the central nervous system of the animal to contact its environment. The skin, therefore, is the *organ of touch*.

The skin is furnished with hair, sebaceous and sweat glands, and blood vessels which *maintain the body temperature* of homeostatic creatures, including our domestic mammals. The blood vessels not only nourish the skin but also serve the vital heat regulating mechanism of the body and, in consequence, the skin possesses a much denser blood vascular system than would be required solely for its nourishment. The numerous networks of cutaneous blood vessels can, depending on the extent to which they are filled, take up a considerable proportion of the total blood volume of the body. The dilatation or constriction of these vessels is automatically regulated by the central nervous system and this action brings about an increase or decrease in heat loss. But also of considerable importance in maintaining body temperature are the thickness and histological structure of the skin, the ratio between surface area and body volume, the increase of the body surface area by skin foldings, the density, structure and colour of hair and the pigmentation of the external layers of the skin. The skin is a poor heat conductor and this is largely due to subcutaneous adipose tissue.

The orientation of the hair on the skin surface and the possible inclusion of air between the two structures, the *passive evaporation* of fluid (perspiratio insensibilis), *active formation of sweat* and its *evaporation* (perspiratio sensibilis) as well as periodic pigmentation, are important physiological adjuncts of thermoregulation.

The skin carries heat-conserving hairs and glands which are characteristic for **mammals**, all of which are haired animals. While the *sweat glands* mainly regulate heat loss (cooling by evaporation) and excretion (discharge of metabolites), the *sebaceous glands* ensure that skin and hair are greased to make them water repellent. Furthermore, the unsaturated fatty acids of the secretion of both sebaceous and sweat glands have an antibacterial action which prevents the accumulation of excessive numbers of bacteria on the skin although, of course, it always carries some microorganisms, even pathogens.

Enlargement or accumulations of *modified sweat* or *sebaceous glands* produce special localised glandular structures which emit odorous substances. These are of great importance for intraspecies communications enabling animals to mark out their territories, offspring to find their dams and mating partners to locate one another.

At all the natural orifices of the body the skin merges with a cutaneous mucosa of very similar structure. This applies to hollow organs (mouth cavity, nasal antrum, anus, vulva) and also to saccular structures (conjunctival sac, prepuce).

The formation of skin folds in certain body regions (prepuce, stifle fold, axilla) allows substantial increases in size or extensive movements.

Finally, extensive keratinization of the limb extremities provides protective cover in the form of the variously-shaped digital organs, the claws, hoofs and pads. Some of these are used as weapons. The horny sheath covering the bony cornual process of ruminants provide both an effective weapon and a head ornament.

Some disease processes are confined exclusively to the skin (eg. mange) but in other generalised diseases (eg. erysipelas, foot and mouth disease) diagnostically important signs occur in the skin. The skin of domestic mammals is often infested with ectoparasites such as fleas, lice and ticks.

It should be mentioned that by salting or dry preservation the skin of slaughtered animals can be turned into *leather*. It thus represents a commercially-important raw material. Leather is produced when animal skin is preserved by tanning, a process which maintains the natural fibre network. Tanning ensures that the skin becomes dry, can no longer rot and has a relatively high degree of heat resistance. Although leather can be produced from the skin of all animals, it is mostly made from the hides of cattle and calves. Sheep and goat hides are also important whereas the skin of horses, pigs, dogs and cats are relatively unimportant.

Fur bearing animals have skin which is covered with very dense wool hairs. Such animals include rabbits, chinchillas, musquash, nutria, beaver, sable, marten, mink, otter, racoon, fox and others.

In grained leather the pattern is due to the arrangement of the hair pores on the superficial layers and this is characteristic for each species. Skivers are produced from the deeper layers of the skin by mechanically splitting thick hides; they thus have no natural grain. In unsplit leather, the grain is retained.

Even with the naked eye one can identify three layers in the **common integument**, the relative thickness of which varies considerably in different parts of the body. These three layers are the *epidermis*, the *corium*, which together form the true skin or *cutis*, and the *subcutis* (tela subcutanea). The last functions as a moveable support for the skin allowing it to glide over the underlying tissues.

The skin of all the domestic animals possesses considerable strength and is usually densely covered with hairs. Even in apparently hairless animals like the African hairless dog, the skin has numerous stunted hairs. On regions where hairs are scanty the skin often has furrows with ridges between them and should these parts reduce in size, the skin tends to become wrinkled.

Individual variation influences the thickness and firmness of the skin and so do species, breed, age and regional differences. They are also affected to some extent by the type of nutrition which the animal obtains and by climatic conditions. As a rule the skin of the back is thicker than that of the belly. The skin is thicker in the ox than in the horse. Those areas of the skin which are more exposed to mechanical stress, such as the lateral walls of the trunk or extensor surfaces of the limbs, are thicker than more protected regions like the lateral surfaces of the abdomen, medial surface of the thigh and medial and flexor aspect of the limbs. Finally, the skin of highly bred and younger animals is thinner than that of older and less intensely selected individuals.

The skin is particularly thick on the dorsal aspect of the tail in the horse, the dewlap of the ox and on the ventral surface of the neck and "shield" of the pig.

In the majority of domestic mammals the colour of the skin is brown, grey or black and this colour depends on the amount of pigment present in the epidermis. Skin pigments are mainly endogenous pigments which develop within the cells. They arise partly from colourless precursors under the influence of oxidizing enzymes. The pigments include the indole-containing melanins and the lipid-containing lipofuscins, the latter often increasing with age. Their colour is reddish-brown to black and the pigment granules are roundish or rod-shaped. On the other hand there are animals without cutaneous pigment and the skin then is a delicate pink or flesh colour. Pigmented and non-pigmented skin areas can alternate in the same animal so as to produce a patchy effect. A total lack of pigmentation (albinism) is usually associated with pigment deficiency of the iris and the pars iridica retinae.

During a clinical examination it is important to pay attention to the skin for a rough, lustreless, shaggy coat suggests that the animal may be ill. Indeed, the skin may be likened to a mirror reflecting the internal condition of the body.

Phylogenesis of skin

The skin of *invertebrates* usually consists only of a single layer of cells (single layered epidermis) which sometimes, as in *insects* and *crustaceans*, forms a noncellular protective layer, known as the cuticle. The single layered skin of *worms* is closely associated with the musculature to form a cutaneomuscular tube.

In *arthropods* the body and limbs are usually surrounded by a chitinous armour made up of rings or segments. The dorsum of *molluscs*, which houses the digestive apparatus, is usually covered by a shell.

Echinoderms have an exoskeleton which consists of calcium lamellae situated in the skin. Their skin may be raised to form pointed prickles.

With the development of a backbone and the reduction of the exoskeleton, the skin assumes new functions and these in turn lead to the formation of further structures. The skin becomes double layered. While the scales of *fish* still recall the erstwhile skeletal function of the skin, a proper double layer is first encountered in *amphibia*: above the relatively thick, tough connective tissue layer there is a multi-cellular epithelium which forms glands but generally remains unkeratinized.

The transition from aquatic to terrestrial life calls for considerably less modifications to the skin than, for example, to the respiratory apparatus. Only the epithelium adapts to life in air and sun; this it does by increasing the number of its cell layers and by keratinization of the outermost cells. The skin of snakes, for instance, has a cornified epidermis in the form of regularly arranged scales. The cornified epidermis of various species is discarded and renewed at regular periods. Animals such as lizards and snakes which have a protective, armoured skin can only grow in the period between discarding the old armour and the solidification of the newly formed one. The epidermis of the snake skin is discarded in one piece and its shedding is under hormonal control. The *slough* or moult (ecdysis) is a periodically repeated process whereas peeling and desquamation of small parts of the cornified layer occur continually.

Scales are considered to be precursors of feathers and hairs. They are skin formations of very varied structure. The scales of butterfly wings, for instance, consist of chitin while the placoid scales of *sharks* are made up of enamel, dentine and cement. The scales of *bony fish* are deeply situated bony plates covered with skin whereas the scales of *reptiles* usually consist of the cornified external layer, or epidermis, of the skin.

Feathers of *birds* are modified scales although these animals still have true scales on the skin of the legs and toes. The skin of reptiles and birds is more or less free of glands.

True scales are encountered in mammals only in the various species of *Manis* (scaly anteaters) and on the tails of beavers and nutria. However, in mammals the outermost layers of epidermis also keratinize and fall off as delicate flakes.

The epithelium of the epidermis of mammals produces various types of skin glands and hairs, the latter being so characteristic that mammals can be differentiated from all other classes of animal by their presence.

Ontogenesis of the skin and its appendages
(351)

The *epidermis* is derived from ectoderm whereas the *corium* and *subcutis* lying below it are mesodermal in origin.

At first the epidermis is formed by a single layer of flat to cuboidal ectoblastic cells. This soon becomes duplicated, the second layer of cuboidal epithelial cells being basally situated and representing the later *germinal* layer. The superficial layer consists of flattened cells which comprise the *primitive periderm*. During subsequent development other cellular layers (intermediate layer) arise between the periderm and germinal layer and thus a multilayered epithelium is formed. The epithelium begins to keratinize during the last third of intrauterine development. Specialized differentiation finally gives rise to the characteristic layers of the stratified squamous epithelium of the epidermis and to the epidermal organs.

Corium and subcutis arise from the subepidermal mesenchyme rather late in embryonic development. This differentiation coincides with the development of hair and skin glands. The corium derives from the dermatome of the somites, that is to say, from the mesoderm. The epithelioid mesoderm cells unite following conversion into a syncytium of mesenchymal cells and they produce the corium and the intermuscular connective tissue and fascia. The innermost layer of the mesoderm of the lateral zone remains epithelial, becoming the endothelium and lining the serous body cavities; the rest of the mesoderm forms the connective tissue of the entire body, including the limbs and their supporting skeleton.

The *mm. arrectores pilorum* arise within the corium from mesodermal elements. The deeper layer of the corium becomes looser in structure and develops into the subcutis which then forms fat cells in the following sequence: steatoblasts – multivacuolar fat cells – univacuolar fat cells. The specialized cutaneous organs are formed during the development of the general integument. These specific organs always arise from the eipidermis but are accompanied by a mesodermal component. Both structures exert a mutual influence on one another *(induction effect)*.

In domestic mammals the first evidence of hair appears on the head (lips, periorbital region, cheeks, chin) where they show as white, slightly raised dots on the otherwise smooth, bare skin. These are the precursors of the *tactile hairs* (vibrissae or sinus hairs). The hairs of other parts of the body are formed later and usually show an elevation of the epidermis.

The first hair anlage appears at the time the epidermis becomes three-layered. The *primitive hair germ* (pre-germ) is formed by proliferation of the basal epithelial cells which take on a cylindrical shape and bulge the basal membrane towards the mesenchyme, this structure then being referred to as the *hair germ*. The mesenchymal cells react to the hair germ formation by becoming more dense; in sinus hairs this process has already occurred by the pre-germ stage. This leads to the formation of a connective tissue *hair papilla*, thus instituting the development of the connective tissue *hair follicle*. The epithelial hair germ becomes lenticular in shape, bulges outwards and its basal cells assume a palisade arrangement. From these cells the hair germ then grows into the corium at an acute angle and becomes the *hair peg*. This oblique growth allows one to differentiate a small angle (anteriorly) and a large one (posteriorly). The direction in which the developing hair grows into the corium determines the future posture of the hair on the skin. During subsequent development the basal cells form the outer layer and polyhedral cells in the centre of the hair peg, the peg being enclosed over its entire length by a mesodermal sheath. At the distal end of the hair peg a nodular swelling now develops and this becomes invaginated by the connective tissue hair papilla. Thus, from the hair peg develops the bulbous peg or hair bulb (bulbus pili). The palisade cells at the end of the bulb represent the matrix for the subsequent hair. In the epidermis above the central cells of the bulbous peg the *hair canal cord* is formed which later, after keratinization, opens to permit passage of the growing hair. Subsequently the basal cells are organized into the *outer epithelial root sheath* and above the papilla they fold in axially, so forming the basis for the *hair cone* which protrudes centrally into the core cells. The hair cone quickly keratinizes, giving rise to the so-called sheath hair. From this arises the actual *hair* (pilus) with its *hair cuticle* and the *inner epithelial root sheath* with the *sheath cuticle*. By multiplication of the matrical cells above the papilla, the tip of the hair and its root sheath push progressively towards the skin surface, following the course of the *hair canal,* and finally erupt. The actual hair first perforates the inner epithelial root sheath which only extends to the point where the sebaceous glands originate.

The eruption of hair on the various body regions occurs at definite times. The various layers of the hair differentiate by further specialization into medulla, cortex, and cuticle, as do the epithelial and connective tissue hair follicle. The individual hairs finally acquire the size and shape characteristic of the species of animal.

Tactile hairs are associated with a *blood sinus* which is located between the inner and outer connective tissue layers of the follicle; this is the reason that they are also known as sinus hairs. They develop before the normal body hairs. The extremities are the last to become haired, development occurring in a proximo-distal direction.

Guide hairs may be arranged, for instance in the cat, in continuous rows, recalling feral markings. Even on goats which do not develop stripes, this natural pattern is recognisable from the pigmentation on the inner surface of the skin. Similar striped markings are also present on the skin of domestic pig embryos and they are reminiscent of the striped pattern found on wild piglets (351).

There is an accumulation of mesenchymal cells on the posterior aspect of the hairs which indicate the development of the arrectores pilorum muscles. An intrauterine replacement of hair known as the loss of laguno hair, takes place in man but does not occur in domestic mammals.

The *apocrine tubular glands* (sweat and scent glands) usually develop before the sebaceous glands. They arise from the columnar basal cells of the hair peg as solid proliferations in which dissolution and absorption of the central cells forms a lumen. They push forward into the subcutis where they become twisted and their blind end forms a coil. These glands often subsequently lose their connection with the hair follicle and they then discharge freely onto the surface. During the development of these glands their epithelium is reduced to two layers of which the inner differentiates into glandular cells and the outer into myoepithelial cells. On the pads and the planum nasale, nasolabiale or rostrale the apocrine tubular glands develop independently of any association with the hair pegs. There are no tubular apocrine glands associated with the sinus hairs.

The first appearance of sebaceous glands is recognised as a single-or multi-layered protrusion of the outer epithelial root sheath below the anlage of the apocrine tubular glands. This grows into a saccular structure, the inner cells of which enlarge and succumb to fatty degeneration. The *tarsal* and *preputial glands* are independently arising sebaceous glands.

Subcutis, tela subcutanea
(336; 365; 383)

The **subcutis, tela subcutanea** or **hypodermis** (336/C, 365/a) consists of irregular bundles of collagenous connective tissue which is freely interspersed with elastic fibres. It forms a loose network binding the skin to the underlying tissue. The more ample the development of the subcutis, the more easily may the skin be moved over its supporting tissue. The connective tissue of the subcutis of different species varies considerably. In horses, oxen and goats the sparse subcutaneous connective tissue is relatively tense but in sheep and carnivores it is loosely structured and plentiful (336). Considerable amounts of subcutis are found in the dewlap (383/d), stifle fold and jowl. The subcutis may be lacking altogether where this is desirable for functional reasons (e.g. on the lips, cheeks, eyelids, external ears, anus) and in these locations the musculature is in direct contact with the skin.

Where the skin overlies protruding parts of bone and a certain amount of mobility is required, a special formation of the subcutis, the *bursae mucosae subcutaneae,* consisting of multilocular spaces lined with villi, is found. These structures are acquired only after birth and develop in response to mechanical influences, particularly pressure. They increase with advancing age and are interpreted as pathological structures (see volume I p. 234 (German Edition) and figs 360 and 361).

In some species there are increased numbers of *fat cells (lipocytes)* (336/h) in the subcutis which appears to have a special predisposition for this phenomenon. This fat accumulation need not be dependent on a calory-rich diet. It effectively protects against heat loss. In the pig this fat forms a more or less solid layer, the *panniculus adiposus*, which is about 2–3 fingers thick and occurs even with normal diets. In the other domestic mammals on a normal diet, fat accumulates only in certain regions such as the lower chest in the ox, the nape in the horse, and the lumbar and inguinal regions in the dog. Accumulations of adipose tissue are *storage organs* of great significance in the body's metabolism.

The accumulation of fat in the subcutis of the pig and dog is usually associated with the formation of a fat store under the superficial layer of the external fascia of the abdomen. Layering of pork fat by the interposition of fasciae may be particularly prominent.

The fat of each species of animal has its own character. Equine fat is yolk yellow and of low melting point and oily consistency. In ruminants the fat is whitish-yellow and of high melting point. In some pathological conditions it may become tallowy and friable. The subcutaneous fat of pigs is greyish-white and firm and its consistency is between that of horses and ruminants. The fat of carnivores is reddish-white and, at room temperature, it is of somewhat oily consistency. Very pronounced cushions of adipose tissue are present in the pads of the toes and sole of carnivores (336); these are called *functional support fat*.

In addition to fat cells the subcutis contains numerous blood vessels, especially venous networks, and nerves which form large meshes. The cutaneous muscles actually lie in the lamina superficialis of the external fascia which is immediately adjacent to the subcutis. Domestic animals living in cold climates are distinguished by having a particularly thick subcutaneous connective tissue. The domestic animals of tropical regions have a thin skin with a poorly developed subcutis.

In the loosely structured subcutaneous connective tissue there is a considerable amount of tissue fluid. This fluid is associated with the cutaneous lymphatic system which thus gives the tela subcutanea a considerable capacity for fluid uptake. This and the rich capillary supply of the subcutaneous connective tissue, is the reason for the efficacy of subcutaneous therapeutic injections and vaccinations.

Corium
(336–340)

The deep layer of the cutis is known as the **corium** (336/*B*; 337/*A*; 339; 340/*b*, *b'*). It is derived from the parietal mesoblast. The thickness of the skin is determined by the thickness of the corium. If one excludes dwarf breeds of dogs and cats, sheep have the thinnest and cattle the thickest corium of the domesticated mammals. The corium is also generally thicker in males than in females. But as a rule the depth of corium depends on the age of the animal and it varies in different body regions. The main layer of the corium is the *stratum reticulare* (336/*g*; 340/*b"*) which is immediately adjacent to the subcutis. This layer consists primarily of delicate bundles of collagen fibres collected into thick cords and interwoven in all directions. Between and, to some extent, around these bundles there is a network of elastic fibres which ensures that the original shape of the skin is regained after temporary distortion. The dense fibre network of this layer is responsible for the firmness of leather.

Above the reticular layer and immediately next to the epidermis there is the *stratum papillare* (336/*f*; 340/*b'*) which is loosely structured and has eminences termed *papillae*. The latter are supplied by delicate, hairpin-like capillary loops and nerve end-plates and they extend into the epidermis forming, in conjunction with connective tissue, the papillary bodies. These papillary bodies form an interdigitating union between the epidermis and corium and because of their relatively great surface area they have a most important function in the nutrition of the epidermis. Their *acid mucopolysaccharide* content, which results in *fluid binding*, is important for maintaining *turgidity* while overdistension is prevented by the tough collagen fibres. At its border with the epidermis the stratum papillare develops a basal membrane which contains reticulin fibres.

The corium has variously-directed lines of tension which can be determined by the cleavage method; when a round needle is inserted into the skin, a slit, not a round hole, results. The alignment of these slits, cleavage or Langer's lines is the same for particular regions of the skin in all individuals. For example, the cleavage lines in the dog coincide with the tension lines of the skin, irrespective of breed, age and sex. From these observations one may conclude that the bundles of collagen fibres of the corium are not randomly interwoven but assume a definite orientation according to their functional requirements. Similarly, the skin does not stretch equally in all directions, so that an incision made in the direction of cleavage will gape less than one made at right angles to it. This phenomenon is of practical importance in surgery.

In histological preparations it is obvious that the papillae of the corium are intimately linked to the stratified squamous epithelium. In the domestic mammals this interdigitation of the epidermis and corium differs in densely haired and hairless regions.

The finer connections between the two layers are achieved by means of delicate cytoplasmic processes from the cells of the stratum basale, the so-called "rootlets", which dip into the superficial reticular network of the corium. The intimacy of this union depends on the density of hair growth. In thickly haired parts of the skin where the epidermis has relatively few layers, the papillary body is also very thin, or present only in the form of a shallow ledge or plinth-like protruberance. Those areas of the skin which carry few or no hairs have numerous tall and closely packed connective tissue pegs on the papillary body. These pegs extend far into the multilayered epidermis. This arrangement ensures not only the adequate nutrition and characteristic innervation of the epidermis but also provides a firm union in an area which is usually exposed to great mechanical stress. It is thus apparent that, depending on the location and function of the particular hairless skin region, the papillary body, and therefore the undersurface of the epidermis, will present a very pleiomorphic appearance. Attempts to separate this union have shown the epidermis and corium to be so tightly linked that a fissure will occur in the epithelial complex before the cells of the stratum basale tear from their basal membrane.

We cannot form a three-dimensional picture of the two contact surfaces simply by studying histological sections; this can only be achieved by examining the apposing surfaces of the epidermis and corium after separating them by maceration (337; 338; 339).

Detailed studies of the surfaces of the epidermis and corium of haired and hairless regions of the mammalian skin have been undertaken by Simon (1952). A variety of troughs and projections can be differentiated on the upper surface of the epidermis; *hummocks* (337/a), *slats* (/c), *beds* (/e), *pits*(/b), *trenches* (/d) and *troughs* (/f). On the undersurface of the epidermis the protrusions are termed *pegs* (/h),

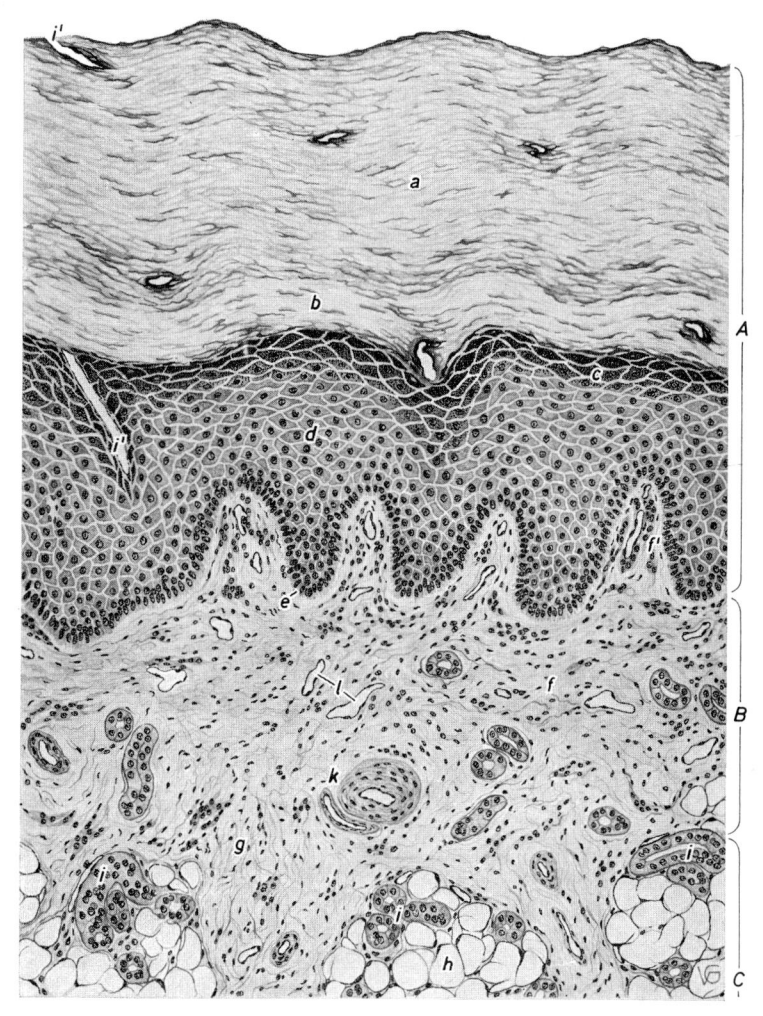

Fig. 336. Sagittal section through the hairless skin of the sole pad of a cat.
(Drawn from a histological section.)

A epidermis; B corium; C tela subcutanea

a stratum corneum; *b* stratum lucidum; *c* stratum granulosum; *d* stratum spinosum; *e* stratum basale; *f* stratum papillare with *f′* tall papillae; *g* stratum reticulare; *h* adipose tissue; *i, i* pad glands; *i′, i′* their efferent ducts; *k* artery and vein; *l* blood capillary

ridges (/k) and *tablets* (/m); depressions are referred to as *caps* (/g), *channels* (/i) or *mortises* (/l). These structures correspond to the appropriate depressions and protrusions on the upper surface of the corium which are the *craters* (/o), *grooves* (/q) and *trays* (/s) or *papillae* (/n), *moats* (/p) and *tenons* (/r). Thus the union between epidermis and corium is such that the *undersurface of the epidermis* (338) forms an exact negative matrix or mould of the *upper surface of the corium* (339). The corium could then be thought of as the patrix or punch. The papillae correspond to the caps, moats or channels whereas the tenons correspond to the mortices. Similarly, the craters and pegs, the grooves and ridges and the trays and tablets fit into one another (337). The depressions and protrusions of the upper surface of the epidermis correspond to the depressions and protrusions of the upper surface of the corium although, on this outer epidermal surface, they are generally indistinct.

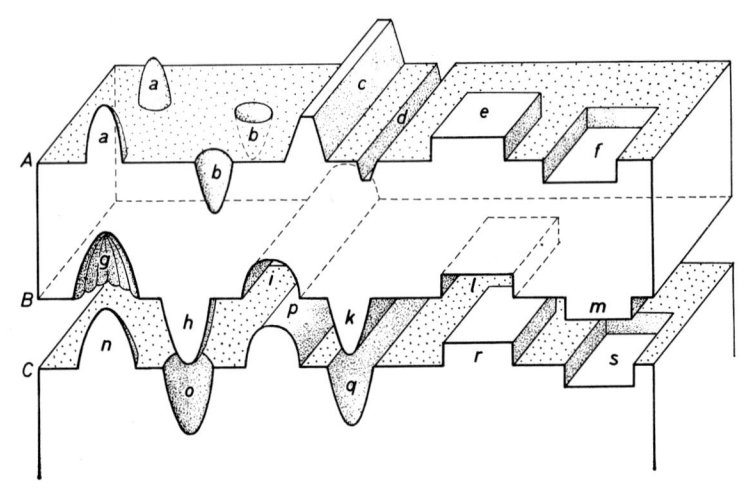

Fig. 337. The interlocking of epidermis and corium in the hair-bearing and hairless skin of domestic mammals. Diagrammatic. (After Simon, 1952).

A upper surface of epidermis; *B* lower surface of epidermis; *C* upper surface of corium

a–f on the upper surface of the epidermis: *a* hummock, *b* pit, *c* slat, *d* trench, *e* bed, *f* through; *g–m* on the undersurface of the epidermis: *g* cap, *h* peg, *i* channel, *k* ridge, *l* mortise, *m* tablet; *n–s* on the upper surface of the corium: *n* papilla, *o* crater, *p* moat, *q* groove, *r* tenon, *s* tray

Epidermis
(336; 337; 338; 340)

The **epidermis** represents the *epithelial* part of the skin. It is subject to continual wear and in some animals (reptiles) its keratinized part is periodically shed. It consists of stratified squamous epithelium the surface of which becomes keratinized, but the thickness and degree of keratinization depend on the wear which that part of the skin is subjected to. When intact, this epithelial body-covering represents a barrier impervious to bacteria. One of the characteristics of the epidermis is that an injury to the skin is covered with new epithelium with great rapidity and this occurs even in physiological exposure such as the raw surface which results when the Cervidae discard their antlers.

The hair-bearing parts of the skin have, as a rule, a thin epidermis with only a moderate degree of keratinization (340/*a*), whereas the hairless areas of the skin – such as the pads (336/*A*), muzzle and snout disc – have a thick epidermis with pronounced keratinization. The greatest amount of keratinization is found in the digital organs (claws, nails, hoof), the horns of ruminants and the chestnuts and ergots of the horse.

The epidermis is derived from the external ectoderm and even during its embryonic stage one can recognise the anlage of three structures which form a genetic and functional unit called by Zietzschmann (1923) the "*epidermal organ complex*". These structures are the *hair* (pilus), the *sebaceous gland* (gld. sebacea) and the *sweat gland* (gld. sudorifera) which extend a variable distance into the corium.

The epidermis is composed of the superficial *horny layer* (str. corneum) (336/*a*) and the deep *germinative layer* (str. germinativum). If the horny layer is removed from the germinal layer, a fluid-filled blister develops. If the epidermis is very thick there are, between these two layers, several rows of cells which contain *keratohyalin granules* and form the *str. granulosum* (/*c*). The keratohyalin granules above the granular layer may liquefy to form *eleidin* and this causes the development of another layer which appears shimmering and translucent and is thus called the *str. lucidum* (/*b*). The most deeply situated layer of the stratum germinativum is the *str. basale* (/*e*) which consists of columnar cells. These columnar cells are firmly attached to the corium by denticulate extremities.

The cells of the germinative layer situated external to the str. basale are large, polygonal epithelial cells which make up the *str. spinosum* (/*d*). They are interlinked by means of particularly prominent desmosomes and are therefore known as the *prickle cells*. They become progressively more flattened towards the horny layer.

The germinative layer continuously produces new cells to replace the keratinized epithelial cells (scales) which have been discarded from the surface of the skin. In pigmented parts of the skin the basal cells contain *melanin granules*. Recent eletronmicroscopic studies have indicated that the epidermis is composed of two fundamentally different cell types: firstly, the ordinary epithelial cells or keratinocytes (see above), and secondly branched or dendritic cells. In the normal epidermis the dendritic cells are situated between the ordinary basal cells and through the action of *tyrosinase* and *dopa*, they are able to form the pigment melanin and are thus known as *melanocytes*. They pass the melanin along their processes and transfer it to the neighbouring epidermal keratinocytes. (This is the *cytocrine secretion* of

Fig. 338. Under surface of the epidermis of the planum rostrale of a domestic pig. There are circular and transverse ridges arranged around the sinus hairs; between them lie the caps. Approx. x 12.
(After Simon, 1952.)

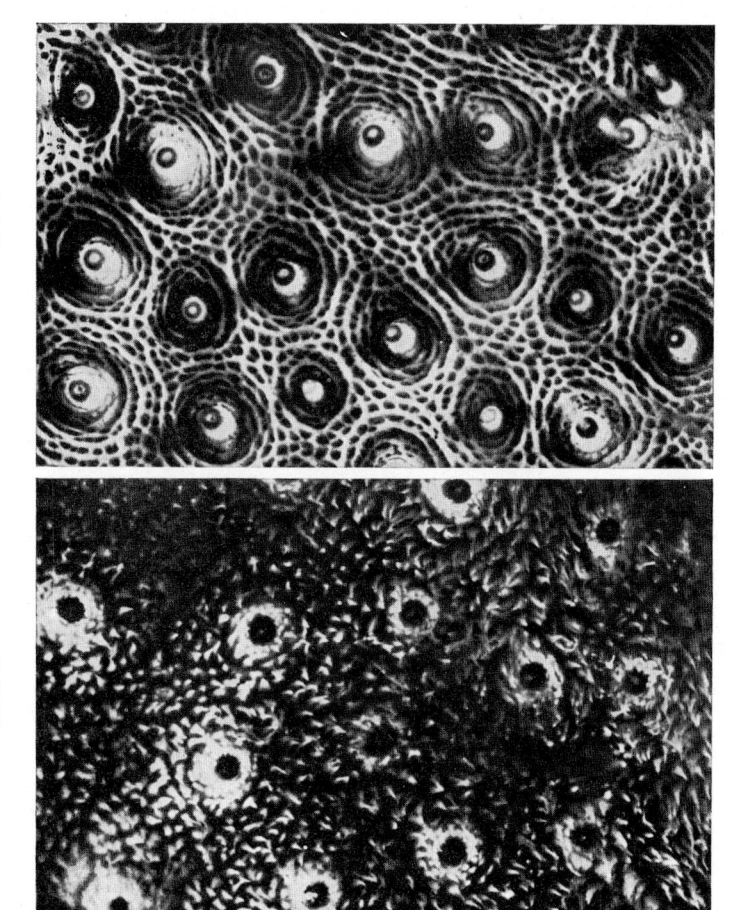

Fig. 339. Corium surface of the planum rostrale of the domestic pig. Arranged around the sinus hairs are rosette-like circular and connecting longitudinal ridges which bear papillae of varying size. Approx. x 12.
(After Simon, 1952)

Masson). As well as these cells, the stratified squamous epithelium contains *non-specific dendritic cells* and *Langerhans cells*. The melanocytes are said to derive from the ectodermal neural ridge and to migrate into the epidermis via the papillary layer of the corium. The genesis and function of the Langerhans cells, which are mainly situated supra-basally, are still in dispute today. They are believed neither to originate in the nervous system nor to be derived from the melanocytes. They are considered very active cells which play a part in the metabolism of the epidermis.

The cells of the epidermis thus arise at the basal layer as active cells which are capable of division and they are discarded at the surface as dead, horny scales. Between 6 and 14 g of these dead scales are discarded each day in man. For this reason a major function of the skin is the production of keratin. Keratinization is a protective mechanism against dessication and keratin formation in the skin is under the influence of vitamin A. A deficiency of this vitamin results in *hyperkeratosis (excessive keratinization)*. The epidermis is devoid of blood vessels, its nutrition being maintained by osmosis and diffusion via the intercellular spaces.

In regions of the skin with poor hair development one can see that the external surface of the epidermis carries raised areas in the shape of cones, slats or tablets and also depressions (337/A) and these make up the surface relief of the skin (see p. 448). Studies of some areas of skin where the surface configurations are particularly distinct, such as the muzzle and snout disc, have shown that there are individual, genetically-determined, differences similar to those of the papillary lines of the human finger tips (*daktyloscopy*). Imprints of these special skin areas are termed *labiograms* or *nasolabiograms* and they can be used for the identification of animals.

Hairs, pili
(340–351; 378; 379)

The **hairs** or **pili** (340/c) are derived from epithelial cells of the epidermis and they represent flexible, *horny fibres* which lie obliquely in the skin. In domestic mammals the thick coat forms an air-retaining cover which is of great significance in thermoregulation. The hair presents the *hair shaft* (scapus pili)

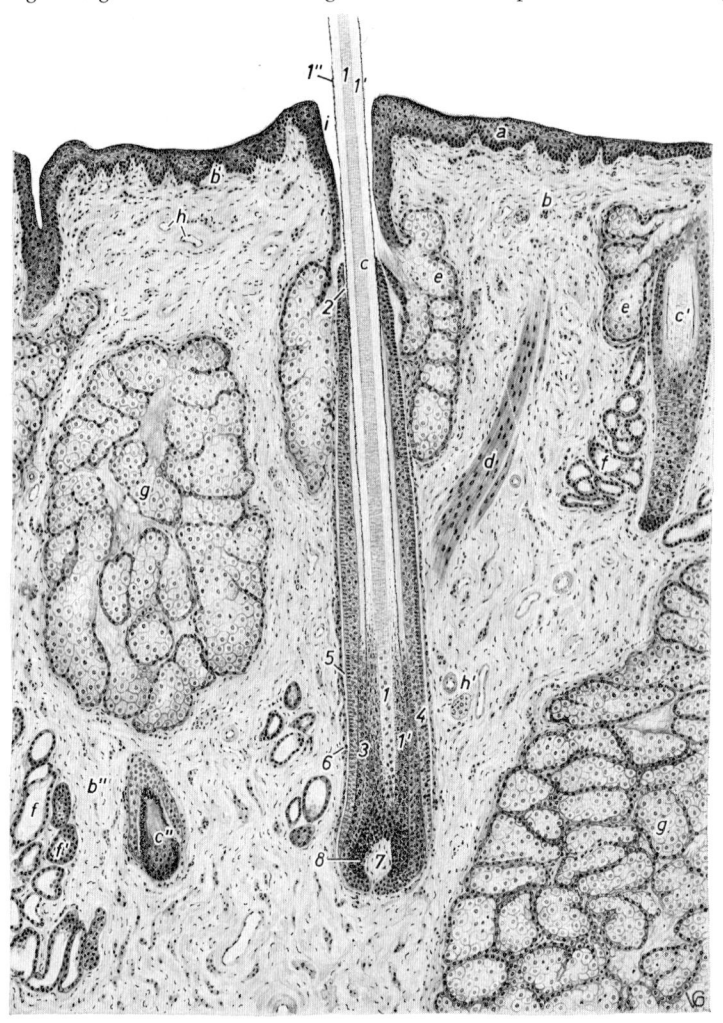

Fig. 340. Sagittal section through the hair-bearing skin in the region of the tail gland of a male cat.
(Drawn from a histological preparation.)

a epidermis; *b* superficial corium layer (str. papillare) with *b'* low papillae, *b''* deep corium layer (str. reticulare); *c* hair in longitudinal section, *c'* hair, oblique section, *c''* hair bulb in oblique section; *d* m. arrector pili; *e, e* hair follicle sebaceous glands; *f, f* coiled tubular glands; *f'* tubular gland in tangential section; *g, g* modified sebaceous glands (scent glands); *h* blood capillaries, *h'* artery, vein, nerve; *i* funnel of the hair follicle

1, 1 medulla pili, *1', 1'* cortex pili; *1'', 1''* cuticula pili; *2* sheath cuticle; *3* internal epithelial root sheath with Huxley's and Henle's layers; *4* outer epithelial root sheath; *5* vitreous membrane; *6* folliculus pili; *7* papilla pili; *8* bulbous pili

(341/2), which projects beyond the surface of the skin, and the *hair root* (radix pili) (/1) which is inserted obliquely into the corium. At its end the hair root is enlarged to form the *hair bulb* (bulbus pili) (340/8) which is indented by the *hair papilla* (papilla pili) (/7), the blood vessels of which nourish the bulb. The hair roots are situated in tubular pockets in the epidermis which extend into the corium and are known as *hair follicles* (folliculi pili) (/6). They have a sack-like base, a constricted neck and a dilated orifice known as the *funnel* of the hair follicle (/i).

The connective tissue sheath of the *hair follicle* is composed of an *outer* and an *inner follicular layer*. The outer layer is made up of longitudinally directed connective tissue fibres and the inner layer of circular fibres which possess contractile properties. Internal to this is the glassy or *vitreous membrane* (/5). The *outer epithelial root sheath* (/4) arises directly from the epidermis; it lies next to the vitreous membrane. The *inner epithelial root sheath* (/3) consists of two layers of keratinized cells (Henle's and Huxley's layers). It is separated from the *hair cuticle* (/1″) by the *inner sheath cuticle* (/2) and the free borders of the cells comprising this cuticle, in contrast to those of the hair cuticle (see below), are directed towards the hair root.

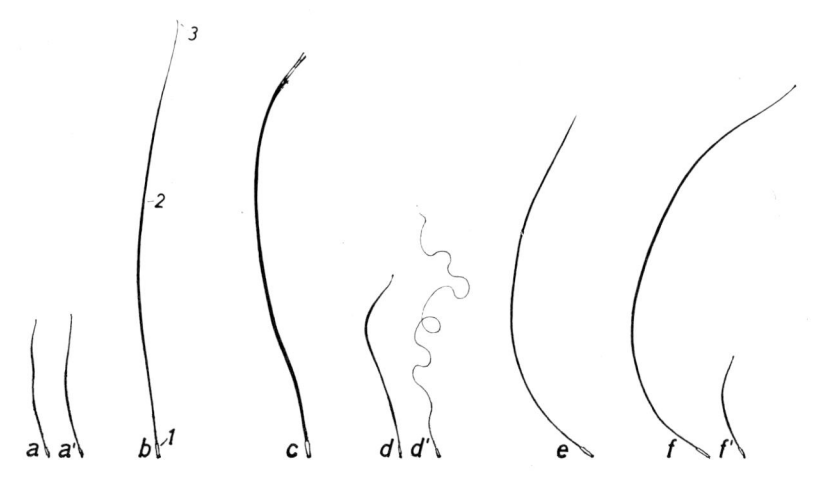

Fig. 341. Hair types in various domestic mammals.

a awn hair (lateral abdomen), *a′* awn wool hair of a boxer; *b* leading hair (lateral abdomen) of a German shepherd dog; *c* back bristle of a wild pig; *d* outer hair (from the limb), *d′* wool hair from the neck of a sheep; *e* outer hair (lateral abdomen) from the ox; *f* long horse hair (fetlock); *f′* outer hair from the croup of a horse

1 hair root (radix pili); *2* hair shaft (scapus pili); *3* tip of the hair (apex pili)

The hairs arise from epithelial cells lying on the apex of the hair papilla. This is known as the *growth point* (matrix pili). The hair grows from the base of the epidermal tubular pocket as a keratinizing cellular strand and is at first accompanied by the inner root sheath. The latter terminates just below the level of the outlet of the sebaceous glands. The inner root sheath may be said to represent an epithelial gliding layer by means of which the hair moves along the outer root sheath.

The hair consists of the *medulla* (medulla pili) (/1), the *cortex* (cortex pili) (/1′) and the *cuticle* (cuticula pili) (1″). Its free tip is known as the *apex pili* (341/3). The *cuticle* of the hair (340/1″) is formed by very thin, transparent, keratinized, anucleate squamous cells, which overlap like roofing slates with their free borders pointing towards the tip of the hair. The number of such cell borders projecting from the hair shaft determines the degree to which the edge of the hair is jagged or serrated. Viewed from the surface, the free cell borders form a system of delicate lines and imprints of them made on gelatine plates can be used in forensic science to *identify* the species from which hair came. However, more recent scanning electron-microscopic examination has shown that the *cuticle cell pattern* alone is not absolutely reliable for the identification of hair.

The *cortex* of the hair (/1′) is made up of a complex of completely keratinized, spindle-shaped cells about 60 μm in length and 5–10 μm in width. They contain pigment in dissolved or granular form.

The *medulla* of the hair (/1) is an axial cord of polygonal, cuboidal or longitudinally flattened cells of 15–20 μm diameter. Gas is sometimes found between the cells and sometimes even within them. Pigment is rather sparse in the medullary cells.

There are numerous species differences in the shape and thickness of the medullary and cortical layers of the hair. The fine wool hair of sheep and the tail hair of horses, for instance, are devoid of medulla. In most domestic mammals the hairs have a slender medulla and a thick cortical layer. Hairs containing much medulla stand erect and are brittle; the more cortex there is in the hairs the stronger they are. The shape and arrangement of the medullary cells may also be used for species identification; (for example, they are large, vesicular and polygonal in the deer but triangular in the goat). The forensic identification of hair makes use of the relative thickness of medulla and cortex, the structure of the medullary cells and the appearance of the free borders of the cuticular cells, but the medulla is the most variable part of the hair.

The term *"hair disc"* has recently been coined to describe a special thick and richly innervated region of epidermis surrounding the orifice of some special hair follicles. Below it lies a well vascularized part of the corium. These special, and usually somewhat larger, hair follicles are regularly distributed in the skin. So far, "hair discs" have been identified in dogs, sheep and rabbits. They are interpreted as especially sensitive receptor organs.

Hairs are raised by means of the arrector muscle (*mm. arrectores pilorum*) (/d) which make the hairs stand on end as, for example, the bristling of hairs and so-called "goose skin", the latter caused by the muscle depressing the epidermis. When the temperature of the environment is low, alteration of the alignment of the hairs causes the *insulating cushion of air* which is trapped between the hair and the surface of the skin, to be increased. A similar procedure is used to make the animals' body appear larger and thus frightening to a potential foe.

In domestic mammals almost the entire surface of the body is covered with closely-placed hairs. They are absent only at the muzzle, anus, vulva and the terminal organs of the toes. There are often striking species and breed differences in hair number and development. Every animal has several types of hair which differ in form according to the body region. Apart from differences in the hair of different species, there are differences within a species which are breed dependent and have largely been artificially selected; for example there are long-haired, rough-haired, wire-haired and short-haired Pointers. There are animals with normal hair cover, with poor hair cover or almost without hair such as the African hairless dog. Especially long-haired goats, cats, rabbits and guinea pigs are given the descriptive prefix "angora" (e. g. Angora goats).

We can differentiate the following types of hair:

Outer hair (Capilli)
(341)

These are the characteristic hairs of the coat of animals, except sheep. They determine the animals colour. These hairs are of varying length and they may be wavy. They are relatively soft with a coarse medulla. They occur in two forms, namely leading hairs and awns.

The non-wavy leading hairs (341/*b*), which are absent in ungulates, are usually stiff and longer and less numerous than awns. They are of almost even width. The awns (/*a*) carry a spindle-shaped thickening, the awn, below the tip. They do not occur in some animals such as the silky-haired dogs.

Wool hair (Underwool, pili lanei)
(341/*d'*)

These hairs vary in length and are usually fine and very wavy. In ungulates they lack a medulla but in carnivores they are medullated. In sheep they form the long-haired fleece which gives the characteristic appearance to the coat of these animals (q. v.). The wool hairs are situated between and below the outer hairs. Their density varies considerably with the seasons. Since wool hair is much longer in winter than in summer, winter pelts, rich in wool hairs, are more valuable than summer pelts with sparse wool hair content. The sea otter has very dense fur and a correspondingly valuable pelt, its skin bearing some 20,000 hairs per square cm.

Fig. 342

Fig. 343

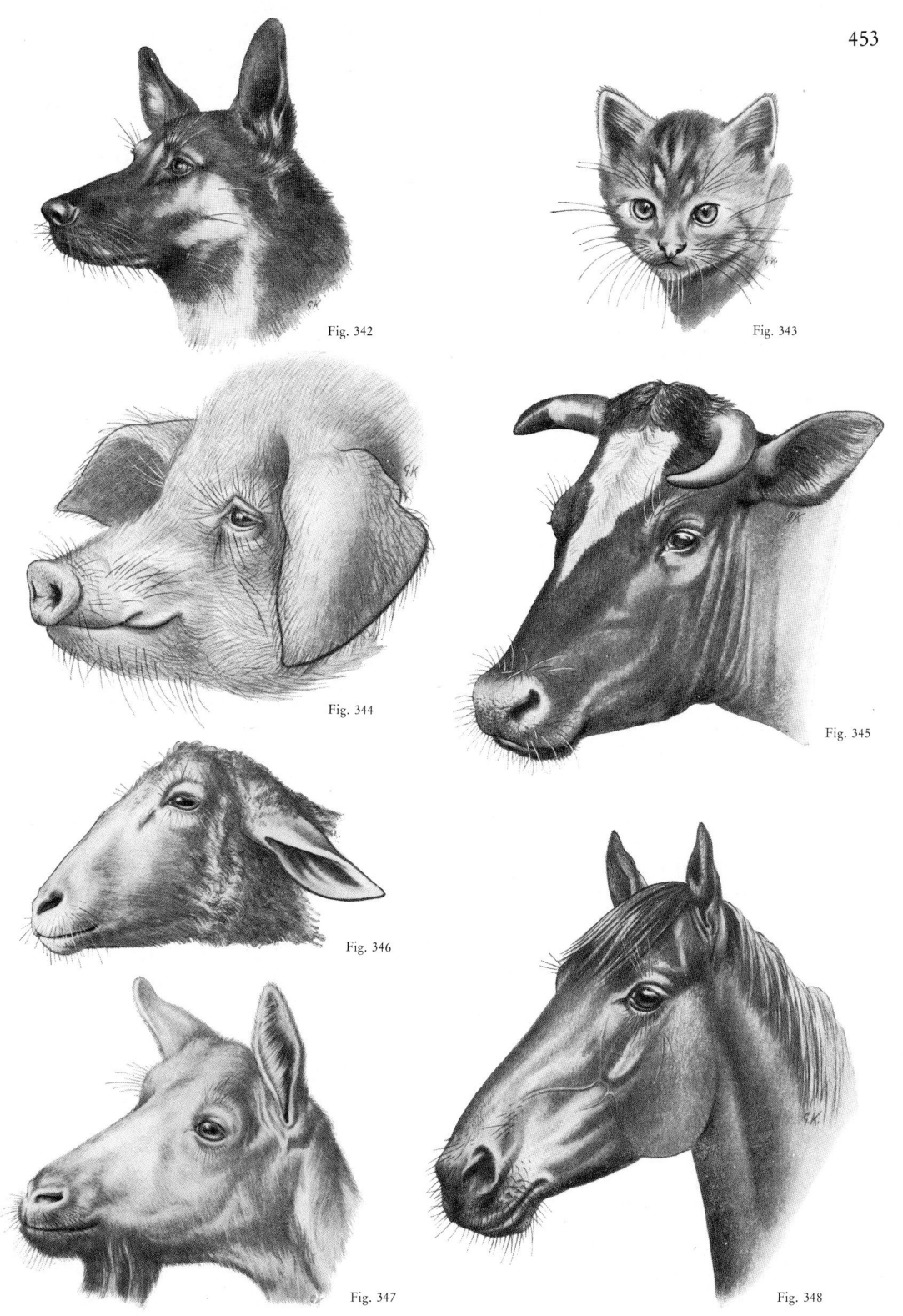

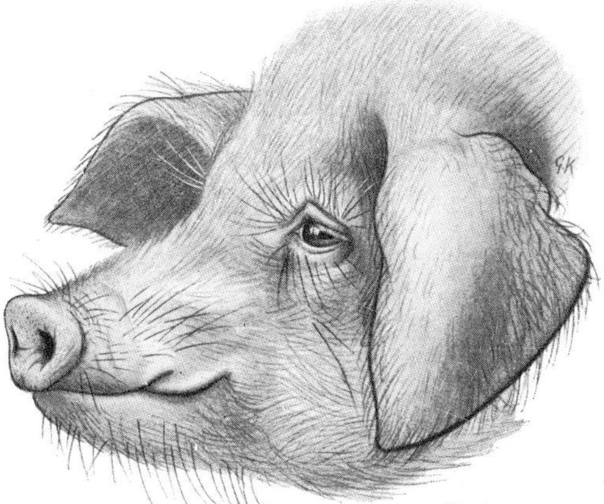

Fig. 344

Fig. 345

Fig. 346

Fig. 347

Fig. 348

Figs 342–348. Heads of domestic mammals showing the typical formation of the skin and arrangement of the tactile hairs in the region of the nares, pili tactiles.

fig. 342 dog with its planum nasale; fig. 343 cat with its planum nasale; fig. 344 pig with its planum rostrale; fig. 345 ox with its planum nasolabiale and cirrus capitis; fig. 346 sheep with its planum nasale and sinus infraorbitalis; fig. 347 goat with its planum nasale and beard (shortened); fig. 348 horse with nostrils, cirrus capitis and juba

Long or horse hairs
(341/f; 349/h–l)

Another type of hair which occurs principally in equines is the long hair or horse hair. This develops great length, is elastic and very lustrous and grows only in certain parts of the body. It may be of different colour to the coat; for example, black long hair occurs in bay horses. These hairs are found in the *forelock* (cirrus capitis) (349/k), *mane* (juba) (/i) and the *tail* (cirrus caudae) (/l). Long hairs are particularly prominent on the palmar or plantar aspect of the fetlock of non-thoroughbreds and heavy draft breeds where they form the *cirrus metacarpeus* (/h) or the *cirrus metatarseus* (/h').

Bristles (setae)
(341; 378; 379)

Bristle hairs form the typical body hair of the pig (378; 379). They are remarkably stiff, thick outer hairs whose tips are split (341/c). They also occur in other animals in certain parts of the body such as the *hairs of the nostrils* (vibrissae), the hairs on the inside of the ears and at the entrance to the *auditory meatus* (tragi), the *eyelashes* (cilia), the *beard hairs* of the goat and the *moustache hairs* of the horse. Vibrissae and tragi form a sort of grille which protects these body orifices against the entry of foreign particles or insects.

Tactile hairs (pili tactiles)
(342–348)

A specialized form of bristle is the *tactile* or *sinus hair* (pili tactiles). These are stiff hairs which protrude, either singly or in several rows, beyond the coat hairs and they have associated *rudimentary sebaceous glands* but not *sweat glands*. The root of this hair and its root sheath is enclosed within a blood sinus which is usually multilocular. The connective tissue outline of the sinus contains numerous *tactile bodies*. In domestic mammals the tactile hairs are found in several horizontal rows on the upper lip (342–348) and they also occur on the lower lip and chin, on the cheek and around the eyes. Any pressure on a tactile hair is transmitted to the blood sinus where it is multiplied by hydraulic effect and passed on to the numerous nerve endings in the sinus wall. The animal thus becomes aware of even the slightest touch in the oro-nasal region.

The following tactile hairs are differentiated according to their location: *tactile hairs of the upper lip* (pili tactiles labiales maxillares); of the *lower lip* (pili tactiles labiales mandibulares); of the *chin* (pili tactiles mentales); of the *cheek* (pili tactiles buccales); of the *zygomatic* region (pili tactiles zygomatici); of the *infraorbital* region (pili tactiles infraorbitales); of the *supraorbital* region (pili tactiles supraorbitales); of the *carpal* region (pili tactiles carpales) (342–348).

Tactile hairs appear prior to pelt hairs during the development of the skin and they are present even in congenital hairlessness.

Arrangement of the hair
(349; 350)

The arrangement of the hair of the domestic mammals is not uniform. Whereas in the horse and ox the coat hairs are arranged in rows evenly distributed over the body (350/i), in the pig and carnivores they occur in groups(/K). Here one can differentiate *central hair*, which is often strong and tough, from the weaker *lateral hair*. If group hairs reach the surface of the skin through a common orifice, one refers to them as hair bundles. The arrangement and distribution of the hair orifices are easily recognised in tanned skin where they are called hair patterns and they may be used to identify the species from which the skin or leather was derived.

In each species of domestic mammal the hairs are arranged in certain patterns. This applies not only to the distribution of the individual types of hairs on the various body regions, which is quite typical, but also to a remarkable constancy in the direction in which hairs are aligned.

The greatest proportion of hairs, especially of the outer hairs, are implanted obliquely into the skin. The direction of the individual hair is determined by the angle of the hair and the edge of its orifice. If the hairs of a certain body region leave the skin in the same direction one speaks of the *hair line*, *hair stream* or *tract* (flumina pilorum) (349). The direction of the hairs is determined in the first place by the direction in which the part of the animal's body normally moves and it thus varies in the different body regions (349). This results in the formation of definite areas or fields where the hairs lie in a certain direction. These fields are bordered by *hair vortices*, *hair partings* or *hair ridges*. The tips of the hairs are directed forwards and downwards on the nose and forehead but in the nuchal and parotid regions and on the neck they are directed towards the chest while on the chest they point towards the abdomen. On

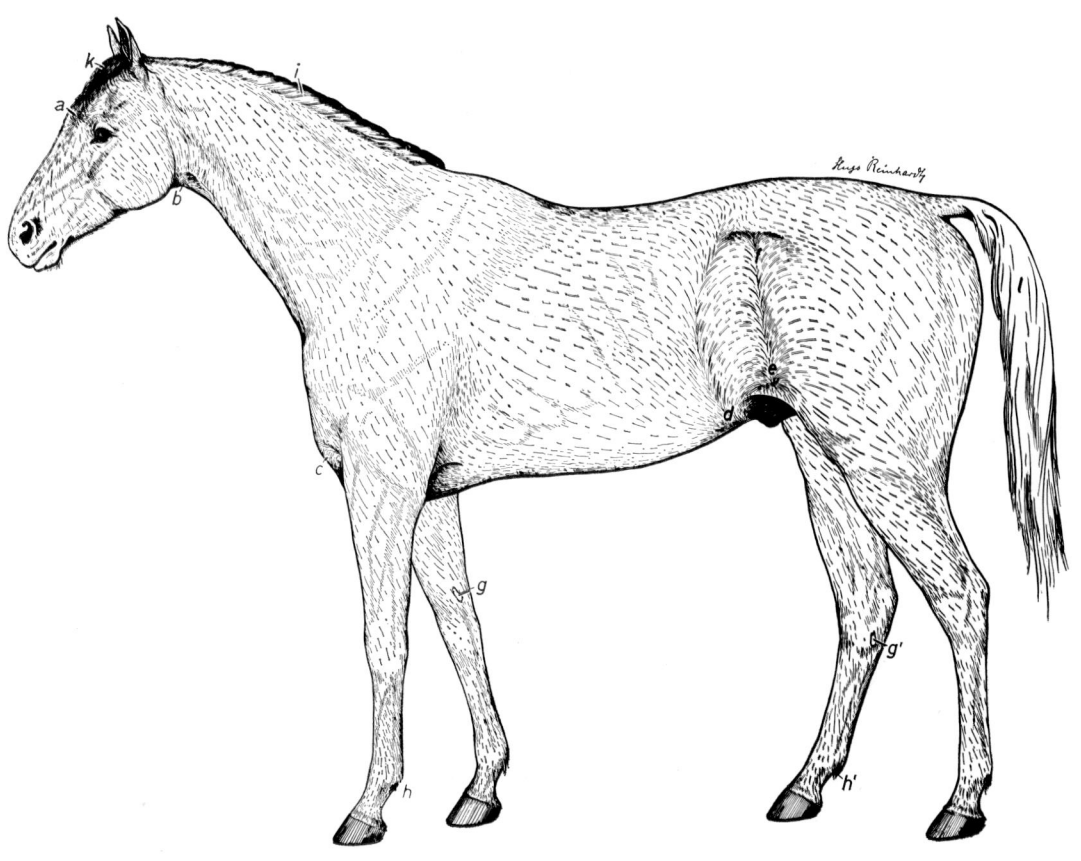

Fig. 349. Hair tracts, fluminae pilorum, and vortices, vortices pilorum, in the horse. (After Martin, 1915).

a forehead vortex; *b* throat vortex; *c* vortex at the front of the chest; *d* vortex at the caudoventral surface of the abdomen; *e* vortex in the region of the stifle fold; *f* vortex in the region of the external angle of the ilium; *g* torus carpeus, *g'* torus tarseus; *h* cirrus metacarpeus, *h'* cirrus metatarseus; *i* juba; *k* cirrus capitis; *l* cirrus caudae

the rump and limbs the hairs are directed backwards and downwards (349). This arrangement prevents the air stream from raising up the hairs when the animal is in forward motion and rain water runs off the slightly greasy hairs without penetrating, at least for a time, the insulating layer of air. The hair direction remains constant throughout life and is not influenced by age, breed and body conformation.

Spirals or *vortices* of *hair* (vortices pilorum) (349) are points of origin or termination of different hair lines. If the hairs of a certain skin region converge on one particular point, then a *convergent vortex* develops (vortex pilorum convergens) (350/*a*, *c*). If, on the other hand, the hairs move out from a common point either in a radial (/*b*) or spiral (/*d*) form, it is referred to as a *divergent hair vortex* or *star* (vortex pilorum divergens) (/*b*, *d*). In most domestic mammals the following divergent spirals of hair occur: one nasal vortix, two orbital vortices, two ear vortices, two vortices on the anterior chest, two vortices in the inguinal region. Species peculiarities are given in the appropriate section.

Hair ridges (combs) (lineae pilorum convergentes) (/e) develop at the border between two apposing streams of hair. In certain regions the hairs may separate in linear fashion so as to form a *parting* (lineae pilorum divergens) (/f). Horizontal, vertical, straight, wavy, oblique and curved partings and ridges may be differentiated according to their position and course.

A *hair cross* (crux pilorum) (/h) is a term applied to an intersection between two hair ridges or partings or the combination of 3 or 4 hair streams impinging upon one another. A *"hair feather"* (penna pilorum) (/g) is a special arrangement of hairs along a hair-covered midline. Some of these specialized hair patterns are found in domestic mammals as a constant feature; others are not invariably present. The latter can, therefore, be used for identifying individual animals. The cause of whorls, ridges and partings is not completely understood.

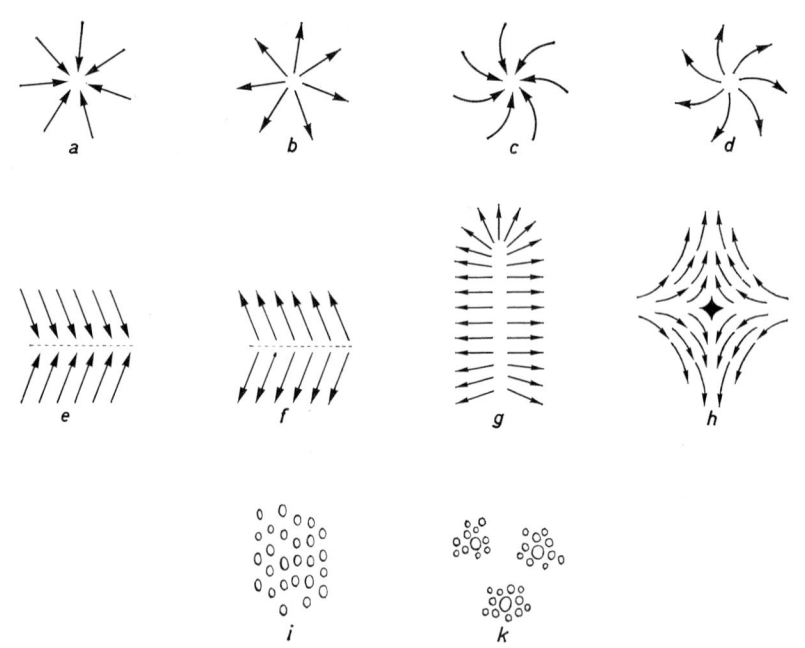

Fig. 350. Diagrammatic presentation of the various hair patterns.

a simple convergent vortex, vortex pilorum convergens simplex; *b* simple divergent vortex, hair star, vortex pilorum divergens simplex; *c* spirally convergent vortex, vortex pilorum convergens contortus; *d* spirally divergent vortex, vortex pilorum divergens contortus; *e* hair ridge, linea pilorum convergens; *f* hair parting, linea pilorum divergens; *g* hair feather, penna pilorum; *h* hair cross, crux pilorum; *i* arrangement of hairs in rows; *k* arrangement of hairs in groups

Hair colour
(351)

The colour of hair is dependent on its *surface structure* and the amount of *pigment* and *air* which it contains. The most important factor is the amount of hair pigment. Without pigment the hairs are white, if only a little is present they are yellow, more colours them red (phacomelanin), then brown while abundant pigment (eumelanin) causes black hair. The pigment occurs mainly in the cortex and to some extent in the medulla and between tho two layers. In light coloured hair the cortical pigment is diffusely distributed while in dark hair the pigment is granular and located in the cortical layer. The deposition of air either between the cells of the medulla or in the spaces between the medulla and cortex can make the hair appear lighter because it reflects light. It is believed that hair becomes grey because it loses pigment from the matrix cells so that the growing hair is colourless. Our knowledge about this process, and the sudden development of white hair in man after severe mental shock, is still not complete.

The colour of mammals depends on the colour of their fur; skin colour need not be the same as hair colour. A true white horse with white hair has dark pigmented skin. Foals of such animals are born with dark coats and only when they reach the age of 3–5 years are the pigmented hairs replaced by nonpigmented ones.

In wild mammals one can detect that the hair is not coloured uniformly throughout its length but is banded. The colouring of the fur is either simple and even or is arranged in *longitudinal* or *cross stripes* and *patches*. Longitudinal striping is said to be the original pattern, the so-called wild or feral pattern. In many young animals we can observe first a longitudinal striping, as in the wild piglet (351), or patches, as in the fawn, which are later replaced by a single colour. Striping or spotting (patching) are a form of protection, camouflaging the young animal so that its colour and pattern blends into the surroundings. Another instance of adaptation of the coat to the environment is the colour change of the hair in summer and winter in some wild mammals (ermine, mountain hare). The cheek, shoulder and back lines (the eel mark of equidae) may be interpreted as remnants of a previous striped coat pattern. Interruption of the stripes can give rise to patchy markings and confluence of the patches to piebald or skewbald patterns.

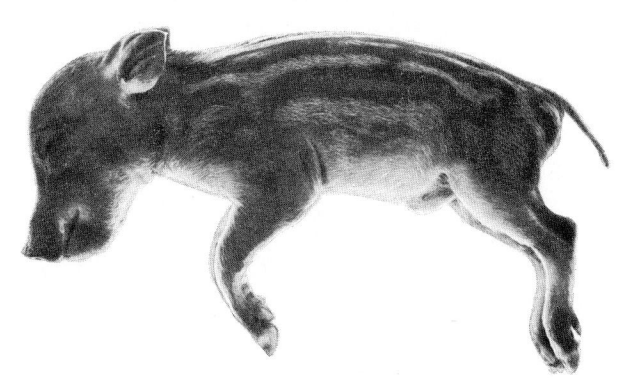

Fig. 351. Coat of a newborn wild piglet with distinct striped pattern (feral or camouflage marking) (Photograph: G. Geiger.)

Adaptation to the environment, including the climate, may also influence the colour of the animal's coat. The variable hair colouring of domestic mammals has resulted from artificial selection and occurs only rarely in wild mammals. Albinism or pigment deficiency is more common in the latter. *Depigmented areas* are probably the results of domestication and, as they do not alter during the animal's lifetime, they can be used for identification. Such non-pigmented regions occur mainly on the head and limbs. *Canitis* is the term used for the appearance of grey hair with increasing age in horses and dogs; it should not be confused with discrete white markings.

Hairs have only a limited life; in man the eyelashes are replaced after 4–5 months while on the scalp each hair persists for $1/2$–4 years, after which period it drops out. Similar investigations on the life span of hair in domestic mammals have been carried out relatively recently.

A special deviation from normal hair pattern is the formation of *curls* which are more common in domestic than in wild mammals. The term curl is applied when variously shaped hairs from one skin area are grouped together. They may occur in dogs, pigs, sheep, oxen, donkeys, horses and man.

True curls are named and classified by furriers according to their various shapes. The cause of the hair curvature, and therefore the formation of curls (*karakul lamb*, *poodle*, *mangalica pig*), must lie in the shape of the follicles. The type of curl formation can be influenced by the formation of skin folds.

Hair replacement

The *replacement* of lost hair is either periodical (animals) or continual (man). The change is initiated by regression of the hair papilla and cessation of the growth of the hair. The matrix cells grow into long keratinized cylinders, so giving rise to the club root, the free end of which later frays. The replacement hairs derive, as did the original hairs, from the remnants of the germinal layer in which a new papilla has developed. The newly formed hair grows up to the point of eruption from the same external root sheath which enclosed the old hair and the latter, having no root, then drops out. A periodic hair change occurs in wild animals which grow longer and thicker coats in the autumn and then change their coats in the spring.

In the domesticated mammals these processes are not so clear cut but here, too, we can differentiate a *summer coat* and a *winter coat*. As a rule there is only one change of coat, which takes place in spring, but the short summer fur increases in length as the colder season sets in. At the same time newly-developed wool hairs push between the outer hairs, so making the pelt thicker. In the spring this winter wool hair then falls out in thick bundles and the long outer hair is replaced by shorter outer hair. It is questionable whether two hair changes occur in the year. Long hair and tactile hairs are not included in the periodic hair replacement.

Skin glands (glandulae cutis)
(336; 340)

The skin of all but a few mammals contains numerous **glands**. These glands are important in *heat regulation*, as *excretory organs*, for *greasing* the hair and skin, keeping certain skin areas *moist*, as *scent organs* for the recognition of species members and to attract the opposite sex during the mating season, as *scent glands* in defense and, modified, as *milk secreting glands* for feeding the young.

The skin glands of mammals belong to the two large groups of *polyptychial* and *monoptychial glands*. They occur as sebaceous, sweat and scent glands and, in certain parts of the body, as special modifications of these. The old belief that sebaceous glands are always alveolar and sweat glands always tubular is no longer tenable.

Sebaceous glands (glandulae sebaceae)
(340)

The **sebaceous glands (gldd. sebaceae)** are generally saccular, *polyptychial* glands which have a *holocrine* type of secretion. They are functionally linked to the hair follicles and have therefore been referred to as hair follicle-sebaceous glands. They form a fatty secretion by the disintegration of their central cells. This secretion is known as the *sebum* and it passes through their wide duct into the hair follicle where it provides fat to protect the hair and surface of the epidermis against the effects of water and air. The sebaceous glands lie fairly superficially and they are arranged in a wreath-like manner encircling the hair follicles. This type of gland is found in all vertebrates except amphibia.

In addition to these hair follicle-associated sebaceous glands, *true* or *free sebaceous glands* occur in certain regions of the skin and are of greater biological significance than the simple sebaceous glands. They have lost their connection with the hair follicle and terminate independently on the surface of the skin. They can form complex *scent organs* which are of importance to the animal during the mating season and, because their secretion has a strong specific odour, it can serve in the recognition of members of the same species or warn the animal that foreign species, particularly predators, are in the vicinity. So-called *"identification glands"* are dealt with later.

The sebaceous glands of sinus hairs become atrophied (e. g. dwarf sebaceous glands of eyelashes) and they are completely lacking from unhaired regions such as the ball of the foot, muzzle, teats, horns and hooves or claws. As a rule sebaceous glands are more widely distributed in mammalian skin than are sweat glands. They are the original elements of the specific skin gland organs.

Sweat glands (glandulae sudoriferae)
(336; 340)

The **sweat glands (gldd. sudoriferae)** are generally *tubular*, *monoptychial* glands. Their efferent ducts may be coiled and their terminal parts are surrounded by *myoepithelial cells*. So far, monoptychial glands have been found only in amphibia and mammals.

In the skin of the higher mammals we can differentiate between *exocrine* and *aprocrine* sweat glands according to the type of secretion they produce.

The small, eccrine sweat glands are also known as skin glands (gldd. glomiformes), because their unbranching terminal part forms a tight clew. They are epidermal in origin and are not connected to hairs so that their ducts perforate the cornfield epidermis in a corkscrew fashion and end free on the body surface as fine openings or pores (336/i'). They are mainly found in regions of the skin which have few or no hairs and they produce a watery secretion, the true *sweat* (sudor). This fluid is not very concentrated and its acidity (pH 4–6) inhibits the growth of bacteria and fungi on the skin (*acid protective coating*). The skin of domestic mammals has few of this type of sweat gland which is, in fact, characteristic of the prioates, particularly man.

The secretion of sweat also plays a part in the body's water and salt balance.

The *apocrine sweat glands* are phylogenetically older structures. They have branched end pieces. They arise from the epithelium of the hair anlage and discharge their secretion into the hair follicles. They comprise the principal type of sweat gland in the hair-covered skin of domestic mammals and they produce a viscous, concentrated secretion which contains *scent* that is characteristic of the individual animal. For this reason they are also referred to as *scent glands* (*gldd.* odoriferae). They may become disassociated from the hair follicle. In some regions of the skin scent glands congregate in large numbers whereas in other parts they are entirely absent. However, this relative distribution varies considerably in the different species (q. v.).

Only in certain species is so much sweat produced that it actually becomes visible and for this to occur extreme heat, exertion or fear are necessary. The sweat of horses, which contains much protein, can be whipped into a lather by continuous movement of the saddle girth or harness leathers. On the other hand, sweat glands are sparsely distributed in the skin of carnivores and in cats they may be only rudimentary structures. In these animals, however, they occur in large numbers in the pads of the feet. In dogs, oxen, sheep and horses sweat production occurs mostly on the flanks, shoulders and lateral and ventral regions of the neck. In pigs, under extreme conditions of heat and humidity, sweat is secreted in the axilla, along the linea alba on the ventral aspect of the abdomen, at the perineum and in the anal region. Cats and rabbits do not produce sweat in the hair-covered parts of the skin.

Apocrine glands usually produce an oily, iron- and cholesterol-containing and scent-binding secretion. Furthermore, they can produce not only protein, as do salivary glands, but in certain circumstances a mucoid secretion (cf. specific glandular organs of the skin).

Anglo-American investigators have recently begun to consider the concept of *"apocrine"* secretion in the classification of tubular glands of the skin inappropriate because unequivocal evidence of a necrobiotic process is lacking. These workers suggest that all tubular exocrine skin glands should be referred to simply as sweat glands until further investigations, possibly of a histochemical nature, have determined the exact mode of secretion; this would then form a sound basis for classifying the different glands.

Blood supply to the skin

The *arteries of the skin* are characterized by the presence of three interlinked networks. The arteries are usually derived from the blood vessels which supply the superficial musculature of the body. Delicate branches issuing from these vessels form a *fascial network* immediately on, or above, the superficial fascia of the body and this network supplies the subcutis and the subcutaneous adipose tissue. The arteries traversing the subcutis follow the larger connective tissue bundles which protect them from undue stretching. In areas where the skin is loose and moveable, the arteries take a meandering course. Delicate branches pass from the fascial network into the deeper layers of the corium where they form a *wide-meshed cutaneous network* which supplies the sweat and scent glands. Small blood vessels arising from the cutaneous network ramify in the upper layers of the corium and form the *close-knit subpapillary network* which provides the blood supply of the hair follicles and sebaceous glands. This net also gives off vessels to the papillae of the corium and, as these vessels have no further connection with other arteries, they are *end-arteries*. Each hair follicle has its own arterial vessel. The capillaries form neat loops and reticulations in the corium and hair papillae. The *avascular epidermis* is nourished by *diffusion* and also by *active transport*, presumably through the intercellular spaces. A capillary network is present in the outer follicular layer of the sinus (tactile) hairs and it communicates to some extent with the inner follicular layer. The *blood sinus* of the tactile hairs is supplied by the latter. Whereas the stratum papillae of the corium has numerous capillaries, the stratum reticulum is said to be devoid of blood vessels.

As well as their direct nutritive rôle, the blood vessels of the skin play a part in regulating blood pressure and body temperature.

There are four *venous networks* in the skin. The first is situated in the basal region of the corium, the second in the middle of the stratum reticulare and the two others close to one another in the stratum papillare. Otherwise the veins follow the same course as the arteries.

Nerve supply of the skin

All the layers of the skin contain sensory and autonomic (sympathetic) nerves and several varieties of nerve endings. As a general rule skin regions which are densely covered with hair are less rich in nerves than poorly haired or hairless areas. *Autonomic nerves* are mainly present in the form of perivascular plexuses in the subcutis and corium; they do not occur in the epidermis.

The *sensory nerve fibres* also form plexuses in the subcutis and corium. The majority of these fibres terminate in *sensory touch receptors*, in the *external epithelial root sheath* of the hairs and *free* in the deeper epidermal layers. The terminal sections of these nerves are non-myelinated but the conducting parts are myelinated. The cutaneous sensory apparatus in its entirety is known as the *organ of touch (organum tactus)*. The organs of surface sensitivity are the first components of the cerebrospinal sensory nerve fibres.

On structural grounds the cutaneous nerve endings can be divided into so-called free nerve endings, those which are connected to the hairs, and the encapsulated nerve endings. We can differentiate pressure, touch, pain and temperature receptors, although not all the varieties of ending have been definitely assigned to a receptor group. Despite their pleiomorphism, one can attribute a definite function to certain types of receptors.

The *sensory organ* of the skin is made up of a specific sensory cell, or exteroceptor, including various ancillary structures, and the sensory nerve itself *(sensory peripheral nerve fibre)* which carries the stimuli created in the *receptor* back to the *sensory centre* of the cerebral cortex.

It is believed that the following are all *pressure* and *touch receptors*:
1. *Cuff of nerves* encircling the hair and the epithelial root sheaths.
2. *Meckel's tactile disks* which are numerous in the deeper layers of the epidermis.
3. *Meissner's touch corpuscles* are pressure receptors that lie singly or in groups in the papillae of the corium immediately below the epidermis.
4. *Vater-Pacini's lamellar corpuscles* are found in the subcutaneous connective tissue. They are larger than any of the other end organs, measuring up to 4 mm in length and 2 mm in width, so that they are visible to the unaided eye.

Tactile receptors appear to be specialized so that they only respond to certain qualities of stimulus and for this reason they are so distributed in the skin surface that each region contains several functional types. For example, there are slow and fast adapting receptors. The *fast adapting receptors* are all sensory fibres which innervate hair follicles whereas the *slow adapting receptors* innervate the epithelial eminences, which are distributed over the entire skin surface, *Meckel's touch cells* and *tactile disks*.

Pain receptors arise from the nerves in the form of fine, non-myelinated, coiled nerve fibrils. They are located in the middle layer of the epidermis where they can be demonstrated by silver methods. These intra-epithelial receptors presumably respond to stimulation by chemical substances produced by epithelial cells which have been damaged by mechanical, thermal or other processes. Not all free nerve endings are pain receptors, however, because some of them are pressure and temperature sensitive. Pain sensitive nerve endings are also found in the capillary-rich subpapillary layer of the corium where they take the form of isolated fibres within the Meissner lamellar bodies.

On the basis of numerous physiological observations it is assumed that different receptors exist for the perception of hot and cold. It is believed that the *cold receptors* lie more superficially than the *heat receptors*.

The *Krause terminal bulbs*, situated at the apex of the connective tissue papillae, are *cold receptors*. *Ruffini's bodies* lie deep in the corium and subcutis and they are believed to be *heat receptors*. The possibility that these various bodies have a double function cannot be excluded. Presumably pain and temperature receptors are evenly distributed over the body surface while pressure receptors are more concentrated in certain areas.

It is obvious that, because of the great difficulties involved in the study of sensory areas in animals, we have to rely to a large extent on analogy with man. The current opinion is that only sympathetic innervation supplies the muscles of the hair follicles, the sweat and sebaceous glands and the cutaneous blood vessels. However, it is possible to demonstrate antagonistic responses between glands and smooth muscle (antagonism within one and the same system). Thus the vasomotor centre of the medulla oblongata regulates the musculature of the vessel wall via stimuli conveyed in the sympathetic nerves and this, together with chemical, mechanical and thermal stimuli, determines the size of the vessel lumen.

Stimuli to the skin (heat rays, mustard poultices, etc.,) can exert their effects on internal organs by reflex routes and, similarly, stimulation of the internal organs may be appreciated as cutaneous sensations. Clinically it is well recognised that inflammatory conditions in certain parts of the intestinal tract can give rise to *hyperaemia* and *hypersensitive reactions* in localised regions of the skin. The concept of *Head's zones* is of importance in medicine and refers to an association between the affected visceral regions and certain skin areas.

Specialized structures of the skin

General skin modification
(342–347; 352; 383)

Around the natural body orifices of the head of domestic mammals the skin has been modified to form structures referred to as the *nasolabial plate (planum nasolabiale)* (345) in the ox, the *rostral plate* in the pig *(planum rostrale)* (344) and the *nasal plate* in small ruminants and carnivores *(planum nasale)* (342; 343; 346; 347). These structures have already been briefly described in volume II. In cattle, sheep, goats and pigs there are large subcutaneous aggregations of glands associated with these structures. These are the glands of the nasolabial, nasal or rostral plates; the *gldd. plani nasolabialis* in the ox, *gldd. plani nasalis* in small ruminants and *gldd. plani rostralis* in the pig. They are coiled, tubular, serous glands, very similar to sweat glands but lacking the characteristic layer of myoepithelial cells. There are no glands in the nasal plate of the dog and cat. The sensory innervation of the nasolabial region is almost identical in cats, dogs, pigs and ruminants; sensory nerve fibres follow a zig-zag course and then terminate in the stratum superficiale of the epidermis. The associated connective tissue contains simple sensory bulbs.

The *dewlap (palear)* (383/d) of the ox and the *collar (plica transversa colli)* on the neck of the sheep are *folds of skin (plica cutis)* in which fat tissue has been deposited.

Tassels (appendices colli) (352) are sometimes found in goats. They are paired cylindrical skin appendages which are situated on the ventral aspect of the throat. Their significance is unknown; sometimes they occur in pigs and, rarely, also in sheep. In the goat they are the size of the little finger and are covered with hair (352). They are composed of connective tissue, a central cartilaginous rod, blood vessels, nerves and sometimes a little muscle. When present in pigs they are a little larger than in goats, sparsely covered with hair and with a rounded bulbous thickening at the free end. They are mainly found in the pigs of southern or south-eastern Europe.

The skin bears special structures in certain parts of the body and these are the *localized special glandular apparatus*, including the *mammary glands*, and the *specific hairless skin organs*.

Localized special glandular apparatus (cutaneous scent glands)
(340; 353–357; 362; 399)

In the hair-covered mammalian skin there are species- and sex-specific glands, the secretion of which has a characteristic scent. They are known as the *cutaneous scent organs*. They are not infrequently associated with pocket-like skin folds and for this reason they were once erroneously thought to function as skin lubricating glands. However, in the majority of cases their secretion embodies a specific scent which facilitates recognition by members of the same species. Thus the cutaneous scent organs are of considerable importance in the social behaviour of mammals. The odour produced by the scent glands of the ano-rectal region is carried by the faeces which then functions as a sort of "visiting card". They are usually apocrine, coiled, tubular glands *(gldd. odoriferae)* or modified sebaceous glands, discretely situated and easily distinguished from the surrounding tissues. They are most frequently found in such exposed parts of the body as the head, ano-genital region, root of the tail or distal parts of the limbs. Frequently the shape, colour and structure of the skin and hair of these regions are distinctly different from that of the surrounding area. The scent organs are often richly supplied with hair follicle muscles, myoepithelial cells and blood capillaries. At times of physical excitement these structures can exert pressure (by contraction of the muscles or by vasodilation) and so quickly eject secretion onto the skin surface.

The secretions produced by the scent organs contain one or more pheromones. *Pheromones* are chemical substances which serve as a mode of communication between individuals of one species, although the effect is said not to be absolutely species specific. The substances are used for marking the animal's territory, either as a deterrent or attractor and even in very low concentrations the signal is instantly detected and interpreted. An inter-relationship has been demonstrated between pheromones and gonad hormones.

The odoriferous substances of those pocket-like scent organs which have few or no hairs (e.g. interdigital organs [356]) are associated with sebaceous secretions and desquamated epithelial scales which both carry and retain the scent.

The secretion of the scent glands is discharged onto the skin or hairs or into storage pouches (e.g. infraorbital organ [353]). However, substantial amounts are continually passed into the animal's environment in deliberately aimed or indiscriminate manner. Indiscriminate, passive dissemination is achieved with the aid of the hairs which, because of their continual movement against one another, massage the scent along to their tips. Alternatively, the scent may pass along the hair by capillary action.

This process has been observed in the *tail glandular* organ (340) of the Canidae. As a general rule, the hairs over the odoriferous skin glands project beyond the level of the neighbouring hairs and this facilitates dissemination of the scent into the environment (e.g. *tail gland* of Canidae and Felidae and the *metatarsal gland* of Cervidae).

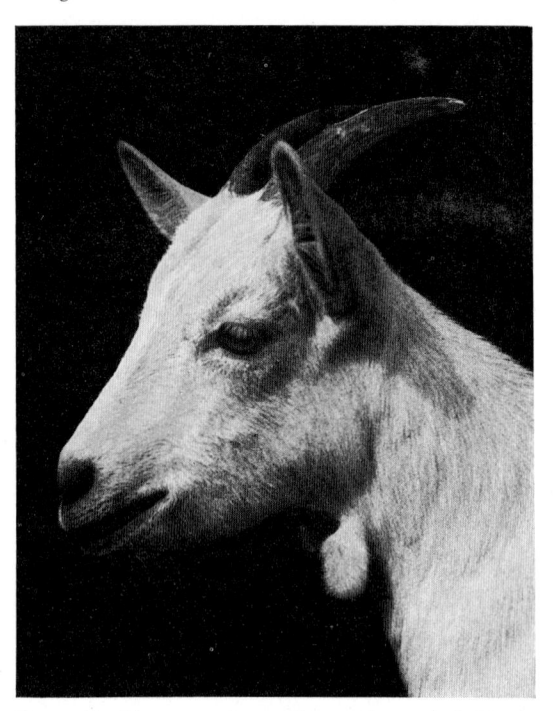

Fig. 352. Tassels in a young male goat with horns. (Photograph: G. Geiger.)

In scent glands which are devoid of hairs or only sparsely covered, dissemination of the scent is brought about by direct skin contact. An example of this is the contact which occurs between the *inguinal organ* (399/f) of the ewe and the head of its lamb. Pressure and massage stimulate secretion in this case.

The following types of odoriferous skin organs are differentiated:
a) *Recognition glands* for conspecific recognition.
b) *Rutting glands* for attracting the sexual partner at the mating season.
c) *Stink glands* for defense.
d) *Marking glands* for communication within the same species.

It may be assumed that cutaneous scent glands containing a large proportion of sebaceous glands, serve mainly to transmit long lasting information to members of the same species. In such cases a more or less weather-resistant and slowly vaporizing scent is placed in carefully selected places during marking; an example is the *anal glands* (357). On the other hand it has been demonstrated that cutaneous scent organs which consist of coiled apocrine glands secreting mainly highly volatile scent (e. g. *carpal organ* [355], *metatarsal brush*), are utilized for only transient communication between members of the same species. They facilitate olfactory contacts between mother and offspring, between sexual partners or between members of a nomadic group like a herd of sheep.

The **specific skin gland organs** are here described collectively for all domestic mammals. There is little doubt that domestication has resulted in some of the cutaneous scent glands partly losing their original significance as organs of communication. Where it is necessary to elucidate the functional significance of individual scent organs, brief references are made to related wild mammals. In many cutaneous scent organs desquamated, keratinized epithelial cells are of some significance as component constituents of the secretion. Specific skin gland organs which consist exclusively of monoptychial tubular glands occur only on parts of the body which are devoid of hair, such as the nose and sole pads. Scent organs made up exclusively of polyptychial glands occur mainly in rodents.

Perioral glands, glandulae circumorale

Perioral glands, (gldd. circumorale) occur only in cats. They are hypertrophic sebaceous glands which occur in the skin around the mouth, especially in the lower lip. These glands are sometimes collectively spoken of as "cleaning glands". Between these enlarged sebaceous glands there are also apocrine scent glands. Their functional significance has not been established.

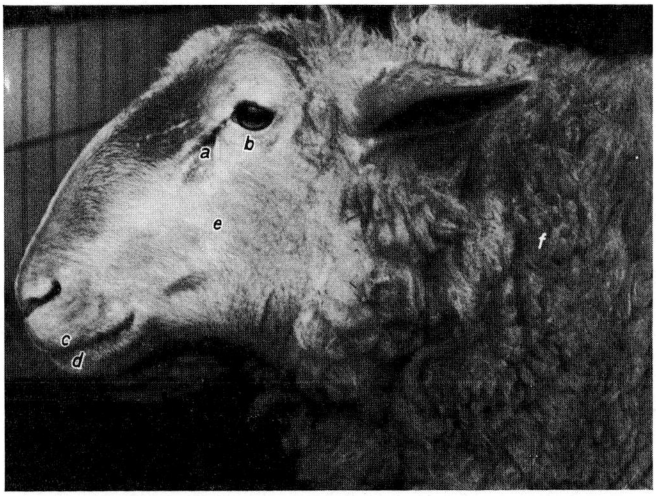

Fig. 353. Position of the infraorbital organ, sinus infraorbitalis, in a ewe. (Photograph: R. R. Hofmann.)

a sinus infraorbitalis; *b* pili tactiles infraorbitales; *c* pili tactiles labiales maxillares; *d* pili tactiles labiales mandibulares; *e* short outer hairs on the head; *f* typical wool hairs in the neck region

Infraorbital organ, sinus infraorbitalis
(353)

In some cloven-hoofed species a collection of glands is situated near the rostral angle of the eye in a depression on the lacrimal bone. These are the *gldd. sinus infraorbitalis* which are also sometimes referred to as the *ante-*, *pre-* or *infra*-orbital organ or the *sinus infraorbitalis*. The erroneous belief that the infraorbital organ served as a tear receptacle, because in Cervidae it is located in a pocket of skin which is connected by a distinct groove to the rostral angle of the eye, had caused it to be named "*tear groove* or *pit*". Of all our domestic animals only the sheep has an infraorbital organ (353/*a*). It presents as a narrow slit about 3 cm long which is a direct continuation of the rostral angle of the eye. It measures 5–12 mm in depth. Internally the organ is made up of a few hairs, numerous well-developed tubular apocrine glands and some large sebaceous glands. The sticky secretion is yellowish-brown and is brushed off onto shrubs, bushes and other objects where it acts as a marker. The infraorbital organ is better developed in males than females and there are considerable breed variations.

Horn gland, glandula cornualis
(354)

The **horn gland** (gld. cornualis) occurs in both male and female goats in which it is found posterior to the base of the horns. It consists of an accumulation of *hair follicle* and *sebaceous glands*. In hornless sheep these glands are located in the same region.

A similarly-located structure occurs in chamois and is under the influence of the oestrus cycle. It also consists of proliferated sebaceous glands. The secretion is deposited on bushes and shrubs and functions as a marker.

Another skin gland of similar structure is found in female and juvenile male Cervidae. It is formed by skin folds and enlarged sebaceous glands situated near where the base of the antlers would be located in adult males. In roebuck a frontal scent organ has also been described; this is lacking in the doe. The "antler gland" develops shortly before and during the rutting period when it appears as a thick, bulging fold of skin between the two antlers. The gland is about 5.5 mm thick and is characterised by the strong odour of the buck. The organ consists of apocrine tubular and sebaceous glands. The apocrine tubular glands are at their maximum development before the rutting period whereas the sebaceous glands are most active during that period. The smell of the secretion before and after rutting is said to be different from that during the heat period. It is assumed that the buck sets its mark on its territory by brushing its head against bushes and small trees and that this warns its rivals against trespass.

Ceruminous glands, glandulae ceruminosae

The **ceruminous glands** (gldd. ceruminosae) are situated in the skin of the external auditory meatus. In all domestic mammals these are supposed to consist of enlarged sebaceous glands and apocrine tubular glands. The *ear wax* or *cerumen* is a mixture of sebaceous secretion and small epidermal scales. The secretion of the tubular apocrine glands is said to make the wax more fluid and aid its removal. As already mentioned, the short hairs at the entrance to the meatus are known as tragi and these, together with the glandular secretion, tend to prevent foreign bodies entering the ear. The ceruminous glands are particularly well developed in carnivores and pigs; in the former they produce a reddish-yellow wax and in pigs a brownish wax.

Mental organ, organum mentale

The **chin gland** or **mental organ** (organum mentale) occurs in both domestic and wild pigs and consists of a wartlike skin eminence situated on the chin. It is about 1.5–2 cm in diameter and 0.5 cm high. On its surface are a few tactile hairs and about 8–10 duct orifices. Its component compound tubular apocrine scent glands and numerous hair follicle-sebaceous glands are located in the underlying corium. Large Meissner's corpuscles and numerous nerve fibres can be demonstrated in the corium papillae. The mental organ has both a tactile and marking function.

Carpal organ, organum carpale
(355; 362)

The **carpal organ** (organum carpale) occurs in domestic and wild pigs in a mediopalmar position above the carpal joint. It presents as several skin pockets which are lined by hairless, keratinized epithelium and surrounded by a highly modified cushion of apocrine tubular glands (gldd. carpeae). The surrounding skin of this region is usually somewhat raised. The organs measures 5.0 cm in length, 2.0 cm in breadth and 0.5–1.0 cm in thickness. There are usually 4 or 5 duct openings or pocket-like invaginations (355/f) but there may be as many as 10. The skin pockets are filled with a greasy mass of fat, hairs, epidermal scales and secretion. The lentil-sized lobes of the gland are clearly separated from one another by adipose and connective tissue. There are numerous smooth muscle fibres in the loose connective tissue between the glandular tubes. As a rule there are no tactile hairs in the neighbourhood of this organ (355/f) so it probably functions primarily as a marking organ. Occasionally, however, tactile hairs with rudimentary sebaceous glands have been observed in the region of the carpal organ so that the possibility of a tactile function cannot be entirely excluded. Contrary to former belief, it is certain that the function of this organ is not to lubricate the carpus. The main function of the scent produced by the carpal organ is sexual stimulation of the mating partner. It can also play a part in territorial marking and in identifying the female partner as the property of the particular male who has marked her by the gripping reflex during mating (Meyer, 1975).

The *carpal organ* of the cat lies about 2.5 cm above the carpal pad and consists of 3–6 non-pigmented sinus hairs (362/f). These sinus hairs may be arranged in two rows on a thickened ridge of skin projecting considerably beyond the body hairs. A few coiled tubular glands may be found in the immediate neighbourhood of the follicles of these sinus hairs; the carpal organ of the cat is thus a touch organ combined with scent glands. It is used mainly in climbing.

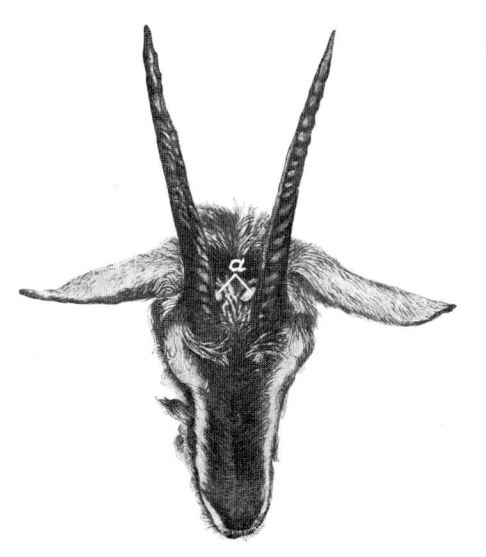

Fig. 354. Horn gland of a 2½ year-old horned female goat. (After Schietzel, 1911.)

a horn gland, glandula cornualis, displayed by removal of the hair normally overlying it

Fig. 355. Carpal organ, organum carpale and hoofs of (A) the left forefoot and (B) the left hindfoot of a pig. Sole aspect. About half natural size.

a, a paries corneus, a' zona alba; b, b solea cornea; c, c torus corneus; d, d spatium interdigitale; e, e accessory hoofs; e', e' bulbs of the accessory hoofs; f ostia glandulae carpeae of the carpal organ; g, g hair-bearing skin

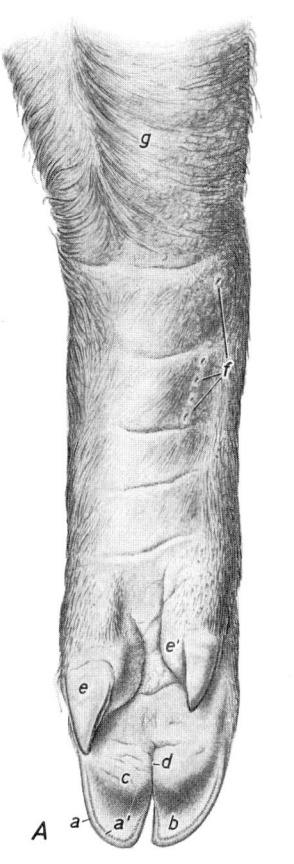

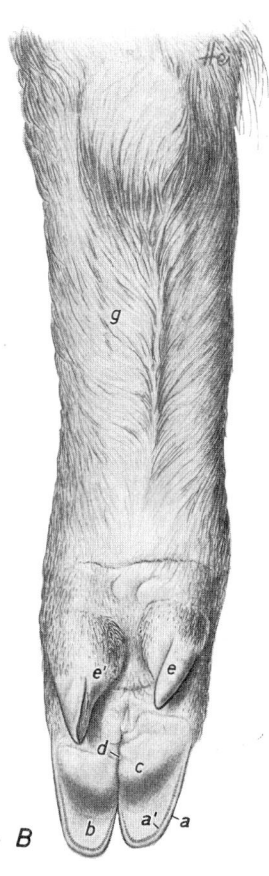

Metatarsal glandular organs, organa metatarsalia

Metatarsal glands (organa metatarsalia) occur in Bovidae and Cervidae. They are raised areas of skin, about 3 cm in diameter, situated at the proximal end of the metatarsus. The hair covering this area is denser and of different colour to the surrounding skin, so that it is sometimes referred to as a metatarsal brush, and in its depths are well-developed hair follicle-sebaceous glands and apocrine scent glands. The efferent ducts of the scent glands also terminate in the hair follicles. The metatarsal glands are used for territorial marking and communication, the scented secretion being brushed onto tall grass or bushes.

Interdigital sinus, sinus interdigitalis
(356)

The skin between the toes may be provided with glands arranged in various patterns. On the dorsal aspect of the interdigital space there are shallow depressions of varying size; these are known as *interdigital glands* (gldd. interdigitales). As a rule they are but sparsely covered with hair and have only a few glands. In other cases they are either deep saccular invaginations or simple grooves with orifices of varying size while yet again they may be simply twisted tubes with dilated ends (356/b). These are the *interdigital sinuses* (sinus interdigitalis).

While in sheep and mufflon (ovis ammon musimon) an interdigital sinus is present on all four limbs, it only occurs on the hind feet in roe deer (*Capreolus capreolus*), red deer (*Cervus elaphus*) and the chamois (*Rupicapra rupicapra*). In the roe deer it is a simple oval sac of about 2.0 cm length and 1.5 cm breadth which is situated further proximally than in the sheep. In the wall of this structure there are apocrine tubular and sebaceous glands. The skin of the cranial and caudal surface of the interdigital space of the forelimb also carries numerous sebaceous glands which secrete scent.

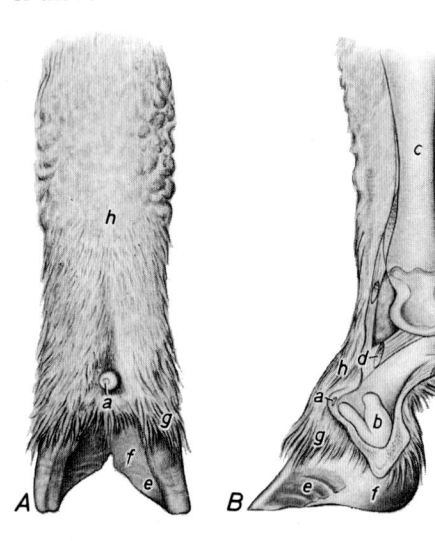

Fig. 356. Interdigital sinus, sinus interdigitalis, of the right forelimb of a sheep.

A dorsal view, orifice of the interdigital sinus displayed by removal of the hairs; *B* lateral view of the unopened sinus after removal of the 3rd digit. About half natural size

a, a orifice; *b* sinus interdigitalis; *c* metacarpus III and IV; *d, d* cut surfaces of tendons and ligaments; *e, e* short hoof plate on the interdigital surface; *f, f* horn bulb in the interdigital region; *g, g* hair covering the coronet; *h, h* hair-bearing skin

The interdigital sinus of the sheep has a suggestion of a sigmoid curve at its blind end. Its overall form is reminiscent of a tobacco pipe (356/b) and it is connected to its surroundings only by loose connective tissue so that it is relatively mobile. The sebaceous gland component is most numerous in the region of the orifice whereas the apocrine tubular glands predominate in the interior of the organ. The circular orifice is about 2–4 mm diameter and leads into a duct 18–20 mm long and 3–4 mm in diameter which, at its deepest part, makes a semicircular curve, turning upwards to form an oval, blind sac 8–10 mm in breadth and about 15 mm in length (356/b). This interdigital organ produces secretion throughout the year and as the animal walks the scent is given off and forms part of its spoor. It thus serves to mark the track; in wild sheep presumably it also marks the territory. It is still unknown whether the adventitial tissue of the interdigital organ of the sheep contains *lamellar bodies* although these are present in this location in the roe deer. In the latter they are said to contribute to the animal's sure-footedness.

Tail gland, organum caudae
(340)

The **tail gland** (gldd. caudae, coccygis) occurs in carnivores. In the sexually mature cat it is located at the root of the tail and is formed by an accumulation of large, very lobulated, hair follicle-sebaceous glands. Amongst them are apocrine scent glands, the secretion of which is also discharged in this region. The tail gland is particularly well developed in the male cat in which it is a scent or marking organ.

A similar structure has long been known in the red fox (*Vulpes vulpes*). It lies above the 7th coccygeal vertebra and its position is identified externally by the presence of a black patch 2–5 cm broad and 1–3 cm long. This patch carries stiff, bristle-like, unpigmented hairs with black tips but there are no intervening wool hairs. The organ itself is oval in outline and about 25–30 mm in length and 5–10 mm in breadth. On its surface there are numerous glandular orifices around which one can see a yellowish, fairly firm secretion. Hairs plucked from this site smell distinctly of violets and hence the German name "Viole". The tail gland of the fox consists of *variously-modified sebaceous glands*, sometimes one may also encounter *true sebaceous glands* and, in the depth of the organ, sparse *apocrine tubular glands*. The primary function of the organ is supposed to be associated with the mating period because it is best developed during heat. However, it may also be used to mark the roof of the passage to the fox's earth so that the animal can quickly recognise its lair even when it is dark. The fox also uses the organ to mark plants when running along, so setting the spoor.

In most breeds of dogs, but especially in long-haired breeds, there is a *rudimentary tail gland*. It too, is characterised by a dark spot on the tail but this mark lies further towards the tip than the organ itself which is always situated over the 9th coccygeal vertebra. In dogs the organ consists of *modified sebaceous glands* of *hepatoid character* which have a *merocrine-holocrine secretion mechanism*. The glands are better developed in old dogs than in young bitches. As in cats and foxes, the tail gland is used for conspecific recognition. During the mating period it is important in intersexual relationships and communications, including *attraction of the mating partner and stimulation of libido*.

Subcaudal gland, glandula subcaudalis

In the goat two glandular pockets termed the **subcaudal gland** (gld. subcaudalis) are formed below the base of the tail and these are said to be responsible for the characteristic smell of the male. As a rule this is a superficially-situated collection of *large sebaceous glands;* in males it can extend to a depth of 1.6 mm. Below or around this group of modified sebaceous glands there is a thin layer of *apocrine tubular glands* interspersed with lobules of adipose tissue. The delicate efferent ducts of these glands terminate far up the hair follicles. In sheep there is said to be a *subcaudal infracaudal organ*, the location of which can be identified by a triangular, sparsely-haired area continuous with the dorsal border of the anus. Its glands are also continuous with the huge *hair follicle-sebaceous glands* of the *circumanal skin* and the underlying coiled *apocrine tubular glands* (scent glands).

In the Cervidae there is a similar structure but it must not be confused with the deeply pigmented circumcaudal organ or the single gland.

Fig. 357. Topography of the anal sacs, sinus paranales, in the dog.

a m. glutaeus medius; *b* m. biceps femoris; *c* m. semitendinosus; *d* m. semimembranosus; *e* tuber ischiadicum; *f* lig. sacrotuberale; *g* m. obturatorius internus; *h* m. levator ani; *i* m. sacrocaudalis dorsalis lateralis; *k* m. intertransversarius caudae; *l* m. sacrocaudalis ventralis lateralis; *m* m. sacrocaudalis ventralis medialis; *n* m. sphincter ani externus, fenestrated at *n'*; *o* m. ischiourethralis; *p* m. ischiocavernosus; *q* m. bulbospongiosus; *r* m. retractor penis

1 right anal sac, sinus paranalis dexter, exposed; *2* orifice of the sinus paranalis in the zona cutanea of the anus; *3* orifice of the efferent ducts of the circumanal glands, glandulae circumanales; *4* transition to finely-haired skin

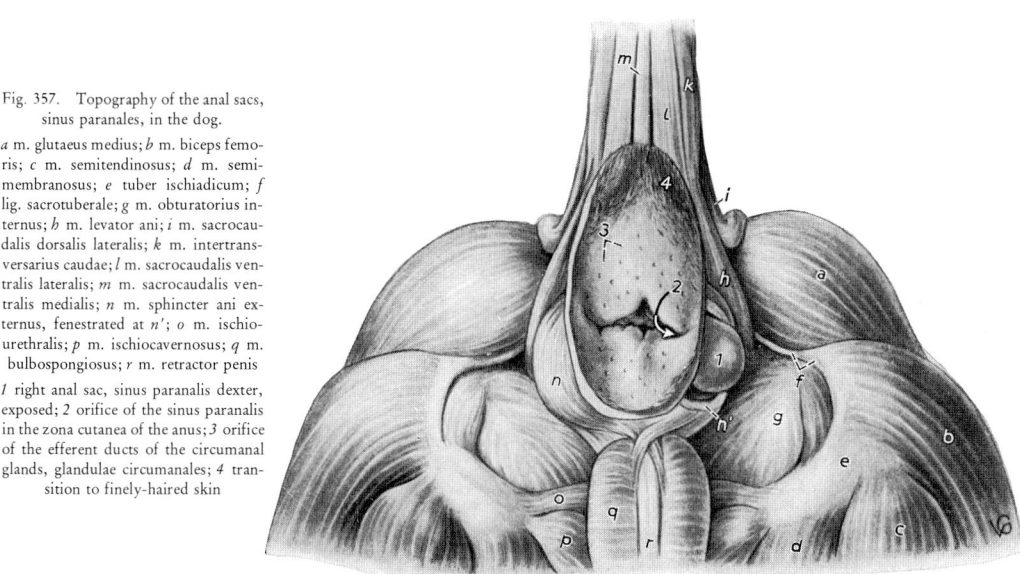

Anal sac, sinus paranalis
(357)

The two **anal sacs** (sinus paranalis) of cats and dogs terminate at the inner border on each side of the anus. They are saccular cavities capable of storing considerable amounts of secretion.

The anal sacs of the cat are spherical or ovoid structures of 6–8 mm diameter. They are lined by a smooth, keratinized, stratified squamous epithelium which is perforated by the efferent ducts of the sebaceous and *apocrine tubular glands* (gldd. sinus paranalis). The narrow efferent ducts of the anal sac are about 3.5 mm in length and they terminate at the transition between anus and skin. The anal sacs are surrounded by both smooth and striated muscles which, when they contract, expel the contents. This discharge is a sero-fatty secretion containing epithelial cell debris which has a much more unpleasant smell than the secretion of the anal sac of the dog. The scent substances adhere to the voided faeces and are utilized for territory marking and individual recognition.

The anal sac of the dog is between 12 and 15 mm (357/1) in diameter and it is surrounded by a thick layer of striated muscle (/n'). It has the same function as the anal sac of the cat. *Apocrine tubular glands* are present in the wall of the sac and only in the vicinity of transition to its duct are there isolated sebaceous glands. These sebaceous glands are supposed to be particularly large during heat. Dogs are frequently seen to rub their anus along the ground, an action which usually results from inflammation of the sac following blockage of this duct and subsequent over-distension of the sac (/2).

Circumanal glands, glandulae circumanales
(357)

In addition to the anal sacs, the dog has **circumanal glands** (gldd. circumanales) right around the anal orifice (/3). Some *apocrine tubular glands* may accompany them. The solid, almost liver-like masses of the circumanal glands are said to derive from sebaceous glands and they are important as scent organs used in communication and resulting in mutual sniffing of the anal region.

In sheep, cattle and horses there are also well-developed sebaceous and apocrine tubular glands in the anal region and these, too, may be referred to as *gldd. circumanales*.

Inguinal sinuses, sinus inguinalis
(399)

Of the inguinal organs of lagomorphs and ungulates, only the **inguinal sinus** (sinus inguinalis) of the sheep (399/f) will be described here. This organ also occurs in the mufflon and consists of a skin invagination on each side of the udder or the base of the scrotum. It contains a greasy, brownish secretion. In the floor of the pouch is a superficial layer of sebaceous glands and a deeper layer of apocrine tubular glands (*gldd. sinus inguinalis*). The secretion contains keratinized epithelial cells. The inguinal pouches are cutaneous scent organs which serve mainly for communication between individuals of the same species. They act as markers indicating, for instance, the location on the ground where the animal has been lying. They probably also guide the young lamb to its mother's udder through the individually-specific scent. The fatty secretion may reduce friction between the lactating udder and the thigh during movement.

Preputial glands, glandulae praeputiales

Preputial glands (gldd. praeputiales) are present in the prepuce of all domestic mammals. As a rule they are composed of *hair-follicle glands*, *free sebaceous glands* (smegma glands) and *alveolar* and *tubular scent glands* and the different types of glands occur in various numbers and combination in the different mammals. In the dog, pig, sheep and goat they are all represented, whereas in cats, cattle and horses sebaceous glands predominate.

Preputial diverticulum, diverticulum praeputiale

In the pig the part of the prepuce which lies against the abdominal wall is invaginated through a narrow orifice to form the "umbilical sac" or preputial diverticulum (diverticulum praeputiale) which is approximately the size of a fist. The wall of this diverticulum contains no glands but at its orifice there are very large sebaceous and apocrine glands. A sickle-shaped fold partially divides the preputial diverticulum into two compartments. These compartments then lie dorsolaterally against the prepuce. The preputial diverticulum communicates with the cranial part of the prepuce through an opening (*ostium diverticuli*) which is large enough to permit the passage of two fingers. Its delicately folded cutaneous mucous membrane produces keratin. The keratinized cells, urine droplets and the secretion of the sebaceous and tubular glands which are situated at the neck of the diverticulum form the greasy, evil-smelling content which is especially unpleasant in the uncastrated male ("boar odour") (cf. volume II, figs 474 and 478 on pages 329 and 332). There are various opinions about the function of the preputial diverticulum. The old concept was that it was a rudimentary secretory organ like the musk gland. Other investigators have considered the diverticulum to be a pressure cushion which surrounds the penis and prevents the backflow of blood during copulation so that the erection is maintained for a longer time. More recent studies suggest that the preputial diverticulum may have a lubricating function during the relatively long copulatory period of the pig. But it is most probable that the material in this organ produces individually-specific olfactory signals which mark the lair and act as a record of possession of the mate.

Mammary gland, mamma

Ontogenesis of the mammary gland

The clearly recognisable first anlage of the mammary gland is the *mammary ridge*. This may extend from the axilla to the inguinal region (pigs, carnivores) or be confined to the area where the mammary gland will later be located – the thoracic region of man, monkey and elephant or the inguinal region of the ruminant and horse.

Its precursor is the "milk line" which is a slightly thickened, barely visible epidermal strip at the edge of the trunk zone or limb ridge of the embryo. The readily-recognisable mammary ridge develops by progressive epidermal proliferation and concomitant thickening of the neighbouring corium. At definite intervals along this ridge there arise small epidermal thickenings known as mammary buds and the remainder of the mammary ridge then regresses. As the lateral body wall grows so the mammary primordium becomes ventrally displaced. An exception among the mammals is the coypu (nutria) in which the mammae are situated on the back.

The mammary buds are precursors of the mammary complexes, the number and position of which is characteristic for each species. Supernumerary mammary buds can give rise to incomplete mammary complexes. If such anomalies are confined to the formation of accessory teats, one speaks of *hyperthelia* but if glandular tissue is also involved then the term *hypermastia* is applied. Such variations are most often encountered in pigs, dogs and cattle but may also occur in other species.

The epithelium of the mammary buds grows into the depth of the tissues forming a bulbous structure while its surface develops a dish-like depression known as the *areolar zone (mammary bud stage)*. This is surrounded by a distinct cutis ridge formed by proliferation of mesenchymal elements. This whole structure gives rise to the teat and its areola. On the surface of the mammary bud a plug of keratin is formed which, when it shrinks, gives rise to the *mammary* or *teat pouch*. The teat also develops from the mammary bud and in the horse and ruminant it develops as a *proliferation teat* whereas in pigs, carnivores and man it forms as an *eversion teat*. At the same time solid epithelial cords, the so-called *primary shoots* or *primary milk ducts*, grow deep into the mesenchyme in numbers corresponding to the future cavity systems typical of each species. Later these give rise to *secondary shoots* and, at the time of puberty or during the first pregnancy, to the *tertiary shoots*. Canalization of these shoots takes place from the primary shoots by dissolution of central cells. Simultaneously the duct system is closed to the exterior by the formation of a keratinous plug at the site of the aperture of the future streak canal.

The primary shoots give rise to the *streak canal* (ductus papillaris) and the *milk sinus* (sinus lactiferus), from the secondary shoots develop the *milk ducts* (ductus lactiferi) while the tertiary shoots form the actual *secreting glandular tissue* of the mamma (gldd. mammariae). Corresponding to the definitive arrangement, the small ruminants develop one mammary bud on each side, whereas the ox develops two buds per side and each side in turn sends one primary shoot into the depth of the gland. In the horse there is one mammary bud on each side and each bud has two primary shoots. In the pig there are 5 to 8 buds, each with 2 to 3 primary shoots. In the cat there are usually 4 buds with 5 to 7 primary shoots on each side and in the dog usually 5 buds per side, each with 8 to 12 primary shoots.

Similar mammary complexes also develop in males but they do not become functional unless hormonal disturbances take place. The primary anlage of the mammary gland and, indeed, its development up to sexual maturity, is similar in both sexes but thereafter the *male gland* (mamma masculina) fails to develop further.

General and comparative considerations
(358–361; 373; 374; 378; 379; 385; 387; 390)

The **mammary gland** (mamma) is a *modified sweat gland* which has been so strikingly specialized that the other components of the epidermal organ complex (page 462) are either only rudimentary (horse, cat) or completely lacking.

The mammary gland is normally fully developed only in the female and it represents an important *secondary sexual* character.

The mammary gland remains in an infantile state until the *first lactation* following the birth of the young when it attains its full size and function. After completion of the suckling period, which varies in duration in the different domestic mammals, milk production ceases and the gland regresses although it never returns to the virginal state. Shortly before the next parturition the mammary gland is again hormonally stimulated to produce milk. In animals which have been specially bred for high milk production (cow, goat, milk sheep), the mammary secretion continues for a much longer period than is biologically necessary. Advancing age is associated with considerable regression of the mamma (*senile involution*) and by this process its function is finally lost entirely. In this aging process, glandular tissue is largely replaced by connective and adipose tissues.

The mammary gland of the domestic animals consists of a variable number of milk gland units which are known as *mammae* or *mammary complexes*. The mammary gland is a bilaterally symmetrical organ which is suspended ventrally on the body wall. Half of it lies on the right and the other half on the left of the ventral midline. In man, horses and small ruminants there is one mammary complex on each side (358/*D*), in the ox there are 2 (/*A*), in the cat 4, in the dog 4 or 5 (/*C*) and in the pig 6 to 8 less commonly 5 or 9 (/*E*). The total number of complexes are not always completely developed. The non-lactating mammary gland is much smaller than the lactating one and, indeed, in the former condition one may often be able to discern only the teats (379).

The mammary gland varies in shape, position and size according to the number of mammary complexes present. In man, elephants and monkeys it is *thoracic*, in cats *thoracoabdominal*, in the dog and pig *thoracoinguinal* (358/*C, E*) and in the horse and ox *inguinal* in position (/*A, B, D*). Thus the mamma of the horse and ox is restricted to the pubic region between the hind limbs. In the horse, ox (/*A*) and sheep (/*D*) it forms an even, hemispherical organ while in the goat (/*B*) it is more sac-like in appearance. In these species the *sulcus intermammarius*, which lies in median position, only indicates a division of the mammary gland into two halves. In the pig (/*E*; 378) and the dog (358/*C*, 373), on the other hand, the lactating mammary gland consists of a left and a right row of more or less distinctly separated glandular units which, lying against the ventral body wall, extend from the thorax to the pubic region. They are separated by a broad sagittal intermediate zone, but at the height of lactation this dividing zone may become obscured by the increase in size of the gland.

Each mammary complex has two component parts: the more or less hemispherical *glandular body* and its papilla-like appendage, the *teat*. The glandular body (corpus mammae) (360/*e*) is composed of glandular parenchyma (*gldd. mammariae*) and its interparenchymal connective tissue in which is the duct system. The whole organ is covered by skin. The teat is distinctly offset.

The *teat* (papilla mammae) (358, 360) projects either abruptly (ox, pig, sheep, carnivores) or more gradually (horse, goat) from the body of the gland. Its shape and covering skin is characteristic for each species. At the apex of the teat there are one, two, three or even more *teat openings* (ostia papillaria) (374/*i*). The cavity of the mammary complexes consists basically of three parts; each ostium papillae is lined by stratified squamous epithelium and leads into a narrow canal, the *teat* or *streak canal* (ductus papillaris) (360/*a*) which has a folded mucous membrane. The teat canal is able to close to prevent polution from the exterior environment and this is aided by a system of circular fibres which are muscular in the dog, ox and goat and elastic in the other domestic mammals. These, together with the conical arrangement of the ostium, bring about a stream of milk during milking.

After a short distance the teat canal dilates to form the *milk sinus* (sinus lactiferus, receptaculum lactis) which serves as a collecting chamber for the milk. A part of this collecting space is situated within the teat and is therefore known as the *pars papillaris* (/*b*); the remainder lies within the body of the gland

and is accordingly termed the *pars glandularis* (/c). These two spaces are usually continuous without a distinct demarcation and they are lined by a pale yellow, double-layered, columnar epithelium. Only in the sheep, and in rare cases the ox, can one discern a circular fold between the two compartments. In the wall of the papillary part of some species, especially the goat, there may be *accessory gland lobules* of varying extent. The milk sinus occupies the greater part of the volume of the collecting space in the goat, ox (359/*b*, *c*; 360/*A*, *C*) and sheep and also in those animals which have only one cavity system in each mammary complex. In the remaining species the milk sinus is but a narrow, elongated structure although it can enlarge considerably during lactation.

The basal portion of the glandular part of the sinus is formed by numerous bays which bulge into the parenchyma of the gland. The large *milk ducts* (ductus lactiferi) (/*d*) enter these bays. Unlike other glandular ducts they are not of uniform diameter but consist of alternating narrow and greatly dilated

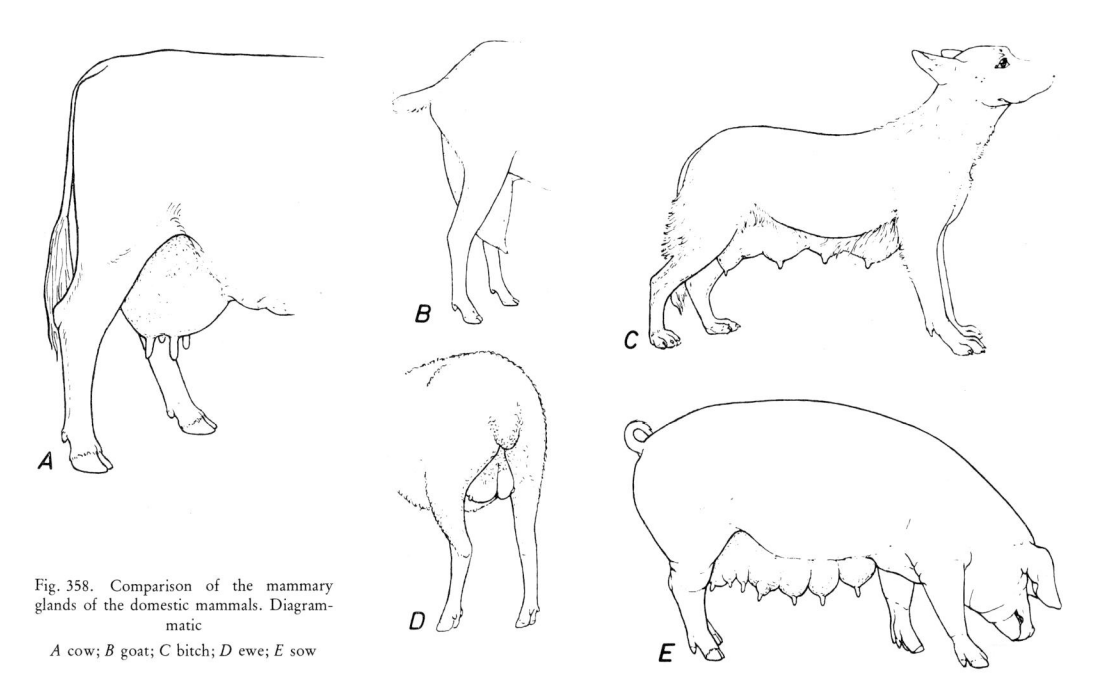

Fig. 358. Comparison of the mammary glands of the domestic mammals. Diagrammatic
A cow; *B* goat; *C* bitch; *D* ewe; *E* sow

short stretches. The milk ducts have a fibroelastic propia containing smooth muscle fibres and on this is a two-layered secretory epithelium. Towards the depth of the glandular parenchyma the ducts progressively branch to form the single-layered *efferent duct* of the milk secreting alveolar glands. In sections of the glandular parenchyma (359/*f*), one can see a distinct *lobulation* caused by the delicate interlobular connective tissue which surrounds groups of such efferent ducts and their secreting glands. The light-coloured connective tissue is continuous with the superficial capsule surrounding the organ (/*g*). When the gland is lactating this connective tissue contrasts with the bright yellow glandular tissue but this distinction becomes less clear as milk secretion regresses.

In the ruminant (360/*A*, *C*) there is only one cavity system in each mammary complex and this system is, therefore, of considerable size. The teat in these animals has only one sinus, one teat canal and one teat orifice. Because of the resultant mechanical demand, ruminants have a relatively thick wall around the cavity system of the teat and this wall contains stout bundles of smooth muscle and thick-walled veins (385/*k*).

In the mare, each mammary complex has two cavity systems (360/*B*) while in the pig there are two or three (/*D*). In the teats of these species there are, therefore, 2 or 3 sinuses and a similar number of teat canals and orifices. In carnivores there are 5 to 7 (cat) or 8 to 12 (dog) (/*E*) punctate teat canal orifices on each teat (374/*i*) which, of course, indicate the presence of an equal number of teat canals and sinuses. Each of these very narrow sinuses receives milk from its afferent milk ducts. As a rule there is no communication with other cavity systems of the same mammary complex. There is an even greater number (15 to 22) of cavity systems to the mamilla of the human breast.

The cut surface of the mammary gland has a granular appearance because its glandular parenchyma is divided by connective tissue into *lobes* (lobi gldd. mammariae) and *lobules* (lobule gldd. mammariae) (387/*f*). In addition to the skin, the mammary gland is covered by the *superficial* and *deep layers* of the *external fascia* of the *trunk* and by a layer of *loose connective tissue* and *adipose tissue* (359/*g*). Between the two halves of the bovine and equine udder there is a connective tissue septum extending from the external deep fascia of the trunk which continues into the *suspensory ligament* of the udder (lig. suspensorium uberis) (385/*e*). This is part of the complex *suspensory apparatus* of the *mammary gland* (apparatus suspensorius mammarum) and it is especially well developed in the udder of the cow (q. v.). As already mentioned, fibres pass between the glandular tissue from the surrounding superficial layers of connective tissue. This interparenchymatous connective tissue carries vessels and nerves into the depth of the organ and the milk ducts also lie in these connective tissue tracts before they open into the milk sinus. Increasing numbers of fat cells are deposited in the connective tissue during the involution phase and with advancing age.

In highly selected breeds of cattle the skin of the mammary gland is thin and has delicate hairs but in other species the covering skin is similar to that of other parts of the body. The teats of the cow and sow have no hairs but those of the mare, small ruminants and cat are sparsely covered with hair. In the bitch hairs are confined to the basal part of the teat. Skin glands are present in the teat but only in association with the hairs.

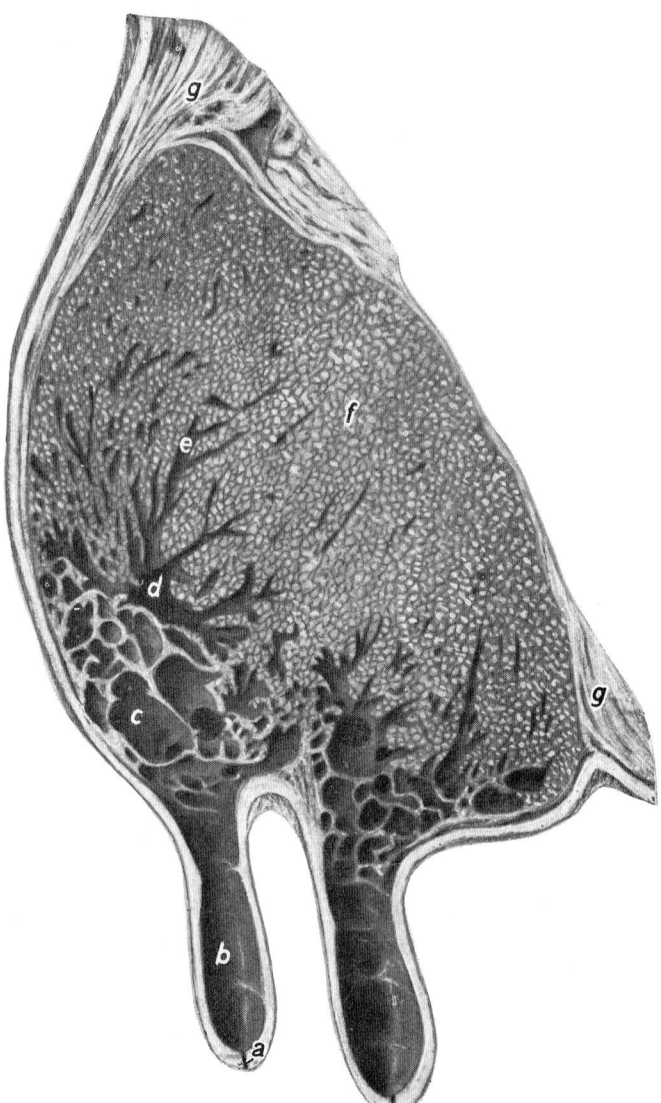

The mammary complex of all the domestic mammals except cows is much larger during lactation than before or after this period. One must, therefore, differentiate the *lactating* and the *non-lactating* (dry) mammary gland; the subsequent description is always based on the lactating mamma of the various species. The more lactating periods an animal has had, the larger will be the mammary body and teats during the non-lactating intervals and this observation may be utilised to some extent in determining the age of an animal.

The *mammary glands of males* (mammae masculinae) are indicated only by the presence of small teats in the appropriate body regions. Rarely does one encounter a complete cavity system and rudimentary glandular tissue in the male despite the fact that hormonal imbalance may induce secretion. Secreting

Fig. 359. Sagittal section through the udder of a cow. The course of the basal line corresponds to its natural position.
(After Paulli from Martin/Schauder, 1938).

a ductus papillaris; *b* pars papillaris sinus lactiferi; *c* pars glandularis sinus lactiferi; *d* large ductus lactiferi; *e* small ductus lactiferi; *f* glandular tissue; *g*, *g* adipose and connective tissue

glands seem to occur particularly frequently in male goats. The teats of male dogs, cats and boars have the same position as the females. In male ruminants the number of teats is usually the same as in females but they are small and situated at the base of the scrotum. However, there may be more or less teats than in the female of the species (390). In the stallion and gelding the rudiment of a mammary gland is seen only in exceptional cases, a small teat then being present on either side of the preputial orifice; in the donkey stallion this is almost invariably present.

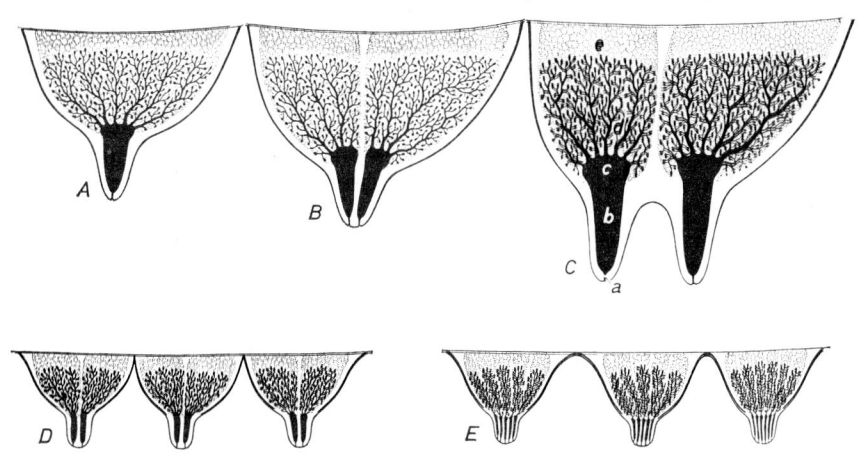

Fig. 360. Diagrammatic representation of the cavity systems of the mammary glands in the different domestic mammals.
A small ruminants; *B* horse; *C* ox; *D* pig; *E* carnivore
a teat canal; *b* teat cistern; *c* gland cistern; *d* milk ducts; *e* glandular tissue

Both in females and males the number of teats can sometimes be increased by the presence of accessory teats which are not connected to any mammary gland tissue. These must not be confused with supernumerary teats which are part of a true mammary complex and which are not uncommon in carnivores and pigs. We speak of *polythelia* when the number of teats is increased and of *polymastia* when there are more mammary complexes than normal. The underdevelopment of a mammary gland is termed *hypomastia*.

In ruminants and horses the *mammary arteries* are derived entirely from the external pudendal artery but in the pig and carnivores they also come from the internal and lateral thoracic arteries. The veins, which have similar names, accompany the arteries. Additional veins occur, especially in ruminants and horses, and further details may be found under the individual species (q. v.).

The numerous lymph vessels drain into the mammary lymph nodes of the superficial or inguinofemoral lymphocentre. In the horse and ox, lymph is then carried further on to the deep inguinal or iliofemoral lymphocentre. In the pig the lymph from the anterior parts of the mammary gland flows to the ventral superficial cervical and the cranial sternal lymph nodes. In dogs and cats some of the lymph goes both to the axillary lymphocentre and through the abdominal wall to the cranial sternal nodes. In pigs, dogs and cats some of the lymph vessels anastomose; further details are given in the chapter on lymph vessels.

The mammary secretion produced in the first few days after parturition is not milk in the accepted sense of the term but is called *colostrum* or *beestings*. This is of different composition from normal milk. Colostrum is of great importance to the neonate because it is rich in salts, vitamins, fats and proteins which are essential nutrients for the newborn animal. It is also laxative and stimulates the expulsion of the meconium and, apart from important nutrients, it contains immunoglobulins which protect the newborn against those infections to which it is most likely to be exposed. The intake of colostrum is particularly important in the pig, ox, small ruminant and horse, because the *epitheliochorial* placenta of these animals does not allow the *in utero* transfer of immunoglobulins from the mother to the foetus. The gammaglobulins taken up in the colostrum produce a passive immunity in the young of the above four species. The *haemochorial* placenta of man and the *endotheliochorial* placenta of carnivores permit the transfer of immune substances from the mother to the foetus during the last weeks of pregnancy. However, in recent years the impermeability of the epitheliochorial placenta to maternal antibodies has been questioned.

Mammogenesis and lactopoiesis

The development, growth and function of the mammary glands are controlled by complicated *neuro-hormonal processes* which influence the female sexual cycle (361). The mammary gland also increases in size to some extent in company with the general growth of the young animal, the teats become longer and adipose tissue, sometimes referred to as space-reserving fat, is deposited where the glandular tissue of the mamma will later develop. With the onset of sexual maturity (puberty) the primary and secondary shoots of the primitive mammary gland which are already present, give rise to progressively more epithelial shoots at each oestrus and, as canalization occurs, they produce an ever more complex system of branching interlobular and intralobular milk ducts.

The formation of the actual glandular tissue of the mamma commences with the eruption of alveoli from the terminal shoots of the milk ducts. These lead to the development of the gland lobules (*f–f'*) and this is stimulated by the first pregnancy. In the cow it is completed by the 7th month of pregnancy. Shortly before parturition the udder enlarges considerably although this is no longer connected with the development of glandular tissue but indicates that milk secretion has commenced and the udder has begun to fill.

Mammogenesis (361), the growth of the mammary gland, is stimulated at the beginning of pregnancy by *oestrogen* and *progesterone* which are initially secreted by the ovaries and subsequently also by the placenta. Our knowledge of mammogenesis during the first half of pregnancy is incomplete and such information as we have is based mainly on experiments with small laboratory animals like rats and rabbits, and on blood hormone analysis in various domestic mammals. Experimental investigations in rats have shown that mammogenesis up to the *prelactation period* requires at least five hormones, the function of which are complexly interrelated. These are *oestrogen*, *progesterone*, *prolactin*, *growth hormone* and *corticosteroids*. Pituitary hormones appear to be particularly significant during the last phase of mammogenesis because none of these five hormones can bring about the complete development of the mammary gland. The "quintet of hormones" is also responsible for the development of the mammary gland of the ox, goat and pig, this having been demonstrated by blood analysis in these species. The mammogenetic processes take place during the first half of pregnancy.

The second phase of development, *lactogenesis* (*lactopoiesis*) occurs progressively during the second half of pregnancy. It has been shown experimentally in rats and rabbits that *prolactin* and *corticosteroids* are also of decisive importance in lactogenesis, whereas *oestrogen* and *progesterone* are more inhibitory in their action. Shortly before birth the placenta, which is no longer very active, begins to loosen and the production of these latter two hormones decreases and this has a favourable effect on milk-secretion because their inhibitory effect is lost. Both the older experimental and more recent biochemical and hormone-level investigations indicate that *glucocorticoids* from the adrenal cortex and *hypophyseal prolactin*, which is stored in the alpha cells, are of the greatest significance to *lactogenesis*. On the other hand, the factor responsible for *galactopoiesis* – that is, the maintenance of milk secretion – are still largely unknown. They appear to differ in the various species. It has been demonstrated, for instance, that hypophysectomized goats require *prolactin*, *growth hormone*, *ACTH* and *thyroid stimulating hormone* for optimal galactopoiesis, while in the hypophysectomized rabbit the same result is achieved by *prolactin* alone.

Milk secretion is maintained as long as the sucking or milking stimulus is present. It can now be stated with certainty that the milk of domestic mammals is secreted continuously during the suckling or milking period and stored in the cavity systems (lactiferous ducts and sinuses). To ensure a continuous flow of milk on demand, both the nervous stimulus which results from the mechanical action of sucking and the posterior pituitary hormone oxytocin are required.

Milk secretion is controlled by a *neurohormonal reflex*. The stimulus of sucking or milking stimulates the *afferent neural limb* of the *reflex arc* and the impulse is then passed to the *oxytocin-producing* neurons in the *paraventricular* and *supraoptic nuclei* of the *hypothalamus*. Activation of these neurones induces liberation of *oxytocin* and small amounts of *vasopressin* from the neurohypophysis, and the *hormonal efferent limb* of the *relfex arc* then commences at the neurohypophysis. The liberated oxytocin reaches the blood stream and is carried to the myoepithelium in the terminal part of the mammary glands. The myoepithelial cells contract, emptying the glandular alveoli and passing more secretion into the milk ducts. These ducts already contain secretion so that the pressure increase and milk flow commences.

Exciting the lactating animal or *pain*, *shock* and *fear*, can cause *sympathetic stimulation* and an increased secretion of *adrenalin*. Adrenalin induces temporary inhibition of oxytocin formation so that the flow of milk is prevented or interrupted.

Mammogenesis

Hereditary factors are also responsible for the development of the mammary gland. In the ox and small ruminants one may encounter a hereditary *hypoplasia* and *aplasia* of individual glandular complexes. In such cases the teats, streak canal and cisterns are normally developed. Aplasia and hypoplasia may occur simultaneously so that various degrees of malformation result.

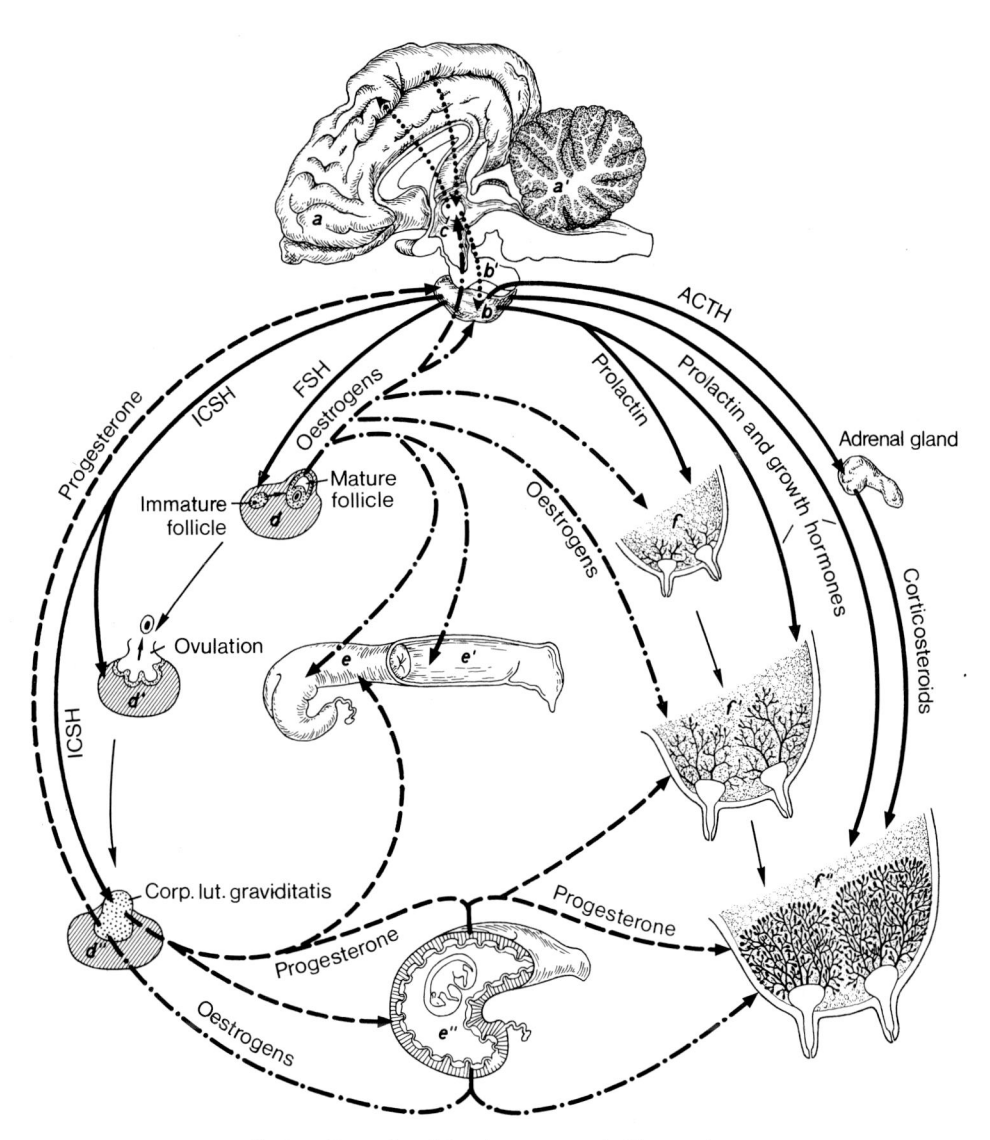

Fig. 361. Hormonal regulation of mammary growth. Diagrammatic.
(After Seiferle, 1949.)

a cerebrum, *a'* cerebellum in longitudinal section; *b* adenohypophysis, *b'* neurohypophysis; *c* diencephalon with genital centre; *d–d"* ovarian cycle; *d* ovary with mature follicle; *d'* ovary with ruptured follicle; *d"* ovary with corpus luteum graviditatis; *e* uterus with vagina exposed (*e'*), *e"* opened gravid uterus; *f–f"* various growth stages of the mammary gland, *f* and *f'* proliferation of the ductus lactiferi, *f"* proliferation of the glandular tissue

solid line: hormones form the adenohypophysis; interrupted lines: corpus luteum hormones; alternating lines and dots: follicular hormones; dotted line: nervous stimulation

FSH = follicle stimulating hormone; ICSH = luteinising hormone; ACTH = adrenocorticotropic hormone

Specific hairless skin organs

Ontogenesis of the specific hairless skin organs

The first anlage of the digital organ is an epidermal thickening at the apex of the limbs. At about the same time, connective tissue papillae and ridges are present in the corium and these stimulate the epidermis to form corresponding horny ridges in the wall and distinct (in the horse) or less distinct (carnivores) horn tubules. At first the *claws* and *hoofs* are more or less spherical and only gradually assume the definitive form. The periderm of their sole (eponychium) is very thick and proliferates to a conical shape. During the entire intrauterine development it retains a rubbery softness which prevents injury to the foetal membranes during the involuntary foetal kicking which takes place in the last few weeks of pregnancy. After birth it dries and is soon discarded as the animal begins to run about. In cloven hoofed animals, but especially in *suidae*, the thick, soft epidermis is distinctly curved upwards at the edge of the sole to form a thickened, beak-like extension of the tip of the claw.

The *chestnuts* and *ergots* are initiated in a manner similar to the hoof.

The *development of the horse's hoof* begins with the growth of the distal phalanx. Commencing from one ossification centre it grows appositionally, leading to a marked increase in length and thickness. In the third month of pregnancy there is accelerated growth of the subcutis and corium in the proximal part of the hoof and this gives rise to the *coronary cushion* and its distinct demarcation against the skin and the other parts of the hoof. In the fourth month of pregnancy *provisional horn* is formed in the coronary region, commencing at the toe and progressing to the heel. This provisional horn grows down in a distal direction pushing the primary epidermis before it. The *epidermis of the wall* (hyponychium) cannot push the cells it has formed further against the pressure of the provisional horn of the coronet. The stratum basale is pressed against the corium of the wall and this causes the first lamellae to be formed in the corium and epidermis.

In the 6th foetal month the pigmented, definitive horn begins to be formed, again commencing over the central part of the coronary corium. As the horn grows downwards (distally) it presses ever more on the hyponychium thus causing new indentations of the stratum basale to be formed on the corium lamellae; these are the secondary lamellae of the epidermis and corium. Those of the epidermis do not become keratinized.

During the 8th foetal month the epidermis above the coronary cushion forms the periople.

During the 10th and 11th months the definitive horn of the *sole* and *frog* are produced. In the newborn foal the wall of the hoof is still thicker proximally than distally because the horn tubules and the intertubular horn in the upper region of the coronary cushion have not yet grown down to the distal part of the wall.

Although the *development* of the *horns* commences during embryonic life, it is not completed until long after birth. On the site where the horn process will later develop, the very vascular corium fuses with the roof of the cranium in the region of the frontal bone. This results in a slightly raised area at this locus even before birth and hair grows here in a whorled manner very early on. Sometimes after birth the epidermis here becomes thickened and keratinized giving rise to a crumbly mass permeated by hairs. With the growth of the special corium papillae, this mass rapidly increases. Since the formation of the bony horn process is somewhat delayed, the small *horn cone* and associated skin can be easily moved over the underlying bone. Finally, as the growth of the bony cornual process begins, the epidermis over the papillary body of the corium forms partly tubular horn.

General and comparative considerations

Under the heading **specific hairless skin organs** one generally includes those specialized structures of the body surface which are characterized by the *absence of hair and glands* and a marked *proliferation* of *highly keratinized epidermis*. These structures include the *pads* of the feet, the *digital organs* in their various forms and the *horns* of ruminants. These organs may be partly covered by hair where they meet the normal hair-bearing skin.

Pads

(336; 362–364; 365; 366; 375; 376;
380; 412; 435)

At the extremities of the limbs of domestic animals there are shock-absorbing, hairless skin organs, the *pads* or tori (pulvini). Apart from a greatly thickened epidermis they are characterized by a thick but soft and elastic keratinous layer, a tall papillary body and a marked proliferation of the subcutis. The subcutaneous connective tissue contains numerous elastic fibres in the meshes of which incompressible addipose cells are deposited. This fat tissue is not depot fat but rather a form of structural fat which functions as a *shock–absorber* and is therefore responsible for the soft, but tough and resilient, consistency of the pad. In the ball of the foot of carnivores (336/C) there are numerous *apocrine tubular glands* but in the frog of the equidae only a few of these glands are present while in ruminants and pigs there are none. When glands are present in the pads, we must interpret them as additional scent or marker organs which give the spoor of the animal a particular odour. In the heat of midsummer the amount of secretion produced by the glands of the dog's pads can be so great that a distinctly wet impression is made. On the finger tips of man and apes the pads also serve as *touch organs* and consequently the epidermis is thinner and keratinization is less. The surface of the pads is either smooth or bears small raised areas with intervening grooves forming, for instance, curved ridges (362; 376). The form and number of the pads is dependent on the number of toes of the species.

In *plantigrade* animals, that is, those which walk on the soles of their feet, the number of pads is more or less complete and according to their position they fall into one of the following three groups. Most distally situated are the *toe* or *digital pads* (tori digitales) 362; 376/c, c). They are associated with the digital organ and their number therefore corresponds to the number of toes. Lying proximal to these at the level of the 1st toe joint in the middle of the sole, are the *intermediate* or *sole pads* (tori metacarpi) (362; 376/b) or metatarsi (362; 376/b'). They are present in carnivores and horses but are lacking in cloven-hoofed animals. The third group are the *carpal* and *tarsal* pads (torus carpeus) (362; 376; 435/a) or tarseus (/a'), which are situated medially on the carpus or tarsus. The development of these pads is even more dependent on the type of foot formation. The carpal pads are present in carnivores and in rudimentary form, as the chestnuts, in the horse but they are absent in ruminants and pigs. In *digitigrade* animals (carnivores) they are thus at least the two distal groups of pads while in *unguligrade* animals (horse, ruminant, pig) at least those pads are represented which are associated with the digital organ (q.v.).

The number of tori corresponds to the number of toes. Among the domestic mammals the following pads, or rudiments thereof, are still functional, that is to say, they are in contact with the ground; the *frog* or *toe pad* of the 3rd toe in equidae (364/e–h), the digital pads of the 3rd and 4th toes in cloven-hoofed species (380/c; 412/b) and in carnivores the digital pads of the 2nd–5th toes and the sole pads (362; 376). There are other pads which only occasionally contact the ground and these include those of the accessory digits of the pig (380), the carpal pads of the cat (362/a) which are used in climbing and, possibly, the *pad rudiment* on the *atavistic hyperdactylic* hind foot of certain breeds of dog such has the St. Bernhard and draught dogs.

The non-functional pad rudiments include the *ergot* (435/b, b') and the chestnut (/a, a') of the equidae, and the pads of the *dew-claws* on the forefoot and the *carpal pads* of the dog (376/a). While the ergot is generally considered to be a rudimentary sole pad of the third digit, opinions vary about the homology of the chestnuts. Some believe them to correspond to the tarsal and metatarsal organs of the Cervidae, while others consider that they are special skin structures or rudimentary tori. Although lacking glands and a subcutaneous cushion, they are generally interpreted as *rudimentary carpal* and *tarsal pads*. The structure of the digital pad is described in the description of the digital organ.

The *tori metarcarpei* and *metatarsei* were originally located between the individual toes on the interdigital connective tissue and accordingly used to be termed the *interdigital* pads. But because of the great reduction in length of the first digit in carnivores, there are now only three such pads. These are distinct in the cat (362/b, b') but even during intrauterine life they fuse into a trilobed, lyre-shaped cushion in the dog (376/b, b'). The sole pads have lost their function in unguligrade species because of the extreme upright position of the foot and in cloven-hoofed species it has consequently completely regressed. In the soliped ungulate it is generally preserved in the form of the ergot but in highly-bred horses it may have completely regressed. Neither the carpal pad nor its rudiment have any function whatsoever in our domestic mammals.

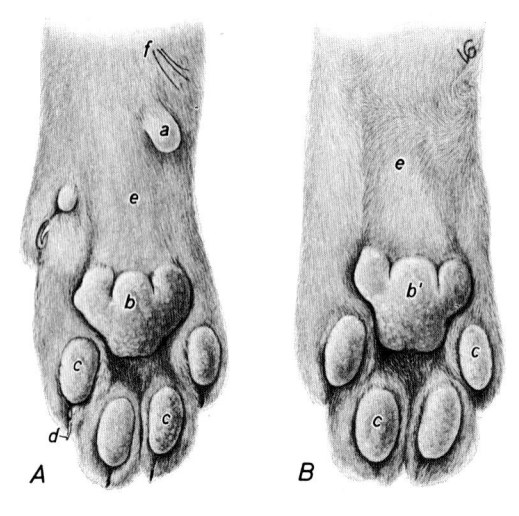

Fig. 362. Pads of (A) the right fore paw and (B) the right hind paw of the cat. Sole view, about half natural size.

a torus carpeus; *b* torus metacarpeus, *b'* torus metatarseus; *c, c'* tori digitales; *d* horn claw; *e* hair-bearing skin; *f* tactile hairs (carpal vibrissae)

Digital organ, organum digitale
(363–366; 375–377; 380–382; 403–417; 422–439)

The keratinized layer of the epidermis increases in thickness wherever skin areas are exposed to excessive mechanical stress, as exemplified by callosities which form on the hands of manual workers and in other Primates. In quadruped mammals the extreme ends of the digits are exposed to the greatest mechanical impact. Evolution acting over a long time, has resulted in a considerable transformation of the digital organ and this has involved not only the epidermis but also the corium and subcutis. The modified, heavily-keratinized parts of the skin, the enclosed part of the toe and the supporting bones constitute the **digital organ** (organum digitale) (363; 365; 366; 380; 403).

These organs are fully adapted to the demands made on the limbs by the way of life of each species and among the domestic mammals we can thus distinguish two groups, the *clawed* animals (Unguiculatae) which include the carnivores, and the *hoofed* aminals (Ungulatae) represented by the pig, ruminants and horse.

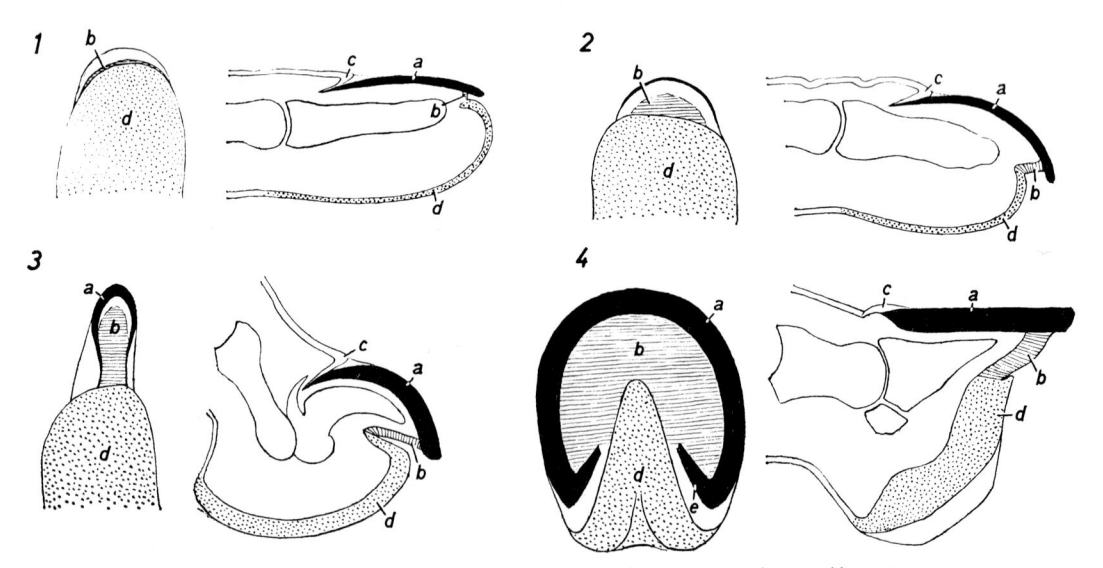

Fig. 363. Median section and palmar view of the digital organs of man (1), ape (2), dog (3) and horse (4). (After Zietzschmann, 1918)

a nail, claw or hoof plate; *b* nail, claw or hoof sole; *c* dorsal part of the nail, claw or hoof vallum; *d* finger tip (man, ape), digital pad (dog), frog (horse); *e* bars of the hoof

The corium of the digital organ usually has a very well developed, and sometimes modified, papillary body (425). In adaptation to special requirements, a shock-absorbing cushion has developed in some regions of the subcutis (365; 366/*d*; *e, e'*) whereas in other areas the subcutis lies directly against the bone and contributes to the development of the periosteum of the terminal phalanx (365).

The digital organ is either a simple *protective* structure for the tip of the limb or has a *shock-absorbing* function. It can also be used for *digging, scratching* and as an organ of *touch*. It occurs in three forms: 1. a *claw* (unguicula) as in carnivores (363/3) and the majority of mammals, 2. a *nail* (unguis) in Primates, (363/1, 2) and 3. a *hoof* (ungula) which is differently shaped in the *single-toed* (Perissodactyla) (/4) and *cloven-hoofed* species (Artiodactyla).

The *claws* of the dog and cat are primarily for the protection of the *distal phalanx* (os unguiculare) but in the dog they may also be used for digging. In the cat the claws are dagger-like curved weapons which are used to good effect in climbing but can be withdrawn when the animal is running and thus do not contact the ground in the latter circumstances. The claws of the dog are blunt because they are worn-down in running. The basic structure in the claw is the distal phalanx and the tendons and ligaments attached to it and these are surrounded by the corium of the horny claw. The springy, elastic, silent tread of the carnivores, especially felines, is possible because of the development of toe and sole pads.

Hoof

The primary purpose of the hoofs in the cloven-hoofed species is a protective capsule of horn which surrounds the terminal phalanges and protects them during progression. Hoofs can be used as weapons but this is of secondary importance. The steep inclination of the phalanges and metacarpals or metatarsals means that, when the foot strikes the ground, some form of shock-absorption is necessary. This is provided in part by the ligaments of the toes which facilitate springing and separation of the toes in the extended position. However, concussion is also mitigated by the structure of the hoof itself because its posterior, softer part and the bulb dilate when pressure is placed on them. Conversely, when relaxed, they return to their normal position.

The best developed *springy-elastic shock absorption* is, however, found in the hoof of the equidae. This is because the horny wall of the hoof becomes thinner in palmar (or plantar) direction and because of the formation of the *bars* (364/*b*), both of which structural arrangements permit the posterior part of the domed sole to expand. However, of even greater importance is the wedge-shaped *frog* which is wider in its posterior part and appears in cross section in the form of a "W" (432/*a*). It consists of relatively soft horn and, together with the underlying *digital cushion* (/*c*), forms a very effective and well-sprung *cushioning mechanism*. Attached to the caudally directed branches of the distal phalanx are the *lateral cartilages* (424/*C*; 432/*B*). These cartilages are sagittally-placed, springy plates which also play a part in hoof mechanics. Horses which walk on asphalt or cobbled surfaces most of their lives are frequently affected by ossification of the lateral cartilage when they become older and this causes a stiff gait. Finally, the presence of extensive vascular networks, especially in the corium (/*h, n*), plays a part in the shock-absorbing mechanism of the hoof.

The nourishment of the thick epidermis and the continuous pressure and tension to which it is exposed during walking, necessitate a very firm connection between epidermis and corium. This leads to striking modifications of the corium of the digital-organ which are known as the corium lamellae and secondary lamellae. Their presence is barely indicated in claws, somewhat better shown in the cloven hoof and developed to the highest degree in the hoof of the solipeds.

It has already been mentioned that, for comparative reasons, the term digital organ is used to include the whole of the third phalanx with its modified skin components, as well as the third toe joint. In the horse, this last toe joint is enclosed by the horny hoof. It is important to appreciate that *claws*, *nails* and *hoofs* do not just consist of the externally-visible horn but include the internal structures. Passing from the centre of the organ to its periphery we can, for descriptive purposes, divide the organ into *layers* consisting of the osseous and connective tissue components and the skin cover, the last comprising the tela subcutanea, corium and epidermis (363; 365; 366; 403). However, the cutaneous layers exhibit such a variable and complex structure in the various parts of the organ, that it is also necessary to look at the organ segmentally.

If we first consider the organization of the digital organ according to its layers, we find that the epidermis is the outermost layer of the claw, nail and hoof. We may think of the epidermal layer as the "mould" for the remaining parts of the organ which are then fitted like a "die" into the interior of this epidermal horn capsule. The outermost surface of this "die" is covered by corium (366/i, i'; 404–406; 425) with a much modified papillary body. Internal to the corium is the subcutis (tela subcutanea) which, in certain regions, is modified into cushions (363/d) while at other sites it becomes the periosteum of the terminal phalanx.

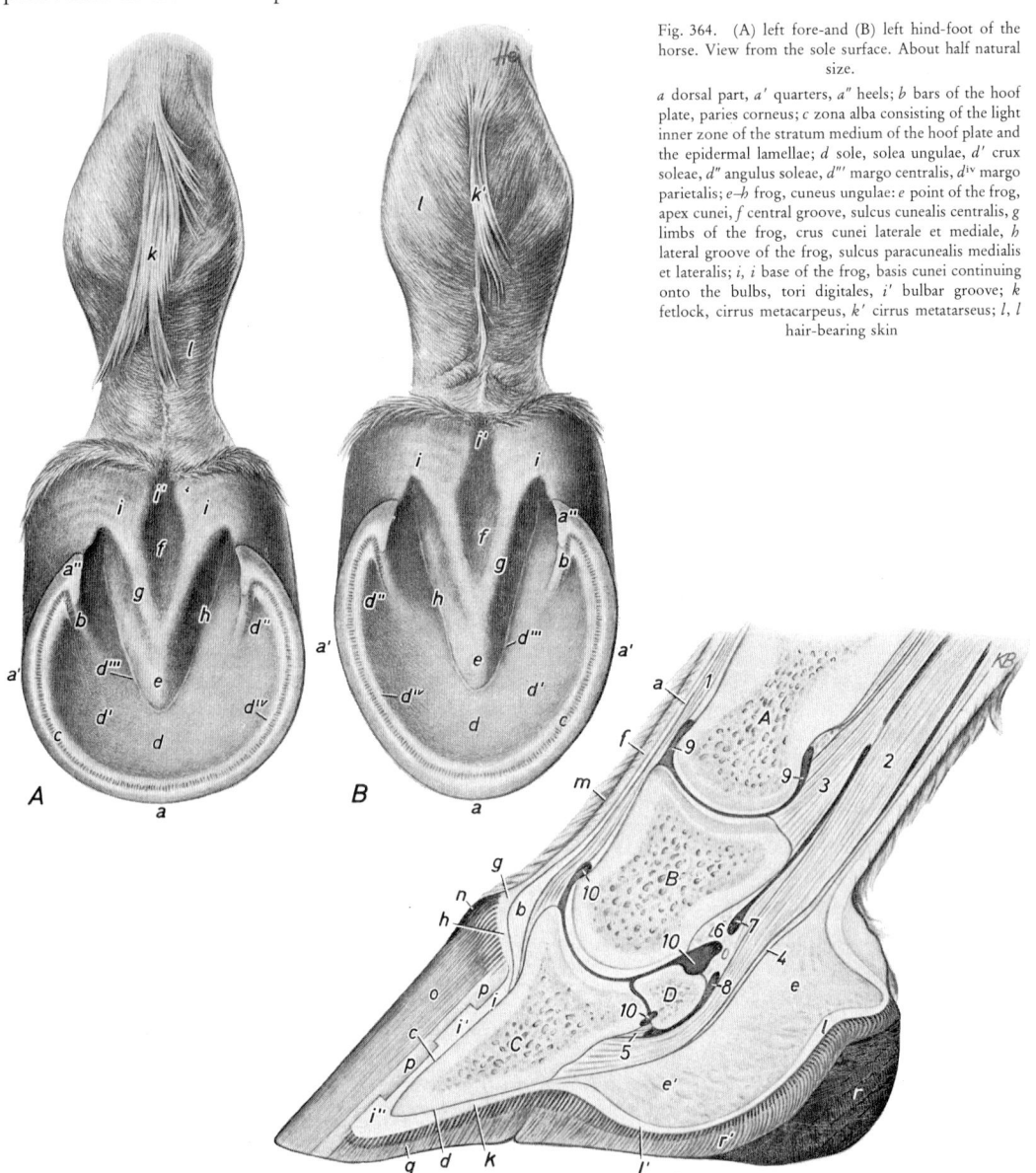

Fig. 364. (A) left fore-and (B) left hind-foot of the horse. View from the sole surface. About half natural size.

a dorsal part, *a'* quarters, *a"* heels; *b* bars of the hoof plate, paries corneus; *c* zona alba consisting of the light inner zone of the stratum medium of the hoof plate and the epidermal lamellae; *d* sole, solea ungulae, *d'* crux soleae, *d"* angulus soleae, *d'"* margo centralis, *d^iv* margo parietalis; *e–h* frog, cuneus ungulae: *e* point of the frog, apex cunei, *f* central groove, sulcus cunealis centralis, *g* limbs of the frog, crus cunei laterale et mediale, *h* lateral groove of the frog, sulcus paracunealis medialis et lateralis; *i, i* base of the frog, basis cunei continuing onto the bulbs, tori digitales, *i'* bulbar groove; *k* fetlock, cirrus metacarpeus, *k'* cirrus metatarseus; *l, l* hair-bearing skin

Fig. 365. Median section through the digital organ of the horse. The somewhat enlarged synovial spaces are shown in black, the joint capsules and the articular cartilages are light. About half natural size.

A phalanx proximalis; *B* phalanx media; *C* phalanx distalis; *D* os sesamoideum distale

a tela subcutanea of the hair-bearing skin; *b* tela subcutanea limbi et coronae; *c* tela subcutanea parietis; *d* tela subcutanea soleae; *e, e'* tela subcutanea tori et cunei; *f* corium of the hair-bearing skin; *g* corium limbi with delicate corial papillae; *h* corium coronae with coarse corial papillae; *i* corium parietis with *i'* lamellae coriales, *i"* distal free end of a corial lamella with papillae; *k* corium soleae with corial papillae; *l, l'* corium tori et cunei with corial papillae; *m* haired epidermis; *n–o* hoof plate: *n* periople, limbus ungulae; *o* hoof wall, paries ungulae; *p* epidermis parietis with epidermal lamellae; *q* sole, solea ungulae; *r* bulb, torus ungulae, *r'* frog, cuneus ungulae

1 tendon of the m. extensor digitalis communis; *2* tendon of the m. flexor digitalis profundus; *3* ligamentum sesamoideum rectum; *4* anular ligament; *5* sesamoid impar ligament, *6* bridge between *7* and *8*; *7* distal tendon sheath of the flexor tendon; *8* bursa podotrochlearis; *9* cavity of pastern joint; *10* cavity of coffin joint

The division of the digital organ is purely theoretical but it represents a subdivision into segments, one of which is orientated dorsally, two laterally and two in a palmar, or plantar, direction. These segments include parts of both "mould" and "die" but they are easier to recognise on the corium-covered "die" than on the epidermal component or "mould". Dorsally and laterally the sequence from above to below is: 1. perioplic segment (425/*b*) immediately continuous with the hair-bearing skin, 2. the coronary segment (/*c*) immediately distal to the foregoing, and 3. the wall segment (/*d*) which is a distal continuation of the second segment. On the palmar (plantar) surface one can recognise 4. the bulb and frog segment (425/*b'*; 423/*f*) which also borders hair-bearing skin and is in contact with the perioplic segment, and 5. the sole segment (423/*g*) which is in contact with the bulb segment and surrounded by the horny wall. Each of these five segments includes the three layers of the skin – epidermis, corium and subcutis. It is difficult to define the dividing line between the dorsal and lateral segments because the distally growing, keratinized epidermis is superficial, forming as it does the horny plate (365/*n–o*). Being in contact behind and below with the sole, the plate constitutes the digital horn capsule organ. The sole is less strongly keratinized than the plate yet it has a clearly defined shape. Detailed descriptions of the hoofs are given for each species.

Fig. 366. Median section through a toe of the fore paw of a dog. About natural size.

A phalanx proximalis; *B* phalanx media; *C* phalanx distalis; *D* os sesamoideum distale; *E* os sesamoideum dorsale; *F* tendon of the m. extensor digitalis communis; *G* tendon of the m. flexor digitalis profundus; *H* tendon of the m. flexor digitalis superficialis; *I* middle anular ligament, transected.

a haired skin, *a'* outer layer of the claw fold; *b* paries corneus, *b'* solea cornea; *c* corium coronae of the dorsal cushion, *c'* corium soleae; *d* groove separating sole from pad; *e* tela subcutanea tori digitalis; *f* epidermis tori digitalis

1 articulatio interphalangea proximalis manus, *1'* dorsal and *1"* palmar pouch of its joint capsule; *2* articulatio interphalangea distalis manus, *2'* dorsal, *2"* palmar pouch of its joint capsule; *3* elastic dorsal ligament of the distal interphalangeal joint; *4* sheath of the deep flexor tendon; *5* crista unguicularis; *6* sulcus unguicularis

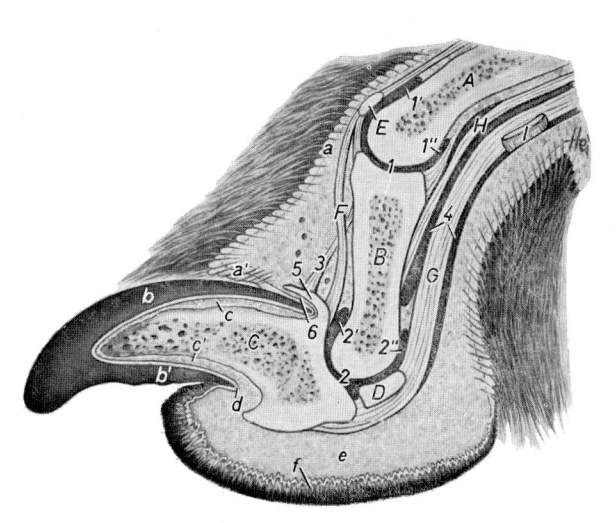

Claw
(363; 366; 375–377)

The **claw** of carnivores (363/3) is the oldest form of mammalian digital organ. Its most prominent part is the horny cone which is shaped to fit the *third phalanx* (os unguiculare) (363; 366). The dorsolateral part of this cone corresponds to the horn plate of the hoof. The epidermis provides the hard, resistant *horn plate* (paries corneus unguiculae) (366/*b*; 375/*a*; 377/*f*), while the corium (corium parietis) supplies a connective tissue support for this horn plate (lectulus parietalis) (366/*c*; 377/*c, c'*). The bed of the horny plate consists of two parts, a proximal *coronary bed* and a distal, more extensive *plate bed*. The coronary bed comprises the *germinative matrix* and it has proliferative epidermal cells which constantly produce new growth of horn. The plate bed, however, is known as the *sterile matrix* because its epidermal cells produce only a small amount of horn which merely acts as a surface over which the new horn, produced by the germinative matrix, can glide as it grows distad. At the distal border of the coronet, the germinative and sterile matrixes gradually merge. In the case of the sole and pad, the *corium* is also known as the *bed*. The sole is, in fact, the palmar or plantar portion of the cone of the claw. Its epidermal part is responsible for the formation of the soft *horn sole* (solea cornea unguiculae) (366/*b'*; 376/*d'*; 377/*h*) and its corium forms the connective tissue *solebed* (lectulus solearis, corium (dermis) soleae) (366/*c'*; 377/*g*).

There is an inconspicuous fold of skin surrounding the claw cone which consists of two parts. Dorsally is the claw fold or vallum (366/*a'*) which covers the root of the horny plate and may bear hairs. The palmar (or plantar) part is the *toe pad* (torus digitalis) (363/*d*) which lies behind the horny sole (cf. p. 447).

Nail
(363)

The **nail** (unguis) of Primates is a horny plate (363/1, 2a) which protrudes at the distal end of the third phalanx from below a crescentic fold of skin, the *nail fold* (363/1, 2c). The nail is thinner at its root than at its free border and is slightly curved across both longitudinal and transverse axes. The fold of skin covers both the root of the plate, as noted above, and its collateral borders where it is termed the nail wall. The inverted part of the nail fold forms a soft horn which lies on the plate and grows along with the nail.

Covered by or distal to the nail fold there is a light crescentic area, the *lunule* which is the location of the active, horn-producing epidermis, the *germinative* part of the nail bed. Below the nail plate, the papillary body of the corium bears small, delicate, longitudinal ridges (*corium lamellae*) which are surrounded by active epithelial cells of the epidermis. These are responsible for the formation of delicate longitudinal ridges (*keratinized epidermal lamellae*) on the undersurface of the nail plate which interdigitate between the corium lamellae. This comprises the *sterile part* of the nail bed which allows the growing nail to glide distally.

The *sole of the nail* (363/1, 2b) is represented by a strip of thin skin, barely 1 mm broad, which connects the undersurface of the projecting free border of the nail plate at the tip of the finger or toe with the pad, or tip, of the finger or toe, The epidermal cells continually produce a colourless crumbly, soft horn which can easily be removed from below the free border of the finger or toe nails.

The pad or tip of the finger (363/1, 2d) is sensitive to touch, having a delicate system of ridges and numerous nerve endings. It arises without any obvious line of demarcation from the nail wall. There is no horn production on the pad of the finger as it is not under any great mechanical stress but the pad of the toe is subject to greater friction and shows some keratinization of the epidermis. The pad of the toe is also elongated so that it completely covers the plantar surface of the third phalanx and even pushes the nail sole apically under the free borders of the nail.

In the nail of man, apes and monkeys only the *horn plate* is fully developed while the sole is reduced to such a small, insignificant structure that it is no longer able to form a continuous horny layer.

As a point of functional morphology, the anatomist has long been interested in how the tubular horn of the wall is pushed progressively distally over the lamellar horn of the wall or over the corium lamellae.

At one time it was believed that the human nail was formed exclusively by the matrix epithelium situated beneath the root of the nail and extending to the distal end to the lunule, while the *hyponychium* and its epithelium situated on the underside of the nail was thought not to participate in its formation. As it grew the nail was supposed to glide over the hyponychium, but the mode by which this gliding was achieved was not understood.

The real answer to this question was not found until Möricke (1954) showed in experiments performed on himself that the hyponychium was not simply a passive guide, but that its uppermost layers grew forward at exactly the same speed as did the nail. He also showed that the growing nail exerted no form of traction but that nail growth depended on the proliferative drive of the epidermis of the wall. One would also assume that the epithelial cells at the basal part, continuously pushed on towards the underside of the nail, must bring about a gradual thickening of the *eponychium* distally. In fact, there is a continuous proximodistal thickening of the hyponychium which therefore cannot act merely as a gliding surface for the nail.

Studies on the horse's hoof have shown that the epidermis of the wall forms the *hyponychium*, a not very conspicuous part of the horny wall but one of considerable functional significance. It forms the connection between the *wall* of the hoof, as it grows down from the coronet (*coronary epidermis*), and the horny sole (*sole epidermis*). One might imagine this junction thus: the proximally situated section of the wall (wall epidermis) produces epidermal material which is gradually pushed further distally by the subsequent production of younger cells which then also keratinize and in turn are pushed on by yet more young cells. The formation of the cells of the wall epidermis leads to an increase in the epidermal material of the hoof plate from coronet to bearing surface. This is largely characterised, however, by an increase in the thickness of the epidermal ridges and a smaller increase in the thickness of the horny lamellae. The keratinized epidermal cells of the wall together with the tubular horn developing over the distal ends of the corium lamellae, constitute a considerable part of the white line of the bearing surface (see below).

The horn of ruminants, cornu
(352; 354; 367–371)

The **horn** (cornu) of domestic ruminants consists, as does the digital organ, of a basic skeletal structure and a covering of skin. The latter is highly keratinized and devoid of hair and glands (367). The horns are retained throughout life. Even hornless breeds of cattle, sheep and goats are not entirely devoid of horn structures. As a rule they are present in both sexes and are unaffected by the sexual cycle. The horns are a non-branching, pointed, conical shape and in males they are generally more strongly developed and broader at the base than in females. The basic osseous structure is the *cornual* or *horn process* (proc. cornualis) of the frontal bone (367/d). It only becomes noticeable some time after birth. In

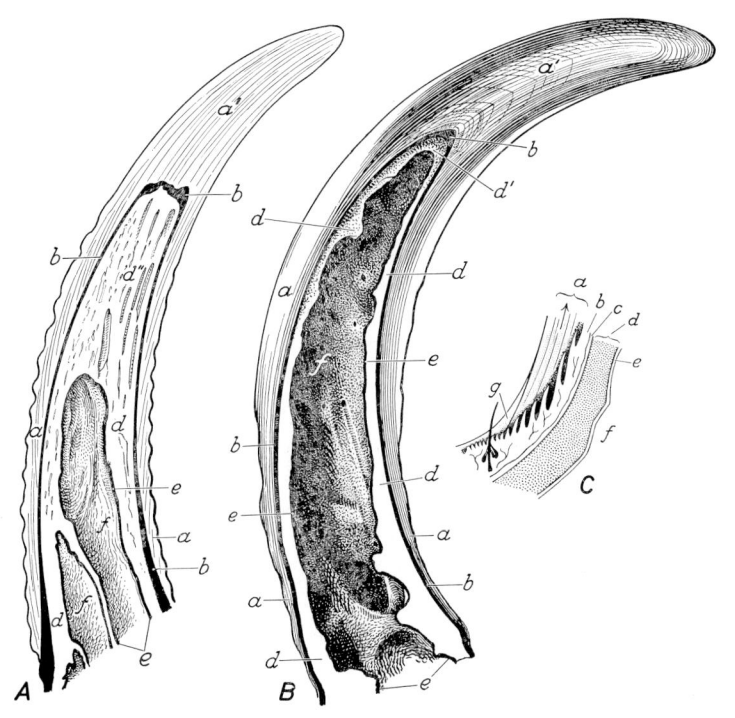

Fig. 367. Longitudinal section through the left horn of (A) a goat and (B) an ox. Diagrammatic representation of a section through the horn root (C). About half natural size.
(After Zietzschmann from Ellenberger/Baum, 1943.)

a, a epidermal horn sheath, *a', a'* its solid tip (in the ox the end is turned upwards and therefore its last 2.5 cm have not been sectioned); *b, b* corium; *c* periosteum (only illustrated in C); *d, d* processus cornualis of the frontal bone – pneumatic in the ox to the very tip (*d'*), in the goat the last 5 cm are solid bone; *e, e* mucous membrane of the frontal sinus; *f, f* sinus frontalis; *g* soft horn at the root of the horn

the ox this process arises as a direct proliferation of the frontal bone and is therefore, according to Zietzschmann's classification, an *exophysis*. In the sheep and goat, on the other hand, the horn process commences development as an isolated periosteal bony nucleus (*os cornu*) or an *epiphysis*. It subsequently unites with the frontal bone. The definitive position of the bony horn process is to the side (temporal) in the ox and more upward-directed (parietal) in the sheep and goat. The shape of the horn process is characteristic of the species and it can thus be utilised for identification and paleo-osteological work.

The horns of the small ruminants lie immediately behind the orbits. Those of the ox are situated at the caudal end of the cranium and they form the lateral border of the protruberatia intercornualis. There is a large protuberance at this location in hornless goats but in hornless sheep it is relatively small. A swelling replaces the horn process in polled cattle. The bony horn process of the ox shows peculiarities in shape according to the animal's breed but its surface is rough, porous and permeated by vascular channels.

The horn is similar in shape to the cornual process and in general the horns of the cow are narrow and long, those of the bull thick and short and those of castrates thick and long. The scabbard-like horns of the goat (352; 354) are only lightly curved as are the underlying horn processes (367/A), the surfaces of which are permeated by narrow vascular channels. The horns of sheep vary greatly according to breed but frequently they take the form of an open spiral which at first bends sharply outwards and backwards, then forwards and outwards.

The cross-sectional outline of the horn process, and therefore of the horn, is round in the ox, triangular in the sheep and elongated oval in the goat.

During the first months of extra-uterine life the horn process is a massive structure which becomes hollowed out (pneumatized) at about 6 months of age. This process of pneumatisation continues with

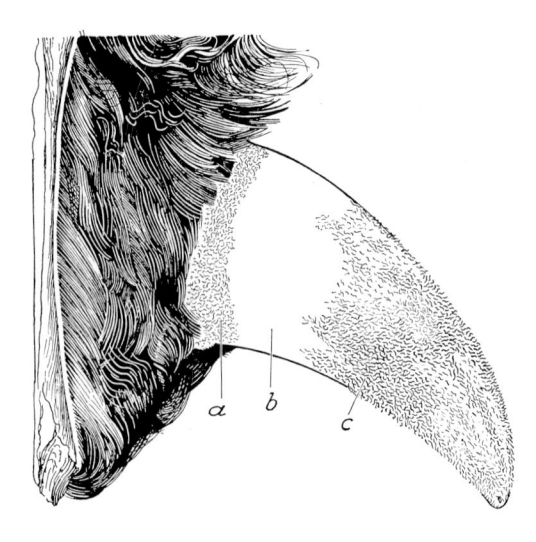

Fig. 368. "Patrice" or die of the left horn of a young ox; the horn tip points forwards. Dorsal view. About half natural size.
(After Zietzschmann, from Ellenberger/Baum, 1943.)

a narrow basal zone of corium with fine corial papillae; *b* middle zone of the corium without papillae and *c* broad apical zone of the corium with stout corial papillae

advancing age until all but the first-formed tip of the horn process is hollow and contains air (/*d'*). Ruminants thus belong to the group of hollow-horned animals (*cavicornia*).

Fractures of the horn process, which not uncommonly occur at the base, should not be considered trivial injuries since in animals more than 7 months old they involve exposure of the frontal sinus. Because of modern intensive methods of husbandry, it is increasingly common for cattle to be surgically dehorned. The horn of adult cattle may be removed (sawn off) using local anaesthesia to block the *r. cornualis* which is a branch of the *n. lacrimalis* of the trigeminal nerve. It runs below the musculature at the lower border of the external frontal crest to the occipital crest and it supplies primarily the skin of the horn process. The more usual practice is to prevent development of the bony horn process and horns by surgical removal of the horn anlage and neighbouring skin of calves.

The surface of the *processus cornualis* is covered by common integument. The thin subcutis becomes, in its entirety, the *periosteum* of the bony horn process. The corium contains the blood vessels and nerves and has a distinct papillary body. The villi (368/*a, c*) of the papillary layer are arranged parallel to the surface at the base of the horn (*basis cornu*) (369/*a*) and at the tip (*apex cornu*) (/*c*). The corium of the middle segment of the horn (*corpus cornu*) (/*b*) has a more or less smooth surface without villi (368/*b*).

The entire epidermis produces abundant horn and forms the characteristically shaped, firm *epidermal horn sheath* (367/*a*; 370/*e*). Horn tubules develop only over the matrix at the tip of the horn process and this region splays into a number of long, very stout and parallel papillae. The latter are many times larger than the corium villi of the horn matrix and only over these large papillae are typical *horn* tubules formed which are thus confined to that region of the horn sheath situated over the end of the horn process matrix. The whole of the remaining horn sheath around the process has modified tubular structure. That is to say, its *lamellar structure* runs more or less parallel to the surface of the horn. Between the closely stacked, delicate, corium villi, solid fibres of keratin develop and these are formed into lamellae by intermediate horn which is more deeply pigmented. The horn grows in length because, due to the special arrangement of the corium villi parallel to the surface, the horn mass is pushed on towards the apex by the productive activity of the epithelial cells. Once the epithelial cells have become keratinized and lost their flexibility, they can no longer stretch to equalise the pressure produced by the continued cell proliferation in the corium and they are therefore displaced towards the apex. Below the old horn there are newly formed layers of horn which also move towards the apex so that horn growth proceeds parallel to the long axis of the processus cornualis. Horn growth is fairly even in the bull and the *surface* of the horn is almost *smooth*. In cows and the small domestic ruminants there are intermittent periods of more intensive horn formation so that *grooves* (369/e) and *ridges* (/d) characterize the surface (/A, B). The production of horn is one of the body's metabolic functions and is therefore dependent on the supply of certain nutritive substances. At times of greater metabolic stress, such as pregnancy, disease or periods of food shortage, groove-like constrictions are left on the horns.

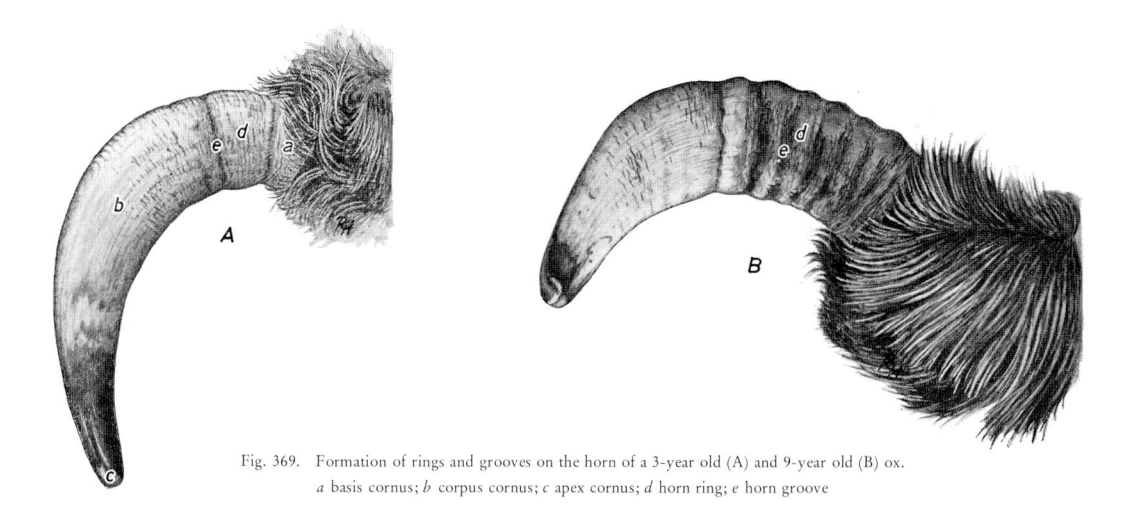

Fig. 369. Formation of rings and grooves on the horn of a 3-year old (A) and 9-year old (B) ox.
a basis cornus; *b* corpus cornus; *c* apex cornus; *d* horn ring; *e* horn groove

In the cow the time of reduced horn production coincides with the last weeks of pregnancy and the lactation period because preference is given to the nutritional requirements of the foetus and milk production. The resulting horn constrictions may be termed *pregnancy grooves* and, assuming an annual pregnancy, the animal's age may be estimated from their number (/A, B). If the first pregnancy occurs at two years of age, then the number of rings plus 2 will indicate the age (/A, B). In chamois and ibex (Capra hircus ibex) sparse food during the winter months reduces horn production so that the number of constrictions is a fair indication of age. Horn ring size can also be used to assess the rate of growth of the horns for this decreases with age.

The growth of the horn sheath results from the formation of layers of horn under or within already existing layers. The formation of new horn follows periods of reduced horn growth and thus the basal rim of the horn sheath is forced free from the hair-bearing skin. In place of this old rim the basal border of newly formed horn becomes visible and forms a funnel over the bony horn process under cover of the old horn sheath. Repetition of this process causes the formation of ring-like growth lines on the surface of the horns. The multitude of horn cones tightly linked one inside the other, makes the apex into a compact mass of horn tissue, while the thickness of the sheath gradually decreases towards the base.

The horn rings caused by constriction are much more numerous and distinct in the sheep and goat (354). 9 to 12 new rings are formed each year.

Under the microscope one can recognise a distinct tubular structure in parts of the keratinized epidermis with radial compression of the horn tubules. As with the perioplic horn on the digital organ, there is a narrow *transitional zone* of skin at the base of the horn which shows progressive loss of hair and increasing epidermal thickening. This zone forms a soft glaze over the base of the horn known as the *epiceras* (367/).

The *blood supply* to the horns is provided by the *cornual arteries* and *veins*. These are terminal branches of the superficial temperal artery and vein.

The horns of chamois, mufflon and ibex have a similar structure to those of domestic ruminants but the antlers of Cervidae differ in several ways. Except for the reindeer (Rangifer rarandus), there are

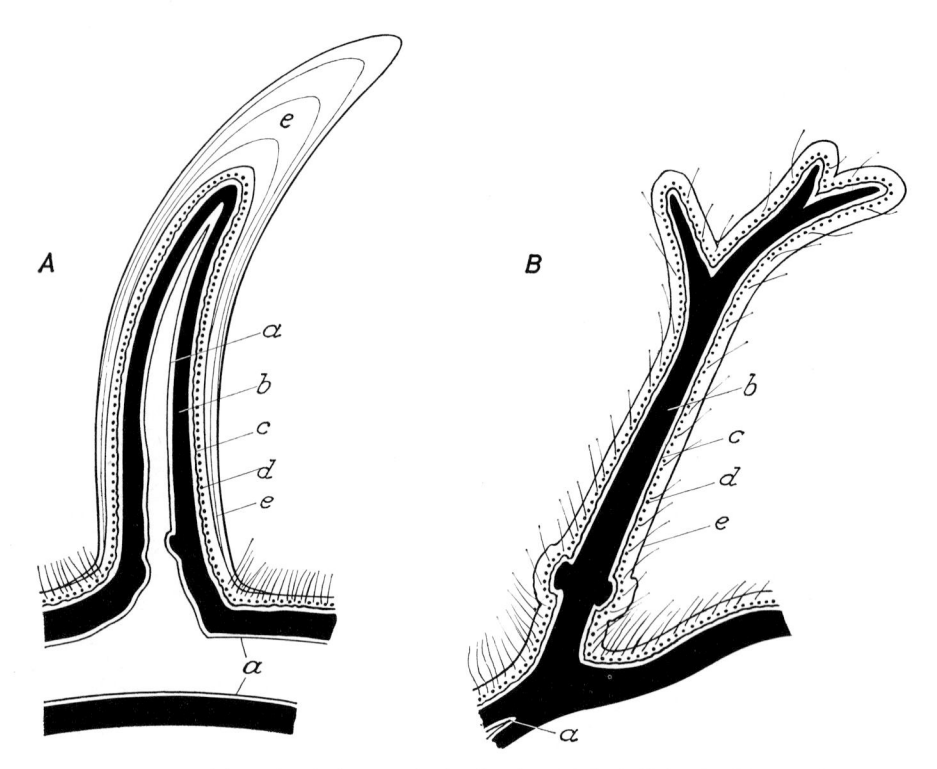

Fig. 370. Horn of the ox (A) and velvet-covered antler of roe deer (B) in longitudinal section. Diagrammatic. (After Zietzschmann, 1942.)

a, a mucous membrane of the frontal sinus; *b, b* processus cornualis; *c, c* periosteum; *d, d* corium; *e, e* epidermis

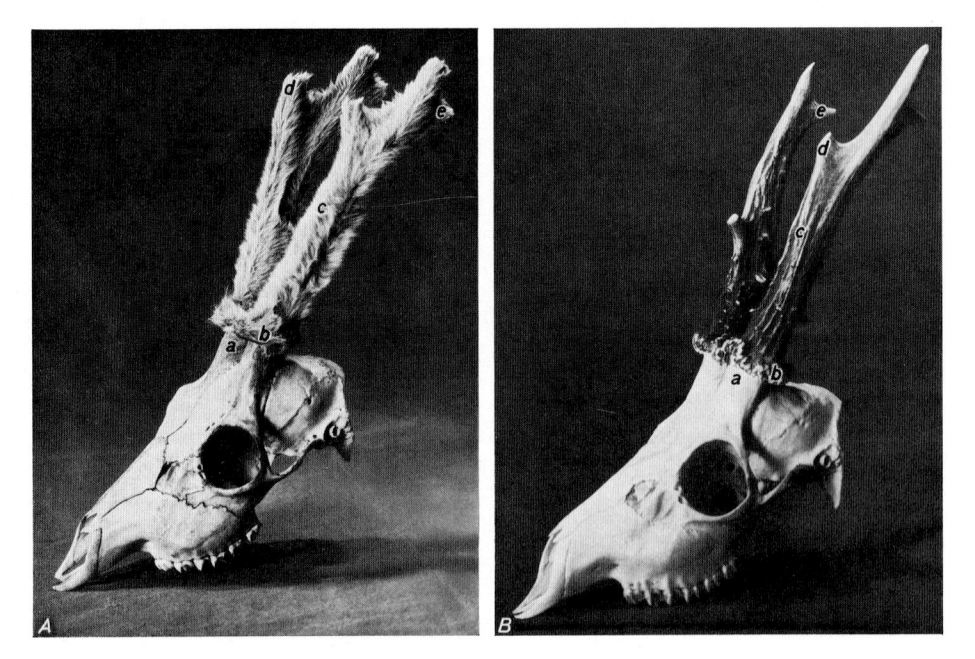

Fig. 371. Antlers of roe deer with velvet (A) and after shedding velvet (B).

The velvet covered antler corresponds morphologically to the horns of domestic ruminants; after the velvet has been shed the antlers resemble the cornual process of domestic ruminants. However, it is a massive structure and is shed and renewed each year.

a pedicle; *b* basal enlargement; *c* stem; *d* anterior tine; *e* posterior tine

antlers only in male Cervidae and they are shed once a year. They are a male secondary sexual character which is controlled by periodic testicular activity. In the course of the year the antlers vary in appearance as they pass through a series of tranformations. The horns of the Cervidae consist of two bony parts. The pedicles (371/*a*) are situated on the skull where they remain throughout life, becoming covered by a hairy skin when the antlers are shed, whereas the antlers themselves (/*c*) are bone temporarily covered by skin and they are shed and replaced annually. The mature antler consists in the main of solid bone (371B/*c–e*) the surface of which bears ridges and excrescences. When developing it is surrounded by a layer of connective tissue (tela subcutanea and corium (370/*c, d*) which in turn is enclosed by a thin epidermis bearing short, soft hairs (/*e*). The skin covering the antlers is termed the "velvet". It is non-glandular. Once the antlers are fully developed, the velvet loses its nutrient supply and is shed. This shedding takes place in the spring in the case of roe deer and in summer in red deer. It is brought about by increased ossification of the pedicle forming a ring of bone which constricts the blood vessels supplying the velvet. Intensive rubbing of the antlers takes place but this lasts only a few hours and the stimulus for it is believed to lie in the male sex hormone because when this hormone is lacking, the velvet is not discarded.

When the velvet (371A) has been shed the definitive antlers (371B) are revealed and they consist of bony stems (371/*c*) and their branches or tines (/*d, e*) and the basal enlargement (/*b*). Upon the loss of these soft tissues the vessels occupying the canals in the superficial dense layers of bone dry up while those in the central, more spongy parts continue to receive blood for only a limited time. Once freed of its velvet and having thus lost its blood supply the antler, unlike the horn of ruminants, is no longer a viable structure and is accordingly discarded annually. This occurs in autumn in the roe deer and in spring in the stag. The pedicle remains and its surface is soon covered with skin. Below the skin growth of a new antler begins by the development of a fibro-cartilaginous process which pushes the newly formed skin outwards. Gradually the antler develops the genetically-determined tines and ossifies, forming a new velvet-covered structure.

Recent studies have shown that the *cortical layer* of the antlers is formed by *desmogene ossification* whereas the primary peg tissue is of cartilage-like material which in its deeper layers is of true hyaline cartilage. In the course of antler growth the interior of the peg shows endosteal apposition and bone reorganization (for further details see Bubenik, 1966).

The skin and its appendages of carnivores

Skin of the dog
(341; 342; 350; 373; 375; 376)

In comparison with other domestic mammals, the **dog's skin** is generally very loose and thus easily movable. This mobility of the skin is plainly seen when a dog is wet and shakes itself. One can easily lift up a large fold of skin on the back of any dog provided it is not too fat. There is also ample subcutaneous adipose tissue. There is more or less dense hair covering the entire skin (373), exceptions being the nose, teats, pads of the feet (376), claws (375) and the anus. In older dogs of large breeds hairless pressure areas (callosities) occur on the elbow joint.

The skin is thicker and the hair denser on the back and dorsum of the neck and tail than on the belly, the flank or the inside of the limbs. The dewlap is the loose skin hanging in the throat region of some breeds.

The integument of the dog, like that of other domestic mammals, consists of *epidermis* and *corium*. It is underlaid by the *tela subcutanea* (336). The epidermis is of uniform thickness ($20\,\mu$) in almost all breeds. The *str. reticulare* and *str. papillare* of the corium are readily differentiated. The *mm. arrectores pilorum* are best developed in the skin of the back as can be seen when the hairs are raised in an imposing or threatening posture. In other parts of the body these muscles are less well developed and may be absent.

It is worth noting that the skin of the dog, unlike that of other domestic mammals, is very susceptible to disease. The pH of the skin surface is above 6 in the dog and below 6 in puppies and it thus provides a relatively favourable medium for the growth of bacteria and fungi. Thus the *acid protective coating* of the dog's skin is less effective than that of man.

In the dog the *hairs*, *pili*, are arranged in groups (350/K) and project in bundles from the funnel-shaped opening of the hair follicle. The individual groups of hairs are made up of one stout *central primary hair* and usually two smaller *lateral primary hairs*. Each of these three *primary hairs* is surrounded by 6 to 12 thinner *secondary hairs*. The primary and secondary hairs together constitute the hair bundle. The outer or pelt hairs determine the coat's characteristic colour. These outer hairs are of two types, the stout main primary hairs, which are straight and pointed leading hairs, and the thinner lateral primary hairs which are slightly wavy *awn hairs* (341/a) with thickened tips. The dinstinctly wavy and very fine secondary hairs provide the *wool hair* (/') which varies in density with breed and season.

The dog's coat has been greatly altered by domestication and intensive genetic selection. The coat of the German shepherd dog (373) may be looked upon as the original type. It consists of moderately long, straight or slightly wavy, coarse outer hairs, the so-called *guard hairs*, and dense wool hairs. This type of pilosity occurs in two forms: 1. a *short guard hair* with dense surrounding awn hairs, the latter being 3 to 4 cm long and sparse *wool hair* and 2. the *long guard hair* with slightly wavy covering hair, the latter 5 to 10 cm long, and dense wool hair. There are transitional forms between these extremes. When the wool hairs grow beyond the covering hairs then a densely packed, felt-like type of hair develops. Examples may be observed in some Hungarian shepherd dogs (Komondor, Puli). In the Newfoundland dog and the German Longhaired Pointer, the outer hairs have become longer, dense and slightly wavy with dense wool hair. If, on the other hand, the wool hair is less well developed and the long hairs are thin and soft the loose, flowing long hair found in the Setter results. If the awn hairs are of even softer consistency this may progress to so-called silk hair (Maltese, Yorkshire, German Spitz).

In long-haired breeds the pelt (outer) hairs are long, soft and flowing. They produce "frills" on the borders of the external ears, "feathers" on the posterior aspect of the limbs, (373) and a "flag" on the ventral surface of the tail (Setter, German Longhaired Pointer).

If the soft and wavy secondary hairs of a hair bundle increase in number and length then soft wavy hair of the kind found in the Borzois results. A more pronounced spiralling of the hair shaft results in the frizzy hair of the poodle. When the hairs are implanted in different directions in the skin one speaks of an "open" coat. It occurs as rough hair in various species of animal and may be classified according to its length, thickness and shape into long, short, stiff, soft, shaggy or frizzy rough hair. Stiff, rough, tousled hair of medium length is sometimes referred to by the cynologist as stubby hair. Short stock hair of greater stiffness is known as wire hair and longer rough hairs are usually concentrated on the face (beard, eyebrows) and the back as in the wire- haired German Pointer or wire-haired Fox Terrier.

Finally the *short guard hair* (see above) can develop into *short* or *smooth* hair by regression of the wool hairs and corresponding reduction in length in the outer hair. This last type of coat is found in the Pinscher, Dachshund, Terrier, German Shorthaired Pointer, Boxer and Dalmatian.

The coat of healthy dogs has a certain sheen except in the felted hair of the corded Poodle, Puli and possibly also the Komondor.

More variable even than the consistency of the canine hair is the colouring of the coat. The original, simple greyish *feral colouring*, which even in wild canines shows variations in colour, has become rare. It can still be seen in the German Shepherd dog, the Husky and the Wolfspitz. Strong colours such as black, pure white or reddish brown and mixtures and variations of these have been brought about by selective breeding. Spotted or pied coat patterns are not uncommon among domestic animals.

It has not been possible to determine definite breed differences in the fine structure of canine hairs. White coats and colourless claws in association with pigmented eyes and skin (*leucodermia*) and *congenital true albinism* (white hair, pink skin, red eyes and unpigmented claws), although occasionally encountered, are considered undesirable in all breeds of dog. Complete or almost complete pigment deficiency is usually associated with a weak constitution and often with functional disturbances of sight, hearing or of the central nervous system (Seiferle, 1949).

Dogs may also have hair vortices (350); they are most prominent in short-haired animals and are poorly developed in long-haired dogs. One may find two diverging vortices on the dorsum of the nose (373), and also around the eyes and ears. With the exception of such dogs as the Ridgeback, differences in the direction or arrangement of the hair due to breed are not generally observed and, indeed, *hair vortices* and *ridges* (350) are fairly constant in most dogs. As a rule there are two hair vortices in the neck region, one in the region of the atlas and the other halfway down the ventral surface. On the lateral surface of the neck there may also be a *hair ridge*. The anterior and ventral aspects of the thorax also carry vortices and ridges. A hair whirl is regularly found on the medial aspect of the forearm and a hair ridge on the caudolateral aspect of the forelimb (373). There is often a poorly defined vortex in the hip region and in the bitch a distinct one is present at the transition between the inner surface of the thigh and the ventral pelvic region. In many bitches there is also a hair ridge in the perineal region; this is usually lacking in males. A vortex is commonly present on the sciatic tuberosity and a ridge often runs from there to the anus.

The dog also has specialized hairs. In addition to the *eyelashes* (*cilia*), there are numerous *tactile* hairs on the head. The roots and sheaths of these tactile hairs lie in a multilocular *blood filled sac* (*sinus*), the walls of which consist of connective tissue. These sinuses are provided with numerous *sensory nerve plexuses*. The dog has the following groups of tactile hairs (342). 1 to 3 tactile hairs situated at the level of the angle of the mouth form the *mental bundle*, while 1 to 3 sinus hairs, usually 3 to 6 cm in length, make up the *cheek bundle*. The follicles of these hairs may be palpated as small prominences. As well as the *eyebrows* (*supercilia*) there are 4 to 8 tactile hairs located above the *medial canthus* of the eye. Four rows of tactile hairs are present on the upper lip and 2 rows on the lower lip and in neither case does their caudal limit exceed the angle of the mouth (angulus oris). There are 30 to 40 on each side of the face. There may be a bundle of sinus hairs in the zygomatic region but the subocular region lacks tactile hairs.

In the dog each *hair follicle* has a sebaceous gland for lubricating the hair and skin. They are more numerous than the sweat glands in most breeds and are particularly numerous in the Spaniel, Rattler, St. Bernhard and Schnauzer.

Although atrophic rudimentary sweat glands are distributed over the entire body surface, they are not capable of secreting any significant amount of sweat. Their ends are twisted but they are not coiled. They are situated in the region of the junction of corium and subcutis and they terminate in the funnel of the hair follicle. Because of the temperature of the skin the secretion of the sweat glands is emitted in gaseous form (*odoriferous gland*) rather than in droplets.

The *coiled glands* of the canine skin also discharge their secretion into the hair follicles; in fact this is a peculiarity of apocrine glands whose function is the production of fat and pheromones. As already mentioned, *eccrine* or true *sweat glands* are rare in the dog. Visible sweat production in the dog is limited to the pads of the feet.

The microscopic organization of the blood vessels in the canine skin follows a general pattern except in certain regions such as the external ear, nasal planum, lips, eyelids, teats, prepuce, anus, vulva and pads. There are three horizontally-orientated layers of *arterial* and *venous networks* situated one above the other.
1. A deep or subcutaneous plexus,
2. an intermediate network lying at the level of or just below the sebaceous glands and
3. a plexus situated in the uppermost layers of the corium which gives rise to numerous capillary loops to the papillary bodies or the papillae.

In various regions of the dog's skin (eyelids, lips, dorsum of the nose, back of the paws, root of the tail, anus), distinctive skin papillae have recently been described which presumably contain slowly adaptive mechanoreceptors that are believed to facilitate reception of stimuli.

Skin of the cat
(336; 340; 343; 350; 362; 372)

In general the **skin** of the cat is similar to that of the dog. It is thickest in the neck and lumbo-sacral regions and thinnest on the lateral aspect of the limbs. The thickness of the skin usually decreases in a dorso-ventral direction on the trunk and in proximo-distal direction on the limbs. The *epidermis* is but a few cells thick (340/a). Since there is no continuous *str. granulosum et lucidum*, the epidermis of the cat consists simply of *str. basale*, *str. spinousm* and *str. corneum*. The papillary body of the *corium* (/b) is relatively low, its presence being indicated only by shallow undulations. Otherwise the corium of the cat shows the usual division into *str. papillare* (/b) and *str. reticulare* (Äb"). The number and arrangement of cells and fibres of the skin show no peculiarities and no differences from those of other domestic mammals (336).

The *subcutis* (*tela subcutanea*) is formed by two morphologically different connective tissue layers. The layer next to the corium is generally rich in adipose cells, especially near the hair roots, and it is therefore also referred to as the *str. adiposum*. This layer is followed by the *str. fibrosum* which is made up of coarse connective tissue and contains the cutaneous muscle. It is possibly identical with the superficial fascia of the body.

The *hairs* (*pili*) of the cat are arranged in groups (350/K) or hair bundles. From the orifice of one follicle arise a centrally placed coarse *leading hair*, a number of fine *guard hairs* and, grouped around these, several fine *secondary hairs*. Each hair bundle has its own *sebaceous gland complex* (340/f). However, leading hairs are less common than other types of hair and during development they are arranged in ridges corresponding to the primitive feral markings. This is still recognisable, even in cats which are not striped, by the pattern of pigmentation on the inner surface of the skin. The awn hairs are shorter than the leading hairs and they show considerable variation in thickness. The *wool hairs* are the shortest and are fine, soft and wavy; they are the commonest type of hair in the cat's pelage. The leading hairs of the cat are on the average 41 mm in length, the awn hairs 37 mm and the wool hairs about 20 mm in length. No awn hairs are present on the head of the cat. The *mm. arrectores pilorum* are well developed, particularly on the hairs of the hairs of the back and tail. Although no characteristics have

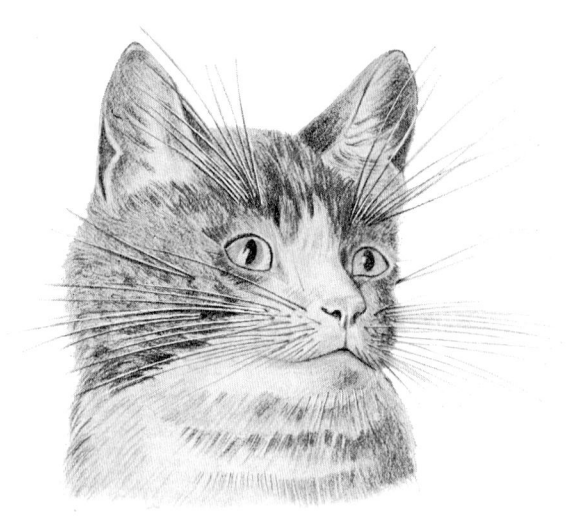

Fig. 372. Sinus hairs on a cat's head (After Müller, 1919).
Long tactile hairs are present on the upper eyebrows, on the cheeks and on the upper and lower lips

so far been found which would differentiate the hairs of individual cats, Siamese cats have shorter hairs and Burmese and Persian cats have longer hairs than common domestic cats. The hair of the Angora cat is particularly long.

Hair colour varies considerably in domestic cats which may be white, black or reddish-yellow and these colours may be combined in a striped or pied pattern. White, black and piebald domestic cats are heritable mutations which recur again and again. Patterns containing three or four colours arise from matings between black-white piebald individuals and reddish, yellowish or feral-coloured animals. Three and four colours occur only in females, males having two colours at most. Despite numerous crossings, the simple speckling of the feral pattern is still to be found. The colour of the skin changes with that of the hair. In feral forms and in feral-coloured domestic cats the skin is uniformly dark. Although rare, lighter areas do occur, even to the extent of complete loss of pigment.

The *colour* of the *planum nasale* is also very variable. In the wild cat it is red; in the dun-coloured cat it is black. Pure white cats invariably have pink noses and in entirely black animals the nose is always black but it is reddish in the natural feral-coloured animal. In spotted animals one nostril may be pink, the other black.

There are two divergent hair vortices (350/b) on the chest and in the inguinal region and similar structures occur in duplicate on the nose, eye and ear.

The following groups of *sinus hairs* (343; 372) are present: 2 *cheek bundles*, 8–12 *tactile hairs* over the eyes, and the tactile hairs on the upper lip known as *whiskers*. The latter are arranged in four rows and on each side of the face there are about 30 such hairs (372). Usually the sinus hairs are white; they are black only in self-coloured black cats. The cat is able to orientate extremely well with the aid of these tactile hairs. The *carpal vibrissae* are discussed on p. 465 and illustrated in fig. 362.

Sweat glands occur predominantly on the back and they terminate, like the *sebaceous glands*, in the funnel of the hair follicles. Sweat glands are especially well developed on the toe pads and sole pads and in the region of the teats but on the remainder of the body they are only rudimentary. Cats do not produce visible sweat. The sebaceous glands are generally small, although more prominent examples are present on the lips, the prepuce and on the dorsum of the root of the tail. Perioral, circumanal and anal glands are dealt with on pages 463, 467 and 468.

Mammary gland of the dog
(358; 360; 373; 374)

The *mammary gland* of the lactating bitch is suspended from the ventral abdominal wall (358; 373). It consists of 4, less often 5 or 6, *mammary complexes (mammae)* (358, 360/*E*; 373) on each side. They are separated medially by a wide sulcus intermammarius. Differences in the number of mammae are in part

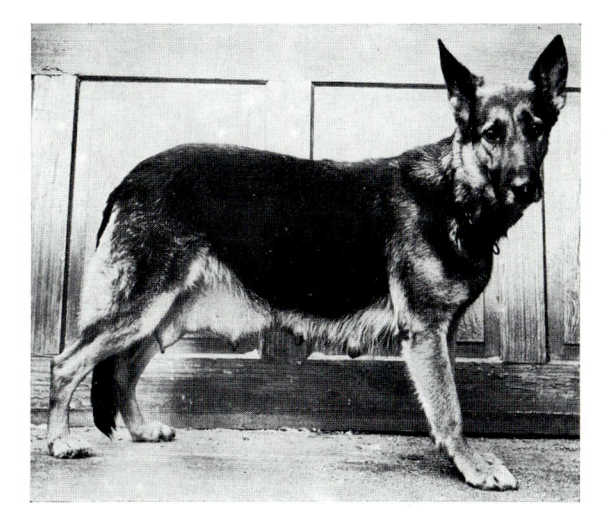

Fig. 373. Lactating mammary gland of a German shepherd dog with 4 pairs of mammae. Lateral view.
(Photograph: G. Geiger.)

breed specific; the number is not dependent on the animal's body size. The number of mammary complexes may vary on the two sides; usually their position alternates so that when the bitch is lying on her side each teat is readily accessible to the pups. The teats are usually cone-shaped and somewhat compressed laterally but the size and shape varies considerably according to the breed. The skin of the mammary gland and the base of the teats carries fine hairs but the teat itself is hairless. The hairs have small sebaceous and large apocrine tubular glands. Except in small breeds of dogs, it is possible to recognise the orifices of the teat canal with the naked eye. Their number fluctuates according to the size of the teat so that between 6 and 20, with a mean of 12 (374/*i*) may be found. All the *ostia papillaria* lie close together on the somewhat flattened tip of the teat, giving it a sieve-like appearance (/*i*). The teat *cisterns* lie parallel and close together in the middle of the teat but diverge distinctly into the short teat canals on the one hand and into the gland cisterns on the other hand (360/*E*). The *teat canal* ist about $1/4$–$1/3$ the length of the teat. Sometimes one teat canal splits into 2 or 3 *cisterns*. It is probable that in the dog, as in the large domestic mammals, the cavity systems of the individual mammae are not interconnected. *Accessory mammary lobules* occur immediately above the papillary duct. The cutaneous mucosa of the teat canals of carnivores has no distinct papillary body.

In the non-lactating bitch the mammary tissue is so poorly developed that it is not normally visible and the teats can then be seen only in shorthaired dogs. The teats of bitches which have been pregnant are always larger and longer than those of the nulliparous female. In males, about the same number of teats is present as in the bitch and, although they are smaller, it is usually possible to palpate them.

A number of vessels are involved in the arterial supply to the mammary gland (374). The thoracic mammae are supplied by the *rr. mammarii* of the *rr. perforantes* (/6) and the *rr. mammarii* of the *a. thoracica interna* (/6) and of the *aa. intercostales* (/8). The blood to the posterior thoracic and the anterior abdominal parts of the mammary gland is derived from *rr. mammarii* from the *a. epigastrica cran. supf.* (/5). the abdominal and inguinal mammary complexes are supplied with blood by the *rr. mammarii* of the *a. epigastrica caud. supf.* (/4'), of the *a. abdominalis cran.* (/9) and the *r. labialis ventr.* of the *a. pudenda ext.* (/4–4"). The latter also vascularizes the lnn. mammarii (lnn. inguinales supff.) which lie caudal to the milk gland. Arterioarterial anastomoses occur.

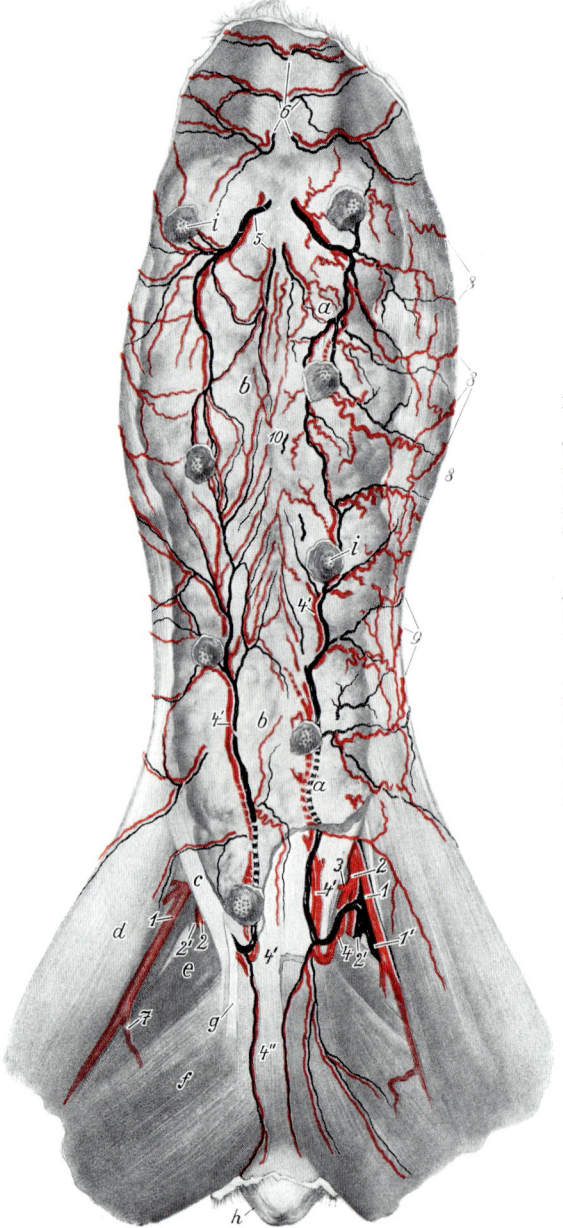

Fig. 374. Arteries and veins of the mammary gland of a bitch. Ventral view of the thorax and abdomen.

The skin has been removed. On the left side a well-developed gland is shown whereas on the right it is less well-developed. Consequently, the almost uninterrupted course of the external pudendal artery can be seen on the right side, while on the left it is interrupted because the artery runs partly within the enlarged mammary parenchyma. Note the alternating arrangement of the mammae.
(After Baum, unpublished.)

a mammae of the left, *b* mammae of the right side; *c* pelvic ligament of the m. obliquus externus abdominis; *d* m. sartorius; *e* m. pectineus; *f* m. gracilis; *g* ligamentum teres uteri (lig. inguinale ovarii) passing through the inguinal canal; *h* vulva; *i* teat with ostia papillaria

1, 1 a. femoralis, *1'* v. femoralis; *2* a. profunda femoris, *2'* v. profunda femoris; *3* a. epigastrica caudalis; *4* a. and v. pudenda externa and its branches: *4'* a. and v. epigastrica caudalis superficialis, *4"* rr. labiales ventrales; *5* rr. mammarii of the a. and v. epigastrica cranialis; *6* rr. mammarii of the rr. perforantes of the a. thoracica interna; *7* a. caudalis femoris media; *8, 8, 8* rr. mammarii of the aa. intercostales; *9, 9, 9* branches of the a. abdominis cranialis supplying the skin and mammary tissue; *10, 10* rr. mammarii of the a. epigastrica caudalis

Venous blood from the caudal part of the 3rd and from the 4th and 5th mammary complexes is drained by the *external pudendal vein* (/4) and that from the cranial region of the 3rd and from the 2nd and 1st mammae by the *superficial cranial epigastric vein* (/5). There are numerous venovenous anastomoses.

The innervation of the mammary gland is provided by branches of the *n. genitofemoris* and the *nn. intercostales*.

Mammary gland of the cat

The **mammary gland** of the cat consists of 4 mammae situated on each side of the midline of the ventral abdominal and thoracic wall. Each mammary unit has a small conical *teat* with rounded apex. Pairs of teats rarely lie exactly opposite one another, being as a rule somewhat displaced so that the kittens can suck conveniently while the cat is lying on her side. In the lactating cat, the small hemispherical mammae are densely covered with hair. The skin of the teats is either white or pigmented depending on the hair colour. It has small wrinkles, is covered by fine hairs and has large sebaceous and sweat glands. The teats of the non-lactating gland are small and often obscured from view but they are palpable about 3 cm from the midline. During the suckling period the teats attain a length of 5 to 9 mm. With the aid of a magnifying glass one can count 5 to 7 *ostia papillaria*; 2 to 3 of these are situated directly on the apex while the remainder are irregularly distributed around the side. The milk duct system is not visible to the naked eye. From the ostia papillaria the *teat canals* and their continuation, the teat sinuses, run obliquely towards the centre of the teats. In the middle of the teats the ducts are parallel and close together as they enter the glandular parenchyma. The cisternae of non-lactating animals show tall longitudinal folds which disappear at lactation. The teat canals may be blind and, like those of the horse, they carry *mammary hairs* and *sebaceous glands*.

The male cat has usually only one small teat on each side in the region of the umbilicus or the xyphoid cartilage.

Vascularization of the feline mammary gland is from branches of the *cranial superficial* and *caudal superficial epigastric arteries* and *veins* and the *lateral* and *internal thoracic arteries* and *veins*.

Innervation is derived, as in the dog, from the genitofemoral and intercostal nerves.

Digital organ of carnivores
(336; 362; 363; 366; 375–377)

The **digital organ** (**organum digitale**) of carnivores is known as the claw (unguicula). Its skeletal supporting structure is the *phalanx distalis* or *os unguiculare*, a bone which is curved along its long axis and generally resembles the claw in shape. In dogs and cats the dorsal convexity of the phalanx carries a longitudinal groove which accommodates the *dorsal cushion* of the *germinative matrix* (377/c').

On the base of the third phalanx there is a bony collar termed the *crista unguicularis* or unguicular crest (366/5) which contacts the skin fold, the claw fold (363/c) that overlies the claw (/a; 366/b).

The claw is lined by the *matrix* (377/c) ("*claw bed*") which covers the dorsal part and sides of the distal phalanx. The *germinative matrix* (/c') is covered by the bony collar and appears proximally as a shallow swelling which is narrow collaterally and on the palmar or plantar aspect but then becomes much thicker on the dorsal part of the claw to form its dorsal cushion (/c'). The latter continues along the dorsal aspect of the phalanx to the tip of the bone, so dividing the sterile matrix more or less completely into two lateral regions. In the dog the dorsal cushion lies with a broad base on the dorsum of the phalanx. Thus the formation of the dorsal cushion displaces the *sterile matrix* of the *claw bed* entirely to the lateral surfaces of the bone. The lateral surface carries very delicate longitudinal ridges which are specialized structures of the papillary body and contact the epithelium on the inner surface of both sides of the claw.

The *sole bed* of the claw (/g) is long and narrow and is confined to the palmar and plantar aspect of the distal phalanges. However, it is not quite as narrow as would appear from the outside. It is covered with coarse papillae (/g), and it pushes far dorsad under the lateral borders of the claw wall (375/a; 376/d; 377/f). It fuses imperceptibly with the sterile part of the claw bed lateral to the phalanx (/c). The *epidermal claw plate*, the claw "mould", (375/a) shows on its inner surface which faces the corium, the exact negative of the underlying matrix, which is thus the "die". The deep dorsal groove in which the dorsal cushion of the germinative matrix is situated is particularly prominent. In a narrow strip of the basal region there are delicate, indistinct openings which correspond to the small papillae on the matrix. These are too short to produce a tubular structure on the claw plate. The horn of the claw grows in layers parallel to the surface, like the human nail. On the inner aspect of the collateral surface of the claw there are delicate, non-keratinized epidermal lamellae which correspond to the lamellae of the sterile matrix.

The shape of the claw may be compared with that of a laterally-compressed cone which is curved along its long axis (366/b; 375/a; 376/d; 377/f). The claws of the dog cannot be withdrawn and accordingly their points become blunted by wear. They are used mainly for scratching and are no longer a true weapon.

The *claw* of the dog is smooth on its surface, shiny and darkly pigmented (366/*b*; 375/*a*). However, in some breeds such as the Dalmatian and Spotted Great Dane, the claws are nonpigmented. In cross-section the claw is approximately round. The *claw plate* is relatively thin laterally and encloses but a narrow germinative matrix and it extends, especially basally, beyond the sole. The horny layer on the dorsum of the claw increases considerably in thickness distally, thus helping to give rigidity to the entire claw (366/*b*). It is situated over the dorsal cushion (/*c*).

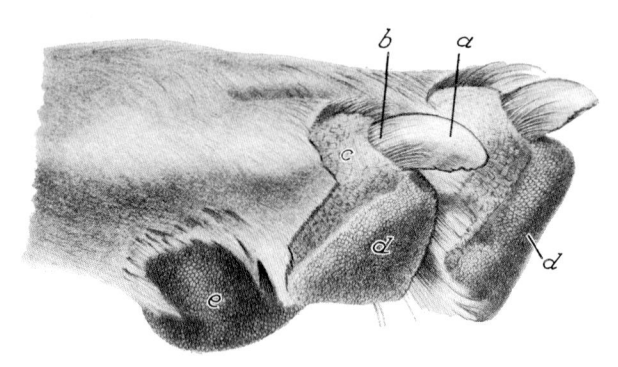

Fig. 375. Right fore paw of a German shepherd dog. Lateral view. Three-quarters natural size.
(After Zietzschmann from Ellenberger-Baum, 1943.)
a paries corneus unguiculae; *b* hairs of the false vallum; *c* clawfold or vallum, clipped; *d* tori digitales; *e* torus metacarpeus

The *epidermal sole* of the claw (376/*d'*; 377/*h*) is only narrow and produces horn which is neither exceptionally hard nor resistant. The sole increases in thickness vertically to its surface, it generally produces no horn tubules and, unlike the plate, does not have the tendency to spread along the surface. The sole of the claw is firmly enclosed by the plate which projects both laterally and apically. Thus an oval area of soft horn is formed behind the tip of the claw. Its inner surface shows the delicate openings for the papillae of the corium of the sole.

Together the *plate* and the *sole* of the claw form the cone-shaped claw capsule which is the *principal part* of the claw, while the so-called *claw vallum* (375/*b*) is a secondary structure. The latter is a ring of skin which follows the base of the claw cone. The vallum consists of two parts: a dorsal and a palmar (or plantar) part, both of which gradually merge with the proximal hair-bearing skin. The dorsal part of this ring of skin lies against the basal part of the claw and forms a fold round it. This fold of skin, also known as the *claw fold* (366/*a'*; 375/*c*), represents the true *claw vallum* (/*b*) and it fuses very firmly with the crista unguicularis of the distal phalanx (366/5) and with the base of the claw. The outer surface of the claw fold may carry hair (375/*c*) but the inflected inner part which lies immediately against and fuses with the plate of the claw, is free of hair and glands. Otherwise the vallum of the claw consists of corium and epidermis. Its function consists not only in covering the root of the claw, but its *epidermal layer*, where it is in direct contact with the claw plate, produces *soft pliable horn*. This forms a protective layer that grows for some distance down the claw plate but as the claw is used it is soon worn down and lost. This horn can be compared with the stratum externum, or glaze, of the hoof.

The vallum completely encompasses the claw capsule at its base and it is separated from the sole by a distinct groove (366/*d*). The *palmar* (or *plantar*) part of the claw vallum is represented by the *toe pad* (*torus digitalis*) (375/*d*; 376/*c*) which projects as a distinct prominence from the surrounding tissues. The toe pad prevents the claw from making direct contact with the ground. Its basic structure is a particularly elastic subcutaneous cushion, the *claw cushion* (*tela subcutanea tori digitalis*) (366/*e*), which forms a perfect shock-absorber for the paw. Usually the skin of the pad is of normal pigmentation (376/*o*) but sometimes it may be non-pigmented or pink (e. g. Dalmatians, Spotted Great Dane). The epidermis of the digital torus (366/*f*) usually bears closely-placed, wart-like prominences which result from papillae on the corium (*papillae coriales tori digitales*). The *surface relief* of the pads cannot be as easily used for identification as the finger prints of man. There are no hairs but numerous large sweat glands are present. The pads support the claw joints; they are triangular with rounded borders (376/*c*) and they are symmetrically arranged adjacent to the *sole pads* (torus metacarpeus (/*b*) and torus metatarseus (/*b'*)). The pad of the first phalanx is only rudimentary on the fore paw and on the hind limb it is either absent or represented by the *dew claw*. There may be two dew claws on each hind limb.

Dew claws are not peculiar to certain breeds of dog but are a characteristic of domesticated dogs in general although they probably occur with greater frequency in closely circumscribed region where inbreeding has occurred for many years (St. Bernhard, highlands of Tibet). The simple dew claw on the hind limb is a form of atavism because they have been almost eliminated by genetical selection.

As the animal gets older the fat cells of the digital pads are replaced by fibrous tissue. The efferent ducts (336/i') of the glands of the pads (/i) extend through the intermediate keratinized epidermis up to the surface of the pads. Cutaneous interdigital webs may be present on the palmar and plantar aspect of the digital pads, these structures being particularly well developed in certain breeds such as the

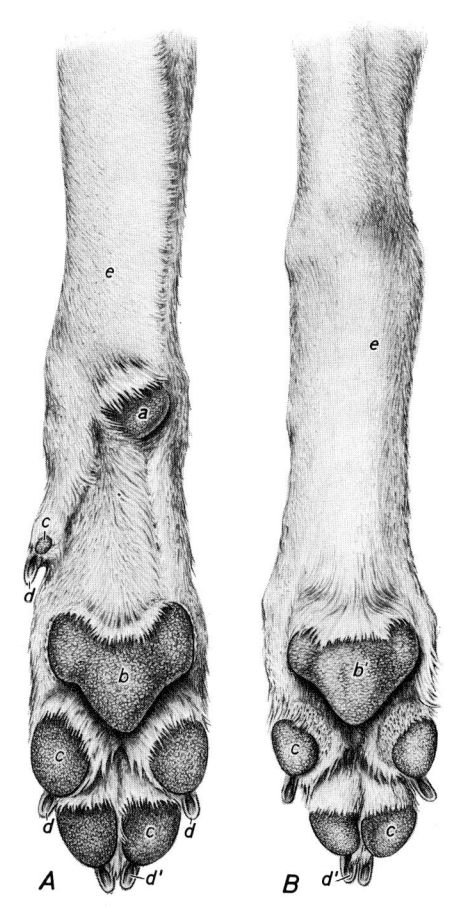

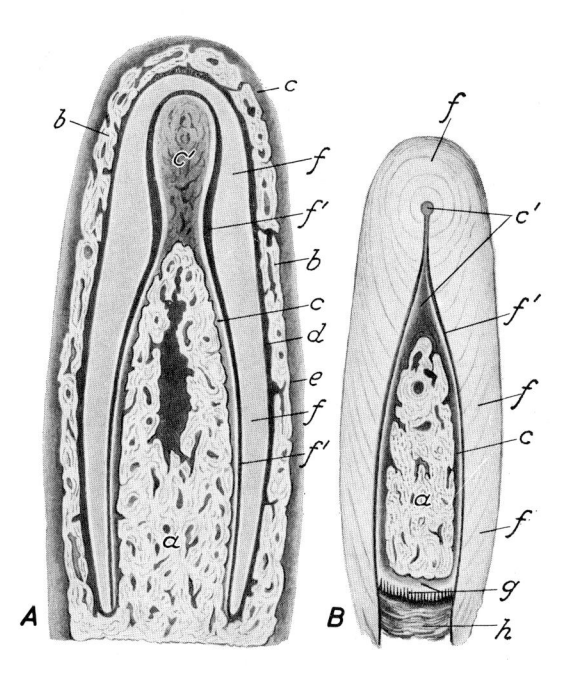

Fig. 377. Cross section through the claw of a cat in the region of the crista unguicularis (A) and near the end of the germinative matrix (B). Magnified several times.
(After Siedamgrotzky, 1870).

a phalanx distalis; *b* crest of distal phalanx; *c* periosteum and corium parietis, sterile matrix, *c'* germinative matrix of the paries corneus of the paries corneus; *d* periosteum lining the sulcus unguicularis; *e* periosteum covering the outer surface of the crista unguicularis; *f* paries corneus, *f'* its active epithelial cells representing the matrice of the claw plate; *g* corium soleae with papillae coriales; *h* solea cornea

Fig. 376. Pads of the right fore-(A) and right hind-(B) paw of a German shepherd dog. Palmar and plantar views. About half natural size.
a torus carpeus; *b* torus metacarpeus; *b'* torus metatarseus; *c, c* tori digitales; *d, d* horny claw, *d', d'* solea cornea; *e* hair-bearing-skin

Newfoundland dog. The formation of encapsulated nerve endings provides the pads of carnivores with additional touch function.

The *claw* of the cat is compressed laterally (377) and the dorsal cushion is distinctly constructed in its entire length (/c'). The dorsal cushion therefore takes on the function of a uniform papilla which extends from the base of the claw far into the well-developed dorsum. The surface of the cat's claw is smooth and generally unpigmented. In self-coloured, dark haired cats the claws are black whereas in light coloured or pure white individuals they are whitish or flesh coloured. Their tips are needle sharp and their lateral borders cut like a pruning knife, so that the claws can be termed "cutting claws" and they are, as is well known, dangerous weapons. In order to protect their sharp points, the claws can be withdrawn into special pockets of skin when the animal is running. This also facilitates walking silently. The cat is able to extend its claws with great rapidity by contracting the digital flexor muscles. The claws of the forepaws are larger, stronger and functionally more important than those of the hind feet. The structure of the cat's claws corresponds in principle to those of the dog but all parts are adapted to its narrower shape (377).

The four *pads* of the 2nd to 5th digits (362/c) are an elongated oval shape and they may be pigmented or unpigmented. They are hairless but have numerous sweat glands (336/i). The *rudimentary pad* of the *1st digit* has a small claw (362).

The essential anatomical features of the sole pads have already been presented in the general introduction to this section (362; 376). The sole pad (362, 376/b, b') is the largest pad of the foot. It lies proximal to the toe pads (362, 376/c) and in the cat (362/b, b') shows even more clearly than in the dog (376/b, b') that it originated from a fusion of three metacarpal, or metatarsal, pads. In the dog (/b, b') the sole pads of the fore paws are somewhat larger than those of the hind paws but in the cat (362/b, b') they are either of equal size or the hind ones are slightly larger. The surface relief is more pronounced and coarser in the dog than in the cat.

Dogs and cats also have a carpal pad (362, 376/a). It is in lateroplantar position and lies distal to the accessory bone of the carpus. It is peg-like and considerably smaller than the digital pads. It no longer makes contact with the ground but may be used in climbing. Neither the dog nor the cat have tarsal pads.

The digital pads of the cat are provided with *Vater-Pacini lamellar corpuscles* and these reach full functional maturity at $3^{1}/_{2}$ months of age. The skin of the pads can either be black or delicate pink depending on the coat colour. Feral-coloured cats always have black pads.

Skin and cutaneous organs of the pig

Skin of the pig
(341; 344; 350; 355; 378; 379)

The **skin** of pigs is fundamentally of similar structure to that of other domestic mammals. European breeds are generally unpigmented although there are exceptions such as the Large Black, Swabian-Halle, Angeln Saddleback, German pasture pig, German Cornwall and Tamworth. The skin varies in thickness in different regions of the body being thickest on the neck, withers and back, moderately thick over the head, lateral aspect of the chest and limbs and thinnest on the belly and inside of the limbs.

An integumental structure peculiar to the pig is the "shield" which is a conspicuous thickened area on the neck, shoulders and lateral aspects of the chest of *sexually mature boars*. The older the animal, the further this thickened skin area extends caudally on the lower chest. It is formed by an increase in tough connective tissue and a consequent loss of subcutis. Since the shield does not develop in males which have been castrated early in life, there would seem to be a connection between its formation and the function of the male sex glands. The thickness of the cutis varies; in the improved German Landrace it is between 1.0 and 2.0 cm and in English pigs between 0.6 and 1.6 cm.

The epidermis is thin in the dorsal region and thicker on the lateral surface of the limbs. Its *stratum corneum* is thickest on the dorsal border of the snout disc and in the interdigital space. The development of the *corium* is subject to considerable individual variation. It is thickest and contains very coarse fibres in unimproved Landraces and it is thinnest in the English pigs. The thickest layers of corium are found on the head, especially the snout disc, and on the neck, particularly its ventral aspect. The corium has a well-developed papillary layer.

The *subcutis (tela subcutanea)* of pigs is very rich in adipose tissue which forms the characteristic layer of fat known as the *panniculus adiposus*. In some breeds this layer is clearly differentiated from the corium but in fat animals it may be 5.0 cm or more in thickness and extend far into the dermis. The panniculus adiposus is connected to the corium by stout fibre bundles. Nowadays it is the practice to select pigs for breeding in which this subcutaneous fat does not exceed 2.0 cm in thickness.

The density and type of hair cover depends on the extent of domestication. While some English and Chinese pig breeds are almost devoid of hair, the Hungarian Mangalitsa pig has hair which resembles the fleece of the sheep. The wild pig has a fairly dense hair covering and the German Improved Landrace pig (378; 379), the Hungarian Steppes pig and the Serbian Highland pig are in an intermediate position. Generally pigs' hairs are white but on pigmented skin areas they are black. Only short hairs are present at the natural body orifices but exceptions to this are the eyelids and the rims of the ears where long hairs are present. There are 2 to 3 rows of eyelashes (cilia) on the upper lid (344) but none on the lower lid.

The heavily keratinized dorsal ridge of the snout disc is of typical tubular horn structure and is hairless but the disc itself has non-medullated *dwarf sinus hairs*. They are implanted at regular intervals and are 2 to 4 mm in length. These sinus hairs are subject to wear. The anterior part of the nasal dorsum immediately behind the disc is free of hairs for a distance of 3 cm and a width of 2 cm (344).

The outer hairs are in the form of stiff, usually fairly long bristles of varying thickness, and generally their tip is frayed into several strands (341/c). These bristles get progressively stiffer and more brittle with increasing age. They are thickest and most densely placed on the nape, back regions and lateral surfaces of the body and limbs (378). Conversely the ventral thorax, the belly and inner surface of the extremities are more sparsely supplied with bristles and these are softer. In young animals the bristle tip is not frayed.

Three groups of hairs arranged in a triangle (350/k) is the commonest type of hair pattern in the pig. The *primary (leading)* hair is inserted into the skin at a more acute angle than the *secondary* hairs (awns). The hair groups are arranged in rows transverse to the long axis of the body. This typical triple grouping is present in young piglets while in older animals two groups are almost equally common and even single bristles occur. Each bristle of the triple group leaves the follicle by its own hair funnel. In cross section the bristle of the domestic pig is approximately circular whereas that of the wild pig is more angular. Furthermore, the bristles show breed differences: in the wild pig they are straight, in Polish pigs slightly curved, in English pigs and most of the Landraces they are bent into almost a semicircle while those of the Mangalitsa pig form several spirals. The tip of the bristle is split into 2 to 4 branches in the Landrace pigs, into 5 branches in the Hungarian pig and into 6 or more branches in the wild pig. This splaying is most marked in the bristles of the withers and back.

Between the bristles more delicate and softer wool hairs may occur, particularly in wild and Mangalitsa pigs. These wool hairs are present in appreciable numbers on the head and limbs, their density being greatest in young animals in cold weather.

In the pig it is easy to identify the *direction* of hair growth and the hair vortices (350). On the dorsum of the nose there is a *divergent* vortex, whence the hairs run parallel to the median plane right along the back. Hairs covering the lateral surface of the head, the neck, trunk and limbs are directed backwards and downwards (378). The anterior aspect of the chest has two *divergent vortices* from which the hair streams run cranially to the neck, caudally onto the trunk and laterally onto the inner surface of the thoracic limb. *Convergent vortices* occur in the throat region, where the bristles from the lower lip meet those of the anterior chest, and in the middle of the abdomen where the hairs from the chest and those from the pubic region converge (378). Further vortices can be found in the inguinal region, on the scrotum, in the elbow region (378; 379) and on the ear. There are also individual variations in the formation of vortices.

Typical groups of sinus hairs occur on the head of the pig (344). Bundles of tactile hairs are present on the chin and cheeks. The *mental bundle* is situated on the throat behind the point of the chin and it consists of 6 to 15 tactile hairs which all originate from a distinctly protruding skin papilla. The *cheek bundle*, also known as the buccal organ, consists of 2 to 3 hairs arising on a raised part of the lateral surface of the face (344). The *eyebrows* are formed by 2 to 3 rows of prominent tactile hairs formed at the base of the upper eyelid; there are more than 40 in all and they are up to 8 cm long. They form into bundles, especially at the medial angle of the eye. Corresponding hairs are less numerous on the lower eyelid where they occur about 1 cm from the edge of the rim (344). There are also about 30 inconspicuous short *tactile hairs* in 4 to 6 rows in the *infraorbital region*. On the *upper lip* there are 5 rows, on the *lower lip* 2 rows, of tactile hairs up to 4 cm in length. Frequently the colourless tactile hairs are no longer than the outer hairs and therefore they are not always easily distinguished. The *carpal organ* (355) of the pig, unlike that of the cat, has no tactile hairs.

In Italian Lancrace pigs and in Balkan breeds the throat is not infrequently adorned by tassels (see general section, p. 461)

The *sebaceous glands* of the bristles are in a rosette arrangement around the hair follicle They vary in shape from semicircular to extremely elongated. The wool hairs have only two apposed sebaceous glands. In sinus hairs these glands are generally very small and in consequence may be referred to as "*dwarf sebaceous glands*". Sebaceous glands unassociated with hairs occur in the eyelids and external auditory meatus.

Sweat glands are relatively large in pigs and they are distributed over the entire body surface. It has been said that there are as many as half a million of these glands and their density is dependent on age. In newborn piglets there are said to be between 550 and 1000 per cubic cm, in one-month old piglets the same area contains only about 185 to 370, while in sows of 2 to 3 years the number of glands is said to be reduced to 10 to 25 per cubic cm. Their mode of secretion is probably *aprocrine* in *summer*, while in the *winter* months they are predominantly *merocrine*. This alteration in mode of secretion is associated with a corresponding change in the structure of the gland. The sweat glands are situated in the region of the border between corium and subcutis, or deeper, and their ends are coiled to varying extents. The largest accumulations of such glands are present on the external ears, the peroneal region, the ventral wall of the thorax and abdomen and in the interdigital skin. In the latter situation they may substitute for the interdigital sac because this is lacking in pigs. In the corium of the *snout disc* there are numerous *compound tubular glands*.

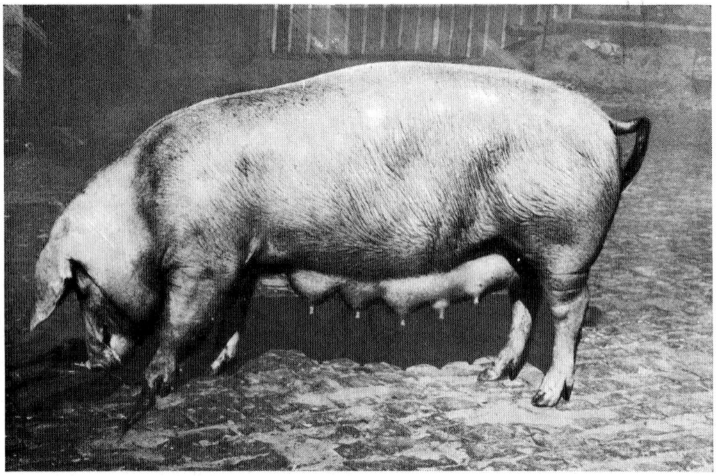

Fig. 378. Improved German Landrace pig with udder in full lactation.
(Photograph: G. Geiger.)

Mammary gland of the pig
(358; 360; 378; 379)

As with the other domestic mammals, this description of the **mammary gland** will be based on the organ in its lactating condition (358/E). The *mamma* of the pig is usually made up of 2 thoracic pairs, 4 abdominal pairs and one inguinal pair of glands which, when fully distended, are in contact with each other (358; 378). Thus there are seven mammary complexes per side, each the size of a man's fist, in the fully lactating mamma. Three of these are generally anterior to the navel, the 4th at umbilical level and the remainder in postumbilical position; they all are equidistant from their neighbours. The most cranial pair of glands lie a little behind the forelimb (378; 379) while the last is inserted between the hind legs (358; 378; 379). The type of alternating arrangement which occurs in carnivores is rarely encountered in pigs. The distance between the right and left mammary complexes is greater in the anterior thoracic region than between the hind limbs. Of the seven pairs of glands the 2nd and 6th pairs vary considerably in development being generally absent in the European wild pig and often absent in unimproved Landraces. The mammary gland has few hairs (378).

Between the mammary gland and the ventral abdominal wall there is a broad zone consisting of connective and adipose tissue. This allows the glands to move fairly freely. The mammary gland is suspended from the abdominal wall in an elastic, springy fashion by strong connective tissue sheets which arise from the fascia of the trunk. This connective tissue envelops the individual glandular units and projects between the glandular tissue itself, carrying with it nerves, blood and lymph vessels. It therefore constitutes the basic framework in which the glandular tissue is embedded.

In nulliparous animals the mammary *parenchyma* consists only of solid cell buds distributed like small islands amongst fat and connective tissue. In the lactating organ the connective tissue is largely replaced by glandular tissue. The *tubular terminal part* of the glands is continuous with *small milk ducts* lined with single or double layered columnar epithelium. They in turn give rise to the *large milk ducts* and these latter finally empty into the gland cisterns. The cisterns are very narrow in the pig and lie above the base of the teat (360/D). The piglets sucking action causes the milk to flow through the *teat cisterna* to the *teat canal* (/D) and so to the exterior. There are at least two cavity systems in each mammary complex each consisting of teat canal, cisterna, milk ducts and the appurtenant glandular tissues (/D). The terminal glandular tissues of those two systems interdigitate as can be demonstrated by injecting dyes up the teat canal. This is particularly so in newly lactating glands. The increasing proliferation causes the terminal piece of one cavity system to push between those of the others. At the teat base the neighbouring cavity systems have a less complex border. The two duct systems of one mammary complex terminate at a variable distance from one another on the apex of the teat. Each *papilla mammae*

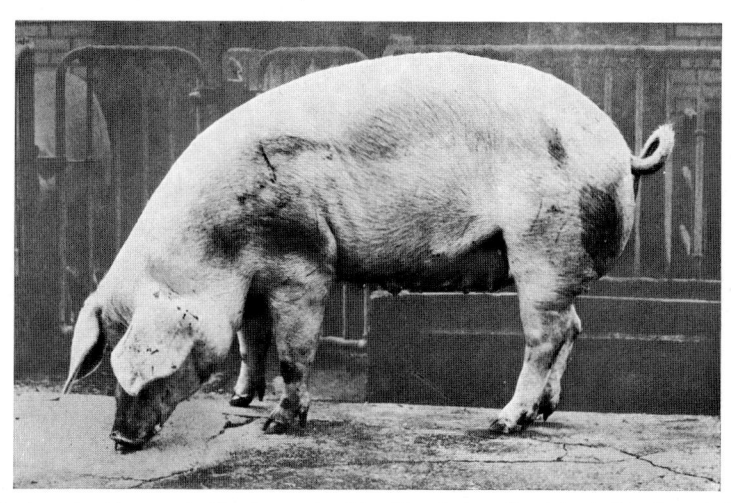

Fig. 379. Improved Landrace pig with regressed udder after weaning piglets. Note the regression of the glandular tissue, the folds in the skin of the mammae and the reduction in size of the teats.
(Photograph: A. Mahler.)

therefore has *two*, or sometimes even *three*, *teat canals* and an equal number of *teat cisterns* (/D). The latter are embedded in connective tissue and smooth musculature and are covered by skin. If three teat canals are present, one usually ends blindly at the base of the teat.

The somewhat wrinkled mammary papillae are without hairs and, depending on the functional status of the gland and the age of the sow, they are between 2 and 3.5 cm in length. They are of cylindrical form. The wall of the teat cistern contains numerous *accessory glands*. The teat canal is only 3 to 4 mm long and tightly closed by longitudinal folds originating from the cisterna. The teat cisterna and teat canal are not distinctly demarcated. There is no muscular sphincter around the opening of the teat canal and its closure, as in the horse, is mainly brought about by elastic fibres. There are no hairs on the skin of the teat and sebaceous and apocrine tubular glands are also lacking. However, at the base of the teat there are hairs with very small sebaceous glands.

Supernumerary and *accessory teats* may occur on the mammary gland of the pig. *Supernumerary teats* are frequently found between the 3rd and 4th mammae, less often between the 4th and 5th and only in exceptional cases between other units. As a rule they are smaller than the others, sometimes they are only unilateral and they usually have no connection with glandular tissue. *Accessory teats* are more common, they are always paired and always vestigial. In female pigs they are situated at the posterior end of the mammary gland, between the thighs, being best seen by caudal inspection. In the boar they are found caudal to the scrotum. There are no sex differences in the occurrence of normal and supernumerary teats.

Small teats can be discerned in young, non-suckling females, in boars and in castrated males, but in older females, especially when they have undergone a lactation, they are always somewhat larger (379).

The *daily milk production* of lactating sows is between 3 and 12 litres. The more piglets there are in the litter, the greater the amount of milk produced by the dam. The *total volume* of milk secreted by a sow during one suckling period is between 100 and 450 litres. If the litters are very small, those mammae which are not accepted and sucked by the young become atrophic and regress (358/E).

Skin and cutaneous organs of the pig

The lactating gland requires a considerable supply of blood and all the vessels of the body wall which approach the skin in the thoracic, abdominal and inter-thigh regions also participate in the supply of the mammae. The *internal* and *lateral thoracic artery* and *vein* supply the anterior pair of thoracic mammae, the *cranial epigastric artery* and *vein* vascularize the two thoracic and anterior abdominal pairs and the *external pudendal artery* and *vein* supply the posterior abdominal and the inguinal pair of mammae.

Digital organ of the pig
(355; 380–382)

The **hoofs** or **claws** (**ungulae**) of the pig are generally similar to those of the small ruminants. They are usually unpigmented and the two hoofs of one limb are almost a mirror image of each other. The *bulbar segment* (355/c; 380/c) of the pig's hoof has a marked distal bulge and occupies more than the posterior half of the ground surface. Nevertheless, in comparison with ruminants, the pig is classed as being "short bulbed". The sole (355/b) encompasses the anterior part of the undersurface of the hoof and is

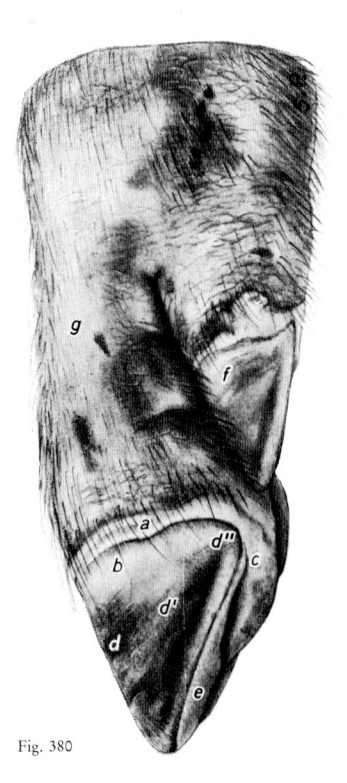

Fig. 380. Digital organ of a pig. Lateral view. (After Geyer, 1974.)

a–e on the main hoof or claw: *a* limbus corneus; *b* margo coronalis; *c* torus corneus; *d–d″* paries corneus: *d* pars dorsalis, *d′* pars collateralis, *d″* margo palmaris lateralis; *e* solea cornea; *f* paries corneus of the accessory hoof; *g* hair-bearing skin

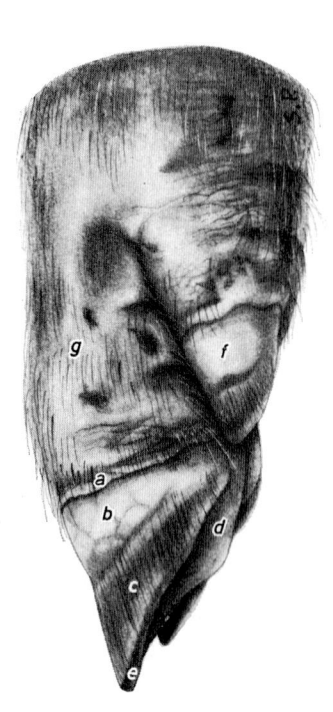

Fig. 381. Digital organ of the pig, after removal of the horny capsule of the main and accessory hoofs. Lateral view. (After Geyer, 1974.)

a–e on the main claw: *a* corium limbi; *b* corium coronae; *c* corium parietis with lamellae coriales; *d* corium tori; *e* corium soleae; *f* corium covering the accessory claw; *g* hair-bearing skin

Fig. 380

Fig. 381

somewhat larger than that of the small ruminants. The *bulbar cushion* forms the foundation for the *bulb*. It consists of connective and adipose tissue and is inserted between the bulbar corium and the deep flexor tendon or onto the third phalanx. Rather similar accumulations of connective tissue form the flat, broad coronary cushion of the pig's hoof (381/b).

The papillae of the *perioplic matrix* (/a) are longer, and thinner than the papillae of the neighbouring skin. They lie vertical to the *epidermis* of the *periople* (380/a) and have a slight distal bend at their apices. The papillae of the *coronary matrix* (381/b) are strikingly short, narrow and distally curved in the proximal germinative zone and they overlap one another like roofing slates. In the middle section of the germinative zone the small papillae are again placed at right angles to their underlying structures, while their apices point in a distal direction. At the transition to the *matrix* of the *wall* the bases of the papillae are extended to form low ridges from which arise thin, delicate papillae which are at first aligned vertically to the epidermis but whose apices are also bent distally. The papillae gradually decrease in number in proximodistal direction until the delicate ridges at the distal border of the germinative matrix are bare. As the *coronary matrix (germinative matrix)* merges into the *matrix* of the *wall (sterile matrix)* (/c), the delicate ridges change into lamellae which occupy the entire length of the sterile matrix. As one can see from figure 381/c the sterile matrix is confined to the distal half of the hoof. As in ruminants, they are only *primary matrix lamellae* (382/c) and their distal extremities are reflected for some distance onto the sole. The matrix lamellae (381/c) which at first are thin and low, later become tall and coarse; they are insinuated vertically between the *epidermal lamellae* (/b). Only in the region of the heel are they reflected onto the palmar (or plantar) aspect. As in the area of the sterile matrix of ruminants, the free border of the lamellae gives rise to long, delicate papillae. Where the lamellae are curved round towards the sole, they are transformed into a row of plump terminal papillae. The papillae of the *sole matrix* (/e) are at first very large and placed side by side in a short row. The remaining papillae of the matrix of the sole are slimmer, shorter and not arranged in rows. The papillae of the *bulbar matrix* (/d) are also not in rows but they are of variable size and may be larger than those of the sole matrix. The size of the papillae of the bulbar matrix decreases in proximal direction so that at the transition to the hair-bearing skin they are only about half as long as those of the surface of the sole. The part of the bulb which contacts the ground is heavily keratinized and it has considerably longer papillae than the part which does not directly bear weight.

Fig. 382. Horizontal section through the protective and parietal layers and the parietal corium in the distal half of the pig's claw. (After Geyer, 1974.)
a stratum medium parietis cornei with tubuli epidermales and intertubular horn; *b* lamellae epidermales of the epidermis parietis; *c* lamellae coriales of the corium parietis

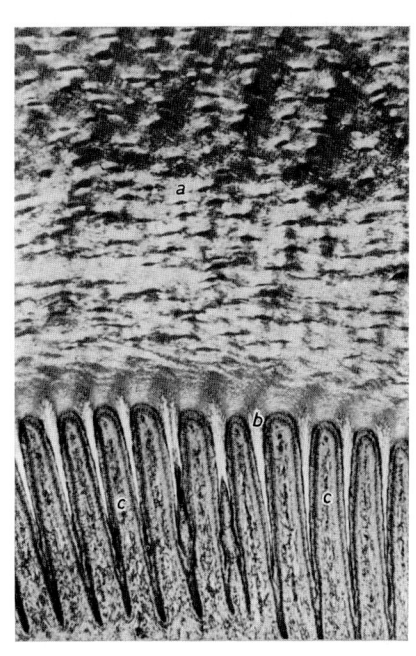

The *horny claw* of the pig is formed by the wall, the sole and the bulb. The *wall of the claw* (380/d–d″) is thick and its lateral surface is slightly depressed proximally and bulges below (/d′) a thick, steep *dorsal part* or toe (*margo dorsalis*) (/d) and a slightly concave *interdigital axial surface*. Both laterally and medially the height of the wall gradually decreases from the toe to the heel (380). Since the horny wall covers only the anterior half of the interdigital surface it is smaller than the lateral wall. On the distal half the interior surface of the wall has tall horny ridges (382/b) which alternate with the matrix lamellae (/c). The distal ends of these lamellae and their papillae are surrounded by tubular horn, the so-called *terminal layers*, which form the *white line* (355/a′) on the ground surface of the hoof. The white line forms the connection between the bearing surface of the wall and the horny sole (/a, b). Only the anterior part of the sole is covered by *horn* (356/b; 380/e). The thick, hard horny sole fills the space between the distal borders (bearing surface) of the wall (355/a). The ground surface of the interdigital walls are short from anterior to posterior whereas this edge is much longer on the outside of the claw (/b). The horny sole continues directly into the horn of the bulb which extends relatively far forward as a tongue-like projection on the interdigital surface (/c). At the level of the sole, the thickness and firmness of the bulbar horn is about the same as that of the horny sole. That part of the horny hoof which is not part of the wall or sole is formed by the bulbar horn. At the base of the interdigital space the bulbs of both main claws fuse with one another and are continuous proximally with the common integument. The *perioplic segment (limbus corneus)* (380/a) is a shallow dorsal swelling which is inserted between the proximal border of the wall and the hair-bearing skin. The *epidermis* of the periople (/a) bulges a little beyond the *coronary epidermis* (/b), and a shallow groove marks the transition. The perioplic horn is loose in structure and extends from the coronary border for about 5 mm distally. The epithelium of the coronary epidermis which produces the horn of the wall, also bulges to some extent due to the underlying connective tissue of the germinative matrix (/b). The epithelium of the *wall epidermis (hyponychium)* produces only few cells which, as the *transitional* or *gliding layer,* grow distally with the wall and form the horn of the distal hyponychium (*horn* of the *terminal layer*). At the same time the hyponychium acts, as in ruminants, as an anchor for the wall. The terminal horn is formed, first and foremost, between the papillae of the lower end of the corium lamellae. The horn wall grows at a rate of 10 mm per month.

The length and thickness of the corium papillae are related to the degree of horn formation. If the papillae are absent or the papillary body consists only of low ridges, then there is little horn formation or only a single layer of cells is produced as, for instance, the gliding layer of the claw. But the gliding surfaces of the horny wall of the hoof carry tall lamellae and this ensures a firm connection which allows the hoof to bear weight.

A horizintal histological section through the horny wall of the pig's hoof (382) shows that the horn tubules of the coronary segment are round in the innermost zone and oval or flattened in all other regions (/a). The horn tubules of the bulbar, sole and perioplic segments are roundish and those of the sole segment are generally smaller than those of the other segments.

The cortex of the horn tubules of all segments is formed by more or less flattened cells and it is not possible to differentiate them exactly from the intertubular horn.

Hoof fissures occur when pigs are kept on slatted floors and they are particularly common where soft and hard horn meet, for example, between wall and sole and between wall and bulb.

The *accessory hoofs* (355/e, e') of the pig are true hoofs since they possess the necessary osseous skeleton. They are less rudimentary than those of ruminants but, because the otherwise complete digital skeleton is reduced in length, they do not reach the ground (379) although in soft ground or bog the accessory hoof comes into its own as an important organ of weight support. The lateral accessory hoof is, as a rule, longer than the medial one (355/e, e'), thus, incidentally, facilitating identification of the right or left foot in forensic cases. The accessory hoofs of the hind limb (355; 379) are shorter and more proximally situated than those of the forelimb.

Blood vessels of the digital organ of the pig

Arteries

The *arcus palmaris supf.* gives rise to two *axial* and *abaxial* arteries for the 3rd and 4th digits. Running along the sides of the toes to the horny hoof, they give off numerous branches at irregular intervals in dorsal and palmar directions and they also anastomose with one another. As they enter the hoof several branches are given off to the bulb. Within the third phalanx the *axial* and *abaxial* arteries of each toe fuse, forming the *arcus terminalis.* In the pig the exit and entry of the canal of the third phalanx are situated on the axial and abaxial surfaces near the sole. Between one and three vessels from the terminal arch supply the apex of the third phalanx and after passing through the bone they supply the networks of the wall, bulb and sole.

The arteries of the third phalanx of the hind foot are similar to those of the forelimb.

Veins

Two *dorsal (axial)* and two *abaxial* veins run to the claw and freely anastomose with each other in the digital region. A stout anastomosis, passing over the dorsal surface of the second phalanx, unites the digital veins and at the same time the anastomosis functions as the *coronary vein.* Each *dorsal digital vein* gives off branches to the *venous reticula* of the *parietal corium* and near the extensor process it forms another anastomosis with the abaxial digital veins. Finally, each dorsal digital vein divides into a slender *distal phalangeal vein* and an *axial marginal vein*. The former passes through the ungular canal to join with the abaxial veins, while the marginal vein follows the axial parietal groove and also links with the abaxial digital veins at the tip of the phalanx. Each of the *abaxial digital veins* divides into a stout *bulbar vein* and a smaller *coronary vein*. The bulbar vein forms the great bulbar network and the coronary vein links with the above-mentioned anastomosis from the dorsal vein and then continues in the abaxial parietal groove to the apex of the claw where it joins the marginal vein.

Skin and cutaneous organs of ruminants

Skin of the ox
(341, 345, 350, 383)

Bovine skin is thicker than that of any other domestic mammals. In calves it varies between 2.0 and 4.8 mm while in adult cattle it is between 3.0 and 12.0 mm thick. Mountain cattle have thicker skin than lowland breeds.

The skin of the calf is thickest in the region of the cheeks, forehead and nape. Increased subcutaneous connective tissue is present in the stifle fold, knee fold, the point of the elbow and the flank and therefore these are the most suitable sites for *subcutaneous injections*.

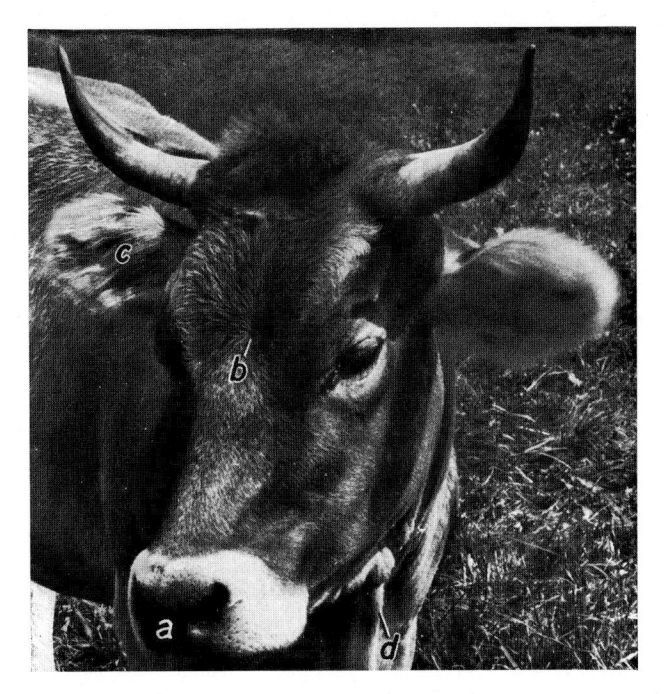

Fig. 383. Head of a young Brown Alpine cow with distinct forelock (cirrus capitis), horns still without rings or grooves. (Photograph: G. Geiger.)
a greyish-blue pigmented planum nasolabiale with lateral sinus hairs and the orifices of the glandulae plani nasolabialis; *b* vortex frontalis; *c* long hairs at the rim and ample hairs on the inside of the ear; *d* dewlap (palear)

Castrated oxen invariably have thicker skin than bulls of the same age. No breed differences in the organization of the different layers of the skin have been recorded. The connective tissue of the corium has larger meshes in calves. The connective tissue is in tighter bundles in this skin than in the thicker skin of adult animals. Otherwise, however, the corium of calves and old cattle tends to have more delicate bundles of connective tissue than in animals of medium age. Both the elastic and collagen fibres of the corium are coarser than in the horse.

It has already been mentioned that there is a median skin fold, the *dewlap (plica colli ventralis)* (383/d), on the anterior aspect of the bovine chest which, although subject to considerable breed variation, contains large amounts of adipose tissue in fat cattle. This fat cushion is permeated by connective tissue and it may be 7.0 cm or more in thickness in well nourished individuals. Calcium is often deposited in the dewlap of older animals.

The external shape of bovine hair shows no particularly characteristic features. The coat consists not only of thick, stiff hairs but also thin *awn hairs* and very fine *wool hairs*. The *outer hairs* (341/e) have a certain similarity to those of the horse but are usually somewhat longer. The rather long outer hairs between the horns are often curled *(forelock)* or increased in number so that they appear bushy (383), particularly in the Spotted and Brown Alpine cattle. Long hairs are present at the tip of the tail where they form the *tassel (cirrus caudae)*. Longer hairs are also present at the edges of the ears and the inner surface of the auricle is densely covered with hairs (/c). Unlike the horse, where the hair colour is not dependent on the breed, the various breeds of cattle have characteristic hair colouring. In Central Europe we therefore differentiate grey, brown, red, yellow, spotted and pied (black pied and red pied) cattle which are given various local names.

The *length* and *thickness* of the hair of cattle are both sex and breed characteristics. As a rule, the coat of bulls is shorter than that of cows but it is longest of all in castrates. In Black Pied Lowland and Simmental Spotted cattle the bulls also have thinner hairs than the cows. The hairs are generally longer than in alpine than lowland breeds. Among the Central European breeds, the red pied cattle have the longest hair (average 63.8 mm) followed, in descending order of hair length, by the Pinzgau, Spotted Alpine cattle, black pied, grey cattle and finally the Murnau-Werdenfels, the hair of which is about 22.5 mm long. Scottish Highland cattle have remarkably long coats. The thickest hairs are found in Murnau-Werdenfelser cattle in which they are 35.6 μm in diameter and the thinnest, mesauring 29.8 μm diameter, occur in the Spotted Alpine breed. Generally their thickness varies between 20 and 50 μm. Bovine hairs have more medulla than the hairs of other domestic mammals.

A striped coat pattern can result when Simmental Spotted cattle are crossed with the Brown Alpine breed. Heavy pigmentation is associated with increased resistance of the skin. Non-pigmented areas of skin are more sensitive to intensive sunlight.

It is said that hairs are longer and coarser when the animals are at pasture and if there is lack of pigmentation. In areas which are exposed to greater pressures from within (bony protruberances), the hairs are shorter and coarser.

As in other domestic mammals, the ox has hair streams, hair crosses and hair vortices in certain parts of the body.

The *hair vortices* (350) of the ox occur on the face (383/b), on the upper lip and on the nape of the neck. The eye (383) and ear hair vortices are paired. Other vortices are found on the elbow and in the axilla and there is a divergent thoracic vortex, a convergent abdominal vortex, a medial vortex on the thigh of males, on the knee fold, on the perineum above the udder and one in the umbilical region. There may be others in some individuals.

The *mental bundle* of *tactile hairs* is almost invariably present (345). It generally consists of 2 or 3 sinus hairs, about 5 cm in length, which are usually directed backwards. The *cheek bundle* is uncommon but when present it consists of 1 or 2 tactile hairs. The *eyebrows* are made up of 8 to 14 isolated tactile hairs at the base of the upper eyelid. The *sinus hairs* of the *upper* and *lower lips* (345) are irregularly arranged and as a rule they are less than 5 cm long. No tactile hairs are present in the regio infraorbitalis (345).

Because they are generally so short and thin, the tactile hairs of cattle are not very distinct. Their colour corresponds to the local skin pigmentation.

The bovine skin is well supplied with *sweat* and *scent glands* and these are lacking only in the skin of the teats and interdigital spaces. There are also a considerable number of *sebaceous glands* with independent openings. The secreting sweat glands are very wide (60–100 μm) and often only slightly undulating but not coiled. Sebaceous glands are more numerous in the following region: anterior end of the nasal dorsum, transition of the haired skin to the planum of the nose, angle of the mouth, base of the horns, at the udder, perineum, anus, vulva, preputial orifices and in the flexor aspect of the pastern.

Bovine hide is the most important raw material for the leather industry. However, it can be so damaged by the larvae of the warble fly (*Hypoderma bovis* and *H. lineatum*) that it loses much of its value.

Skin of the goat
(347; 350; 352; 354)

The **skin** of the goat is considerably thinner than that of the ox but it is thicker, tougher and more elastic than that of the sheep. Its thickness varies in different regions of the body and there are only slight sex differences. Only in the *epidermis* of the lips, nasal planum and coronary border is there a *str. lucidum*. In all other respects the structure of the skin corresponds to that of the other domestic mammals.

The thin, long, smooth and medullated *leading hairs* of the goat project distinctly beyond the rest of the hairs. The shorter, slightly wavy and medullated *awn hairs* are very numerous (352). Thin, delicately waved and non-medullated *wool hairs* are interspersed in the coat but, as a rule, they occur only during the winter.

In goats the *coat* shows considerable breed variation. The German Toggenburg goat has the longest awn hairs and the shortest wool hairs of all the domestic mammals. The wool hairs are longest in the White German Improved goat and the awn hairs of this animal are shorter than any other German breed of goat. The thickest wool hair is found in the Pied German Improved goat which has a deer-coloured coat with a distinct eel mark on the back and black haired limbs. The beard, when present, also consists of black hairs. While the outer hairs are generally isolated, the wool hairs are usually arranged in bundles.

Particularly long hairs are found in the *beard (barba)* (347) of the throat region. This is more pronounced in male than female goats. Between the follicles of these beard hairs there are sebaceous glands with long, branched efferent ducts. In goats the finest hairs are present on the udder.

In addition to the beard, other specialized cutaneous structures on the head are the *tassels* and the *horns*. Some breeds have only one of these structures, whereas others have two or all three (352).

The *hair vortices* (350) of the goat are arranged in about the same manner as the sheep. There are two vortices on the chest, lumbar region, above the eye and on the ear and one on the nose and on the nape.

The goat has no *tactile hairs* on the *chin* and *cheek*. There are approximately 25 tactile hairs in the *eyebrows* distributed over the entire upper eyelid in four irregular rows (347). The *lower eyelid* bears 10 to 20 sinus hairs (347) in two rows. On the *upper* and *lower lips* they have a patchy distribution and can attain a length of 4 to 6 cm, but because they are so delicate, they are not easily recognised (347).

Typical sebaceous glands are distributed over the entire skin but in addition there are very large, branched sebaceous glands on the coronary border of the claws, at the base of the horns and ears and in the perineal region. During the breeding season sebaceous glands all over the body, but especially on the head and neck, show a marked increase in size. This glandular enlargement is accompanied by an alteration in the chemical composition of the lipids of the skin. Presumably these hypertrophied sebaceous glands are responsible for the characteristic smell of male goats at that time.

No such seasonal alterations occur in the size of the sweat glands; they are distributed over the whole skin and are tubular, apocrine, coiled glands *(scent glands)*. The sweat glands are largest on the teats, the udder, the scrotum and in the perineal region whereas they are smaller on the outer ear and the eyelids than in the skin covering the remainder of the body. The planum of the nose contains compound tubular and serous glands.

The horn glands (354) and tassels (352) have already been discussed on pages 465 and 462.

Histological studies of the skin of the roe buck have revealed seasonal changes in its structure brought about by a neurohormone dependent on the sexual cycle and development of the antlers. The skin is thinnest during the period of antler development which occurs from December to February. From March onwards there is a distinct thickening of the skin, enlargement of the skin glands and development of the summer coat. From September to December the involution processes take place resulting in regression of the various layers of the skin and growth of the winter coat. No corresponding studies have been carried out on the goat's skin.

Skin of the sheep
(341; 346; 353)

The **skin** of the sheep is thinner than that of the goat. In adult animals its average thickness is 2.5 mm. It is thickest on the forehead and dorsolateral part of the trunk. The thickness of the whole skin and of its various layers varies with age. There are also sex differences, the ram having much thicker skin than the ewe or wether. It is thicker in coarse-haired than in fine-haired and Merino sheep.

The long, thin, curled and usually medullated *wool hairs* (or fibres) (341/*d'*) form the sheep's *fleece* (353/*f*). Between the wool hairs there are isolated stiff, thick and more or less coiled *awn hairs* which are generally medullated. Short, straight outer hairs (341/*d*) are present on the face (353/*e*) and limbs and they extend, depending on the breed, a variable distance proximally (356).

The hair follicles of sheep occur in *groups* which contain both primary and secondary hair follicles. The primary hair follicles have both sebaceous and tubular glands as well as follicular muscles; the secondary follicles only have sebaceous glands. The density of follicles varies considerably in newborn lambs. In Stara-Sagosa lambs, for example, the average number of follicles per square mm is: in single females 174.9, in twin females 200.7, in single males 162.7 and in twin males 193.0. This follicular density generally decreases with advancing age and at 18 months it is about 69.5 per mm^2 of skin in both males and females.

There is a topographical correlation between the hair groups and the fibre structures of the skin.

When young, many breeds of sheep have wavy body hairs which are referred to as curls. The most pronounced *curl formation* is seen in *Karakul lambs* and various patterns such as "*mixed*", "*lyre*", "*fir tree*" and "*chess board*" patterns can be differentiated. In some instances the curls may have an asymmetrical or even feral pattern. The curls of the Karakul sheep are mainly of "tube" form. The curling of the hair gradually regresses with advancing age and is finally lost altogether.

Two *divergent hair vortices* are seen on the chest, lumbar region, eyes and ears respectively of the sheep and one divergent vortex occurs on the nose and nape of the neck.

The sheep, like the goat, lacks bundles of tactile hairs on the chin and cheek. The *eyebrow* consists of a loose bundle of 8 to 15 sinus hairs situated on the anterior half of the *upper eyelid* (346). The tactile hairs of the *lower eyelid* are arranged in two rows near the rim of the lid. Finally, the *upper* and *lower lips* carry numerous tactile hairs, some of which are arranged in irregular rows (346; 353). They are not always easily recognised because they are short and very thin.

The *sweat glands* of sheep are twisted but their ends are not coiled. They are particularly large and numerous on the ventral surface of the tail. The complement of *sebaceous glands* remains constant throughout the animal's life while the sweat glands increase in number with age.

The specialized skin glands of the sheep have been discussed on pages 463, 466 and 468.

The prepared sheep skin of the Karakul lamb is known as *Persian lamb*. A large number of factors determine the eventual value of the lamb's fleece but the thickness and length of the hairs is of primary importance. White hairs are, as a rule, longer and thinner than black ones.

The clipped hair of the sheep is known as the fleece and this, of course, forms the raw material for the wool industry. Greater development of hair medulla and a relative reduction in cortex decreases the quality of the wool. The sheen of wool is dependent on the fatty secretion of the sebaceous glands; this secretion protects the wool against injury and can be up to 60% of the clipped weight. Weathering of the wool or "dryness" is due to insufficient sebaceous secretion. We speak of "mixed wool" when awn and wool hairs are clearly distinguished from one another and of "uniform wool" when they are indistinguishable. Merino wool consists entirely of wool hair.

Mammary gland of the cow
(358–360; 384–394)

The **mammary gland** of the domestic cow is of particular significance, since its product not only nourishes its own young but is of great importance as human food. We shall therefore describe it in somewhat greater detail. The size and structure of the udder of domestic ruminants varies considerably being dependent on several factors such as age, breed, nutritional status and phase of lactation. The present description is based on the lactating organ.

The *udder (uber)* of the cow is a very large, hemispherical, glandular body (*corpus mammae*) (358/*A*; 384) which consists of four *quarters* (*mammae*) each with a *teat* (*papilla mammae*) (358/*A*; 384). The very impressive size of the cow's udder has been achieved by selective breeding. In good milch cows it is a pendulous organ situated in the inguinal region and extending cranially to the navel; caudally it may almost reach the vulva (386).

The mammary gland is covered by thin, easily-moved skin which bears sparse, thin hairs. The superficial veins (384) of the udder are therefore often visible through the skin. On the caudal surface of the udder there is a double hair vortex. The size and shape of the udder is not a reliable indication of its milk-producing capability. The skin of the teats is tightly adherent to the underlying tissues and, in fact, it represents a significant component of the teat wall.

The udder of the cow is firmly attached to the ventral abdominal wall by ligaments and lamellae. This *suspensory apparatus (apparatus suspensorius mammarum)* (385/e, f) arises from the deep layer of the superficial fascia of the trunk which, in herbivores, contains numerous elastic fibres giving it the yellow appearance from which its name *tunica flava* (/f) derives. It is tightly fused with the oblique external abdominis muscle. The suspensory apparatus consists of four primary and numerous secondary sheets. The four primary sheets are applied to the lateral (/f) and medial (/e) surface of each half of the udder and therefore represent the *lateral* and *medial suspensory ligaments* of the udder *(laminae laterales et mediales apparati suspensorii mammarum)*. These ligaments unite at the base of the teats and disappear in the teat wall. They comprise the *capsule* of the udder *(capsula uberis)*.

The suspensory ligaments emerge from the yellow fascia, the lateral ones above and lateral to the *external inguinal ring*, the medial ones immediately beside the *linea alba*. The medial ligaments form into the *double-layered, highly elastic middle suspensory ligament* of the udder *(ligamentum suspensorium uberis)* (/e). This lies between the two halves of the udder and, because it is attached to their medial surfaces, it contributes to the formation of the *intermammary groove (sulcus intermammarius)*. The caudal part of the lig. suspensorium uberis originates from the prepubic tendon. The four primary sheets split, not only at the base but also on the medial and lateral surfaces, into 7 to 10 secondary sheets *(lamellae suspensoriae)* which enter the glandular tissue and subdivide it into lobes.

The *line of origin* of the lig. suspensorium uberis is of particular interest because this structure carries the main weight of the udder. Its caudal section branches from the ventral abdominal wall before the

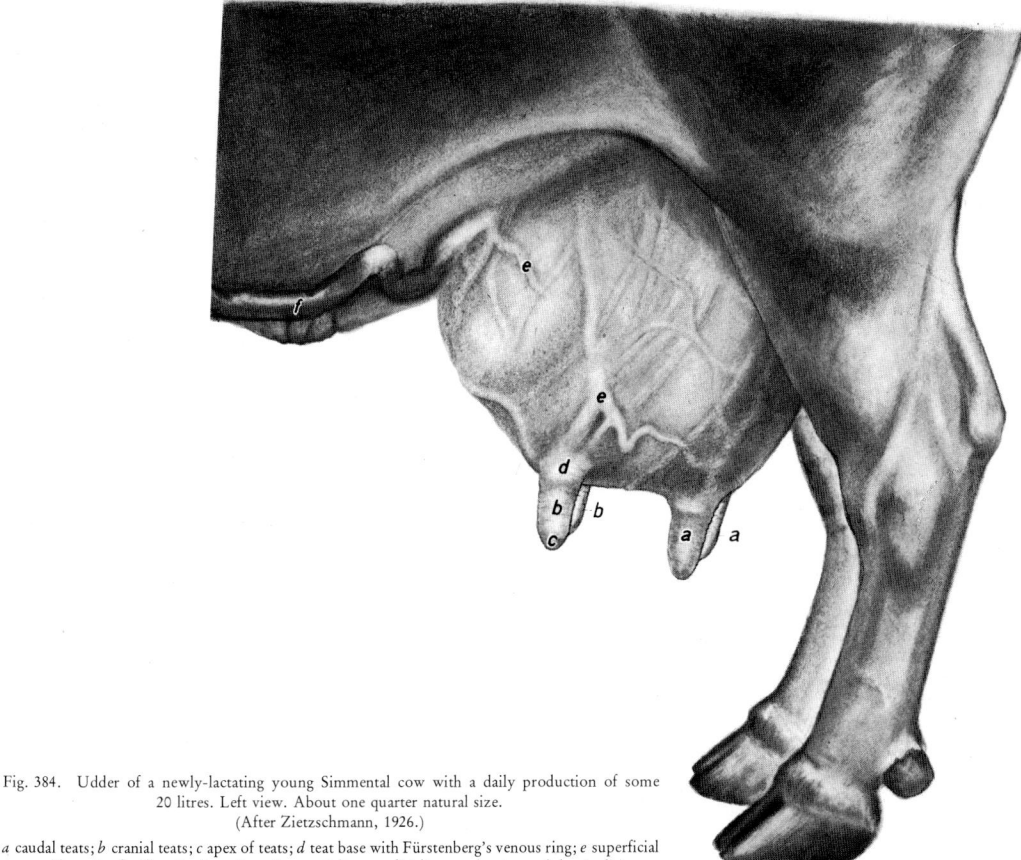

Fig. 384. Udder of a newly-lactating young Simmental cow with a daily production of some 20 litres. Left view. About one quarter natural size.
(After Zietzschmann, 1926.)

a caudal teats; *b* cranial teats; *c* apex of teats; *d* teat base with Fürstenberg's venous ring; *e* superficial udder vein; *f* milk vein, (v. epigastrica cranialis superficialis, v. subcutanea abdominalis)

latter becomes fused to the pecten of the pubis. Thus the udder is mainly suspended from the flexible abdominal wall and only indirectly, through the prepubic tendon, from the bony pelvic floor; skeletal jolting during locomotion thus has little effect on the mammary gland.

This splitting of the primary sheets into secondary lamellae ensures that the two halves of the udder do not simply lie in rigid connective tissue sacks. They are individually suspended because of the alternating arrangement of connective tissue lamellae and glandular lobes. This prevents the glandular parenchyma being subjected to excessive pressure. The elastic elements in the connective tissue ensure that the latter are not torn during locomotion.

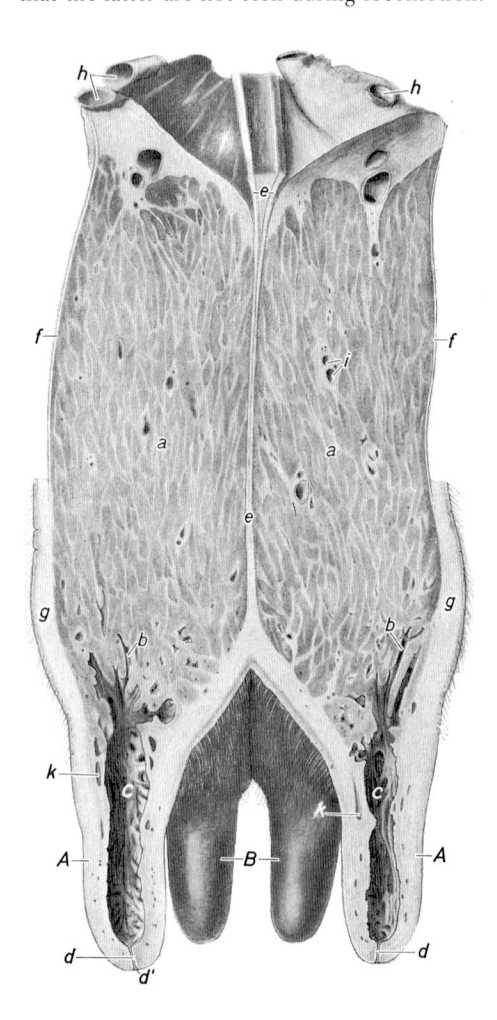

The shape and size of the bovine udder may vary greatly. As well as the normal udder (386/a) other forms are described which, in part at least, may be breed differences. A mammary gland which is smaller than normal may be referred to as a *primitive udder* (/b). If, when looking at the cow in profile, the bulk of the udder is found to lie in front of the hind limb, it is termed an *abdominal udder* (/c) or a *thigh udder* (/d) if the condition is the opposite. Deficient development of the fore- or hind-quarter is termed *hypoplasia* of the respective quarter (/e, f). In the so-called *goat udder* (/h) the teats arise, as in the goat, in a more or less continuous line from the udder.

Fig. 385. Cross section through the udder of a cow at the level of the cranial pair of teats. Cranial view. About one third natural size.
(After Zietzschmann, 1926.)

A cranial teats; *B* caudal teats

a lobi glandulae mammariae of the two forequarters: *b* large ductus lactiferi; *c* pars papillaris sinus lactiferi with wrinkled mucous membrane; *d* ductus papillaris, *d'* ostium papillare; *e* ligamentum suspensorium uberis; *f* sheet of tunica flava abdominis covering the outer surface of the mammary body; *g* skin covering the udder; *h* basal vein of the udder; *i* vessels in the interior of the glandular parenchyma; *k* vv. papillares

The well-developed udder of a lactating cow weighs approximately 5–10 kg depending on its content of blood and milk. The full udder should be firm but not hard whereas after milking it is soft and flabby and its skin shows longitudinal folds, especially on the caudal surface. Such European breeds as the Black or Red Variegated Lowland cattle have been so intensively selected for high milk production that the udders of some individuals are excessively large and the tips of the teats are only about 10 cm from the ground when the animal is standing.

The *mammary gland* consists of *four quarters,* each quarter having *one teat* (384). The *intermammary groove* indicates the border between the two halves of the udder. The two quarters on the same side are at the most only indistinctly demarcated externally, the line of separation of the fore and rear quarters sometimes being called the udder yoke (387). Despite this indistinct demarcation, the cavatiy systems and the glandular lobes of the two quarters are completely separated from one another, as can be demonstrated by injecting a differently coloured substance into each teat (387). This is is of practical

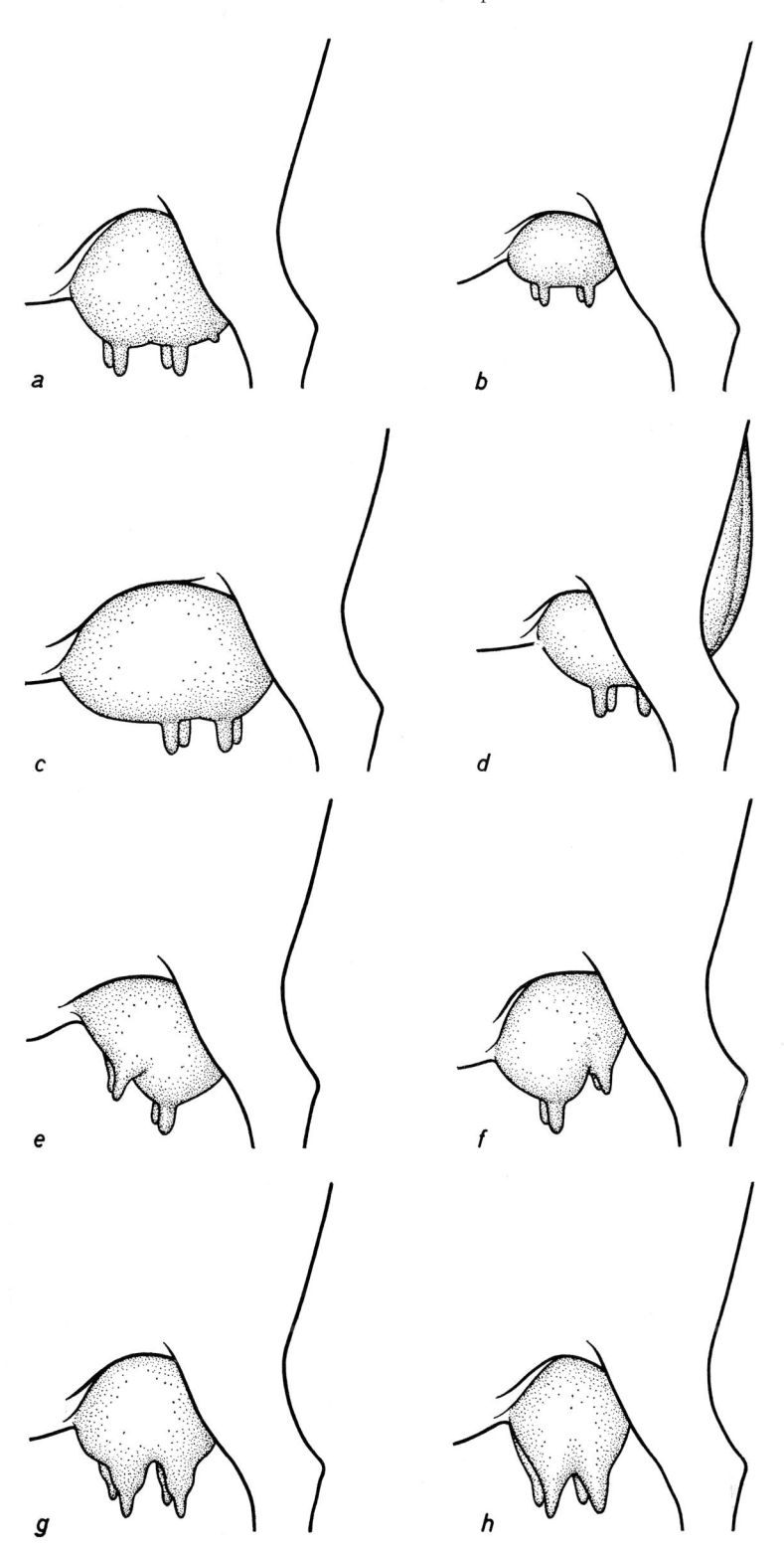

Fig. 386. Diagram of various forms of udder in the cow. Lateral view.
a normal udder with posteriorly directed caudal teats, *b* small or primitive udder, *c* abdominal udder (rare); *d* thigh udder; *e* hypoplasia of the forequarter; *f* hypoplasia of the hind quarter (rare); *g* udder with dilated teats; *h* goat udder, occurring in old, high-yielding cows

significance in "milking out" and in udder diseases. The border line between the two quarters of the same side is rather irregular because their glandular parenchyma overlaps. The cranial (fore) quarters are generally somewhat smaller than the caudal or hind quarters (387). The same terminology is also applied to the respective teats (385/*A*, *B*). In the infantile udder the incompletely developed glandular systems of the individual quarters are separated by adipose tissue (389/*a*).

The *teats (papillae mammae)* (384/*a*, *b*) of normal individuals are cylindrical, peg-like appendages of the udder with rounded tips. Because of an abundance of muscular veins, they have erectile capacity. They are 7–9 cm in length but teats as short as 2.5 cm and as long as 14 cm have been reported. The long axis often deviates in a craniolateral direction, especially when the cisterns are full of milk. The base, or root, of the teat (/*d*) is that region which contains the widest part of the cistern. As a rule, it is found at the transition between the hair-bearing skin of the udder and the hairless skin of the teat (385).

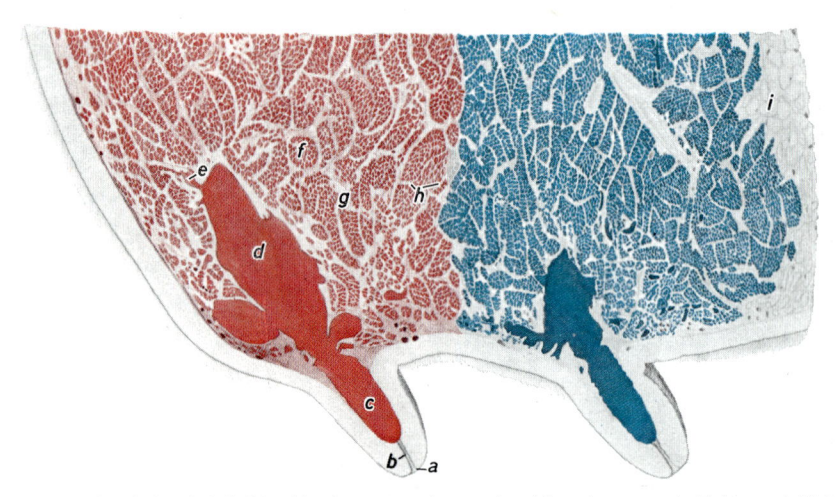

Fig. 387. Sagittal section through the right half of the udder of a cow. Note the separation of the cavity systems: the hind quarter is filled with red and the fore quarter with blue gelatine. About one third natural size.
(After Zietzschmann, 1926.)

a ostium papillare; *b* ductus papillaris; *c* pars papillaris sinus lactiferi; *d* pars glandularis sinus lactiferi; *e* ductus lactiferi; *f* lobus glandulae mammariae, composed of lobuli glandulae mammariae; *g* interlobular connective tissue; *h* intralobular connective tissue; *i* adipose tissue

Each bovine *teat* has only one *teat* or *streak canal (ductus papillaris)* (385/*d*; 387/*b*), the punctiform opening of which *(ostium papillare)* (385/*d'*; 387/*a*) is surrounded by an epithelial wall 0.5–1 mm in height. Its white mucous membrane is arranged in delicate longitudinal folds and is lined by stratified keratinizing epithelium which has a prominent stratum granulosum (388A/*b*). The proximal end of the canal is clearly demarcated from the mucosa of the cisterna by a slightly projecting fold (Fürstenberg's rosette).

The cavity immediately proximal to the teat canal is known as the *teat cistern (pars papillaris sinus lactiferi)* (385/*c*; 387/*c*). In the cow (385/*c*) and goat (397/*b*) it is large and elongated whereas in the sheep it is much smaller. It continues far into the glandular parenchyma of the udder (360/*c*) as the *gland cistern (pars glandularis sinus lactiferi)* (387/*d*). Its thin mucous membrane consists of two-layered columnar epithelium (388/*h*). It is yellow and, when empty, exhibits a delicate pattern of net-like ridges and folds. Its wall, especially the dorsal part, contains millet-to hempseed-sized units of yellow lactiferous gland tissue. The wall of the teat cistern consists of very *muscular* and *vascular connective tissue* (/*d'*) surrounded externally by cutis (/*e'*, *f'*) which is devoid of hair and glands but is richly supplied with sensory nerves. There is no true subcutis. While the coarser muscle fibres form a net-like, interlinked, spiral system, the finer muscle tracts frequently terminate in elastic fibres.

The *propria mucosa* of the teat wall consists of collagenous and elastic connective tissue and contains numerous bundles of smooth muscle which concentrate into the *m. sphincter papillae* at the *ostium papillare*. The propria also contains numerous *thick-walled veins* which form a long-meshed *erectile body (plexus venosus papillaris)* and which is characteristic of the cow (392/*p*). This functions as a "*haemostatic apparatus*" which is important in "holding back" the milk under certain physiological and psychic influences. At the transition between the teat and glandular parts of the cistern there is usually a distinct constriction. This is caused by the formation of a circular fold 2 to 6 mm in thickness. It consists of firm connective tissue and circularly arranged veins *(Fürstenberg's venous ring)* (393/o). This venous ring and the elastic-muscular fibres around the teat canal prevent the outflow of milk except during sucking or milking.

Difficulties in milking may be due to various morphological alterations in the teat. These include kinked teat canal and hyperplasia of the keratinized teat canal epithelium, both of which cause stenosis of the canal. Compression or constriction of the canal by nodules of squamous epithelium is also not uncommon, while stenosing circular folds can occur in the teat itself.

The glandular cistern is divided by tall folds of mucous membrane into bays in which terminate the 5 to 17 large openings of the many large *milk ducts (ductus lactiferi)* (385/b). The capacity of the bovine

Fig. 388. Cross section through the teat of a young cow in the region of the teat canal (A) and in the region of the teat cistern (B). (Photomicrograph).

a ductus papillaris with plug of keratin; *b* stratified squamous epithelium of the ductus papillaris; *c* m. sphincter papillae; *d, d'* fibro-muscular lamina propria of the teat wall with blood vessels and nerves; *e, e'* corium of the hairless skin of the teat; *f, f* epidermis of the hairless skin of the teat; *g* pars papillaris sinus lactiferi; *h* its epithelial lining; *i, i* thick-walled vv. papillares

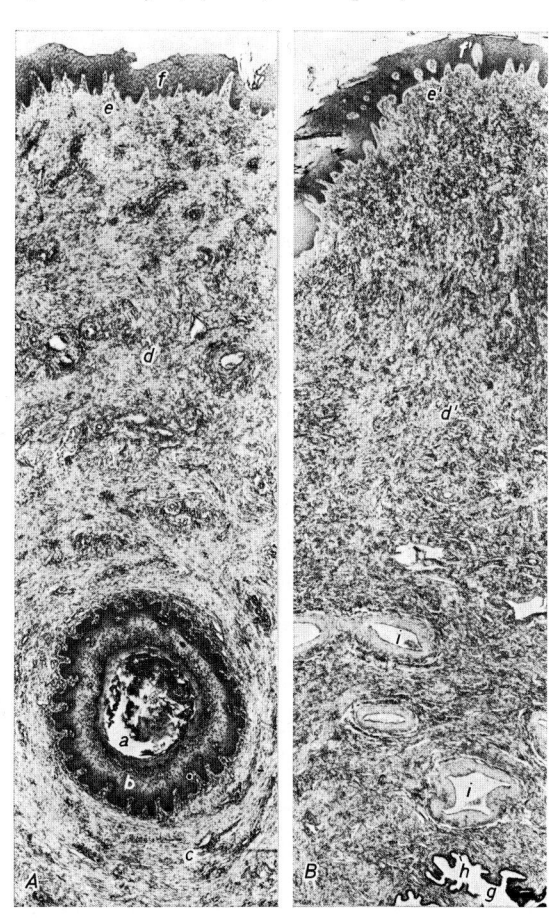

cistern is about 500 ml whereas that of the entire cavity system of an udder of average size is about 10 litres. From this one can conclude that the total capacity of the cavity system is usually greater than the milk produced during one milking.

The number of large milk ducts (387/e) varies from quarter to quarter; there are usually between 8 and 12 ducts per quarter. In the forequarter they run mainly along the lateral surface and in the hindquarters along the caudal surface. Their average distance from the skin is only between 9 and 12 mm. The position of these large milk ducts is of importance, because the depth from the surface at which they are situated means that the pressure of the medial surfaces of the pelvic limbs on the udder is not transmitted directly to them. They usually join one another at a fairly acute angle of between 20° and 45° although, rarely, they may form a 90° junction.

The cut surface of a lactating udder shows numerous irregularly round or angular areas having a somewhat granular, yellow appearance. These represent the *glandular lobules (lobuli gld. mammariae)*

512 Skin and cutaneous organs of ruminants

(359/f) which are separated by delicate, whitish-yellow interlobular connective tissue networks. The latter contain many elastic fibres and are continuous not only with the intralobular connective tissue but also with that which surrounds the mammary gland itself. The *connective tissue support* of the *mammary gland* (387/g, h) has considerable expansive capability and forms a closed functional unit. The ratio of glandular tissue to connective tissue varies between individuals. The lactating udder (389/b) always contains less connective tissue than the non-lactating gland (/c). A lactating udder which has more

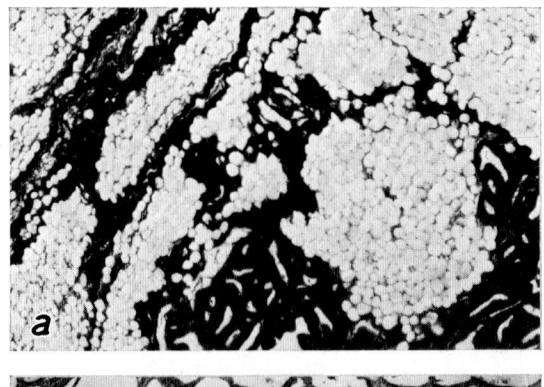

Fig. 389. Histological sections of the mammary gland of the cow.

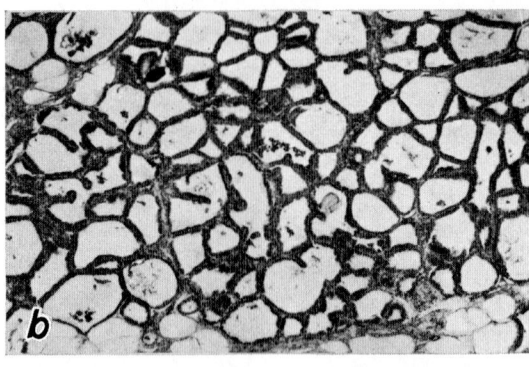

a. Section of the mammary anlage in a calf. Dark: islets of glandular tissue; light: space-occupying adipose tissue.

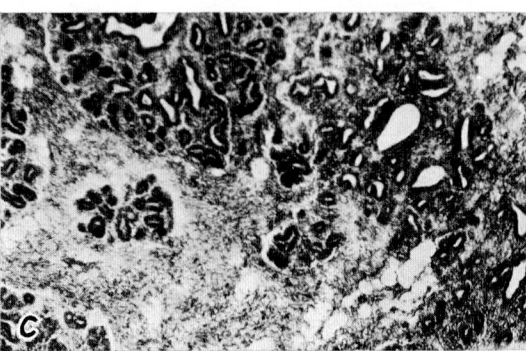

b. Part of a lactating mammary gland of a cow. Dilated acini with epithelial cells in various stages of secretion; there is no adipose tissue.

c. Section of a non-lactating udder of a dry cow. The glandular tissue has regressed, the acini are atrophied and there is an increase in connective and adipose tissue

supporting connective tissue than glandular parenchyma is referred to as a *"fleshy udder"* and although it may be large, it produces little milk. Unlike glandular udders, such fleshy udders are still large after milking and feel firm and hard on palpation.

Within the *supporting tissue* of the udder are the interlobular milk ducts (359/d). These are lined by one or two layered columnar epithelium and accompanied by numerous blood and lymph vessels (385/i), nerve fibres and isolated smooth muscle fibres.

Each *mammary gland lobule (lobulus gld. mammariae)* is made up of closely placed *glandular acini (gld. mammariae)*. These are linked to the *intralobular ducts* and, like them, they are surrounded by contractile *myoepithelial cells*, very fine connective tissue fibres and blood capillaries. As a rule the epithelium of the gldd. mammariae is only one layer thick but the cells can vary considerably in height from low cuboidal to tall columnar, depending on the secretory state and the degree of fullness of the udder (389/b). Tall columnar cells with secretory apices are seen immediately preceding and during the onset of milking. The cell nuclei are mainly situated basally and lipid droplets occur in the cytoplasm. According to recent studies, the glandular terminal segments of the udder show *branching alveolar* form. The individual glandular acini are, like the pulmonary alveoli, separated from one another by thin septa. This contributes to an increase of surface area and gives the mammary gland the structure of an *apocrine retention gland* which is able to store the secretion (Ziegler and Mosiman, 1960). The term "*apocrine*" indicates a form of secretion which is accompanied by loss of part of the living cell. However, the concept of apocrine secretion as a form of necrobiosis resulting in separation of the apical part of the cell is erroneous because it is really the separation of a membrane-covered vesicle, the content of which is the true secretion and only the membrane-envelope is part of the living cell. This is the method by which milk fat is secreted. It necessitates a continual replacement of the cell tissue.

Additional teats are found on the udder of bovines. They are known as accessory teats and are usually not connected to the glandular tissue. They are most commonly located behind the posterior teats (386/a) but may be situated between the two pairs of normal teats or in front of the fore teats. The frequency of occurrence of accessory teats varies in different breeds and this has been particularly studied in some Central European breeds. They occur in 52–54% of Simmenthaler Fleckvieh; 36–37% of Vogelsberger Höhenvieh; 30% of Schwarzbuntes Niederungsvieh. In bulls and castrated oxen accessory teats usually occur anterior to the base of the scrotum (390).

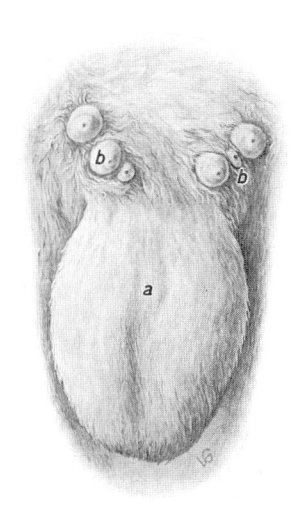

Fig. 390. Accessory teats at the base of the scrotum in a bull calf. Cranial view. Half natural size.
a hair-bearing skin of the scrotum; *b* accessory teats of variable size

The milk produced by the glandular acini is white and opaque. Milk production is normally continued for as long after birth as is necessary for the nourishment of the young but in domestic ruminants whose milk secretion is of economic importance, the lactation period is artificially prolonged. In the cow this is about 300 days.

Cow's milk consists of 84–90% of water and 10–16% dry matter. The latter is made up of 2.8–4.5% fat, 3.3–3.95% total protein (casein, albumin, globulin), 3–5.5% lactose, 0.7–0.8% salts (ash).

Goat's milk has 87.15% water and 12.85% dry matter of which 4.1% is fat, 3.75% total protein, 4.2% lactose and 0.8% ash.

The fat is not in solution but in an emulsion of suspended droplets 3–4 μm in diameter. Vitamin A and D and their precursors are present in milk fat together with other fat soluble vitamins such as E, F, K_1–K_6 and the water soluble vitamins B_1, B_2, B_6, B_{12}, C, H, p-aminobenzoic acid, nicotinamide, pantothenic acid and folic acid.

Milk contains the following minerals: calcium, phosphorus, potassium and, in small amounts, sodium chloride and iron with traces of zinc, copper, aluminium, lead, manganese, silicon and iodine.

Good milch cows of the Black-flecked Lowland breed produce about 30–40 litres of milk daily, although even up to 60 litres is not too exceptional, with a butterfat content of more than 4%. This gives an annual production figure of more than 6000 litres containing 270–300 kg of fat[*].

---

[*] A record production achieved in Germany was in 1968 when an "Angler" cow, "Intermezzo" the daughter of "Freikönig", produced 10,592 kg milk with 5.44% butterfat in the test year. This corresponds to a year's fat production of 576 kg.

Blood vessels of the udder of the cow

Arteries
(391–394)

The **arterial** supply to the bovine udder is mainly derived from the *external pudendal artery* and from a few smaller branches of the *internal pudendal artery*. In lactating cows the former vessel may be 2 cm in diameter. As it passes through the inguinal canal the *external pudendal artery* is accompanied cranially by the external pudendal vein (392/a') and caudally by the main lymph vessels of the udder (/W). After passing through the inguinal canal, the external pudendal artery (/a) approaches the base of the udder and divides, above the posterior teat, into the *cranial* and *caudal mammary arteries* (391/b, c). Before reaching the base of the udder it makes a sigmoid bend (392/a). The external pudendal artery often gives off a posterior basal branch (r. basalis caud.) (391/d) before entering the mammary tissue and this vessel supplies the caudolateral parts of the udder and the udder lymph nodes.

There are many possible deviations from this pattern. Cases have been described where the external pudendal artery does not divide into the cranial and caudal mammary arteries until after entering the udder. The caudal basal ramus may also arise from the caudal mammary artery (/d).

The *cranial mammary artery* (/b; 392/b) runs in a cranioventral direction within the mammary parenchyma and gives rise firstly to one or more aa. lateralis sinus caud. (391/1) vascularizing the cranial part of the hindquarter. Numerous branches originate from this vessel to supply the parenchyma, one of which is the *papillary artery* (/1') to the posterior teat.

The cranial mammary artery subsequently gives off several *cranial lateral sinus arteries* (/2; 393/d) to the lateral region of the forequarter; one of these goes to the fore teat as the *papillary artery* (391/2'). Smaller dorsal branches (/3) of the cranial mammary artery supply the parenchyma at the base of the forequarter. Communicating branches are given off this vessel to the *saphenous* (/4) and *deep circumflex iliac arteries* (/5). The *cranial mammary artery* corresponds to the caudal part of the *superficial caudal epigastric* artery (/6) which, accompanied by its satelite vein (393/h), anastomoses with the *superficial cranial epigastic* artery.

The caudal mammary artery (391/c) runs caudoventrally in the hindquarter, giving off the caudal basal ramus (/d), except in those cases where this branch originates directly from the external pudendal artery. The caudal basal ramus supplies several branches to the *mammary lymph nodes* (/11). The caudal mammary artery vascularizes the parenchyma at the base of the posterior quarter through various dorsal branches (/9). Several caudal lateral sinus arteries (/7) pass through the mammary parenchyma to reach the ventrolateral region of the caudal quarter. One of these branches, the *a. papillaris* (/7'), extends beyond the root of the teat and supplies the caudal teat. From the terminal division of the caudal mammary artery, some dorsal branches finally reach the caudodorsal part of the hindquarter and establish an anastomosis with the caudal basal ramus or the *dorsal labial* and *mammary ramus* of the internal pudendal artery (/10). The *a. caudalis sinus caud.* (/8) is given off in the intermammary groove, but in rare cases the latter can also give off a papillary artery (/8') to the caudal teat.

A third important vessel supplying the udder is the *a. mammaria media* (/e; 394/1). There are individual differences in the origin of this artery. It can arise from the cranial mammary (391/b), the caudal mammary (/c) or from the point of bifurcation of the external pudendal artery into the two former vessels. After a short but undulating ventral course, the middle mammary artery divides into a *cranial* (/e') and a *caudal* (/e") ramus. These supply the medial regions of both fore and hind quarters. The middle mammary artery may be absent, in which event these two rami can arise from either the cranial or caudal mammary arteries. The cranial ramus of the middle mammary artery has several *cranial medial sinus arteries* (/12) to the medial region of the posterior mamma. Finally the cranial ramus is continued as the *medial cranial basal ramus* (/13) and it courses along the ventral abdominal wall to the umbilical region. The caudal ramus of the middle mammary artery gives rise to several *caudal medial sinus arteries* (/14) to supply the caudomedial section of the anterior and the medial region of the caudal quarters. There may be connections with the dorsal labial and mammary ramus of the internal pudendal artery (391/O).

The papillary artery (391) is the only artery supplying the teat and, as recorded above, it may originate from various parent vessels. In the teat wall it takes a lateral, caudal or medial course depending from which mammary artery, or from which of that artery's branches, it stems. The *a. papillaris* (/1', 2', 7', 8', 12') runs from the base to the tip of the teat near the inner surface of the wall, passing between the

Udder of the cow, blood suply 515

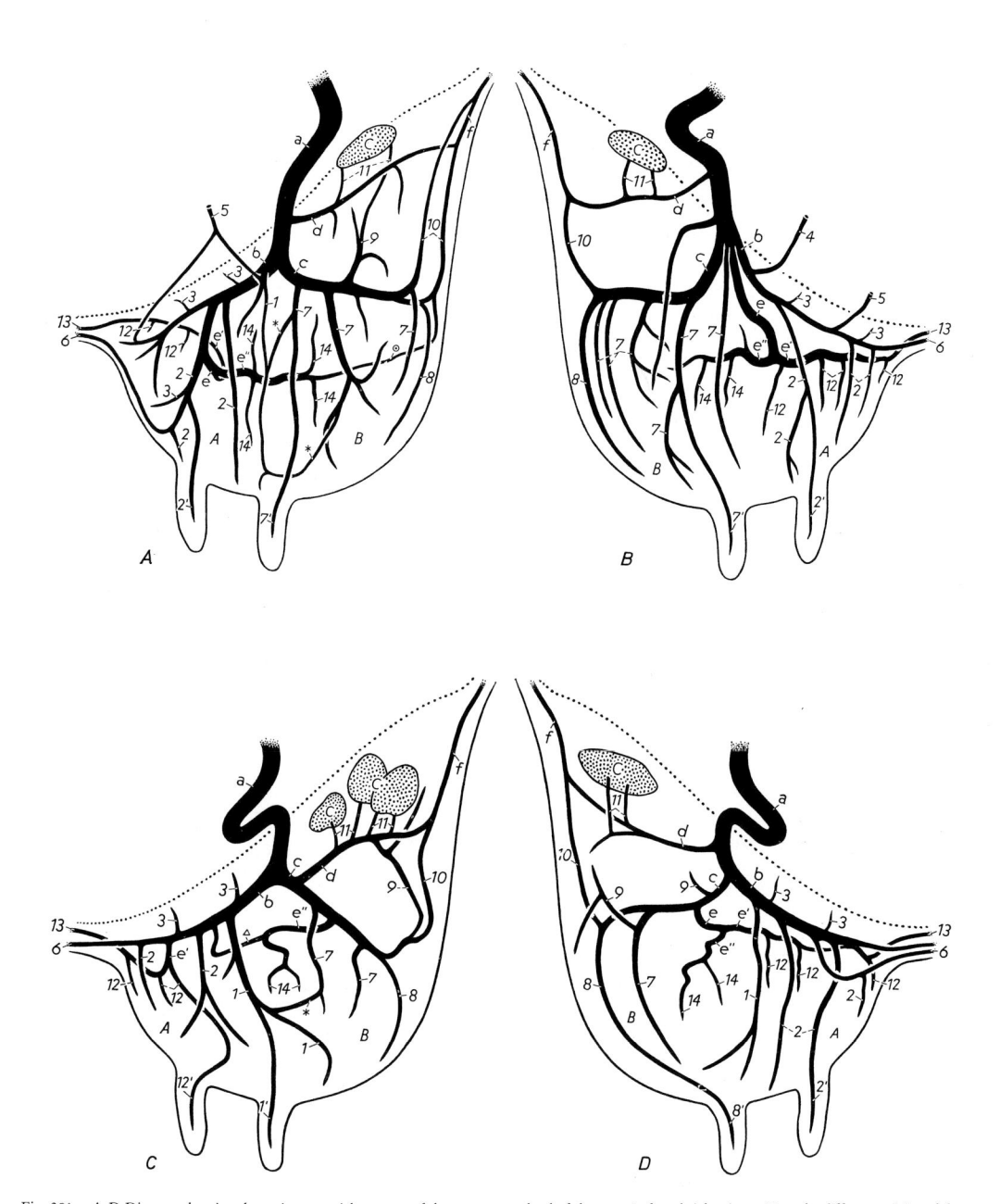

Fig. 391. A-D Diagram showing the various arterial patterns of the mammary gland of the cow. Left and right views. Note the different origins of the a. papillaris.
(After Le Roux and Wilkens, 1959.)

A fore quarter; *B* hind quarter; *C* lymphonodus mammarius

a a. pudenda externa; *b* a. mammaria cranialis (a. epigastrica caudalis superficialis); *c* a. mammaria caudalis (r. labialis ventralis et mammarius); *d* r. basalis caudalis; *e* a. mammaria media (Fürstenberg's artery), *e'* its r. cranialis, *e"* its r. caudalis; *f* r. labialis dorsalis et mammarius of the a. pudenda interna

1 a. lateralis sinus caudalis of the a. mammaria cranialis, *1'* a. papillaris; *2* aa. laterales sinus cranialis, *2'* a. papillaris; *3* rr. dorsales of the a. mammaria cranialis; *4* connecting branch to the a. saphena; *5* connecting branch to the r. superficialis of the a. circumflexa ilium profunda; *6* a. epigastrica caudalis superficialis; *7* aa. laterales sinus caudalis of the a. mammaria caudalis, *7'* a. papillaris; *8* a. caudalis sinus caudalis; *8'* a. papillaris; *9* rr. dorsales of the a. mammaria caudalis; *10* r. labialis ventralis et mammarius of the a. pudenda interna; *11* branches supplying the lymphonodus mammarius; *12* aa. mediales sinus cranialis, *12'* a. papillaris; *13* r. basalis cranialis medialis; *14* aa. mediales sinus caudalis; ⊙ connecting branches to the r. labialis ventralis et mammarius; *,* connecting branches

516   Skin and cutaneous organs of ruminants

large and greatly branched veins to which it is linked in the distal regions of the teat. In addition to the papillary artery, there are other, smaller vessels which supply the skin. The net-like connections of these superficial arteries can simulate an arterial vascular ring at the base of the teat.

Arterio-arterial anastomoses occur between vessels of the same side but arterial cross-links between the two halves of the udder are of functional significance. These occur in the first place between the caudal basal rami of the two sides provided that these are linked with the internal pudendal artery through the dorsal labial and mammary ramus. A superficially-situated anastomosis between the external pudendal arteries courses round the caudal border of the suspensory ligament, to which it gives off branches. The middle mammary arteries may be linked through the medial suspensory ligament.

In company with the homonymous vein, (392/*r*; 394/5) the *dorsal labial* and *mammary ramus* (391/*f*) of the internal pudendal artery runs in the subcutaneous connective tissue of the intermammary groove.

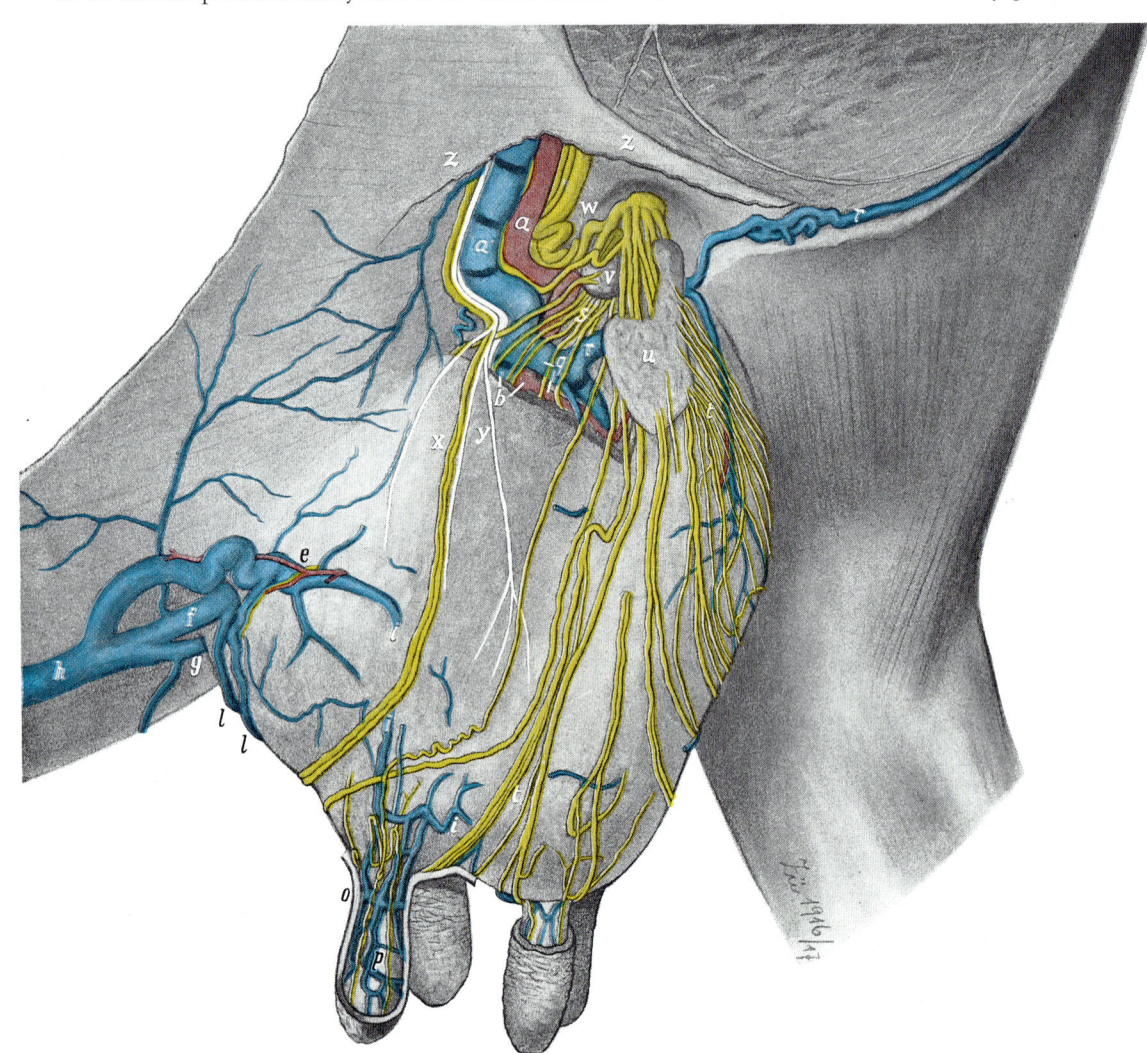

Fig. 392. Topography of the superficial blood and lymph vessels and nerves of the left half of the udder of a cow. The left hind limb has been removed at the hip joint. Lateral view. About one third natural size.
(After Zietzschmann, 1917.)

red: arteries, *blue*: veins, *yellow*: lymph vessels, *white*: nerves

a, a' a. and v. pudenda externa with valves showing through; *b* a. and v. mammaria cranialis; *e, f, g* lateral, middle and medial connecting branches with the *h* v. epigastrica cranialis superficialis (v. subcutanea abdominis); *i* superficial lateral udder vein; *l, l* superficial medial udder vein; *o* Fürstenberg's venous ring at the base of the teat; *p* plexus venosus papillaris; *q, r* a. and v. mammaria caudalis or v. labialis ventralis, anastomosing with the v. labialis dorsalis et mammaria of the v. pudenda interna; *s* deep, *t* superficial vasa afferentia lymphonodi mammarii; *u* superficial, *v* deep mammary lymph node; *w* vasa efferentia lymphonodi mammarii; *x* a superficial lymph vessel which bypasses the udder lymphnodes; *y* superficial branches of the n. genitofemoralis; *z* incised leaf of the fascia trunci profunda which runs from the lateral layer of the anulus inguinalis externus to the lateral surface of the udder

Udder of the cow, veins 517

It is interesting to note that the mammary vessels of the left side are usually thicker than those of the right.

Veins
(392–394)

A continuous, rich blood flow is essential for the normal physiological function of the lactating mammary gland. Stoppage of the blood flow, such as might occur due to venous compression when the animal is lying down, is effectively prevented by the development of alternative routes for blood

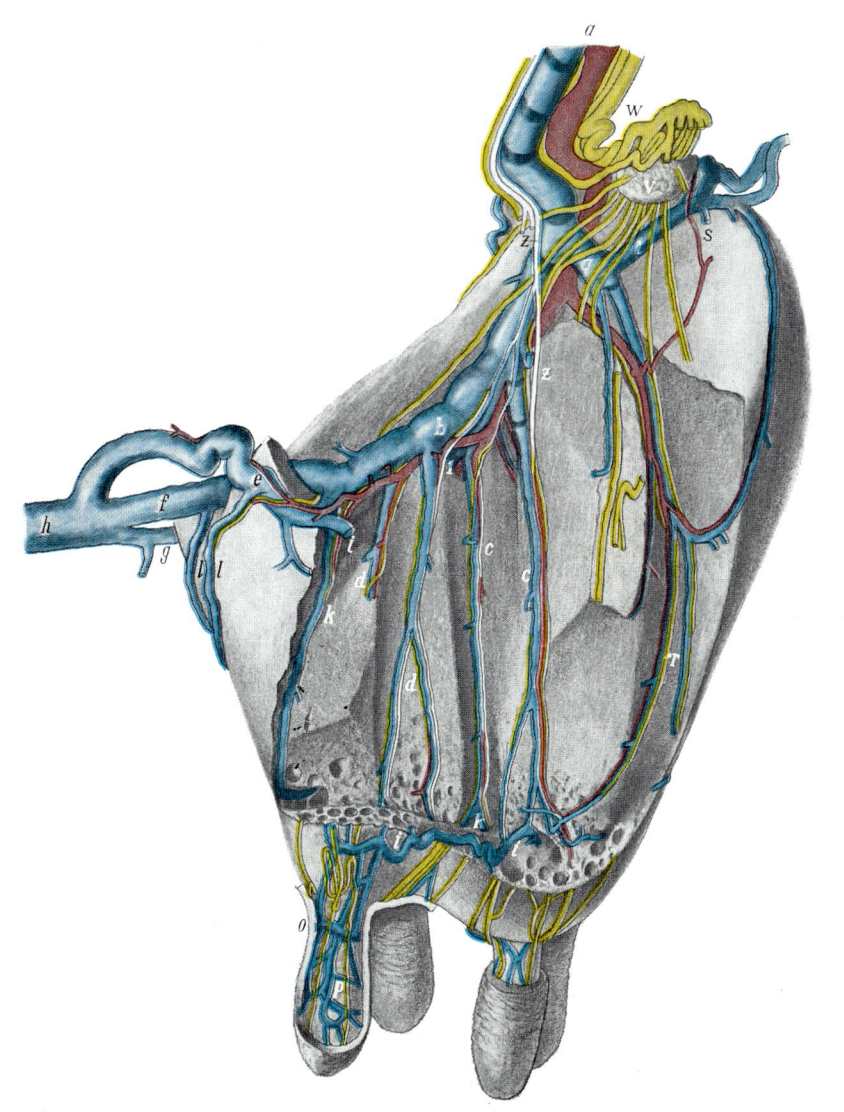

Fig. 393. Topography of the deep blood and lymph vessels and the deep nerves of the left half of the udder of a cow. Lateral view. About one third natural size.
(After Zietzschmann, 1926).

red: arteries, *blue*: veins, *yellow*: lymph vessels, *white*: nerves

a a. and v. pudenda externa; *b* a. and v. mammaria cranialis; *c* aa. and vv. laterales sinus caudalis; *d* a. and v. lateralis superficialis sinus cranialis; *e* lateral, *f* middle, *g* medial connecting branches to the *h* v. epigastrica cranialis superficialis; *i* v. sinuum superficialis lateralis; *k* a. and v. lateralis profunda sinus cranialis; *l* superficial veins joining the v. basalis cranialis and the v. mammaria cranialis; *o* circulus venosus papillae; *p* vv. papillares; *q*, *t* v. mammaria caudalis and v. labialis ventralis; *r* a. and v. caudalis profunda sinus caudalis; *s* artery supplying the udder lymph nodes; *v* lymphonodus mammarius with deep afferent lymph vessels; *w* vasa efferentia from the udder lymph nodes, running towards the inguinal canal; *z* rr. genitales of the n. genitofemoralis

1 a. and v. mammaria media

drainage. From the *erectile body* of the teat *(plexus venosus papillaris)* blood passes through numerous thick-walled and very muscular teat veins *(vv. papillares)* (392; 393/*p*). These veins form several freely anastomosing layers in the vascular layer of the teat wall but ultimately they join the circle of veins situated at the base of the teat. This is *Fürstenberg's venous ring (circulus venosus papillae)* (393, 394/*o*). Thence most of the blood is carried to the base of the udder by the meandering *vv. sinuum supff. latt.* (393, 394/*i*). This vein lies immediately subcutaneously and is clearly visible in good milch cows. The veins forming in the interior of the udder run dorsally in company with the arteries of the same name to enter the *cranial* (393/*b*) and *caudal* (/*q*) mammary veins at the base of the udder. Cross anastomoses join these veins with the corresponding vessels from the other side to form the *circulus venosus mammae*. Several vessels can carry the blood from this venous circle:

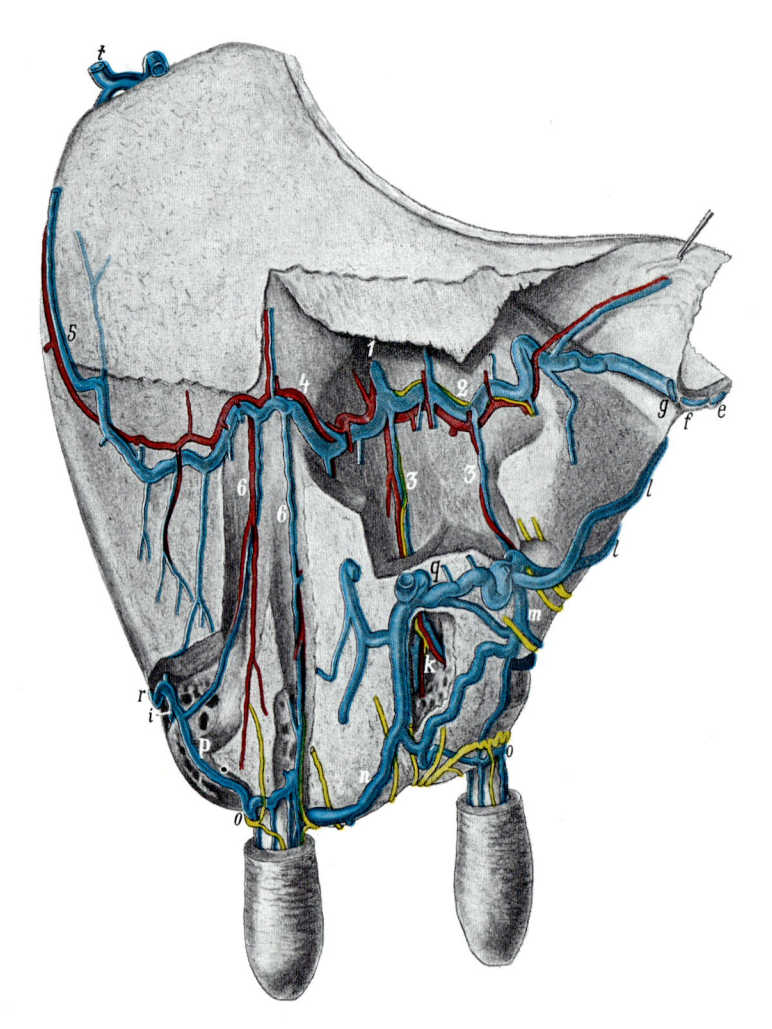

Fig. 394. Topography of the superficial and deep blood and lymph vessels of the left half of the udder of a cow. Medial view. About one third natural size. (After Zietzschmann, 1917.)

red: arteries, *blue*: veins, *yellow*: lymph vessels

e lateral, *f* middle, *g* medial connecting branch with the v. epigastrica cranialis superficialis; *i* v. sinuum superficialis lateralis; *k* a. and v. lateralis profunda sinus cranialis; *l* superficial venous branches to the v. basalis cranialis; *m* v. medialis sinus cranialis; *n* branch to the cisterna of the hind quarter; *o* circulus venosus papillae; *p* branch of the v. sinuum superficialis lateralis to Fürstenberg's venous ring; *q* v. basalis cranialis; *r* v. caudalis profunda sinus caudalis; *t* v. basalis caudalis

1 a. and v. mammaria media, *2* its rr. craniales; *3* aa. mediales sinus cranialis, *4* its rr. caudales; *5* vein running between the two halves of the udder to anastomose with the v. pudenda interna; *6* vv. mediales profundae sinus caudalis

1) the external pudendal vein (392/*a'*; 393/*a*) which passes through the inguinal space into the pudendo-epigastric vein,
2) the *dorsal labial* and *mammary vein* (392/*r*) which runs caudodorsally over the ischiatic notch into the internal pudendal vein that goes towards the pelvic cavity,
3) the usually voluminous *milk vein (v. epigastrica cran. supf., = v. subcutanea abdominis* (392, 393/*h*) which carries the blood in a cranial direction and clearly bulges the abdominal skin.

The latter is the thickness of the thumb and usually passes through the abdominal wall between the xyphoid cartilage and the 8th costal cartilage to discharge into the cranial vena cava by way of the internal thoracic and subclavian veins. Its point of penetration of the abdominal wall can be palpated with the finger and is sometimes known as the "milk well". The size of this aperture is sometimes considered an indication of the potential for milk production. Anastomoses between the *superficial cranial epigastric (subcutaneous abdominal) vein* and the *saphenous vein* are not uncommon in the ox, indeed, *veno-venous anastomoses* are generally quite numerous in the udder.

Opinions still differ on these routes of blood drainage from the bovine udder. Recent studies suggest that the drainage area of the *dorsal labial* and *mammary vein* (392/*r*) is not confined to the caudal part of the udder but includes the skin of the medial aspect of the thigh which is adjacent to the udder, and the skin covering the caudal aspect of the mammary gland. The blood from these regions may be carried to the udder but from the vulval region blood drains to the *internal pudendal vein*. In this vein, therefore, the blood flows in both directions. Thereafter the venous blood from the udder is drained by the *external pudendal vein* (393/*a'*; 394/*a*) and by the *superficial cranial epigastric (subcutaneous abdominal) vein* (392, 393/*h*) and the latter also carries blood from the skin and subcutaneous tissue of the ventral abdominal wall. Other investigations indicate that only the *external pudendal vein* carries blood from the udder, while the *milk vein* serves to carry blood from the ventral abdominal wall and the *dorsal labial* and *mammary vein* carry it from the perineal region to the udder. In older animals the valves in the milk vein are supposed to be entirely insufficient, so that the venous blood will flow anteriorly in the standing animal and towards the udder when the animal is recumbent. The arrangement of the valves of the caudal mammary vein is subject to individual variation. (see p. 240).

In good milking cows the udder veins are very wide and in old animals they are meandering and thin walled. In emergencies, these veins, but especially the milk vein, can be used for intravenous injections.

The capacity of the udder veins is about fifty times greater than that of the arteries. This reduces the speed of the blood flow and allows the blood constituents which are necessary for milk formation to be transported into the glandular epithelium. About 400 litres of blood must flow through the udder to produce a litre of milk and to facilitate this exchange of substances, the milk producing terminal pieces of the glands are surrounded by networks of fine capillaries.

Lymph vessels

A subcutaneous network of lymph vessels situated at the base of the udder collects lymph from this organ. This network gives rise to larger lymph collecting vessels which run to the udder lymph nodes *(Ln. mammarii)* which are part of the inguinofemoral lymphocentre. These nodes can be palpated above and caudal to the hindquarters. Other lymph collecting vessels pass directly through the inguinal canal to the *medial iliac lymphocentre* and yet other lymph vessels empty into the *subiliac node* (for further details see lymph vessel system).

Nerves

The udder is well supplied by sensory and autonomic nerves. The **sensory innervation,** which is of importance to the function of the mammary gland, is dependent on the following spinal nerves: *rr. cutanei ventrr.* of the *iliohypogastric* and of the *ilioinguinal nerves,* which provide sensory fibres for the skin of the forequarters and the cranial part of the base of the udder; the *genitofemoral nerve* which innervates the skin, the teats and the glandular tissue except the caudal regions of the hindquarter; finally, the *r. mammarius* of the *pudendal nerve* which is responsible for supplying the skin of the caudal region of the hindquarters to just above the caudal teats. The **autonomic innervation** is supplied mainly by *sympathetic* fibres of the *caudal mesenteric ganglion*. These pass through the inguinal canal to the udder in company with the genitofemoral nerve, and are supposed to extend to the lobules of the

Mammary gland of the goat
(358; 360A; 395–398; 402)

In relation to its body size, the goat has a relatively large **udder** (395) which consists of two *mammary complexes* (mammae) situated in the inguinal region. The cone-shaped, elongated, pendulous glandular body of each side (358/B) gives rise to a *teat* (395) which projects in a craniolateral direction. In primiparous individuals they are of slender form and are distinctly demarcated from the more spherical

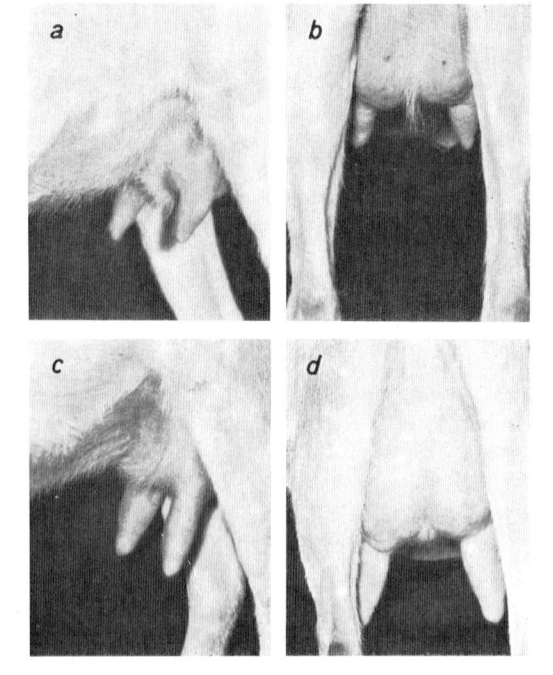

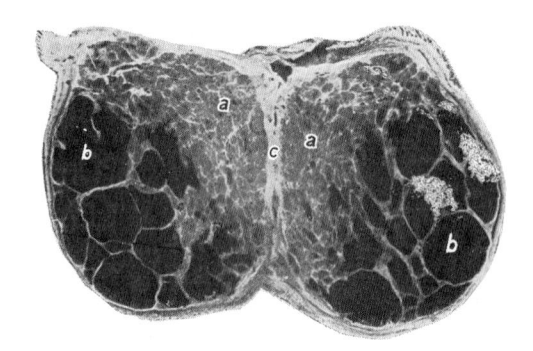

Fig. 396. Cross section through the udder of a goat. The anterior surface is at the top of the photograph. About half natural size.
(After Martin and Schauder, 1939.)

Craniomedially (a) is the glandular tissue with its small and medium sized lactiferous ducts, caudolaterally (b) there are the large milk ducts filled with gelatine. Between the two halves of the udder are the cut vessels and the suspensory ligament (c).

Fig. 395. Udder of a young (a, b) and an older (c, d) goat in lateral and caudal view. Note the difference in shape and size of the mammae and of the teats.

mamma (395/*a*, *b*; 402/*c*). In older goats which have lactated more frequently, the teats are large and "wide-bellied" and appear as if undemarcated and continuous with the body of the gland (/*c*, *d*). However, in the transition area between the body of the gland and the base of the teat there is often an indistinct circular constriction. In white breeds the skin of the udder and teats is non-pigmented but in fawn or darker breeds it is brown.

The cavity system of the udder corresponds fairly closely to that of the cow. Not infrequently the *intralobular efferent* ducts and, indeed, the *interlobular collecting ducts,* show large cavernous dilatations. The 6 to 9 large *ductus lactiferi* (396/*b*; 397/*c*) are situated superficially in the caudolateral region of the udder (396/*b*) and they terminate ventrally in the common milk collecting sinus (397/*b'*) of the appropriate side; this may be as large as a child's fist. This lactiferous sinus of older goats extends caudally immediately beneath the skin (389/*c*, *c'*) where it can be palpated (397/*b'*). The voluminous *teat cistern* fills the teat almost completely (/*b*; 389/*d*, *d'*) and if measured in a standing animal in full lactation it is 7 cm long and 2.5 cm broad. The *teat canal* (397/*a*) is only 0.5 to 0.7 cm long and the basal half of its lumen is constricted by the presence of longitudinal folds. Distally it merges with the conical *ostium papillare*. If the cavity system is opened (397) the border between the white teat canal epithelium and the more yellow epithelial covering of the teat cistern can be clearly identified. The teat canal is lined by stratified keratinizing epithelium whereas the cistern is lined by double-layered columnar epithelium.

The structure of the wall of the teat is essentially similar to that of the cow. In the middle layer there are thick-walled veins with valves. There is no subcutis. The cutis has many hairs and is rich in sebaceous and coiled scent glands. Hair and glands are absent only at the tips of the teats. As a rule there is a small accessory teat, 0.5 to 1.0 cm in length, at the base of each udder.

Accessory teats are often found in males. They are 2.0 to 6.0 cm in length and are located anterior to the base of the scrotum. These accessory teats may be connected to glandular tissue and sometimes have been observed to secrete a milk-like fluid; up to 500 ml of secretion per day has been reported. Active accessory teats have not been reported in bulls and rams. The accessory teats of castrated goats are usually larger than in entire animals.

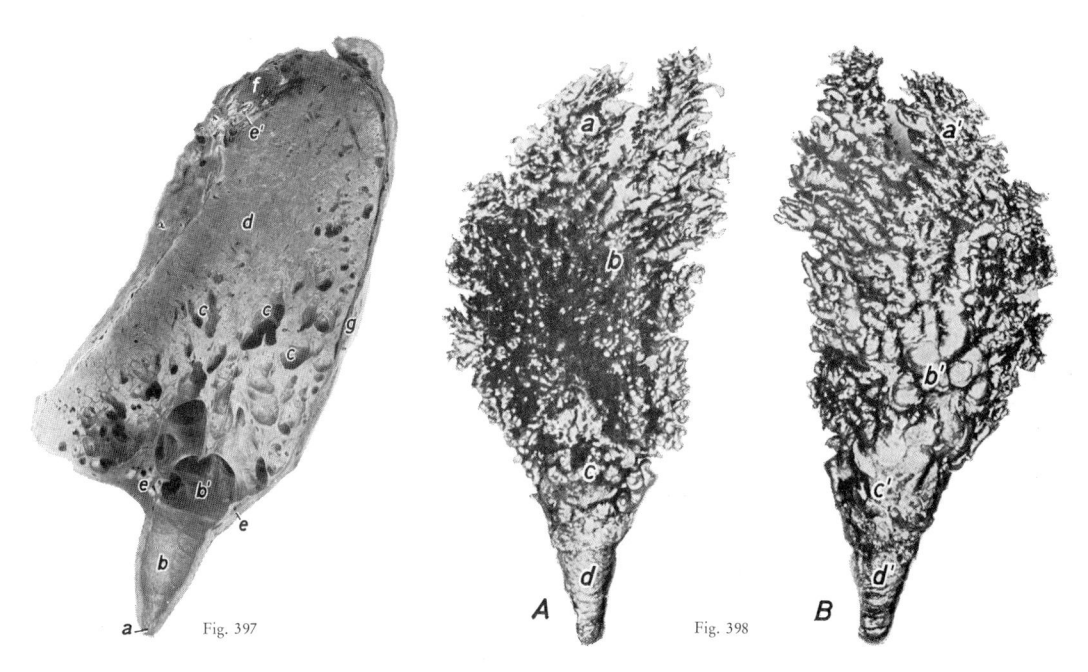

Fig. 397. Sagittal section through the right half of the udder of an older goat which was formalin-fixed with the animal in the standing position.
(After Schauder, 1951.)

a ductus papillaris; *b* pars papillaris, *b'* pars glandularis sinus lactiferi; *c* ductus lactiferi; *d* lobi glandulae mammariae; *e* veins at the base of the teat, *e'* vessels at the base of the udder; *f* lymphonodus mammarius; *g* skin bearing delicate hairs

Fig. 398. Milk duct system of the udder of the goat. Metal corrosion preparation.
(After Martin-Schauder, 1938.)

A cranial view: *a* lobuli glandulae mammariae; *b* small ductus lactiferi; *c* pars glandularis; *d* pars papillaris sinus lactiferi
B caudal view: *a'* lobuli glandulae mammariae; *b'* large ductus lactiferi; *c'* pars glandularis; *d'* pars papillaris sinus lactiferi

Mammary gland of the sheep
(358; 360A; 399)

The **udder** of the sheep is also found in the inguinal region and it is shaped like a flattened hemisphere (358/D). It consists of two halves separated by a well developed *intermammary groove* (/D; 399/d) which can be readily distinguished on external inspection. Each half of the udder consists of one *mammary complex* (360/A) which, however, is much smaller than that of the goat. The cone-shaped *teats* (358/D) are small (1–3 cm long) and laterally directed and their tips point craniolaterally. The skin of the udder is usually brown and rarely unpigmented. The orifice of the teat canal (399/c) is easily recognised at the tip of the teat. While the udder parts bordering on the inner surface of the thigh have, like the teats, only fine hairs, the rest of the udder is densely covered with wool (358/D; 399/d).

The internal structure of the sheep's udder corresponds closely to that of the goat. The mucous membrane of the teat canal is darkly pigmented and in longitudinal folds. The teat wall contains numerous elastic fibres while the smooth musculature is but poorly developed. There is no papillary sphincter muscle; the closure of the teat canal is achieved by a dense network of elastic fibres. The *teat cistern* of the sheep is much smaller than that of the goat, its distal part being very narrow and its proximal part having a saccular form. The glandular cistern is the size of a walnut and is distinctly constricted at the transition to the teat cistern. The glandular parenchyma and the milk ducts are like those of the cow. The lactation period lasts about 130 to 140 days in both goats and sheep. During this period the goat will produce some 600 litres and a "milk sheep" 500 litres of milk.

As a rule the sheep does not have *accessory teats*. The ram has two accessory teats on each side laterocranial to the scrotum. The cranial of these male accessory teats is about 0.5 cm in length and the caudal is 1.5–2.5 cm in length. Between the udder, or the scrotum, and the inner surface of the thigh the sheep has *inguinal pouches (sinus gld. inguinalis)* (399/*f*) (see p. 468).

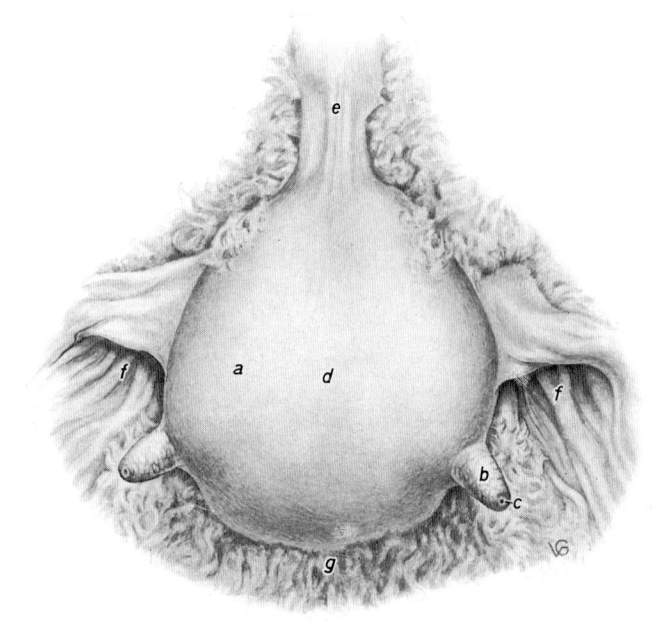

Fig. 399. Lactating mammary gland of the sheep. Caudoventral view. About half natural size.

a hemispherical corpus mammae; *b* papilla mammae; *c* ostium papillare; *d* sulcus intermammarius; *e* perineal fold without hairs; *f, f* sinus inguinalis; *g* hair-bearing skin

Blood vessels of the udder of small ruminants

Arteries
(400–402)

The udder of the small ruminants is supplied only by the *external pudendal artery* (400/*a*; 402/*1*). This vessel arises from the pudendoepigastric trunk and passes through the inguinal canal to reach the base of the udder. Shortly before entering the caudal section of the base of the ovine udder, it gives off the *r. labialis ventralis* (400/*b*) which supplies branches to the mammary lymph nodes. In the goat there is a special lymph node branch (402/*9*) in addition to the ventral labial artery (/*8*), and therefore, in this species, the ventral labial ramus supplies only the caudodorsal third of the udder.

Immediately after entering the mammary parenchyma the external pudendal artery gives off a *caudal ramus* (400/*e*; 402/*4*) which vascularizes the caudal region of the udder. Shortly afterwards the external pudendal artery divides into the *middle mammary* (400/*c*, *n*; 402/*7*, *7'*) and the *cranial mammary arteries* (400/*d*, *o*; 402/*2*, *3*).

The *middle mammary artery* (400/*c*; 402/*7*) generally gives rise to the *medial sinus artery* (400/*f*) which forks, usually at the level of the teat base, into two *papillary arteries* (/*h*, 401/*b*). These subdivide further and form the *plexus arteriosus papillae* (400/*i* 401/*c*) at about the middle of the teat, and the *plexus arteriosus ductus papillaris* (400/*k*; 401/*d*) at the level of the teat canal.

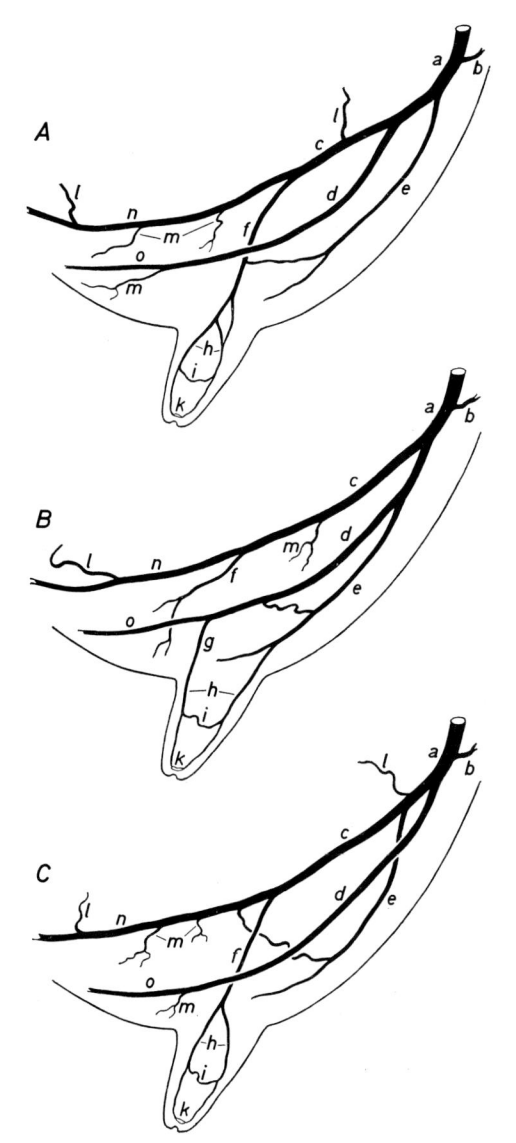

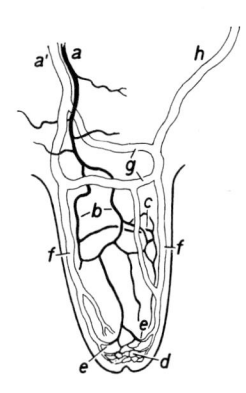

Fig. 401. Blood vessels of the teat of the sheep. Semidiagrammatic. About natural size.
(From a plastic corrosion preparation made at the Institute by Stojanovic, 1975.)

a a. medialis sinus; *a'* v. medialis sinus; *b* aa. papillares; *c* plexus arteriosus papillae; *d* plexus arteriosus ductus papillaris; *e* probably arterio-venous anastomoses; *f* vv. papillares; *g* circulus venosus papillae; *h* v. lateralis sinus

Fig. 400. A–C. Semidiagrammatic representation of the variation in the arterial pattern of the sheep's udder. Left lateral view.
(After Stojanovic, Anatomical Institute, Giessen, 1975.)

a a. pudenda externa; *b* r. labialis ventralis with branch to lymph nodes; *c, n* a. mammaria media; *d, o* a. mammaria cranialis (a. epigastrica caudalis superficialis); *e* r. caudalis; *f* a. medialis sinus; *g* a. lateralis sinus; *h* aa. papillares; *i* plexus arteriosus papillae; *k* plexus arteriosus ductus papillaris; *l* rr. communicantes; *m* branches to the glandular tissue

As a variant of this vascular pattern, the *caudal ramus* (400/e) of the sheep may arise from the *cranial* (400B/e) or the *middle* (400C/e) *mammary arteries*. Anastomoses can occur between the main arterial branches. Unlike the arrangement in cattle, there may be cross connections between the arteries of the two halves of the udder through the *suspensory ligament* and these occur mainly in the cranial region of the udder and less frequently in its caudal part. These are, in the one case, branches of the *middle mammary artery*, and in the other case, small vessels originating from the *ventral labial branch*. Having passed through the median septum, they link up with branches of the corresponding arteries of the other side.

Veins
(401–402)

The main venous drainage from the udder is via the *external pudendal vein* (402/10). This vessel receives a *ventral labial vein* (/17) from the mammary lymph nodes but otherwise the disposition of the venous branches is similar to that of the arteries. The smaller veins are usually more numerous than the corresponding arteries.

The venous blood from the teat wall is drained through capillary networks and arterio-venous anastomoses. The *vv. papillares* (401/*f*; 402/*16*) terminate at the level of the teat base in the *circulus venosus papillae* (401/*g*; 402/*15*). Thence the blood may be carried either via the *medial sinus vein* to the *middle mammary vein* (402/*12, 12'*), or via the *lateral sinus vein* (401/*h*; 402/*14*) to the *cranial mammary vein* (402/*11, 11'*). The latter route is shorter. Both the *medial mammary vein* (/*12, 12'*) and the *cranial mammary vein* (/*11, 11', 13, 13'*) can empty into the *superficial cranial epigastric vein*.

The *innervation* of the udder resembles that of the large ruminant.

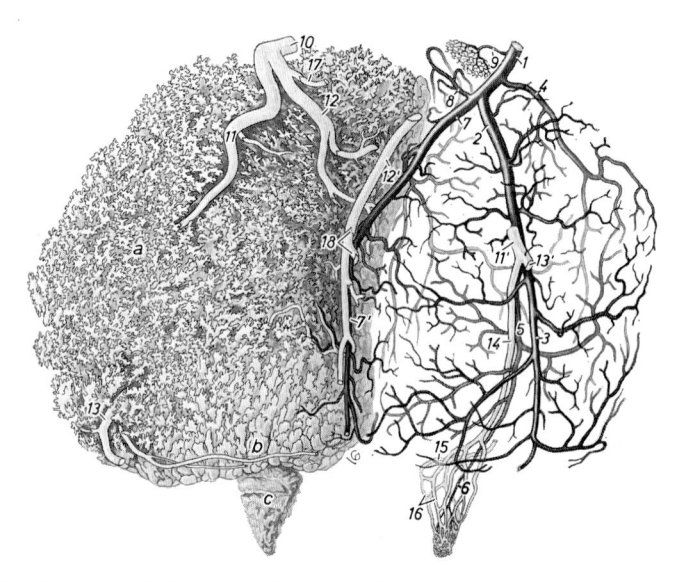

Fig. 402. Broad-based udder of a young goat. Craniodorsal view. On the right half of the udder the cavity system and the veins are shown, on the left the arteries. From a plastic corrosion preparation.

Dark: arteries, light: veins.

a lobuli glandulae mammariae; *b* pars glandularis, *c* pars papillaris sinus lactiferi;

1 a. pudenda externa; *2, 3* a. mammaria cranialis (a. epigastrica caudalis superficialis); *4* r. caudalis; *5* a. lateralis sinus; *6* a. papillaris; *7, 7'* a. mammaria media; *8* r. labialis ventralis; *9* branch to the udder lymph node; *10* v. pudenda externa; *11, 11', 13, 13'* v. mammaria cranialis or v. epigastrica caudalis superficialis; *12, 12'* v. mammaria media in the right half of the udder at its transition into the v. epigastrica cranialis superficialis (v. subcutanea abdominis); *14* v. lateralis sinus; *15* circulus venosus papillae (Fürstenberg's venous ring); *16* vv. papillares; *17* v. labialis ventralis; *18* valves in the veins

Digital organ of the ox
(403–413)
General considerations

The **claw (hoof, ungula)** is the special type of organ of the *even-toed ungulates* (artiodactyla). Each foot has two main and two accessory claws (412). When in close apposition the two main claws do not appear dissimilar from the horse's single hoof.

By the term "claw" is meant the *distal phalanx* and its *skin covering*, the epidermis of the latter forming the claw capsule. The *central supporting* structures include the distal phalanx (403/*D*), the distal part of the second phalanx (/*C*), the distal sesamoid bone (/*E*), the joint ligaments, the terminal parts of the extensor (/*4–6*) and flexor tendons (/*9, 10*) and the podotrochlear bursa (/*16*).

It has already been pointed out in the introduction to this section that the skin covering digital organs can be considered both by layers and segments. Accordingly we can distinguish in the claw the *tela subcutanea ungulae*, the *corium ungulae* and the *epidermis ungulae* (403) which correspond to the three layers of the skin. Similarly there are *perioplic, coronary, parietal, sole* and *bulbar* segments. The three layers of the skin can be demonstrasted in all these segments (403). The claw has neither a *frog* nor *bars*.

Fig. 403. Left forefoot of an ox. Sagittal section through the lateral primary toe. Lateral view. The papillary body of the corium is not shown. (After Wilkens, 1964.)

A metacarpus IV; *B* phalanx proximalis; *C* phalanx media; *D* phalanx distalis; *E* os sesamoideum distale; *F* os sesamoideum proximale mediale; *G* lateral accessory claw

a epidermis limbi, *a'* corium limbi with perioplic fold overlying the tela subcutanea limbi; *b* epidermis tori, *b'* corium tori, *b''* tela subcutanea tori; *c* epidermis coronae, *c'* corium coronae, *c''* tela subcutanea coronae; *d* epidermis parietis, *d'* corium parietis; *e* epidermis soleae, *e'* corium soleae

1 articulatio metacarpophalangea, *1'* dorsal, *1''* palmar extremity of the joint capsule; *2* articulatio interphalangea proximalis manus, *2'* dorsal, *2''* palmar extremity of the joint capsule; *3* articulatio interphalangea distalis manus, *3'* dorsal, *3''* palmar extremity of the joint capsule; *4* tendon of the m. extensor digiti III proprius; *5* tendon of the m. extensor digitalis communis; *6* tendon of the m. extensor digiti IV proprius; *7–8* m. interosseus medius; *7* middle plate; *8* connecting plate to the tendon of the m. flexor digitalis superficialis; *9* tendon of the m. flexor digitalis profundus; *10* tendon of the m. flexor digitalis superficialis, *10'* its cuff around the deep flexor tendon; *11* palmar anular ligament; *12* digital anular ligament; *13* ligamenta sesamoidea decussata; *14* axial palmar ligament of the pastern joint; *15* common sheath of the flexor tendon of the digit and its pouches; *16* bursa podotrochlearis; *17* venous arcus palmaris distalis; *18* arterial arcus palmaris distalis

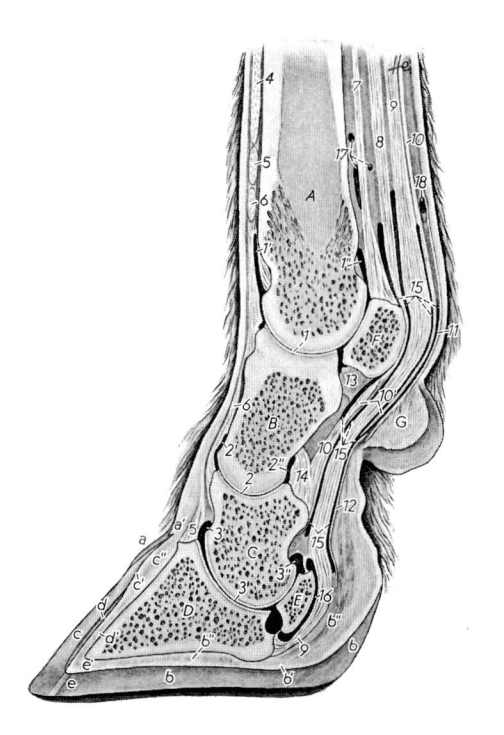

Subcutis of the claw (tela subcutanea ungulae)

The **subcutis** of the claw (tela subcutanea ungulae) covers the central supporting structures and it shows a variable development in the five segments of the claw. In the perioplic region it forms the *perioplic cushion* (403/*a'*) which broadens out in the palmar and plantar direction to fuse with the *bulbar cushion* (/*b''*). On the axial (interdigital) surface the perioplic subcutis is but poorly developed.

The *tela subcutanea coronae* (/*c''*) forms the slightly protruding *coronary cushion* which gradually increases in thickness as it spreads from the dorsum of the toe in the palmar and plantar direction. At the *laminar* and *sole segments* the subcutis forms part of the periosteum of the distal phalanx, thus binding the corium firmly to the central supporting structures. This union is firm at the apical region of the distal phalanx (/*e'*).

The subcutis is most abundant in the bulbar segment where it forms the *bulbar cushion (tela subcutanea tori)* (/*b''*). This structure has a springy, elastic and shock-absorbing action when weight is placed on the claw. In the palmar and plantar regions it is up to 1.5 cm thick and occupies the entire breadth of the claw (/*b''*). On the other hand, the bulbar cushion gradually decreases in thickness and becomes flatter towards the point of the toe. It extends a considerable distance along the palmar surface of the claw and finally merges, without a definite demarcation, with the *tela subcutanea soleae*. This subcutis of the sole is thin and lies in immediate contact with the distal phalanx (/*D*).

Corium of the claw (corium ungulae)

The *corium* and *epidermis* of the claw comprise the *cutis* of the claw. The *corium ungulae* overlies the subcutis. Together with its underlying structures, including the central support structures, the corium forms the patrice (or die) which has a very characteristic surface relief. In the perioplic, coronary, sole and bulbar segments it bears papillae whereas in the parietal segment it forms lamellae (404–406).

The *perioplic corium (corium limbi)* (404/*a*) with its *papillae coriales*, appears as the elevated perioplic cushion. The amount of the outer wall which it occupies varies for it is 5–6 mm in breadth dorsally, 4–7 mm laterally and 8 mm in breadth on the palmar or plantar surfaces. A shallow groove separates it from the corium of the hair-bearing skin (404; 405). In the palmar and plantar regions the perioplic corium broadens out as it merges with the bulbar corium (404–406/*b*). A distinct *fold* or *vallum* (404/*1*)

526 Skin and cutaneous organs of ruminants

separates the perioplic corium (/a) from the coronary corium (404, 405/c). This is particularly prominent on the outer (abaxial) wall. The length of the perioplic papillae varies from 1.0 to 1.8 mm, the largest always being situated on the free border of the fold. There are about 20–30 papillae per mm².

The *coronary corium* (*corium coronae*) (404, 405/c) forms the germinative bed of the plate of the claw. The coronary corium borders proximally on the groove formed under the perioplic fold (404/2). It is underlaid by the *coronary cushion* (403/c″) which is a relatively low, raised area. The breadth of the coronary corium on the outer wall is as follows: – dorsally 3 cm, laterally 2.5–3 cm and in the region of the heel 1.5–2 cm. On the interdigital wall it is 2–2.5 cm broad dorsally, 1–1.5 cm in the middle and at the heel 0.5 cm (404, 405). The papillae are 0.2–0.3 mm long and their ends are either conical, rounded or pointed. Lamellae covered by delicate papillae (404/c′) can be seen at the transition to the parietal

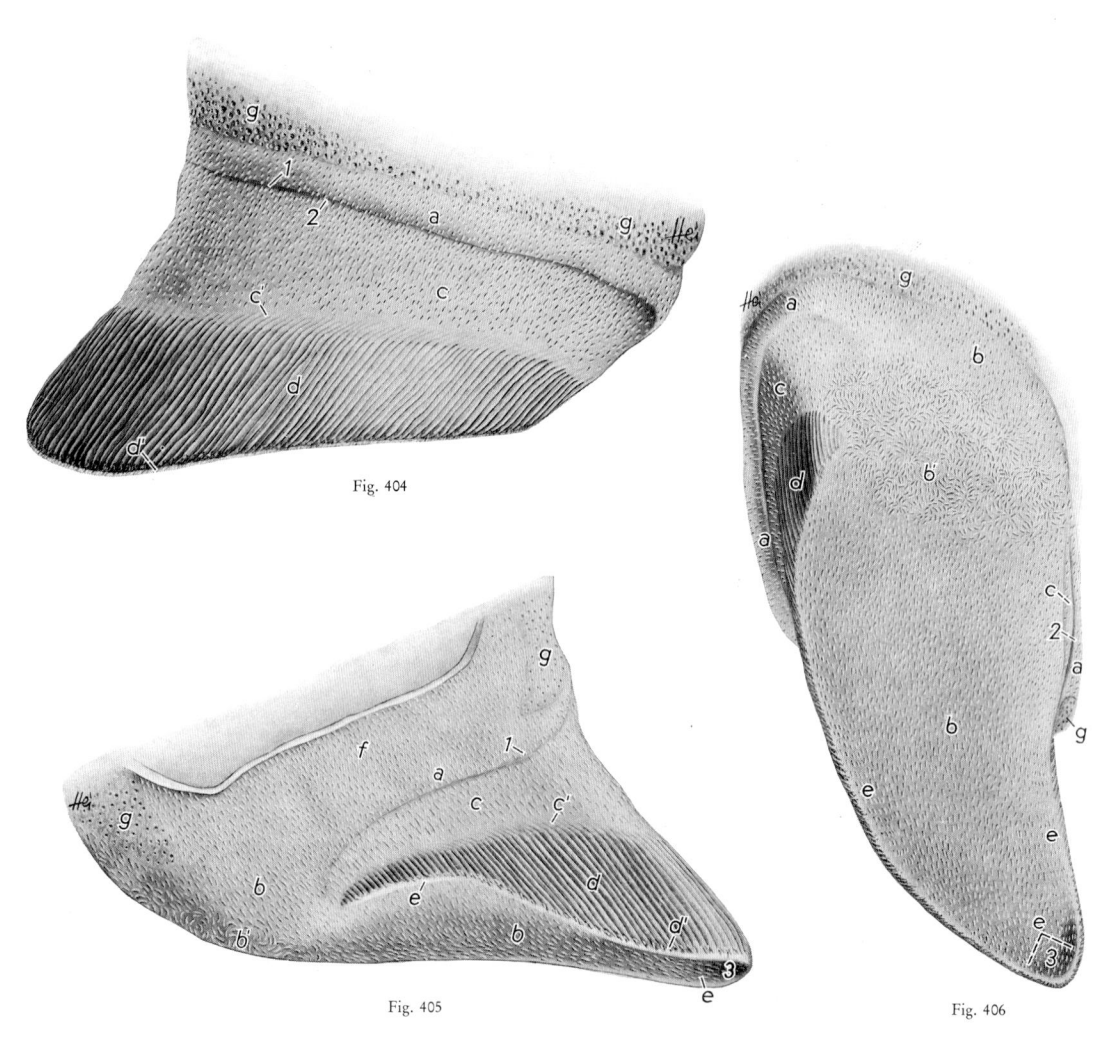

Fig. 404

Fig. 405

Fig. 406

Figs 404–406. Patrice and corium of the outer claw of the left forefoot of the ox. The papillary body is somewhat diagrammatic.
(After Wilkens, 1964.)

Fig. 404: outer surface
Fig. 405: interdigital surface
Fig. 406: ground surface of the patrice

a corium limbi with papillae coriales; *b* corium tori with papillae coriales, *b′* bulbar swelling; *c* corium coronae with papillae coriales, *c′* low lamellae, covered by small, delicate papillae, in the distal part of the coronary segment; *d* corium parietis with lamellae coriales, *d′* distal end of the lamellae covered with papillae; *e* corium soleae with low, papillae-covered lamellae; *f* corium of the hairless skin of the interdigital space, carrying papillae coriales; *g* corium of the hairy skin

1 perioplic fold of the corium limbi; *2* sulcus coronalis; *3* small depression in the solar corium at the point of the claw

corium and these lamellae gradually merge with the corionic lamellae (404, 405/d). This transitional region may be marked by a shallow groove, especially on the outer wall (see distal phalanx). As there are no bars in the ox's foot the corresponding part of the coronary corium is missing.

Distal to the coronary corium is the *parietal corium (corium parietis)* (404, 405/d) which represent the *sterile matrix* of the *horny capsule*. It is somewhat less broad than the coronary corium (404, 405/c). Since the subcutis of the wall forms part of the periosteum of the third phalanx, it takes on the shape of the distal phalanx and continues onto the bearing surface and for a little distance onto the sole surface (406/e). The *laminae* of the *parietal corium* are shorter than in the horse's hoof and they have no secondary lamellae. They vary in length from 0.9 mm at the heel to 2.5 mm dorsally and laterally on the outer wall. They decrease in length from dorsal to palmar (or plantar) (404/d); the thickness of the parietal corium increases in the same direction being between 2–4 mm in the region of the toe and about 7 mm at the bulb. The number of laminae per unit area is greater, especially at the toe, than in the horse. Altogether there are about 1300 laminae covering the laminae corium, which itself has an area of about 14.5 cm^2.

The very narrow *sole corium (corium soleae)* (406/e) occupies only the peripheral areas of the sole surface. The free border of the laminae of the sole corium bears papillae. These laminae can be looked upon as the continuation of the parietal laminae that are reflected onto the sole surface. The papillae are therefore arranged in distinct rows. At the point of the claw there is a concavity the size of a finger tip in the sole corium (/3).

The *bulbar corium (corium tori)* (404–406/b) extends far towards the point of the claw along the bearing surface and makes direct contact with the perioplic corium in a proximo-palmar position (406/b). It is underlaid by the *bulbar cushion* (/b') which flattens off towards the sole segment. Here the bulbar corium (/b) merges, without any demarcation, with the corium of the sole (/b, e). The corium of the bulbs of the two neighbouring toes are often connected. Proximal to this connecting bridge and under the interdigital skin there is a cushion of adipose tissue which reduces friction between the claws during locomotion.

The long, thin and pointed papillae of the bulbar corium are placed close together and form an acute angle with the bearing surface at the tip of the claw (404/b). They are almost vertical in the palmar and plantar regions of the bulb (/b). Their length varies between 0.1 and 1.5 mm and their thickness also varies considerably. The papillae of the bulbar corium are, as a rule, also arranged in rows and in the palmar and plantar areas of the claw they form peculiar whorls (406/b'). This must influence the direction of the horn tubules of the epidermal bulbar segment.

Epidermis of the claw (epidermis ungulae)

The *epidermis* of the claw consists of a stratified squamous epithelium characterized by the multiplicity of its layers and its pronounced keratinization. Its inner surface resembles the outer surface of the corium, every indentation of which it follows like an exact mould. The epidermis forms the horny capsule of the claw, which also has five segments and forms the protective cover of the digital organ. As in the equine hoof, the perioplic, coronary and parietal horn grow in a proximo-distal direction and so form the claw plate. This plate is laid around the central axis of the digit in such a fashion that dorsally a rounded edge is produced (412/a). The plate has a dorsal part or *toe* (407/1), a slightly convex *outer wall* (/2) and a mildly concave *interdigital wall* (409/2') which is, of course, one side of the interdigital cleft (412/e). The *outer* and *interdigital wall* of the plate can be divided into the anterior region or the *quarters*, and the posterior region towards the bulbs, referred to as the *heel*. Distally the toe turns in towards the interdigital space (412/e) and this curvature is more pronounced on the medial than the lateral claw, thus making it possible to distinguish the right foot from the left. The ungulae of the forefoot (/A) are broader, blunter and shorter than those of the hind foot (/B) and the pair of claws of each forefoot has a potentially wider interdigital cleft than has the hind foot. These characteristics help to differentiate the fore and hind feet.

The thickness of the claw plate decreases from the dorsal to plantar (or palmar) aspect but from proximal to distal it increases (403). In the middle of the quarters it is 7 mm (abaxially) and 5 mm (axially) thick.

The tall papillary body (404–406) results in a firm connection being formed between the multilayered, keratinized epidermis of the claw and the corium. At the same time the extensive surface area of these

528 Skin and cutaneous organs of ruminants

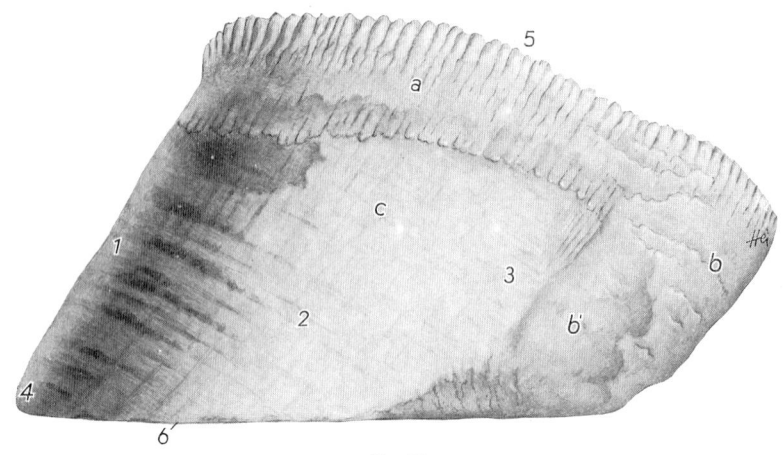

Fig. 407

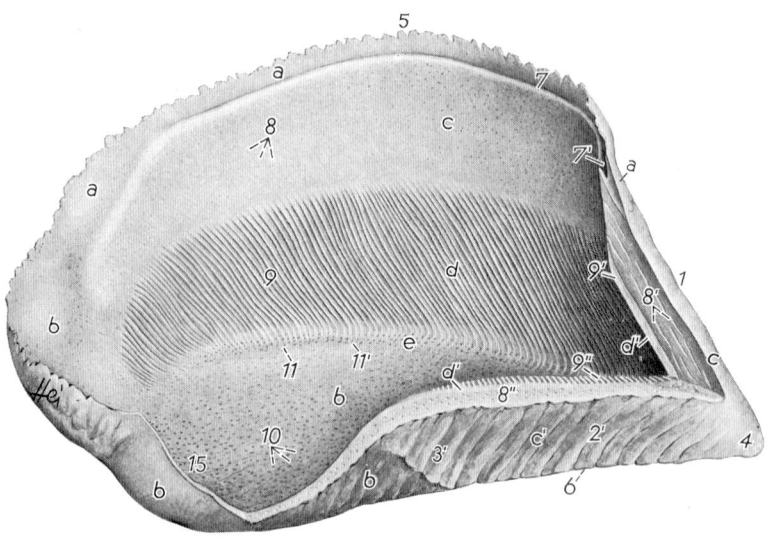

Fig. 408

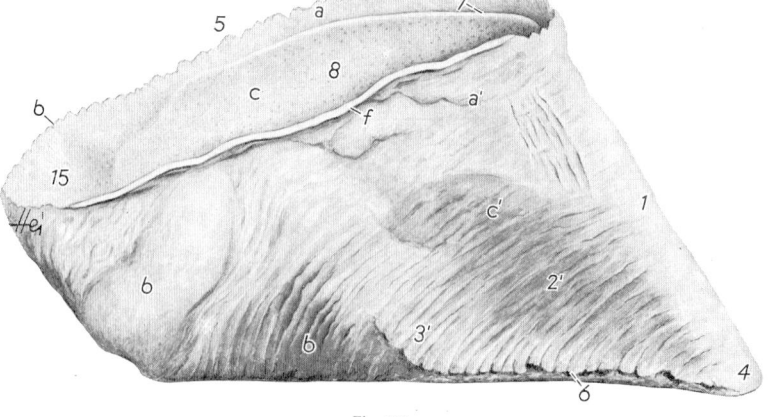

Fig. 409

Fig. 410

Figs. 407–411. Epidermal capsule of the outer claw of the left forefoot of the ox. Internal relief and ground surface are shown in semi-diagrammatic form.
(After Wilkens, 1964.)

Fig. 407: outer wall, lateral view; Fig. 408: outer wall, after substantial removal of the interdigital wall and part of the bulbar epidermis, medial view; Fig. 409: interdigital wall, medial view; Fig. 410: interdigital wall after substantial removal of the outer wall, lateral view; Fig. 411: ground surface of the epidermal claw capsule

a stratum externum parietis cornei lateralis, *a'* stratum externum parietis cornei interdigitalis; *b* epidermis tori, *b'* its swelling extending onto the outer wall; *c* stratum medium parietis cornei lateralis; *c'* stratum medium parietis cornei interdigitalis; *d* stratum internum parietis cornei lateralis, *d'* stratum internum parietis cornei interdigitalis; *e* limb of the sole epidermis bordering on the outer wall, *e'* limb of the sole epidermis bordering on the interdigital wall; *f* epidermis of the cutis in the spatium interdigitale

1 pars dorsalis, *2* pars lateralis, *3* pars palmaris (heels) of the outer wall of the plate; *3'* pars palmaris of the interdigital wall of the plate; *4* point of the claw; *5* margo coronalis; *6* margo soleae; *7* sulcus limbi showing holes for papillae; *7'* groove for perioplic fold; *8* sulcus coronalis with holes for papillae, *8'* horn tubules in longitudinal section, *8"* horn tubules in cross section in the stratum medium parietis cornei (protecting layer), *8'''* ends of horn tubules in the margo solearis; *9* lamellae epidermales of the stratum internum parietis cornei (connecting layer), *9'* longitudinally cut, *9"* transversely cut epidermal lamellae, *9'''* distal ends of the horny lamellae; *10* holes for the papillae in the epidermis tori, *10'* ends of horn tubules on the ground surface of the bulbar segment, *10"* tubules showing through in the palmar region of the epidermis tori; *11* rows of holes for papillae and *11'* epidermal lamellae of the sole epidermis, *11"* ends of the horn tubules on the ground surface of the sole segment; *12* spur; *13* zona alba; *14* the heel part of the wall is slightly curved inwards as a hint of the bar; *15* bulbar "cup" (which covers the bulbar swelling)

Fig. 411

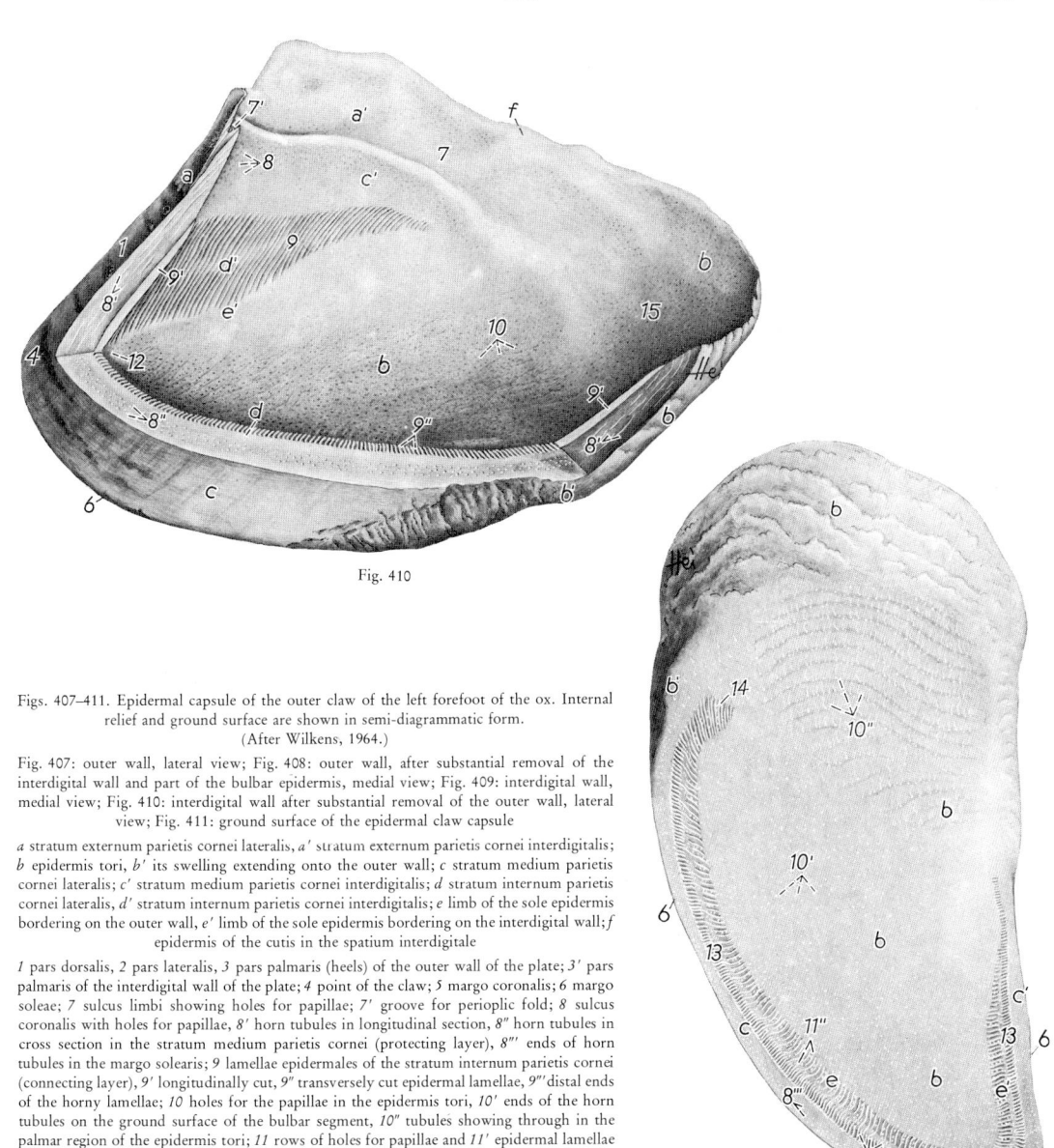

interdigitations ensures adequate nutrition to the epidermis. *Horn tubules* are produced over the papillae of the corium. The *cortex* of these tubules is formed from the *circumpapillary epidermal cells* and the *medulla* of the tubules arises from the *suprapapillary cells*. Between the tubules are the *interpapillary* regions of the corium and the *intertubular horn*. Between the lamellae the active epidermal cells produce the *horn lamellae* which connect the wall segment to the corium (408/*d*). Neither of these lamellae have secondary lamellae; they are non-pennate.

The soft *perioplic horn* is produced by the *perioplic epidermis* (*epidermis limbi*) (403/*a*) and it is confined to the proximal quarter of the parietal wall. Distally it is irregularly demarcated. Its outer wall appears striped (407/*a*). The *protective layer* of the *claw plate* is produced by the epidermis of the *coronet* (*epidermis coronae*) (403/*c*) and it consists of very resistant and hard *coronary horn* (407/*c*; 408/*c'*). In the heel region it is covered by the bulging bulbar horn (407, 408/*b*). On the interdigital surface it forms a free border distopalmarly (or distoplantarly), which folds over the bulbar horn (/*b*).

The general surface of the coronary horn is fluted to a variable degree and these grooves diverge slightly in dorsopalmar direction (407/c). On its interdigital surface the coronary horn is fissured (409/c'), its inner surface, where it lies against the coronary cushion, forms a shallow, broad coronary groove (410/c'). But distal to this region it is covered by the lamellae of the parietal horn (/9). The small holes which receive the little papillae of the coronary corium increase in number in the distal third of the coronary groove, and form rows which run proximodistally between the delicate horn lamellae (/8). The largest horn tubules are found in the middle layer of the coronary epidermis which, as a rule, is non-pigmented.

The lamellae of the parietal epidermis are without secondary lamellae and keratinize only in their central portion (408/d). As a whole the lamellae form the parietal horn and their large epidermal cells intimately contact the lamellae of the parietal corium. The horny lamellae are very short proximally but they quickly increase in size, attaining their full height before half their length is reached (/d). Figure 410/d' illustrates the extent of the parietal epidermis on the interdigital wall. In the last two thirds of the parietal segment, horn is produced along the free borders of the corium lamellae. This horn is pushed between the epidermal lamellae so increasing in mass distally. The horny substance of the parietal segment is only slightly thicker towards the bearing surface. From this one must conclude that horn is produced proximally and that it is pushed over the large epidermal cells of the parietal segment by the downward-growing protective layer of the coronary segment (403/d). The term *sterile matrix* is justified for the parietal epidermis because it produces so little horn.

The distal free ends of the corium lamellae merge into papillae (404, 405/d') and this part of the epidermis then produces tubular horn. On the *bearing surface (margo solearis)* (407/6) the keratinized parietal epidermis forms the *white line* in the claw just as it does in the equine hoof (411/13; 412/d') but it does not usually appear so distinctive against the protective layer because the latter is usually unpigmented in the ox. Keratinization of the superficial layers of cells of the *epidermis* of the *sole (epidermis solearis)* (411/e, e') gives rise to the sole horn. In the bovine claw the latter forms a relatively small part of the *horny sole (solea cornea)* (412/c) and it is difficult to demarcate it from the bulbar horn in poorly maintained claws. It forms two narrow *limbs (crura soleae)* along the *zona alba* (411/e, e''). The sole horn has a tubular structure (/e), borders peripherally on the parietal horn (/c) and merges axially and palmarly (or plantarly) with the bulbar horn (/b). In the calf it is easily recognised as a narrow strip along the white line. It is of about equal width to the white line.

The *epidermis* of the *bulb (epidermis tori)* (407–411/b) produces the bulbar horn by keratinization of its epidermal cells. At the quarters and particularly on the bearing surface of the claw, the bulbar horn extends far towards the tip (/b) and it therefore occupies the greater part of the surface of the sole. The superficial layers of the horny sole are discarded in large flakes.

At the palmar (or plantar) aspect the bulbar horn forms a rounded swelling which represents the limit of the claw (407, 408/b). Between the limbs of the horny sole, the bulbar horn is hard but caudally it is of softer consistency. For this reason the hard bulbar horn and the sole horn were once referred to as the "horny sole of the claw". Although this is incorrect from the morphological viewpoint, the phrase is still used in clinical descriptions.

Unlike the sole of the hoof, the surface of the sole of the claw is not arched but flat (412/c). The inner surface of the palmar (plantar) region of the bulbar horn shows a depression, the bulbar "cup", which corresponds to the bulbar cushion (409/15). At the proximopalmar limit the bulbar horn is directly continuous with the perioplic horn (*epidermis limbi*) (408/a). Reflecting the superficial structure of the bulbar corium, the horn of the bulb consists of tubular and intertubular horn.

Histologically, the *epidermis* of the *coronary* and *parietal* segments shows no discernible str. granulosum either in the juvenile or adult stage. The cells of the superficial layers of the str. spinosum are very flattened and merge immediately with the str. lucidum which is followed by the str. corneum. There is a granulosa layer in the perioplic and bulbar segments.

In the region of the bulbs and the interdigital wall there is a continual distal movement of the horny layers and this is supposed to be the reason for the overlapping of these layers (409/a').

The accessory claws (412, 413) are small and consist, like the main claws, of corium and keratinized epidermis. The latter can often become very long if the tip is not worn by contacting the ground. These accessory claws are attached to the metacarpophalangeal joint proximally by the fascia pedis and the palmar anular ligament of the fetlock in such a way that their dorsal part is turned outwards and its bulbar region faces the pedal axis (412/g). There are additional attachments through the tendons of the accessory claw which join with the fasciae of the pedal joint and with the bulbar cushion. The pronounced protrusion of the perioplic corium is very striking (413/e), as is the well developed perioplic horn (/a) which overlaps the coronary horn (/b) for an appreciable distance. Since the perioplic horn merges with the bulbar horn (/c) without any distinct delineation, the accessory claws are often cylindrical in structure. In other respects its layers are similar to those of the main claws.

The *eponychium* of the claws of newborn calves is bright yellow and soft. It is 1 to 2 cm in length. It dries quickly after birth since it contains much water and within 3 to 24 hours, depending on how much the animal moves about, it is discarded.

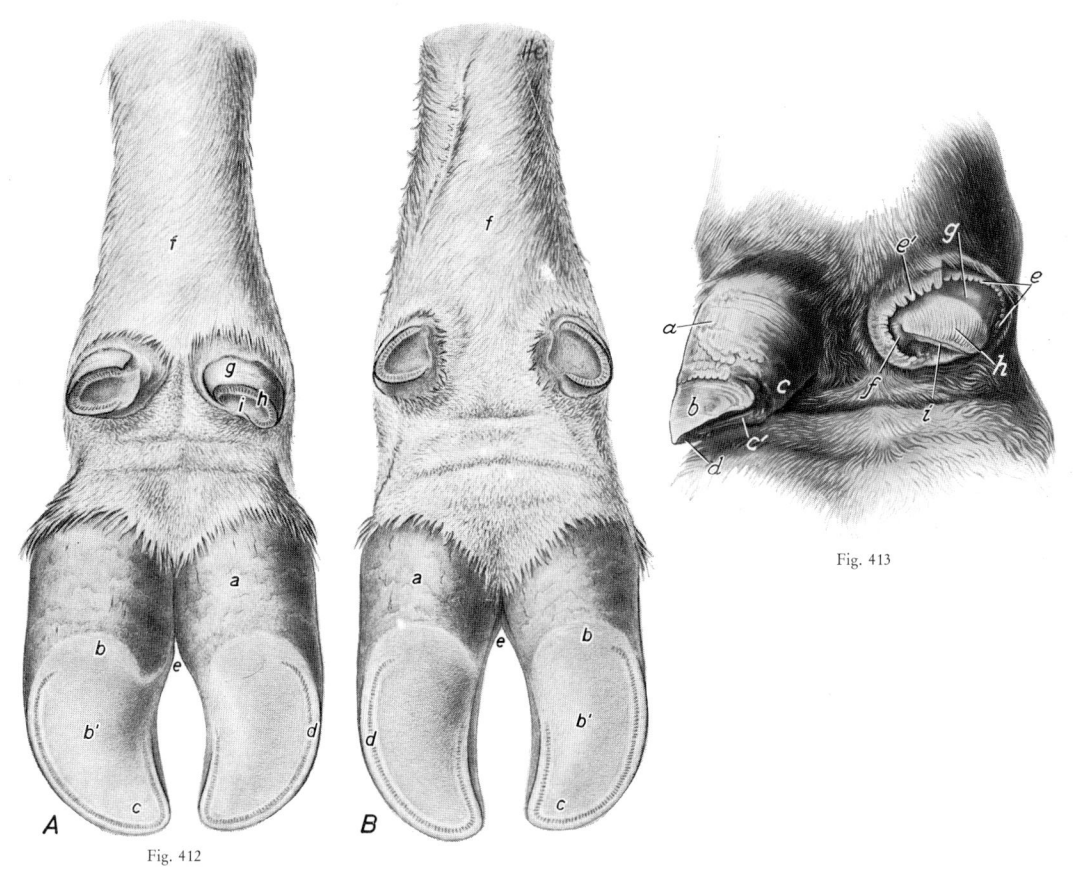

Fig. 412. View of the hoofs of the left fore-(A) and the left hind-(B) foot of the ox looking towards the sole. The primary and accessory claws have been trimmed. About half natural size.

a claw plate; *b* torus corneus, *b'* horny bulb extending into the sole region; *c* solea cornea; *d* margo solearis with zona alba; *e* spatium interdigitale; *f* hair skin; *g* accessory claw; *h* zona alba; *i* solea cornea of the accessory claw

Fig. 413. Accessory claws of the forefoot of the ox. The capsule of the medial accessory claw has been removed. About half natural size.
(After Zietzschmann from Ellenberger-Baum, 1943.)

a bulging covering layer; *b* paries corneus; *c* torus corneus; *c'* bulbar horn extending towards the sole; *d* solea cornea; *e* corium limbi with papillae, *e'* remnants of covering epithelial and horn tissue; *f* corium tori; *g* slightly bulging corium cornae (fertile bed); *h* lamellae-carrying corium parietis (sterile bed); *i* region of the corium soleae

Wilkens (1964), utilizing *polarization* and *electron microscopic* studies, produced a model to illustrate the fine structure of the tubules of the claw. They are likened to the appearance of a pine cone. The *medulla* of the *claw tubules* corresponds to the *central (axial) spindle* of the cone around which the flattened and dish-like, curved *epidermal cells* of the *cortex* are arranged in the form of *scales*. These scales are more or less turned towards the axis of the tubule in the more distal parts. The epidermal cells of the claw tubules are closely interdigitated and joined by desmosomes. The *tonofilaments* of the epidermal cells are arranged in all three directions but they do not extend to the neighbouring cells.

The ability of the horny wall to resist wear is reflected in both the number of horn tubules per unit area and the amount of pigment.

Digital organ of the small ruminants
(414; 415)

The **claws** of sheep and goats are similar in structure to those of pigs. The *horn capsule* has a slightly convex *outer* and somewhat more concave *interdigital wall*. At the *dorsum* (415/a) these two regions meet at an acute angle and form a narrow ridge. The *horny wall* is highest somewhat caudaul to the dorsum (/a). At the *point* of the *toe* (/e) the surface of the sole (/8) is raised so that the wall is shorter in the toe region. The outer wall which covers the whole of the abaxial surface of the distal phalanx decreases only slightly in height towards the palmar (or plantar) region (/a, c, d). The interdigital (axial) wall, on the other hand, reduces much more and covers only the cranial two thirds of the interdigital surface.

Next to the distal rim of the wall is the *white line (zona alba)* which, as in the pig, is formed by the outermost protective layer and the distal end of the horny lamellae of the lower surface of the horn wall. In the goat there is usually only a narrow strip of sole horn (/e) between the white line and the bulbar horn. In the small ruminants the *bulb* displaces the true sole horn so much that the ground surface is formed almost entirely by bulbar horn (/b, e). The bulb gradually increases in breadth in the palmar (or plantar) direction (/b) and, axially and abaxially, it extends steeply upwards at the heels to form the

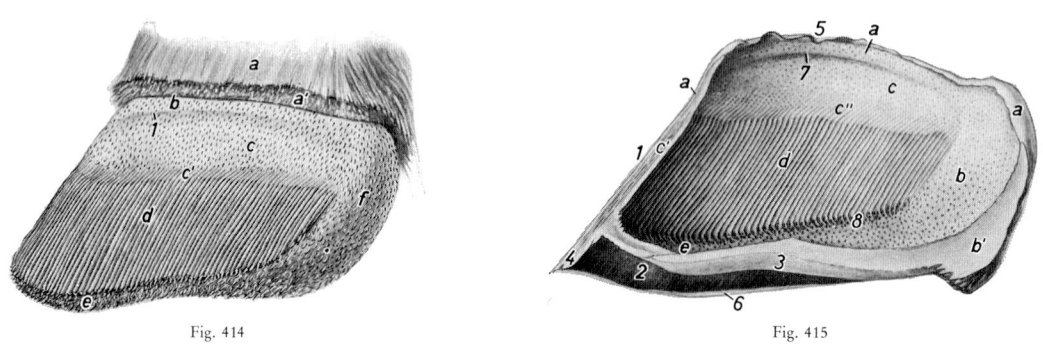

Fig. 414

Fig. 415

Fig. 414. Patrice with corium segments on the outer claw of the forefoot of a sheep. Papillary body somewhat diagrammatic. About natural size.

a hairy skin, *a'* papillary body of the skin; *b* corium limbi with papillae coriales; *c* corium coronae with papillae coriales; *c'* low lamellae, bearing delicate papillae, in the distal part of the coronary segment; *d* corium parietis with lamellae coriales; *e* corium soleae with tall papillae; *f* corium tori with papillae

1 fold of the perioplic segment of the corium

Fig. 415. Epidermal capsule of the right primary claw of the forefoot of a sheep. Interior surface of the outer wall after removal of substantial parts of the interdigital wall. Papillary body somewhat diagrammatic. About natural size.

a epidermis limbi of the outer wall; *b* epidermis tori with holes for the papillae, *b'* cut surface of the bulbar horn; *c* epidermis coronae of the outer wall with holes for the papillae, *c'* tubules in longitudinal section, *c"* transition of tubular horn into laminar horn of the epidermis parietis; *d* epidermis parietis of the outer wall with epidermal lamellae; *e* limb of the sole epidermis which borders on the outer wall and has holes to receive the papillae

1 dorsal part; *2* quarter of the outer wall projecting beyond the sole surface; *3* sole part of the bulbar horn; *4* point of the horny capsule; *5* margo coronalis; *6* margo solearis; *7* sulcus limbalis; *8* papillary holes and epidermal lamellae of the sole epidermis arranged in rows

posterior limit of the claw (/b). The bulb merges with the haired skin without contacting the horny bulb of the neighbouring toe. The bulbar horn of small ruminants is more strongly keratinized (/b') than in the pig and it merges with the horn of the quarters without a demarcation. The solid horn of the wall continues proximally into the narrow, soft perioplic horn (/a), which clearly protrudes above the level of the haired skin. In the interdigital space the two toes are joined by a fold of skin which lies above the periople at the transition of the axial wall into the bulb.

In the goat the hair-bearing skin shows a slight convexity as it merges with the narrow perioplic epidermis (415/a), from which the non-keratinized epithelium of the plate bed is demarcated by a *groove (sulcus limbalis)* (/7). The horn plate is divided into the proximal matrice, or mould, (/c), then followed by the *hyponychium* (/d) and then the distal terminal layer (/e). On the interdigital side the matrice occupies the proximal quarter of the claw and on the outer side the proximal third. It reduces in height not only towards the heel but also towards the toe. The hyponychium shows a similar pattern. Where it becomes narrower, the bulbar epidermis (/b) becomes broader. The claw plate is extraordinarily rigid; in the goat its protective layer is 2 to 3 mm and the connecting layer 1 or 2 mm in thickness. In these animals, too, the thickness of the layers decreases from dorsal to palmar (or plantar). The *ground border* (/6) extends considerably beyond the surface of the sole; this is especially so in animals which have been kept indoors with the result that wear is reduced and the hard axial and abaxial walls may bend over the sole (/6). In the goat the soft bulbar horn does not extend so far towards the apex of the claw as it does in the ox, so that a distinct area of hard sole horn can be identified at the tip of the claw. This is more easily appreciated in the corium where the sole segment (414/e) forms a triangular area at the tip of the claw. This area is clearly demarcated from the posterior bulbar corium (414/f).

The *corium papillae* of the hair-bearing skin of the feet are plump (/a') whereas the *perioplic papillae* (/b) are elongated and thin and their apices are directed slightly distally.

The *papillae* of the *corium* (/c) in the proximal region are also thin but somewhat shorter than those of the perioplic corium. The more distally placed papillae are similar to those of the pig although in the small ruminants they are arranged in regular rows.

The *lamellae* of the *parietal corium* (/d) are arranged in the same direction as the rows of papillae of the coronary corium. Only in the distal region do they carry delicate, distally-pointing papillae. The lamellae finally terminate in a row of long, stout papillae. The number of corium lamellae in the sheep is 550–700 and, as in the ox, secondary lamellae are absent in both sheep and goats.

Papillae of the *bulbar corium* (/f) are of variable length and they are placed in rows only where the bulbar corium borders on the parietal corium. There are *papillae* of the *sole corium* (/e) lying between the bulbar corium and the lower rim of the wall, but they are hardly distinguishable from those of the bulbar corium.

Blood vessels of the digital organ of ruminants
(416; 417)

Arteries
(416)

The *a. digitalis palm.* (or *plant.*) *propr. axialis et abaxialis* of the IIIrd and IVth digits (416/2–5) are primarily responsible for the blood supply to the claws. The dorsal arteries of the toes (*aa. digitales dorss. propr. III* and *IV axiales*) (/7) are of less importance. The palmar (or plantar) digital arteries arise from special vascular arches and from the *a. digitalis palm.* (or *plant.*) *comm. III* (/1) (see pp. 98 and 151).

The palmar (or plantar) and the dorsal vessels are linked in the toe region by the *aa. interdigitales*. The palmar (or plantar) and the dorsal digital arteries give off branches to each phalanx and these are known respectively as *rr. palmares* (or *plantares*) and *dorsales phalangia prox., med.* and *dist*. They are also linked by means of anastomoses. The smaller *aa. digitales palmm.* (or *plantt.*) *proprr. abaxiales* (/2, 5) terminates by forming a network in the bulb of the same side to which the *a. digitalis palm* (or *plant. com.* (/1) contributes branches known as the *rr. tori digitales* (/9, 9').

The larger *aa. digitales palmm.* (or *plantt.*) *proprr. axiales* of the *III*rd and *IV*th toes (/3, 4), give off the *rr. palmares* (or *plantares*) (/14) and then run dorsad in the interdigital space, finally entering the horn capsule near the dorsal contour of the claw. At the last location each gives off a stout *a. coronalis* (/11) which divides into one deep and two superficial vessels for the coronary cushion and its skin covering. The axial digital arteries then continue as the *a. phalangis distalis* (/13) and enter the distal phalanx through the axial foramen. Before doing so, they give off a vessel (/12) to the extensors of the digit and the dorsal aspect of the distal interphalangeal joint. The distal phalangeal artery runs through the ungular canal parallel to the axial parietal groove until it almost reaches the tip of the phalanx then, making an acute angled turn, it continues parallel to the abaxial parietal groove in a palmar (or plantar) direction and emerges again from the abaxial foramen. The part of the vessel which runs in the ungular canal of the third phalanx is known as the arcus terminalis (/15), because the vessel turns back as it leaves the canal and anstomoses with the bulbar arteries (/17) and the terminal branches of the proper abaxial palmar (or plantar) digital artery of the IIIrd and IVth toes (/10, 10'). The arcus terminalis is therefore an arch-like link between the axial and abaxial digital arteries which run down the outside and inside of the toes. Within the angular canal the arch gives off numerous small branches which perforate the bone en route to the corium of the coronet, wall, bulb and sole. A stouter, more proximal branch (/18) forms an anastomosis with the deep branch of the *coronal artery* (/11) and also provides several small branches to the parietal corium. Two further branches (/15') go to the tip of the toe where they ramify in the corium of the sole and in the axial and abaxial parietal corium and then anastomose with the *a. marginis solearis* (/16). One stout and several small arteries run parallel to the surface of the sole to reach the walls of the claw; secondary branches turn off distally to the ground surface where some of them join together to form an arcade-like pattern. These arched anastomoses are collectively referred to as the artery of the rim of the sole, *a. marginis solearis* (/16). Other thicker branches supply the corium of the axial and abaxial wall, of the sole and of the bulb.

The accessory claw always has an *axial* vessel whereas the *abaxial* vessel is not invariably present.

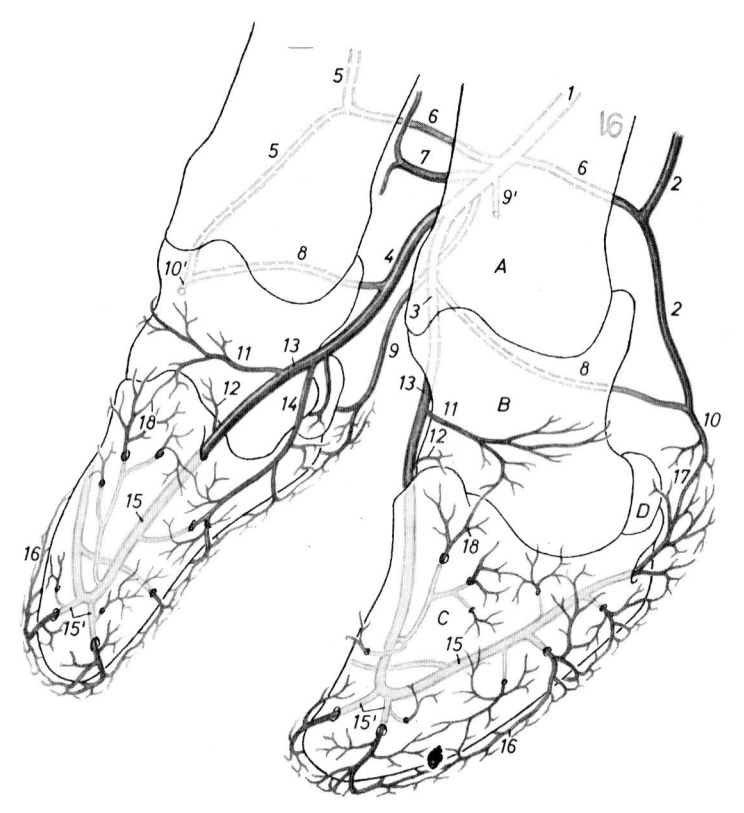

Fig. 416. Arteries of the claw of the right forefoot of the ox, somewhat diagrammatic. Craniomedial view. The claws are maximally spread. Drawn from a plastic corrosion preparation. About natural size.

A phalanx proximalis; *B* phalanx media; *C* phalanx distalis; *D* os sesamoideum distale

1 a. digitalis palmaris communis III; *2* a. digitalis palmaris propria III abaxialis; *3* a. digitalis palmaris propria III axialis; *4* a. digitalis palmaris propria IV axialis; *5* a. digitalis palmaris propria IV abaxialis; *6* anastomosing rr. palmares phalangium proximalium; *7* a. interdigitalis III; *8* rr. palmares phalangium mediarum; *9, 9'* rr. tori digitales of the axial digital arteries, at 9' cut off; *10, 10'* rr. tori digitales of the abaxial digital arteries, cut off at 10'; *11* rr. dorsales phalangium mediarum with aa. coronales; *12* branch of the a. phalangis distalis to the extensors of the toe; *13* a. phalangis distalis; *14* r. plantaris; *15* arcus terminalis; *15'* its branches to the tip of the claw; *16* a. marginis solearis; *17* anastomoses between the arcus terminalis and the arterial bulbar network; *18* connecting branches between the arcus terminalis and the aa. coronales

Veins
(417)

Unlike the arteries, which supply each individual claw by means of one large vessel only, the venous blood is collected from each claw by three veins. These are referred to as the dorsal (main drainage vessel) and two lateral veins of the digit.

In the forelimb the bulk of the blood is drained by an *anastomosis* (417/9) between the third common dorsal digital vein *(v. digitalis dors. com. III)* (/1) and the third common palmar digital vein *(v. digitalis palm. com. III)* (/2). There is no such anastomosis in the hind limb.

The dorsal digital vein *(v. digitalis dorsalis prop. axialis)* of each major claw (/7, 8) arises from the third common dorsal digital vein (/1) and runs abaxially towards the dorsum of the claw, giving off the *r. dorsalis phalangis mediae* (/7', 8'). This ramus runs towards the coronary border in the dorsal region of the horny claw but divides before it is reached. Its two arched branches continue in superficial position both along the axial and the abaxial surface of the coronary swelling, to a palmar (or plantar) position. These vessels may therefore be referred to as the *v. coronalis supf. axialis et abaxialis* (/11, 11'). Both these vessels participate in the formation of the superficial coronary and parietal networks and freely anastomose with the vessels of, respectively, the axial or abaxial digital veins. The abaxial superficial coronary vein (/11) also sends a slender branch through the foramen on the proximal part of the abaxial surface of the third phalanx into the depth of the bone.

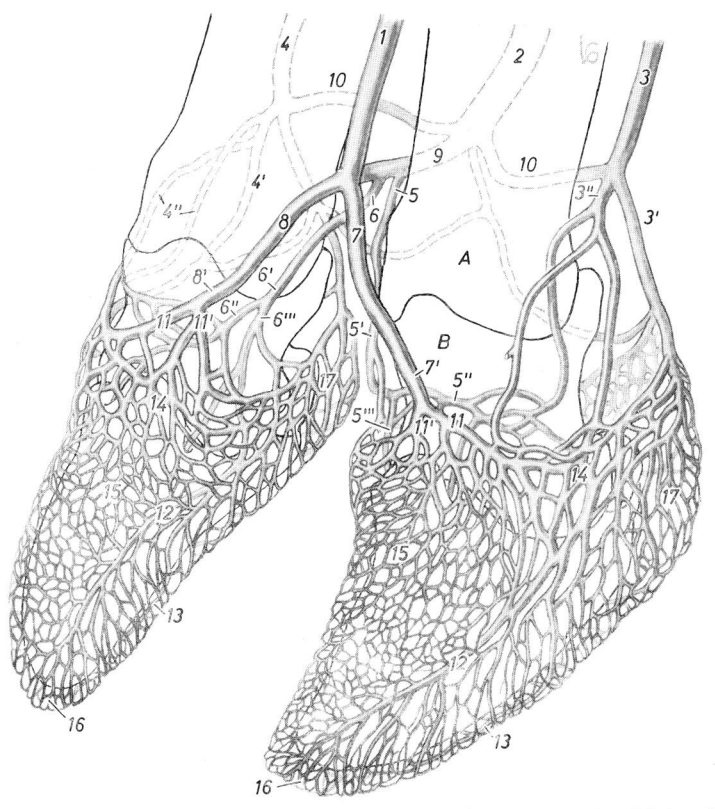

Fig. 417. Veins and venous plexuses of the hoof of the right forefoot of the ox, somewhat diagrammatic. Craniomedial view with the claws maximally spread. The venous networks have been simplified. Drawn from a plastic corrosion preparation. About natural size.

A phalanx proximalis; *B* phalanx media

1 v. digitalis dorsalis communis III; *2* v. digitalis palmaris communis III; *3* v. digitalis palmaris propria III abaxialis; *3'* its bulbar branch, v. tori digitalis, *3"* its bifurcation into the r. dorsalis phalangis mediae and collateral vv. coronales; *4* v. digitalis palmaris propria IV abaxialis, *4'* its bulbar branch v. tori digitalis, *4"* its bifurcation into the r. dorsalis phalangis mediae and collateral vv. coronales; *5, 5', 5"'* v. digitalis palmaris propria III axialis, *5"* v. coronalis profunda, *6, 6', 6"'* v. digitalis palmaris propria IV axialis, *6"* v. coronalis profunda; *7* v. digitalis dorsalis propria III axialis, *7'* r. dorsalis phalangis mediae; *8* v. digitalis dorsalis propria IV axialis, *8'* r. dorsalis phalangis mediae; *9* v. interdigitalis III; *10* rr. palmares phalangium proximalium; *11* v. coronalis superficialis, abaxial branch, *11'* v. coronalis superficialis, axial branch; *12* r. dorsalis phalangis distalis; *13* v. marginis solearis; *14* venous networks of the coronary corium; *15* venous networks of the parietal corium; *16* venous networks of the sole corium; *17* venous networks of the bulbar corium

From their network the *v. coronalis supf. axialis et abaxialis* (/11, 11') each give off a fairly large vessel which descends about half the height of the wall to form an anastomosis with a corresponding branch of the abaxial digital vein. This anastomotic vessel runs parallel to the bearing surface along the axial and abaxial parietal grooves as the parietal collecting vein (*v. dorsalis phalangis digitalis*) (/12). It progresses towards the tip of the phalanx where it joins the sole network. This collecting vein receives blood from both the proximal and distal regions of the parietal corium. All the veins which join the collecting vein from distal may be linked with one another on the border of the sole by anastomoses to form the slender vein of the sole border *(v. marginis solearis)* (/13). From the two lateral veins of the toe the axial digital veins of each claw originate via the stout anastomosis (/9) between the dorsal and palmar common vein of the third digit (/1, 2). They continue as the axial palmar proper veins of the IIIrd and IVth digits (*v. digitalis palm. prop. III. axialis*) (/5) and *v. digitalis palm. prop. IV. axialis* (/6)) to the axial surface of the claw. Here they divide into a *v. coronalis prof.* (/5″, 6″) and the *v. phalangealis dist.* (/5‴, 6‴).

The *distal phalangeal vein* (/5‴, 6‴) gives off some branches to the coronary cushion and to the parietal (/15) and bulbar (/17) corium.

The *deep coronary vein* (/5″, 6″) also divides into an axial and an abaxial branch which pass under the superficial coronary vein in a palmar direction. They anastomose with those branches which form the deep coronary and parietal networks (/14, 15).

In the palmar region of both the coronet and the wall, the branches of the dorsal and axial digital veins link up with the corresponding branches of the abaxial digital vein and their terminal ramifications form the bulbar venous network (/17). Reference has already been made to the participation of the *v. digitalis palm. prop. III abaxialis* (/3) and the *v. digitalis palm. propr. IV. abaxialis* (/4) in the formation of the *axial* and *abaxial collecting veins* of the wall of the claw.

The collecting veins of the wall *(vv. dorsales phalangis distalis)* (/12) are, as a rule, thicker than the veins of the margin of the sole (/13).

Each of these large veins gives rise to a larger number of smaller veins which join to form the large-meshed *networks* of the *sole* (/16) and *parietal* (/15) *corium*. Peripherally these branches also form another, denser, precapillary network, so that the corium of the claw contains a coarse inner and a fine outer venous reticulum.

The following venous networks can thus be differentiated in the bovine claw:

1. The *venous networks* of the *parietal corium* (/15), which are in two layers. Their drainage is via the dorsal (/7, 8) and, to a lesser extent, via the axial (/5, 6) and abaxial (/3, 4) digital veins.

2. The *venous sole networks* (/16), which are duplicated at the tip of the toe but are otherwise only single. Their blood is discharged into the axial (/5, 6) and abaxial (/3, 4) digital veins.

3. The *networks* of the *bulb* (/17), which carry blood through the *vv. tori digitales* (/3′, 4′) and other branches. They mainly empty into the axial (/5, 6) and abaxial digital veins (/3, 4).

4. *Networks* of the *coronary region* (/14) which join up to form the large axial and abaxial superficial coronary veins (/11, 11′). They discharge their blood via these collecting trunks into the dorsal, axial and abaxial digital veins.

5. The *venous network* of the *distal phalanx*. This is not very distinct in the ox but it is well developed in the small ruminants, especially the goat.

The networks of the parietal and sole corium are joined to the plexus of the pedal bone by special channels. This is again more pronounced in the small ruminants than in the ox. This network at the tip of the phalanx forms the drainage route for the *inner venous sole network*.

In the claws of the hind feet, the proper dorsal digital veins resemble the analogous vessels of the forelimb. At the level of the accessory claw the *arcus venosus metatarsalis plant.* (see. p. 255) gives rise to the *vv. digitales plantt. proprr.* The last-named veins then form the *arcus venosus digitalis plant.* which also receives the *v. digitalis plant. comm.* The axial digital veins arise from this latter arch and run in the interdigital ligament and in the adipose tissue of the digital cushion towards the bulb where they fuse with branches of the bulbar vein.

The superficial coronary, the bulbar, the distal phalangeal and the veins to the skin of the claw are similar to those of the forelimb.

In all parts of the corium of the claw there are venous valves; they are particularly numerous in the veins and venous plexuses of the coronary rim. As in the equine hoof, there are *throttle veins* and *arteries* in the venous system of the claw. *Arteriovenous anastomoses* occur throughout the corium of the claw where they take the form of marginal loops with a peripheral (in the papillae) and a central (in the lamellae) capillary network. A continuous blood flow is ensured by an arteriovenous pressure gradient in the anastomoses and the capillaries and this is maintained by venous valves and by movement of the structures within the claw when the animal places weight on it.

The pattern of the *blood capillaries* of the *corium* is largely dependent on the *shape* and *size* of the *papillae* and *lamellae*. However, there are also other vascular patterns. As a rule the shape of the papillary body and the capillary pattern are dependent on the function of the individual parts of the digital organ. The germinative matrices have better developed vascular networks than the sterile matrices, for the latter have a lower functional requirement.

In principle the organization of the blood vessels of the digital organ of the pig, ox and small ruminant is fairly uniform.

Skin and cutaneous organs of the horse

Skin of the horse

(341; 348–350; 418)

The **skin** (*cutis*) usually closely follows the contours of the horse's body, though in most regions it readily glides over the underlying tissues. There are constant folds of skin between the chest and the forelimb, and between the abdominal wall and the knee, known respectively as the axillary and the knee folds, which permit the skin to be freely moved by the associated cutaneous musculature. In areas where this musculature is well-developed, as over the chest, the abdomen, the scapula and the lower arm, the skin can be vigourously twitched as a defence against biting insects or to shake off dust or water.

The *epidermis* lacks a *str. lucidum*, and its surface layers are continually desquamated as fine, light-coloured or grey scales, which, apart from dust, form the main ingredient of scurf.

The corium of the horse has an average thickness of 3.8 mm, which is thinner than in cattle. It is thickest on the head and back, less thick on the abdomen and chest wall, and thinnest on the udder, the inner surface of the thigh, and the external genitalia.

Young individuals have a finer and more vascular skin than older animals, and their coats are smoother and more glossy. However, the fine, elastic, smooth and pliant nature of the skin also depends on the health of the animal, its breed, how well it is cared for, and on the climate in which it lives.

The contours of the bones in the distal limbs can often be recognised in fine-skinned horses such as thoroughbreds. Similarly the profiles of various muscles and tendons, and superficial blood vessels such as the facial vein and its branches, the external thoracic vein, and the superficial veins of the udder may be easily seen. Other skin veins on the head, shoulder, lower arm, cannon and abdomen become prominent after prolonged exercise.

In addition to the thick, elastic *long hairs* previously mentioned (341/*f*), and the thick, stiff *awn hairs* (11–17 mm) with long tips and even shafts (/*f'*), horses also possess long, thin, slightly-coiled *awn hairs* with *short tips*. Between these are found the very thin, short, wavy *wool hairs*, whose shafts are of an even thickness. Generally, the hairs are finer and less closely-packed around the eyes and the external genitalia, and the anal and perineal region.

The outer hairs become long and rough with constant exposure to the cold, as in Northern climates and in cold, draughty stabling, while in ponies they can be twice as long as in other breeds of horses. During winter too, the outer hairs usually become longer than in summer.

Thoroughbreds often have fine, glossy hair, but it is not possible to make a positive identification of the breed on the basis of length, thickness and scale size of the hair cortex, or the shape of its medulla. From birth to about 8 weeks old, the hair of horse foals shows a slight curl formation which in donkey foals is very distinct (cf. p. 457). Mane and tail hairs of both foal types show little tendency to curl and they have no sheen at all. They are replaced towards the end of their first year by permanent long hairs.

Horses may be identified by their *coat colour* and their markings, which can be areas of congenitally non-pigmented hairs on the head and limbs, or acquired areas of pigment loss on other parts of the body caused by injuries, or saddle or harness pressure.

The most important basic colours that are recognised are chestnut, black, brown and grey. The *chestnut* horse for instance, has body hairs of various shades of red or liver, and long hairs which are various shades of chestnut but not black. In *black* horses on the other hand, both the body and long hairs are black, while in *brown* individuals, the body hairs are brown and the long hairs black. *Grey* horses have white hairs over the entire body, though they can occasionally be born with white outer hair and a lack of pigment in the skin, the hoofs and, rarely, the iris. Albinos, however, usually have a pink skin and a pink iris. Genuine greys can sometimes be born with dark hairs which later change to white (see p. 456), and though at that time their dark outer hairs may be mixed with white, the skin, hoofs and iris are always pigmented.

Various secondary colours and combinations of colours exist as, for example, in bays, duns and roans. In greys, the colours may be flecked, dappled or patchy, the last being known as piebald if the patches are black and skewbald if the colour is other than black. Patchily-distributed non-pigmented areas can also occur on the lips or other parts of the head, where they are known as stars, blazes, etc. or when on the limbs, as socks or stockings.

Traces of feral markings can still be recognised in some horses. They are most noticeable and common in duns, whose long hair, like that of brown horses, is black. These feral marks occur with decreasing frequency in chestnuts, creams and greys. They take the form of lines down the back, when they are known as eel marks, or as shoulder, neck or lumbar lines, and possibly as cross stripes on the limbs. The base of the tail may also be striped, and this usually appears as four transverse lines which interrupt the median eel mark.

The horse exhibits a number of diverging hair vortices – one on the upper and the lower lip, and two in both the thoracic and inguinal regions (349/*f*), while one or more vortices can be present on the forehead and forelock. In other parts of the body, vortices may occasionally be found at the level of the manubrium (/*c*), and in the elbow regions, the scrotum, umbilicus and ischiatic tuber etc., but these are usually *converging vortices* (349).

Tactile hairs are rarely found around the chin or the cheeks of the horse (348), but some 2 to 5 sinus hairs are present over the eyes. There are 9 to 18 tactile hairs (348), some of which may be as long as 12 cm, arranged in two rows on the lower eyelid, whilst as many as 50 sinus hairs have been counted on both the *upper* and *lower labial regions*. These are arranged in groups on either side, but they do not extend beyond the commissures of the lips. In addition to the sinus hairs, the lips present tactile hairs, which are basically ordinary coat hairs with a specialized innervation. Otherwise, the colour of both types is the same as that of the coat, or perhaps somewhat darker.

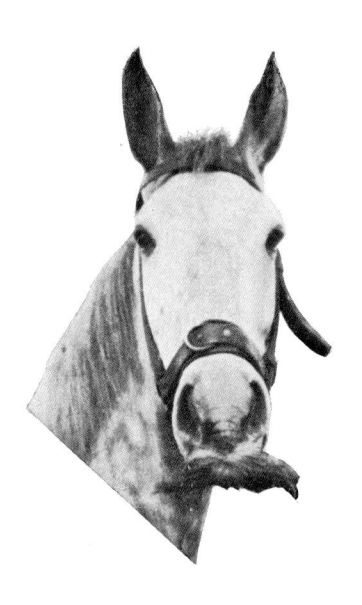

Some 2.5% of all horses develop **moustaches** on the upper lip (418). These are most commonly met with in heavy bay draught horses, but they are seldom seen in thoroughbreds, ponies, donkeys, mules and zebras, and there is considerable individual variation in the position, shape, colour, length and thickness of the moustaches which occur in both sexes. Moustache hairs represent intermediate forms of coat and long hairs, and they are never shed when the coat moults. The tendency to develop a moustache stays with the animal throughout its life, and this can be an important factor for purposes of identification.

Fig. 418. Well developed moustache in a thoroughbred horse. (Photograph: R. Rudofsky.)

Sebaceous and *sweat glands* have an ubiquitous distribution throughout the horse's skin. There is, however, a characteristic concentration of sebaceous glands in the perineal and anal regions, and there are tubular glands in the frog stay, the *gldd. tori*, the secretion of which is used for marking trails (see p. 466).

The blood supply to the horse's skin arises from branches of the arteries serving the superficial muscle layers of the body, and the skin veins drain into the veins of the same layers (see above). Arterio-arterial and veno-venous anastomoses are found everywhere, and arterio-venous anastomoses occur in the region of the ears, around the coronary rim and in the corium of the hoof (see p. 557).

Mammary gland of the horse
(419–421)

The lactating **mammary gland** of the horse takes the form of a flattened hemisphere situated in the inguinal region, and it comprises a right and left *glandular body* (mamma) (419/*a*). Each mamma bears a single, laterally-compressed, blunt, cone-shaped *teat* (/*b*; 420/*a*). The two mammae are separated by a broad, median *sulcus intermammarius* (/*c*), the skin of which has numerous sebaceous glands whose dark-grey, greasy secretion protects the two halves of the udder when rubbing against each other in locomotion. Otherwise, the skin of the mammary gland and teats bears many apocrine tubular glands and fine hairs. Its colour is usually black, though in piebald or striped animals, it is either non-pigmented or pigmented in patches.

Each *mammary complex* consists of *two cavity systems*. These are not visible in the live animal, but the cranial one is the larger (421). The apex of each teat bears a shallow depression which contains two, or occasionally three, *teat canal orifices (ostia papillaria)*, placed one behind the other (420/*b*). A cluster of 5–8 hairs projects from these orifices in newly-born fillies, but as they are only loosely attached, they are absent in udders that have lactated. The teat canal is 5–10 mm long (421/*h*, *h'*). Its mucosa is darkly pigmented and it is thrown into prominent longitudinal folds. The epithelium is keratinized stratified squamous, and the transition to the columnar epithelium of the *teat cistern* is gradual, which is at variance with the situation in ruminants and cats. The teat cisterns (/*g*, *g'*) take the form of dilated canals which pass up the teat to end in their appropriate cranial and caudal *glandular cisternae* (/*f*, *f'*). Any

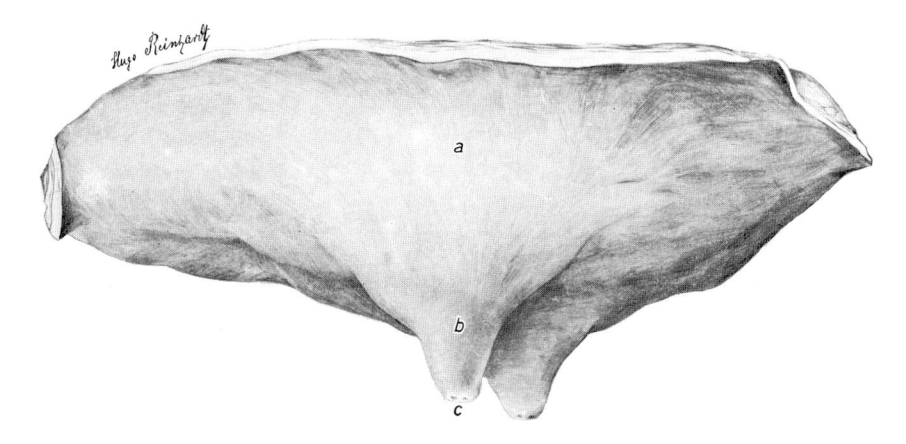

Fig. 419. Mammary gland of a mare. Lateral view.
(After Martin, 1915.)
a corpus mammae; *b* papilla mammae; *c* ostia papillaria

accessory teat cisterns which may be present communicate directly with the glandular parenchyma above. The mucosa of the teat cisterns bears many longitudinal and transverse folds. The middle layer, containing muscle and connective tissue, is well-developed, as are the deep layers of the skin, which are especially rich in elastic fibres, but there is no readily-discernible teat sphincter. At the same time, the vascularization of the teat is relatively poor, the veins – unlike those of the cow – having no valves and a noticeably thin media. A suckling mare will produce about 10 litres of milk per day.

Accessory teats are rarely found in the mare, and they are not at all common in the stallion or gelding. Two are regularly found in the donkey stallion in which, when the penis is retracted, each lies caudo-laterally to the preputial orifice, about 4–5 cm cranial to the scrotum. Any accessory teats are cone-shaped, and about 1–1.5 cm long and 0.5–1.0 cm in diameter. They usually have two ostia at the apex.

Blood vessels of the mammary gland of the horse

Arteries

The *external pudendal artery*, the calibre of which is about 5–7 mm, accompanies a thin vein through the inguinal canal before dividing into a stout cranial branch, which passes between the abdominal wall and the udder, and a smaller caudal branch. Both vessels run some 3–4 cm from the linea alba, where they can be termed the *cranial* and *caudal mammary arteries*. Both give off many tributaries to the udder and the teats. The cranial branch, however, supplies mainly the udder and the skin as far forward as the umbilicus, whilst the caudal branch also supplies the mammary lymph nodes, before anastomosing with the *obturator artery*.

Veins

The short, stout external pudendal vein runs between the gracilis and pectineus muscles, 4–5 cm caudal to the artery of the same name. Ventral to the pubis, the vein communicates with its neighbour on the other side, then it forms either a trunk or a coarse plexus of vessels between the ventral abdominal wall and the udder, before giving rise to several large branches which run to the mammary gland and mammary lymph nodes. Cranially, these trunks or plexuses are continuous with the *superficial cranial epigastric vein (v. subcutanea abdominis)*, and caudally with the *obturator*, or the *dorsal labial* and *mammary vein*, which are branches of the *internal pudendal vein*. Small twigs also unite with the previously-mentioned vein which accompanies the external pudendal artery.

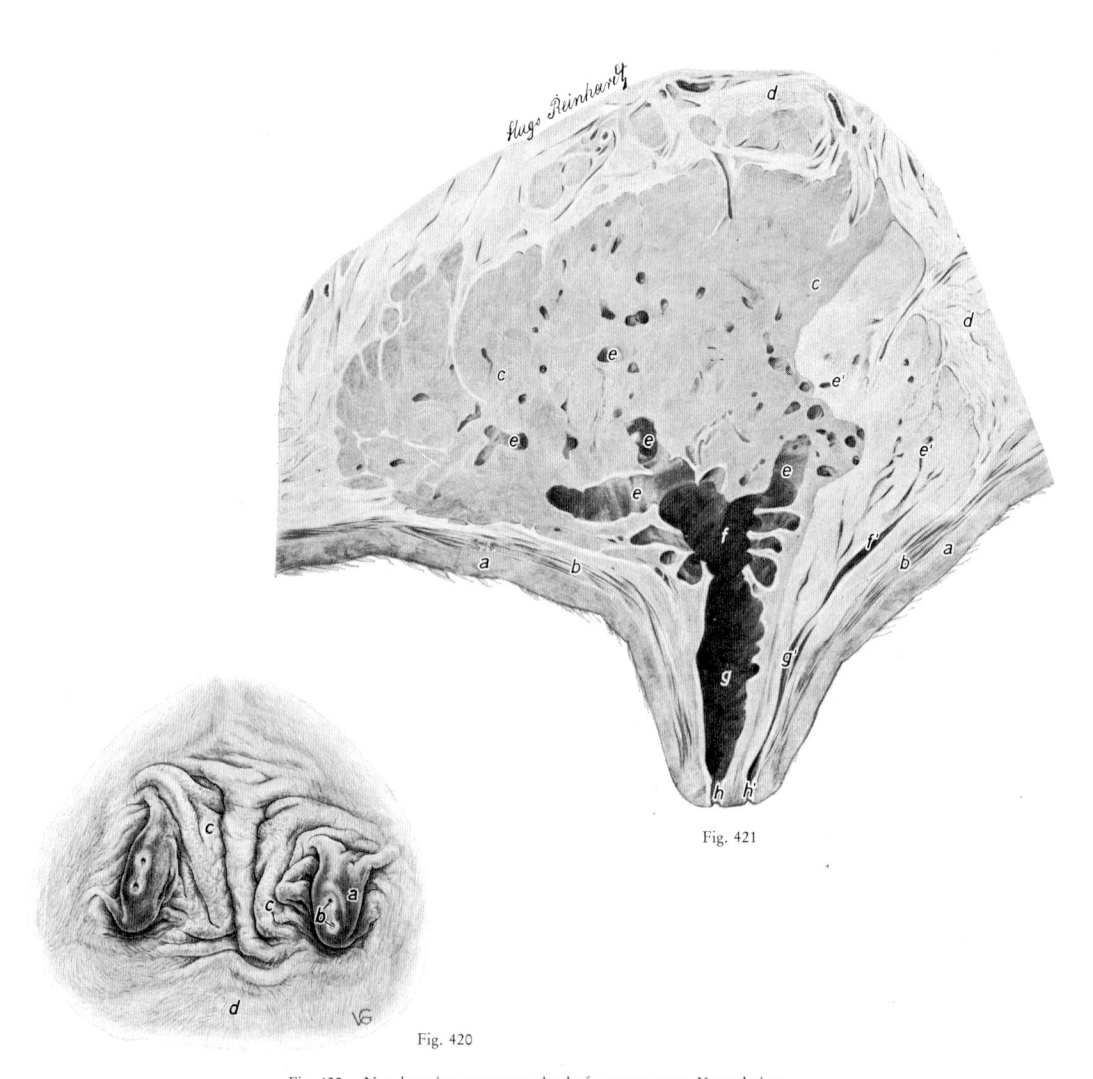

Fig. 421

Fig. 420

Fig. 420. Non-lactating mammary gland of a young mare. Ventral view.
a papilla mammae; *b* ostia papillaria; *c, c* skin area containing sebaceous glands, lying between the two halves of the udder; *d* delicately haired skin

Fig. 421. Sagittal section through half of a mare's udder; one of its quarters (e–h) was filled with mucilage, so as to visualise its duct system. The unfilled quarter (e'–h') appears somewhat lighter and its duct system is only partly visible.
(After Martin, 1915.)

a cutis; *b* tela subcutanea; *c* glandula mammaria; *d* adipose tissue; *e, e'* ductus lactiferi in section; *f, f'* pars glanularis, *g, g'* pars papillaris sinus lactiferi; *h, h'* ductus papillaris

The digital organ of the horse
General considerations

The **digital organ** of the horse, the *hoof (ungula)*, is the modified distal extremity of the single-toed foot. During phylogenesis, it increased in size as a four-toed structure before evolving into one sculpted around the single third digit.

Topographically, the hoof is divided into six regions: the *periople (limbus ungulae)* (365/n), the *coronet (corona ungulae)* (/h), the *wall (paries ungulae)* (/o), the *sole (solea ungulae)* (/q), the *frog (cuneus ungulae)* (/r'), and the *bulb (torus ungulae)* (/r).

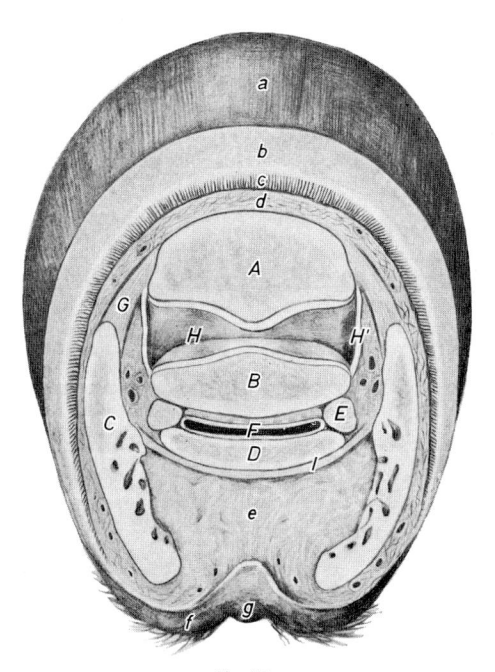

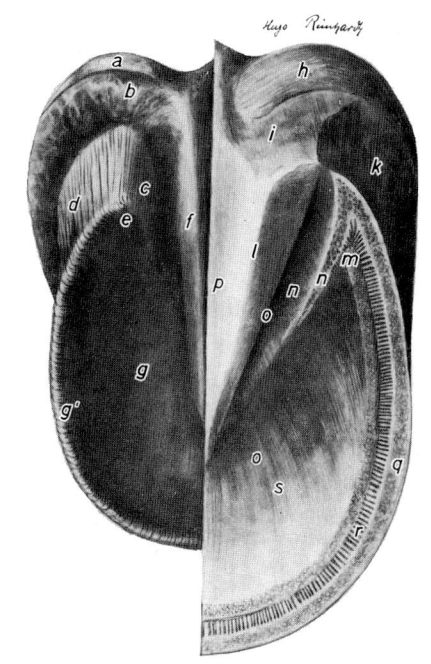

Fig. 422. Transverse section through the hoof of a horse cut in a slightly oblique plane and tilted towards the bulbs. (After Martin, 1915.)

A phalanx distalis; *B* os sesamoideum distale; *C* cartilago ungularis; *D* tendon of the m. flexor digitalis profundus; *E* suspensory ligament of the navicular bone; *F* bursa podotrochlearis; *G* colateral ligament of the coffin joint; *H* articular surfaces of the navicular and pedal bones, *H'* capsule of the coffin joint; *I* anular ligament of the digit

a paries corneus; *b* tubuli epidermales coronae; *c* lamellae epidermales et coriales; *d* corium parietis; *e* tela subcutanea cunei; *f* torus corneus; *g* median tip of the bulbar horn

Fig. 423. The left half of the equine hoof has been removed. The left shows the parts of the corium, the right the regions of the horny capsule. Sole aspect. (After Martin, 1915.)

a corium limbi; *b* tela subcutanea coronae with corium coronae; *c* lamellae coriales of the bar; *d* lamellae coriales of the parietal corium; *e* parietal corium at the angle of the heel; *f* corium cunei; *g* corium soleae, *g'* transition from the lamellae of the parietal matrix to the papillae of the sole matrix; *h* torus corneus; *i* transition from the horny bulb into the horny frog; *k* horn plate; *l* crus cunei; *m* horn capsule inflected at the heel; *n* bar region of the horn plate; *o* sulcus paracunealis; *p* sulcus cunealis centralis; *q* margo solearis; *r* zona alba; *s* solea cornea

The skeleton of the digital organ (see Vol. I, Passive Locomotor Apparatus), comprises the distal coronary bone (middle phalanx) (/B), the pedal bone (distal phalanx) (/C), and the navicular bone (distal sesamoid) (/D). The hoof cartilages (422/C), the ligaments (365/3, 5), the flexor (/2) and extensor (/1) tendons, and the navicular bursa (bursa podotrochlearis), (/8), are regarded as accessory supporting structures. All are covered by common integument, which has become highly modified. Hair and sebaceous glands, for instance, are absent and modified apocrine tubular glands are strictly confined to the frog.

The *subcutis (tela subcutanea ungulae)* (/a–e'), which immediately overlies the skeleton and accessory structures, shows considerable variation in structure. In areas where it is directly applied to the hard tissues of the hoof, such as the parietal and sole surfaces of the pedal bone, or to the hoof cartilages, it takes over the function of periosteum or perichondrium respectively (/c, d). At the same time, in other regions the subcutis acquires added fat and connective tissue whereby perioplic, coronary, cuneate, digital and bulbar cushions are formed, which give the hoof its characteristic shape. These cushions provide a functional transition between the haired skin above and the digital organ below. They are also important factors which contribute to the overall resilience of the hoof and ensure its ability to absorb concussion.

The *corium* of the skin above (/f), is continuous with that of the hoof (*corium ungulae*) (/g–l'), and again it is named according to the regions of the hoof in which it is found. Thus there is *perioplic* (/g), *coronary* (/h), *parietal* (/i), *sole corium* (/k), *cuneate* (/l'), and *bulbar corium* (/l).

The epidermal regions of the hoof correspond to those of the corium. Accordingly, the *epidermis ungulae* (/n–r'), is recognized as being *perioplic* (/n), *coronary* (/o), *parietal* (/p), *sole* (/q), *cuneate* (/r'), and *bulbar* (/r). These regions give rise to the horn of the hoof or the hoof *capsule* (*capsula ungulae*), which, depending on the surface configuration of the underlying corium, can be *tubular* (426/d), *laminar* (/e), or *intermediate horn* (/d'). Reflecting growth from the different regions of the corium, epithelial horn is also recognised as being perioplic (432/k), coronary (430/d), parietal (432/g), sole (/e), cuneate (/a), and bulbar (430/b).

The *horn sole* of the hoof is regarded as being separate from the *horn plate* (*horn wall*), which includes the dorsal segment (toe), the lateral and medial walls (quarters), and the heels and bars of the horn capsule. The *horn* or *hoof plate* (363/a; 429), is formed from above to below by the keratogenous cells of the perioplic, coronary and parietal epidermis (430/a″, d, f). The outermost layer, or *glaze*, is formed by the perioplic epidermis. The middle, and chief or *protective* layer, develops from the large keratogenous cells of the coronary epidermis, whilst the innermost connecting layer is produced by the parietal epidermis.

Despite its apparent rigidity, the *hoof capsule* possesses considerable elasticity because of the specialized nature of the posterior parts of the hoof. The wedge-shaped digital cushion (422/e) which is inserted from behind between the horn sole (423/s) and the skeleton of the hoof (422/A), contributes to this resilient mechanism. At the same time, the digital cushion, together with the inclination of the joints and the specialized structure of the posterior parts of the hoof (heels and bars), aid considerably in the dissipation of the concussion which occurs when the limb comes into contact with the ground (*shock absorption*). The common integument of the hoof is regarded as being formed by both the corium and the epidermis.

Subcutis of the hoof (tela subcutanea ungulae)

The posterior region of the hoof presents two proximal prominences – the medial and lateral parts of the bulb (*partes latt. et medd. torus ungulae*) (364/i), which are separated by the *bulbar groove (fossa intratorica)* (/i'). They are covered in part by haired skin above and partly by the keratinized bulbar epidermis below (365/r). The sponge-like *bulbar cushion (tela subcutanea tori)* (365/e) lies underneath, and it continues forward into the sole region as the aforementioned *digital cushion*, which then spreads medially and laterally as far as the *hoof cartilages* (432/B). The bulbar cushion also plays a significant role in shock absorption because its connective tissue is rich in elastic fibres.

The *digital cushion (tela subcutanea cunei)* (365/e') is a wedge-shaped elastic cushion which forms the base of the frog (*cuneus ungulae*). Its proximal portion borders the palmar fascia whilst its distal surface is covered by the corium of the frog (/l'). There is a median sulcus bordered by two ridges which divide the cushion into the limbs of the frog (*crura cunei*) (428/c). The sulcus is continued caudally, as the digital cushion forms the previously-mentioned *bulbar cushion (tela subcutanea tori)* (365/e), underlying the bulb (364/i). The apex of the digital cushion takes the form of a cellular or fibrous fan which is inserted under the apex of the frog. Otherwise, the cushion is poorly supplied with vessels and its structure comprises a feltwork of collagen and elastic fibres, in the meshes of which fat cells and glandular tissue are embedded (424/B).

At the junction of hair-bearing skin and hoof, the subcutaneous tissue is also modified to form a slender *perioplic cushion (tela subcutanea limbi)*, and a more prominent *coronary cushion (tela subcutanea coronae)* (365/b). The *subcutis* of the wall (*tela subcutanea parietis*) (/c), and of the *sole (tela subcutanea soleae)* (/d) on the other hand, forms the *periosteum* of the *pedal bone* and the *perichondrium* of the *hoof cartilages* (422/C).

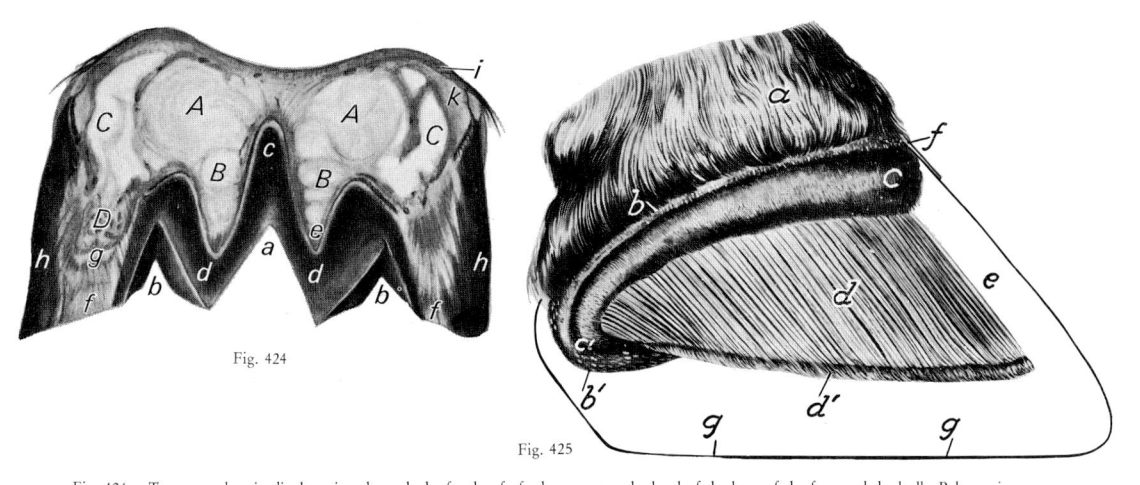

Fig. 424. Transverse longitudinal section through the forehoof of a horse cut at the level of the base of the frog and the bulb. Palmar view.
A tela subcutanea tori; B tela subcutanea cunei; C cartilago ungularis; D processus palmaris
a sulcus cunealis centralis; b sulcus paracunealis lateralis et medialis; c spina cunei ("frog-stay"); d epidermis cunei; e corium cunei; f epidermis soleae; g corium soleae; h hoof plate; i epidermis, k corium of the hairy skin

Fig. 425. Corium of the equine hoof. Lateral view. Horny wall is indicated in outline. About three-fifths natural size.
(After Nickel, 1938.)

a hairy skin; b corium limbi, b' corium tori with enlarged papillae; c corium coronae, c' pars inflexa of the corium coronae; d corium parietis, d' papillae at the free distal border of the lamellae coriales; e stratum medium parietis cornei; f stratum externum parietis cornei; g margo solearis shown as outline

Corium of the hoof

The *corium* of the *hoof* (*corium ungulae*) (425) consists largely of connective tissue rich in blood vessels and nerves. Its main function is to supply nutrition to the epidermal cells which are closely applied to its surface. By virtue of its pliability and rich vascularity, it can also be assumed that the corium has a subsidiary shock-absorbing function. Representing the connecting junction between the horn capsule and the supporting skeleton of the hoof, the *papillary body* (*corpus papillaris*) (425) is prominent in comparison with that in other regions of the common integument and bears numerous *papillae* or *lamellae* (425).

The various parts of the corium can be readily demonstrated when the epidermal horn capsule is removed by macerating with heat. Separation, however, does not occur along the junction between corium and epidermis, but in the region of the active epidermal cells because their basal layers firmly adhere to the corium by means of hemidesmosomes.

The *perioplic corium* (*corium limbi*) (425/b) is a shallow furrow, some 4–6 mm wide, which lies between the hair-bearing skin above and the coronary cushion below. It is clearly demarcated from the coronary corium (/c) by the coronary fold. In the palmar (or plantar) region, the perioplic corium continues as bulbar corium (/b') which gradually becomes wider before uniting with that of the other side in the bulbar groove (364/i'). Its surface is covered with fine papillae (*papillae coriales*) (365/l) which, measuring 1–2 mm in length, are shorter than those of the coronary corium. The superficial epidermal cells here form the perioplic horn (*str. corneum epidermis limbi*) (430/a).

The *coronary corium* (*corium coronae*) (425/c) covers the coronary cushion (365/b) which is 7–8 mm thick. Distally, it follows the same course as the perioplic corium (425/b). On the dorsal aspect, the coronary corium covers the extensor tendon and its insertion into the extensor process of the pedal bone (365/l). Laterally, it is in contact with the middle phalanx (/B), and the hoof cartilages (432/B), whilst in a palmar (plantar) direction it is continuous with the corium covering the two limbs of the frog. It is widest (1.3–1.5 cm) dorsally over the extensor process of the distal phalanx (365/C), but it gradually narrows as it passes medially and laterally. The coronary corium bears papillae 4–6 mm in length, which contain blood vessels (/h). The papillae shorten and become thinner at the parieto-corial junction (425/d). They take the form of a strip, 4–5 mm in width, as they extend into the medial and lateral paracuneate grooves, and, at the corium of the bars, they continue as the corium of the sole on either side of the frog. The papillae are arranged in rows at the junction with the laminar region of the parietal corium. In the toe of the hoof, they are perpendicular whilst in the quarters and the heels, they are inclined backwards towards the heels (365/*h*). The epidermal cells of the *coronary horn* (str. *corneum epidermis coronae*) (430/*c*, *d*) are formed superficial to the coronary corium.

The *corium* of the *wall* (*corium parietalis*) (425/*d*) is the distal continuation of the coronary corium (/*c*) and, extending from the coronet to the bearing surface (431/*C*), it is applied to the pedal bone (/*B*) and the base of the hoof cartilages. On the palmar (plantar) aspect, it bends acutely on either side of the cuneate corium to continue towards the sole, forming the *pars inflecta* of the *parietal corium* (423/*e*; 428/*g*). On the bearing surface (425/*g*), the parietal corium (423/*d*) is continued as the corium of the sole (/*g*). The outer surface bears fine *lamellae* (*lamellae coriales*) (423/*d*) which contain capillaries, and which are distributed from the coronet to the ground surface. The parietal corium decreases in length and breadth from before backwards and its lamellae are separated by deep, narrow grooves which interdigitate with the horny lamellae (429/*g*).

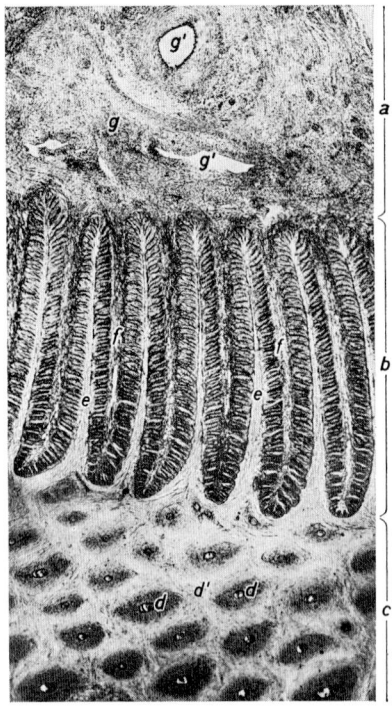

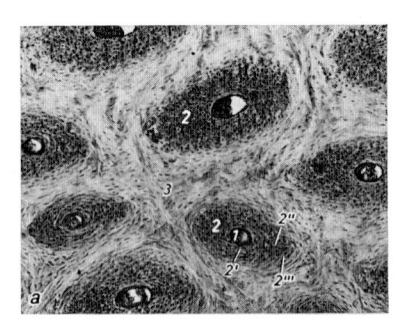

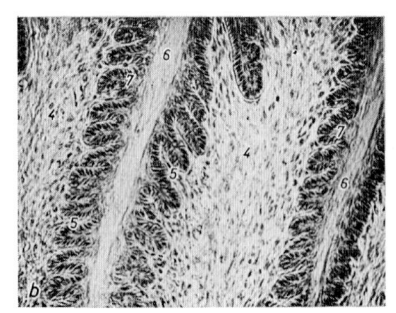

Fig. 426

Fig. 427

Fig. 426. Horizontal section through the epidermis and parietal corium of a horse's hoof cut immediately below the coronary cushion. The pedal bone, periosteum and the glaze layer are not shown, the protective layer is depicted only in part.
(Photomicrograph.)

a corium parietis; *b* stratum internum parietis cornei (connecting layer); *c* stratum medium parietis cornei (protective layer); *d* horn tubules, *d'* intertubular horn; *e* horny lamellae; *f* corium lamellae; *g* connective tissue part of the corium with vessels (*g'*)

Fig. 427. Enlarged portions of Fig. 426.

a horizontal section through the tubular horn of the protective layer of the horny wall:

1 medulla of tubule (suprapapillary horn); *2* cortex of tubule (circumpapillary horn) with *2'* inner zone, *2"* middle zone, *2'''* outer zone; *3* intertubular (interpapillary) horn with holes for the papillae

b horizontal section through epidermal and corium papillae of the connecting layer of the horny wall:

4 primary lamellae of the parietal corium with vessels; *5* secondary lamellae of the parietal corium; *6* primary lamellae of the epidermis (horny lamellae) with unkeratinized epithelium of the secondary lamellae (*7*) on both sides

Close to the coronet, the lamellae are very narrow. They gain their maximum height about half-way down and continue thus to the ground surface (365/*i*). The height of the parietal lamellae varies from 1 to 4 mm. They are between 0.05 and 0.2 mm thick, and they number about 600 per hoof. Histologically, their surface area is increased by the presence of secondary lamellae (427/*5*), each primary lamella being said to carry some 100–200 secondary lamellae. The latter project from the free border and surfaces of the primary lamellae, giving the characteristic feathered appearance of the equine parietal corium (426/f; 427/4). The primary lamellae carry 4–6 mm long papillae at their distal ends (365/i″; 425/d′); these are similar to those occurring at their free ends in the heel region.

In the region of the toe, near the ground surface, the parietal corium has a shallow depression to accommodate the toe of the pedal bone and here the lamellae are also lined with numerous papillae. As the lamellae of the corium become thinner towards the ground surface, the keratinized epidermal lamellae correspondingly increase in thickness. The presence of the secondary lamellae ensures considerably greater adhesion between the corium and the epidermal horn than is found in the claw of the cloven-hoofed species. The *epidermal cells* of the *lamellae* of the *parietal corium* produce *parietal horn (str. corneum epidermis parietis)* in the form of *horny lamellae*(430/f), which act as the connecting layer between the horn capsule and the parietal corium. The epidermal cells of the papillae at the distal end of the corium lamellae produce the interlaminar horn which, like that of the horny lamellae

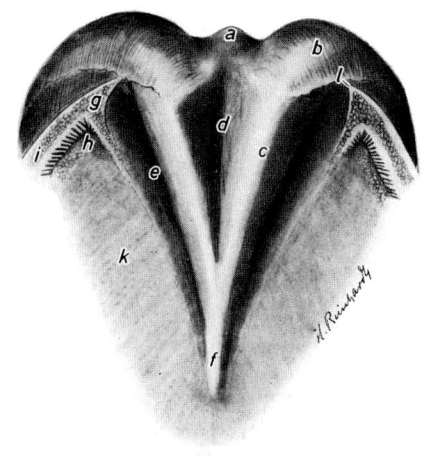

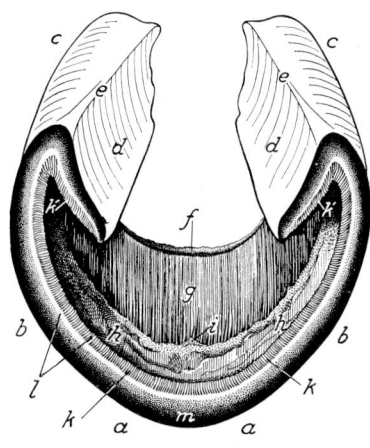

Fig. 428. Horny bulb, horny frog, bars and part of the horny sole of the equine hoof. Sole surface.
(After Martin, 1915.)

a medial tip of the bulbar horn; *b* torus corneus; *c–f* cuneus corneus: *c* crus cunei, *d* sulcus cunealis centralis, *e* sulcus paracunealis, *f* apex cunei, *g* pars inflexa (bar); *h* angulus partis inflexae (angle of the wall); *i* margo solearis of the paries corneus; *k* solea cornea; *l* margo palmaris or plantaris of the hoof plate

Fig. 429. Isolated plate of the left fore hoof of a horse after removal of the horny sole, the bulb and frog. The bar portion at the coronet has been somewhat contracted during drying. Sole surface. About half natural size.
(After Zietzschmann from Ellenberger-Baum, 1943.)

a, *a* pars dorsalis (toe); *b*, *b* pars collateralis (quarters), *c*, *c* heel part, and *d*, *d* bars of the hoof plate; *e*, *e* margo palmaris (angle of the heel); *f* sulcus coronalis; *g* lamellae epidermales on the inside of the hoof plate; *h* remains of the detached sole; *i* spur of the sole; *k*, *k* lamellae epidermales marginis solearis, *k′*, *k′* lamellae epidermales on the bar portion of the plate; *l* zona alba; *m* stratum medium parietis cornei of the margo solearis

themselves, is unpigmented, and which gives rise to the *white line* (zona alba) (364/c) on the ground surface of the wall.

The *corium* of the *sole (corium soleare)* (365/k), which is often patchily-pigmented, is closely applied to the distal surface of the pedal bone (431/B). Towards the axis of the foot, it continues as the cuneate corium (424/e) and peripherally, at the ground surface, as the parietal corium (422/d). The corium of the bars (425/c′) forms the junction between the coronary corium and the corium of the sole. The corium of the sole is relatively thin. It carries numerous long papillae which are directed obliquely downwards. By virtue of the insertion of the frog from behind, it is *semi-lunar in shape* (423/g) with its angles (anguli soleae) situated at the inflections of the bars.

The *epidermal cells* of the *papillae* of the corium of the sole produce the *horny sole (str. corneum epidermis soleae)* (430/g).

The *corium* of the *frog (corium cunei)* (365/l′) is 2–4 mm thick, and it covers the digital cushion (/e′) to which it is firmly attached. It is lighter in colour than the corium of the sole, and the short, crowded papillae carry blood vessels. On the palmar (plantar) aspect, the cuneate corium (/l′, 423/f) is continuous on either side with the bulbar corium (365/l; 425/b′), which in turn is confluent with the perioplic corium (365/g; 423/a). The corium of the frog is in contact with that of the bars on both sides (425/c'). Its shape corresponds to that of the digital cushion, and it presents for description a *medial* and *lateral limb* (crus cunei med. et lat.) (423/l), a *central groove* (sulcus cunealis centralis) (/p) and two *paracuneate grooves* (sulcus paracunealis med. et lat.) (/o).

The epidermal cells of the surface of the corium produce the *horn of the frog* (str. corneum epidermis cunei) (430/i).

The *bulbar corium* (corium tori) (425/b') covers both parts of the bulb and bears extremely delicate papillae. The epidermal cells of the proximal region form haired skin above, and below, the very thin, soft *bulbar horn* (str. corneum epidermis tori) (430/b).

The corium of the hoof is rich in elastic and connective tissue fibres and, like the corium of the common integument generally, it is divided into a *str. reticulare* and a *str. papillare*. The elastic fibro-reticular layer, which is very similar to that of the integument, is highly vascular and can accordingly also be termed the *str. vasculare*. It is relatively thick in the coronary region and on the ground surface, and thinner below the frog. It blends with any subcutaneous cushions or periosteum with which it comes into contact.

The *str. papillare et lamellatum* bears villus-like papillae on the perioplic, coronary, sole, cuneate and bulbar corium, and lamellae on the corium of the wall and the bars, which are visible to the naked eye.

Epidermis of the hoof (epidermis ungulae)

The **epidermis of the hoof** (*epidermis ungulae*) covers all parts of the corium, and so it assumes a similar shape. The two are intimately attached to each other by interdigitating lamellae, papillae and tubules.

According to the different regions of the corium, the hoof capsule, which is formed by the epidermis of the hoof, is divided into the following segments:

1. *perioplic horn* (432/k);
2. *coronary horn* (430/c);
3. *parietal horn* (428/i);
4. *sole horn* (432/e);
5. *cuneate horn* (428/c–f);
6. *bulbar horn* (428/b).

The perioplic, coronary and parietal horn together form the *hoof plate* (paries corneus) (429/a–d). This presents an outer convex surface (433/l) and an inner concave one, which bears horny lamellae (/h), a *coronary rim* (margo coronalis) (/k) and a *bearing surface* (margo solearis) (423/q). At the angle of the wall (angulus partis inflexae) (428/h), the caudal part of the plate turns inwards and forwards to form the bars (pars inflecta) (429/d). These run along the paracuneate groove (423/o) and gradually merge with the sole (364/d; 423/s). The frog (364/e–h) is inserted into the space between the bars.

The *coronary rim* (margo coronalis) (433/k) takes the form of an open oval, the open portion being directed towards the palmar (plantar) aspect. Within, the rim presents the *perioplic groove* (sulcus limbi), and immediately below, the *coronary groove* (sulcus coronalis) (430/3; 433/i). Both grooves have small openings which permit the insertion of the papillae of the perioplic and coronary corium (430/C). Caudally, the coronary groove broadens out in the bulbar region, forming a wide bilateral groove which receives the digital cushion and the cuneate corium (433/c).

The *bearing surface* (margo solearis) (429/m) of the hoof capsule describes a wider arc than the coronary rim (433/k). The *angle of the wall*, angulus partis inflexae (angulus parietalis [428/h; 433/f]) is found where the palmar (plantar) border of the hoof (428/l; 429/e) turns in towards the axis of the foot.

The wall itself presents an *inner surface* (facies interna) (/g), and an *outer surface* (facies externa) (433/l). Each comprises a *dorsal* or *toe part* (pars dorsalis) (429/a), two *quarters* (partes collaterales latt. et medd.) (/b) and the *heels* (margines palmares) (plantares) (428/l; 429/e). Like the coronary groove (430/c), the upper border of the bars (/c') is punctate within the hoof to accommodate the papillae on the bar portion of the coronary corium. The distal border of the hoof plate is the *bearing surface*, and it projects beyond the level of the sole. Its axial surface faces the paracuneate groove and is joined by horny lamellae to the surface apposing the corium of the bars.

The *colour* of the *hoof plate* may be whitish-yellow, black or striped. The plate comprises the three previously-mentioned layers: 1. the very thin *covering layer* or *glaze*, which is produced by the perioplic keratogenous epidermal cells (365/n); 2. the very thick *protective layer* (/o) which consists of

Fig. 430. Hoof capsule of the horse with one side removed. Interior surface as seen from the left side. Half natural size.
(After Nickel, 1938.)

a epidermal periople which widens towards the heel (*a'*) and bears holes for papillae, *a"* stratum externum parietis cornei; *b* epidermis tori; *c* sulcus coronalis, *c'* flattened bar part of the coronary groove, both with holes for papillae; *d* stratum medium parietis cornei, *d'* its inner pigment-free and *d"* outer pigmented zones; *e* outer aspect of the wall at the quarters, *f* lamellae epidermales of the hoof plate, *f'* lamellae of the bar, inner view, *f"* in longitudinal section at the toe, *f'''* in cross section at the quarters; *g* epidermis soleae with holes for papillae, *g'* their comb-like median protrusion towards the dorsal part of the wall, *g"* crus of the sole; *h* ridges formed by bar and frog; *i* epidermis cunei with holes for papillae; *k* spina cunei; *l* sulcus cunealis centralis; *m* bulbar cup

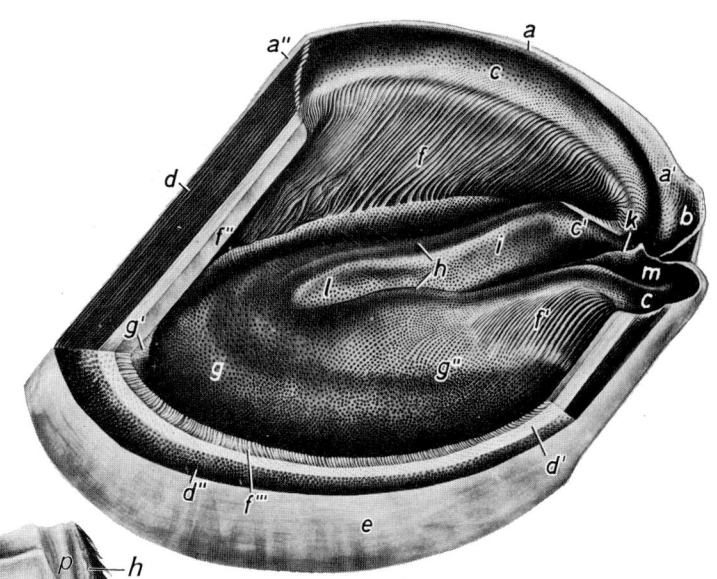

Fig. 431. Transverse longitudinal section through the fore hoof of a horse at the level of the apex of the frog. Palmar view.

A phalanx media; *B* phalanx distalis; *C* cartilago ungularis

a solea cornea; *b* cuneus corneus; *c* sulci paracuneales; *d* zona alba; *e* margo solearis; *f* paries corneus; *g* limbus corneus; *h* cutis; *i* corium soleae with venous plexus; *k* corium cunei; *l* corium parietis; *m* corium coronae; *n* corium limbi; *o* articulatio interphalangea distalis; *p* ligamenta collateralia; *q* ligamenta chondrocoronalia; *r* vessels of the distal phalanx

Fig. 432. Transverse longitudinal section through the fore hoof of a horse at the middle of the frog. Palmar view.

A processus palmaris; *B* cartilago ungularis; *C* deep flexor tendon, *C'* its terminal limbs; *D* the sheath of its terminal tendon

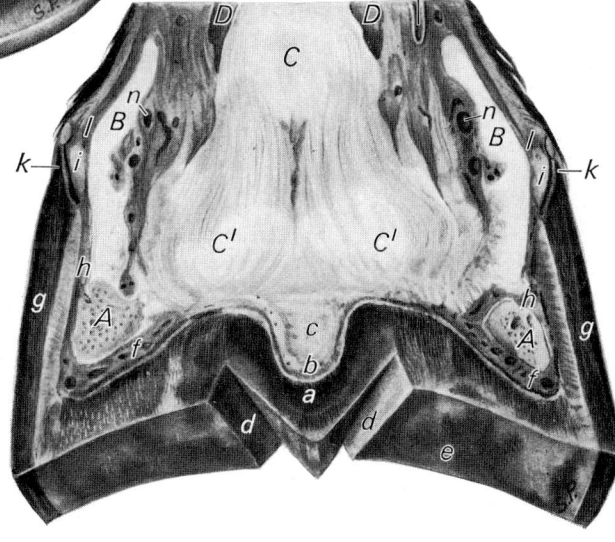

a epidermis cunei; *b* corium cunei; *c* tela subcutanea cunei; *d* sulci paracuneales; *e* epidermis soleae; *f* corium soleae with venous plexuses; *g* epidermis parietis; *h* corium parietis with venous networks; *i* corium coronae; *k* epidermis limbi; *l* corium limbi; *m* a. digitalis; *n* venous plexuses on the inner surface of the hoof cartilage

tubular horn situated over the coronary corium, and 3. the *connective layer* (/p) which, in the form of primary horn lamellae, is produced by the primary and secondary lamellae of the parietal corium. All three epidermal segments form a continuous unit (/n–p).

The *glaze* or *outer covering layer* (*str. ext. parietis*) (/n), consists of glossy, elastic horn which, if immersed in water, swells and becomes brittle and opaque in appearance. In the palmar (plantar) region, it covers the bulb as the *bulbar epidermis* (*epidermis tori*) forming the *bulbar horn* (*torus corneus*) (428/b). The bulbar horn turns inwards towards the axis of the foot, forming the *bulbar groove* (*sulcus tori*) which is continued behind as the *bulbar fossa* (*fossa tori*) (364/i'), and in front, as the *central sulcus* of the *frog* (*sulcus cunealis centralis*) (/f). The glaze is well-developed in neonatal foals, but in older horses it is well worn, and all but completely lost. The glaze gives the horn wall its smooth outer surface and protects the hoof against moisture.

The *middle* or *protective layer* of the horn wall (*str. medium parietis cornei*) (365/o; 426/c; 430/d) is the strongest and thickest layer of the wall. It consists of "fibre-containing" tubular (426/d) and intertubular (/d') horn, and it grows distally from the coronary border to the bearing surface. The thicker outer zone is heavily-pigmented (430/d''); the thinner and softer inner zone is non-pigmented (/d') forming a light rim around the white line (364/c) at the bearing surface.

The outer surface of the protective layer, and possibly the glaze, shows faint, semi-circular transverse lines which run parallel to the coronary rim. These are caused by fluctuations in the nutrition of the epidermis and they represent the so-called *growth rings*.

The *horn tubules* (*tubuli epidermales*) (426/d) present a cortex (427a/2), and a medulla (/1). The cortex consists of keratinized epithelial cells (/2–2''). At the coronet, the lumina of the horn tubules accommodate the papillae of the corium. The spaces between the horn tubules are also occupied by keratinized cells which make up the intertubular horn (426/d'; 427a/3). These cells are derived from the epidermal cells found between the papillae of the corium.

The *lamellar* or *connecting layer* (*str. int. parietis cornei*) (426/b) is the innermost layer of the wall; it is invariably unpigmented and it carries the *horny lamellae* (*lamellae epidermales*) (/e; 427b/6) which are congruent with the lamellae of the corium (426/f; 427b/4). Like those of the corium, the horny lamellae have secondary lamellae (427b/5, 7) which, however, are not keratinized. At the bearing surface, the horny lamellae merge into the white line. The str. internum forms an intimate connection between the keratinized wall of the hoof (426/b, c) and the parietal corium (/a). The inner parts of the hoof are thus, in essence, 'suspended' within the horn capsule, so that the sole, bulb and frog only bear a small amount of the body weight. If the adhesion between wall and corium is disturbed by pathological processes, the pedal bone drops and the sole bulges outwards (e. g. laminitis).

The *epidermis* of the *sole* (*epidermis soleae*) (424/f) covers the corium of the sole and, as the hoof sole (364/d), it is situated between the wall of the hoof (423/k), the bars (/n) and the frog (/l). It is subdivided into a *body* (*corpus soleae*) (364/d) which lies in front of the apex of the frog (/e), two *limbs* (*crura soleae*) (/d') and two *angles* (*anguli soleae*) (/d'') which lie between the wall of the heel (/a'') and the bars (/b).

The outer surface of the horny sole (*facies externa*) (432/e) is concave, with the inner convex surface directed towards the pedal bone. This concavity is more marked in the hind foot than in the fore. The deepest part of the concavity is near the apex of the frog (431/b). A neglected sole, for instance, one which has not been cleaned or pared, appears fissured and rough and it continually sheds flat pieces of horn of varying size. Although the deeper layers of the horny sole are somewhat more dense than the middle layers of the hoof wall, they are softer and thus sharp objects such as nails, splinters of glass and wire can readily penetrate the sole.

The outer surface of the sole being concave, it has a correspondingly convex inner surface (*facies interna*) (432/e). It bears numerous small excavations which accommodate the papillae of the corium of the sole (430/g). The thickness of the horny sole varies considerably. It is thinnest at the apex of the frog and thickest near the wall of the hoof. The horny sole is comprised of horn tubules, which run parallel to the hoof wall, and intertubular horn. Normally it is greyish-black in colour though occasionally it has a flecked appearance or may even be pigment-free. It is united with the hoof wall (364/a–a'') and the bars (/b) by the so-called white line (/c). Its transition to the horny frog is gradual and there is apparently no demarcation between these two parts of the hoof.

The *white line* (*zona alba*) (364/c; 423/r; 429/l) is confined to the hoof wall and the bars. There is an outer line on the wall and an inner line on the bars which resemble white wax (/l). This corresponds to the deep, unpigmented zone of the protective layer. There follows another more yellow and brittle layer which is formed by the *horny lamellae* of the *connecting layer* of the wall, which do not have secondary lamellae (/l). The spaces between are occupied by young, yellowish horn which is formed by the epidermal cells of the secondary lamellae of the corium. Such "interlamellar horn" consists of horn tubules which are arranged in obliquely-directed rows.

The zona alba gives an indication of the angles at which nails have to be driven during shoeing.

The wedge-shaped *frog (cuneus ungulae)* (364/e–h) consists of *cuneate horn (epidermis cunei)*. It is inserted into the horny sole (/d) from behind, between the two bars (428/g), and it covers the cuneate corium (423/f). In cross section, it takes the shape of a 'W' (424/c, d), and it consists of soft, elastic

Fig. 433. Internal view of the hoof capsule of a horse, seen from above. About half natural size. (After Martin, 1915.)

a spina cunei (floor of the central sulcus of the frog); *b* floor of the paracuneal (collateral) sulci; *c* groove for the crus of the frog; *d* apex cunei; *e* lamellae epidermales of the bar; *f* angle of the heel; *g* facies interna of the solea cornea; *h* lamellae epidermales of the wall at the quarters; *i* sulcus coronalis which encloses the tela subcutanea coronae; *k* margo coronalis; *l* facies externa parietis cornei

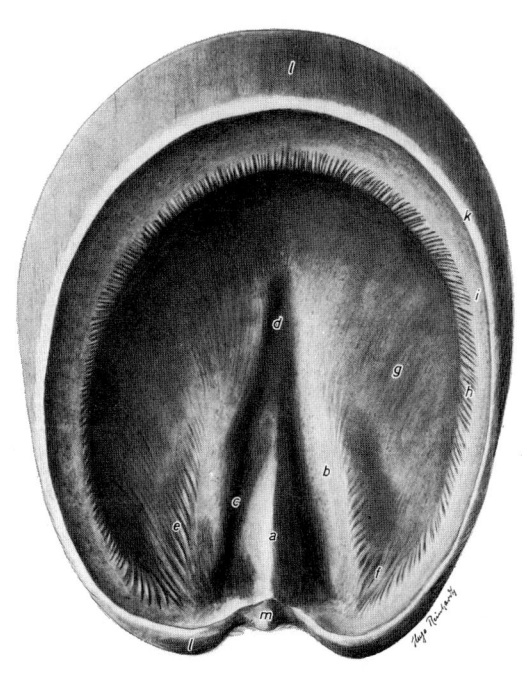

tubular horn. It is an important shock-absorbing structure in the hoof. In front, it blends with the horny sole (364/d) without obvious demarcation. Behind, it merges with the horny bulb (/i) whilst on either side it flanks the inner margin of the bars (/b) and the margo centralis of the horny sole (/d'''). In the normal hoof, the *ground surface (facies externa)* of the frog is on the same level as the bearing surface of the hoof wall, and it thus helps support the weight of the body. The *central groove (sulcus cunealis centralis)* (/f; 428/d) divides the frog into two *limbs (crus cunei lat. et med.)* (364/g; 428/c). The outer surfaces of the limbs together with the bars and the central edges of the sole form the collateral sulci of the frog *(sulcus paracunealis med. et lat.* [364/h; 428/e]). The blunt tip of the frog *(apex cunei)* (364/e; 428/f) lies above the level of the bearing surface, while its caudal end *(basic cunei)* continues into the bulb (364/i; 428/b). The corial surface *(facies interna)* of the horny frog (433/a–d) has two deep depressions or grooves which accommodate the limbs of the cuneate corium (/c). The two grooves are separated by a rounded ridge *(spina cunei)* (/a) which reaches the level of the ridge of the bars. The inner surface of the frog is usually darkly-pigmented and has numerous small excavations (430/i) which lodge the papillae of the corium. The elastic, horny frog consists of tubular and intertubular horn. Its W-shaped cross-sectional structure (424/c, d) helps to give it its characteristic resilience and this is reinforced by the buffering effect of the digital cushion (/B). When pressed down the 'W' is flattened, thereby exerting outwards pressure on the bars (364/b), the hoof cartilages (424/C), and the wall of the heels (/h). When the weight is lifted, the structures all regain their original positions because of their own inbuilt resilience. The wall in the toe region does not alter its shape during the process.

Differences between the hoofs of the fore- and hind-limbs

The ratio of the height of the wall at the toe to the height at the heels is 3:1 in the fore foot and 2:1 in the hind foot. The angle formed by the dorsal wall and the ground surface is 45–50° in the fore-, and

50–55° in the hind-hoof, the toe of the latter thus being steeper. The outline of the bearing surface (364) shows particularly important differences. In the fore foot, it is semi-circular in the toe region and widest at the quarters (364/A). In the hind-hoof on the other hand, the anterior part of the bearing surface (364/B) is pointed and the posterior part wider. The outline of the bearing surface of the hoof of the fore foot can perhaps best be compared to the blunt end of a hen's egg, and that of the hind foot to the pointed end of the egg (364/A, B). In normal hoofs the medial quarter of the hoof plate is steeper than the lateral one, affording a very straightforward means of determining whether a hoof has come from the near or the off side.

The *growth rate* of the hoof horn is about 8–10 mm a month. The replacement of the entire wall at the toe thus requires 12 months, at the quarters 6–8 months and at the heels 4–5 months. The sole and the frog are replaced every two months.

Histological structure of the horn tubules

The *horn tubules* of the hoof (434C/e) are hollow in the distal regions of the wall, the medulla being only represented by cellular debris (427a/1; 434C/a'). Thus this part of the horn tubules has no functional significance. The *cortex* of the horn tubules (427a/2; 434C/b) on the other hand, is under mechanical stress. It consists of spirally-arranged cell cords (434C/b'–b''') with the long margin of the individual cells facing the direction of pressure and their tonofibrils interlocked at desmosomes. The *tubular cortex* consists of three differently-arranged layers; the *inner* (427a/2'; 434C/b'); the *middle* (427a/2''; 434C/b''), and the *outer zone* (427a/2'''; 434C/b'''). Under an evenly-distributed load, the horn tubules appear circular in cross section (434/A, B), and under uneven pressure, they are oval or triangular.

The *mechanical significance* of the horn tubules is reflected by their structural differences (434/A, B). When the limb is bearing weight, pressure is exerted in a proximo-distal direction, which is opposed by a similar force from the ground. This bi-directional pressure is distributed throughout the horn capsule of the hoof. The intertubular horn, which has a functional association with the epidermal lamellae, receives *vertical pressure* in the form of *tension*, and this is then passed on to the horn tubules from the wall as *radial pressure*, and, in the long axis, as *axial pressure*. The tubules are also subjected to a certain amount of bending. The horn tubules which are mainly arranged in steep spirals (434/A) are more resistant to axial pressure than those with flat spirals (434/B). The former are found in the toe and in the protective layer of the inner part of the quarters. The latter are found mainly in the outer parts of the protective layer, the remaining portions of the hoof plate and all other hoof segments. In the hoof plate, the transition from one form into the other is gradual, from inside out, and from dorsal to palmar (plantar), with a gradual loss of the steeply-coiled components, and a concomitant reduction in size of the horn tubules (Nickel, 1938).

The structure of the hoof wall is fundamentally the same in domestic and wild equidae. There are certain variations in respect of the size of the horn tubules, and the arrangement of the individual layers of the coronary epidermis. Rapid wear induces the horn tubules to become more crowded and thus increase the resistance of the wall, which, in the main, is determined by the number of tubular cortices present.

Chestnuts and ergots
(349; 364; 435)

The *chestnut* (*torus carpeus*; *torus tarseus*) is a horny excresence with a very thickened, keratinized epidermis, overlying a portion of corium, which is devoid of glands. Very tall, thin papillae extend from the corium and thus tubular horn is formed within the epidermis. On the fore limb, the *chestnut* is situated medial to and above the *carpus* (349/g; 435/a), but on the hind limb it lies medial to and below the *tarsus* (349/g'; 435/a'). The horny material of the chestnut is desquamated as scales from the surface. There is considerable variation in the size and the shape of the chestnuts. The breadth ranges from 0.5 to 4.5 cm, the length from 1.0 to 10 cm and the height from 1.0 to 9.0 cm. The chestnuts of the fore limb are usually the larger, and occasionally they may be absent from the hind limb.

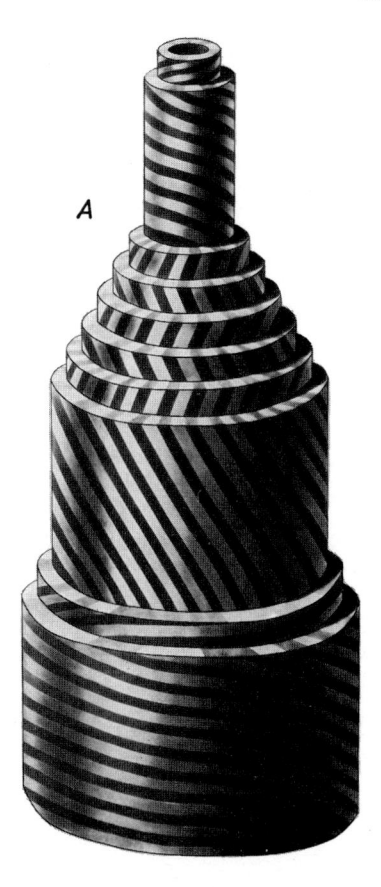

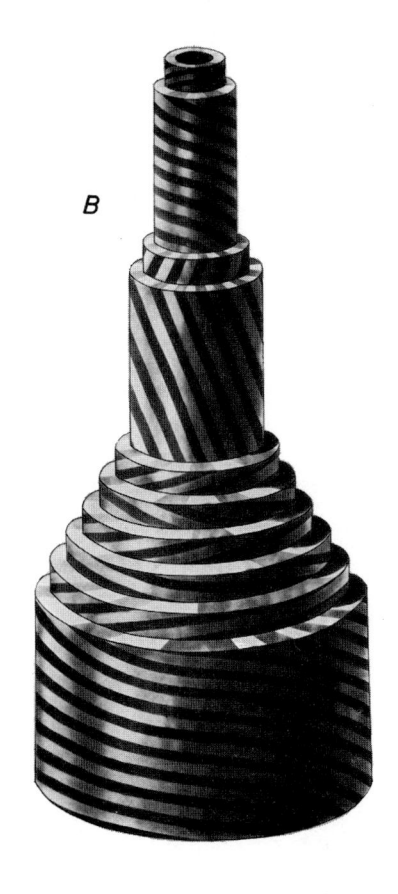

Fig. 434. A–C. Structure of the horn tubules of the hoof wall (A, B) and semidiagrammatic illustration of the epidermis and corium of the hoof in sagittal section (C).
(After Nickel, 1938.)

A Diagram of the structure of a round horn tubule of mainly steeply-spiral type. The thin outer layer is of low spirals, the thick middle layer of steep spirals and the thin inner layer of low spirals

B Diagram showing the structure of a round horn tubule of mainly low-spiral type. Here there is a thick outer layer of low spirals, a thin middle layer of steep spirals and a thin inner layer of low spirals

C *1* stratum basale; *2* stratum intermedium; *3* stratum corneum of the epidermis; *4* corium

a circumpapillary, *a'* suprapapillary tubular epithelium (medullary epithelium); *b* cortex of the epidermis tubules pushed up by the circumpapillary epithelium, *b'* inner, *b''* middle, *b'''* outer zone of an epidermal tubule with variable spiral winding; *c* interpapillary horn remaining in horizontal direction; *d* vascular stratum reticulare of the corium; *d'* corium papilla; *e* total extent of a horn tubule

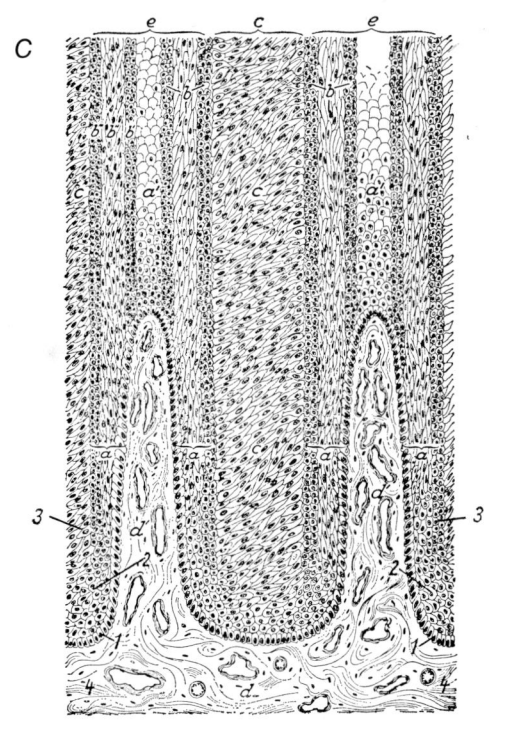

552 Skin and cutaneous organs of the horse

The chestnuts of heavy horses are generally larger than those of light breeds, and they can develop into relatively bizarre structures. Their size also varies in the different breeds. There are neither sweat nor sebaceous glands in the region of the chestnuts, and their functional significance and homology have still not been adequately explained (see p. 477).

In donkeys, mules and zebra, the chestnuts are round, flat, soft and black. As a rule they are absent from the hind limbs, but on the fore limbs they are relatively larger than those of horses. They are most heavily-pigmented in the zebra and mule.

The *ergot* (*calcar*) (435/*b*, *b'*) is a small, wart-like projection on the palmar (plantar) surface of the fetlock. It is generally hairless and thickly keratinized. As a rule, it is considered to represent a rudimentary sole pad. The base of the ergot is round or oval, and it measures between 0.5 and 3.2 cm (/*b*). There are numerous long hairs around the ergot, and they are known collectively as the *feathers* (*cirrus metacarpeus*) (349/*h*; 364/*k*), or *cirrus metatarseus* (349/*h'*; 364/*k'*). The ergots are particularly well-developed in heavy draught horses. Their function, and that of the feathers, is to ensure that the hollow of the heel, which is sensitive to the effects of water and rain, is kept dry. The donkey has both fore and hind ergots and, like those of the zebra, they appear as low, flat, heavily-pigmented plates. The mule has ergots which can occasionally grow to more than 2 cm long.

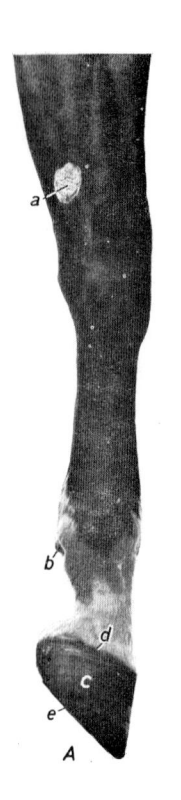

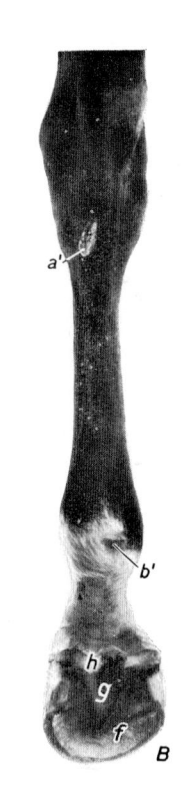

Fig. 435.   Chestnut and ergot of the fore-(A) and hind-(B) limb of the horse. The forelimb is shown in medial and the hindlimb in plantar view. About one-eighth natural size.
(Photogreaph: G. Geiger.)

a torus carpeus, *a'* torus tarseus; *b* calcar metacarpeum, *b'* calcar metatarseum, both exposed by clipping fetlock hair; *c* hoof plate; *d* margo coronalis; *e* margo solearis; *f* horny sole; *g* horny frog; *h* horny bulb

Blood vessels of the digital organ of the horse
(436–439)

Arteries

The digital organ of the horse is supplied by the *lateral* and *medial palmar* (*plantar*) *digital arteries* (436/*a*), whose origins in the fore- and hind-limbs have already been described on pages 99 and 154 respectively. Partially covered by the superficial flexor tendon, they run distally over the collateral surfaces of the fetlock joint, accompanied by satellite veins and nerves. In their subsequent course, they pass deep to the hoof cartilages and the two parts of the bulb until they terminate within the hoof. They give off the same branches to lateral and medial aspects before forming both a dorsal and a palmar (plantar) anastomosis. The larger arteries of the hoof are so disposed that they are protected from pressure and tension. The blood supply (both arterial and venous), however, is very similar in the fore-and hind-limbs, so it is convenient to discuss them together.

The *a. digitalis palmaris* first gives off the *bulbar artery* (*a. tori digitalis*; *a. pulvinalis*) (436, 437/*c*) in the hollow of the heel at the proximo-palmar (proximo-plantar) angle of the hoof cartilage. This divides into a peripheral (436, 437/*c'*) and an axial (436, 437/*c''*) branch. The former supplies the frog sulcus, the

bars and the wall of the heels, together with the corium of the periople and the coronet (436, 437/c').
The axial branch follows the limb of the frog to the apex. Other small branches of the bulbar artery pass
to the digital cushion, the hoof cartilage, the deep flexor tendon, the distal sesamoid, the podotrochlear
bursa and the distal interphalangeal joint (436/c–c''). The next branch of the palmar digital artery is the *a.
coronalis* (436/d), which provides a lateral trunk and branches which supply the heel and the quarters
(436/d–d'''). Arising somewhat more distally from the digital artery, the *a. dorsalis phalangis mediae*
(436/e–e''') runs first along the inner surface of the hoof cartilage, then turns upwards and forwards
before crossing under the extensor tendon and anastomosing with the corresponding vessel of the other
side. At the dorsal border of the hoof cartilage, it gives off a dorsal trunk (436/e') to the periople and

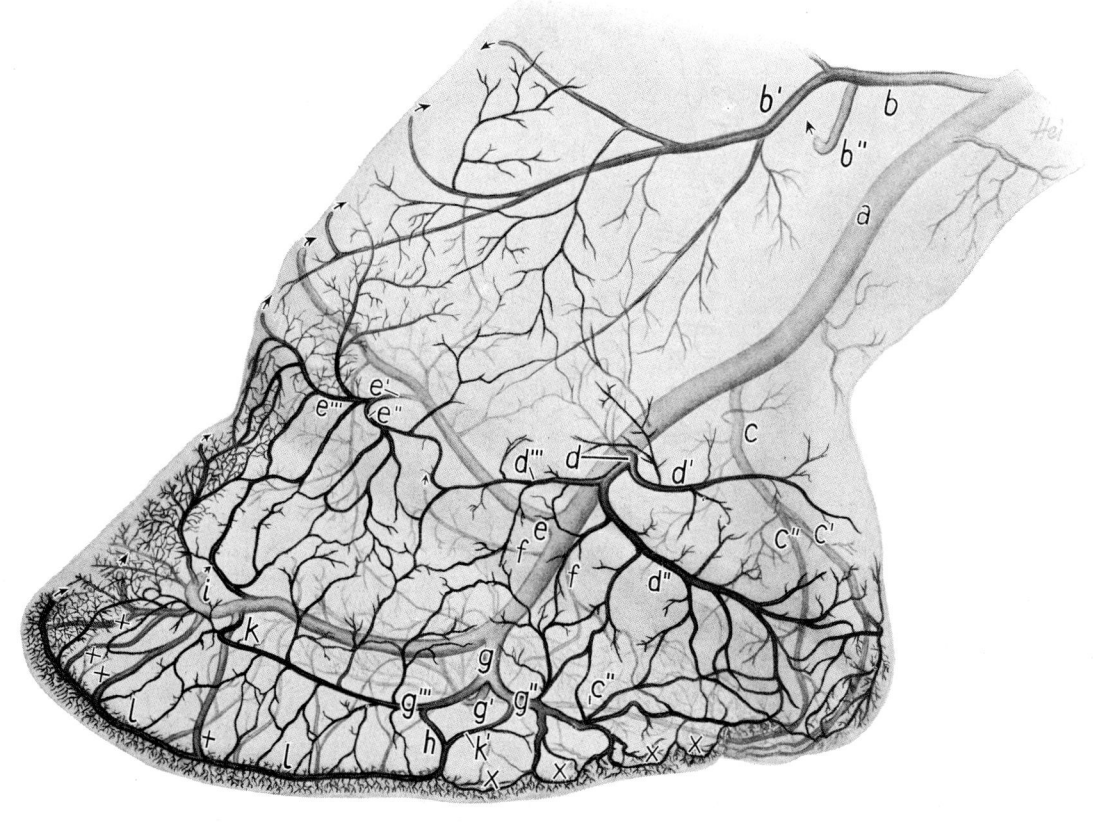

Fig. 436. Arteries of the digital organ of the forelimb of the horse. Lateral half. Drawn from a plastic corrosion preparation. About natural size. Superficial vessels are darker, deeper vessels lighter in tone.
(After Schummer, 1951.)

a a. digitalis palmaris lateralis; *b* common stem of origin of the r. dorsalis (*b'*) and the r. palmaris phalangis proximalis (*b''*); *c* a. tori digitalis with peripheral (*c'*) and axial (*c''*) branches; *d* main trunk of the a. coronalis, *d'* branch supplying the skin proximal to the coronet in the heel region, *d''* heel part and collateral part of the a. coronalis; *e* a. dorsalis phalangis mediae, *e'* its r. coronalis with connecting branches *e''* and *e'''*; *f* a. palmaris phalangis mediae with rr. articulares to the pedal joint; *g* common origin of the a. dorsalis phalangis distalis (hoof wall artery) and the a. palmaris phalangis distalis (*g'*) with rr. cunei, *g''* palmarly directed branches of the hoof wall artery with arterial arches (*x, x*) to the border of the sole, *g'''* collateral part of the hoof wall artery; *h* connecting branch to the a. marginis solearis; *k* branch of the arcus terminalis to the collateral section of the a. dorsalis phalangis distalis; *k'* branch of the palmar segment of the hoof wall artery; *l* a. marginis solearis; +, + branches of the arcus terminalis to the a. marginis solearis; *i* arcus terminalis

coronet. At about the same level, the digital artery gives rise to the *a. palmaris (plantaris) phalangis
mediae* (436/f) which unites with the vessel of the opposite side to supply the second phalanx, the distal
sesamoid bone, the distal interphalangeal joint, the digital cushion and the cranial parts of the frog.

The *a. dorsalis phalangis distalis* (436/g) branches off the digital artery at the foramen (or, as the case
may be, the notch) of the palmar (plantar) process. The vessel then divides into a medial and a lateral
branch. The former, the *a. palmaris phalangis distalis* (436, 437/g') supplies the digital cushion and the
cuneate corium. The lateral branch (436, 437/g''') passes through the foramen or notch in the palmar
(plantar) process to divide into a dorsal and a palmar (plantar) vessel. The latter (436, 437/g'') runs

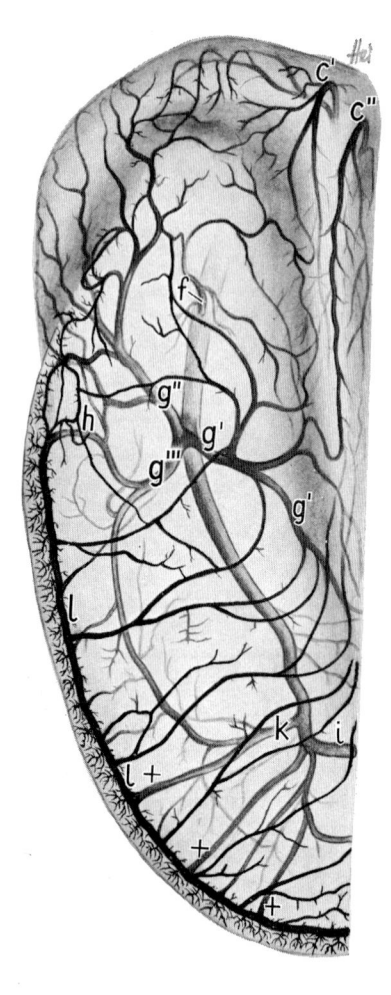

Fig. 437. Arteries of the digital organ of the forelimb of the horse. Viewed from the sole. Drawn from a plastic corrosion preparation. About natural size. Superficial vessels are darker, deep vessels lighter in tone.
(After Schummer, 1951.)

c' peripheral, *c''* axial branches of the a. tori digitalis; *f* a. palmaris phalangis mediae; *g'* a. palmaris phalangis distalis; *g''* heelward, *g'''* collateral part of the hoof wall artery, a. dorsalis phalangis distalis; *h* its branch to the a. marginis solearis; *i* arcus terminalis; *k* connecting branch between the arcus terminalis and the hoof wall artery; *l* a. marginis solearis; +, + branches of the arcus terminalis to the marginal artery of the sole

towards the heels and divides up to supply the heels and the quarters. The vessel supplying the dorsal part of the hoof is the lateral branch of the dorsal artery of the distal phalanx (436, 437/*g'''*), which runs in the parietal groove of the pedal bone. Proximally, this unites by means of several branches with vessels from the coronary artery (436/*d*); distally it unites with branches of the artery of the rim of the sole (436, 437/*h*).

After the origin of the dorsal artery (436/*g*), the digital artery continues in the sole groove of the pedal bone to provide vessels which supply the distal sesamoid bone and the frog. As it does so, it passes into the sole canal where it forms the *arcus terminalis* (436, 437/*i*) with the corresponding vessel of the other side.

The terminal arch gives off some 8–10 vessels of varying sizes which perforate the dorsal part of the pedal bone and emerge through the parietal foramina. A further vessel (436, 437/*k*), running along the border between the dorsal and lateral (medial) face of the pedal bone, also joins that part of the vascular arch formed by the lateral part of the dorsal artery. All other branches supply the skin of the dorsal part of the hoof and join up with tributaries of the coronary and sole margin arteries.

In a distal direction, the terminal arch provides 4–5 vessels which, after an initially straight course, emerge from the foramina at the rim of the pedal bone and join the artery of the sole margin (436, 437/*l*) at almost right-angles.

The *a. marginis solearis* (436, 437/*l*) traverses the corium of the sole a few millimetres from the rim of the pedal bone. This vessel is formed by a number of large arteries which spring from the terminal arch, and the lateral portion of the dorsal artery of the distal phalanx (436, 437/+). The artery of the margin of the sole is a stout vessel and it curves around the entire rim of the pedal bone. At the junction between the pedal bone and the hoof cartilage, it ends by uniting with a connecting branch from the lateral portion of the dorsal artery (436/*k'*). At the heel region of the pedal bone, the function of the artery of the sole rim is taken over by individual branches of the palmar (plantar) segment of the dorsal artery (436, 437/*g''*).

Some 8–10 proximal branches (436/*x*) arise from the artery of the sole margin on each side. These anastomose with corresponding branches of the dorsal and collateral segments of the dorsal artery and with another 8–10 vessels running towards the toe, which unite with similar branches from the other side, as well as with vessels from the ramus of the frog. Numerous bundles of small branches are distributed throughout the corium of the border of the sole. All the arteries of the hoof are interconnected by many arterio-arterial anastomoses (436, 437).

Veins

The *vv. digitales palmares latt. et medd.* (438/*a*) arise from the *median* and *radial* veins. The *vv. digitales plantares latt. et medd.* of the hind limb originate from the *lateral* and *medial plantar veins* (see p. 214 and 256). They run towards the hoof cartilages and divide, forming individual networks.

At the level of the ergot, the two digital veins anastomose on the palmar (plantar) aspect. Branches from this anastomosis supply the ergot or unite within the digital cushion with branches from veins which themselves originate more distally. About 2–3 cm above the proximal border of the hoof cartilage, the digital veins usually divide into a dorsal and a palmar (plantar) trunk (/*a*) which are linked on the inner surface of the cartilage by 1 or 2 transverse vessels.

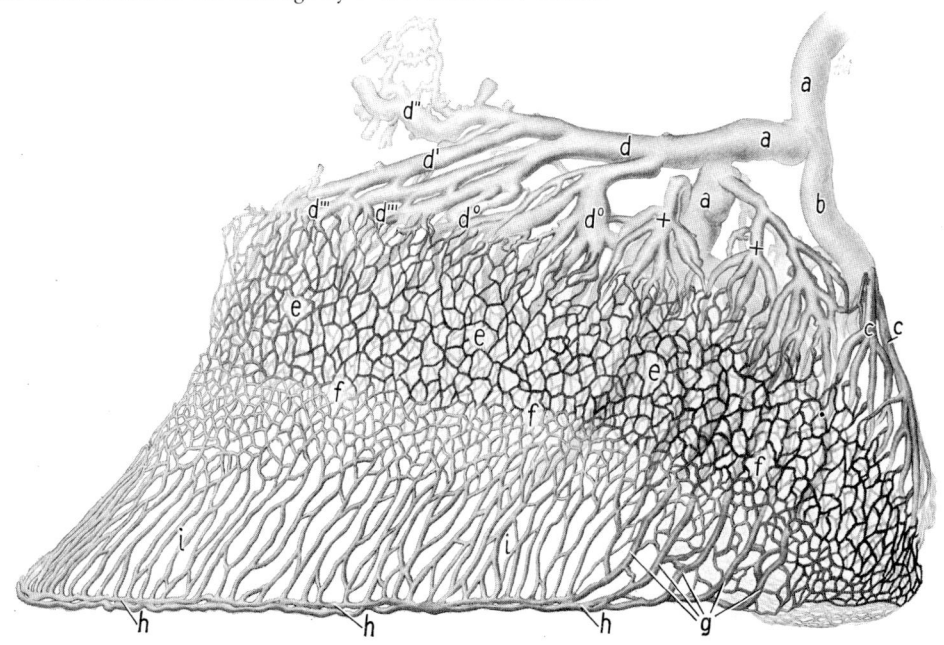

Fig. 438. Veins and subcutaneous venous plexuses of the digital organ of the forelimb of the horse. Lateral view. Drawn from a plastic corrosion preparation. About natural size. Superficial vessels are darker, deep vessels lighter in tone.
(After Schummer, 1951.)

a v. digitalis palmaris lateralis; *b* v. tori digitalis, *c* its heelward branches; *d, d″* v. dorsalis phalangis mediae; *d′* vv. coronales, *d‴* its dorsal, *d°* its lateral branches; + rr. coronales arising from the venous plexus at the inner surface of the hoof cartilage; *e* superficial and deep subcutaneous venous network of the periople-coronary segment; *f* border region between the venous plexus of the periople, coronary and wall segments; *g* branches of the plexus at the inner surface of the hoof cartilage to the v. marginis solearis; *h* v. marginis solearis; *i* subcutaneous venous network

Usually the palmar (plantar) branch gives rise to the *bulbar vein, v. tori digitalis (v. pulvina)* (/*b*), which anastomoses with the vein from the other side.

A few centimetres after its origin, the bulbar vein gives off several branches (/*c*) which are directed towards the heel. They form a fine double meshwork of vessels which drains the haired skin of the perioplic-coronary junction.

In its proximal portion, the lateral palmar (plantar) digital vein lies parallel to the hoof cartilage and follows a dorsal course to give rise to a vessel of similar calibre, the *v. dorsalis phalangis mediae* (/*d, d″*). The latter divides at the border of the extensor tendon into the *vv. coronales* (/*d′*) and a deeper branch (/*d″*). In the sub-tendinous connective tissue, the latter vessel forms a plexus, also uniting with branches from the other side, and with the continuation trunk of the digital vein of the same side. The coronary veins lie on the extensor tendon where they are linked proximally with the venous plexus of the hair-bearing skin above. The main branches of the coronary veins pass distally, and in the perioplic-coronary region they form a double network of vessels (/*e*), the *rr. dorsales* (/*d‴*). The coronary veins give off collateral branches to the hoof wall (/*d°*) before dividing into a superficial and a deep branch. A stout anastomosis which supplies branches to the pedal bone, connects the dorsal vein of the middle phalanx from either side.

After giving rise to the dorsal vein (/d), the digital vein forms a venous plexus on the inner surface of the hoof cartilage from which the *continuation trunk* of the digital vein re-emerges at the palmar (plantar) border of the pedal bone. This trunk follows the sole groove in the pedal bone, dividing into two branches at the level of the sole foramen and then entering the foramen accompanied by the satellite artery. Before uniting with its counterpart from the outer side, the more axial of these two vessels gives rise to a stout branch which provides the venous plexus of the distal sesamoid bone.

In the sole canal, the digital veins of the two sides from the *arcus terminalis venosum*, which establishes the venous plexus of the pedal bone. It connects with the parietal plexus of the corium by means of numerous small branches. These branches accompany the corresponding arteries arising from the *arterial terminal arch*, and they wind around the arteries forming a vascular sheath.

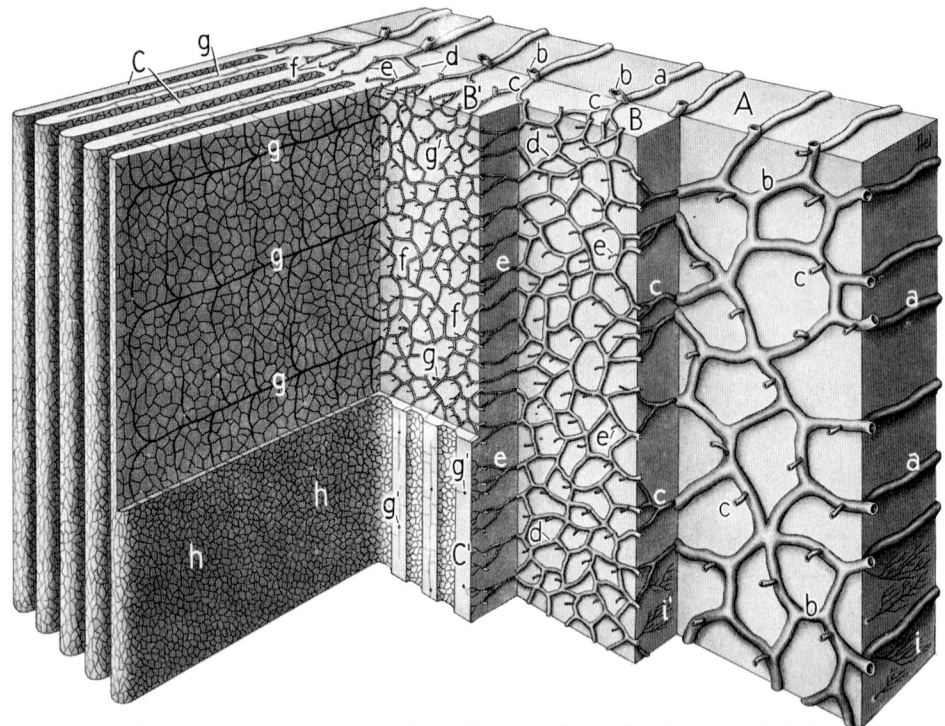

Fig. 439. Diagrammatic presentation of the arterial networks of part of the wall segment of the hoof.
(After Schummer, 1951.)

A subcutis (stratum periostale); *B* and *B'* corium; *C* lamellae coriales, *C'* lamellae coriales, cut off at their base
a afferent vessel; *b* subcutaneous plexus; *c* connecting branches; *d* deep corial network; *e* connecting branches; *f* subpapillary network; *g* aa. lamellares, *g'* aa. lamellares on the cut surface; *h* subepithelial capillary plexus; *i* capillaries of the subcutis; *i'* capillaries in the corium (the smaller meshed venous plexuses are of similar organization)

The digital vein forms a coarse plexus of vessels on the inner surface of the hoof cartilage, and from this gives rise to various vessels (/+). In the axial plane there is the stout *v. palmaris (plantaris) phalangis mediae*, which describes an arch over the distal sesamoid bone, joining a corresponding vessel from the other side. The same plexus gives rise to another branch which conjoins the dorsal vein of the middle phalanx along the inner surface of the hoof cartilage. Several medium-sized branches are also given off which reach the perioplic and coronary swellings, completing the palmar (plantar) part of the coronary vein (/+). On the inner aspect of the hoof cartilage, the plexus further provides several branches (/g) to the *v. marginis soleae* (/h), and the latter is linked, in turn, to the single-layered venous plexus of the wall segment (/i). About mid-way down the hoof, the subcutaneous venous plexus of the perioplic-coronary segment merges with those of the wall segment (/f). In the palmar (plantar) region, the venous networks finally unite with one another and form a single plexus which runs distally as the so-called "*internal*" veins of the hoof. Their function is to drain the corium of the bulb, frog, bars, sole and wall, and also the pedal bone, distal sesamoid, pedal joint, the podotrochlear bursa and the sheath of the deep flexor tendon.

There are numerous veno-venous shunts and *arterio-venous anastomoses* in the corium of the hoof. These are especially present in the large papillae at the edge of the sole, where they join the papillary arteries and veins at the tips of the papillae. They form a direct connection between the arteries and the veins at the edge of the sole, and their function is to stimulate the circulation of the hoof (Schummer, 1951).

The vascular networks are necessary prerequisites to supply the relatively large areas involved in the structures of the hoof. Recent studies contradict the once-held opinion that, together with the hoof mechanism, the vascular networks have the effect of a suction and pressure pump in stimulating and maintaining blood flow. The mechanism of the hoof certainly plays a small part in stimulating the circulation. The flow of blood, however, is maintained not only by the fact that the blood pressure gradient is directed away from the heart, but also by the presence of specialized structures within the vascular system itself, such as bypasses, "cushion" arteries, "throttle" veins and venous valves.

Within the hoof, the arterial networks are arranged in layers (439). They include a *subcutaneous* (/b), a *deep corial* (/d) and a *superficial corial* or *subpapillary* (/f) network. These networks ensure that the vessels of the skin of the hoof are in direct communication in both the horizontal and vertical planes.

The *aa. papillares* arise from the subpapillary arterial network. These supply the papillae and give rise to the *aa. lamellares* (/g) which vascularize the lamellae of the corium, forming a subepithelial capillary network (/h). The presence of these networks or plexuses and their specialized angioarchitecture ensures the maintenance of an adequate blood supply throughout all phases of the mechanical demands of the digital organ.

All hoof segments have characteristic subcutaneous venous networks which can be classified in three ways:

1. Venous plexus of the *perioplic-coronary segment* (438/e)
2. *wall and sole network* (/i), which is conjoined in the marginal veins of the sole (/i), and
3. the plexuses of the *bar* and *bulbar-frog segment* which empty their blood into the internal veins of the hoof.

The subcutaneous plexuses give rise to the deep plexuses of the corium. These in turn provide the superficial networks which give off the papillary and lamellar veins. The distal sesamoid and pedal bone have strikingly well-developed venous networks. Some veins of the hoof are valved.

Venous blood is carried from the hoof by several routes, as follows:

1. From the subcutaneous networks of the perioplic-coronary segment (438/e) via the dorsal ramus of the coronary vein (/d''') and thence by way of the dorsal vein of the second phalanx (/d) to the digital veins (/a);
2. from the parietal and sole networks (/i) through the veins of the margin of the sole (/h) to the digital veins (/a), and
3. from the bars, the frog and the bulb, as well as from the internal veins of the hoof, to the plexus situated on the inner aspect of the hoof cartilage and thereafter to the digital veins (/a).

Bibliography*

Circulatory system

Blood vascular system

Handbooks, textbooks, monographs

Akajevskii, A. I., und M. I. Lebedev (1971): Anatomy of the domestic animals. Part 3: cardiovascular, endocrine and nervous systems, skin and poultry. (Russian) Izdatel'stvo Vyss. Schkola, Moskva.

Bargmann, W. (1964): Histologie und mikroskopische Anatomie des Menschen. 5. Aufl. G. Thieme, Stuttgart.

W. Bargmann und W. Doerr (1963): Das Herz des Menschen. Bd. I und II. Thieme, Stuttgart.

Barone, R. (1957): Appareil circulatoire. In: R. Tagaud et R. Barone: Anatomie des équidés domestiques. Vol. 2, tome 4. Toulouse, Lab. d'Anat. École Nat. Vét.

Begemann, H., H.-G. Harwerth (1971): Praktische Hämatologie. 5. Aufl. G. Thieme, Stuttgart.

—, J. Rastetter (1972): Atlas der Klinischen Hämatologie. 2. Aufl. J. Springer, Berlin, Heidelberg, New York.

Benninghoff, A., K. Goertler (1971): Lehrbuch der Anatomie des Menschen. 2. Bd. Urban und Schwarzenberg.

Berg, R. (1973): Angewandte und topographische Anatomie der Haustiere. VEB G. Fischer Verlag, Jena.

Bradley, O. Ch. (1920): The topographical anatomy of the limbs of the horse. W. Green and Son, Edinburgh.

— (1922): The topographical anatomy of the thorax and abdomen of the horse. W. Green and Son, Edinburgh.

— (1923): The topographical anatomy of the head and neck of the horse. W. Green and Son, Edinburgh.

— (1959): rev. by T. Grahame: Topographical anatomy of the dog. 6th rev. ed. Oliver and Boyd, Edinburgh—London.

Bressou, C. (1964): Le porc. 2e éd. In: L. Montané, E. Bourdelle et C. Bressou: Anatomie régionale des animaux domestiques. Vol. 3. J.-B. Baillière et Fils, Éd., Paris.

Bucher, O. (1970): Cytologie, Histologie und mikroskopische Anatomie des Menschen. 7. Aufl. H. Huber, Bern, Stuttgart, Wien.

Canossi, C. C., M. Dardari, N. Cortesi, B. Brunelli und C. Pasquinelli (1968): Vascular anatomy of the dog. Technique and atlas. (French) Vigot Frères, Paris.

Clara, M. (1956): Die arteriovenösen Anastomosen. 2. Aufl., J. Springer, Wien.

Crouch, J. E. (1969): Text-atlas of cat anatomy. Lea and Febiger, Philadelphia.

Dobberstein, J., und G. Hoffmann (1964): Lehrbuch der vergleichenden Anatomie der Haustiere. 3. Bd.: Das Blutgefäßsystem. 2. Aufl. Verlag S. Hirzel, Leipzig, 1—74.

Ellenberger, W., und H. Baum (1891): Systematische und topographische Anatomie des Hundes. Verlag Paul Parey, Berlin.

—, — (1894): Topographische Anatomie des Pferdes. II. Teil: Kopf und Hals. Verlag Paul Parey, Berlin.

—, — (1897): Topographische Anatomie des Pferdes. III. Teil: Der Rumpf. Verlag Paul Parey, Berlin.

—, — (1943): Handbuch der vergleichenden Anatomie der Haustiere. 18. Aufl. Verlag J. Springer, Berlin.

Field, H. E., and M. E. Taylor (1969): An atlas of cat anatomy. Univ. Chicago Press, Chicago (and London).

Frick, H. (1956): Morphologie des Herzens. In: Handbuch der Zoologie, Bd. 8/7/5. Walter de Gruyter, Berlin.

Ghetie, V., E. Pastea si I. Riga (1955): Anatomie topografica a calului. Bucuresti, Ed. Agro-Silvica De Stat.

Grau, H., P. Walter (1967): Grundriß der Histologie und vergleichenden mikroskopischen Anatomie der Haussäugetiere. Paul Parey, Berlin und Hamburg.

Hafferl, A. (1933): Das Arteriensystem. 1. Die Arterien des Kiemen- und Körperkreislaufes. In: L. Bolk, E. Göppert, E. Kallius und W. Lubosch (Hrsg.): Handbuch der vergleichenden Anatomie der Wirbeltiere. 6. Bd. Verlag Urban und Schwarzenberg, Berlin—Wien, 563—677.

Haltenorth, Th. (Hrsg.) (1971): Die Säugetiere. In: Gessner, F. (Hrsg.): Handbuch der Biologie VI., 3. Akad. Verlagsges. Athenaion, Frankfurt/M.

Heberer, G., G. Rau und W. Schoop (1974): Angiologie. Grundlagen, Klinik und Praxis. G. Thieme, Stuttgart.

---

* The titles of German, English and most French papers are reproduced in the original language but titles of publications in other languages are translated into English.

HOPKINS, G. S. (1914); A guide to the dissection of the blood vessels and nerves of the pectoral and pelvic limbs of the horse. 3rd ed. W. F. Humphrey, Geneva, N. Y.
— (1925): Guide to the dissection and study of the blood vessels and nerves of the limbs, thorax and abdomen of the horse. 2nd ed. Publ. by author, Cornell Univ., Ithaca.
HORSBURGH, D., and J. HEATH (1938): Atlas of cat anatomy. Stanford Univ., California.
KOCH, T. (1970): Lehrbuch der Veterinäranatomie. 3. Bd. 2. Aufl. VEB G. Fischer Verlag, Jena.
KRAUSE, C. (1933): Lehrbuch der Sektion der Haustiere. Urban und Schwarzenberg, Wien.
KRÖLLING, O., H. GRAU (1960). Lehrbuch der Histologie und vergleichenden mikroskopischen Anatomie der Haustiere. 10. Aufl. Paul Parey, Berlin und Hamburg.
LESBRE, F.-X. (1923): Précis d'anatomie comparée des animaux domestiques. 2e vol.: Appareil de la circulation. J.-B. Baillière et Fils, Paris, 254—422.
MANNU, A. (1930): Apparecchio vascolare. In: U. ZIMMERL, A. C. BRUNI, G. B. CARADONNA, A. MANNU e L. PREZINSO: Trattato di anatomia veterinaria. Vol. 3. Casa Ed. Dott. Fr. Vallardi, Milano.
MAREK, J., J. MÓCSY (1956): Lehrbuch der klinischen Diagnostik der inneren Krankheiten der Haustiere. 5. Aufl. G. Fischer, Jena.
MARTIN, P. (1915): Die Blutgefäße. In: P. MARTIN: Lehrbuch der Anatomie der Haustiere, 2. Bd., 2. Hälfte. 2. Aufl. Verlag von Schickhardt und Ebner, Stuttgart, 121—206.
— (1923): Gefäßsystem der Fleischfresser. A. Blutgefäße. In: P. MARTIN: Lehrbuch der Anatomie der Haustiere. 4. Bd. 2. Aufl. Verlag von Schickhardt und Ebner, Stuttgart, 240—265.
—, W. SCHAUDER (1938): Das Blutgefäßsystem der Wiederkäuer. In: P. MARTIN und W. SCHAUDER: Lehrbuch der Anatomie der Haustiere. 3. Bd., 3. Teil. 3. Aufl. Verlag von Schickhardt und Ebner, Stuttgart, 378—427.
MAY, N. D. S. (1964): The anatomy of the sheep. 2nd ed. Univ. Queensland Press, St. Lucia, Brisbane, Queensland.
McCLURE, R. C., M. J. DALLMANN and Ph. G. GARRETT (1973): Cat anatomy. Lea and Febiger, Philadelphia.
MILLER, M. E., G. C. CHRISTENSEN and H. E. EVANS (1964): Anatomy of the dog. W. B. Saunders Company, Philadelphia—London.
MONTANÉ, L., et E. BOURDELLE (1913): Anatomie régionale des animaux domestiques. 1er vol.: Cheval. J.-B. Baillière et Fils, Paris.
—, — (1917): Anatomie régionale des animaux domestiques. 2e vol.: Ruminants. J.-B. Baillière et Fils, Paris.
—, —, C. BRESSOU (1953): Anatomie régionale des animaux domestiques. 4e vol.: Carnivores. Chien et chat. J.-B. Baillière et Fils, Paris.
MUELLER, C. (1873): Das Blutgefäßsystem. In: A. G. T. LEISERING und C. MUELLER: E. F. GURLT'S Handbuch der vergleichenden Anatomie der Haussäugethiere. 5. Aufl. Verlag A. Hirschwald, Berlin.
NIEPAGE, H. (1974): Methoden der praktischen Hämatologie für Tierärzte. Paul Parey, Berlin und Hamburg.

NOMINA ANATOMICA (1966): 3rd ed. Excerpta Med. Found., Amsterdam — New York — London — Milan — Tokio — Buenos Aires.
NOMINA ANATOMICA VETERINARIA (1973): Publ. by the Int. Committee on Vet. Anat. Nomenclature of the World Ass. of Vet. Anat., 2nd ed. Wien.
PIERARD, J. (1972): Anatomie appliquée des carnivores domestiques, chien et chat. Éd. S. A. Maloine, Paris. Somabec Lee St. Hyacinthe, Que.
POPESKO, P. (1961): Atlas der topographischen Anatomie der Haustiere. 1. Teil. VEB G. Fischer Verlag, Jena.
— (1963): Atlas der topographischen Anatomie der Haustiere. 2. Teil. VEB G. Fischer Verlag, Jena.
— (1968): Atlas der topographischen Anatomie der Haustiere. 3. Teil. VEB G. Fischer Verlag, Jena.
RATSCHOW, M. (1974): Angiologie. Hrsg. von G. Heberer, G. Rau und W. Schoop, 2. Aufl. Thieme, Stuttgart.
REIGHARD, J., and H. S. JENNINGS (1935): Anatomy of the cat. 3rd ed. H. Holt and Comp., New York.
ROONEY, II, J. R., W. O. SACK and R. E. HABEL (1967): Guide to the dissection of the horse. Publ. by W. O. Sack. Distr. by Edwards Brs Inc., Ann Arbor, Michigan.
SCHALM, O. W. (1965): Veterinary Haematology. 2. Aufl. Lea & Febiger, Philadelphia.
SCHEUNERT, A., A. TRAUTMANN (1965): Lehrbuch der Veterinär-Physiologie. 5. Aufl. Paul Parey, Berlin and Hamburg.
SCHMALTZ, R. (1927): Atlas der Anatomie des Pferdes. 4. Teil: Die Eingeweide. Verlagsbuchhandlung R. Schoetz, Berlin.
— (1928): Anatomie des Pferdes. 2. Aufl. Verlagsbuchhandlung R. Schoetz, Berlin.
— (1929): Atlas der Anatomie des Pferdes. 5. Teil: Der Kopf. R. Schoetz, Berlin.
— (1939): Atlas der Anatomie des Pferdes. 2. Teil: Topographische Myologie. 5. Aufl. Verlagsbuchhandlung R. Schoetz, Berlin.
— (1940): Atlas der Anatomie des Pferdes. 3. Teil: Die Lage der Eingeweide. 2. Aufl. Verlagsbuchhandlung R. Schoetz, Berlin.
SCHWARZE, E. (1964): Kompendium der Veterinär-Anatomie. 3. Bd.: Das Blutgefäßsystem. VEB G. Fischer Verlag, Jena, 3—105.
SISSON, S., and J. D. GROSSMAN (1953): The anatomy of the domestic animals. 4th ed. W. B. Saunders Company, Philadelphia—London.
STRUSKA, J. (1903): Lehrbuch der Anatomie der Hausthiere. W. Braumüller, Wien—Leipzig.
STUBBS, G. (1766): The anatomy of the horse. J. Purser, London. With a modern Paraphrase by J. McCUNN and C. W. OTTAWAY. J. A. Allen and Co, Ltd., London (1965).
TAYLOR, J. A. (1954): Regional and applied anatomy of the domestic animals. Part 1: Head and neck. Oliver and Boyd, Edinburgh.
— (1959): Regional and applied anatomy of the domestic animals. Part 2: Thoracic limb. Oliver and Boyd, Edinburgh.
— (1970): Regional and applied anatomy of the domestic animals. Part 3: Pelvic limb. Oliver and Boyd, Edinburgh.
ZIETZSCHMANN, O. (1943): Die Arterien. Die Venen. In: W. ELLENBERGER und H. BAUM: Handbuch

der vergleichenden Anatomie der Haustiere. 18. Aufl. Verlag J. Springer, Berlin, 627—743.

ZIMMERL, U., A. C. BRUNI, G. B. CARADONNA, A. MANNU e L. PREZINSO (1930): Trattato di anatomia veterinaria. Casa Ed. Dott. Fr. Vallardi, Milano.

Blood vessels, general; blood

ÁBRAHÁM, A. (1953): Die Innervation der Blutgefäße. Acta Biol. 4, 69—160.

ASCHOFF, L. (1925): Das reticulo-endotheliale System. Erg. inn. Med. Kinderheilk. 26. 1—118.

BARGMANN, W. (1958): Über die Struktur der Blutkapillaren. Dtsch. Med. Wschr. 83, 1704—1710.

BAUM, H. (1889): Die Arterienanastomosen des Hundes und die Bedeutung der Collateralen für den thierischen Organismus. Dtsch. Z. Thiermed. vergl. Path. 14, 273—316.

BECHER, H. (1932): Praktische wichtige Kapitel aus der Anatomie der Kreislauforgane. In: Herzneurosen und Moderne Kreislauftherapie. IX. Fortbildungslehrg., Bad Nauheim, 131—140. Th. Steinkopff, Dresden und Leipzig.

BENNINGHOFF, A. (1927): Über die Formenreihe der glatten Muskulatur und die Bedeutung der Rouget'schen Zellen an den Capillaren. Z. Zellforsch. mikr. Anat. 4, 125—170.

— (1927): Über die Beziehungen zwischen elastischem Gerüst und glatter Muskulatur in der Arterienwand und ihre funktionelle Bedeutung. Z. Zellforsch. 6, 348—396.

BLIN, P. C. (1963): Plasticité et dynamique vasculaires. „La circulation collatérale expérimentale". (With extensive references). Extr. de Economie et Medicine animales 4, 273—319.

BONGARTZ, G. (1958): Über die Struktur und Funktion der V. cava caudalis bei Rind, Schaf, Pferd, Schwein und Hund. Z. Zellforsch. 48, 24—50.

BOSTROEM, B., P., W. SCHNEIDER, W. SCHOEDEL (1953): Über die Durchblutung der arteriovenösen Anastomosen in der hinteren Extremität des Hundes. Pflügers Arch. ges. Physiol. 256, 371—380.

BOUCEK, R. J., R. TAKASHITA, R. FOJACO (1964): Functional anatomy of the ascending aorta and the coronary ostia (dog). Amer. J. Anat. 114, 273—282.

CLARA, M. (1956): Über die Morphologie der epitheloiden Zellen in der terminalen Strombahn. Acta neuroveg. 14, 3—15.

CONTI, G. (1953): Über das Vorkommen von Sperrvorrichtungen in Arterien mit spezieller Berücksichtigung der „gestielten Polster". Acta Anat. 18, 234—255.

DRAGENDORFF, O. (1911): Über die Formen der Abzweigungsstellen von Arterien bei den Wirbeltieren. Anat. H. 42, 737—803.

DZIALLAS, P. (1949): Über das Vorkommen von Klappen in den kleinsten Venen beim Menschen. Z. Anat. 114, 309—315.

EL ETREBY, M. F. (1963): Zur Orthologie und Pathologie der Glomerula digitalia, der sog. arterio-venösen Anastomosen in den Extremitätenenden des Hundes. Diss. med. vet., München.

FISCHER, H. (1951): Über die funktionelle Bedeutung des Spiralverlaufes der Muskulatur in der Arterienwand. Morph. Jb. 91, 394—445.

FREERKSEN, E. (1943): Gestalt, Anordnung und Einbauweise der Blutgefäße als funktionsfördernde Faktoren (Teil I). Z. Anat. Entwckl. 112, 304—318.

GRAU, H. (1933): Beiträge zur vergleichenden Anatomie der Azygosvenen bei unseren Haustieren (Pferd, Hund, Rind, Schwein) und zur Entwicklung der Azygosvenen des Rindes. Z. Anat. Entw. 100, 119—148, 256—276, 295—329.

— (1943): Allgemeines über den Kreislaufapparat. In: Ellenberger-Baum, Handbuch der vergleichenden Anatomie der Haustiere. 13. Aufl. Verl. J. Springer, Berlin.

GRIGOR'EVA, T. A. (1962): The innervation of blood vessels. Pergamon Press, New York.

GROSSER, O. (1902): Über arteriovenöse Anastomosen an den Extremitätenenden beim Menschen und den krallentragenden Tieren. Arch. mikr. Anat. 60, 191.

HAMMERSEN, F. (1970): Morphologische Befunde zur Ernährung der Gefäßwand. In: Lokalisierende Faktoren für Arterien- und Venenverschlüsse. Hrsg. von W. Rotter, H. Kief, D. Gross. Schattauer, Stuttgart.

— (1974): Endstrombahn, Mikrozirkulation. Allgemeiner Teil: Das Muster der terminalen Gefäße, S. 611—615. Zur Onthologie des Wandbaues und der Histophysiologie terminaler Gefäße, S. 615—633. Wege und Barrieren des transkapillaren Stoffaustausches, S. 633 bis 637. In Angiologie. Grundlagen. Klinik und Praxis. Hrsg. von G. Heberer, G. Rau und W. Schoop. G. Thieme, Stuttgart.

HAVLICEK, H. (1929): Vasa privata und Vasa publica. Hippokrates 2, 105—127.

— (1935): Die Leistungszweiteilung des Kreislaufes in Vasa privata und Vasa publica. Verh. dtsch. Ges. Kreisl.-Forsch. 8, 237—245.

HENNING, A. (1957): Modellversuch zur arteriovenösen Koppelung. In: T. v. Lanz, Anatomisches Seminar, München.

HENNINGSEN, B. (1969): Zur Innervation arteriovenöser Anastomosen. Z. Zellforsch. 99, 139 bis 145.

HETT, J. (1943): Zur feineren Innervation der arterio-venösen Anastomosen in der Fingerbeere des Menschen. Z. Zellforsch. 33, 151—156.

HOYER, H. (1877): Über unmittelbare Einmündungen kleinster Arterien in Gefäßäste venösen Charakters. Arch. mikr. Anat. 13, 603—644.

HYRTL, J. (1873): Die Korrosionsanatomie und ihre Ergebnisse. Wien.

ILLIG, L. (1961): Die terminale Strombahn. Capillarbett und Mikrozirkulation. Pathologie und Klinik in Einzeldarstellungen. Bd. X. Springer, Berlin, Göttingen, Heidelberg.

KNOCHE, H. (1958): Untersuchungen über die feinere Innervation der arterio-venösen Anastomosen. I. Mitteilung. Z. Zellforsch. 120, 379 bis 391.

KÜGELGEN V., A. (1951): Über den Wandbau der großen Venen. Morph. Jb. 91, 447—482.

— (1958): Die Venenwand als Gesamtkonstruktion. 3. Internat. Tag. der Dtsch. Arbeitsgemeinsch. für Phlebologie, Leverkusen.

LANZ v. T. ET AL. (1936/7): Über den funktionellen Einbau peripherer Venen. Anat. Anz. (Erg. H.) 83, 51—60.

—, A. KRESSNER, R. SCHWENDEMANN (1938): Der Einbau der oberflächlichen und der tiefen Ve-

nen am Bein, morphologisch und konstruktiv betrachtet. Z. Anat. Entw. 108, 695 bis 718.
LASSMANN, G., R. GOTTLOB (1970): Über die Bildung von epitheloidzellhaltigen Sperrpolstern in der Wand kleiner venöser Anastomosen im Bereich des Fußrückens bei Hunden. Act. Anat. 75, 47—53.
LEHMANN, W. (1909): Über Bau und Entwicklung der Wand der hinteren Hohlvene des Rindes und Venenklappen bei Pferd und Rind. Diss. Bern.
LOWENSTEIN, L. M. (1959): The mammalian reticulocyte. Int. Rev. Cytol. 8, 136—174.
LUCKNER, H. (1955): Die Funktion der arteriovenösen Anastomosen. In: Bartelsheimer — Küchenmeister; Kapillaren und Interstitium. G. Thieme, Stuttgart.
MAXIMOW, W. (1927): Bindegewebe und blutbildende Organe. In: Handbuch der mikroskopischen Anatomie des Menschen. Bd. II/1, 232 bis 583, Springer.
MAYERSBACH, H. (1956): Der Wandbau der Gefäßübergangstrecken zwischen Arterien rein elastischen und rein muskulösen Typs. Anat. Anz. 102, 333—360.
MILLEN, J. W. (1948): Observation of the innervation of blood vessels. J. of Anat. 82, 68—80.
MOLYNEUX, G. S. (1970): Innervation of arteriovenous anastomoses. J. Anat. (Lond.) 106, 203.
MOORE, D. H., H. RUSKA (1957): The fine structure of capillaries and small arteries. J. Biophysic. and Biochem. Cytol. 3, 457—461.
ORTMANN, R. (1959): Allgemeine Anatomie der Herz- und Gefäßnerven. Verh. dtsch. Ges. Kreisl. Forsch. 25, 15—36.
PALADE, G. E. (1953): Fine structure of blood capillaries. J. Appl. Physics 24, 1424—1445.
RACHMANOW, A. W. (1901): Zur Frage der Nervenendigung in den Gefäßen! Anat. Anz. 19, 555—558.
REALE, P., H. RUSKA (1966): Die Feinstruktur der Gefäßwand. In: Morphologie und Histochemie der Gefäßwnd. Hrsg. von M. Comel, L. Laszt: Karger, Basel.
ROLLHÄUSER, H. (1959): Die Morphologie der Kapillaren. In: Angiologie von M. Ratschow, S. 73—82. G. Thieme, Stuttgart.
ROTTER, W., W. BÜNGELER (1955): Blut und Blutbildende Organe. In: Lehrbuch der speziellen patholog. Anatomie. Bd. I., 414—834. Springer.
ROUILLER, CH., W. G. FORSSMANN (1969): Morphologie der arteriellen Gefäßwand. In: Arterielle Hypertonie. Hrsg. von R. Heinz, G. Loose. G. Thieme, Stuttgart.
RUHENSTROTH-BAUER, G. (1957): Die Struktur der Säugererythrozyten. In: Handbuch der gesamten Hämatologie. Bd. I/1, Urban und Schwarzenberg.
SCHAEWEN, H. v. (1969): Normwerte hämatologischer Merkmale beim Hund. Diss. med. vet. Berlin FU.
— (1971): Die Morphologie der Thrombocyten bei Mensch und Tier. P. Parey, Berlin. 86 S.
SCHENK, E. A., A. EL BADAWI (1868): Dual innervation of arteries and arterioles. Z. Zellforsch. 91, 170—177.
SCHÖNBERGER, F. (1960): Über die Vaskularisation der Rinderaortenwand. Helv. physiol. pharmacol. Acta 18. 136—150.

SCHORN, J. (1955): Zur normalen und pathologischen Anatomie der sogenannten „arterio-venösen Anastomosen" in den Endgliedern der Finger und Zehen des Menschen. Habil. Schr., Med. Fak. Gießen.
SCHUMMER, A. (1949): Zirkulationsfördernde Einrichtungen am Zehenendorgan des Pferdes. Dtsch. Tierärztl. Wschr. 56, 36—38.
— (1954): Morphologische und funktionelle Betrachtung zum peripheren Blutkreislauf. Tierärztl. Umsch. 9, 377—385.
— (1961): Das Blutgefäßsystem als Gegenstand anatomischer Forschung. Nachrichten der Gießener Hochschulges. 30, 35—50.
SPALTEHOLZ, W. (1941): „Endarterien", historische und kritische Studie. Erg. Anat. 33, 21—30.
SPANNER, R. (1932): Neue Befunde über die Blutwege der Darmwand und ihre funktionelle Bedeutung. Gegenbaurs Morph. Jb. 69, 394—454.
— (1952): Zur Anatomie der arteriovenösen Anastomosen. Verh. Dtsch. Ges. Kreislaufforsch. 18, 257—277.
STAUBESAND, J. (1949): Über den Wandbau der arterio-venösen Anastomosen und die Bedeutung der epitheloiden Zellen. Ärztl. Forsch. 3, 78—86.
— (1950): Über verschiedene Typen arterio-venöser Anastomosen. Anat. Anz. (Ergh.) 97, 68—75.
— (1955): Zur Morphologie der arterio-venösen Anastomosen. In: H. Bartelsheimer und H. Küchenmeister; Kapillaren und Interstitium. G. Thieme, Stuttgart.
— (1956): Eigenarten des Gefäßmusters bei räumlicher und bei flächenhafter Ausbreitung der arteriellen Strombahn in Organen. Verh. dtsch. Ges. Kreisl. Forsch. 22, 263 bis 267 (Darmstadt).
—, W. RULFFS (1958): Die Klappen kleinerer Venen. Z. Anat. 120, 392—423.
— (1959): Anatomie der Blutgefäße. In: M. Ratschow: Angiologie. G. Thieme, Stuttgart.
— (1959): Über die Versorgung der Arterienwand. Anat. Anz. 107, 332—339.
— (1963): Anatomische Befunde zur Ernährung der Gefäßwand. Verh. dtsch. Ges. Kreisl-Forsch. 29, 1—16.
— (1968): Zur Orthologie der arterio-venösen Anastomosen. In: Die arterio-venösen Anastomosen. Hrsg. von F. Hammersen. D. Gross, Huber, Bern.
— (1974): Normale Anatomie (der Blutgefäße). In: Angiologie. Grundlagen, Klinik und Praxis. S. 1—39. Begr. von M. Ratschow, Hrsg. von G. Heberer, G. Rau und W. Schoop. 2. Aufl. G. Thieme, Stuttgart.
STENIUS, P. I. (1928): Untersuchungen zur Kenntnis der Altersveränderungen an den Blutgefäßen des Hundes. Diss. med. vet. Leipzig.
STÖHR, PH. jr. (1925): Über den formgestaltenden Einfluß des Blutstromes. Würzburger Abhandl. 22, 269—282.
THIENEL, M. (1903): Vergleichende Untersuchungen über den mikroskopischen Bau der Blutgefäße der Schultergliedmaßen von Pferd, Esel, Rind, Kalb, Schaf, Schwein und Hund. Diss. Bonn.
TISCHENDORF, F. (1948): Bau und Funktion der arterio-venösen Anastomosen. Dtsch. med. Rdsch. 2, 432—435.
WATZKA, M. (1936 a): Über Gefäßsperren und arterio-venöse Anastomosen. Z. mikrosk. anat. Forsch. 39, 521—544.

Yoffey, J. M. (1950): The mammalian lymphocyte. Biol. Rev. 25, 314—343.
Zweifach, B. W. (1939): Character and distribution of blood capillaries. Anat. Rec. 73, 475—495.

Heart

Aagard, O. C., H. C. Hall (1915): Über Injektionen des Reizleitungssystems und der Lymphgefäße des Säugetierherzens. Anat. H. 51, 357 bis 427.
Ábrahám, A., L. Erdélyi (1957): Über die Struktur und die Innervation des Reizleitungssystems im Herzen der Säugetiere. Acta. Biol. 3, 275.
Ackerknecht, E. (1918): Die Papillarmuskeln des Herzens. Untersuchungen an Karnivorenherzen. Arch. Anat. Physiol. 63—136.
— (1941): Der Säugetierherz-Mechanismus. VI. Beitrag zur „Anatomie für den Tierarzt". Dtsch. Tierärztl. Wschr. 49, 301—307.
— (1943): Das Herz. In: Ellenberger-Baum: Handbuch der vergl. Anatomie der Haustiere. 18. Aufl. J. Springer, Berlin.
Albrecht, R. (1957): Zur Anatomie des Bovidenherzens (Untersuchungen am Yak, Wisent, Bison, indischen Büffel, Zebu, Zwergzebu und Steppenrind). Morphol. Jb. 59, 574—605.
Angst, J. (1928): Das Herz des Hausschafes (Ovis aries L.). Diss. med. vet. Zürich.
Aschoff, L. (1910): Nervengeflechte des Reizleitungssystems des Herzens. Dtsch. med. Wschr. 36, 104.
Balmer, J. (1937): Über Herzgewichte gesunder und nierenkranker Hunde. Diss. med. vet. Bern.
Bargmann, W. (1963): Bau des Herzens. In: Das Herz des Menschen. Bd. 1, 88—118, G. Thieme, Stuttgart.
Barone, R., R. Malavieille (1951): Les vaisseaux du cœur des équidés. Recueil Med. Vet. 77, 513 bis 529.
—, A. Colin (1951): Les artères du cœur chez les ruminants domestiques. Rev. Méd. Vét. 102, 172 bis 181.
Benninghoff, A. (1930): Blutgefäße und Herz. In: v. Möllendorf's Handbuch der mikroskopischen Anatomie des Menschen. II/1, 1—225. J. Springer, Berlin.
— (1933): Herz. In: L. Bolk, E. Göppert, E. Kallius und W. Lubosch, Handbuch der vergleichenden Anatomie der Wirbeltiere. 6. Bd. 467—556. Urban und Schwarzenberg, Berlin und Wien.
— (1948): Anatomische Beiträge zur Frage der Verschiebung der Ventilebene im Herzen. Ärztl. Forsch. 2, 27—32.
Berg, R. (1962): Untersuchungen über das Verhalten der Coronargefäße beim Hausschwein im Hinblick auf das Herztodproblem. Vorl. Mitt. Mh. Vet. Med. 17, 469—472.
— (1962): Das makroskopisch-anatomische Verhalten der Aa. coronariae und ihrer Äste beim Hausschwein im Vergleich zum Menschen. Mh. Vet. Med. 17, 628—635.
— (1963): Über das Auftreten von Myokardbrücken über den Koronargefäßen beim Schwein (Sus scrofa dom). Anat. Anz. 112, 25—31.
— (1964): Über den Entwicklungsgrad der Koronargefäßmusters beim Hausschwein (Sus scrofa dom.). Anat. Anz. 115, 193—204.
— (1964): Beitrag zur Phylogenese des Verhaltens der Koronararterien zum Myokard beim Hausschwein (Sus scrofa dom.). Anat. Anz. 115, 184 bis 192.
— (1965): Zur Morphologie der Koronargefäße des Schweines unter besonderer Berücksichtigung ihres Verhaltens zum Myokard. Arch. exper. Vet. Med. 19, 1145—1307.
Bettinger, H. (1932): Beiträge zur Pathologie des Ductus Botalli. Cbl. allg. Path. path. Anat. 54, 289—295.
Bhargava, I., C. Beaver (1970): Observations on the arterial supply and venous drainage of the bovine heart. Anat. Anz. 126, 343—354.
Blair, E. (1961): Anatomy of the ventricular coronary arteries in the dog. Circulat. Res. 9, 333—341.
Blum, S. (1925): Beiträge zu den Maß- und Gewichtsverhältnissen des Pferdeherzens. Diss. med. vet. Budapest.
Böhme, G. (1964): Die Herzbeutel-Zwerchfell-Verbindung beim Hund. Anatom. Anz. 115, 83—88.
Booth, N. H. et al. (1966): Postnatal changes in the ventricles of the pig. Proc. Soc. exper. Biol. Med. 122, 186—188.
Boucek, R. J., Fojaco, R. Takashita (1964): Anatomic considerations for regional intimal changes in the coronary arteries (dog). Anat. Rec. 148, 161—169.
Brown, R. E. (1965): The pattern of the microcirculatory bed in the ventricular myocardium of domestic mammals. Amer. J. Anat. 116, 355 bis 373.
Bucher, O. (1945): Sondervorrichtungen an Kranzgefäßen. Schweiz. Med. Wschr. 75, 966—969.
Chiodi, V. (1932): Il nodo seno-atriale del cuore dei mammiferi. La Clinica Vet. 55, 689—705.
— (1957): Le strutture profonde del cuore in canidi. Atti. Acad. Sci. Bologna 245, 59—72.
Christensen, G. C., F. L. Campeti (1959): Anatomic and functional studies of the coronary circulation in the dog and pig. Amerik. J. vet. Res. 20, 18—26.
— (1962): The blood supply to the interventricular septum of the heart. Amer. J. veterin. Res. 23, 869—874.
Corodan, G., C. Radu, L. Radu (1966): Investigations of the capillary supply to the heart in mammals. (Rumanian) Ser. Med. veterin. 9, 87—89.
Daasch, T. (1927): Die Herzknochen beim Schweine. Diss. med. vet. Berlin.
Davies, F., E. T. B. Francis, D. R. Wood, E. A. Jonson (1959): The atrioventricular pathway for conduction of the impulse for cardiac contraction in the dog. Trans. roy. soc. Edinb. 63, 71—84.
Didion, H. (1942): Über die Persistenz des Ductus Botalli im höheren Alter. Zbl. allg. Path. path. Anat. 80, 55—56.
Fehn, P. A., B. B. Howe, R. R. Pensinger (1968): Comparative anatomical studies of the coronary arteries of canine and porcine hearts. II. Interventricular septum. Acta. Anat. 71, 223—228.
Filho, A. F. (1969): Beitrag zum Studium des Sinusknotens beim Vollblutpferd. Rev. Fac. Vet., Sao Paulo 8, 43—58.
Fuchs, J. (1954): Der Feinbau der Koronargefäße bei Pferd und Rind. Diss. med. vet. Zürich.
Glaus, A. (1958): Systematische und statistische Untersuchungen am Schweineherz. Diss. med. vet. Zürich.

GOERTTLER, K. (1951): Die Bedeutung der funktionellen Struktur der Gefäßwand. I. Untersuchungen an der Nabelschnurarterie des Menschen. Morph. Jb. **91**, 368—393.

GROSSMANN, H. E. (1923): Über Herzknochen. Verh. zool. Ges. **28**, 41—42.

GSCHWED, T. (1931): Das Herz des Wildschweines. VI. Beitrag zur Anatomie von Sus scrofa L. und zum Domestikationsproblem. Diss. med. vet. Zürich.

HABERMEHL, K. H. (1956): Die Verlagerung der Bauch- und Brustorgane des Hundes bei verschiedenen Körperstellungen. Habilschr. Gießen 1953, in Zbl. Vet. med. **3**, 1—43 und 172—204.

— (1959): Die Blutgefäßversorgung des Katzenherzens. Zbl. Vet. med. **6**, 655 bis 680.

— (1964): Zur Technik der intrakardialen und intrapulmonalen Injektion beim Fleischfresser. Sonderdruck aus „Die Blauen Hefte" für den Tierarzt **1**, 13 S.

— (1966): Morphologie und Funktion der Herzeigengefäße. Zbl. Vet. Med. A. **13**, 111—138.

— (1967): Zur Variationsbreite des Koronarvenenmusters bei Mensch und Haussäugetier. Zbl. Vet. Med. A **14**, 777—788.

HAHN, A. W. (1908): Beitrag zur Anatomie der Kammerscheidewand unserer Haustiere. Diss. med. vet. Bern.

HAMLIN, R. L. (1960): Radiographic anatomy of heart and great vessels in healthy living dogs. J. Amer. veterin. med. Assoc. **136**, 265—273.

HARMS, D. (1966): Über den Bau und Verschluß des Ductus arteriosus Botalli der Rinder. Z. Zellforsch. **72**, 344—363.

HAUSOTTER, E. (1924): Das Herzskelett der Haussäuger Pferd, Rind, Schaf, Schwein, Hund und Katze. Diss. med. vet., Wien, 1923. Wien. Tierärztl. Mschr. **11**, 311.

HEGAZI, A. EL H. (1958): Die Blutgefäßversorgung des Herzens von Rind, Schaf und Ziege. Diss. med. vet. In: Zbl. Vet. Med. **5**, 776—819.

HIRSCH, S. (1949): Grundsätzliches zur Frage der Regulationseinrichtungen im Coronarkreislauf. Acta. Anat. **8**, 168—184.

HOFFMANN, V. (1960): Die Blutgefäßversorgung des Pferdeherzens. Diss. med. vet. Gießen.

HUWYLER, B. (1926/27). Zur Anatomie des Schweineherzens. Untersuchungen des Kammerinneren bei Sus scrofa domesticus. Anat. Anz. **62**, 49 bis 76.

ILLY, F. (1956): Beiträge zur Kenntnis der Maß- und Gewichtsverhältnisse des Rinder- und Schweineherzens. Diss. med. vet. Bundapest.

JANSEN, H. H. (1963): Innervation des Herzens. In: Das Herz des Menschen. Bd. 1., 228—255, G. Thieme, Stuttgart.

JARISCH, A. (1913): Die Pars membranacea septi ventriculorum des Herzens. Sitzungsber. Kaiserl. Akad. Wiss. Wien **121**, 187—207.

KÁDÁR, F. (1956): Topographische Beziehungen zwischen arteriellen und venösen Kranzgefäßen des Herzens. Anat. Anz. **103**, 112—115.

— (1963): Die topographischen Verhältnisse zwischen Gefäßen und Muskelfasern des Herzens. Anat. Anz. **113**, 381—386.

KATSCHINSKY, P. (1923): Die Herzknorpel des Pferdes. Diss. med. vet. Bern.

KEITH, A., M. W. FLACK (1906): The auriculoventricular bundle of the human heart. Lancet II. 359—364.

—, — (1907): The form and the nature of the muscular connections between the primary divisions of the vertebrate heart. J. Anat. Physiol. **41**, 172—189.

KLUMP, W. (1910): Die Bewegung des Herzens und der großen Gefäße. Diss. med. vet. München.

KNESE, K.-H. (1963): Topographie des Herzens. In: Das Herz des Menschen. Bd. 1, 260—308, G. Thieme, Stuttgart.

KOCH, W. (1913): Zur Entwicklung und Topographie des spezifischen Muskelsystems im Säugetierherzen. Med. Klin. **9**, 77—78.

KRETZ, I. (1927): Über die Bedeutung der Venae minimae Thebesii für die Blutversorgung des Herzmuskels. Virchows Arch. path. Anat. **266**, 647—675.

KRIPPENDORF, W. (1923): Die Größenverhältnisse des Herzens bei verschiedenen Hunderassen. Diss. med. vet. Berlin.

KÜLBS, F. (1912): Vergleichende Anatomie und Histologie des His'schen Bündels. Med. Klin. **8**, 1294—1295.

KUNZE, G. (1932): Messungen am Hundeherzen. Diss. med. vet. Gießen.

KUVŠYNOV, J. A. (1965): Form und Größe der atrio-ventrikulären Öffnungen und Klappen beim Pferdeherz. Veterynarija, Kyiv, 63—69.

— (1965): Die Herzform beim Pferd. Veterynarija, Kyiv, 60—62.

LECHNER, W. (1942): Vorkammermuskulatur und große Herzvenen bei Säugern. Z. Anat. **111**, 545 bis 571.

— (1942): Herzspitze und Herzwirbel. Anat. Anz. **92**, 249—283.

LÜCKE, R. (1955): Blutgefäßversorgung des Hundeherzens. Diss. med. vet. Hannover.

LUKASZEWSKA-OTTO, H. (1968): Subepikardiales lymphatisches Netzwerk des Herzens bei Mensch und Schwein. Fol. morph., Warszawa **27**, 453 bis 456.

— (1968): Die linke Atrioventrikularklappe beim Hund. Fol. morph. Warszawa **27**, 115—128.

— (1968): Die Mitralis beim Kalb und Ochsen. Fol. morph., Warszawa **27**, 233—247.

— (1968): Die Klappen der V. cava caudalis und des Koronarsinus der Schweine, Rinder und des Rotwildes. Fol. morph. V., Warszawa **27**, 441 bis 446.

— (1968):Die Klappen der V. cava caudalis und des Koronarsinus am Herzen des Hundes. Fol. morph., Warszawa **27**, 447—452.

MARTINI, E. (1965): Die arterielle Gefäßversorgung des Herzens einiger Haussäugetiere. Arch. ital. Anat. Embriol. **70**, 351—380.

MCKIBBEN, J. S., G. C. CHRISTENSEN (1964): The venous return from the interventricular septum of the heart. Amer. J. veterin. Res. **25**, 512 bis 517.

—, R. GETTY (1968): A comparative study of the cardiac innervation in domestic animals. The canie. Amer. J. Anat. **122**, 533—543.

—, — (1968): A comparative morphologie study of the cardiac innervation in domestic animals. II. The feline. Amer. J. Anat. **122**, 545—553.

—, — (1969): Innervation of heart of domesticated animals: Horse. Amer. J. veterin. Res. **30**, 193 bis 202.

—, — (1969): Innervation of heart of domesticated animals: Pig. Amer. J. veterin. Res. **30**, 779 bis 789.

—, — (1969): A comparative study of the cardiac innervation in domestic mammals: Sheep. Acta. anat., **74**, 228—242.

—, — (1970): A comparative study of the cardiac innervation in domestic animals: The goat. Anat. Anz. **126**, 161—171.

Melka, J. (1926): Beiträge zur Kenntnis der Morphologie und der Obliteration des Ductus arteriosus Botalli. Anat. Anz. **61**, 348—361.

Meinertz, Th. (1966): Eine Untersuchung über den Sinus coronarius cordis (v. cava. sin.), die V. cordis media und den Arcus aortae sowie den Ductus (Lig.) Botalli bei einer Anzahl von Säugetierherzen. Morphol. Jb. **109**, 473—500.

— (1975): Weitere Untersuchungen über den Sinus coronarius cordis, die V. cordis media und den Arcus aortae sowie den Ductus (Lig.) Botalli bei einer Anzahl von Säugetierherzen. Morphol. Jb. **121**, 139—154.

Meyling, H. A., H. Ter Borg (1957): The conducting system of the heart in hoofed animals. Cornell Vet. **47**, 419—447.

Michel, G. (1962): Zur mikroskopischen Anatomie der Purkinjefasern im Herzen des Schweines und des Hundes. Mh. Vet. Med. **17**, 848—850.

— (1963): Zum Bau des Reizbildungs- und Erregungsleitungssystems bei Haus- und Wildschwein. Arch. exp. Vet. Med. **17**, 1049—1080.

— (1963): Zum Bau der Herzmuskulatur bei Haus- und Wildschweinen. Zbl. Vet. med. A **10**, 381 bis 396.

— (1966): Zum Bau der Herzmuskulatur bei Haus- und Wildschwein sowie beim Rind. Arch. exper. Vet. Med. **20**, 1071—1076.

Mühlenbruch, H. G. (1970): Zum Bau des Herzens des Göttinger Miniaturschweines unter besonderer Berücksichtigung der Herzeigengefäße. Diss. med. vet. München.

Müller, G., E. Wernicke (1969): Das Relief der Trabeculae carneae der Herzhöhlen. Anat. Anz. **125** Ergh., 75—78.

Muir, A. R. (1954): The development of the ventricular part of the conducting tissue in the heart of the sheep. J. Anat. (Lond.) **88**, 381 bis 391.

— (1957): Observations on the fine structure of the Purkinje fibres in the ventricles of sheep's heart. J. Anat. (Lond.) **91**, 251 bis 258.

Nandy, K., G. H. Bourne (1963): A study of the conducting tissue in mammalian hearts. Acta. anat. **53**, 217—226.

Ottaway, C. W. (1944): The anatomical closure of the Foramen ovale in the Equine and Bovine Heart: A comparative study with observations on the foetal and adult states. Vet. J. **100**, 111 bis 118, 130—134.

Ottolenghi, M., P. Sartoris (1929): Topografia Toraco-Cardiaca del Cane. Nuovo Ercolani, Torino, 1—31.

Palmgren, A. (1928). Herzgewicht und Weite der Ostia atrioventricularia des Rindes. Anat. Anz. **65**, 333—342.

Petersen, G. (1918): Über das atrioventrikulare Reizleitungssystem bei den Haussäugetieren. Arch. wiss. Tierheilk. **44**, 97—113.

Pianetto, M. B. (1939): The coronary arteries of the dog. Amer. Heart J. **18**, 403—410.

Poláček, P. (1959): Über die myokardialen Bündel, die den Verlauf der Koronararterien überbrücken. Anat. Anz. **106**, 386—395.

—, L. Steinhart, J. Endrys, J. Vyslouźil (1962): Muskelbrücken und Fesseln auf Kranzarterien im Coronariogramm. Českoslov. Morfol. **10**, 251—258.

Preuss, F. (1955): Zur Nomenklatur am Herzen. Anat. Anz. **103**, 20—37.

— (1955): Einheitliche Benennung am Herzen der Tiere und des Menschen. Zbl. Vet. Med. **2**, 802 bis 805.

Puff, A. (1960): Der funktionelle Bau der Herzkammern. Verl. G. Thieme, Stuttgart.

— (1960): Die funktionelle Bedeutung des elastischmuskulären Systems der Kranzarterien. Morph. Jb. **100**, 546—558.

— (1964): Funktionelle Besonderheiten im Wandbau der Herzvenen. Verh. Anat. Ges. **59**, 282 bis 284.

—, J. Bernardi (1965): Die mechanische Bedeutung der Koronararterien für die diastolische Entfaltung der Herzkammern. Morphol. Jb. **107**, 399—414.

Quiring, D. P., and R. J. Baker (1953): The equine heart. Amer. J. Vet. Res. **14**, 62—67.

Racknitz, v. W. (1964): Untersuchungen zur Vaskularisation der normalen und der fibrotischen Herzklappen des Hundes. Diss. med. vet. München.

Rickert, J. (1955): Blutgefäßversorgung des Schweineherzens. Diss. med. vet. Hannover.

Röse, C. (1890): Beiträge zur vergleichenden Anatomie des Herzens der Wirbelthiere. Morphol. Jb. **16**, 27—96.

Rühl, B. (1971): Gewichte, Faserdicken und Kernzahlen des Herzmuskels und deren Beziehungen zu Körpergewicht und Skelettmuskelmasse bei 205 Tage alten, 5 Rassen zugehörigen Schweinen. Zbl. Vet. Med. A **18**, 151—173.

Scaglia, G. (1927): L'apparato nervoso contenuto nel sistema atrioventricolare di Bos taurus. Arch. ital. Anat. Embriol **24**, 658—696.

Schaller, O. (1958): Korrosionsanatomie des Pferdeherzens. Zbl. Vet. Med. **5**, 152—170.

— (1962): Die arterielle Gefäßversorgung des Erregungsleitungssystems des Herzens bei einigen Säugetieren. I. Die arterielle Gefäßversorgung des Nodus sinu-atrialis beim Hunde (Canis familiaris). Morph. Jb. **102**, 508—540.

— (1962): Die arterielle Gefäßversorgung des Erregungsleitungssystems des Herzens bei einigen Säugetieren. II. Die arterielle Gefäßversorgung des atrioventriculären Anteiles des Erregungsleitungssystems beim Hunde (Canis Familiaris). Morph. Jb. **102**, 541—569.

Schauder, W. (1918): Makroskopische Darstellung des atrioventrikularen Verbindungsbündels im Herzen des Pferdes. Arch. wiss. prakt. Tierheilk. **44**, 371—380.

Schiebler, T. H. (1953/54): Herzstudie. I. Mitteilung. Histochemische Untersuchungen der Purkinjefasern von Säugern. Z. Zellforsch. **39**, 152 bis 167.

— (1955/56): Herzstudie. II. Mitteilung. Histologische, histochemische und experimentelle Untersuchungen am Atrioventrikularsystem von Huf- und Nagetieren. Z. Zellforsch. **43**, 243 bis 306.

— (1961): Histochemische Untersuchungen am Reizleitungssystem tierischer Herzen. Naturwiss. **48**, 502—503.

—, W. Doerr (1963): Orthologie des Reizleitungs-

systems. In: Das Herz des Menschen. Bd. 1, 165 bis 221, G. Thieme, Stuttgart.
SCHMACK, K.-H. (1974): Die Ventilebene des Herzens bei Pferd, Rind und Hund. Diss. med. vet. Giessen.
SCHMALTZ, R. (1886): Die Purkinje'schen Fäden im Herzen der Haussäugetiere. Arch. wiss. prakt. Tierheilk. 12, 161—209.
SCHMIDT, D., B. HOHAUS, F. RÖDER (1967): Offener Ductus arteriosus (Botalli) beim Hund. Berl.-Münch. tierärztl. Wschr. 9, 168—171.
SCHRÖDER, F. (1921): Die Größenverhältnisse am Herzen beim Schwein und Schaf und über den Einfluß der Kastration auf die Entwicklung des Herzens. Diss. med. vet. Leipzig.
SCHUBERT, F. (1909): Beiträge zur Anatomie des Herzens der Haussäugetiere. Diss. med. vet. Leipzig.
SCHWARZ, G. (1910): Untersuchungen über das Sinusgebiet im Wiederkäuerherzen. Diss. med. vet., Giessen.
SCIACCA, A. (1952): Topografia delle fibre muscolari del fascio atrioventricolari di Bos taurus. Atti. Soc. ital. Anat. 60, 314.
SEMMLER, A. (1923): Untersuchungen über Größenverhältnisse von Herz und Lunge gegenüber Größe, Lebend- und Schlachtgewicht bei zwei verschiedenen Schweinerassen. Diss. med. vet. Bern.
SICHERT, E. (1935): Zur vergleichenden Anatomie des Herzens der Katze (Felis domestica Briss.). Diss. med. vet. Budapest.
SIMIC, V. (1938): Zur Anatomie des Carnivorenherzens (Untersuchungen an Feliden, Hyäniden, Caniden, Procyoniden und Musteliden). Morph. Jb. 82, 499—536.
— (1964): Herzvasographie bei den Haustieren und beim Menschen. Verh. Anat. Ges. 59, 334 bis 351.
SLEZÁČEK, L., P. ZUBAL (1968): Die Kranzarterien des Schafherzens. Acta Univ. Agric., Brno, Fac. agron. 16, 282—291.
SPALTEHOLZ, W. (1924): Die Arterien der Herzwand. Anatomische Untersuchungen an Menschen- und Tierherzen. Leipzig, S. Hirzel.
— (1934): Die Thebesischen Venen. Anat. Anz. 79, 212—216.
STEINMÜLLER, G. (1910): Segel- und Taschenklappen unserer Haussäugetiere. Diss. med. vet. Bern.
STIÉNON, L. (1925): Recherches sur l'origine du systéme purkinien dans le cœur des mammifères. Arch. Biol. 35, 89—115.
— (1926): Recherches sur l'origine du nœud sinusal dans le cœur des mammifères. Arch. Biol. 36, 523—539.
STROH, G. (1923): Foramen ovale. Münch. tierärztl. Wschr. 293.
STRUBELT, H. (1925): Anatomische Untersuchungen über den Verschluß und die Rückbildung des Ductus Botalli bei Kälbern und Rindern. Diss. med. vet. Berlin.
STÜNZI, H., E. TEUSCHER und A. GLAUS (1959): Systematische Untersuchungen am Herzen von Haustieren. 2. Mitt. Schwein. Zbl. Vet. Med. 6, 640—654.
SUMMERFIELD KING, T. J. B. COAKLEY (1958): The intrinsic nerve cells of the cardiac atria of mammals and man. J. Anat. 92, 353—376.

SUSSDORF, V. M. (1923): Anatomische Vorbemerkungen über die Lage des Herzens. Aus Lehrb. der klin. Untersuchungsmethoden F. Enke, Stuttgart.
TAWARA, S. (1906): Das Reizleitungssystem des Säugerherzens. Eine anatomisch-histologische Studie über das Atrioventrikularbündel und die Purkinjeschen Fäden. G. Ficher, Jena.
TCHENG, K. T. (1951): Innervation of the dog's heart. Amer. Heart. J. 41, 512—524.
TER BORG, H. (1937): Untersuchungen über das Vorkommen von Purkinje-Zellen in den Herzvorkammern unserer Haustiere unter besonderer Berücksichtigung des Pferdes! Acta neerl. morphol. 1, 64—67.
THEBESIUS, A. G. (1709): Disputatio medica de circulo sanguinis in corde. Lugduni Batavorum.
UNGER, K. (1934/35): Die Venae minimae und die Foramina venarum minimarum (Thebesii) des Herzens. Z. Kreislforsch. 26, 27, 57—93, 865 bis 877.
— (1938): Beitrag zur Kenntnis der Vv. cordis minimae (Thebesii) des menschlichen Herzens. Z. Anat. Entw. 108, 356—375.
VAERST, G. (1888): Vorkommen, anatomische und histologische Entwicklung sowie physiologische Bedeutung der Herzknochen bei Wiederkäuern. Dtsch. Z. Thiermed. vergl. Path. 13, 46—71.
VALLET, L.-P. (1951): Les Artères Coronaires Cardiaques chez les Carnivores. These med. vet. Lyon.
VAU, E. (1968): Über die Variation der Koronararterien im Schafherzen. Truy po veterinarii, Tartu, 57, 35—39.
WAHLIN, B. (1935): Das Reizleitungssystem und die Nerven des Säugetierherzens. Diss. Uppsala.
WELSCH (1921): Herzknorpel von Hund und Katze. Diss. med. vet. Berlin.
WENSING, C. J. G. (1965): Das Erregungsleitungssystem und seine Nervenkomponenten im Schweineherz. Tijdschr. Diergenees. 90, 765 bis 777.
— (1965): Innervation des atrioventriculären Reizleitungssystems beim Schwein. Zbl. Vet. Med. A 12, 531—533.
WITZEMANN, S. (1923): Über die Noduli valvularum semilunarium und ihre physiologische Bedeutung bei unseren Haustieren. Diss. med. vet. Bern.
ZIMMERL, U. (1911): Topografia Toraco-Cardiaca degli Equidi. Arch. Scient. della Reale Societa Naz. Veterin. Torino, 1—41.
ZIMMERMANN, A. (1923): Das Reizleitungssystem des Herzens bei Equiden. Anat. Anz. (Erg. H.) 57, 252—258.
— (1924): Das Reizleitungssystem des Herzens bei Haussäugetieren. Berl. Tierärztl. Wschr. 39, 39 bis 41.
ZINCK, K. H. (1941): Weiteres über Sondervorrichtungen an Kranzgefäßen. Klin. Wschr. 20, 1032.
ZÖLCH, K. (1967): Korrosionsanatomische Untersuchungen an den Herzeigengefäßen des Hausschweines (Sus scrofa dom.) Unter Berücksichtigung des Kapillarsystems. Diss. med. vet. Giessen.
ZYPEN, E. VAN DER (1974): Über die Ausbreitung des vegetativen Nervensystems in den Vorhöfen des Herzens. Eine enzymhistochemische und elektronenmikroskopische Untersuchung. Acta Anat. 88, 363—384.

Arteries, veins

General

Barone, R. (1954): Les anomalies artérielles chez les équidés domestiques. Bull. Soc. Sci. vét. Lyon 1954, 1—9.
Baum, H. (1889): Die Arterienanastomosen des Hundes und die Bedeutung der Collateralen für den tierischen Organismus. Diss. phil. Erlangen.
Blin, P.-C. (1963): Plasticité et dynamique vasculaires. La circulation collatérale expérimentale. Econ. Méd. anim. 4, 273—319.
Bressou, C. (1932): Anastomose artério-veineuse chez un cheval. Recl Méd. vét. 108, 401—403.
Burrows, C. F. (1973): Techniques and complications of intravenous and intraarterial catheterization in dogs and cats. J. Am. vet. med. Ass. 163, 1357—1363.
Bourdelle, E. (1899): Anomalie de l'artère collatérale du canin. Revue Méd. vét. Toulouse 24, 479—483.
Faujour, R. (1923): Contribution à l'anatomie du système artériel du chat. Thèse doct. vét. Lyon.
Horowitz, A. (1967): Remarks on the arteriae bovis. Produced as manuscript for the discussions on nomenclature.
Horvath, E. (1934): Das arterielle System der Hauskatze. Diss. med. vet. Budapest.
Krestev, L. (1948): Beitrag zur Erforschung der Arterien der Ziege. Jb. Univ. Sofia, Vet. Med. Fak., 24, 511—520.
Pohle, C. (1920): Das Venensystem des Hundes. Diss. med. vet. Leipzig.
Schmaltz, R. (1898): Über die Beschreibung der Venen. Berl. tierärztl. Wschr. 1898, 193—195.
Simic, V., et V. Ghetie (1939): Des variations dans la division de quelques artères importantes chez le cheval. Revue Méd. Milit., No. 4.
Smallwood, J. E., and R. F. Sis (1973): Selective arteriography in the cat. Am. J. vet. Res. 34, 955—963.
Wachtel, W. (1966): Kreislauf des Schweines. Arch. exp. Vet. Med. 20, 1005—1113.
Zimmermann, A. (1930): A vénás rendszerről. (The venous system) Természettudományi Közlöny, Budapest.

Trunk

Anderson, W. D., and W. Kubicek (1971): The vertebral-basilar system of dog in relation to man and other mammals. Am. J. Anat. 132, 179—188.
Barone, R., et Cl. Pavaux (1959): Veine cave céphalique gauche chez une vache. C. r. Ass. Anat. 82, —.
Bartels, J. M., and J. T. Vaughan (1969): Persistent right aortic arch in the horse. J. Am. vet. med. Ass. 154, 406—409.
Bassett, E. G. (1965): The anatomy of the pelvic and perineal regions of the ewe. Aust. J. Zool. 13, 201—241.
— (1971): The comparative anatomy of the pelvic and perineal regions of the cow, goat and sow. N. Z. Vet. J. 19, 277—290.
Berg, R. (1958): Vergleichende anatomische Messungen an der Vena cava caudalis unserer Haustiere. Diss. med. vet. Humboldt-Univ. Berlin.
— (1961): Systematische Untersuchungen über das Verhalten der Äste der Aorta abdominalis bei Felis domestica. Anat. Anz. 110, 224—250.
— (1962): Systematische Untersuchungen über das Verhalten der Äste der Aorta abdominalis bei Canis familiaris. Mh. Vet. Med. 17, 307—315.
—, A. Smollich (1961/62): Systematische Untersuchungen über die Aufzweigung der Aa. subclaviae bei Canis familiaris. Anat. Anz. 110, 410—416.
Beron, A. (1964): Contribution à l'étude de la vascularisation interne des vertèbres cervicales du chien. Thèse doct. vét. Alfort.
Biermann, A. (1953): Blutgefäßversorgung des Zwerchfells beim Schwein. Diss. med. vet. Hannover.
Blin, P.-C., et A. Beron (1964): Vascularisation artérielle du segment vertébral cervical chez le chien. Econ. Méd. anim. 5, 426—437.
Bohn, F. K. (1970): Beitrag zur Diskussion von Fällen mit Ductus arteriosus persistens. Tierärztl. Umschau 25, 301—303.
Bordoni, A., e J. A. D. Morees Pessamilio (1974): Observações sobre a veia ázigos em bovinos (Bos taurus L.). Rev. Med. Vet. 10, 139—152.
Bory, G. (1917): Az arteria thoracica externa rendellenes eredése kutaában. (The irregular origin of the a. thoracica externa of the dog.) Állatorvosi Lapok XL 50, 323.
Bressou, C. (1919): Présence d'une jugulaire antérieure chez le cheval, accompagnée d'une anastomose jugulo-carotidienne. Bull. Soc. Cent. Méd. vét. 1919, 147—.
Brown, R. E., and R. E. Carrow (1963): Vascular anatomy of the bovine tail. J. Am. vet. med. Ass. 143, 1214—1215.
Buergelt, C.-D., and L. G. Wheaton (1970): Dextroaorta, atopic left subclavian artery, and persistant left cephalic vena cava in a dog. J. Am. vet. med. Ass. 156, 1026—1029.
—, P. F. Suter and W. J. Kay (1968): Persistent truncus arteriosus in a cat. J. Am. vet. med. Ass. 153, 548—552.
Çalislar, T. (1968): Distribution of the cervical and thoracic arteries of the sheep. (Turkish) Vet. Fak. Derg. Ankara Univ. 15, 250—265.
Chambers, G., E. Eldred and C. Eggett (1972): Anatomical observations on the arterial supply to the lumbosacral spinal cord of the cat. Anat. Rec. 174, 421—433.
Czembirek, H., G. Freilinger, L. Gröger, H. Mandl und H. Zacherl (1974): Zur Gefäßversorgung der Bauchhaut des Schweines. Acta anat. 87, 146—153.
Daigo, M., Y. Sato, M. Otsuka, T. Yoshimura, S. Komiyama and Y. Ogawa (1973): Stereoroentgenographical studies on the peripheral arteries of the udder of the cow. Bull. Nippon vet. zootech. Coll. No 22, 31—39.
Davis, D. M. (1910): Studies on the chief veins in early pig embryos, and the origin of the vena cava inferior. Am J. Anat. 10, 461—472.
Deniz, E., und K. H. Wrobel (1964): Über eine Vena cava cranialis sinistra persistens beim Esel. Zbl. Vet. Med. A 2, 358—362.
Duvernoy, H., Cl. Maillot et J. G. Koritke (1970): La vascularisation de la moelle épinière chez le chat (Felis domestica). Les artères extramédullaires postérieures. J. Hirnforsch. 12, 419—437.

FARKAS, D. (1929): A ló vénás törzseiről. (The venous trunks of the horse.) Diss. med. vet. Budapest.
FERNANDES FILHO, A. (1958—1959): Note on the origin of the common carotid arteries in Sus scrofa domesticus. Folia Clin. Biol. 28, 100—102.
—, V. BORELLI (1970): Wichtige Kollateralen des Aortenbogens bei der Katze. (port.) Revta Fac. Med. Vet., Univ. S. Paulo 8, 385—388.
GETTY, R., and N. G. GHOSHAL (1967): Applied anatomy of the sacrococcygeal region of the pig as related to tail-bleeding. Vet. Med. small Anim. Clin. 62, 361—367.
GHOSHAL, N. G., and R. GETTY (1967): Applied anatomy of the sacrococcygeal region of the ox as related to tail-bleeding. Vet. Med. small Anim. Clin. 62, 255—264.
GLÄTTLI, H. (1924): Anatomie des Venensystems des Kuheuters. Diss. med. vet. Zürich.
GOMERČIĆ, H. (1967): Persistent vena cardinalis cranialis sinistra in a dog. (Croatian) Vet. Arh. 37, 307—314.
GRAU, H. (1933): Beiträge zur vergleichenden Anatomie der Azygosvenen bei unseren Haustieren (Pferd, Hund, Rind, Schwein) und zur Entwicklungsgeschichte der Azygosvenen des Rindes. Z. Anat. Entwicklungsgesch. 100, 119—148; 256 bis 276; 295—330.
— (1944): Über die venöse Versorgung der präkardialen Rumpfwand bei unseren Haussäugetieren, insbesondere über die V. intercostalis suprema und V. vertebralis thoracica. Morph. Jb. 89, 481—498.
GREIFENHAGEN, U. (1973): Arterien der Körperwand des Pferdes. Diss. med. vet. Hannover.
HABEL, R. E. (1966): The topographic anatomy of the muscles, nerves, and arteries of the bovine female perineum. Am. J. Anat. 119, 79—96.
HABERMEHL, K.-H. (1951): Das Verhalten der V. cava caudalis (postrenaler Abschnitt) und ihres visceralen Zuflußgebietes bei der Katze (Felis domestica). Anat. Anz. 98, 295—308.
HAMMOND, W. S. (1937): The developmental transformations of the aortic arches in the calf (bos taurus), with especial reference to the formation of the aorta. Am. J. Anat. 62, 149—177.
HARE, W. C. D. (1961): Radiographic anatomy of the cervical region of the canine vertebral column. I. Fully developed vertebrae. II. Developing vertebrae. J. Am. vet. med. Ass. 139, 209—216; 217—220.
HÜTTEN, H., und F. PREUSS (1953): Blutentnahme beim Schwein. Berl. Münch. Tierärztl. Wschr. 66, 89—90.
HUGHES, T. (1967): The aorticopulmonary artery of the cat — its location and postnatal closure. Anat. Rec. 158, 491—499.
HUTTON, P. H. (1969): The presence of a left cranial vena cava in a dog. Br. vet. J. 125, 21—22.
INGHAM, B. (1969): An unusual configuration of the posterior vena cava in a beagle. Z. Versuchstierk. 11, 276—278.
IVANOV, S. (1947): Über die Variabilität von Vena azygos bei den Haustieren. Jb. Univ. Sofia, Vet. Med. Fak., 23, 289—342.
—, K. DIMITROV und D. DINOV (1964): Variability of the v. azygos in domestic animals. IV sheep. (Bulgarian) Nauchni Trud. vissh vet.-med. Inst. Prof. G. Pavlov 13, 25—30.
—, L. KRESTEV, K. DIMITROV und A. TODOROV (1950): Über die Variabilität von Vena azygos bei den Haustieren. II. Untersuchungen am Rind. Jb. Univ. Sofia, Vet. Med. Fak., 26, 185—200.
KÄHLER, W. (1960): Arterien der Körperwand des Schweines. Diss. med. vet. Hannover.
KADLETZ, M. (1928): Über eine Mißbildung im Bereiche der Vena cava caudalis beim Hunde. Z. Anat. Entwicklungsgesch. 88, H. 3 und 4.
— (1931): Die Venen der Thoracolumbalgegend eines Hundeembryos von 12 mm S.-S.-L. und über eine zweite Mißbildung im Bereiche der Vena cava caudalis beim Hunde. Z. Anat. Entwicklungsgesch. 94, H. 2—5.
KAYANJA, F. I. B. (1971): The blood supply to the lumbar vertebrae of the cat. Zbl. Vet. Med. A 18, 219—224.
KNELLER, S. K., R. E. LEWIS and R. B. BARRETT (1972): Arteriographic anatomy of the feline abdomen. Am. J. vet. Res. 33, 2111—2119.
KNIGHT, D. H., D. F. PATTERSON and J. MELBIN (1973): Constriction of the fetal ductus arteriosus induced by oxygen, acetylcholine and noerepinephrine in normal dogs and those genetically predisposed to persistent patency. Circulation Res. 47, 127—132.
KÖSTERS, W. (1967): Sulcocommissuralgefäße bei Wiederkäuern und Pferd. Diss. med. vet. Hannover.
KOSTYRA, J. (1953): Żyła nieparzysta u owcy. (The vena azygos of the sheep.) Annls Univ. Mariae Curie-Skłodowska, Sect. DD 8, 87—102.
KOSYKH, A. P., und V. V. PETROV (1959): Topography and technique for puncturing the a. carotis of the ox. (Russian) Trudy Buryat. zoovet. Inst. 14, 175—204.
KOWATSCHEV, G. (1968): Über die Variabilität der Äste der Brust- und Bauchaorta bei Schafföten. Anat. Anz. 122, 37—47.
KRAHMER, R. (1964): Über eine paarige V. cava cranialis beim Schäferhund. Anat. Anz. 115, 354—357.
— (1966): Ein Beitrag zum Verhalten der V. cava caudalis und ihres viszeralen Zuflußgebietes bei der Katze. Anat. Anz. 118, 310—316.
— (1966): Über die sogenannte „Verdoppelung" der V. cava caudalis im postrenalen Abschnitt bei Katzen (Felis domestica). Anat. Anz. 119, 436—443.
— (1968): Über die funktionelle Bedeutung der Kollateralen der V. cava caudalis beim Rind. Wiss. Z. Karl-Marx-Univ. Leipzig 17, 171—174.
—, M. GÜNTHER (1967): Über die funktionelle Bedeutung der Kollateralen der V. cava caudalis bei Rind und Schwein. Arch. exp. Vet. Med. 21, 475—482.
LAZORTHES, G., A. GOUAZÉ, G. BASTIDE, L.-H. SOUTOUL, O. ZADEK et J.-J. SANTINI (1966): La participation des artères radiculaires lombosacrées à la vascularisation fonctionelle du renflement lombaire. Bull. Ass. Anat. 51e Réun., 580—588.
LESCHKE, U. (in Vorbereitung): Venen der Körperwand des Pferdes. Diss. med. vet. Hannover.
LEVINGER, I. M., and N. APPEL (1966): The anastomoses between the vertebral artery and the rete

mirabile epidurale in cattle. Refuah vet. 23, 241—244.

LOEFFLER, K. (1966): Zur Blutgefäßversorgung der Haut des Rindes. Berl. Münch. tierärztl. Wschr. 79, 365—367.

LOGINOVA, L. A. (1970): Sravnitel'naya kharakteristika krovosnabzheniya pozvonochnykh venoznykh spletenii tscheloveka i sobaki. (Comparative characteristics of the blood supply to the vertebral venous plexuses in man and the dog.) Arkh. Anat. Gistol. Embriol. 59, 50—55.

MANNU, A. (1914): Considerazoni sulla morfologia delle arterie vertebralis e occipitalis in alcuni mammiferi. Arch. ital. Anat. Embriol. 12, 434—442.

— (1914): Variazioni dell'arteria vertebralis nell' uomo e nei mammiferi. Arch. ital. Anat. Embriol. 13, 79—113.

MARIN, D. R. (1972): Aportaciones al conocimiento de la vascularización en la columna vertebral. An. Anat. (Zaragoza) 21, 557—569.

MARTHEN, G. (1939): Über die Arterien der Körperwand des Hundes. Diss. med. vet. Hannover.

MAY, N. D. S. (1960): Absence of the prerenal segment of the posterior vena cava of the dog. Aust. vet. Inl. Feb. 1960, 67—68.

MÜNTER, U. (1962): Arterien der Körperwand des Schafes. Diss. med. vet. Hannover.

NITSCHKE, Th., und F. PREUSS (1971): Die Hauptäste der A. iliaca interna bei Mensch und Haussäugetieren in vergleichend-anatomisch häufiger Reihenfolge. Anat. Anz. 128, 439—453.

OPITZ, M. (1961): Arterien der Körperwand der Katze. Diss. med. vet. Hannover.

OTSUKA, J. (1969): Studies of the vascular channels in the costal cartilage of the goat and ox. (Japanese) Bull. Fac. Agric. Kagoshima Univ. No. 19, 21—29.

OTTO, E. (1961): Arterien der Körperwand der Ziege. Diss. med. vet. Hannover.

PAIVA, O. M. (1948): Dois casos de a. subclavia dextra como última colateral do arcus aorticus no cao. Revta Fac. Med. Vet., Univ. S. Paulo 3, 203—222.

— (1953/54): A. subclavia dextra como última colateral do arcus aorticus em sus scrofa domestica. Revta Fac. Med. Vet., Univ. S. Paulo 5, 5—16. Folia Clin. Biol. 22, 190—292.

—, P. PINTO E SILVA (1958—59): Aspects of the distribution of the truncus omocervicalis in the dog. Folia Clin. Biol. 28, —.

PALIC, D. (1954): Vascularisation des Schafeuters. Acta Vet. 4, Fasc. 2.

PARKER, A. J. (1973): Distribution of spinal branches of the thoracolumbar segmental arteries in dogs. Am. J. vet. Res. 34, 1351—1353.

PARSONS, F. G. (1902): On the arrangement of the branches of the mammalian aortic arch. J. Anat. Physiol. (N. S.) 16, 389—399.

PEARL, R. (1908): An abnormality of the venous system of the cat, with some considerations regarding adaption in teratological development. Arch. Entwicklungsmech. 25, 648—654.

PETERS, K. H. (1967): Sulcocommissuralgefäße bei Hund und Katze. Diss. med. vet. Hannover.

PETIT, M. A. (1929): Les veines superficielles du chien. Revue Méd. vét. 81, 425—437.

PUGET, E., et M. TOTY (1956): Sur la circulation artérielle de la mamelle chez la chienne. Revue Méd. vét. 1956, 84—93.

RAUHUT, D. (1962): Venen an der Körperwand der kleinen Wiederkäuer: Ziege und Schaf. Diss. med. vet. Hannover.

RICHMOND, B. T. (1968): A case of persistent right aortic arch in the cat. Vet. Rec. 83, 169 —.

ROOT, C. R., and R. J. TASHJIAN (1971): Thoracic and abdominal arteriography in calves. Am. J. vet. Res. 32, 1193—1205.

ROUX, J. M. W. LE, und H. WILKENS (1959): Beitrag zur Blutgefäßversorgung des Euters der Kuh. Dtsch. tierärztl. Wschr. 66, 429—435.

SCHALLER, O. (1955): Die V. cava cranialis sinistra persistens bei unseren Haussäugetieren, insbesondere den Fleischfressern. Z. Anat. Entwicklungsgesch. 119, 131—155.

SCHAUDER, W. (1951): Die Blutgefäße des Euters der Ziege. Tierärztl. Umsch. 6, 71.

SCHRÖDER, L., und R. KRAHMER (1966): Über die funktionelle Bedeutung der Kollateralen der V. cava caudalis bei den Fleischfressern. Arch. exp. Vet. Med. 20, 443—450.

SCHWARZ, R., und H. BADAWI (1961): Eine doppelte V. cava caudalis bei einem Ziegenbock. Anat. Anz. 110, 52—62.

—, — (1962): Unterschiede in der Einmündung der V. spermatica interna und V. circumflexa ilium profunda sowie Besonderheiten im Entstehungsgebiet der V. cava caudalis bei den Haussäugetieren. Dtsch. tierärztl. Wschr. 69, 498—501.

SEIDLER, D. (1966): Arterien und Venen der Körperwand des Rindes. Diss. med. vet. Hannover.

SKODA, K. (1912): Eine seltene Anomalie des Carotidenursprunges — Mangel des Truncus bicaroticus — beim Pferd. Anat. Anz. 40, Nr. 19 und 20.

SMIRNOV, G. N. (1928): The anatomy of the aortic arch. (Russian) Utschenye Zapiski Kasansk. Univ. 88, 49—52.

SMITH, H. W. (1909): On the development of the superficial veins of the body wall in the pig. Am. J. Anat. 9, 439—462.

SMOLLICH, A. (1959): Ursprungsvariationen der Kopf- und Schlüsselbeinarterien beim Hund. Anat. Anz. 106, 6—10.

—, R. BERG (1959): Beobachtungen über das Verhalten der Äste des Aortenbogens bei Canis familiaris, Felis domestica und Sus scrofa domesticus. Anat. Anz. 107, 309—316.

—, R. BERG (1960): Systematische Untersuchungen über den Ursprung und Aufzweigung der Äste des Aortenbogens beim Hausschwein (Sus scrofa domesticus). Mh. Vet. Med. 14, 489—492.

—, H. J. FRANZKE (1959): Ursprungsanomalie der Arteria carotis communis sinistra beim Hund. Anat. Anz. 107, 187—189.

SOLIS, J. A., and C. P. MAALA (1973): Intrathoracic vessels of the Philippine carabao (Bos bubalis). Philipp. J. vet. Med. 12, 1—11.

SOUZA GARCIA, O. DE (1963): Origem das artérias pudenda externa e epigástrica caudal profunda no cão-tronco pudendo-epigástrico. Arqs Esc. Vet. 15, 153—166.

— (1965): Estudo anatômico acêrca de um caso de persistência da veia precardinal esquerda em equino. Arqs Esc. Vet. 17, 71—73.

STAROSTINAS, V. (1967): Some veins of the thoracic

cavity of the horse and their valves. (Lithuanian) Trudy Litovsk. vet. Akad. 8, 39—47.
STEFANOWSKI, T. (1971): Tetnice przepony piersiowej u zwierzat miesozernych. (Arteries of the thoracic diaphragm in carnivores. (Polish) Polskie Archwm wet. 14, 623—643.
TELSER, R. (1971): Angiographie der A. carotis communis und der A. vertebralis beim Hund. Diss. med. vet. München.
TSOLOV, S. (1966): Variations in the branching of the truncus brachiocephalicus communis in sheep embryos. (Bulgarian) Nauchni Trud. vissh. vet.-med. Inst. Prof. G. Pavlov 17, 237—248.
VAU, E. (1959): Blutversorgung des Euters des Schweines. Zborn. nautsch. trud. eston. sel'sk. akad. 8 —.
— (1960): Die Blutabflußwege des Kuheuters. Wiener tierärztl. Mschr., Festschr. Prof. Schreiber, 312—319.
VERGNAUD, P. (1966): Contribution à l'étude de la vascularisation interne des vertèbres dorsales du chien. Thèse doct. vét. Alfort.
VITUMS, A. (1962): Anomalous origin of the right subclavian and common carotid arteries in the dog. Cornell Vet. 52, 5—15.
— (1969): Development and transformation of the aortic arches in the equine embryos with special attention of the formation of the definitive arch of the aorta and the common brachiocephalic trunc. Z. Anat. Entwicklungsgesch. 128, 243—270.
— (1970): Abnormal origin of the carotid arteries in a Shetland pony. Anat. Anz. 126, 284—288.
— (1972): Anomaly of the vena cava caudalis in a dog. Zbl. Vet. Med. C 1, 149—152.
WAIBL, H. (1973): Linke Vena cava cranialis ohne entsprechende Venen auf der rechten Seite bei der Hausziege. Berl. Münch. tierärztl. Wschr. 86, 171—174.
WAKURI, H., and Y. KANO (1960): Study on the aortic arch and the branches arising from it in the Japanese domestic cat. Bull. Azabu vet. Coll., Japan, No 7, 125—133.
—, — (1961): Study on the aortic arch and its branches in the pig. Bull. Azabu vet. Coll., Japan, No 8, 57—66.
WEIR, E. C. (1970): Venous anomalies in the abdomen of a dog. Vet. Rec. 86, 582 —.
WESZELY, E. (1925): A juh truncus brachiocephalicus communisa és ágai. (The truncus brachiocephalicus and its branches in the sheep.) (Hungarian) Diss. med. vet. Budapest.
WIEBOLDT, A. (1966): Venen der Körperwand des Hundes und der Katze. Diss. med. vet. Hannover.
WILKENS, H., und G. ROSENBERGER (1957): Betrachtungen zur Topographie und Funktion des Oesophagus hinsichtlich der Schlundverstopfung des Rindes. Dtsch. Tierärztl. Wschr. 64, 393 bis 396.
WISSDORF, H. (1970): Die Gefäßversorgung der Wirbelsäule und des Rückenmarkes vom Hausschwein (Sus scrofa F. domestica L., 1758). Zbl. Vet. Med., Beih. 12, 1—104.
WOLFF, K. (1963): Venen der Körperwand des Schweines. Diss. med. vet. Hannover.
WORTHMANN, R. P. (1956): The longitudinal vertebral venous sinuses of the dog. I. Anatomy. II. Functional aspects. Am. J. vet. Res. 17, 341—363.
WYROST, P. (1968): A rare case of left anterior vena cava (vena cava cranialis sinistra persistens) in a dog. Fol. Morph. 27, 129—133.
YASUDA, M. (1949): Studies on Vv. thoracicae longitudinales of mammalia. 1. Studies on Vv. thoracicae longitudinales of dog. Jap. J. zootech. Sci. 19, 39—40.
ZAKIEWICZ, M., B. KORZYBSKA-BLENAU und H. ZEMBRZYCKA (1965): Arcus aorticus dexter persistens in a dog. (Polish) Medycyna wet. 21, 11—13.
ZIETZSCHMANN, O. (1917): Die Zirkulationsverhältnisse des Euters einer Kuh. Dtsch. tierärztl. Wschr. 25, 361—365.
ZIMMERMANN, G. (1933): Topographisch-anatomische Untersuchungen mit besonderer Berücksichtigung des Vorkommens von Vena cava cranialis sinistra beim Hund. Közlemények az összehasonlító élet- és kórtan köréből 30, 306 —.

Head

ADAMS, W. E. (1957): On the possible homologies of the occipital artery in mammals, with some remarks on the phylogeny and certain anomalies of the subclavian and carotid arteries. Acta anat. 29, 90—113.
BAIER, W. (1929): Über Venennetze am Speiseröhreneingang bei den Haussäugetieren. Berl. tierärztl. Wschr. 45, 625—626.
BALDWIN, B. A. (1964): The anatomy of the arterial supply to the cranial regions of the sheep and ox. Am. J. Anat. 115, 101—118.
—, F. R. BELL (1963): The anatomy of the cerebral circulation of the sheep and ox. The dynamic distribution of the blood supplied by the carotid and vertebral arteries to cranial regions. J. Anat. Lond. 97, 203—215.
BECKER, H. (1960): Arterien und Venen am Kopf des Schweines. Diss. med. vet. Hannover.
BENVENUTI, C., und M. FEDRIGO (1969): Observations on the arterial blood supply to the mandible of the dog. (Italian) Ann. Fac. Med. Vet. Pisa 21, 190—204.
BESSAGUET, P. (1969): Vascularisation artérielle de la moelle épinière des ongulés domestiques. Thèse Doct. vét. Toulouse.
BINEV, K., N. BODUROV und C. GADEV (1970): Röntgenologische Untersuchungen über die arterielle Blutversorgung der Hörner beim Rind. Anat. Anz. 127, 290—295.
BOCCADORO, B. (1964): Radiological investigations of the intra- and extra-cranial arterial system in the dog. (Italian) Veterinaria, Milano, 13, 463—480.
BRÜCKNER, C. (1909): Die Kopfarterien des Hundes unter spezieller Berücksichtigung derer des Bulbus und der Schädelhöhle. Diss. med. vet. Zürich.
CANOVA, P. (1909): Die arteriellen Gefäße des Bulbus und seiner Nebenorgane bei Schaf und Ziege. Diss. med. vet. Zürich. Anat. 1909, 5—52.
ČERNÝ, H., and R. NAJBOT (1970): Contribution to morphology and arterial supply to rete mirabile epidurale in the calf. Acta Vet. Brno 39, 367—375.
ČERVENY, C., und J. KAMAN (1962): Zur Innervation und Blutversorgung des Hornes beim Rind. Veterinářství 12, 73—75.
CHADZYPANAGIOTIS, D., and A. KUBASIK (1968):

Arteries supplying blood to the brain in the cat. Fol. Morph. 27, 411—421.

CHOMIAK, M., und J. WELENTO (1968): Arteries of the brain in the calf. (Polish) Polskie Archwm wet. 11, 185—190.

CHRISTENSEN, G. C., and S. TOUSSAINT (1957): Vasculature of external nares and related areas in the dog. J. Am. vet. med. Ass. 131, 504—509.

DAIGO, M., Y. SATO, M. OTSUKA and Y. OGAWA (1968): Stereoroentgenographical and dimensional studies on the physical structure of the dog. V. Organs and arteries of the head. VI. Peripheral arteries of the stomach. Bull. Nipp. vet. zootechn. Coll. No 17, 1—9; 10—17.

DENNSTEDT, A. (1903): Die Sinus durae matris der Haussäugetiere. Diss. med. vet. Gießen.

DIWÓ, A., und J. ROTH (1913): Die Kopfarterien des Schweines. Österr. Wschr. Tierheilk. 38, 437—440.

DRÄGER, K. (1937): Über die Sinus columnae vertebralis des Hundes und ihre Verbindung zu Venen der Nachbarschaft. Morph. Jb. 80, 579—598. Diss. med. vet. Hannover.

DZIALLAS, P. (1952): Die Entwicklung der Venae diploicae beim Haushunde und ihr Einschluß in das knöcherne Schädeldach. Morph. Jb. 92, 500—576.

FLECHSIG, G., und I. ZINTZSCH (1969): Die Arterien der Schädelbasis des Schweines. Anat. Anz. 125, 206—219.

FLORENTIN, P., et R. FLORIO (1956): Veines auriculaires et injections par voie intraveineuses chez les bovins. Revue Méd. Vét. 1956, 34.

FRENZEL, K. (1967): Venen am Kopf der Katze. Diss. med. vet. Hannover.

GASTINGER, W., und E. HENSCHEL (1960): Vorläufige Mitteilung über die röntgenologische Gefäßdarstellung der Kopfarterien beim lebenden Tier, insbesondere beim Hunde. Zbl. Vet. Med. A 7, 984—990.

GILLILAN, L. A. (1974): Blood supply to brains of ungulates with and without a rete mirabile caroticum. J. comp. Neurol. 153, 275—290.

GODYNICKI, S. (1972): Morfologia prównawcza akładu głownych tętnic głowy u niektorych zwierzat parzystokopytnych (Artiodactyla). (Comparative morphology of the system of head arteries in some members of the Artiodactyla.) (Polish) Rocz. AR, Poznań, H. 36, 1—60.

GROSSER, O. (1907): Die Elemente des Kopfvenensystems der Wirbeltiere. Verh. anat. Ges. 21, 179—192.

HAINES, D. E., K. R. HOLMES and J. A. BOLLERT (1969): The occurrence of a common trunk of the anterior cerebral artery in dog. Anat. Rec. 163, 303 —.

HEESCHEN, W. (1958): Arterien und Venen am Kopf des Schafes. Diss. med. vet. Hannover.

HEGEDUS, S. A., and R. T. SHACKELFORD (1965): A comparative anatomical study of the craniocervical venous systems in mammals, with special reference to the dog: relationship of anatomy to measurements of cerebral blood flow. Am. J. Anat. 116, 375—386.

HEGNER, D. (1962): Das Blutgefäßsystem der Nasenhöhle und ihrer Organe von Canis familiaris, gleichzeitig ein Versuch der funktionellen Deutung der Venenplexus. Diss. med. vet. Gießen.

—, B. SCHNORR und A. SCHUMMER (1964): Korrosionsanatomische Untersuchungen der Blutgefäße des harten Gaumens von Schaf und Ziege. Z. wiss. Mikr. mikr. Techn. 65, 458—471.

HEINZE, W. (1961): Die Kopfvenen des Schweines unter besonderer Berücksichtigung der venösen Organversorgung. Wiss. Z. Humboldt-Univ. 10, 641—688.

— (1961): Systematische Untersuchungen über den Ursprung der V. reflexa und der V. buccinatoria sowie über das Auftreten eines Anastomosenastes zwischen den beiden Vv. nasofrontales des Schweines. Anat. Anz. 110, 30—40.

—, D. LINDNER (1963): Makroskopische und mikroskopische Untersuchung der V. facialis des Rindes — ein Beitrag zum Problem der Muskelvenen. Anat. Anz. 112, 362—376.

HÜRLIMANN, R. (1911): Die arteriellen Kopfgefäße der Katze. Diss. med. vet. Zürich. Int. Mschr. Anat. Physiol. 29, 1—74 (1912).

JAMES, C. W., and B. F. HOERLEIN (1960): Cerebral angiography in the dog. Vet. Med. 55, 45—56.

JANKOVIC, Z. (1953): Einige interessante Variationen der A. carotis interna, A. occipitalis und ihrer Äste beim Pferde. Acta vet., Beogr., 2, H. 2.

JENKE, W. (1919): Die Gehirnarterien des Pferdes, Hundes, Rindes und Schweines, verglichen mit denen des Menschen. Diss. med. vet. Leipzig.

KOPER, S. (1966): Radiological investigation of the course of the a. alveolaris mandibulae in the ox. (Polish) Annls Univ. Mariae Curie-Skłodowska Sect. DD 21, 175—180.

LÄNGLE, D. (1973): Korrosionsanatomische Untersuchungen am Blutgefäßsystem des Encephalon und der Meninges bei Capra hircus. Diss. med. vet. München.

LECHNER, W. (1941): Die A. alveolaris mandibulae beim Wiederkäuer. Anat. Anz. 91, 273—320.

LEE, R., and I. R. GRIFFITHS (1972): A comparison of cerebral arteriography and cavernous sinus venography in the dog. J. small Anim. Pract. 13, 225—238.

MARTÍNEZ, P. (1965): Le système artériel de la base du cerveau et l'origine des artères hypophysaires chez le chat. Anat. anat. 61, 511—546.

MAY, N. D. S. (1967): Arterial anastomoses in the head and neck of the sheep. J. Anat. Lond. 101, 381—387.

— (1968): Experimental studies of the collateral circulation in the head and neck of sheep (Ovis aries). J. Anat. Lond. 103, 171—181.

MIA, A., and R. F. SIS (1970): The arterial supply to the salivary glands of the cat. Archs oral Biol. 15, 1—10.

MOBILIO, C. (1909): Della circolazione venosa della testa, con speciale riguardo ai rapporti fra quella intra ed extra-craniane negli equini. Tesi lib. doc. Torino.

MÖCKEL, O. (1909): Die Venen des Kopfes des Pferdes und ihre Variationen. Diss. med. vet. Leipzig.

MOLENDA, O. (1970): Arteries of the parotid gland in sheep. Fol. Morph. 29, 187—195.

— (1973): Arteries supplying the mandibular gland in sheep. Fol. Morph. 32, 185—193.

MOSKOV, M. (1939): Über die Variationen in der Verzweigung der oberflächlichen Kopfvenen der Schafsembryonen. Jb. Univ. Sofia, Vet. Med. Fak., 15, 337—351.

NICKEL, R., und R. SCHWARZ (1963): Vergleichende

Betrachtung der Kopfarterien der Haussäugetiere (Katze, Hund, Schwein, Rind, Schaf, Ziege, Pferd). Zbl. Vet. Med. A 10, 89—120.

Oliviera, A. de, und I. P. Neves (1972): Morphology of the craniovertebral venous system of bovine foetuses. (Portuguese) Arqs Univ. Fed. Rur. Rio de Janeiro 2, 71—75.

Popović, S. (1964): Arteriovenous anastomoses between the aa. carotides internae and the vv. maxillares internae of pigs. (Serbian) Acta vet., Beogr., 14, 45—48.

— (1965): Ungewöhnliche Erscheinungen extrakranialer arteriovenöser Anastomosen zwischen den Aa. carotides internae und den Vv. maxillares internae sowie Anomalien gewisser Blutgefäße beim Schwein. Acta anat. 61, 469—.

— (1967): Anatomical and radiological study of the blood supply to the pig's nasal mucosa. (Croatian) Acta vet., Beogr., 17, 445—458.

—, D. Jojić (1973): Arterial blood supply to the pig's tongue (Slovenian) Acta vet., Beogr., 23, Suppl., 111—116.

Porhajmova, J. (1963): Beitrag zur arteriellen Versorgung der Nasenhöhle des Schweines. Diss. med. vet. Brno.

Preuss, F. (1954): Gibt es eine V. reflexa? Tierärztl. Umsch. 9, 388—389.

Prichard, M. M. L., and P. M. Daniel (1953): Arterio-venous anastomoses in the tongue of the dog. J. Anat. 87, 66—74.

Prince, J. H., C. D. Diesem, I. Eglitis and G. L. Ruskell (1960): Anatomy and histology of the eye and orbit in domestic animals. Blackwell Scient. Publ. Ltd., Oxford.

Reinhard, K. R., M. E. Miller and H. E. Evans (1962): The craniovertebral veins and sinuses of the dog. Am. J. Anat. 111, 67—87.

Richter, E. (1962): Das Blutgefäßsystem der Nasenhöhle und ihre Organe von Felis domestica, gleichzeitig ein Versuch der funktionellen Deutung der Venenplexus. Diss. med. vet. Gießen.

Roux, J. M. W. le (1959): Die Venen am Kopf des Rindes. Diss. med. vet. Hannover.

—, H. Wilkens (1972): Zur Angiographie der Kopfarterien des Rindes. Dtsch. tierärztl. Wschr. 79, 342—346.

Rümpler, G. (1967): Venen am Kopf des Hundes. Diss. med. vet. Hannover.

Ruedi, M. (1922): Topographie, Bau und Funktion der Arteria carotis interna des Pferdes. Diss. med. vet. Zürich.

Sauerländer, R. (1971): Die makroskopisch-präparatorische Darstellung der Arterien und Venen des äußeren Ohres des Hausschweines (Sus scrofa f. domestica L., 1758). Diss. med. vet. Zürich.

Schmidt, K. (1910): Die arteriellen Kopfgefäße des Rindes. Diss. med. vet. Zürich.

Schnorr, B., und D. Hegner (1967): Gefäßarchitektur der Nasenhöhle bei Schaf und Ziege. Zbl. Vet. Med. A 14, 445—468.

Schummer, A., und G. Zimmermann (1937): Weitere Untersuchungen über die Sinus durae matris, Diploe- und Kopfvenen des Hundes mittels der Korrosionsmethode. Z. Anat. Entwicklungsgesch. 107, 1—6.

Schwarz, R. (1959): Arterien und Venen am Kopf der Ziege. Diss. med. vet. Hannover.

Shahrasebi, H., und B. Radmehr (1974): Investigation of the vessels of the brain of Iranian ruminants (ox, sheep, goat). (Persian) Revue Fac. Vét. Univ. Tehran 29, 41—51.

Sharma, D. N., Y. Singh and L. D. Dhingra (1974): The vascular supply and innervation of the horn of buffalo (Bubalus bubalis). Haryana Agric. Univ. J. Res. 3, 224—224 d, 225.

Shimizu, E. (1968): Stereological studies on several ducts and vessels by injection method of acrylic resin. XX. On the ethmoidal artery in some mammals. Okajimas Folia Anat. Jap. 45, 99—141.

Shust, I. V. (1959): Blood supply to the occipital region of the pig. (Hungarian) Nauk. Pratsi L'viv. zoovet. Inst. 10, 428—433.

Steven, D. H. (1964): The distribution of external and internal ophthalmic arteries in the ox. J. Anat. Lond. 98, 429—435.

Suzuki, T. (1967): The vascular system of the neck in the dog. II. On the vascular supply of the pharynx and larynx. Ann. Rep. Tokyo Univ. Agric. Technol., No 10, 99 —.

Ueshima, T., and Y. Suenaga (1972): Arteries of the basal region of the brain in the dog. I. Origins of main arteries. II. Anatomical structures and courses of main arteries. J. Fac. Agric., Tottori Univ. 7, 38—46; 47—56.

Virat, P. (1972): Arteries of the canine head. (French) Thèse doct. vét. Alfort.

Vitums, A. (1954): Nerve and arterial blood supply to the horns of the goat with reference to the sites of anesthesia for dehorning. J. Am. vet. med. Ass. 125, 284—286.

Wiland, C. (1973): Variation of the basal arteries of the brain in dogs. Folia morph. (engl. ed.) 32, 63—70.

Zietzschmann, O. (1912): Zur Vaskularisation des Bulbus und seiner Nebenorgane. Anat. Anz. 41, Erg.-H., 107.

— (1912): Die Orbitalarterien des Pferdes. Arch. vergl. Ophthal. 3, 129—210.

Zimmermann, A. (1916): A 16 fejartériájának rendellenességei. (Anomalies of the head arteries in the horse.) Közlemények az összehasonlító élet- és kórtan köréből. 13, 53.

— (1925): Adatok a belső fejarteria összehasonlító anatomiájáról. (The comparative anatomy of the internal head arteries.) Matematikai és természettudományi Éertesitő 47, 46.

— (1937): Összehasonlító vizsgálatok a kemény agyvelőburok vénás öbleiről, különös tekintettel a vizsgálati módszerekre. (Comparative anatomical studies of the sinus system of the cranial cavity.) Közlemények az összehasonlító élet- és kórtan köréből. 28, 269.

Zimmermann, G. (1936): Über die Dura mater encephali und die Sinus der Schädelhöhle des Hundes. Z. Anat. Entwicklungsgesch. 106, 107—137.

Pectoral and pelvic limbs

Aureli, G., B. Boccadoro, R. Calvari und L. Leonardi (1964): Anatomical and radiological studies in the dog. Arteriography of the limbs in flexion and extension. (Italian) Veterinaria, Milano, 13, 481—491.

Baum, H. (1907): Die Benennung der Hand- und Fußarterien des Menschen und der Haussäugetiere. Anat. Anz. 31, 428—448.

GHOSHAL, N. G., and R. GETTY (1967): The arterial supply to the appendages of the goat (Capra hircus). Iowa State Univ. Vet. 29, 123—144.
—, — (1968): The arterial supply of the appendages of the sheep (Ovis aries). Iowa State J. Sci. 42, 215—244.
—, — (1968): The arterial blood supply to the appendages of the ox (Bos taurus). Iowa State J. Sci. 43, 41—70.
—, — (1968): The arterial blood supply to the appendages of the domestic pig (Sus scrofa domesticus). Iowa State J. Sci. 43, 125—152.
—, — (1968): The arterial blood supply to the appendages of the horse (Equus caballus). Iowa State J. Sci. 43, 153—181.
HABEL, R. E. (1950): The nerves and arteries of the bovine foot. Proc. Bks Am. vet. med. Ass., 78th meet., Miami Beach.
HEINZE, W., B. RICHTER und P. RIESSNER (1973): Morphologische Untersuchungen an den Venen der Vorder- und Hintergliedmaße des Rindes im Hinblick auf den Blutrückfluß. I. Mitt. Einführung, Material und Methodik, das Venensystem der Vordergliedmaße. Anat. Anz. 134, 20—37.
—, —, — (1973): Morphologische Untersuchungen des Rindes im Hinblick an den Venen der Vorder- und Hintergliedmaße auf den Blutrückfluß. II. Mitt. Das Venensystem der Hintergliedmaße, Teildiskussion, zusammenfasesnde Diskussion, Literaturverzeichnis. Anat. Anz. 134, 186—208.
HERTSCH, B. (1973): Zur Arteriographie der Zehe des Pferdes. Berl. Münch. tierärztl. Wschr. 86, 461—465.
KORTUM, M. (1934): Untersuchungen über die Hautvenen der Gliedmaßen mit besonderer Berücksichtigung der Verhältnisse beim Rinde. Diss. med. vet. Hannover.
KRÜGER, G. (1933): Über die Blutgefäßversorgung der Zehe und besonders der Zehenendorgane des Pferdes. Diss. med. vet. Gießen.
LAUWERS, H., en N. R. DE VOS (1967): Systematic and topographic description of the veins of the fore- and hind-feet of the ox. Vlaams diergeneesk. Tijdschr. 36, 81—90.
LECHNER, W. (1934): Die Blutgefäßnetze in den Zehenenden einiger Paarzeher, ihre Beziehung zum Zehenendorgan und zu den analogen Gefäßen der Unpaarzeher und des Menschen. Z. Anat. Entwicklungsgesch. 102, 594—622.
MOSKOV, M. (1940): Über die Variationen in der Verzweigung der oberflächlichen Venen der Extremitäten der Schafsembryonen. Jb. Univ. Sofia, Vet. Med. Fak. 16, 235—242.
PORCHER, —, et — FORGEOT (1902): Étude radiographique des artères du pied chez le cheval. Bull. Soc. Sc. Vét. Lyon 1902, 7.
PRENTICE, D. E., and G. WYN-JONES (1973): A technique for angiography of the bovine foot. Res. vet. Sci. 14, 86—90.
PREUSS, F., und W. MÜLLER (1965): Die Ursprungsgefäße der Vasa digitalia des Hundes, ein Beitrag zur vergleichend-anatomischen Bezeichnung der Hand- und Fußgefäße. Berl. Münch. tierärztl. Wschr. 78, 281—283.
RICHTER, B., und P. RIESSNER (1973): Morphologische Untersuchungen an den Venen der Vorder- und Hintergliedmaße des Rindes im Hinblick auf den Blutrückfluß. Diss. med. vet. Humboldt-Univ. Berlin.
RUBELI, O. (1929): Zur Benennung der Extremitätenarterien bei den Haussäugetieren. Baum-Festschrift, Verlag M. und H. Schaper, Hannover, 257—272.
SCHUMMER, A. (1951): Blutgefäße und Zirkulationsverhältnisse im Zehenendorgan des Pferdes. Morph. Jb. 91, 569—649.
SUSSDORF, M. VON (1889): Die Verteilung der Arterien und Nerven an Hand und Fuß der Haussäugetiere. Festschr. 25j. Regierungsjubiläum S. M. König Karl von Württemberg. Verlag W. Kohlhammer, Stuttgart.
TZSCHACHEL, C. (1953): Darstellung der Arterien an der Extremität des Pferdes im Röntgenbild. Diss. med. vet. Leipzig.
ZIMMERMANN, A. (1922): A patások végtag-arteriáinak összehasonlitó anatomiájához. (Comparative anatomy of the arteries of the ungulate foot.) Állatorvosi Lapok 55, 199.

Pectoral limb

BADAWI, H. (1959): Arterien und Venen der Vordergliedmaße des Schweines. Diss. med. vet. Hannover.
—, H. WILKENS (1961): Zur Topographie der Arterien an der Schultergliedmaße des Rindes, unter besonderer Berücksichtigung der Versorgung des Vorderfußes. Zbl. Vet. Med. A 8, 533—550.
—, W. MÜNSTER und H. WILKENS (in Vorbereitung): Venen der Schultergliedmaße und des Vorderfußes der Haussäugetiere.
BEGO, U. (1960): Die komparativen Verhältnisse der Blutgefäße und Nerven der vorderen Extremitäten bei Kamel, Lama, Giraffe und Rind. Acta anat. 42, 261—262.
BLIN, P.-C. (1963): Radiographie des artères de la région du coude chez le chien. Econ. Méd. anim. 4, 68.
BOSSI, V. (1902): Contributo alla morfologia delle arterie dell'arto toracico nei mammiferi domestici. Tip. Simoncini, Pisa.
DAIGO, M., S. MORITA, G. KAWAHARA and A. KAGAMI (1965): Individual deviation of peripheral terminal branch running beneath the nail and the courses of running of the arteriae digitales propriae of the anterior and posterior extremity in the dog. Bull. Nippon vet. zootech. Coll. 14, 64—82.
DALLMAN, M. J., and R. C. MCCLURE (1967): Nomenclature of the brachial artery branches in the antebrachium of the domestic cat and dog. Anat. Rec. 157, 354.
—, — (1970): Nomenclature of the brachial artery branches in the antebrachium of the domestic cat and dog. Zbl. Vet. Med. A 17, 365—377.
DAVIS, D. D. (1941): The arteries of the forearm in carnivores. Pap. Mammal. 17, 137—227.
DE VOS, N. (1961): Topography of the arteries of the forelimb in the sheep. Mededel. Veearteseneijschool Rijksuniv. Gent. 7, 1—43.
— (1963): Topography of the arteries of the forelimb of the dog. Vlaams diergeneesk. Tijdschr. 32, 185—207 en 318—330.
— (1964): Comparative study of the arteries of the forelimb in the domestic animals. Mededel. Veeartsenijschool Riksuniv. Gent 8, 1—176.
FREWEIN, J. (1963): Die Vv. communicantes an den Schultergliedmaßen einiger Säugetiere (Rind,

Pferd, Schwein, Hund und Katze). Verh. Anat. Ges., Jena, **59**, 304—309.
— (1967): Die Faszien an den Schultergliedmaßen von Schwein, Rind und Pferd. Anordnung, Struktur und Bedeutung für den Einbau der Leitungsbahnen. Acta anat., Suppl. **53**.
—, M.-B. Morcos (1962): The arteries of the forefoot of the ox. Vlaams diergeneesk. Tijdschr. **31**, 161—170.
Ghoshal, N. G. (1972): The arteries of the thoracic limb of the cat. Anat. Anz. **131**, 259—271.
—, R. Getty (1970): Comparative morphological study of the major arterial supply to the thoracic limb of the domestic animals (Bos taurus, Ovis aries, Capra hircus, Sus scrofa domestica, Equus caballus). Anat. Anz. **127**, 422—443.
Giese, G. (1941): Über die Arterien des Halses und der Vordergliedmaße beim Hund, insbesondere ihr topographisches Verhalten. Diss. med. vet. Hannover.
Gomerčić, H. (1969): The comparative relationship of blood vessels and nerves in the thoracic limb of some felidae. (Slovanian) Biol. Glasn. **21**, 9—19.
Göppert, E. (1904): Die Beurteilung der Arterienvarietäten der oberen Gliedmaße bei den Säugetieren und beim Menschen auf entwicklungsgeschichtlicher und vergleichend-anatomischer Grundlage. Erg. Anat. Entwicklungsgesch. **14**, 170—233.
Horowitz, A. (1964): The veins of the thoracic limb of the ox. Speculum, Ohio, **17**, 21—30.
—, L. M. Bixby, E. W. Moss and B. Wurtz (1971): Median cubital vein of man and domestic animals. Proc. XIX. World Vet. Congr., Mexico City.
Kayanja, F. I. B. (1970): The postnatal development of the blood supply of the humerus of the cat. Anat. Anz. **127**, 354—366.
Lechner, W. (1933): Besonderheiten der Arteria mediana und ihrer Äste bei einem Pferde. Anat. Anz. **76**, 417—456.
Müller, W., und F. Preuss (1966): Zur Benennung einiger Armgefäße des Hundes. Anat. Anz. **118**, 209—218.
Münster, W., und R. Schwarz (1968): Venen der Schultergliedmaße des Rindes. Zbl. Vet. Med. A **15**, 677—717.
Nickel, R., und H. Wissdorf (1964): Vergleichende Betrachtung der Arterien an der Schultergliedmaße der Haussäugetiere (Katze, Hund, Schwein, Rind, Schaf, Ziege, Pferd). Zbl. Vet. Med. A **11**, 265—292.
Nickel, W. (1962): Arterien und Venen der Vordergliedmaße der Ziege. Diss. med. vet. Hannover.
Paulick, H.-J. (1967): Venen der Vordergliedmaße des Hundes. Diss. med. vet. Hannover.
Peduti Neto, J., A. Fernandes Filho y V. Bobelli (1971): Origin of the medial and lateral deep volar metacarpal arteries in the donkey. (Portuguese) Revta Fac. Med. Vet., Univ. S. Paulo **8**, 625—629.
—, — y A. A. D'Errico (1972): Ursprung der tiefen volaren Metakarpalarterien bei Vollblütern. Revta Fac. Med. Vet., Univ. S. Paulo **9**, 55—62.
Sapra, R. P., and L. D. Dinghra (1973): The blood vessels of the thoracic limb of buffalo (Bubalus bubalis). The digital veins. Anat Anz. **134**, 45—50.
—, — (1973): The blood vessels of the thoracic limb of buffalo (Bubalus bubalis). The metacarpal veins. Anat. Anz. **134**, 94—98.
—, — (1973): The blood vessels of the thoracic limb of buffalo (Bubalus bubalis). The superficial system of veins. Anat. Anz. **134**, 134—138.
—, — (1973): The blood vessels of the thoracic limb of buffalo (Bubalus bubalis). The deep system of venous drainage. Anat. Anz. **134**, 269—277.
—, — (1974): The blood vessels of the thoracic limb of buffalo (Bubalus bubalis). Anat. Anz. **135**, 116—139.
Speed, J. G. (1943): The thoraco-acromial artery of the dog. Vet. J. **99**, No 6.
Starostin, V. K. (1958): I. Variation in the course and branching of the v. brachialis of the horse with consideration of age changes and valves. II. Technique for the preparation of veins in the fore limb of the horse. (Russian) Trudy Litovsk. vet. Akad. **4**, 171—178, 179—187.
Wasiljewa, Z. A. (1973): Gewisse Besonderheiten der Arterien der Brustextremität der Wiederkäuer in der postnatalen Periode. Nautsch. tr. Omsk. vet. in-ta **29**, 21—25.
Wilkens, H. (1955): Arterien des Unterarms in vergleichender Betrachtung beim Menschen und bei unseren Haussäugetieren. Zbl. Vet. Med. A **2**, 193—198.
Wissdorf, H. (1961): Arterien und Venen der Schultergliedmaße des Schafes. Diss. med. vet. Hannover.
—, (1963): Arterien an der Schultergliedmaße der Katze und des Löwen. Kleintier-Prax. **8**, 159 bis 166.
— (1965): Die Venensysteme an der Schultergliedmaße der Katze. Kleintier-Prax. **10**, 101—109.

Pelvic limb

Badawi, H., und R. Schwarz (1963): Venen der Beckengliedmaße der Ziege. Morph. Jb. **104**, 125—140.
Bassett, F. H., J. W. Wilson, B. L. Allen Jr. and H. Azuma (1969): Normal vascular anatomy of the head of the femur in puppies with emphasis on the inferior retinacular vessels. J. Bone Jt Surg. **51 A**, 1139—1153.
Bego, U., i M. Zabundžija (1968): Komparativni odnosi krvnih žila i živaca stražnjih ekstremiteta nekih zvijeri (Malajski i tibetanski medvjed, vuk, tigar i pas). (The comparative relationship of blood vessels and nerves in the pelvic limb of some predators [Malayan and Himalayan bears, wolf, tiger, dog].) Biol. Glasn. **21**, 1—8.
Bickhardt, K. (1961): Arterien und Venen der Hintergliedmaße des Schweines. Diss. med. vet. Hannover.
Biel, M. (1966): Arterien und Venen der Beckengliedmaße der Katze. Diss. med. vet. Hannover.
Cherepakhin, D. A. (1972): Epiphyseal veins of the bovine femur. (Russian) Sb. Nauchn. trud. Mosk. Vet. Akad. **62**, 91—92.
Cummings, B. C. (1961): Collateral circulation of the canine pelvic limb. Small anim. Clin. **1**, 260; 264—267 and 20 a.
Daigo, M., S. Morita, G. Kawahara and A. Kagami (1965): Stereoroentgenographical and topographical studies on the anatomy of peripheral blood vessels in domestic animals and

domestic fowls. 12. Individual deviation of peripheral branch running beneath the nail and the courses of running of the arteriae digitales propriae of the anterior and posterior extremity in limbs in the dog. 13. Dorsal and plantar arteries of hind limbs in the dog. Bull. Nippon vet. zootech. Coll. 14, 64—82; 83—103.

DE Vos, N. (1964): Description topographique des artères du pied chez le boeuf. Econ. Méd. anim. 5, 367—401.

—, M.-B. Morcos (1960): The arteries of the hind foot of the ox. (Dutch) Vlaams diergeneesk. Tijdschr. 29, 241—246.

ELEK, P. (1938): The vessels of the hock joint (Hungarian) Állatorvosi Lapok. 46. Ref.: Jber. Vet. Med. 64, 521 —.

FITZGERALD, T. C. (1961): Blood supply of the head of the canine femur. Vet. Med. 56, 389—394.

FREYTAG, K. (1962): Arterien und Venen an der Beckengliedmaße des Schafes. Diss. med. vet. Hannover.

GHOSHAL, N. G. (1972): The arteries of the pelvic limb of the cat (Felis domestica). Zbl. Vet. Med. A 19, 78—85.

— (1973): Significance of the so-called perforating tarsal artery of domestic animals. Anat. Anz. 134, 289—297.

HERRMANN, G. (1940): Über die Arterien der Hintergliedmaße des Hundes, insbesondere ihr topographisches Verhalten. Diss. med. vet. Hannover.

HOWLETT, C. R. (1971): Anatomy of the arterial supply to the hip joint of the ox. J. Anat. 110, 343—348.

IPPENSEN, E. (1969): Venen der Beckengliedmaße des Rindes. Diss. med. vet. Hannover.

KANE, W. J., and E. GRIM (1969): Blood flow to canine hind-limb bone, muscle, and skin. J. Bone Jt Surg. 51 A, 309—322.

KÖNIG, H. E. (1970): Die Arteria poplitea einiger Haussäugetiere. Zbl. Vet. Med. A 17, 644—651.

MÜNSTER, W., H. BADAWI und H. WILKENS (in Vorbereitung): Venen der Beckengliedmaße und des Hinterfußes bei den Haussäugetieren.

NITSCHKE, Th. (1971): Zur Frage der Arteria profunda femoris und der Arteriae circumflexae femoris bei Mensch, Hund und Schwein. Acta anat. 79, 239—256.

PAROUTI, J.-P. (1962): Contribution à l'étude de la vascularisation interne du fémur du chien. Thèse doct. vét. Toulouse.

PINEY, G. (1972): The interosseous arterial vascularization of the tibia and fibula of the rabbit. (French) Thèse doct. vét. Alfort.

POHLMEYER, K., und H. WISSDORF (1975): Die arterielle Gefäßversorgung des Musculus pectineus et adductor longus beim Hund. Kleintier-Prax. 20, 73—108.

PREUSS, F. (1942): Arterien und Venen des Hinterfußes vom Hund, vorzüglich ihre Topographie. Diss. med. vet. Hannover.

SALAMANCA, M. E. DE, und R. SCHWARZ (1960): Die Arterien an der Beckengliedmaße der Ziege. Wien. tierärztl. Mschr., Festschr. Prof. Schreiber, 102 bis 114.

TAMM, R. H. (1953): Untersuchungen über das Verhalten der arterio-venösen Anastomosen in der hinteren Hundeextremität. Diss. med. Göttingen.

VITUMS, A. (1972): Abnormal development of the cranial and caudal tibial arteries in a horse. Anat. Anz. 131, 487—490.

WILKENS, H., und H. BADAWI (1962): Beitrag zur arteriellen Blutgefäßversorgung vom Fuß der Beckengliedmaße des Rindes. Berl. Münch. Tierärztl. Wschr. 75, 471—476.

WILSON, J. W., B. L. ALLEN and F. H. BASSETT (1967): Normal vascular supply of the femoral head in young pups and revascularization following experimental aseptic necrosis. Anat. Rec. 157, 342—343.

WÜNSCHE, A. (1966): Die Nerven des Hinterfußes vom Rind und ihre topographische Darstellung. Zbl. Vet. Med. A 13, 428—443.

Organs of the thoracic cavity

ASSALI, N. S., N. SEGHAL and S. MARABLE (1962): Pulmonary and ductus arteriosus circulation in the fetal lamb before and after birth. Am. J. Physiol. 202, 536—540.

AWTOKRATOW, D. M. (1930): Zur Frage nach dem Vorhandensein einer Längskommissur zwischen den visceroventralen Bogengefäßen bei Säugetieren. Anat. Anz. 69, 7—12, 282—284.

BARER, G. R. (1966): Bronchopulmonary anastomoses in foetal, newborn and adult animals. Q. J. exp. Physiol. 51, 103—111.

BARONE, R. (1953): Arbre bronchique et vaisseaux sanguins des poumons chez les Equidés domestiques. Recl Méd. vét. 129, 545—564.

— (1956): Bronches et vaisseaux pulmonaires chez le boeuf. C. r. Ass. Anat., Lisbonne.

— (1957): Arbre bronchique et vaisseaux pulmonaires chez le chien. C. r. Ass. Anat., Leiden, 132.

— (1958): Bronches et vaisseaux pulmonaires chez le porc. C. r. Ass. Anat., Gand, 143.

BÜHLING, H. (1943): Die Venae pulmonales des Rindes. Diss. med. vet. Hannover.

CAŁKA, W. (1967): Bronchial arteries with extrapulmonary course in domestic cattle. Fol. Morph. 26, 359—367.

— (1969): Precapillary anastomoses between the bronchial and pulmonary arteries in domestic cattle. Fol. Morph. 28, 60—68.

— (1969): The blood supply of the lungs through direct branches of the aorta in domestic cattle. Fol. Morph. 28, 442—450.

CASTIGLI, G. (1954): I vasi sanguigni del polmone di Bos taurus. Arch. ital. Anat. 59, 283—322.

CHAUDHRY, M. S. (1964): A study of the bronchopulmonary vasculature in postnatal growth of the dog. Diss. Abstr. 25, 2163.

COTOFAN, V., und I. COZARIUC (1972): Circulatory system of the lung in pigs. (Rumanian) Lucr. sti. II. Zooteh. Med. vet. Inst. agron. Ion Ionescu Brad, Iasi, 99—106.

DAWES, G. S. (1966): Pulmonary circulation in the foetus and the newborn. Br. med. Bull. 22, 61—65.

EHRSAM, H. (1957): Die Lappen und Segmente der Pferdelunge und ihre Vaskularisation. Diss. med. vet. Zürich.

FISCHER, A. (1942): Die Bronchialgefäße und ihre Anastomosen mit dem Pulmonalgefäßsystem beim Pferd. Diss. med. vet. Hannover.

FIZE, M. (1965): Anatomy of the lung and distribution of the bronchial vessels in ruminants. (French) Thèse doct. vét. Lyon.

GADEV, CHR. (1954): Über einige Variationen in

den nutritiven Gefäßen der Lunge beim Pferd. Wiss. Arb. Tierärztl. Hochsch. Sofia, 3, 67—77.
Härtl, H. (1942): Über die Bronchialgefäße und ihre Anastomosen mit dem Pulmonalgefäßsystem bei Schaf und Ziege. Diss. med. vet. Hannover.
Heuser, Ch. H. (1924): The bronchial vessels and their derivates in the pig. Contrib. Embryol., Washington, 77, 123—139.
Kaman, J., und Č. Červený (1968): Akzessorische Lungenarterien beim Schwein. Anat. Anz. 122, 60—67.
Kuwilski, S. (1945): Beziehungen des nutritiven zum funktionellen Gefäßsystem der Hundelunge. Diss. med. vet. Hannover.
Moriconi, A., und S. Lorvik (1960): Origin of the bronchial arteries in the ox. (Italian) Atti Soc. ital. Sci. vet. 14, 504—508.
Radu, C., und L. Radu (1969): Comparative anatomy of the vascularization of the lung in domestic animals and poultry. (Rumanian) Lucr. sti. Inst. agron. Rim., Ser. Med. vet. 12, 89—104.
Schorno, E. (1955): Die Lappen und Segmente der Rinderlunge und deren Vaskularisation. Diss. med. vet. Zürich.
Silva, P. (1938): Arterias bronquicas do Cao. Med. contemp. Nr. 20.
Simić, V., und D. Jojić (1967): Arterial blood supply to the oesophagus of the dog. (Croatian) Acta vet., Beogr., 17, 27—33.
Steinbrecher, H. (1942): Das nutritive Gefäßsystem der Lunge des Schweines und seine Verbindungen zu den Pulmonalgefäßen. Diss. med. vet. Hannover.
Stitz, B. (1936): Anatomische Untersuchungen über den Verlauf der Aa. und Vv. bronchiales des Hundes und über ihre Anastomosen mit dem Pulmonalsystem. Diss. med. vet. Hannover.
Varićak, T. (1969): Verschiedene Muster der Anordnung der Zweige der Lungenvenen beim Rind. Biol. Glasn. 21, 21—23.

Organs of the abdominal and pelvic cavities

Anderson, W. D., and A. F. Weber (1969): Arterial supply to the ruminant (ovine) stomach. J. Anim. Sci. 19, 183.
Arnautović, I. (1962): Die Vaskularisation der Niere bei Haustieren. Biol. Glasn. 15. —
—, M. Bevandić (1964): Nomenclature of the arterial system of the kidney of domestic animals. (Croatian) Veterinaria, Sarajewo, 13, 389—396.
Ashdown, R. R. (1958): The arteries and veins of the sheath of the bovine penis. Anat. Anz. 105, 222—230.
Audron, P. (1934): Des veines portes accéssoires et collatérales. Thèse doct. vét. Toulouse.
Babić, K., and H. Gomerčić (1971): A contribution to the knowledge of the variation of the arterial supply of the colon in the dog. Abstracta. 14. kongr. Udruzenja anat. Jugoslav. Beograd.
Baird, D. T., and R. B. Land (1973): Division of the uterine vein and the function of the adjacent ovary in the ewe. J. Reprod. Fert. 33, 393—397.
Bardin, J. (1953): Vascularisation de l'estomac chez les équidés domestiques. Lyon, Annequin.
Barone, R. (1956): Les vaisseaux sanguins des reins chez les équidés. Bull Soc. Sc. Vét. Lyon 1956, 237.
— (1957): La vascularisation utérine chez quelques mammifères. C. r. Ass. Anat. Leiden 1957, —.
—, H. Burel (1957): Les vaisseaux sanguins du tractus génital chez la vache. Revue Méd. vét. 1957, 382.
—, B. Blavignac (1964): Les vaisseaux sanguins des reins chez le boeuf. Bull. Soc. Sc. Vét. Lyon 66, 113.
—, Cl. Pavaux (1962): Les vaisseaux sanguins du tractus génital chez les femelles domestiques. Bull. Soc. Sc. Vét. Lyon 64, 33—52.
—, —, P. Frapart (1962): Les vaisseaux sanguins de l'appareil génital chez la truie. Bull. Soc. Sc. Vét. Lyon 64, 337.
—, H. Schwarzenbart (1952): Les vaisseaux sanguins du tractus génital de la jument. Revue Méd. vét. 1952, 833.
Barpi, U. (1906): Contributo alla conoscenza dei vasi aberranti del fegato in alcuni animali domestici. Nota II. Mon. Zool. It. 17, 8, 235.
Bauer, F, W. (1968): The aortic origin of renal arteries in man and other mammals. Archs. Path. 86, 230—233.
Bego, U., and K. Babić (1969): On some more fundamental characteristics in the constitution and ramification of kidneys of blood vessels in some carnivores. 13. Kongr. anat. Ohrid 6, —.
Bellamy, J. E. C., W. K. Latshaw and N. O. Nielsen (1973): The vascular architecture of the porcine small intestine. Can. J. comp. Med. 37, 56—62 .
Beutler, O. (1922): Das Verhalten der Arteria spermatica interna im Hoden der Haussäugetiere (Rind, Schaf, Pferd, Schwein, Hund und Katze). Diss. med. vet. Hannover.
Bevandić, M., and I. Arnautović (1964): A contribution to the arterial system of the kidney in domestic animals. Veternaria, Sarajewo, 13, 389—396.
Bignardi, C. (1948): Sul comportamento dei vasi nella tuba della bovina. Atti Congr. Int. Fecond. Artif.
Blavignac, B. (1964): Investigations of the blood and nerve supply to the kidneys of the ox. (French) Thèse doct. vét. Lyon.
Borisevich, V. B. (1966): Collateral blood circulation of the bovine testis. (Hungarian) Visn. silhospod. Nauki 9, 106—108.
Boye, H. (1956): Vergleichende Untersuchungen über die arterielle Gefäßversorgung des Uterus von Wild- und Hausschweinen. Z. Tierzücht. Zücht. Biol. 67, 259—296.
Bremer, J. L. (1915): The origin of the renal artery in mammals and its anomalies. Am. J. Anat. 18, 179—200.
Bressou, C., et J. le Gall (1936): Contribution à l'étude de la vascularisation de l'utérus des ruminants. Recl Méd. vét. 112, 5—9.
Burel, J. (1957): Les vaisseaux sanguins du tractus génital de la vache. Thèse doct. vét. Lyon.
Busch, Chr. (1973): Gefäßversorgung der Magenwand vom Schwein. Diss. med. vet. Hannover.
Cadette, Leite, A. (1973): The arteries of the pancreas of the dog. An injection-corrosion and microangiographic study. Am. J. Anat. 137, 151—157.
Campos, V. J. M. (1973): Sobre a existência da artérial vesical ventral no cão (Canis familiaris). Revta Med. vet. S. Paulo 8, 227—239.

— Contribução ao estudo da artéria umbilical (A. umbilicalis) no cao adulto (Canis familiaris). Rev. Med. Vet. 10, 106—132.

CARDOSO, F. M., und H. P. GODINHO (1972): Parenchymal ramifications of the a. testicularis in sheep and goats. (Portuguese) Arqs Esc. Univ. Fed. Minas Gerais 24, 11—20.

CHAHRASBIE, H., und I. POUSTIE (1971): The parenchymal distribution of the splenic artery in ruminants and pigs. (Persian) Revue Fac. Vét. Univ. Teheran, 27, 89—96.

CHATELAIN, E. (1973): Vascularisation artérielle et veineuse des organes digestifs abdominaux et de leurs annexes chez le porc (Sus scrofa domesticus). I. Artère coeliaque (A. coeliaca). Ann. Rech. vét. 4, 437—455.

— (1973): Vascularisation artérielle et veineuse des organes digestifs abdominaux et de leurs annexes chez le porc (Sus scrofa domesticus). II. Artères mésentériques craniale et caudale (A. mesenterica cranialis, A. mesenterica caudalis) et système veineux. Ann. Rech. vét. 4, 457—485.

CHEETHAM, S. E., and D. H. STEVEN (1966): Vascular supply to the absorptive surfaces of the ruminant stomach. J. Physiol. Lond. 166, 56—58.

CHRISTENSEN, G. C. (1954): Angioarchitecture of the canine penis and the process of the erection. Am. J. Anat. 95, 227—262.

COLLIN, B. (1972): Renal blood vessels in the dog. (French) Annls Méd. Vét. 116, 631—646.

— (1973): La vascularisation artérielle du testicule chez le cheval. Zbl. Vet. Med. C 2, 46—53.

COUDERT, S. P., G. D. PHILIPPS, C. FAIMAN, W. CHERNECKI and M. PALMER (1974): A study of the utero-ovarian circulation in sheep with reference to local transfer between venous and arterial blood. J. Reprod. Fert. 36, 319—331.

CUQ, P., P.-C. BLIN et A. BÉRENGER (1965): Topography of the intrahepatic vein in the dog. (French) Recl. Méd. vét. 141, 5—15.

—, — (1965): Topographie artérielle du foie du chien. Recl Méd. vét. 141, 123—135.

DELANEY, J. P. (1967): Arteriovenous anastomoses in the mesenteric organs of the dog. Diss. Abstr. 27 B, 4537.

DELLBRÜGGE, K. F.-W. (1940): Die Arterien des weiblichen Geschlechtsapparates vom Hunde. Diss. med. vet. Hannover. Morph. Jb. 85, 30 bis 48.

DEL CAMPO, C. H., and O. J. GINTHER (1972): I. Anatomy of utero-ovarian vasculature of laboratory species. II. Anatomy of utero-ovarian vasculature of mares, ewes and sows. J. Anim. Sci. 35, 1117—1119.

—, — (1973): Vascular anatomy of the uterus and ovaries and the unilateral luteolytic effect of the uterus: horses, sheep, and swine. Am. J. vet. Res. 34, 305—316.

—, — (1974): Arteries and veins of uterus and ovaries in dogs and cats. Am. J. vet. Res. 35, 409—415.

—, W. P. STEFFENHAGEN and O. J. GINTHER (1974): Clearing technique for preparation and photography of anatomic specimens of blood vessels of female genitalia. Am. J. vet. Res. 35, 303—310.

DRAHN, F. (1924): Varietät der Arteria bronchooesophagea beim Pferd. Anat. Anz. 58, 173—174.

ENGELMANN, K. (1971): Beitrag zur Anatomie der Baucheingeweide des Göttinger Zwergschweines unter besonderer Berücksichtigung ihrer Blutgefäßversorgung. Diss. med. vet. München.

FISCHER, K. (1949): Die Darmvenen der Katze unter gleichzeitiger Berücksichtigung der Resorptionsverhältnisse im Mastdarm. Diss. med. vet. Hannover.

FLORENTIN, P., et M. NAGHAVI (1960): Particularités anatomiques du système porte du chien. Recl Méd. vét. 136, 85—94.

FORGEOT, —, et — GRAS (1903): Le système veinaux de la verge chez les animaux domestiques. J. Méd. vét. Lyon 1903, 11 und 71.

FRANZKE, H.-J. (1958): Über eine Gefäßvariation im Bereich der Aorta abdominalis beim Schaf (A. coeliaca-mesenterica). Anat. Anz. 105, 332 bis 334.

FRAPART, P. (1963): La vascularisation du tractus génital de la truie. Thèse doct. vét. Lyon.

FULLER, P. M., and D. F. HUELKE (1973): Kidney vascular supply in the rat, cat and dog. Acta anat. 84, 516—522.

GADEV, C. (1966): Über die Blutversorgung des Eierstocks bei der Stute und bei der Eselstute. Wiss. Arb. Tierärztl. Hochschulinst. Sofia 16,

— (1968): Über die Vaskularisation des Mesometriums bei der Stute und der Eselstute. Anat. Anz. 122, 391—402.

— (1972): Blood vessels of the uterus and placenta of sheep. (French) Revue Méd. vét. 123, 1095 bis 1104.

—, N. BODUROV und K. BINEV (1974): Röntgenologische Untersuchungen der arteriellen Blutversorgung der Gebärmutter bei der Büffelkuh. Anat. Anz. 135, 321—326.

GEOROCEANU, P., und C. DUCA (1970): Visceral collateral arteries rising to abnormal levels from the abdominal aorta in a sheep. (Rumanian) Lucr. şti. Inst. agron. Cluj, Ser. Med. vet. Zooteh. 26, 37—41.

GHEȚIE, V., P. OPRIŞESCU, V. NICOLESCU, M. PANAITESCU, A. HILLEBRAND und I. MICLĂUS (1965): Studies on the blood vascular and autonomic nervous system in the pelvic cavity of the pig. (Rumanian) Lucr. şti. Inst. agron. N. Bălcescu Ser. C 8, 89—98.

GINTHER, O. J., and C. H. DEL CAMPO (1973): Vascular anatomy of the uterus and ovaries and the unilateral luteolytic effect of the uterus: areas of close apposition between the ovarian artery and vessels which contain uterine venous blood in sheep. Am. J. vet. Res. 34, 1387—1393.

—, — (1974): Vascular anatomy of the uterus and ovaries and the unilateral luteolytic effect of the uterus: cattle. Am. J. vet. Res. 35, 193—203.

—, M. C. GARCIA, E. L. SQUIRES and W. P. STEFFENHAGEN (1972): Anatomy of vasculature of uterus and ovaries in the mare. Am. J. vet. Res. 33, 1561—1568.

GODINA, G. (1936): Les artères utérines de la vache pendant et après la grossesse. Arch. It. Anat. Embriol. 37, 371—410. Nuova Ercol. 41, 138—146.

— (1937): L'artère utérine moyenne de la vache pendant et après la grossesse. Arch. It. Anat. Embriol. 38, 459—492. Nuova Ercol. 43, 213—215.

GODINHO, H. P. (1964): Estudo anatômico da terminacao e anastomoses da A. lienalis e as zonas (segmentos) arteriais lienais em canis familiaris. Arqs Esc. Vet. Minas Gerais 16, 163—196.

—, J. F. do NASCIMENTO (1962): Nota anatômica sôbre a sintopia hepato-cava em capra hircus. Arqs. Esc. Vet. Minas Gerais 14, 133—137.

GODYNICKI, S. (1976): Das Blutgefäßsystem der Magenwand der Katze. Zbl. Vet. Med. C, im Druck.

GOMERČIĆ, H., and K. BABIĆ (1972): A contribution to the knowledge of the variations of the arterial supply of the duodenum and the pancreas in the dog (Canis familiaris). Anat. Anz. 132, 281—288.

GRÄVENSTEIN, H. (1938): Über die Arterien des großen Netzes beim Hund. Diss. med. vet. Hannover. Morph. Jb. 82, 1—26.

GRAHAM, T., and P. G. D. MORRIS (1957): Comparison of the vascular supply to the virgin and post gravid uterus of the pig, ox and sheep. Br. vet. J. 113, No 12.

GROTTEL, K. (1971): Arteries of the middle part of the celiac plexus in the dog. Folia morph. (engl. ed.) 30, 488—496.

GÜNTHER, E. (1957): Zur Vaskularisation der Uterus-Karunkel des Schafes. Diss. med. vet. FU Berlin.

GUDEV, KH. (1966): Vascularization of the oviduct of the cow and donkey. (Bulgarian) Nauchni Trud. vissh vet.-med. Inst. Prof. G. Pavlov 17, 215—224.

GYÜRÜ, F., und GY. KOVÁCS (1967): Die Beckenarterie (A. hypogastrica) der Haussäugetiere. Acta Vet. Acad. Sci. Hung. 17, 371—399.

HAPKE, H.-J. (1957): Die Pfortader des Schweines. Diss. med. vet. Hannover.

HAPPICH, A. (1961): Blutgefäßversorgung der Verdauungsorgane in Bauch- und Beckenhöhle einschließlich Leber, Milz und Bauspeicheldrüse beim Schaf. Diss. med. vet. Hannover.

HARLÉ, H.-F.-C. (1964): Anatomie du système porte du chat; ses particularités. Thèse doct. vét. Alfort.

HEATH, T. (1968): Origin and distribution of portal blood in the sheep. Am J. Anat. 122, 95—106.

HENNAU, A., et B. COLLIN (1973): Les vaisseaux sanguins du rein chez le chien. Acta vet. Beogr. 23, 33—42.

HILLIGER, H.-G. (1957): Zur Uterus-Karunkel des Rindes und ihrer Vascularisation unter Berücksichtigung der zuführenden Uterusgefäße. Diss. med. vet. FU Berlin. Zbl. Vet. Med. 5, 51—82 (1958).

HODSON, N. (1968): On the intrinsic blood supply to the prostate and pelvic urethra in the dog. Res. vet. Sci. 9, 274—280.

HOFMANN, R. (1960): Die Gefäßarchitektur des Bullenhodens, zugleich ein Versuch ihrer funktionellen Deutung. Zbl. Vet. Med. A 7, 59—93.

HÖFLIGER, H. (1943): Die Ovarialgefäße des Rindes und ihre Beziehungen zum Ovarialzyklus. Berl. Münch. tierärztl. Wschr. 1943, 179.

HOLLE, U. (1964): Das Blutgefäßsystem der Niere von Schaf (Ovis aries) und Ziege (Capra hircus). Diss. med. vet. Gießen.

HOROWITZ, A. (1965): The distribution of the blood vessels to the postdiaphragmatic digestive tract of five mature female goats. Diss. Abstr. 26, 1278.

—, W. G. VENZKE (1965): The distribution of the blood vessels to the postdiaphragmatic digestive tract of the goat. J. Am. vet. med. Ass. 147, 1659.

—, — (1966): Distribution of blood vessels of the postdiaphragmatic digistive tract of the goat. Celiac trunk — gastroduodenal and splenic tributaries of the portal vein. Am. J. vet. Res. 27, 1293—1315.

IPPENSEN, E., CH. KLUG-SIMON und E. KLUG (1972): Der Verlauf der Blutgefäße vom Hoden des Pferdes im Hinblick auf eine Biopsiemöglichkeit. Zuchthyg. 7, 35—45.

IWAKU, F., S. MORI and S. TOMITA (1971): Blood vessels and bile ducts of the liver of the dog. (Japanese) Acta Anat. Nippon 46, 259—274.

JANKOVIC, Z. (1954): Ein Beitrag zur Kenntnis der Lebervenen bei den Hunden. Acta vet. Beogr. 4, Fasc. 4.

JANTOŠOVIČOVÁ, J. (1969): I. Contribution to the study of the veinal system of the testis and epididymis of rams, boars and stallions. II. Anastomoses of the arteries of ram, boar and stallion testis and epididymis. III. The intraorganic arterial system of the testes of the sheep, pig and horse. (Slovak) Folia vet. 13, 13—20; 21—26; 26—31.

KAMAN, J. (1962): Die Blutversorgung der Leber des Schweines. Diss. med. vet. Brno.

— (1965): The extra-hepatic branches of the hepatic artery of the pig. (Czech) Sb. vys. Šk. zeměd. Brně, Ser. B 13, 447—464.

— (1966): Die Grobramifikation der Leberblutgefäße des Schweines. Zbl. Vet. Med. A 13, 719—745.

KHAN, J. R., and A. VITUMS (1971): Portosystemic communications in the cat. Res. vet. Sci. 12, 215—218.

KOVÁCS, G., und F. GYÜRÜ (1967): Recent observations on the blood vascular system of the pelvic organs in the domestic animals. (Hungarian) Magy. Allatorv. Lap. 22, 216—220.

KRATOCHVIL, M., J. PAYER und J. RIEDEL (1957): Das System der Leberarterie und ihr Verhältnis zum Pfortadersystem in der Leber des Hundes. Acta anat. 31, 246—260.

KUDO, N. (1973): Studies on the alterations of the ovarian veins in goats. (Japanese) Acta Anat. Nippon. 48, 152—153.

KÜHN, H., und R. ROTHKEGEL (1962): Beitrag zur makroskopischen Anatomie der V. portae des Schafes (Ovis aries). Anat. Anz. 110, 312—326.

LAMOND, D. R., and M. DROST (1974): Blood supply to the bovine ovary. J. Anim. Sci. 38, 106—112.

LANGE, H. (1959): Neue Untersuchungen zur Vaskularisation des Schweineeuterus. Diss. med. vet. FU Berlin.

LASSERRE, R., et F. ARMANGAUD (1934): Anatomie des vaisseaux testiculaires chez le cheval et applications à la pathologie chirurgicale. Revue Méd. vét. 86, 13—38.

LIBERSA, C., und M. LAUDE (1965): Anatomical studies on variations of the veins of the splenic hilus in the dog. (French) Recl Méd. vét. 141, 1055—1064.

MAGILTON, J. H., and R. GETTY (1969): Blood supply to the genitalia and accessory genital organs of the goat. Iowa State J. Sci. 43, 285—305.

MIA, M. A. (1969): The posterior mesenteric circulation in the goat. Pakist. J. vet. Sci. 3, 127—131.

MIYAGI, M. (1966): Changes in the arteria uterina

media of cows caused by pregnancy. Jap. J. vet. Res. 13, 137—138.
MICLEA, M., und H. POP (1965): Variations in origin of the branches of the a. coeliaca and a. mesenterica in the sheep. (Rumanian) Lucr. şti. Inst. agron. Cluj, Ser. Med. vet. Zooteh. 21, 23—26.
MOZES, E. (1943): Die Venenklappe der hinteren Hohlvene bei der Leber. Közlemények az összehasonlító élet- és kórtan köréból 31, 310. Ref.: Jber. Vet. Med. 71, 370 —.
NASCIMENTO, J. F., and H. P. GODINHO (1960/61): The relations between the vena cava caudalis and the liver in ovis aries. Arqs Esc. Vet. Minas Gerais 13, 249—254.
NEIDER, CH. (1951): Zur Gefäßversorgung des Hundeuterus nebst Angioarchitektur seiner Wandabschnitte. Diss. med. vet. FU Berlin.
NICKEL, R. (1937): Die Haemorrhoidalvenen des Hundes und ihre Bedeutung bei der Resorption im Mastdarm. Dtsch. tierärztl. Wschr. 42, 595 bis 596.
NITSCHKE, TH. (1966): Zur Frage der Vena profunda glandis des Rüden. Zbl. Vet. Med. A 13, 474—476.
NUNEZ, Q., and R. GETTY (1969): Arterial supply to the genitalia and accessory genital organs of swine. Iowa State J. Sci. 44, 93—126.
—, — (1970): Blood vessels of the genitalia and accessory genital organs of swine (Sus scrofa domesticus). II. Veins. Iowa State J. Sci. 45, 297—315.
OLIVEIRA, A. de (1956): The portal venous district in sus scrofa domesticus. Arqs Esc. Vet. 9, 141—160.
— (1960): Die Zusammensetzung des Stammes der Vena portae bei Canis familiaris. Wien. Tierärztl. Mschr., Festschr. Prof. Schreiber, 88—97.
OTTOLENGHI, M. (1957): Le variazioni delle arterie renali nel cane studiate col metodo statistico seriale. Nuova Ercol. Riv. Med. vet. 15, 1—11.
OXENREIDER, S. L., R. C. MCCLURE and B. N. DAY (1965): Arteries and veins of the internal genitalia of female swine. J. Reprod. Fert. 9, 19—27.
PAECH, C.-D. (1962): Die arterielle Blutgefäßversorgung der Bauch- und Beckenhöhle bei Schwein und Schaf. Diss. med. vet. FU Berlin.
PANIGEL, M., and H. LEFREIN (1960): Preliminary note on the vascular anatomy of the cotyledon in cattle. C. r. Ass. Anat. No 108, 577—580.
PAVAUX, CL., et J. DESCAMPS (1966): Sur la vascularisation artérielle de l'oviducte des mammifères domestiques. Bull. Soc. Sci. Vét. Méd. comp. Lyon 1966, 343.
PETER, A. (1929): Die Arterienversorgung von Eierstock und Eileiter. Untersuchungen bei Hund und Katze. Diss. med. vet. Zürich. Z. Anat. Entwicklungsgesch. 89, 763 —.
PFÖRRINGER, L. (1971): Die arterielle Versorgung des Ductus choledochus. Acta anat. 79, 389—408.
POPESKO, P. (1965): Vascularization of the testis in the bull: a. spermatica interna. (Slovak) Folia vet. 9, 137—146.
POPOVIC, N. A., and J. F. MULLANE (1972): Common renal vein in the dog. Vet. med. Small Anim. Clin. 67, 558—559.
POTT, G. (1949): Die arterielle Blutgefäßversorgung des Magen-Darmkanales, seiner Anhangdrüsen (Leber, Pancreas) und der Milz bei der Katze. Diss. med. vet. Hannover.
PREUSS, F. (1959): Die A. vaginalis der Haussäugetiere. Berl. Münch. Tierärztl. Wschr. 72, 403—406.
RAUCH, R. (1962): Beitrag zur arteriellen Versorgung der Bauch- und Beckenhöhle bei Katze und Hund. Diss. med. vet. FU Berlin.
RESOAGLI, E. H., y R. L. GIMÉNEZ (1967): Double renal artery in the dog. (Spanish) Gac. vet. 29, 341—345.
—, — R. A. MOREIRA (1972): Renal artery in the dog; its possible variations. (Spanish) Gac. vet. 34, 590—599.
SACK, W. O. (1972): Das Blutgefäßsystem des Labmagens von Rind und Ziege. Zbl. Vet. Med. C 1, 27—54.
SAJONSKI, H. (1955): A. lienalis als Ast der A. mesenterica cranialis und Truncus bicaroticus beim Hund. Anat. Anz. 101, 243—246.
SCHILTSKY, R. (1966): Arterien der Verdauungsorgane in Bauch- und Beckenhöhle einschließlich Leber, Bauchspeicheldrüse und Milz des Schweines. Diss. med. vet. Hannover.
SCHMALTZ, R. (1898): Bemerkungen über die Gefäße des Penis beim Pferde. Berl. tierärztl. Wschr. 1898, 254—257.
SCHMITZ, A. (1910): Die Pfortader des Pferdes, Rindes und Hundes und ihr mikroskopisches Verhalten beim Pferd. Diss. med. vet. Leipzig.
SCHNORR, B., und B. VOLLMERHAUS (1968): Das Blutgefäßsystem des Pansens von Rind und Ziege. IV. Mitteilung zur funktionellen Morphologie der Vormägen der Hauswiederkäuer. Zbl. Vet. Med. A 15, 799—828.
SCHUMMER, A., und B. VOLLMERHAUS (1960): Die Venen des trächtigen und nichtträchtigen Rinderuterus als blutstromregulierendes funktionelles System. Wien. Tierärztl. Mschr., Festschr. Prof. Schreiber, 114—138.
SCHWARZENBART, H. (1952): Les artères du tractus génital de la jument. Thèse doct. vét. Lyon.
SCUPIN, E. (1960): Blutgefäßversorgung der Verdauungsorgane in Bauch- und Beckenhöhle einschließlich Leber, Milz und Bauchspeicheldrüse bei der Ziege. Diss. med. vet. Hannover.
SHURBENKO, A. (1955): Zur Frage der Blutversorgung der Gebärmutter bei der Stute. Wiss. Abh. Beloruss. Landw. Akad. 21, 82—97.
SIEBER, H. F. (1903): Zur vergleichenden Anatomie der Arterien der Bauch- und Beckenhöhle bei den Haussäugetieren. Diss. philos. Zürich.
SIMIĆ, V. (1953): Die Arterien der Geschlechtsorgane des Schafes und der Ziege. Acta vet. Beogr. 3, Fasc. 1.
—, R. ANDRIĆ (1967): Vascularization of the ovary, oviduct, infundibulum and uterine horns of the cat in comparison with that of the bitch. (Croatian) Acta vet. Beogr. 17, 3—16.
—, H. GADEV (1968): Anatomical and radiological studies on the arterial vascularization of the ovary, oviduct and anterior uterine horn in domesticated equidae. (Croatian) Acta vet. Beogr. 18, 101—118.
SLEIGHT, D. R., and N. R. THOMFORD (1970): Gross anatomy of the blood supply and biliary drainage of the canine liver. Anat. Res. 166, 153—160.
STARFLINGER, F. (1971): Zum Bau des Begattungsorgans beim Ziegenbock mit besonderer Berücksichtigung der Angioarchitektonik. Diss. med. vet. München.

TANUDIMADJA, K., and R. GETTY (1970): Arterial supply of the digestive tract of the sheep (Ovis aries). Iowa State J. Sci. 45, 275—295.
—, —, N. G. GHOSHAL (1968): Arterial supply to the reproductive tract of the sheep. Iowa State J. Sci. 43, 19—39.
TAUSCHER, W. (1922): Über Besonderheiten an den Arterien der Ligamenta lata weiblicher Haustiere. Diss. med. vet. Wien.
THAMM, H. (1941): Die arterielle Blutversorgung des Magendarmkanals, seiner Anhangsdrüsen (Leber, Pankreas) und der Milz beim Hunde. Diss. med. vet. Hannover. Morph. Jb. 85, 417 bis 446.
TUFFLI, G. (1928): Die Arterienversorgung von Hoden und Nebenhoden. Untersuchungen bei Hund und Katze mit Hilfe Spalteholz'scher Aufhellung an Injektionspräparaten. Diss. med. vet. Zürich.
VAERST, L. (1937): Über die Blutversorgung des Hundepenis. Diss. med. vet. Hannover. Morph. Jb. 81, 307—352 (1938).
VITUMS, A. (1959): Portal vein in the dog. Zbl. Vet. Med. A 6, 723—741.
— (1959): Portosystemic communications in the dog. Acta anat. 39, 271—299.
— (1963): Die Anastomosen zwischen der Pfortader und dem Hohlvenensystem unter Berücksichtigung ihrer funktionellen Bedeutung bei den Haustieren, insbesondere beim Hund. Berl. Münch. Tierärztl. Wschr. 76, 335—339.
VOLLMERHAUS, B. (1962): Die Arteria und Vena ovarica des Hausrindes als Beispiel einer funktionellen Koppelung viszeraler Gefäße. Verh. Anat. Ges., Genua, 258—264.
— (1964): Gefäßarchitektonische Untersuchungen am Geschlechtsapparat des weiblichen Hausrindes (Bos primigenius f. taurus L., 1758). Zbl. Vet. Med. A 11, 538—646.
VRZGULOVÁ, M., B. HÁJOVSKÁ und J. JANTOŠOVIČOVÁ (1965): The occurrence of accessory testicular arteries in the bull. (Slovak) Folia vet. 9, 165—171.
WELLER, U. (1964): Das Blutgefäßsystem der Niere des Pferdes (Equus caballus). Diss. med. vet. Gießen.
WILLIAMSON, I. M. (1969): Some responses of bovine mesenteric arteries, veins and lymphatics. J. Physiol. Lond. 202, 112—113.
WROBEL, K.-H. (1961): Das Blutgefäßsystem der Niere von Sus scrofa dom. unter besonderer Berücksichtigung des für die menschliche Niere beschriebenen Abkürzungskreislaufs. Diss. med. vet. Gießen.
YAMAUCHI, S., and F. SASAKI (1970): Studies on the vascular supply of the uterus of a cow. Jap. J. vet. Sci. 32, 59—67.
ZHURBENKO, A. M. (1966): The vascular system of the sheep's uterus. (Russian) Veterinariya, Kiev, No 10, 132—138.

Endocrine organs

BABIĆ, K., and H. GOMERČIĆ (1971): Variations of the arterial supply of the adrenal gland in the dog (Canis familiaris). 7. Congr. Ass. Vet. Anat. Bologna, 3—4.
BARONE, R. (1956): Les artères des glandes surrénales chez le cheval. Bull. Acad. Vét. Fr. 29, 77—78.
BENNETT, H. S., and L. KILHAM (1940): The blood vessels of the adrenal gland of the adult cat. Anat. Rec. 77, 447—472.
BERNHARDT, S. (1959): Die Blutgefäßversorgung der Schilddrüse des Pferdes. Diss. med. vet. Hannover.
CAPUTO, G. (1964): Blood supply to the thyroid gland of the sheep. (Italian) Acta med. vet. Napoli 10, 499—512.
COTOFAN, V., O. COTOFAN and I. COZARIUC (1970): Cercetari privind vascularizatta tiroidei si paratiroidei la pasari. (Studies on the vascularization of the thyroid and parathyroid glands.) Inst. agron. Ion Ionescu Brad Iasi Lucr. sţi. II Zooteh. Med. Vet., 145—152.
DENIZ, E. (1964): Die Blutgefäßversorgung des Thymus beim Kalb. Zbl. Vet. Med. A 11, 749 bis 759.
ERICHSEN, C. P. (1957): Die Blutgefäßversorgung der Schilddrüse beim Schwein. Diss. med. vet. Hannover.
GROTTEL, K. (1971): The suprarenal arteries in dogs and their extravisceral and intracapsular connections. Folia morph. (engl. ed.) 30, 497—509.
HARRISON, F. A., and I. R. McDONALD (1965): The arterial supply to the adrenal gland of the sheep. J. Anat. 100, 189—202.
HELM, F. CHR. (1957): Die Gefäßverzweigung in der Schilddrüse des Rindes. Zbl. Vet. Med. A 4, 71—79.
KRÖLLING, O. (1939): Über die Venenversorgung der Schilddrüse beim Hund. Wien. Tierärztl. Mschr. 26, 689—698.
— (1951): Über die Venenversorgung der Schilddrüse bei den Raubtieren (Feliden und Ursiden). Acta anat. 11, 479—489.
LOEFFLER, K. (1955): Blutgefäße der Schilddrüse des Hundes. Diss. med. vet. Hannover.
NEGREA, A., und H. E. KONIG (1970): Contributil la sudiul vascularizatiei suprarenalei la unele specii de mamifere domestice. (Studies on the vascularization of the adrenal glands in some species of domestic animals.) Inst. agron. Ion Ionescu Brad Iasi Lucr. sţi. II Zooteh. Med. Vet., 153—158.
OLIVEIRA, M. C., S. MELLO DIAS, P. PINTO-SILVA e A. M. ORSI (1974): Sull'origine e frequenza delle arterie tiroidee craniali e caudali nel porco (Sus scrofa domestica). Arch. vet. ital. 25, 71—78.
OTTOLENGHI, M. (1932): Le vene tiroidee e paratiroidee in alcuni mamifere domestici. Ric. morf. 13, 221—225.
PASTEA, E. (1973): Contribution à l'étude macroscopique de l'innervation et de la vascularisation des glandes surrénales chez le boeuf. Anat. Anz. 134, 120—126.
PEDUTI NETO, J., und V. BORELLI (1970): A common trunk of origin for the coeliac and cranial mesenteric arteries in the domestic cat. (Portuguese) Revta Fac. Med. Vet. Univ. S. Paulo 8, 395—398.
PUNTO E SILVA, P., M. C. OLIVEIRA E V. ROSSI (1973): Frequencia e origem das artérias tiroideas caudalis (Aa. thyreoideae caudales) no cão (Canis familiaris). Revta Med. vet. 9, 25—37.
RUSSO, E., und G. V. PELAGALLI (1972): The macro- and micro-circulation of the adrenal gland of the small ruminants as studied in sheep and goats. (French) Acta anat. 82, 179—197.
SINGH, Y., D. N. SHARMA and L. D. DHINGRA (1973): Anatomical study on the vessels of the

thyroid gland of the buffalo (Bos bubalis). Philipp. J. vet. Med. **12**, 20—26.

ZIMMERMANN, A. (1942): The vessels of the thymus gland. (Hungarian) Közlemények az összehasonlitó éket. és kórtan köréból 30, 225—230. Ref.: Jber. Vet. Med. **70**, 514 —.

Lymphatic system

Handbooks, textbooks and monographs

ABRAMSON, D. I. (ed.) (1962): Blood vessels and lymphatics. Academic Press, New York.

ALLEN, L. (1970): Abdominal lymphaticovenous communications as species characteristics and anomalies. In: Progress in Lymphology II., hrsg. von VIAMONTE, M. et al., Thieme, Stuttgart.

BARGMANN, W. (1943): Der Thymus. In: Handbuch der mikroskopischen Anatomie des Menschen. Bd. VI, 1—172, hrsg. von W. v. MÖLLENDORF, Springer, Berlin.

BARTELS, H. (1968). Die Untersuchung der Schlachttiere und des Fleisches. Paul Parey, Berlin u. Hamburg.

BARTELS, P. (1909): Das Lymphgefäßsystem. Gustav Fischer, Jena.

BAUM, H. (1912). Das Lymphgefäßsystem des Rindes. A. Hirschwald, Berlin.

— (1918): Das Lymphgefäßsystem des Hundes. A. Hirschwald, Berlin.

— (1928): Das Lymphgefäßsystem des Pferdes. Springer, Berlin.

— (1928): Zur Technik der Injektion der Lymphgefäße. In: Handbuch der biolog. Arbeitsmethoden Abt. VII. Urban & Schwarzenberg, Berlin, Wien.

—, und H. GRAU (1938): Das Lymphgefäßsystem des Schweines. Paul Parey, Berlin.

—, und A. TRAUTMANN (1933): Das Lymphgefäßsystem der Säugetiere. In: BOLK — GÖPPERT — KALLIUS — LUBOSCH, Handbuch der vergleichenden Anatomie der Wirbeltiere, **IV**, 758—842, Urban & Schwarzenberg, Berlin, Wien.

BERNHARD, W., and R. LEPLUS (1964): Structure fine du ganglion humain normal et malin. Fine structure of the normal and malignant human lymph node. Pergamon Press, Oxford, Gauthier-Villars, Paris, Macmillan, New York.

BURKE, J. F., and L. V. LEAK (1970): Lymphatic capillary function in normal and inflamed states. In: Progress in Lymphology II., 81—85, hrsg. VIAMONTE, M. et al., Thieme, Stuttgart.

CASLEY-SMITH, J. R. (1970): How the lymphatic system overcomes the inadequacies of the blood system. In: Progress in Lymphology II, 51—54, hrsg. von VIAMONTE, M. et al., Thieme, Stuttgart.

— (1973): The lymphatic system in inflammation. In: ZWEIFACH, B. W., L. GRANT, R. T. MCCLUSKEY (ed.): The inflammatory process. Sec. Ed., Vol. II, 161—204, Academic Press, New York and London.

COURTICE, F. C. (1972): The Chemistry of Lymph. In: Handbuch der Allgemeinen Pathologie, III/6, 311—362, Springer, Berlin — Heidelberg — New York.

DEFENDI, D., and D. METCALF (ed.) (1964): The thymus. Philadelphia, A Wistar Institute Monograph No. 2, Wistar Institute Press.

DRINKER, C. K., and J. M. YOFFEY (1941): Lymphatics, lymph and lymphoid tissue. Cambridge, Harvard University Press.

DUMONT, A. E., and P. E. PETERS (ed.) (1968—75): Lymphology. Official organ of the International Society of Lymphology. Vol. 1—8.

FIORE-DONATI, L., and M. G. HANNA jr. (1969): Lymphatic tissue and germinal centers in immune response. Plenum Press, New York.

FÖLDI, M. (1972): Physiologie und Pathophysiologie des Lymphgefäßsystems. In: Handbuch der Allgemeinen Pathologie, III/6, 239—310, Springer, Berlin — Heidelberg — New York.

GERTEIS, W. (1972): Darstellungsmethoden des Lymphgefäßsystems und praktische Lymphographie. In: Handbuch der Allgemeinen Pathologie Bd. III/6, 595—636, Springer, Berlin — Heidelberg — New York.

GOOD, R. A., and A. E. GABRIELSEN (1964): The thymus in immunbiology. Hoeber medical Division, Harper u. Row Publ., New York.

GRAU, H. (1963): Die Mandeln im Rahmen des Lymphapparates. In: Lymphsystem und Lymphatismus, hrsg. von M. J. ZILCH. J. A. Barth, München.

— (1972): Vergleichende Anatomie des Lymphgefäßsystems. In: Handbuch der Allgemeinen Pathologie, III/6, 39—88, Springer, Berlin — Heidelberg — New York.

— (1974): Vergleichende Darstellung des Lymphgefäßsystems der Säugetiere. Fortschritte der Veterinärmedizin. Beihefte zum Zentralblatt für Veterinärmedizin, **19**, Paul Parey, Berlin u. Hamburg.

— und J. BOESSNECK (1960): Der Lymphapparat. In: HELMCKE — LENGERKEN — STARCK, Handbuch der Zoologie, **8**, 1—74, Berlin.

HARTMANN, A. (1930): Die Milz. In: Handbuch der mikroskopischen Anatomie des Menschen, Bd. VI/1, 397—563, hrsg. von W. v. MÖLLENDORFF, Springer, Berlin.

HELLMAN, T. (1927): Der lymphatische Rachenring. In: Handbuch der mikroskopischen Anatomie des Menschen, Bd. V/1, 245—289, hrsg. von W. v. MÖLLENDORFF, Springer, Berlin.

— (1943): Lymphgefäße, Lymphknötchen und Lymphknoten. In: Handbuch der mikroskopischen Anatomie des Menschen, Bd. VI/1, 233—396, Springer, Berlin, 1930. Bd. VI/4, 173—201, Springer, Berlin.

HERRATH, E. von (1958): Bau und Funktion der normalen Milz. de Gruyter, Berlin.

HUNTINGTON, G. S. (1911): The anatomy and development of the systemic, lymphatic vessels in the domestic cat. Memoirs of the Wistar Institute of Anatomy and Biology No. 1, Philadelphia, PA.

ISHIDA, O., H. UCHIDA, Y. TAJI and S. SONE (1970): Lymphatic-venous anastomoses — experimental study. In: Progress in Lymphology II, hrsg. von M. VIAMONTE et al. Thieme, Stuttgart.

JOSSIFOW, G. M. (1930): Das Lymphgefäßsystem des Menschen mit Beschreibung der Adenoide und der Lymphbewegungsorgane. Gustav Fischer, Jena.

KAMPMEIER, O. F. (1969): Evolution and comparative morphology of the lymphatic system. Charles C. Thomas, Springfield, III.

KRÖLLING, O. (1930): Retikulo-endotheliales System. In: STANG-WIRTH, Tierheilkunde und Tierzucht,

VIII, 542—549, Urban & Schwarzenberg, Berlin, Wien.
LEAK, L. V. (1972): The fine structure and function of the lymphatic vascular system. In: Handbuch der Allgemeinen Pathologie, III/6, 149—196, Springer, Berlin — Heidelberg — New York.
LEIBER, B. (1961): Der menschliche Lymphknoten. Anatomie, Physiologie und Pathologie nach Ergebnissen der vergleichenden klinischen und histologischen Zytodiagnostik. Urban & Schwarzenberg, München und Berlin.
LENNERT, K. (1961): Lymphknoten. In: Handbuch der speziellen pathol. Anat. Histol., Bd. I/3 A, hrsg. von E. UEHLINGER, Springer, Berlin.
LIMBORGH, J. VAN (1966): Mikroskopische Anatomie der Lymphgefäßwand. In: COMÈL, M., und L. LACZT (ed.): Morphologie und Histochemie der Gefäßwand, Teil II, 309—324. Karger, Basel.
MALÉK, P. (1972): Lymphaticovenous anastomoses. In: Handbuch der Allgemeinen Pathologie, III/6, 197—218, Springer, Berlin — Heidelberg — New York.
MILLER, J. F. A. P., und P. DUKOR (1964): Die Biologie des Thymus nach dem heutigen Stand der Forschung. Akademische Verlagsgesellschaft Frankfurt a. M.
MISLIN, H. (1972): Die Motorik der Lymphgefäße und die Regulation der Lymphherzen. In: Handbuch der Allgemeinen Pathologie, III/6, 219 bis 238, Springer, Berlin — Heidelberg — New York.
MÖLLER, G. (ed.) (1975): Subpopulation of B lymphocytes. In: Transplantation Reviews 24, Munksgaard, Copenhagen.
— (ed.) (1975): Separation of T and B lymphocyte subpopulations. In: Transplantation Reviews 25, Munksgaard, Copenhagen.
MÜLLER, B. (1970): Lymphgefäße. In: JOEST, E.: Handbuch der speziellen pathologischen Anatomie der Haustiere, II. Bd., 3. Aufl. Paul Parey, Berlin u. Hamburg.
OTTAVIANI, G., und G. AZZALI (1966): Ultrastructure des capillaires lymphatiques. In: COMÈL, M., und L. LACZT (ed.): Morphologie und Histochemie der Gefäßwand, Teil II, 325—360. Karger, Basel.
REBUCK, J. E. (ed.) (1960): The lymphocyte and lymphocytic tissue. Hoeber, New York.
RÉNYI-VÁMOS, F. (1960): Das innere Lymphgefäßsystem der Organe. Anatomie, Pathologie, Klinik. Verlag der Ungarischen Akademie der Wissenschaften, Budapest.
RÖHRER, H. (1970): Lymphknoten. In: JOEST, E.: Handbuch der speziellen pathologischen Anatomie der Haustiere, II. Bd., 3. Aufl. Paul Parey, Berlin und Hamburg.
RUSZNYÁK, I., M. FÖLDI und G. SZABÓ (1969): Lymphologie. Physiologie und Pathologie der Lymphgefäße und des Lymphkreislaufes. 2. dtsch. Auflage, Fischer, Stuttgart.
—, —, — (1960): Lymphatics and lymph circulation. 4th Ed. English translation by A. DEÁK and J. FESÜS New York, Pergamon Press.
SKODA, K. (1929): Lymphknoten, Lymphonodi. In: STANG-WIRTH, Tierheilkunde und Tierzucht, VI, 647—659, Urban & Schwarzenberg, Berlin, Wien.
TISCHENDORF, F. (1956): Milz. In: Kükenthals Handbuch der Zoologie (hrsg. v. J.-G. HELMCKE und H. v. LENGERKEN). VIII/5 (2). 1—32. De Gruyter & Co., Berlin.
— (1969): Die Milz. In: Handbuch der mikroskopischen Anatomie des Menschen, hrsg. von W. v. MÖLLENDORFF und W. BARGMANN, Bd. VI/6. Erg. VI/1. Springer, Berlin — Heidelberg — New York.
TÖNDURY, G. (1967): Embryology and topographic anatomy of the lymphatic system. In: Progress in Lymphology. Hrsg. von A. RÜTTIMANN, Thieme, Stuttgart.
—, und S. KUBIK (1972): Zur Ontogenese des lymphatischen Systems. In: Handbuch der Allgemeinen Pathologie, III/6, 1—38, Springer, Berlin — Heidelberg — New York.
WELLAUER, J. (1967): The lymphatic system in history. In: Progress in Lymphology. Hrsg. von A. RÜTTIMANN, Thieme, Stuttgart.
WELLER, C. V. (1938): The hemolymph nodes. In: DORONEY, Handbook of hematology, vol. III, 1759—1787.
WENZEL, J. (1972): Normale Anatomie des Lymphgefäßsystems. In: Handbuch der Allgemeinen Pathologie, III/6, 89—148, Springer, Berlin — Heidelberg — New York.
WIRTH, W., und S. KUBIK (1974): Anatomie, Topographie und funktionelle Aspekte des Lymphsystems. In: Atlas der Lymphographie. Hrsg. von A. RÜTTIMANN, M. VIAMONTE et al., Thieme, Stuttgart.
WOLSTENHOLME, G. E. W., und J. KNIGHT (ed.) (1963): The immunologically competent cell: its nature and origin. J. and A. Churchill, Ltd., London.
YOFFEY, J. M., and F. C. COURTICE (1956): Lymphatics, lymph and lymphoid tissue. 2nd ed. Edward Arnold Publ., London.
—, — (1970): Lymphatics, lymph and the lymphomyeloid complex. Academic Press, London and New York.
ZARIBNICKY, F. (1911): Über die chemische Zusammensetzung der Pferdelymphe. Wurst, Wien.
ZIETZSCHMANN, O. (1958): Das Lymphsystem von Schwein, Rind und Pferd. In: Die Ausführung der tierärztlichen Fleischuntersuchung mit besonderer Berücksichtigung der anatomischen Grundlagen und der gesetzlichen Bestimmungen. F. SCHÖNBERG und O. ZIETZSCHMANN, 5. Aufl. Paul Parey, Berlin und Hamburg.
ZILCH, M. J. (1963): Lymphsystem und Lymphatismus. A. J. Barth, München.

Lymphatic tissue, including tonsils and lymph nodes; RES, immunity

ARNSDORFF, A. (1923): Die Noduli aggregati bei den Fleischfressern. Diss. med. vet. Berlin.
ASCHOFF, L. (1924): Das Retikulo-endotheliale System. Ergebn. inn. Med. Kinderheilk. 26, 1—118.
— (1926): Die lymphatischen Organe. Med. Klin. 22, Beih. 1, 1—22.
BARONE, R., L. JOUBERT, STAGNARA et VALENTIN (1957): Immunologie des hétérogreffes artérielles et osseuses. Colloque sur les greffes, Rennes.
BAUM, H. (1911): Die Lymphgefäße der Mandeln des Rindes, zugleich ein Beitrag zur Beurteilung der Mandel als Eingangspforte für Infektionserreger. Zschr. f. Infektionskrankh. d. Haust. 9, 157—160.

BIGGS, P. M. (1956): Lymphoid and haemopoietic tissue. Vet. Rec. 68, 525—526.
BURNET, F. M. (1968): Evolution of the immune process in vertebrates. Nature 218, 426—430.
CHIODI, V. (1958): Il cosi detto sistema reticolo endoteliale nell' apparato cutaneo degli animali. Atti Acc. Scien. Ist. Bologna, V, 5—8.
COHRS, P. (1931): Knochenmark und Körperlymphknoten. Arch. Tierheilk. 64, 152—159.
CULZONI, V. (1961): La bourse de Fabricius en quelques oisseaux de cage et de volière. La nuova Veter. 37/12, 257—261.
DAHMEN, E. (1970): Die embryonale Entwicklung des Waldeyer'schen Rachenringes beim Rind. Diss. med. vet. München.
DUBIEZ, R. (1967): Contribution à l'étude de la formule leucocytaire et de la numération globulaire du porc. Diss. med. vet. Lyon.
ERENCIN, Z. (1945): Die Untersuchungen über das Retikulo-endotheliale System. Acta Vet. Turcica 13, 55—62.
FEHER, G., und Z. A. NAGY (1972): Histometrische Analyse der Hühnermilz während der primären Immunitätsreaktion gegenüber löslichem Rinderserumalbumin. Mathematisch-histometrische Methode zur Bestimmung quantitativer Veränderungen von Thymus- bzw. Bursa-abhängigen Lymphozyten. Z. f. Immunitätsforsch., exp. u. klin. Immunol. 143, 245—251.
FREEMAN, L. W. (1942): Lymphatic pathways from the intestine in the dog. Anat. Rec. 82, 543—550.
FRIESS, A. E. (1969): Fluoreszenzmikroskopische Untersuchungen an Lymphozyten. Zbl. Vet. Med. A 16, 341—353.
FUJITA, T., M. MIYOSHI and T. MURAKAMI (1972): Scanning Electron Microscope Observation of the Dog Mesenteric Lymph Node. Z. Zellforsch. mikr. Anat. 133, 147—162.
GIURGEA, R. (1973): Veränderungen an der Bursa fabricii und am Thymus bei den Küken nach der Milzexstirpation. Zbl. Vet. Med. A 20, 677—682.
—, und V. TOMA (1975): Reaktionen der Thymusdrüse und der Bursa Fabricii auf Verabreichung von ACTH bei einer ontogenetischen Unterfunktion der Nebennieren. Zbl. Vet. Med. A 22, 485—492.
—, und G. SIMU (1975): Das Verhalten von Thymus und Bursa Fabricii bei Hühnern mit nicht-tumorösen Formen von Infektionen mit dem Rous-Sarkom-Virus. Zbl. Vet. Med. B 22, 448 bis 454.
GORGOLLON, P., and J. KRSULOVIC (1973): Ultrastructure of the lymph nodes in the dog. Anat. Anz. 134, 239—252.
GRAU, H. (1954): Über die Herkunft der Lymphozyten. Tierärztl. Umschau, 21/22, 392—396.
— (1955): Über das lymphoretikuläre Gewebe. Berl. Münch. Tierärztl. Wschr. 23, 404—406.
— (1965): Das Lymphgewebe des Organismus in neuerer Sicht. Zbl. Vet. Med. A 12, 479—492.
GRUNDMANN, E. (1958): Die Bildung der Lymphozyten und Plasmazellen im lymphatischen Gewebe der Ratte. Beitr. path. Anat. 119, 217—262.
HABERMEHL, K. H. (1969): Das lymphatische Gewebe — ein Stoffwechselapparat. Schweiz. Arch. Tierheilk. 111, 501—517.
HASHIMOTO, Y., and Y. EGUCHI (1957): Studies on the intra-embryonic haematopoietic tissue of the cattle foetus. 4. various haematopoietic tissues, except the liver, spleen and bone marrow, with special reference to the thymus and lymph node. Jap. J. of Vet. Sci. 19, No. 4.
HASSA, O. (1955): Histomorphologischer Charakter der Bursa fabricii. Diss. med. vet. Ankara.
— (1955): Über die Ontogenie und hematopoetische Funktion von Bursa fabricii bei den Haushühnern. Ankara Üuniversitesi Veteriner Fakültesi yayinlari 70.
HEBEL, R. (1960): Untersuchungen über das Vorkommen von lymphatischen Darmkrypten in der Tunica submucosa des Darmes von Schwein, Rind, Schaf, Hund und Katze. Anat. Anz. 109, 7—27.
—, und H.-G. LIEBICH (1969): Elektronenmikroskopische Untersuchungen an kleinen Lymphozyten aus dem Ductus thoracicus der Ratte. Z. Zellforsch. 93, 232—248.
HILLE, R. (1908): Untersuchungen über das Vorkommen der Keimzentren in den Lymphknoten von Rind, Schwein, Pferd und Hund und über den Einfluß des Lebensalters auf die Keimzentren. Diss. med. vet. Leipzig.
HÖLSCHER, H. (1925): Das Vorkommen lymphatischer Herde in der Thyreoidea trächtiger Tiere. Diss. med. vet. Berlin.
HULLIGER, L. (1959): Über die unterschiedlichen Entwicklungsfähigkeiten der Zellen des Blutes und der Lymphe in vitro. Virchows Arch. path. Anat. 329, 289—318.
KELLER, L. (1951): Der Bau des Lymphknotens. Verh. Anat. Ges. (Jena) 48, Erg.-H. zu Anat. Anz. 97, 92—94.
KESSLER, H. (1955): Zur Histologie der Lymphknoten. Zbl. allg. Path. path. Anat. 93, 139—143.
KEYE, W. (1922): Die natürliche Abwanderung des Pigments aus der Haut in die Lymphdrüsen bei Pferden. Diss. med. vet. Berlin.
KIHARA, T. (1956): Entwicklungsgeschichtliche und experimentelle Untersuchungen über die Retikulumfasern. Bull. Osaka med. Sch. Suppl. 1, 1—19.
— (1956): Das extravaskuläre Saftbahnsystem. Folia anat. jap. 28, 601—621.
KOBOSIL, K. (1973): Versuche zur Wiederherstellung der humoralen Reaktionsfähigkeit immunologischer defekter Hühner. Diss. med. vet. München.
KOCK, G. DE (1929): A study of the reticulo-endothelial system of the sheep. 13th + 14th Repts. of the Dir. of Vet. Education and Research I, 647.
KÖHLER, H. (1958): Das Retikulo-Histiozytäre System (RHS) in der Veterinärpathologie. Wien. Tierärztl. Mschr. 45/3, 155—168.
KREHAHN, P. (1921): Die Verteilung und Anordnung des zytoblastischen Gewebes in der Choanengegend beim Schwein, Kalb, Rind und Pferd. Diss. med. vet. Leipzig.
KRÖLLING, O. (1928): Über das retikulo-endotheliale System. Wien. Tierärztl. Mschr. XV, 459 bis 463.
KÜRZ, E. (1921): Die Verteilung und Anordnung des zytoblastischen Gewebes in der Choanengegend bei Schaf, Hund und Katze. Diss. med. vet. Leipzig.
LAULANIE, P. (1880): Expériences sur la reconstitution des globules rouges du sang après les hémorragies abondantes. Rev. Vét. Toulouse, 400.
— (1881): Sur le passage des globules rouges dans

la circulation lymphatique. Rev. Vét. Toulouse, 65.
LEMM, E. (1921): Die Lymphdrüsen am Darm des Pferdes — Anzahl, Gestaltung, Gewicht, Verteilung. Diss. med. vet. Berlin.
LIEBICH, H.-G. (1970): Zur Morphologie kleiner Lymphozyten. Ergh. Anat. Anz. 126, 381—385.
— (1970): Elektronenmikroskopische Untersuchungen an kleinen Lymphozyten. Zbl. Vet. Med. A 17, 97—119.
— (1971): Zur Feinstruktur elektrophoretisch getrennter Zellen des Ductus thoracicus. Anat. Anz. Ergh. 65, 281—287.
— (1973): Experimentell-morphologische Untersuchungen an immunkompetenten Zellen. Habilitationsschrift München.
— und R. HEBEL (1969): Elektronenmikroskopische Untersuchungen an Zellen aus dem Ductus thoracicus des Hundes. Z. ges. exp. Med. 151, 308 bis 320.
MASUI, K. (1926): Preliminary note on the effect of gonadectomy upon the weight of the kidney, thymus and spleen of mice. Proc. Imp. Acad. 2, 33—35.
— and Y. TAMURA (1926): The effect of gonadectomy on the weight of the kidney, thymus and spleen of mice. British J. Exp. Biol. 3, 207—223.
MAY, S. N. (1903): Vergleichende anatomische Untersuchungen der Lymphfollikelapparate des Darmes der Haussäugetiere (Pferd, Esel, Rind, Schaf, Ziege, Schwein, Hund, Katze). Diss. med. vet. Gießen.
MESIPUU, I. (1973): Lymphovenöse Anastomose zur Langzeitgewinnung von Lymphe aus dem Ductus thoracicus bei Schafen und Kälbern. Zschr. f. Versuchstierk. 15, 199—203.
MOVAT, H. Z., and N. V. P. FERNANDO (1965): The fine structure of the lymphoid tissue during antibody formation. Exp. Molec. Path. 4, 155—188.
NAGY, Z. A., und G. FEHER (1972): Histometrische Analyse der Hühnermilz während der primären Immunitätsreaktion gegenüber löslichem Rinderserumalbumin. I. D. Beziehungen zwischen quantitativen Veränderungen von Thymus- bzw. Bursa-abhängigen Lymphozyten in der Milz und der Splenomegalie. Z. f. Immunitätsforsch., exp. u. klin. Immunol. 143, 223—244.
—, — (1972): Histometrische Analyse der Hühnermilz während der primären Immunitätsreaktion gegenüber löslichem Rinderserumalbumin. III. Der Einfluß der Antigendosis auf die Proliferation immunkompetenter Zellen bei optimalen und größeren Antigenmengen. Z. f. Immunitätsforsch., exp. u. klin. Immunol. 143, 323—332.
PAERTAN, J., and N. THUMB (1958): Studies on lymphocytic function. Blood 13, 417—426.
PATZELT, V. (1933): Die Entwicklung der Peyer'schen Platten und die Beziehungen des Epithels zum lymphoretikulären Gewebe. Wien. kl. Wschr. 15, 461—462.
PISCHINGER, A. (1951): Über den Bau des lymphoretikulären Gewebes und die Genese der Lymphozyten. Verh. Anat. Ges. Erg.-H. z. Anat. Anz. 98, 49—53.
— (1954): Über den Bau des Lymphgewebes und die Vermehrung der Lymphozyten. Z. Zellforsch. 40, 101—116.
RICHTER, J. (1901): Vergleichende Untersuchungen über den mikroskopischen Bau der Lymphdrüsen von Pferd, Rind, Schwein und Hund. Diss. med. vet. Erlangen.
SCHNAPPAUF, H., und B. SCHNORR (1968): Zur Natur der stark basophilen Zellen in der Ductus thoracicus-Lymphe. Acta Haemat. 39, 282—290.
SCHUHMACHER, A. (1962): Elektronenmikroskopische Untersuchungen an Plasmazellen in Lymphknoten und Milz der Ratte. Diss. med. vet. Wien.
TOMA, V., und R. GIURGEA (1974): Dynamik der Nukleinsäuren und des Eiweißgehaltes im Thymus und in der Bursa fabricii der Hühnchen unter dem Einfluß von Cortisol. Zbl. Vet. Med. A 21, 506—513.
TRAUTMANN, A. (1926): Die Lymphknoten (Lymphonodi) von Sus scrofa, insbesondere deren Lymphstrom-, Färbungs- und Rückbildungsverhältnisse. Zschr. Anat. 78, 733—755.
VARICAK, T., und A. FRANK (1966): Das histiozytäre System der Lymphknoten während der Hypothermie, Reanimation und Posthypothermie. Bull. sci. Acad. RSF Yougosl. A 11/10/12, 248.
VIERTEL, W. P. (1973): Untersuchungen über das Auftreten pyrinophiler Zellen bei mit Rotlaufimpfstoffen behandelten Schweinefeten unter besonderer Berücksichtigung der Lymphknoten. Diss. med. vet. Berlin.
VOGEL, K., und J. BEYER (1975): Die immunologische Bedeutung von Bursa Fabricii und Thymus des Huhnes. Monatshft. Vet. Med. 30, 386—394.
VOLLMERHAUS, B. (1957): Über tonsilläre Bildung in der Kehlkopfschleimhaut des Rindes. Berl. Münch. Tierärztl. Wschr. 70, 288—290.
— (1959): Zur vergleichenden Nomenklatur des lympho-epithelialen Rachenringes der Haussäugetiere und des Menschen. Zbl. Vet. Med. A 6, 82—89.
WAGNER, G. (1973): Untersuchungen von Graft versus Host reaktiven Lymphozyten mit Hilfe der trägerfreien Elektrophorese. Diss. med. vet. München.
WIRTZ, A. S. (1972): Entwicklung und Morphologie der Bursa Fabricii und ihre Rolle im immunologischen System. Diss. med. vet. Hannover.
ZIMMERMANN, A. (1941): Die Veränderungen der Lymphknoten im hohen Alter. Közlemények az összehasonlitó élet- és kórtan köréböl 31, 245.
ZIMMERMANN, G. (1932): Über den Waldeyerschen lymphatischen Rachenring. Allatani Közlemények XXIX, 126—137.
— (1933): Über den Waldeyer'schen lymphatischen Rachenring. Arch. wiss. prakt. Tierheilk. 67, 141—153.

Haemolymph nodes

BAUM, H. (1907): Rote Lymphknoten. Dtsch. Tierärztl. Wschr. 34, 477—480.
ERENCIN, Z. (1948): Hemolymph nodes in small ruminants. Am. J. Vet. Res. IX, 291—295.
— (1951): Die Zytologie der Haemallymphknoten von Wiederkäuern (Schaf und Ziege). Acta. Anat. (Basel), Seperatum 11, 401—413.
— (1952): Haemallymphknoten. Ankara Üniversitesi-Vet. Fakültesi Yayinlari: 34 Calismalar: 18 Ankara Üniversitesi Bas mevi.
KARPFER, K. (1927): Über die Blutlymphknoten. Allatorvosi Lapok L, 159.
KELLER, O. (1922): Om Haemolymphoglandler. En Anatomisk Studie. Københaben.

KOCK, G. DE (1929): Hemo-lymphoid-like nodules in the liver of ruminants a few years after splenectomy. 15th Rept. of the Dir. of Vet. Services, II, 577.
KUDO, N. (1953): Studies on the red Lymphonodus I. Macroscopical observations on the red Lymphonodus in goats. Jap. J. Vet. Res. 1, 97—110.
— (1953): Studies on the red Lymphonodus II. Microscopical observations on the peripheral sinus of the red Lymphonodus in goats. Jap. J. Vet. Res. 1, 157—166.
— (1954): Studies on the red Lymphonodus III. About the agyrophilic fibers on the peripheral sinus of the red Lymphonodus in goats. Jap. J. Vet. Res. 2, 117—128.
MEYER, A. W. (1908): The haemolymph glands of the sheep. Anat. Rec. 2, 62—64.
OLAH, J., und J. TÖRÖ (1970): Blutlymphknoten der Ratte. Cytobiologie (Stuttgart) 2, 376—386.
PILTZ, H. (1907): Über Hämolymphdrüsen. Berl. Tierärztl. Wschr. 27, 518—520.
— (1909): Ein Beitrag zur Kenntnis der roten Lymphknoten. Diss. med. vet. Berlin.
SCHMALTZ, R. (1907): Blutlymphdrüsen. Berl. Tierärztl. Wschr. 47, 853.
SCHUHMACHER, S. v. (1912): Über Blutlymphdrüsen. Verh. d. Anat. Ges., 131—139.
— (1913): Bau, Entwicklung und systematische Stellung der Blutlymphdrüsen. Arch. mikr. Anat. 81, 92—150.
TURNER, D. R. (1969): The vascular tree of the hemal node in the rat. J. Anat. (London) 104, 481—493.
VARICAK, T., und A. FRANK (1966): Die Haemalknoten der Ziegen unter normalen Bedingungen sowie während der Hypothermie, Reanimation und Posthypothermie. Vet. archiv. 36/11/12, 334 bis 336.
VINCENT, S., and S. HARRISON: On the hemolymph glands of some vertebrates. J. Anat. Phys. 31, 176—198.
ZIMMERMANN, A. (1916): Von den Blutlymphknoten. Allatorvosi Lapok XXXIX, 179.

Spleen

BARGMANN, W. (1941): Zur Kenntnis der Hülsenkapillaren der Milz. Z. Zellforsch. 31, 630—647.
BORTOLAMI, R., et S. LOMBARDO (1952): Osservazioni sullo sviluppo delle fibre elastische nella capsula e nelle trabecole della milza in feti di Bos taurus. Atti Soc. It. Scien. Veter. 6, 324—327.
—, — (1953): Dello svolgimento e della fine struttura della capsula lienis in feto di Bos taurus. La nuova Veterinaria 29, 37—40.
BRINKMANN, A. (1958): Die Arterien und Venen der Rindermilz unter Berücksichtigung ihres Einbaues in das Trabekelsystem. Diss. med. vet. Gießen.
CURSON, H. H. (1930): Accessory spleens in a horse. 16th Report of the Director of vet. Services of South Africa, 875—877.
DIRSCHLMAYER, K. (1936): Beitrag zur vergleichenden Anatomie und Histologie der Milz bei den Wiederkäuern. Diss. med. vet. Wien.
DOOLEY, P. C., J. F. HECKER and M. E. D. WEBSTER (1972): Contraction of the sheep's spleen. Austr. J. Exp. Biol. Med. Sci. 50, 745—755.

FILLENZ, M. (1970): The innervation of the cat spleen. Proc. Roy. Soc. London, B. 174, 459—468.
FRANK, A., und J. VARICAK (1966): Morphologisch-funktionelle Abhängigkeit der Zellenelemente und Aa. folliculares in den Folliculi lymphatici lienales. Bull. Sci. Acad. RSF Yougoslavie A 11, 10/12, 249, Zagreb.
GODINHO, H. P. (1963): Anatomical studies about blood circulation of the dog's spleen. I. Venous drainage: venous lienal zones. Arq. Esc. Vet. 15, 63—72.
— (1964): Anatomical studies on the termination and anastomoses of the a. lienalis and arterial lienal segments in the dog. Arq. Esc. Vet. 16, 163—196.
GOSCH, L. (1931): Über das Vorkommen und die Gestalt glatter Muskelzellen im Parenchym der Milz einiger Säugetiere. Z. mikr.-anat. Forsch. 25, 455—495.
GRAHAME, T., and J. TEHVER (1931): The capsule and trabeculae of the spleens of domestic animals. J. Anat. (Lond.) 65, 473—481.
HARTWIG, H. (1950): Die makroskopischen und mikroskopischen Merkmale und die Funktion der Pferdemilz in verschiedenen Lebensaltern und bei verschiedenen Rassen. Z. mikr.-anat. Forsch. 55, 287—409.
HASHIMOTO, Y., and Y. EGUCHI (1957): Studies on the intra-embryonic haematopoietic tissue of the cattle foetus. 2. Haematopoiesis in the spleen. Jap. J. of Vet. Sci. 19, No. 2.
HERRATH, E. v. (1935): Anatomische Bemerkungen zur Frage der Blutspeicherfunktion der Milz. Dtsch. Med. Wschr. 48, 1924—1933.
— (1935): Vergleichend-quantitative Untersuchungen an acht verschiedenen Säugermilzen. Z. mikr.-anat. Forsch. 37, 389—406.
— (1935): Bau und Funktion der Milz. Z. Zellforsch. 23, 375—430.
— (1935): Über einige Beobachtungen bei der Durchspülung verschiedener Säugermilzen. Anat. Anz. 80, 38—44.
— (1936): Einiges über die Beziehungen zwischen Bau und Funktion der Säugermilz. Anat. Anz. Erg.-H. 81, 182—186.
— (1937): Experimentelle Untersuchungen über die Beziehungen zwischen Bau und Funktion der Säugermilz. 1. Der Einfluß des Lauftrainings auf die Differenzierung der Milz heranwachsender Tiere. a) Hunde. Z. mikr.-anat. Forsch. 42, 1—32.
— (1938): Experimentelle Ergebnisse zur Frage der Beziehungen zwischen Bau und Funktion der Säugermilz. Anat. Anz. Erg.-H. 85, 196—207.
— (1938): Zur vergleichenden Anatomie der Säugermilz und ihrer Speicher- und Abwehraufgaben. Zugleich ein Beitrag zur Typologie der Milz und zum Problem der artlichen und individuellen Milzgröße. Med. Klin. 34, 1355—1359.
— (1939): Experimentelle Untersuchungen über die Beziehungen zwischen Bau und Funktion der Säugermilz. I. Der Einfluß des Lauftrainings auf die Differenzierung der Milz heranwachsender Tiere. b) Hunde. Z. mikr.-anat. Forsch. 45, 111—156.
— (1939): Die Milztypen beim Säuger. Anat. Anz. Erg.-H. 87, 247—254.
— (1941): Milz und Wärmeregelung. Anat. Anz. 91, 20—31.

— (1947): Beiträge und Fragestellungen zu einigen anatomischen Problemen des peripheren Kreislaufs. Med. Rdsch. **1**, 140—149.
— (1953): Zur Morphologie des Retothelialen Systems. Verh. Dt. Ges. Pathol. **37**, 13—25.
— (1955): Experimentelle Untersuchungen über die Beziehungen zwischen Bau und Funktion der Säugermilz. 2. Der Einfluß der Außentemperatur auf die Differenzierung der Milz heranwachsender Tiere (Hunde, Katzen, Kaninchen). Bemerkungen über das Verhalten der Gewichte wachsender Organe unter Außentemperatur- und Trainingseinfluß. Gegenb. Morph. Jb. **96**, 162—208.
— (1958): Bau und Funktion der Milz. De Gruyter & Co, Berlin.
— (1963): Zur Frage der Typisierung der Milz. Anat. Anz. **112**, 140—149.
IMAI, M. (1956): Histological study on the sheathed tissue (the ellipsoid body) and sheathed artery of the spleen. 1. A new fact on the structure of the sheathed artery. J. Vet. Med. Tokyo **186**; Japanisch.
— (1957): Histological study on the sheathed tissue (the ellipsoid body) and sheathed artery of the spleen. 2. On the sheathed tissue. J. Vet. Med. Tokyo **209**; Japanisch.
JACQUIN, A. (1953): Etude anatomique de la rate des Equides domestiques. Diss. med. vet. Lyon.
KÖNIG, H. E., und P. CURA (1971): Eine Nebenmilz beim Pferd. Anat. Anz. **128**, 489—490.
LANGER, P. (1941): Die Altersveränderungen der Milz beim Pferd mit besonderer Berücksichtigung der Gitterfasern. 5. Beitrag zur Altersanatomie des Pferdes. Diss. med. vet. Hannover.
MALL, F. P. (1903): On circulation through the pulp of the dog's spleen. Am. J. Anat. **2**, 315—332.
OBIGER, L. (1940): Untersuchungen über die Altersveränderungen der Milz bei Hunden. (2. Beitrag zur Altersanatomie des Hundes.) Diss. med. vet. Hannover.
POPESCU, P. (1937): Beitrag zum Studium der Topographie und der Punktionstechnik der Milz beim Rinde. Diss. med. vet. Bukarest.
REISSNER, H. (1929): Untersuchungen über die Form des Balkengerüstwerks der Milz bei einigen Haussäugetieren, sowie über die Verteilung von elastischem und kollagenem Bindegewebe und glatter Muskulatur in Kapsel und Trabekel. Z. mikr.-anat. Forsch. **16**, 598—626.
RIEDEL, H. (1932): Das Gefäßsystem der Katzenmilz. Z. Zellforsch. **15**, 459—529.
ROBINSON, W. L. (1930): The venous drainage of the cat spleen. Am. J. Path. **6**, 19—26.
SCHABADASCH, A. (1935): Beiträge zur vergleichenden Anatomie der Milzarterien. Versuch einer Analyse der Evolutionsbahnen des peripheren Gefäßsystems. Zschr. Anat. Entw.-gesch. **194**, 502—570.
SCHLÜNS, J. (1964): Untersuchungen zur Histotopochemie der alkalischen Phosphatase in der Milz einiger Säugetiere. Acta histochem. **19**, 201—233.
— (1964): Über den Nachweis einer γ-Glutamyltranspeptidase-ähnlichen Enzymaktivität in den Schweiger-Seidelschen Kapillarhülsen der Milz des Schweines. Tierärztl. Umsch. **4**, 183—188.
SCHÖNBERG, F. (1926): Über Nebenmilzen bei 8 Schweinen mit gleichzeitiger Einsprengung von Pankreasläppchen in das Milzgewebe. Berl. Tierärztl. Wschr. **26**, 428—430.
SCHULZ, P. (1956): Maße und Gewichte der Milzen unserer Schlachttiere. Dtsch. Schlacht. u. Viehhof Ztg. **56**, 86—88.
SCHWARZE, E. (1937): Über Bau und Leistung der Milzkapsel unserer Haussäugetiere. Berl. Tierärztl. Wschr. **34**, 521—522.
SCHWEIGER-SEIDEL, F. (1863): Untersuchungen über die Milz. Abt. II Virch. Arch. pathol. Anat. Physiol. **27**, 460—504.
SNOOK, T. (1950): A comparative study of the vascular arrangements in mammalian spleens Am. J. Anat. **87**, 31—78.
STEGER, G. (1939): Die Artmerkmale der Milz der Haussäugetiere (Pferd, Rind, Schaf, Ziege, Schwein, Hund, Katze, Kaninchen und Meerschweinchen). Diss. med. vet. Leipzig, 1938.
— (1939): Die Artmerkmale der Milz der Haussäugetiere. Gegenb. Morph. Jb. **83**, 125—157.
— (1938): Zur Biologie der Milz der Haussäugetiere. Dtsch. Tierärztl. Wschr. **39**, 609—614.
— (1939): Die tierartlichen Merkmale der Haussäugermilzen bezüglich Form, Hilus und Gefäßen. Dtsch. Tierärztl. Wschr. **21**, 325—327.
TISCHENDORF, F. (1948): Beobachtungen über die feinere Innervation der Säugermilz. Klin. Wschr. **26**, 125.
— (1951): Die Pulpamuskulatur der Milz und ihre Bedeutung. Z. Zellforsch. **36**, 2—44.
— (1953): Über die Elefantenmilz. Zschr. Anat. Entw.-gesch. **116**, 577—590.
— (1956): Milz. In: Kükenthals Handbuch der Zoologie, hrsg. von J.-G. HELMCKE und H. v. LENGERKEN, VIII/5, 1—32, De Gruyter & Co., Berlin.
— (1956): Neue Beobachtungen zur Frage der arteriellen Endigungen in der menschlichen Milz. Anat. Anz. **103**, 437—442.
— (1956): Die Innervation der Säugermilz. Ein Beitrag zur neurohistologischen Analyse funktioneller Organstrukturen. Biol. lat. (Milano) **9**, 307 bis 342.
— (1958): Über die Hippopotamidenmilz. Ein Beitrag zur Typen- und Altersanatomie der Milz. Z. mikr.-anat. Forsch. **64**, 228—257.
— (1959): Untersuchungen über die terminale Strombahn im Bereich der Pars subcapsularis der menschlichen Milz. Z. Zellforsch. **50**, 369—414.
— (1969): Die Milz. In: v. MÖLLENDORF/BARGMANNS Handbuch der mikroskopischen Anatomie des Menschen. VI/6, Erg. VI/I, Springer, Berlin — Heidelberg — New York.
— und A. LINNARTZ-NIKLAS (1958): Autoradiographische Untersuchungen zur Frage des Eiweißstoffwechsels in den lymphoretikulären Organen. Experientia **14**, 379—383.
TURNER, A. W., and V. E. HOGETTS (1959): The dynamic red cell storage function of the spleen in sheep. I. Relationship to fluctuations of jugular haematocrit. Austr. J. exp. Biol. **37**, 399—420.
VEREBY, K. (1943): Vergleichende Untersuchungen über die Kapsel, Trabekel und Gefäße der Milz. I. Die Milz des Schafes und Rindes. Zschr. Anat. Entw.-gesch. **112**, 634—652.
WAGEMEYER, M. (1956): Über den Einbau des Gefäßsystems der Milz in die Trabekelarchitektur und dessen funktionelle Bedeutung. Diss. med. Mainz.

WINQVIST, G. (1954): Morphology of the blood and the hemopoietic organs in cattle under normal and some experimental conditions. Acta Anat. (Basel) Suppl. 21 ad 22, 7—159.

Thymus

ANDREASEN, E. (1943): Studies on the thymolymphatic system. Acta path. microbiol. scand., Suppl. 49, 1—171.
ARNASON, G., B. D. JANKOVIĆ and B. H. WAKSMAN (1962): A survey of the thymus and its relation to lymphocytes and immune reaction. Blood 20, 617—628.
BEVANDIC, M., and I. ARNAUTOVIC (1966): The thymus of the ewe from its birth till sexual maturity. Veterinaria 15/1, 51—56.
—, — (1965): Der Thymus des Lammes bis zur Geschlechtsreife. Bericht der Jugosl. Anatomen Ges. erschienen in: Acta Anat. 61, 456.
BIMES, C. H., P. DE GRAEVE, S. AMIEL et al. (1975): Beziehungen zwischen Thymus und Geschlechtshormonen beim Meerschweinchen. Zbl. Vet. Med. C 4, 162—171.
BURNET, F. M. (1962): The thymus gland. Sci. Am. 207, 50—57.
DENIZ, E. (1964): Die Blutgefäßversorgung des Thymus beim Kalb. Zbl. Vet. Med. A 11, 749—759.
FUJISAKI, S. (1966): The fine structure of Hasall's corpuscles and reticular cells in the mouse thymus. Acta. Med. Biol. 14, 107.
HAGSTRÖM, M. (1921): Die Entwicklung des Thymus beim Rind. Anat. Anz. 53, 545—566.
HOSHINO, I., M. TAKEDA, K. ABE and T. ITO (1969): Early development of thymic lymphocytes in mice, studied by light and electron microscopy. Anat. Rec. 164, 47—66.
JAROSLOW, B. N. (1967): Genesis of Hassall's corpuscles. Nature 215, 408—409.
KINGSBURY, B. F. (1936): On the mammalian thymus, particulary thymus IV: the development in the calf. Am. J. Anat. 60/1, 149—183.
KÖHLER, H. (1975): Zum Auftreten tödlicher Verblutungen im Thymusrestgewebe bei Hunden. Wien. Tierärztl. Mschr. 62, 341—345.
LATIMER, H. B. (1954): The pernatal growth of the thymus in the dog. Growth 18, 71—77.
LEE, D. G., and W. J. LENTZ (1947): The tonsillar tissue of the dog. University of Penna. Vet. Ext. Quart. 105, 23—26.
LIEBICH, H.-G. (1974): Elektronenmikroskopische Untersuchungen zur Differenzierung von Thymus-Lymphozyten. Berl. Münch. Tierärztl. Wschr. 87, 122—125.
LUCKHAUS, G. (1966): Ein Beitrag zur Entwicklungsgeschichte des Schafsthymus. Berl. Münch. Tierärztl. Wschr. 79, 183—188.
— (1966): Die Pars cranialis thymi beim fetalen Rind. Morphologie, Topographie, äußere Blutgefäßversorgung und entwicklungsgeschichtliche Betrachtungen. Zbl. Vet. Med. A 13, 414—427.
METCALF, D., and M. BRUMBY (1966): The role of the thymus in the ontogeny of the immune system. J. Cell. Physiol. 67, 149—168.
METTLER, F. (1975): Thymome bei Hund und Katze. Schweiz. Arch. Tierheilk. 117, 577—584.
MILLER, J. F. A. P. (1961): Immunological function of the thymus. Lancet 11, 748—749.
— (1964): The thymus and the development of immunological responsiveness. Science 144, 1544—1551.
PAPP, E., und W. G. VENZKE (1958): Beobachtungen an zellulären Bestandteilen der Thymusdrüse in Gewebekulturen. Wien. Tierärztl. Mschr. 56/7, 411—418.
PHILIPP, A. (1967): Zur Frage der Herkunft der Thymozyten nach Untersuchungen am Material vom Rind. Diss. med. vet. München.
RUTTANAPHANI, R. (1965): Histology of the canine thymus gland at various ages. M. S. Thesis, Cornell University.
RYGAARD, J., and C. W. FRIJS (1974): Die Zucht kongenital thymusloser Mäuse (nude Mäuse). Zschr. f. Versuchstierk. 16, 1—10.
SCHNEEBELI, S. (1958): Zur Anatomie des Hundes im Welpenalter. 2. Beitrag: Form und Größenverhältnisse innerer Organe. Diss. med. vet. Zürich.
VARICAK, T. (1938): Thymus aus der Gegend der zweiten Schlundtasche. Zschr. Anat. Entw.-gesch. 108, 394—397.
WHITE, J. B. (1942): Growth changes of the thymus of the dog (Canis familiaris). M. S., Ames/Iowa.
ZIMMERMANN, A. (1940): Die funktionelle Anatomie der Arterien der Thymusdrüse. Közlemények az összehasonlitó élet-és kórtan köréból 30, 225.
— (1942): Über Thymus-Retikulum. Matematikai és Természettudomanyi Ertesító 62, 201.

Lymphovascular system

ANDERSON, D. H. (1926): Lymphgefäße des Ovars beim Schwein. Contr. Embryol. Carneg. Instn. 17, 107.
APOSTOLEANO, E. (1925): Contribution à l'étude du système lymphatique mammaire chez les carnivores domestiques. Diss. med. vet. Alfort.
— (1925): Système lymphatique mammaire chez les carnivores. Diss. med. vet. Toulouse.
— (1925): Perfectionnement du matériel employé pour les injections des lymphatiques (Procédé Gérota). Bull. Soc. Centr. Méd. Vét. 78, 104—106.
— et M. A. PETIT (1925): A la recherche des lymphatiques du pied du cheval. Bull. Soc. Centr. Méd. Vét. 78, 288—292.
AUER, J. A. (1974): Die Lymphographie der Beckengliedmaße des Pferdes. Diss. med. vet. Zürich.
BÄRISWYL, K. (1960): Das Lymphsystem und seine Beziehungen zur Fettspeicherung und zum Fetttransport in der Rindermilchdrüse. Diss. med. vet. Bern.
BALANKURA, K. (1950/51): Entwicklung des Ductus thoracicus bei den Säugern. Diss. med. vet. Cambridge.
BALAZSY, J. L. (1934): Über die Herstellung von Lymphgefäßpräparaten. Allattani Közlemények XXXI, 56—64.
BARONE, R., M. BERTRAND et R. DESENCLOS (1950): Recherches anatomiques sur les ganglions lymphatiques des petits rongeurs de laboratoire (cobaye, rat, souris). 4 planches horstexte. Rev. Méd. Vét., 423—437.
—, ARNULF, BENICHOUX, LOSSON et MORIN (1954): Documents expérimentaux et cliniques sur la lymphographie. Presse Médicale 78, 1631—1633.
—, —, —, — (1955): Données expérimentales sur la ligature des lymphatiques étudiée par la lymphographie. Minerva Cardioangiologia Europea, I, 2—12.

— und H. Grau (1971): Zur vergleichenden Topographie und zur Nomenklatur der Lymphknoten des Beckens und der Beckengliedmaße. Zbl. Vet. med. A **18**, 39—47.

—, — (1970): Sur la topographie comparée et la nomenclature des nodules lymphatiques du bassin et du membre pelvien. Rev. Méd. Vét. **121**, 649—659.

Baum, H. (1911): Übertreten von Lymphgefäßen über die Medianebene. Dtsch. Tierärztl. Wschr. **26**, 401—402.

— (1911): Die Lymphgefäße der Muskeln und Sehnen der Schultergliedmaße des Rindes. Anat. Hefte **44**, 623—656.

— (1911): Die Lymphgefäße der Gelenke der Schultergliedmaße des Rindes. Anat. Hefte **44**, 439 bis 456.

— (1911): Können Lymphgefäße direkt in Venen einmünden? Anat. Anz. **39**, 593—602.

— (1911): Die Lymphgefäße der Pleura costalis des Rindes. Zschr. f. Infektionskrankh. d. Haust. **9**, 375—381.

— (1911): Können Lymphgefäße, ohne einen Lymphknoten passiert zu haben, in den Ductus thoracicus einmünden? Zschr. f. Infektionskrankh. d. Haust. **9**, 303—306.

— (1911): Die Lymphgefäße der Milz des Rindes. Zschr. f. Infektionskrankh. d. Haust. **10**, 397 bis 407.

— (1912): Zur Technik der Lymphgefäßinjektion. Anat. Anz. **40**, 303—309.

— (1912): Die Lymphgefäße des Thymus des Kalbes. Zschr. f. Tiermed. **16**, 13—16.

— (1912): Die Lymphgefäße der Harnblase des Rindes. Zschr. f. Fleisch- und Milchhyg. **XXII**, 101—103.

— (1912): Welche Lymphknoten sind regionär für die Leber. Zschr. f. Fleisch- und Milchhyg. **XXIII**, 121—124.

— (1912): Die Lymphgefäße des Nervensystems des Rindes. Zschr. f. Infektionskrankh. d. Haust. **12**, 387—396.

— (1916): Können Lymphgefäße direkt in das Venensystem einmünden? Anat. Anz. **49**, 407 bis 414.

— (1916): Die Lymphgefäße der Gelenke der Schulter- und Beckengliedmaße des Hundes. Anat. Anz. **49**, 512—520.

— (1916): Die Lymphgefäße der Leber des Hundes. Zschr. f. Fleisch- und Milchhyg. **XXVI**, 225—228.

— (1917): Die Lymphgefäße der Skelettmuskeln des Hundes, ihrer Sehnen und Sehnenscheiden. Bericht über die Tierärztliche Hochschule in Dresden.

— (1917): Die Lymphgefäße der Haut des Hundes. Anat. Anz. **50**, 1—15.

— (1918): Die im injizierten Zustande makroskopisch erkennbaren Lymphgefäße der Skelettknochen des Hundes. Anat. Anz. **50**, 521—539.

— (1918): Das Lymphgefäßsystem des Hundes. Arch. wiss. prakt. Tierheilk. **44**, 521—650.

— (1918): Lymphgefäße der Skelettknochen und und Hufe des Pferdes. Berl. tierärztl. Hochschule, Dresden.

— (1918): Lassen sich aus dem anatomischen Verhalten des Lymphgefäßsystems einer Tierart Schlüsse auf dasjenige anderer Tierarten ziehen? Unterschiede im Lymphgefäßsystem zwischen Rind und Hund. Anat. Anz. **51**, 401—420.

— (1920): Die Lymphgefäße der Gelenke und der Schulter- und Beckengliedmaße des Pferdes. Anat. Anz. **53**, 37—46.

— (1922): Über die Einmündung von Lymphgefäßen der Leber in das Pfortadersystem. Anat. Verhandl., Erg.-Bd. z. Anat. Anz. **55**, 97—103.

— (1923): Die Kommunikation der Lymphgefäße der Prostata mit denen der Harnblase, Harnröhre, Samenblase Bulbourethraldrüse. Anat. Anz. **57**, 17—27.

— (1925): Die Lymphgefäße der Faszien des Pferdes. Zschr. Anat. **77**, 266—274.

— (1925): Lymphgefäße der Leber des Pferdes. Zschr. Anat. Entw.gesch. **76**, 645—652.

— (1925): Allgemeines über das Lymphgefäßsystem der Haustiere, insbesondere Unterschiede im makroskopischen Verhalten des Lymphgefäßsystems verschiedener Tierarten. Z. Fleisch- u. Milchhyg. **36**, 49—54.

— (1926): Die Lymphgefäße der Lungen des Pferdes, Rindes, Hundes und Schweines. Zschr. Anat. **78**, 714—732.

— (1926): Folgen der Exstirpation normaler Lymphknoten für den Lymphapparat und die Gewebe der Operationsstelle. Dtsch. Z. Chir. **195**, 241—266.

— (1926): Die Benennung der Lymphknoten. Anat. Anz. **61**, 39—42.

— (1927): Die Lymphgefäße der Schultergliedmaßen des Pferdes. Anat. Anz. **63**, 122—131.

— (1927): Die Lymphgefäße der Beckengliedmaßen des Pferdes. Berl. Tierärztl. Wschr **35**, 581—584.

— (1927): Lymphgefäße der Gelenke der Schulter- und Beckengliedmaße der Haustiere. Zschr. Anat. Entw.gesch. **84**, 192—202.

— (1927): Die Lymphgefäße des Euters der Haustiere (Rind, Pferd, Schwein, Hund). Dtsch. Tierärztl. Wschr. **35**, 413—415.

— (1928): Zu dem Artikel von J. M. Josifoff: „Die tiefen Lymphgefäße der Extremitäten des Hundes", im Anat. Anz. Bd. 65, S. 65. Anat. Anz. **65**, 421—428.

— (1928): Die Lymphgefäße des Kehlkopfes der Haustiere (Pferd, Rind, Schwein und Hund). Festschrift f. Eugen Fröhner, Stuttgart, Enke Verlag.

— (1929): Die Lymphgefäße des Kniegelenkes, Tarsalgelenkes und der Zehengelenke des Menschen. Anat. Anz. **67**, 301—318.

— (1929): Zum Kapitel Reißmannsche Drüse und rechte obere Bronchialdrüse. Z. Fleisch- und Milchhyg. **XXXIX**, 3—8.

— (1929): Betrachtungen über die Arbeit von Potsma: „Das Lymphgefäßsystem des Schweines." Z. Fleisch- u. Milchhyg. **XXXIX**, 133—140.

— (1929): Nach der Tierart verschiedenes Verhalten der Lymphgefäße der Serosa der Leber und der Lunge. Anat. Anz. **67**, 88—98.

— (1930): Das Verhältnis der Lymphgefäße der Nierenkapseln zueinander und zu denen der Nierensubstanz. Berl. Tierärztl. Wschr. **40**, 673 bis 678.

— (1930): Lymphgefäße der Nieren. Berl. Tierärztl. Wschr. **46**, 673—693.

— (1930): Lymphgefäße des Magens und der Milz des Schweines. Berl. Tierärztl. Wschr. **46**, 375 bis 384.

— (1932): Ist es berechtigt von Schaltlymphknoten zu sprechen? Anat. Anz. **74**, 154—166.

— und T. Kihara (1929): Untersuchungen über den

Bau der Lymphgefäße und den Einfluß des Lebensalters auf diese. Z. mikrosk.-anat. Forschung 18, 159—198.
— und A. TRAUTMANN (1926): Die Lymphgefäße in der Nasenschleimhaut des Pferdes, Rindes, Schweines und Hundes und ihre Kommunikation mit der Nasenhöhle. Anat. Anz. 60, 161—181.

BARTELS, H., und R. HADLOCK (1964): Die Untersuchung der Lymphknoten am Kopf des Schweines im Rahmen der amtlichen Fleischuntersuchung. Fleischwirtsch. 16, 189—191.

BASSET, J. (1920): Relations des ganglions lymphatiques du bœuf. Bull. Soc. Cent. Méd. Vét. 476 bis 484.

BENOIT, J. (1947): La circulation lymphatique à travers le diaphragme chez les animaux domestiques. Rev. Méd. Vét., 49—58.

BODA, J. (1929): Die abdominalen Lymphknoten der Schafe. Diss. med. vet. Budapest.

CASLEY-SMITH, J. R. (1962): The identification of chylomicra and lipoproteins in tissue sections and their pasage into jejunal lacteals. J. Cell. Biol. 15, 259—277.
— (1967): The fine structure, properties and permeabilities of the lymphatic endothelium. Experientia (Basel), Suppl. 14, 19—39.
— (1968): How the lymphatic system works. Lymphology 1, 77—80.
— (1969): The structure of large lymphatics: How this determines their permeabilities and their ability to transport lymph. Lymphology 2, 15 bis 25.

DANESE, A., R. BROWER and J. M. HOWARD (1962): Experimental anastomoses of lymphatics. Arch. Surg. 84, 6—9.

DAVISON, A. (1903): Lymphgefäßsystem an den Extremitäten der Katze. Anat. Anz. 22, 125 bis 128.

DESENCLOS, R. (1949): Recherches sur la topographie des ganglions lymphatiques du rat et de la souris. Diss. med. vet. Lyon.

EGEHÖJ, J. (1934): Das Lymphsystem des Kopfes beim Rinde. Dtsch. Tierärztl. Wschr. 42, 333 bis 336.
— (1936): Untersuchungen über das Verhalten einiger Lymphknoten am Kopf und am Halse des Schweines. Dtsch. Tierärztl. Wschr. 44, 287—289 und 319—322.
— (1937): Das Lymphgefäßsystem des Schweines. Z. Fleisch- u. Milchhyg. 47, 273—280, 293—298, 313—315, 333—341, 353—360, 372—378.

FABIAN, G. (1969): Zur Darstellung der Lymphkapillaren mittels Patentblau-Violett und Tusche. Berl. Münch. Tierärztl. Wschr. 82, 113—116.

FÖLDI, M., A. GELLERT, M. KOZMA, M. POBERAI, Ö. T. ZOLTAN und E. CSANDA (1966): Neue Beiträge zu den anatomischen Verbindungen zwischen Gehirn und Lymphsystem. Acta anat. (Basel) 64, 498—505.

FORGEOT, E. ((1908): Les ganglions lymphatiques des ruminants. Journ. Méd. Vét. Lyon, 666—669.

FORSTNER, V. v. (1974): Zur makroskopischen Anatomie der Lymphknoten und Lymphgefäße am Magen und Darm der Ziege. Diss. med. vet. München.

GOONERATNE, B. (1972): Lymphatic system in the cats outlined by lymphography. Acta Anat. 81, 36—41.

GRAU, H. (1931): Ein Beitrag zur Histologie und Altersanatomie der Lymphgefäße des Hundes. Z. mikrosk.-anat. Forsch. 25, 207—237.
— (1933): Die Lymphgefäße der Haut des Schafes (Ovis aries). Zschr. Anat. Entw.gesch. 101, 423 bis 448.
— (1934): Die Lymphgefäße der Schultergliedmaßenmuskeln des Schafes (Ovis aries). Morph. Jb. 75, 62—91.
— (1941): Zur Benennung der Lymphknoten. Hier: Die Lymphknoten des Beckeneinganges und der Beckenhöhle. Berl. Münch. Tierärztl. Wschr. 57, 237—241.
— (1942): Zur Benennung der Lymphknoten. Hier: Die Lymphknoten der Beckenwand und des Brusteinganges. Berl. Münch. Tierärztl. Wschr. 58, 180—181.
— (1960): Prinzipielles und Vergleichendes über das Lymphgefäßsystem. Verhandlungen der Deutschen Gesellschaft für innere Medizin. 66. Kongreß. München, Verlag J. F. Bergmann.
— (1965): Die Lymphgefäße, ein Sonderdrainagesystem der Bindegewebsräume. Wien. Tierärztl. Mschr. 52, 353—359.
—, und A. KARPF (1963): Das innere Lymphgefäßsystem des Hodens. Zbl. Vet. Med. A. 10, 553 bis 557.
—, und U. MEYER-LEMPENAU (1965): Das innere Lymphgefäßsystem der Leber. Zbl. Vet. Med. A 12, 232—242.
—, und J. SCHLÜNS (1962): Experimentelle Untersuchungen zum zentralen Chylusraum der Darmzotten. Anat. Anz. 111, 241—249.
—, und M. TAHER (1965): Das innere Lymphgefäßsystem von Pankreas und Milz. Berl. Münch. Tierärztl. Wschr. 78, 147—152.

GREGOR, P. (1914): Lymphknoten und Lymphbahnen am Kopf und Hals des Schweines. Diss. med. vet. Berlin.

GRODZINSKY, E. (1922): Entwicklung des Ductus thoracicus beim Schwein. Bull. Inter. Acad. Sci. Krakau, 183—185.

HADLOK, R. (1974): Die für die amtliche Fleischuntersuchung im nationalen und internationalen Fleischhygienerecht vorgesehenen Lymphknoten. Fleischwirtschaft 54, 1621—1622.

HAMPL, A. (1965): Lymphonodi intramammarii der Rindermilchdrüse. I. Makroskopisch-anatomische Verhältnisse. Anat. Anz. 116, 281—298.
— (1965): Lymphonodi intramammarii der Rindermilchdrüse. II. Mikroskopisch-anatomische Verhältnisse. Anat. Anz. 117, 129—137.
— (1967): Die Lymphknoten der Rindermilchdrüse. Anat. Anz. 121, 38—54.
—, J. BARTOŠ und R. ZEDNÍK (1967): Lymphonodi supramammarii der Schafmilchdrüse. Zbl. Vet. Med. A 14, 570—577.

HARAZDY, K., und J. MOHACSY (1916): Die Lymphknoten des Rindes. Husszemle XI, 21—25.
—, — (1916): Vom Lymphgefäßsystem. Allatorvosi Lapok XXXIX, 143.

HARTUNG, K., H. M. BLAUROCK und W. CLAUSS (1968): Zur Technik der Lymphographie beim Hunde. Berl. Münch. Tierärztl. Wschr. 81, 254 bis 256.

HIGGINS, G. M., und A. S. GRAHAM (1929): Lymphdrainage aus der Peritonealhöhle des Hundes. Arch. Surgery 19, 453.

HORSTMANN, E. (1950): Beobachtungen an den Lymphgefäßen des Mesenteriums. Anat. Nachr. 1, 90—91.

— (1951): Über die funktionelle Struktur der mesenterialen Lymphgefäße. Morph. Jb. 91, 483 bis 510.
— (1959): Beobachtungen zur Motorik der Lymphgefäße. Pflüg. Arch. ges. Physiol. 269, 511—519.
— (1961): Die Motorik der Lymphgefäße. Europ. Konf. Mikrozirkulation, Hamburg 1960. Bib. Anat. 1, 306—308.
— (1968): Die Lymphgefäße. Bild der Wissenschaft 9, 765—773.
—, und H. BREUCKER (1972): Über die Lymphkapillaren in den Darmzotten von Meerschweinchen u. Affe. Z. Zellforsch. mikr. Anat. 133, 551—557.
HOYER, H. (1934): „Das Lymphgefäßsystem der Wirbeltiere vom Standpunkt der vergleichenden Anatomie." Extrait des Mémoires de l'Académie Polonaise des Sciences et des Lettres, Classe de Médicine, Krakau.
HUBER, F. (1909): Der Ductus thoracicus von Pferd. Rind, Hund und Schwein. Diss. med. vet. Dresden.
IWANOFF, St. (1947/48): Über die Anatomie und Topographie der Lymphknoten und großen Lymphgefäße bei der Ziege. Jb. d. Universität Sofia, 24, 551—571.
JELÍNEK, K. (1975): Das innere Lymphgefäßsystem der Gebärmutter der Kuh. I. Lymphkapillaren des Perimetrium. Anat. Anz. 138, 281—287.
— (1975): Das innere Lymphgefäßsystem der Gebärmutter der Kuh. II. Lymphkapillaren und Lymphgefäße des Myometrium. Anat. Anz. 138, 288—295.
— (1975): Das innere Lymphgefäßsystem der Gebärmutter der Kuh. III. Lymphkapillaren des Endometrium. Anat. Anz. 138, 296—306.
—, und V. KACER (1973): Die Lymphkapillaren der Portio vaginalis uteri der Kuh. Anat. Anz., Jena, 133, 431—440.
JOSSIFOW, J. M. (1928): Tiefe Lymphgefäße der Extremitäten des Hundes. Anat. Anz. 65, 65—76.
— (1932): Das Lymphgefäßsystem des Schweines. Anat. Anz. 75, 91—104.
KARBE, E. (1965): The development of the cranial lymph nodes in the dog. Anat. Anz. 116, 155 bis 164.
KARPF, A. (1965): Das innere Lymphgefäßsystem der Lunge. Anat. Anz. 116, 442—451.
—, und E. S. TAHER (1965): Untersuchungen über das innere Lymphgefäßsystem des Hodens, des Ovars, der Lunge und des Pankreas. Zbl. Vet. Med. A 12, 553—558.
KISS, Z. (1958): Lymphgefäßuntersuchungen bei der Katze. Diss. med. vet. Budapest.
KRAUS, H. (1955): Zur Lymphgefäßversorgung des Dünndarms bei Schweinen. Tierärztl. Umschau 10, 8—10.
— (1957): Zur Morphologie, Systematik und Funktion der Lymphgefäße. Z. Zellforsch. 46, 446 bis 456.
KRETSCHMANN, M. J. (1958): Die morphologisch-funktionellen Beziehungen zwischen Aorta und Trunci lumbales, Cisterna chyli, Ductus thoracicus beim Hund. Morph. Jb., 99, 662—678.
KUBIK, I., T. VIZKELETY und J. BÁLINT (1956): Die Lokalisation der Lungensegmente in den regionalen Lymphknoten. Anat. Anz. 104, 104—121.
KUBIK, I., und T. TÖMBÖL (1958): Über die Abflußfolge der regionären Lymphknoten der Lunge des Hundes. Acta Anat. 33, 116—121.

KUBIK, S. (1969): Die normale Anatomie des Lymphsystem. Fortschr. Röntgenstr. Beilage Dt. Röntgenkongreß 1968, 110, 87—88.
— (1971): Morphologische Grundlagen des Lymphsystems. Diagnostik 4, 477—480.
KUPRIANOV, V. V. (1969): Some features of the initial lymphatic vessels in their interrelation with blood capillaries. Acta Anat. 73, 69—80.
LEAK, L. V. (1971): Studies on the permeability of lymphatic capillaries. J. Cell. Biol. 50, 300—323.
MEYER, A. W. (1906): An experimental study on the recurrence of lymphatic gland and regeneration of lymphatic vessels in the dog. Johns Hopkins Hosp. Bull. 17, 185—192.
— (1906): An experimental study on the recurrence of lymphatic gland and regeneration of lymphatic vessels in the dog. J. Am. Vet. Med. Assoc. 140, 943—947.
MISLIN, H. (1961): Experimenteller Nachweis der autochthonen Automatie der Lymphgefäße. Seperatum Experientia. Mschr. f. das gesamte Gebiet der Naturwissenschaften, 17, 29—30.
MOSLER, U. (1973): Lymphographic diagnosis of the large afferent lymphatic ducts (thoracic duct). Med. Welt 24, 2026—2028.
NAUWERK, G. (1964): Eine photographische Studie über die Untersuchung von geschlachteten Rindern mit kritischen Anmerkungen. Diss. med. vet. München.
NAVEZ, O. (1927): Le système lymphatique de l'espèce bovine. Annales de Med.-Vet. Oct.
— (1927): Le système lymphatique du chien. Annales de Med.-Vet. Déc.
— (1927): Le système lymphatique des animaux domestiques. Annales de Med.-Vet. Août-Sept.
— (1929): Le système lymphatique du cheval. Annales de Med.-Vet. Janv., Fév., Mars.
— (1939): Le système lymphatique du porc. Annales de Med.-Vet. Mars.
NICKEL, R. (1939): Blut- und Lymphgefäßsystem des Darmes als Infektionspforte. I. Bestehen direkte Verbindungen zwischen den Darmlymphgefäßen und der Pfortader? Dtsch. Tierärztl. Wschr. 47, 91—93.
—, und W. GISSKE (1939): Blut- und Lymphgefäßsystem als Infektionspforte. II. Dringen Bakterien vom Darm in die Pfortaderkapillaren ein? Dtsch. Tierärztl. Wschr. 47, 434—435.
—, — (1941): Blut- und Lymphgefäßsystem des Darmes als Infektionspforte. Zschr. Fleisch- und Milchhyg. 51, 225, 239, 257.
—, und H. WISSDORF (1966): Die Topographie des Ductus thoracicus der Ziege und Operationsbeschreibung zur Lymphgewinnung aus seinem Endabschnitt. Zbl. Vet. Med. A 13, 645—648.
NORÉN, S. (1939): Beitrag zur Kenntnis über die Lymphgefäße vom Spatium retromucosum in der Luftröhre des Rindes. Skand. veterinärtidskr. 781—787.
ONNO, L. (1940): Le système lymphatique du boeuf. Bull. Acad. Vét. France 93/13, 113—115.
PAPP, M., P. RÖHLICH, J. RUSZNYÁK und J. TÖRÖ (1962): An electron microscopic study of the central lacteal in the intestinal villus of the cat. Z. Zellforsch. 57, 475—486.
PETIT, M. A. (1925): Sur la présence de lymphatiques dans le pied du cheval. Bull. Soc. Centr. Méd. Vét. 78, 74—76.
POSTMA, H. (1928): Das Lymphgefäßsystem des Schweines. Z. Fleisch-Milchhyg. 38, 354—362.

PRIER, J. E., B. SCHAFFER and J. F. SKELLEY (1962): Direct lymphangiography in the dog. Am. J. Vet. Med. Assoc. 140, 943—947.

PÜSCHNER, J. (1974): Einiges über das Blut- und Lymphsystem. Rundschau für Fleischbeschauer und Trichinenschauer 26, 115—118.

ROMSOS, D. R., and A. D. MCGUILLARD (1971): Preparation of thoracic and intestinal lymph duct shunts in calves. J. Dairy Sci., 53, 1275—1278.

ROOS, H., und J. FREWEIN (1974): Die Lymphknoten und Lymphgefäße des Beckens und der Beckengliedmaße der Ziege. Berl. Münch. Tierärztl. Wschr. 87, 101—105.

ROY, P. (1947): Recherches sur la topographie des ganglions lymphatiques du cobaye. Diss. med. vet. Lyon.

SAAR, L. I., and R. GETTY (1961/62): The lymphatic system. A neglected area in veterinary research. I. S. U. Vet. 24/3, 146—151.

—, — (1962): Nomenclature of the lymph apparatus. I. S. U. Vet. 25/1, 23—29.

—, — (1962/63): Lymph nodes of the head, neck and shoulder region of swine. I. S. U. Vet. 25/3, 120—134.

—, — (1964): The interrelationship of the lymph vessel connections of the lymph nodes of the head, neck und shoulder regions of swine. Am. J. Vet. Res. 25/100, 618—636.

—, — (1964): The lymph nodes and the lymph vessels of the abdominal vall, pelvic wall and the pelvic limb of swine. I. S. U. Vet. 27/2, 97—113.

—, (1964): The lymph vessels of the thoracic limb of swine. I. S. U. Vet. 26/3, 161—168.

SAUER, J. (1965): Das innere Lymphgefäßsystem der Nebenniere. Diss. med. vet. München.

SCHAUDER, W. (1920): Über die oberflächlichen Lymphgefäße der Widerrist-, Schulter-, Oberarmgegend und angrenzenden Brustgegenden des Pferdes nach klinischen Befunden. Monatshefte f. Tierheilk. 30, 88—92.

— (1949): Über die Lymphgefäße und Lymphknoten des Euters der Ziege. Dtsch. Tierärztl. Wschr. 56, 41—42.

SCHMALTZ, R. (1927): Zur Benennung der Lymphdrüsen. Anat. Anz. 63, 170—171.

SCHNEPPE, K. (1912): Die Lymphgefäße der Leber und die zugehörigen Lymphdrüsen. Diss. med. vet. Berlin.

SCHNORR, B., D. WEYRAUCH und A. HILD (1975): Die Feinstruktur der Lymphgefäße in der Pansenwand der Ziege. Anat. Anz. 138, 271—280.

SHDANOV, D. A. (1962): Zur Lösung der Streitfragen über die funktionelle Morphologie des Lymphgefäßsystems Anat. Anz. 111, 17—50.

SOMERS, R. K. (1951): The lymph gland of Cattle, Dogs and Sheep. Circular Nr. 866, Washington D. C.

SPIRA, A. (1961): Die Lymphknotengruppen (Lymphocentra) bei den Säugern — ein Homologisierungsversuch. Diss. med. vet. München.

SUGIMURA, M., N. KUDO and K. TAKAHATA (1955): Studies on the lymphonodi of cats. I. Macroscopical observations on the lymphonodi of heads and necks. Jap. J. Vet. Res. 3 (2), 90—105.

—, —, — (1956): Studies on the lymphonodi of cats. II. Macroscopical observations on the lymphonodi of the body surfaces, thoracic and pelvic limbs. Jap. J. Res. 4 (3), 101—115.

—, —, — (1958): Studies on the lymphonodi of cats. III. Macroscopical observations on the lymphonodi in the abdominal and pelvic cavities. Jap. J. Vet. Res. 6 (2), 69—90.

—, —, — (1959): Studies on the lymphonodi of cats. IV. Macroscopical observations on the lymphonodi in the thoracic cavity and supplemental observations on those in the head and neck. Jap. J. Vet. Res. 7 (2), 27—53.

—, —, — (1960): Studies on the lymphonodi of cats. V. Lymphatic drainage from the peritoneal and pleural cavities. Jap. J. Vet. Res. 8 (1), 35—49.

SUNDERVILLE, E. (1910): The lymphatics of cattle. N. Y. S. Vet. Med. Soc. Proc., 47—56.

— (1915): The location of the accessible lymph glands in cattle with reference to physical diagnosis. Cornell Vet., 269—276.

TAGAND, R., E. BARONE et Ch. SOURD (1946): Le système lymphatique du lapin. Rev. Méd. Vét., 116, 167.

—, (1948): Sur la topographie et la nomenclature de quelques groupes ganglionaires lymphatiques. Bull. Soc. Sc. Vét. Lyon, 10.

TAHER, E. S. (1965): Das innere Lymphgefäßsystem der Niere. Diss. med. vet. München.

— (1965): Zur Technik der Lymphgefäßdarstellung. Zbl. Vet. Med. A 12, 501—508.

TANUDIMADJA, K., and N. G. GHOSHAL (1973): The lymph nodes and lymph vessels of the thoracic wall of the goat. Iowa State J. of Res. 47 (4), 229—243.

—, — (1973): The lymph nodes and lymph vessels of the neck and thoracic limb of the goat. Anat. Anz. 134, 64—80.

—, — The lymph nodes and lymph vessels of the head of the goat. Am. J. Vet. Res. 34 (7), 909—914.

—, — (1973): The lymph nodes and lymph vessels of the thoracic viscera of the goat (Capra hircus). Zbl. Vet. Med. C 2, 316—326.

TODD, G., and G. BERNARD (1973): The symphathetic innervation of the cervical lymphatic duct of the dog. Anat. Rec. 177, 303—316.

VERMEULEN, H. A. (1911): Een en ander over het systema lymphaticum. Tijdschr. v. Veeartsenijkunde 1911, 24, 1.

WENZEL, N. (1965): Vergleichende Untersuchungen über den Wandbau des Ductus thoracicus bei Schaf und Hund. Diss. med. vet. München.

WILKENS, H., und W. MUENSTER (1972): Eine vergleichende Darstellung des Lymphsystems bei den Haussäugetieren (Hund, Schwein, Rind und Pferd). Dtsch. Tierärztl. Wschr. 79, 574—581.

WOLF, H. (1920): Der histologische Bau des Ductus thoracicus von Ziege, Schwein und Hund. Diss. med. vet. Leipzig.

ZIEGLER, H. (1959): Das Lymphgefäß-System der Rindermilchdrüse und dessen Bedeutung für die Milchsekretion. Bull. Schweiz. Akad. med. Wiss. 15, 105—120.

— (1959): Der Fettkörper der Rindermilchdrüse und seine Beziehung zum Lymphapparat. Verhandl. Anat. Ges., Zürich, 237—240.

ZIMMERMANN, A. (1915): Zur Geschichte der Anatomie des Lymphgefäßsystems. Husszemle X. 7. 25; 9. 33.

— (1915): Zur vergleichenden Anatomie des Lymphgefäßsystems. Allatorvosi Lapok, XXXVIII, 157.

Skin and cutaneous organs
Handbooks and textbooks

Bargmann, W. (1967): Histologie und mikroskopische Anatomie des Menschen. 6. Aufl. G. Thieme, Stuttgart.

Benninghoff, A., und K. Goerttler (1967): Lehrbuch der Anatomie des Menschen. Bd. 3, 8. Aufl. Urban u. Schwarzenberg, München, Berlin, Wien.

Bloch, B., F. Pinkus und W. Spalteholz (1927): Anatomie der Haut. In: J. Jadassohn: Handbuch der Haut- und Geschlechtskrankheiten. Julius Springer, Berlin.

Brink, F. H. van den (1972): Die Säugetiere Europas westlich des 30. Längengrades. 2. Aufl. Paul Parey, Hamburg u. Berlin.

Bolk, L., E. Göppert, E. Kallius und W. Lubosch (1931): Handbuch der vergleichenden Anatomie der Wirbeltiere. Bd. I. Urban und Schwarzenberg, München, Berlin, Wien.

Bubenik, A. B. (1966): Das Geweih. Entwicklung, Aufbau und Ausformung der Geweihe und Gehörne und ihre Bedeutung für das Wild und für die Jagd. Paul Parey, Hamburg u. Berlin.

Cowie, A. T. (1973): In: Hormones in Reproduction. Cambridge University Press 106—143.

Dabelow, A. (1957): Die Milchdrüse, in: W. v. Möllendorf und W. Bargmann: Handbuch der mikr. Anat. des Menschen. Bd. III, 3. Teil. J. Springer, Berlin.

Ellenberger, W., und H. Baum (1943): Handbuch der vergleichenden Anatomie der Haustiere. 18. Aufl. (von O. Zietzschmann, E. Ackerknecht, H. Grau). J. Springer, Berlin.

Friedenthal, H. (1911): Tierhaaratlas. G. Fischer, Jena.

Fürstenberg, M. H. F. (1868): Die Milchdrüsen der Kuh, ihre Anatomie, Physiologie und Pathologie. Leipzig.

Gegenbaur, C. (1874): Grundriß der vergleichenden Anatomie. W. Engelmann, Leipzig.

Grau, H., und P. Walter (1967): Grundriß der Histologie und vergleichenden mikroskopischen Anatomie der Haussäugetiere. Paul Parey, Berlin und Hamburg.

Hofmann, R. R. (1972): Zur funktionellen Morphologie des Subauricularorganes des ostafrikanischen Bergriedbockes, Redunca fulvorufula chanleri (Rothschild, 1895). Berl. Münch. Tierärztl. Wschr. 85, 470—473.

Ihle, J. E. W., P. N. van Kampen, H. F. Nierstrasz und J. Versluys (1927): Vergleichende Anatomie der Wirbeltiere. J. Springer, Berlin.

Kampfe, L., R. Kittel und J. Klapperstück (1970): Leitfaden der Anatomie der Wirbeltiere. 3. Auflage. G. Fischer, Stuttgart.

Karg, H. (1972): Hormonale Regulation der Milchdrüsenentwicklung und der Milchbildung. In: W. Lenkeit und K. Breirem: Handbuch der Tierernährung, Bd. II. Paul Parey, Berlin u. Hamburg.

Koch, T. (1970): Lehrbuch der Veterinäranatomie. Bd. III, 2. Aufl. VEB G. Fischer, Jena.

Kolb, E. (1962): Lehrbuch der Physiologie der Haustiere. VEB G. Fischer, Jena.

Krölling, O., und H. Grau (1960): Lehrbuch der Histologie und vergleichenden mikroskopischen Anatomie der Haustiere. Paul Parey, Berlin u. Hamburg.

Litterscheid, F., und H. Lambardt (1921): Die Erkennung der Haare unserer Haussäugetiere und einiger Wildarten. Reimann u. Co., Hamm.

Löffler, K. (1970): Anatomie und Physiologie der Haustiere. E. Ulmer, Stuttgart.

Martin, P., und W. Schauder (1938): Lehrbuch der Anatomie der Haustiere, Bd. III, 3. Aufl. Schickhardt u. Ebner, Stuttgart.

Masson, P. (1948): Pigment cells in man. In: „Biology of Melanomas". M. Gordon et al. New York Academy of Sciences, Spec. Publ. 6, 15—51.

Nickel, R., A. Schummer und E. Seiferle (1968): Lehrbuch der Anatomie der Haustiere. Bd. I, 3. Aufl. Paul Parey, Berlin u. Hamburg.

—, — (1975): Lehrbuch der Anatomie der Haustiere. Bd. IV. Paul Parey, Berlin u. Hamburg.

Nusshag, W. (1949): Lehrbuch der Anatomie und Physiologie der Haustiere. S. Hirzel, Leipzig.

Romer, A. S. (1966): Vergleichende Anatomie der Wirbeltiere. 2. Aufl. Paul Parey, Berlin u. Hamburg.

Sajonski, H., u. A. Smollich (1972): Mikroskopische Anatomie. Mit besonderer Berücksichtigung der landwirtschaftlichen Nutztiere. S. Hirzel, Leipzig.

—, — (1973): Zelle und Gewebe. Eine Einführung für Mediziner und Naturwissenschaftler. 2. Aufl. Dr. D. Steinkopf, Darmstadt.

Schaffer, J. (1940): Die Hautdrüsenorgane der Säugetiere. Urban u. Schwarzenberg, Berlin u. Wien.

Schaller, O., R. E. Habel und J. Frewein (1973): Nomina Anatomica Veterinaria. 2. Aufl. A. Holzhausen Nachf., Wien.

Scheunert, A., und A. Trautmann (1965): Lehrbuch der Veterinär-Physiologie. 5. Aufl. Hrsg. von Brüggemann, J., Hill, H., Horn, V., Kment, A., Moustgaard, J., Spörri, H. Paul Parey, Berlin u. Hamburg.

Schumacher v. Marienfrid, S. (1956): Jagd- und Biologie, ein Grundriß der Wildkunde. 2. Aufl. Wagner, Innsbruck.

Seiferle, E. (1949): Kleine Hundekunde. A. Müller, Rüschlikon/ZH.

Sisson, S., and J. D. Grossmann (1938): The anatomy of the domestic animals. 3. Aufl. W. B. Saunders Company, Philadelphia u. London.

Steiniger, Fr. (1940): Erbbiologie und Erbpathologie des Hautorganes der Säugetiere. Aus: „Handbuch der Erbbiologie des Menschen". Hrsg. von G. Just. 3. Bd. J. Springer, Berlin.

Tänzer, E. (1932): Haar- und Fellkunde. Der Rauchwarenmarkt, Leipzig.

Toldt, K. (1935): Aufbau und natürliche Färbung des Haarkleides der Wildsäugetiere. Dtsch. Ges. f. Kleintier- u. Pelztierzucht, Leipzig.

Trautmann, A., und J. Fiebiger (1941): Lehrbuch der Histologie und vergleichenden mikroskopischen Anatomie der Haustiere, 7. Aufl. Paul Parey, Berlin.

Ziegler, H., und W. Mosimann (1960): Anatomie und Physiologie der Rindermilchdrüse. Paul Parey, Berlin u. Hamburg.

Zietzschmann, O. (1926): Bau und Funktion der Milchdrüse. In: Grimmer: „Lehrbuch der Chemie und Physiologie der Milch". 2. Aufl. Paul Parey, Berlin.

—, und O. Krölling (1955): Lehrbuch der Entwicklungsgeschichte der Haustiere. 2. Aufl. Paul Parey, Berlin u. Hamburg.

Skin, hair, glands

Baker, K. P. (1974): Hair growth and replacement in the cat. Brit. veter. J. London 130, 327—335.

Baumann, E. T. (1965): Untersuchungen der Feinstruktur von Rinderhaaren zur Möglichkeit einer Rassendifferenzierung. Diss. med. vet. München.

Bethcke, Fr. (1917): Das Haarkleid des Rindes. Diss. med. vet. Leipzig.

Bittner, H. (1928): Haut als Industrieartikel. Tierhlkd. u. Tierzucht V. 176—195.

Bloch, B. (1917): Chemische Untersuchungen über das spezifische pigmentbildende Ferment der Haut, die Dopaoxydase. Z. f. physiol. Chemie 98, 226—254.

Blümel, B. (1965): Untersuchung der Feinstruktur von Ziegenfellhaaren zur Möglichkeit einer Rassendifferenzierung. Diss. med. vet. München.

Bosch, E. (1910): Untersuchungen über die Ursachen der Haarwirbelbildungen bei den Haustieren mit besonderer Berücksichtigung des Gesichtswirbels und dessen praktische Bedeutung für Beurteilung, Leistung und Zucht der Haustiere. Jb. f. wiss. u. prakt. Tierzucht.

Brinkmann, A. (1912): Die Hautdrüsen der Säugetiere (Bau und Sekretionsverhältnisse). Ergeb. Anat. Entw. 20, 1173—1231.

Claussen, A. (1933): Mikroskopische Untersuchungen über die Epidermalgebilde am Rumpf des Hundes mit besonderer Berücksichtigung der Schweißdrüsen. Anat. Anz. 77, 81—97.

Ebner, H., und G. Niebauer (1967): Elektronenoptische Befunde zur Funktion der Langerhans-Zelle. Z. Haut- u. Geschl.krkh. 42, 677—684.

Edelmann, K. (1940): Die Haut des Schweines als Leder. Dtsch. Tierärztl. Wschr. 31—32.

Englert, H. K. (1936): Über die Vererbung der Haarfarben beim Hund. Diss. med. vet. München.

Ewert, H. (1944): Über den Spaltlinienverlauf in der Haut der Haustiere. Arch. wiss. u. prakt. Tierhlkd. 79, 99—120.

Feder, F.-H. (1964): Untersuchungen der Feinstruktur von Pferdehaaren zur Möglichkeit einer Rassendifferenzierung. Diss. med. vet. München.

Fuchs, F. (1934): Mikroskopische Untersuchungen über die Epidermalgebilde an Kopf und Gliedmaßen des Hundes. Inaug.-Diss. med. vet. Berlin.

Goldsberg, St., and M. L. Calhoun (1959): The comparative Histology of the skin of Hereford and Aberdeen Angus cattle. J. Veter. Res. Vol. 20, 74, 61—68.

Habermehl, K. H. (1950): Untersuchungen über das Vorkommen des Schnurrbartes beim Pferd. Tierärztl. Umschau 5, 453—458.

Hebel, R. (1974): Neue Erkenntnisse über den Tastsinn. Eine Gegenüberstellung neurophysiologischer und morphologischer Befunde aus den letzten Jahren. Berl. Münch. Tierärztl. Wschr. 86, 81—84.

Heck, H. (1936): Bemerkungen über die Mähne der Urwildpferde. Zool. Garten N. F. 8, 179 bis 189.

Heide, H. (1938): Anfall und Verwertung der Schweineborsten in Deutschland. Diss. med. vet. Gießen.

Herre, W., und H. Wigge (1939): Die Lockenbildung der Säugetiere. Kühn-Archiv 52, 233 bis 254.

Hirschfeld, W. K. (1937): Genetische Untersuchungen über die Haarfarbe beim Hunde. Diss. phil. Gießen.

Hirt, E. O. (1923): Makroskopische Untersuchungen über das Verhalten der Haarwurzeln und des Schweißdrüsenapparates des Hundes. Diss. med. vet. Bern.

Höfliger, H. (1931): Haarkleid und Haar des Wildschweines. Inaug.-Diss. med. vet. Zürich.

— (1937): Über die Haarbalgmuskulatur des Schweines. Anat. Anz. 85, 1—14.

Hoffmann, R. (1938): Untersuchungen über die Hauttemperatur des Schafes mit dem Thermoelement. Inaug.-Diss. med. vet. Hannover.

Hohenstein, von (1914): Ein Beitrag zur Streifenzeichnung beim Rind. Dtsch. Landw. Tierzucht 9, 105 ff.

Holm, J. P. (1964): Untersuchungen der Feinstruktur von Katzenfellhaaren zur Möglichkeit einer Rassendifferenzierung. Inaug.-Diss. med. vet. München.

Hoppe, H. (1950): Über die Wasserstoffionenkonzentration (pH) der Hautoberfläche gesunder Hunde. Inaug.-Diss. med. vet. Gießen.

Hornitschek, H. (1938): Bau und Entwicklung der Locke des Karakul-Schafes. Kühn-Archiv 47, (12. Sonderheft f. Tierzucht) 81—174.

Hughes, H. V., and J. W. Dransfield (1959): The blood supply to the skin of the dog. Brit. Veterin. J. 115, 229—310.

Irwin, D. H. G. (1966): Tension line in the skin of the dog. J. small animals Pract. 7, 593—598.

Jabonero, V., und J. Moya (1971): Studien über die sensiblen Endausbreitungen. Acta anat. 78, 488—520.

Jäkel, H. (1940): Mikroskopische Untersuchungen über die Epidermalgebilde an verschiedenen Körperstellen mehrerer Hunderassen. Diss. med. vet. Wien, 1940 u. Wien. Tierärztl. Mschr. 27, 458—459.

Jenkinson, D. Mc Ewan, P. S. Blackborn and R. Proudfoot (1967): Seasonal changes in the skin glands of the goat. Brit. Veter. J. 123, 541—549.

— (1967): On the classification of sweat glands and the question of the existence of an apocrine secretory process. Brit. Veter. J. 123, 311—316.

Jess, P. (1896): Beiträge zur vergleichenden Anatomie der Haut der Haussäugetiere. Diss. med. vet. Basel—Leipzig.

Kakarov, J. (1970): Veränderungen der Haarfollikel von der Geburt bis zum Alter von 18 Monaten beim feinwolligen Stara-Sagora-Schaf. Zivot nuvudni nauki, Sofija 7, 28—30.

Kanter, M. (1965): Zur Morphologie der Hautrezeptoren. Zb. Vet. Med. Reihe A, 12, 493 bis 500.

Kormann, B. (1906): Über die Modifikationen der Haut und die subkutanen Drüsen in der Umgebung der Mund- und Nasenöffnungen, die Formationes parorales et paranasicae der Haussäugetiere. Anat. Anz. 28, 113—137.

Kozlowski, G. P., and M. L. Calhoun (1969):

Microscopic anatomy of the integument of the sheep. Amer. J. veter. Res. 30, 1267—1279.

Kränzle, E. (1912): Untersuchungen über die Haut des Schweines. Arch. mikroskop. Anat. 79, 525 bis 559.

Krüger, G. (1949): Die Bedeutung der Haarwirbel für die Signalementsaufnahme bei Trabern. Mhefte Vet. Med. 4, 147—151.

Küpper, W., und M. Hundeiker (1973): Möglichkeiten einer vergleichenden Oberflächenmorphologie der Haarkutikula. Berl. Münch. Tierärztl. Wschr. 86, 125—129.

Lambardt, H. (1921): Ein Beitrag zur Erkennung der Haare unserer Haussäugetiere und verschiedener Wildarten. Inaug.-Diss. med. vet. Gießen.

Laszlo, F. (1935): Über die Schildbildung der Eber. Dtsch. Tierärztl. Wschr. 790.

Link, L. (1962): Eigenartige Hautpapillen an der Schwanzwurzel des Hundes. Z. Zellforschg. 56, 143—148.

— (1974): Über das Vorkommen von „Haarscheiben" in der Haut von Säugetieren. Berl. Münch. Tierärztl. Wschr. 87, 127—129.

Lyne, A. G., and H. B. Chase (1967): Branched-cells in the Epidermis of the sheep. Landw. Zbl. 06—0027.

Malinovský, L. (1966): Variabilität der Tastkörperchen in der Nasenhaut und im Bereich des Sulcus labiomaxillaris bei Katzen. Folia. morphol. Praha 14, 417—429 (Landw. Zbl. 1968, 04—0032).

Marcarian, H. Q., and M. L. Calhoun (1966): Microscopic anatomy of the integument of adult swine. Amer. J. veter. Res. 27, 765—772.

Minder, K. (1930): Die natürlichen Körperöffnungen des Wildschweines. Diss. med. vet. Zürich.

Mohr, E. (1952): Ungewöhnliche Streifung bei Pferden. Zool. Anz. 148, 303—305.

Müller, H. (1919): Über das Vorkommen von Sinushaaren bei den Haussäugetieren. Inaug.-Diss. med. vet. Zürich.

Müller, W. (1965): Untersuchung der Feinstruktur von Hundehaaren zur Möglichkeit der Rassendifferenzierung. Diss. med. vet. München.

Naaktgeboren, C., und W. van den Driesche (1962): Beiträge zur vergleichenden Geburtskunde. Z. Säugetierkd. 27, 83—110.

Neurand, K., und R. Schwarz (1969): Lichtmikroskopische Untersuchungen an der Haut der Katze (Epidermis, Corium, Subcutis). Dtsch. Tierärztl. Wschr. 76, 521—527.

Niedoba, Th. (1917/18): Untersuchungen über die Haarrichtungen der Haussäugetiere. Anat. Anz. 50, 178—192 u. 204—216.

Novotný, E., und J. Holmann (1960): Die histologische Zusammensetzung der Kälberhaut mit Hinblick zur subkutanen Injektion größerer Flüssigkeitsmengen. Acta univ. agricult. Brno.

Pasečnik, N. M. (1972): Der Bau der Faserstrukturen in der Haut von grobwolligen, dünnwolligen und Kreuzungsschafen. Ref. Z. Moskva Zivot novodstro i. Veter. 1.58 (S. 15).

Pavlović, M. B. (1967): Histophysiologische Untersuchungen der Haut des Rehbockes. Acta veter. Beograd 17, 215—225.

Rast, A. (1911): Studien über das Haarkleid, den Haarwechsel und die Haarwirbel des Pferdes. Inaug.-Diss. med. vet. Bern.

Reinhardt, V. (1940): Beitrag zur Kenntnis der Häuteschäden. Diss. med. vet. Gießen.

Rudzinski, K. J. (1944): Untersuchungen über die Hauttemperatur bei Tieren des Rindergeschlechtes, gemessen mit dem Thermoelement und ihre Beeinflussung durch die Umgebungstemperatur. Inaug.-Diss. med. vet. Zürich.

Samandari, F. (1973): Die Mechanik der Hautleisten- und Tiradienbildung auf Palma und Planta. Anat. Anz. 134, 484—496.

Sar, M., and M. L. Calhoun (1966): Microscopic anatomy of the integument of the common American goat. Amer. J. veter. Res. 27, 444 to 456.

Schäfer, H. (1975): Untersuchungen am Haarkleid eintägiger Karakullämmer. — Eine Bilanz 10jähriger Forschungsarbeit. Dtsch. tierärztl. Wschr. 82, 264—267.

Schaller, R. (1972): Licht- und elektronenmikroskopische Untersuchungen am Grannenhaar der Katze. Inaug.-Diss. med. vet. Hannover.

Schaller, R., und R. Schwarz (1972): Licht- und elektronenmikroskopische Untersuchungen am Mark vom Grannenhaar der Katze. Dtsch. tierärztl. Wschr. 79, 588—590.

Schauder, W. (1919): Über die dunkle Streifenzeichnung („Wildzeichnung") beim Pferd. Berl. Tierärztl. Wschr. XXXV, 29.

Schieferdecker, P. (1922): Die Hautdrüsen des Menschen und der Säugetiere, ihre biologische und rassenanatomische Bedeutung sowie die Muscularis sexualis. Zoologica 27, 1—154.

Schläfli, W. (1950): Untersuchungen über Ursachen der Haarformen und vergleichende Studien über Haar und Horn beim Simmentaler Rind. Inaug.-Diss. med. vet. Bern.

Schmid, W. (1967): Untersuchung der Feinstruktur von Hundehaaren zur Möglichkeit einer Rassendifferenzierung. Diss. med. vet. München.

Schmidt, W., J. Richter und R. Geissler (1974): Die dermoepidermale Verbindung. Untersuchungen an der Haut des Menschen. Z. Anat. Entw. 145, 283—297.

Schnorr, B. (1972): Dendritenzellen im pigmentierten Plattenepithel des harten Gaumens vom Hund. Berl. Münch. Tierärztl. Wschr. 85, 474 bis 476.

Schönberg, Fr. (1929): Über die Bildung und Lagerung des Oberhaut- und Haarpigmentes in der braunen Pferdehaut. Berl. Münch. Tierärztl. Wschr. 45, 173—176.

Schotterer, A. (1933): Vergleichende Hautuntersuchungen bei Rindern. Z. Züchtg. 26, 203—218.

Severnjuk, L. O. (1975): Altersabhängige Veränderungen im Aufbau der Haut und in der Entwicklung der Haarfollikel bei Lämmern aus Kreuzungen mit Marschschafen. Ref. Landw. Zbl. 20, Heft 6.

Siegel, R. (1907): Anatomische Untersuchungen über die äußere Haut des Hundes. Inaug.-Diss. med. vet. Leipzig/Dresden.

Sokolowski, A. (1933): Das Haarkleid der Säugetiere in biologischer Beziehung. Dermat. Wschr. I, 373—377.

Spichtig, M. (1974): Stereologische Untersuchungen der Schweißdrüsen und anderer Hautstrukturen des Hundes. Diss. med. vet. Bern.

Sprankel, H. (1955): Die fibrilläre Architektur von Epidermis und Sinushaaren der Rüsselscheibe des Hausschweines (Sus scrofa domesticus), erschlossen aus der Polarisationsoptik. Z. Zellforschg. 41, 236—284.

STAHL, W. (1947): Die Schweinehaut als Industrierohstoff. Diss. med. vet. Gießen.
STEPHAN, E., und R. REDECKER (1970): Die Rolle der Haut bei der Thermoregulation von Haustieren. Dtsch. Tierärztl. Wschr. 77, 628—631.
STRAILE, W. E. (1961): The morphology of „tylotrich" follicles in the skin of the rabbit. Amer. J. Anat. 109, 1—7.
STRICKLAND, J. H., and M. L. CALHOUN (1963): The integumentary system of the cat. Amer. J. Veter. Res. 24, 1018—1029.
TALUDKAR, A. H., M. L. CALHOUN and A. L. W. STINSON (1970): Sensory endorgans in the upper lip of the horse. Amer. J. veter. Res. 31, 1751 to 1754.
—, — (1972): Specialised vascular structures in the skin of the horse. Amer. J. veter. Res. 33, 335 to 338.
VULOV, T. (1969): Altersbedingte Veränderungen und Geschlechtsunterschiede in der Mikrostruktur der Haut bei 12 bis 18 Monate alten Zigaja-Schafen. Veterinarno medicinski nauki Sofija 6, 33—42.
WAHODE, E. (1927): Biometrische Untersuchungen über Länge und Dicke am Deckhaar des Rindes. Inaug.-Diss. med. vet. Leipzig.
WALTHER, A. R. (1913): Die Vererbung unpigmentierter Haare (Schimmelung) und Hautstellen („Abzeichen") bei Rind und Pferd als Beispiels transgressiv fluktuierender Faktoren. Habil.-Schrift agr. Gießen.
WALTER, P. (1956): Sinneshaare im Bereich der Pferdelippe. Zbl. f. Vet.-Med. III, 599—604.
— (1958): Die Innervation der Hautmodifikationen bei Haussäugetieren. Acta Neurovegetativa XVIII, 60—66.
— (1960): Die sensible Innervation des Lippen-Nasenbereiches von Rind, Schaf, Ziege, Schwein, Hund und Katze. Z. Zellforschg. 53, 394—410.
WALTERFANG, E. (1950): Der Rohstoff „Haut". Eine veterinärwirtschaftliche Studie. Inaug.-Diss. med. vet. Gießen.
WROBEL, K. H. (1965): Bau und Bedeutung der Blutsinus in den Vibrissen von Tupaia glis. Zbl. Vet. Med. Reihe A, 12, 888—899.
ZIETZSCHMANN, O. (1904): Vergleichende histologische Untersuchungen über den Bau der Augenlider der Haussäugetiere. Von Graefes Arch. Ophthalm. 58, 61—122.
— (1943): Die allgemeine Decke. In: W. ELLENBERGER und H. BAUM: Handbuch der vergleichenden Anatomie der Haustiere. 18. Aufl. J. Springer, Berlin, 1028—1072.
ZÜBLIN, H. (1947): Wesen und Ursachen der Schimmelbildung beim Pferd. Inaug.-Diss. med. vet. Bern.
ZURBENKO, A. M. (1969): Postnatal development of the sweat glands of the pig. (Ukrainian) Veterinarija Kyiv. 21, 98—104.

**Specialized glands
(scent glands)**

ACKERKNECHT, E. (1939): Zur Frage der Rudimentärorgane. Dtsch. Tierärztl. Wschr. 86—88.
CLAUSSEN Cl. P., and H. JUNGIUS (1973): On the Topography and Structure of the so-called Glandular Subauricular Patch and the Inguinal Gland in the Reedbuck. Z. f. Säugetierkd. 38, 97—109.
GERSTENBERGER, Fr. (1919): Die Analbeutel des Hundes und ihre Beziehungen zum Geschlechtsapparat. Inaug.-Diss. med. vet. Dresden.
GREER, M. B., and M. L. CALHOUN (1966): Anal sacs of the cat (Felis domesticus). Amer. J. Veter. Res. 27, 773—781.
HAUSENDORFF, E. (1949): Duft- und Hautdrüsenorgane als Markierungs-, Brunft- und Abwehrdrüsen. Wild u. Hund 12.
KARLSON, P., und D. SCHNIEDER (1973): Sexualpheromone der Schmetterlinge als Modelle chemischer Kommunikation. Nat.-Wiss. 60, 113 bis 121.
KRAGE, P. (1907): Vergleichende histologische Untersuchungen über das Präputium der Haussäugetiere. Diss. med. vet. Zürich.
KRÖLLING, O. (1927): Entwicklung, Bau und histologische Bedeutung der Analbeuteldrüsen bei der Hauskatze. Z. Anat. Entw. 88, 22—69.
— (1955): Duftdrüsen-Morphologie und -Physiologie. Jb. d. Arbeitskreises f. Wildtierforschg. S. 1—11.
KUONI, F. (1922): Das Karpalorgan des Schweines, seine Entwicklung und sein Bau. Inaug.-Diss. med. vet. Zürich.
MEYEN, J. (1958): Neue Untersuchungen zur Funktion des Präputialbeutels des Schweines. Inaug.-Diss. med. vet. Berlin.
MEYER, P. (1971): Das dorsale Schwanzorgan des Hundes, Glandula caudae s. coccygis (Canis familiaris). Zbl. Vet.-Med. Reihe A, 18, 541 bis 557.
—, und H. WILKENS (1971): Die Viole des Rotfuchses (Vulpes vulpes L.). Zbl. Vet.-Med. Reihe A, 18, 353—364.
— (1976): Innerartliche Kommunikation durch Hautduftorgane. Zbl. Vet.-Med. Beiheft Nr. 20.
MLADENOWITSCH, L. (1907): Vergleichende anatomische Untersuchungen über die Regio analis und das Rectum der Haussäugetiere. Diss. med. vet. Leipzig.
OEHMKE, P. (1897): Anatomisch-physiologische Untersuchungen über den Nabelbeutel des Schweines. Arch. wiss. prakt. Tierhlkd. 23, 146.
OHE, H. v. D. (1927): Über das Vorkommen und den Bau der Zirkumoraldrüse der Katze. Inaug.-Diss. med. vet. Hannover.
RIECK, W. (1934): Die Hautdrüsen, jagdkundlich bedeutungsvolle Organe unseres Wildes. Dtsch. Jagd. Nr. 22.
SCHALLER, O., J. FREWEIN und J. LEIBETSEDER (1961): Geschlechtsunterschiede an den Extremitätenenden des Rehes (Capreolus capreolus L.). Wien. tierärztl. Mschrft. 48, 415—433.
SCHIETZEL, O. (1911): Die Horndrüse der Ziege. Diss. med. vet. Leipzig.
SCHUMACHER, S. v. (1936): Das Stirnorgan des Rehbockes (Capreolus capreolus L.), ein bisher unbekanntes Duftorgan. Z. mikroskop.-anat. Forschg. 39, 215—230.
TEMPEL, M. (1897): Die Drüsen in der Zwischenklauenhaut der Paarzeher. Diss. med. vet. Leipzig.
WALLENBERG, A. (1910): Die Carpal- und Mentalorgane der Suiden. Inaug.-Diss. med. vet. Bern.
ZIETZSCHMANN, E. H. (1903): Beiträge zur Morphologie und Histologie einiger Hautorgane der Cerviden. Z. wiss. Zool. 74, 1—63.
ZIMMERMANN, A. (1909): Über das Klauensäckchen

des Schafes. Öster. Mschrft. Tierheilkd. **34**, 145 bis 154.
ZIMMERMANN, K. W. (1904): Untersuchungen des Analintegumentes des Hundes. Inaug.-Diss. Bern und Arch. wiss. prakt. Tierheilkd. **30**, 472—515.

Mammary gland

ADAMIKER, D., und E. GLAWISCHNIG (1967): Elektronenmikroskopische Untersuchungen an der Schweinemilchdrüse. Teil I. Befunde an Drüsen virgineller, gravider und laktierender Tiere. Wien. Tierärztl. Mschrft. **54**, 507—518.
ANDREAE, U., und F. PANDZA (1969): Versuch einer objektiven Erfassung der inneren Struktur des Kuheuters durch morphologische und histologische Merkmale. Z. Tierzüchtg. u. Züchtgsbiol. **85**, 325—337.
BALMYŠEV, N. P. (1971): Zur Innervation der Euterzitzen bei Kühen, Schafen und Ziegen. Ref. Z. Moskva Zivotnovodstro i. Veter. 12.58.73, 10.
BOMMELI, W. (1972): Die Ultrastruktur der Milchdrüsenalveole des Rindes, insbesondere die Basalfalten des Epithels und der Mitochondrien-Desmosomen-Komplex. Zbl. Vet.-Med. Reihe C, **1**, 299—325.
COMURI, N. (1972): Untersuchungen über zyklusabhängige Strukturveränderungen am distalen Gangsystem der Milchdrüse des Rindes. Inaug.-Diss. med. vet. Gießen.
DERENDINGER, H. (1974): Die topographisch-anatomischen Grundlagen zu den Operationen in der Inguinalgegend und im Bereich des Gesäuges des Hundes mit besonderer Berücksichtigung der Prostatektomie. Inaug.-Diss. med. vet. Zürich.
EL HAGRI, M. A. A. M. (1945): Study of the arterial and lymphatic system in the udder of the cow. Vet. J. **101**, 27—33, 51—63, 75—88.
GLÄTTLI, H. (1924): Anatomie des Venensystems des Kuheuters. Inaug.-Diss. med. vet. Zürich.
HABERMEHL, K.-H. (1970): Form und Funktion des Gesäuges beim Hausschwein. Schweiz. Milchzeitung **96**, 89—90.
HAMPL, A. (1965): Lymphonodi intramammarici, neue Euterlymphknoten beim Rind. Veterinarstvi **15**, 468—472.
— (1968): Beitrag zur Frage der regionalen Zugehörigkeit der Intramammarlymphknoten und ihre Beziehung zu den Supramammarlymphknoten beim Rind. Acta univ. agricult. Brno **16**, 293—298.
HARRIS, G. W. (1958): The central nervous system, new-hypophysis and milk ejection. Proc. Roy. Soc. B **149**, 336—353.
HENNEBERG, B. (1905): Abortivzitzen des Rindes. Anat. Hefte I, **25**.
HÖFLIGER, H. (1952): Drüsenaplasie und -hypoplasie in Eutervierteln des Rindes — eine erblich bedingte Entwicklungsanomalie. Schweiz. Arch. Tierhlkd. **94**, 824—833.
JURKOV, M. J., L. J. CHOLODOVA und V. J. NIKITIN (1971): Anatomie der Arterien des Schafeuters in der Norm und Pathologie. Ref. Z. Moskva Zivotnovodstro i. Veter. 8.58.53. S. 6.
KAEPPELI, F. (1918): Über Zitzen- und Zisternenverhältnisse der Haussäugetiere. Inaug.-Diss. med. vet. Zürich.
KÄSTLI, P. (1953): Die Ausscheidung von toxisch wirkenden Stoffen durch die Milchdrüse mit besonderer Berücksichtigung der Insektizide. Schweiz. Arch. Tierheilkd. **95**, 171—187.
KOCH, T. (1956): Die Milchdrüse (Glandula lactifera, Mamma) des Rindes. Monatshefte Vet.-Med. **11**, 527—532.
KOLB, E. (1958): Zur Biochemie der Milchsekretion beim Rind. Mhefte Vet.-Med. **5**, 129—134.
KRÄHENMANN, A. (1971): Zur Involution des Gems-, Hirsch- und Rehgesäuges. Schweiz. Arch. Tierhlkd. **113**, 504—516.
KREIKENBAUM, K., und A. KÖNIG (1974): Neuere Erkenntnisse der Endokrinologie der Fortpflanzung bei Haustieren. 7. Folge. Endokrinologie der Geburt und Laktation. Dtsch. Tierärztl. Wschr. **17**, 409—412.
KRÜGER, W. (1953): Begünstigen bestimmte Zitzen und Euterformen die Ausbildung von Euterentzündung beim Rinde? Tierärztl. Umschau 23/24.
KÜNG, W. B. (1956): Weiterer Beitrag zur Kenntnis einer erblich bedingten Drüsenaplasie und -hypoplasie in Eutervierteln des Rindes. Inaug.-Diss. med. vet. Zürich.
LEBEDEWA, N. A. (1960): Die Klappen in den Venen des Euters bei einigen Haustieren. Schreiber-Festschrift Wien. Tierärztl. Mschr. 358—365.
LE ROUX, J. M. W., und H. WILKENS (1959): Beitrag zur Blutgefäßversorgung des Euters der Kuh. Dtsch. Tierärztl. Wschr. **66**, 429—435.
LINZELL, L. J. (1960): Valvula incompetence in the venous drainage of the udder. J. Physiol. (London) **153**, 481—491.
LOPPNOW, H. (1959): Über die Abhängigkeit der Melkarbeit vom Bau der Zitze. Dtsch. Tierärztl. Wschr. **66**, 88—97.
MAINZER, G. (1939): Ein Beitrag zur Morphologie der Milchgänge im Euter der Kuh. Z. mikr.-anat. Forschg. **45**, 443—460.
MEISSNER, R. (1964): Beiträge über den anatomischen Bau des elastisch-muskulösen Systems der Rinderzitze. Diss. med. vet. Berlin (Ost).
MICHEL, G., und B. SCHNEIDER (1975): Histologische und histochemische Untersuchungen zur Innervation der Milchdrüse vom Rind (Bos taurus L.). Z. mikrosk.-anat. Forsch. Leipzig **89**, 231—238
MOSIMANN, W. (1949): Zur Anatomie der Rindermilchdrüse und über die Morphologie ihrer sezernierenden Teile. Diss. med. vet. Bern 1949 u. Acta anat. **8**, 347—378.
— (1957): Das Volumen der Zellkerne im Epithel der Milchdrüse in Abhängigkeit vom Funktionszustand und bei Stilboestrol-Zufuhr (Ziege, Ratte). Z. mikr.-anat. Forschg. **63**, 303—316.
— (1969): Zur Involution der bovinen Milchdrüse. Schweiz. Arch. Tierheilkd. **111**, 431—439.
NEUHAUS, U. (1956): Die Bedeutung des Oxytocins für die Milchsektretion. Dtsch. Tierärztl. Wschr. **63**, 467—469.
NÜESCH, A. (1904): Über das sogenannte Aufziehen der Milch bei der Kuh. Inaug.-Diss. med. vet. Zürich.
RENK, W. (1959): Zur Pathologie der Milchsekretions- und Abflußstörungen. Berl. Münch. Tierärztl. Wschr. **72**, 41—44 u. 64—66.
RICHARDSON, K. C. (1947): Some structural features of the mammary tissues. Brit. Med. Bull. **5**, 1099.

RICHTER, J. (1931): Mehrzitzigkeit beim männlichen und weiblichen Rind. Diss. med. vet. Leipzig.
ROTARU (1924): Zitzenzahl der Hündinnen. Diss. med. vet. Bukarest.
RUBELI, O. (1913): Besonderheiten im Ausführungsgangsystem der Milchdrüsen des Rindes. Mittlg. nat. forsch. Ges. Bern.
— (1914): Bau des Kuheuters. Verlag Art. Inst. Orell Füssli, Zürich.
RUOSS, G. (1965): Beitrag zur Kenntnis der Euterarterien des Rindes mit besonderer Berücksichtigung der Beziehung zwischen Feinbau und Funktion. Inaug.-Diss. med. vet. Zürich.
SCHMALSTIEG, R. (1958): Die Strukturverhältnisse der Milchdrüse des schwarzbunten Rindes und ihre Beziehungen zu Euter und Leistungsmerkmalen. Z. Tierzüchtg. u. Züchtgsbiol. **72**, 113 bis 150 u. 196—224.
SCHAUDER, W. (1951): Die Blutgefäße des Euters der Ziege. Tierärztl. Umschau **5/6**, 77.
SEIFERLE, E. (1949): Neuere Erkenntnisse über Bau und Funktion der Milchdrüse der Kuh. Schriften der Schweiz. Vereinigung für Tierzucht, Euter und Milchleistung. Banteli AG, Bern-Bümpliz.
SKJERVOLD, H. (1961): Überzählige Zitzen bei Rindern. Hereditas, Lund **46**, 1960; Landw. Zbl. S. 1156.
STOJANOWIĆ, V. (1975): Die Blutgefäßversorgung des Euters vom Schaf. Anat. Anz. **138**, 240—250.
TGETGEL, B. (1926): Untersuchungen über den Sekretionsdruck und über das Einschießen der Milch in das Euter des Rindes. Diss. med. vet. Zürich.
TURNER, C. W. (1934): The causes of the growth and function of the udder of cattle. Agricult. Exper. Station, Univ. of Missouri, Bul. 339.
USUELLI, F. (1948): I fattori ormonici e nervosi che spiegano gli effeti della gimnastica funzionale della mammella. Revista di zootecnica XXI. Bd. 6.
VAU, E. (1960): Die Blutabflußwege des Kuheuters. Schreiber-Festschrift Wien. Tierärztl. Mschrft. S. 312.
VENSKE, C. E. (1940): A histological study of the teat and gland cisterns of the bovine mammary gland. J. Am. Vet. Med. Assoc. **96**, 170.
VIERLING, R. (1956): Das Zwischenhirn-Hypophysensystem und die Laktation. Z. Tierzücht., Zücht.-Biol. **66**, 317—322.
VYAS, K. N. (1971): On the individuality and number of the mammary components draining through a teat of the mare. Nord. Veterinaermed. **23**, 244—245.
ZIEGLER, H. (1941): Zur baulichen Eigenart der Milchgänge. Schweiz. Arch. Tierheilkd. **83**, 47 bis 52.
— (1954): Zur Hyperthelie und Hypermastie (überzählige Zitzen und Milchdrüsen) beim Rind. Schweiz. Arch. Tierheilkd. **96**, 344—350.
ZIETZSCHMANN, O. (1917): Anatomische Skizze des Euters der Kuh und die Milchströmung. Schweiz. Arch. Tierheilkd. **12**, 645—667.
— (1917): Die Zirkulationsverhältnisse des Euters einer Kuh. Dtsch. Tierärztl. Wschr. **25**, 1—29.
ZWART, S. G. (1911): Beiträge zur Anatomie und Physiologie der Milchdrüse des Rindes. Inaug.-Diss. med. vet. Bern.

Specialized hairless organs of the skin (claws, hoofs and horns)

BAIER, W. (1950): Über die Beziehung zwischen Epidermis und Korium an Huf und Klauen. Berl. Münch. Tierärztl. Wschr. **63**, 59—63.
BONADONNA, T., L. PECHCIAI und A. SFERCO (1957): Sulle caratteristiche esteriosi ed istologiche delle cosidette „castagnette" nel cavallo, nell'asino de nei loro ibsidi. Zootecn. e Veterin. **12**, 86—117.
BUTLER, W. F. (1967): Innervation of the horn region in domestic ruminants. Veterin. Rec. **80**, 490—492.
ČERVENÝ, Č. und J. KAMAN (1963): Zur Innervation und Blutversorgung des Rinderhornes. Veterinarstvi **12**, 73—75.
DOBLER, Chr. (1969): Papillarkörper und Kapillaren der Hundekralle, Schweine- und Ziegenklaue. Morph. Jb. **113**, 382—428.
ERNST, R. (1954): Die Bedeutung der Wandepidermis (Hyponychium) des Pferdehufes für die Hornbildung. Inaug.-Diss. med. vet. Bern u. Acta anat. **22**, 15—48.
FESSL, L. (1967): Untersuchungen von Klauenkapseln heimischer Rinderrassen. Ref. Landw. Zbl. 02—0020.
FREI, O. (1928): Bau und Leistung der Ballen unserer Haussäugetiere. Jb. Morph. u. mikrosk. Anat. **59**, 253—296.
GEYER, H., J. POHLENZ und H. K. SPÖRRI (1974): Die Morphologie der normalen Schweineklaue im Hinblick auf die Entstehung pathologischer Veränderungen. Vortrag gehalten auf dem IX. Kongreß der Europ. Vereinigung der Vet.-Anatomen in Toulouse.
HARTWIG, H., und J. SCHRUDDE (1974): Untersuchungen zur Bildung der primären Stirnauswüchse beim Reh. Z. Jagdwiss. **20**, 1—13.
HEINZE, W., und H. KANTOR (1972): Morphologisch-funktionelle Untersuchungen über das Blutgefäßsystem der Rinderklaue. Morph. Jb. **117**, 472—482, 1971/72 u. **118**, 139—159.
HERTSCH, B. (1973): Zur Arteriographie der Zehe des Pferdes. Berl. Münch. Tierärztl. Wschr. **86**, 461—465.
HOHMANN, H. (1901): Untersuchungen über die Klauenlederhaut des Rindes. Inaug.-Diss. med. vet. Bern.
HORSTMANN, E. (1955): Bau und Struktur des menschlichen Nagels. Z. Zellforsch. **41**, 532—555.
KAMEYA, T., S. YOSHIDA, K. KIRYU und S. YAMAOKA (1971): Morphological studies on the chestnut of the horse. Exp. Rep. equine Health Labor Tokyo **8**, 10—25.
KIND, H. (1961): Vergleichende Untersuchungen über die Abnutzung der Hufe einiger Equiden auf Grund der Struktur der Hufkapselwand. Diss. med. vet. Berlin.
KRÜGER, G. (1934): Über die Blutgefäßversorgung der Zehe und besonders des Zehenendorganes des Pferdes. Morph. Jb. **74**, 639—669.
LECHNER, W. (1934): Die Blutgefäßnetze in den Zehenenden einiger Paarzeher, ihre Beziehung zum Zehenendorgan und zu den analogen Gefäßen der Unpaarzeher und des Menschen. Z. f. ges. Anat. I. Abtlg. **102**, 594—622.
LOJDA, Z. (1950): Histogenesis of the antlers of our Cervidae and its histochemical picture. Čsl. Morfologie **IV**, 42—62.

Malinovský, L. (1966): Die Variabilität in den Nervenendigungen in den Fußballen einer Hauskatze. Acta nat. 64, 82—106.

Möricke, K. D. (1954/55): Das Verhalten des Hyponychiums beim normalen Nagelwachstum. Verhdlg. Anat. Ges. Münster, Erg. Heft z. Anat. Anz. Bd. 101, 289—293.

Müller, Fr. (1936): Der Pferdehuf im sagittalen Axialschnitt. Arch. wiss. prakt. Tierhlkd. 70, 296—301.

Nickel, R. (1938): Über den Bau der Hufröhrchen und seine Bedeutung für den Mechanismus des Pferdehufes. Morph. Jb. 82, 119—160.

— (1939): Untersuchungen über den Bau des Pferdehufes mit besonderer Berücksichtigung des Hufmechanismus und von Hufkrankheiten. Dtsch. Tierärztl. Wschr. 47, 521—524.

— (1949): Anordnung des Zwischenhornes an Trachte und Eckstrebe der Hufplatte. Dtsch. Tierärztl. Wschr. 56, 34—36.

Olt, A. (1921): Innersekretorischer Einfluß der Hoden auf die Entwicklung des Cervidengeweihes. Dtsch. Jägerztg. 76, 28/29.

Rhumbler, L. (1931): Ergänzende Mitteilungen über den Aderverlauf im Kolbengeweih der Hirsche an Hand einiger Diapositive. Zool. Anz. Suppl. — Bd. 5, 171—178.

Schälicke, H. (1932): Über die Verwertbarkeit von Ballenabdrücken für den Identitätsnachweis bei Hunden. Inaug.-Diss. med. vet. Berlin.

Schmidt, W. J., und H. Sprankel (1954): Bildet sich im Stratum corneum des Rinderhornes Röhrchenstruktur aus? Z. Morph. u. Ökol. Tiere 42, 449—470.

Schröder, H. D. (1961): Untersuchungen über die Struktur des Klauenhornes bei einigen exotischen Rinderrassen aus dem Tierpark Berlin unter besonderer Berücksichtigung der Abnutzungsverhältnisse. Diss. med. vet. Berlin.

Schumacher, S. v. (1936): Die sog. Ballen an den Pfoten des Hasen. Anat. Anz. 82, 102—112.

Schummer, A. (1949): Zirkulationsfördernde Einrichtungen am Zehenendorgan des Pferdes. Dtsch. Tierärztl. Wschr. 56, 36—38.

— (1951): Blutgefäße und Zirkulationsverhältnisse im Zehenendorgan des Pferdes. Morph. Jb. 91, 568—649.

Seiferle, E. (1927): Atavismus und Polydaktylie der hyperdaktylen Hinterpfoten des Haushundes. Morph. Jb. 57, 3.

— (1928): Wesen, Verbreitung und Vererbung hyperdaktyler Hinterpfoten beim Haushund. Schweiz. Arch. Tierheilkd. 70.

Siedamgrotzky, O. (1870): Die Krallen der Fleischfresser. Bericht Vet.-Wesen Könige. Sachsen 15, 135—150.

Smith, R. N. (1954): The Chestnuts and ergots of the horse. Association of Vet. Stud. Journal 14.

Wilkens, H. (1964): Zur makroskopischen und mikroskopischen Morphologie der Rinderklaue mit einem Vergleich der Architektur von Klauen- und Hufröhrchen. Zbl. Vet. Med., Reihe A, 11, 163—234.

Wintzer, H. J. (1971): Zur arteriellen Blutversorgung des Strahlbeines und der Gleichbeine beim Pferd. Zbl. Vet. Med., Reihe A, 18, 646 bis 652.

Wolf, J., and S. Hanšusová (1965): The transport of the nailplate. Fol. morph. Czech. Akad. Sci. Prague 14, 283—307.

Ziegler, H. (1954): Die Bildung des menschlichen Nagels und des Pferdehufes. Z. mikroskop.-anat. Forsch. 60, 556—572.

Zietzschmann, O. (1915): Beiträge zur Entwicklung von Hautorganen bei Säugetieren. I. Die Entwicklung der Hautschwielen (Kastanie u. Sporn) an den Gliedmaßen der Equiden. Arch. mikroskop. Anat. 86, 371—434.

— (1917): Betrachtungen zur vergleichenden Anatomie der Säugetierkralle. Morphol. Jb. 50, 433 bis 453.

— (1918): Das Zehenendorgan der rezenten Säugetiere: Kralle, Nagel, Huf. Schweiz. Arch. Tierheilkd. 6, 241—272.

— (1942): Horn und Geweih. Dtsch. Tierärztl. Wschr. 50, 55—57.

Zimmermann, A. (1913): Die Kastanien des Pferdes. Z. f. Tiermed. 17, 1—16.

Index

The letters preceding page numbers refer to the animals: C. = cat, Cn. = carnivore, D. = dog, G. = goat, H. = horse, O. = ox, P. = pig, R. = ruminant, S. = sheep. Entries of a general nature have no such letters.

Accessory claws P. 502; O. 530
Accessory teats 473; P. 499; O. 513; G. 521; H. 539
Adrenal vessels, arterial, possible sources 175
Adventitial cells 12
Albinism 457
Anal sac Cn. 467
Anisocytosis 4
Antlers 485
Antler velvet 487
Angulus partis inflexae H. 546
— venosus dexter 306
— — sinister 306
Anuli fibrosi arteriosi 20
— — arterioventriculares 20
Anulus fibrosus aortae 71
Aorta 16, 71
— abdominalis 72, 126
— —, visceral arteries 159
— ascendens 71
— descendens 71
— thoracica 72, 120
— —, visceral arteries 123
Apex cordis 16
— cunei H. 549
— pili 451
Apocrine tubular glands 445
Appendices colli 461
Apparatus suspensorius mammarum 472; O. 507
Arachnoid cell accumulations 275
Arcus aortae 71, 72
— dorsalis superficialis C. 86, 93; Cn. 95
— palmaris profundus 91, 92; Cn. 94; P. 95; R. 98; H. 99
— — superficialis 91, 92, 93; Cn. 94; P. 95; R. 98; H. 99
— plantaris profundus 92; Cn. 150; P. 150; R. 151; H. 154
— — distalis 93
— — superficialis 94
— terminalis 94, P. 502; R. 533; H. 580
— (venosus) dorsalis profundus 93; Cn. 251
— (—) — superficialis 93; C. 211; D. 254
— (—) hyoideus Cn., P. 222
— (—) — profundus Cn. 222
— (—) laryngeus caudalis 218

Arcus (venosus) palmaris profundus 93
Cn. 209; P. 211; R. 214; H. 214
— (—) — profundus distalis 93; P. 211; O. 214
— (—) — superficialis 93, 206; Cn. 210; P. 211
— (—) plantaris profundus 93, 244; Cn. 251; P. 254; R. 255; H. 256
— (—) — profundus distalis 93; P. 254; R. 255; H. 256
— (—) — superficialis 93; Cn. 251; P. 254
— (—) terminalis 94
Arteries 8, 71
Arteria, Arteriae
— abdominalis caudalis 135
— — cranialis 72; Cn., P. 130
— alveolaris mandibularis 111
— angularis oculi 108
— — oris 106
— antebrachialis superficialis cranialis 86
— arcuata D. 93, 150
— auricularis caudalis 108
— — profunda 109
— — rostralis 110
— axillaris 77
— basilaris 74
— bicipitalis 83; Cn. 85; R. 89
— brachialis 83
— — superficialis 83, 85
— broncho-oesophagea 72, 123
— buccalis 112
— bulbi penis 158
— — vestibuli 158
— caecales C. 170
— caecalis 170, 173
— — lateralis H. 173
— — medialis H. 173
— carotis communis 73, 99
— — — dextra 73, 99
— — — sinistra 73, 99
— — externa 102
— — interna 101
— caudales femoris 138
— caudalis dorsolateralis 159
— — femoris distalis 144
— — — media Cn. 144
— — — proximalis Cn. 144
— — lateralis (a. caudalis lateralis superficialis) 159

Arteria, *Continued*
— — mediana 159
— — ventralis Cn. 159
— — ventrolateralis 159
— centralis retinae 113
— cervicalis profunda 74
— — superficialis 74, 77
— ciliares anteriores 114
— — posteriores breves 113
— — — longae 113
— circumflexa femoris lateralis 142
— — — medialis 137
— — humeri caudalis 81, 82
— — — cranialis 81, 82
— — ilium profunda 72, 131
— — — superficialis Cn. 142
— — scapulae 80, 81, 82
— clitoridis 158
— — media H. 158
— coeliaca 72, 159, 160
— colica dextra 174
— — media 174
— — sinistra 174
— collateralis media 82
— — radialis 82; H. 83
— — ulnaris 83
— comitans n. ischiadici 157
— — n. tibialis (a. recurrens tibialis) 145
— condylaris 102
— conjunctivales anteriores 113; P. 115
— — posteriores 114
— cornualis R. 109
— coronalis 94; R. 533; H. 553
— coronariae 38
— coronaria dextra 71
— — — dorsalis 168
— — — ventralis 168
— — sinistra 71
— — — dorsalis 168
— — — ventralis 168
— costoabdominalis dorsalis 72, 121
— cremasterica 135
— cystica R. 162
— digitales dorsales communes Cn., P., R. 87, 93; Cn. 95, 150; P. 98; R. 98, 99, 154
— — — propriae 95; Cn. 95, 150; P. 98, 151; R. 99
— — palmares communes 93; Cn. 94; P. 95; R. 98; H. 99

Arteria, *Continued*
— — — propriae 93; Cn., P. 95; R. 98; H. 99
— — plantares communes 93; Cn. 150; P. 150; R. 151; H. 154
— — — propriae 93; Cn. 150; P. 151; R. 151; H. 154
— — propriae 93
— digitalis dorsalis I abaxialis C. 87, 93
— — — V abaxialis 93; Cn. 95, 150
— — — propria III axialis R. 151
— — — — IV axialis R. 151
— — palmaris I abaxialis 93; Cn. 94
— — — V abaxialis 93; Cn. 94
— — — lateralis H. 99
— — — medialis H. 99
— — plantaris lateralis H. 154
— — — medialis H. 154
— — — propria II abaxialis Cn. 150
— — — — V abaxialis 93
— — — — I axialis Cn. 150
— diverticuli P. 161
— dorsalis clitoridis 158
— — nasi 108; G. 109; Cn. 115
— — — rostralis D. 120
— — pedis 148
— — penis 158
— — phalangis mediae H. 553
— ductus deferentis 177
— epigastrica caudalis 135
— — — superficialis 137; D. 492; C. 493; O. 514
— — cranialis 77
— — — superficialis 77; D. 492; C. 493; P. 500; O. 514
— episclerales 114
— ethmoidalis externa 113
— facialis 103
— femoralis 140
— gastrica dextra 165
— — sinistra 161
— gastricae breves 161, 166, 168
— gastroduodenalis 165
— gastroepiploica dextra 166
— — sinistra 167
— genus descendens 144
— — distalis lateralis 145
— — — medialis 145
— — media 145
— — proximalis lateralis 145
— — — medialis 145; C. 148
— glutaea caudalis 157
— — cranialis 156
— hepatica 162
— — hepatic branches 162
— ilei 170
— ileocolica 170
— iliaca externa 72, 133
— — interna 72, 155
— — — visceral arteries 176
— iliacofemoralis 142, 157
— iliolumbalis 157
— infraorbitalis 115
— intercostales D. 491
— — dorsales 72, 120
— intercostalis suprema 73, 76
— interdigitales 94; Cn. 94, 150; P. 95; R. 99, 151

Arteria, *Continued*
— interosseae 83, 90
— — caudalis 90
— — communis 83, 90
— — cranialis 90
— — cruris P., O. 145
— — ischiadica 145, 156
— jejunales 170
— labialis mandibularis 106
— — maxillaris 107
— lacrimalis 115
— laryngea cranialis 101
— laterales nasi P. 120
— lateralis nasi 108; Cn. 120
— — — caudalis 108
— — — rostralis 108
— lienalis 161
— lingualis 103
— lumbales 72, 127
— malaris 115
— malleolaris caudalis lateralis H. 145
— — cranialis lateralis P., O. 148
— — — medialis P., O. 148
— mammaria caudalis H. 137, 539; O. 514; R. 137
— — cranialis H. 137, 539; O. 514; R. 137
— — media O. 514; R. 522
— marginis solearis R. 534; H. 554
— masseterica Cn., P., O. 111
— maxillaris 110
— mediana 83, 91
— meningea caudalis 102
— — media R. 102; 111
— — rostralis D., H. 120
— mentalis R., H. 111
— mesenterica caudalis 72, 174
— — cranialis 72, 168, 169
— — metacarpeae dorsales C. 92, 93; Cn. 95; P., R. 98; H. 99
— — palmares 92; Cn. 94; P. 95; R. 98; H. 99
— metatarseae dorsales 93; Cn. 150; P. 151; R. 151; H. 154
— — plantares 92; Cn. 150; P., R. 151; H. 154
— musculophrenica 76
— nervomedullaris 121
— nutriciae / a. interossea communis 90
— nutricia fibulae P. 148
— — humeri 82, 83
— — radii 90
— — scapulae 82
— — tibiae H. 145; P., R. 148
— — tibiae et fibulae Cn. 148
— — ulnae 90
— obturatoria 156
— occipitalis 102
— ophthalmica externa 113
— — interna 114
— ovarica 72, 176
— palatina ascendens 103
— — descendens 120
— — major 120
— — minor 120
— palmaris phalangis mediae H. 553
— palpebrae tertiae 115

Arteria, *Continued*
— palpebralis inferior lateralis Cn., R. 109; P., H. 115
— — — medialis 115
— — superior lateralis Cn., R. 109; P., H. 115
— — — medialis P. 115
— pancreaticoduodenalis caudalis 169
— — cranialis 165
— papillaris O. 514; R. 522
— parotidea Cn. 102
— penis 158
— — cranialis H. 137; 158
— — media H. 158
— pericardiacophrenica 76
— perinealis dorsalis Cn. 157; R. 183
— — ventralis 158
— phalangis distalis R. 533
— pharyngea ascendens 101
— phrenica caudalis 72, 129; P., R. 159
— — craniales 72, 122
— plantaris lateralis 144
— — medialis 144
— poplitea 145
— profunda antebrachii 91
— — brachii 83
— — clitoridis 158
— — femoris 135
— — linguae 103
— — penis 158
— — prostatica 177
— — pudenda externa 135; P. 500; O. 514; R. 522; H. 539
— — interna 158; O. 514
— — — visceral arteries of the – 176
— — —, short type P., R. 156, 158
— — —, long type Cn., H. 156, 158
— pulmonalis dextra 71
— — sinistra 71
— radiales superficiales 85
— radialis 92
— — proximalis H. 92
— rectalis caudalis 158; R. 183
— — cranialis 175
— — media 177, 183
— — recurrens interossea 90
— — tibialis cranialis 148
— — ulnaris 91
— renalis 72, 175
— reticularis 8
— — accessoria S., G. 162
— — ruminalis dextra 168
— — sinistra 168
— sacralis mediana 72, 159
— saphena 142
— scapularis dorsalis 74, 75
— sigmoideae 174
— sphenopalatina 115
— stylomastoidea P. 102; 108
— — profunda 102
— subclavia 72
— — sinistra 72
— sublingualis 103
— submentalis 103
— subscapularis 81

Index

Arteria, *Continued*
— supraorbitalis 115
— suprarenales craniales 159
— — mediae P. 72, 175
— suprarenalis media Cn. 72, 175
— suprascapularis 80
— supratrochlearis 115
— tarsea lateralis 148
— — medialis 148
— — perforans 148
— — — distalis 93; P. 148
— — — proximalis 93; P. 148
— temporales profundae 111
— temporalis profunda S., G. 111
— — — caudalis 111
— — — rostralis 111
— — superficialis 109
— testicularis 72, 176
— thoracica externa 79
— — interna 74, 76; D. 491; P. 500
— — lateralis Cn., P. 79; C. 493
— thoracodorsalis 81, 82
— thyreoidea caudalis 100
— — — dextra 74
— — cranialis 100
— tibialis caudalis 145
— — cranialis 148
— tori digitales R. 533; H. 552
— transversa cubiti 88
— — faciei 109
— tympanica caudalis D.102; H. 108
— — rostralis Cn., H. 111
— ulnaris 91
— umbilicalis 176
— urethralis 183
— uterina 177; Cn. 183
— vaginalis 183
— vertebralis 74
— — thoracica 74;76
— vesicalis caudalis 177, Cn. 183
— — cranialis 176
— — media Cn., P. 135
— vestibularis O. 183
Arteries, forefoot 92; Cn. 94; P. 95; R. 98; H. 99
—, —, dorsal 93; Cn. 95; P., R. 98; H. 99
—, —, palmar 92; Cn. 94; P. 95; R. 98; H. 99
—, head 99
—, heart 17, 24, 38; Cn. 46; P. 52; O. 58; H. 64
—, hindfoot 92; Cn. 148; P. 150; R. 151; H. 154
—, —, dorsal 93; Cn. 150; P. 151; R. 151; H. 154
—, —, plantar 93; Cn. 148; P. 150; R. 151; H. 154
—, neck 99
—, pectoral limb 77
—, pelvic 155
—, pelvic limb 137
—, precapillary 7, 8, 11
—, pulmonary circulation 71
—, tail 155
Arterial structure 8, 9
Arterioles 7, 8
Arterio-venous anastomoses 12
Artiodactyla 479
Atrioventricular node 35

Atrioventricular valve, left 33
—, right 30
Atrium dextrum 25
— left 26
— right 25
— sinistrum 26
Auricula cordis s. atrii 16, 24
Awns 452; H. 537
Azygos veins, segmental vessels of 187

Bars 479; H. 546
Basis cordis 16
— cunei H. 549
B-cells 275
Bearing surface of the hoof H. 546, 550
Blood 1
— cells 2
— —, development 6
— —, number 5
— coagulation 2
— flow regulating mechanism 8
— formation 6
— lymph nodes 278
— vascular system 1
Blood vessels
— —, acropodium 93
— —, autopodium 92
— —, cardiac 38, Cn. 46; P. 52; O. 54; H. 64
— —, —, structure of 40
— —, chemoreceptors 15
— —, function of 7
— —, general considerations 7
— —, metapodium, deep 92
— — —, superficial 93
— —, nutrition of 13
— —, pressoreceptors 15
— —, structure of 7
— —, vasoconstrictors 14
— —, vasodilators 14
— —, vasomotor 14
Blood vessel wall, nutrition 13
Blood-thymus barrier 285
Blood-tissue barrier 12
B-lymphocytes 275
Bone marrow, red 6
— —, yellow 6
Bridge anastomosis 12
Bristles 454
Bulb and frog segment 481
Bulbar corium P. 500; O. 522; R. 533; H. 546
— cushion P. 500; O. 525; H. 542
— epidermis 477; H. 456
— fossa H. 548
— horn P. 501; O. 530; R. 532; H. 546
— rudiment 477
— segment O. 524
Bulbus aortae 32, 71
— pili 444, 451
Bursa mucosa subcutanea 445
By-pass vessels 12

Calcar H. 552
Callosities D. 487
Canities 457
Capilli 452

Capillaries 11
—, adventitial cells 11
—, basal membrane 11, 12
—, endothelium 11
—, pericytes 11
—, sinusoids 11
Carpal pads Cn. 495
Cartilago cordis 21
Cavicornia 484
Cavum pericardii 15, 16
Cerumen 464
Ceruminous glands 464
Chemoreceptors 15
Chestnut 448; H. 477, 550
Chiasma anuli fibrosi arteriosi 20, 36
Chordae tendineae 30, 33
Chyle 292
Cilia 454; D. 489
Circulus arteriosus cerebri 111
— venosus mammae O. 518
— — papillae O. 518; R. 548
Circumanal glands 468
Cirrus capitis H. 454
— caudae H. 454
— metacarpeus H. 454, 552
— metatarseus H. 454, 552
Cisterna chyli 294, 295, 330; D. 353; C. 364; P. 382; O. 404; S. 419; G. 419; H. 438
Claw, claws 479; Cn. 481, 493; C. 495
— bed (matrix) Cn. 493
— cone Cn. 481; D. 493
— corium 481
— —, dorsal cushion of Cn. 493
— cushion D. 493
— die Cn. 493
— epidermis 481
— fold Cn. 481; D. 493, 494; O. 525
— mould Cn. 493
— plate Cn. 493
— sole D. 494
— vallum Cn. 494
Cloven hoofed species 479
Colostrum 473
Communication, organ of 461
Conducting vessels 295, 301
Connective layer H. 548
Conus arteriosus 16, 27, 71
Cor, see heart 15
Cords, tendinous 30, 33
Corium 446, 480; D. 487; P. 496; O. 525; H. 543
— coronae O. 526; H. 543
— cunei H. 545
— lamellae 479; S. 533; H. 544
— limbi O. 525; H. 543
— parietis Cn. 481; O. 527; H. 544
— soleae O. 527; H. 545
— tori O. 527; H. 545
— ungulae 525; H. 543
Cornu R. 483
Coronary corium P. 501; O. 526; H. 543
— cushion O. 526; H. 542
— epidermis P. 502; O. 529
— groove H. 546
— groove (heart) 16
— horn O. 529; H. 542, 546
— rim H. 546
— segment 481; O. 524

Corona ungulae H. 541
Corpuscula thymi 284
Corpus mammae O. 506
Cortex pili 451
Corticosteroids 474
Covering layer, glaze H. 546
Crista terminalis 25
— unguicularis 493
Crura cunei H. 549
Crux pilorum 456
Cuneus ungulae H. 541, 549
Curls, formation of 457; S. 506
Cuspes valvae atrioventricularis dextrae 30
— — — sinistrae 33
Cutaneous scent glands 458
Cuticle cell pattern 451
Cuticula pili 451
Cutis 441; H. 537
Cytocrine secretion 449
Cytopempsis 12, 13

Daktyloscopy 450
Dendritic cells 449
Dermis 481
Desmosomes 448
Dewlap 461; D. 487; O. 504
Die 480, 481
Digital cushion 479; H. 542
Digital organ 448, 476, 478; Cn. 493; P. 500; O. 524; R. 532; H. 541
— —, division into layers 479
— —, division into segments 481
— —, ontogenesis 476
Digital pads 477
Diverticulum prepuciale P. 468
Drainage area 307
„Drosselarterien" 9
Ductus arteriosus (Botalli) 26, 71
— lymphaticus dexter 295, 306, 314; D. 354; P. 383; O. 404; H. 440
— thoracicus 294, 295, 306; D. 352; C. 364; P. 382; O. 403; S. 419; G. 419; H. 438
— venosus (Arantii) Cn., R. 261
Ductus thoracicus 322
Dwarf sebaceous glands 458; P. 497

Ecdysis 443
Eelmark 457
Eleidin 448
Endocardium 20
Endothelium 8, 11
Epicardium 16, 19
Epiceras 485
Epidermal organ complex 448
Epidermis 448, 479; D. 487; C. 489; P. 517; H. 537
— coronae O. 529
— cunei H. 530
— limbi O. 529
— parietis O. 530
— soleae O. 530; H. 542
— tori O. 530
— ungulae O. 524, 527; H. 542, 546
Eponychium 476; O. 531
Ergot 448, 477; H. 550
Erythroblasts 6
Erythropoiesis 6

Erythrocytes 2, 6
Excitation and conducting system 34
Expulsion route 27, 32
Extravascular circulation 296

Facies atrialis 16
— auricularis 16
Fascia endothoracica 16
Fat 445
Fat marrow 6
Feathers 454, 552
Feral pattern 457; H. 537
Fibrin 2
Fibrinogen 2
Filum tendineum intermedium 20
Finger tip 482
Fleece 452; S. 506
Fleshy udder O. 512
Flumina pilorum 455
Follicles, secondary 276
Folliculi lymphatici aggregati 277
— — solitarii 276
Folliculus pili 451
Foramen ovale 26
— venae cavae caudalis 233
Foramina venarum minimarum 26
Forelock 454
Frizzy hair D. 488
Frog 479; H. 549
—, apex of H. 549
—, corium H. 545
—, cushion H. 542
—, epidermis H. 549
—, groove H. 549
—, horn H. 549
—, limb H. 549
Fürstenberg's venous ring O. 511, 518

Ganglion sinuatriale 35
Germinative matrix P. 501; O. 526
Giant capillaries 11
Glandula, glandulae
— caudae C. 466
— ceruminosae 464
— circumanales 468
— circumorales C. 463
— cornualis G. 463
— cutis 458
— glomiformes 458
— interdigitales 465
— odoriferae 459
— praepuciales 468
— sebaceae 458
— sinus paranalis 467
— subcaudalis G. 467
— sudoriferae 458
Glandular udder O. 512
Glomus anastomoses 13
Glomus organs 13
Goose skin 452
Granulocytes 4, 7
—, basophil 4
—, eosinophil 4
—, neutrophil 4
—, polymorphonuclear 7
Growth hormone 474
Guard Hair D. 488

Haemal nodes 280
— —, lymphoid 280
— —, splenoid 280
Haemocytoblasts 6, 7
Haemoglobin 3
Haemolysis 3
Hair, hairs 444, 450; D. 488; C. 490; P. 497; O. 504; G. 505; S. 506; H. 537
— anlage 444
—, arrangement of 454
— bulb 444, 451
— bundle 454
— canal 444
— colour 456; C. 490; O. 504; H. 537
— comb 456
— cortex 451
— cross 456; O. 504
— curl 457
— cuticle 444, 451
— disc 452
— follicle 444, 451
— funnel 451
— medula 451
— outer 452
— papilla 444, 451
— peg 444
— primordium 444
— replacement 457
— ridges 456
— root 451
— shaft 450
— spiral 456
— star 455
— stream 455
— tract 455
— types 452
— vortex 455, 456; D. 488; C. 490; P. 497; O. 504; G. 505; S. 506; H. 538
— wool 452
Hassal's corpuscles 284
Head's zones 461
Heart 15; Cn. 42; P. 49; O. 54; S. 58; G. 58; H. 62
—, anuli fibrosi 20
—, apex 17
—, arteries 38; Cn. 46; P. 52; O. 58; H. 64
—, atrium dextrum et sinistrum 16, 23
—, auricula atrii 16
—, base 16
—, blood vessels 38; Cn. 46; P. 52; R. 58; H. 64
—, bone of 21
—, cartilage of 21
—, chambers 23
—, chordae tendineae 30, 33
—, conformation 16
—, conus arteriosus 17, 27
—, coronary groove 16
—, crista terminalis 25
—, endocardium 20
—, epicardium 19
—, excitation and conducting system 34
—, expulsion route 27
—, facies auricularis 16

Heart, *Continued*
—, — atrialis 16
—, fasciculus atrioventricularis 34
—, foramen ovale 26
—, foramina venarum minimarum 26
—, ganglion sinuatriale 35
—, inflow route 27
—, innervation 37
—, limbus fossae ovalis 26
—, lymph vessels 41
—, margo ventricularis dexter 16
—, — — sinister 16
—, musculature 21
—, mm. papillares 22, 30
—, — pectinati 22, 26
—, myocardium 19
—, nerves 37
—, nodus atrioventricularis 35
—, — sinuatrialis 34
—, os cordis 21
—, ostia venarum pulmonalium 28
—, ostium aortae 33
—, — atrioventriculare dextrum 23, 27
—, — — sinistrum 32
—, venae cavae caudalis 25
—, — — — cranialis 25
—, pars membranacea septi 21
—, position 17; D. 44; P. 51; O. 57; H. 63
—, "powerhouse" of 23
—, septum interatriale 23
—, — interventriculare 27, 32
—, sinus coronarius 25
—, — venarum cavarum 19, 25
—, size, weight measurements 41; D. 43; C. 45; P. 49; O. 57; H. 63
—, skeleton 20
—, species characteristics 41; D. 68; P. 69; R. 69; 0. 70; H. 70
—, sulcus coronarius 16, 23
—, — interventricularis paraconalis 17
—, — — subsinuosus 17
—, — terminalis 25
—, trabecula septomarginalis 30, 33
—, trabeculae carneae 22
—, tuberculum intervenosum 26
—, valva aortae 33
—, — atrioventricularis dext. 30
—, — — sin. 33
—, — trunci pulmonalis 31
—, veins 40; Cn. 48; P. 53; O. 62; H. 65
—, ventricle, right 27
—, —, left 32
—, ventriculus cordis dexter 27
—, — — sinister 32
—, vortex 22

Heels of the hoof H. 546
Horn, horns 448; R. 476; 483
Horn bulb 532
Horn capsule P. 501; R. 532; H. 542
Horn development 476
Horn glands G. 463, 505
Horn grooves O. 485
Horn lamellae H. 548
Horn plate 481; H. 541, 548

Horn process 483
Horn production 485
Horn rings 485
Horn sheath, epidermal 484
Horn tubules H. 548
Horny sole Cn. 481; O. 530; R. 532; H. 542
Hoof 479, H. 541
— bulb H. 542
— capsule H. 542
— corium 481; H. 542, 543
— coronet H. 542
— frog H. 542
— periople H. 541
— plate H. 546
— sole H. 542, 548
— subcutis H. 542
— tubules H. 542, 548
— wall H. 542, 546
Horse hair 454
Hyperkeratosis 449
Hypodermis 445
Hypomastia 473
Hyponychium 476, 482; R. 532

Immune system 270
— —, classification of organs 275
Immunity 270
—, active 272
—, adaptive 272
—, adoptive 272
—, passive 272
Immunocompetent cells 272
Immunocytes 274
Immunoglobulin 473
Incisura apicis 16
Inflow route 27, 32
Infraorbital organ 463
Inguinal sinus S. 468
Injection, intravenous 215
Innervation, blood vessels 14
Innervation, heart 37
Integumentum commune 441
Interdigital gland 465
Intermediate horn H. 542
Intima 7, 10
Intimal swellings 10

Juba 454

Keratinocytes 449
Keratohyalin granules 448

Lactopoiesis 474
Lamellar horn H. 548
Lamellae coriales 543
— epidermales H. 548
Lamina subendothelialis 8
Langerhans cells 449
Leading hairs 452
Lectulus parietalis Cn. 481
— solearis Cn. 481
Leucocytes 4
Leucodermia D. 488
Lien 281
Ligamentum arteriosum 71
— phrenicopericardiacum 16
— sternopericardiacum 16
— suspensorium uberis 472; O. 507

Limbus fossae ovalis 26
— ungulae H. 541
Linea pilorum 456
Liquor pericardii 16
Littoral cells 272, 278
Lunula 482
Lymphangion 301
Lymphatic organs 269
— —, fixed cells 272
— —, free cells 273
— —, peripheral organs 275
— —, phylogenesis 269
— system 269
— —, discovery of 300
— tissue 275
— — diffuse 275
Lymph capillaries 295, 297, 298
— —, fine structure 296
— nodes (s. nodi lymphatici) 278
— —, ontogenesis 294
Lymph collecting ducts 305; D. 352; C. 364; P. 382; O. 403; S. 419; G. 419; H. 438
Lymph, formation of 298
Lymph hearts 293
Lymph nodes, regional 307
Lymphocentrum 308
Lymphocentrum axillare 314, 318; D. 342; C. 356; P. 370; O. 388; S. 408; G. 408; H. 424
— bronchale 321; D. 345; C. 359; P. 372; O. 391; S. 411; G. 411; H. 428
— cervicale profundum 313, 315; D. 342; C. 356; P. 369; O. 387; S. 407; G. 407; H. 423
— — superficiale 312, 315; D. 341; C. 355; P. 368; O. 386; S. 407; G. 407; H. 422
— coeliacum 325; D. 346; C. 360; P. 374; O. 393; S. 412; G. 412; H. 430
— iliofemorale 333; D. 350; C. 363; P. 379; O. 400; S. 417; G. 417; H. 436
— iliosacrale 331; D. 350; C. 362; P. 377; O. 399; S. 415; G. 415; H. 435
— inguinale profundum 333; D. 350; C. 363; P. 379; O. 400; S. 417; G. 417; H. 436
— — superficiale 333; D. 351; C. 363; P. 380; O. 401; S. 417; G. 417; H. 436
— inguinofemorale 333; D. 351; C. 363; P. 380; O. 401; S. 417; G. 417; H. 436
— ischiadicum 335; C. 363; P. 380; O. 402; S. 417; G. 417; H. 437
— lumbale 323; D. 346; C. 360; P. 373; O. 393; S. 412; G. 412; H. 429
— mandibulare 309; D. 337; C. 354; P. 365; O. 383; S. 405; G. 405; H. 420
— mediastinale 320; D. 344; C. 359; P. 372; O. 390; S. 410; G. 410; H. 427

Index

Lymphocentrum, *Continued*
— mesenterericum caudale 330; D. 358; C. 362; P. 377; O. 398; S. 415; G. 415; H. 433
— — craniale 328; D. 348; C. 361; P. 375; O. 397; S. 415; G. 415; H. 432
— parotideum 308; D. 337; C. 354; P. 364; O. 383; S. 405; G. 405; H. 420
— popliteum 335; D. 352; C. 364; P. 381; O. 403; S. 419; G. 419; H. 438
— retropharyngeum 310; D. 340; C. 355; P. 366; O. 384; S. 406; G. 406; H. 422
— thoracicum dorsale 317; D. 344; C. 357; P. 370; O. 389; S. 410; G. 410; H. 425
— — ventrale 319; D. 344; C. 358; P. 372; O. 390; S. 410; G. 410; H. 426
Lymphoblasts 276
Lymphocytes 5, 7, 273, 275
Lymphonodi s. nodi lymphatici 278
Lymphonodi haemales 280
Lymphovenous anastomoses 305
Lymph vessels 292, 301
— —, afferent vessels 301, 307
— —, central nervous system 305
— —, circulatory and defense system 305
— —, digestive system 304
— —, efferent vessels 301, 307
— —, endocrine system 305
— —, heart 41
— —, locomotor system 303
— —, ontogenesis 293
— —, phylogenesis 293
— —, respiratory system 304
— —, serous membranes 304
— —, skin 305
— —, structure and function 294
— —, urogenital system 304

Macroblasts 6
Macrophages 274
Mamma, mammary complex 469, 470; D. 491; P. 498; O. 506; G. 521; H. 539
Mammary bud 469
Mammary gland, mammary glands 469; D. 491; C. 493; P. 498; O. 506; G. 520; S. 521; H. 538
— —, ductus lactiferi 471; O. 511; G. 520
— —, — papillaris 421; D. 491
— —, lactiferous sinus O. 510
— —, — duct 471; O. 511; G. 520
— —, ontogenesis 469
— —, parenchyma P. 498
— —, sinus lactiferus O. 510
— —, tubular terminal part P. 498
Mammogenesis 474
Mane 454
Margo coronalis H. 546
— ventricularis dexter 16
— — sinister 16
Marking glands 462

Markings H. 537
Matrix pili 451
Meconium 473
Mediastinum 15
Mediator cells 274, 275
Medulla ossium flava 6
— — rubra 6
— pili 451
Megakaryoblasts 7
Melanin 442
Melanocytes 449
Mental organ P. 464
Metatarsal glands 465
Micropinocytosis 12
Milk ducts 471; P. 499; O. 511; S. 522
Milk ridge 469
Milk secretion 474
Milk spots 275
Milk vein 240; O. 519
Milk well 195; O. 519
Moderator band 33
Monoblasts 7
Monocytes 5, 7
Mould 480, 481
Moustache 454; H. 538
Musculi arrectores pilorum 444, 452; D. 487
— papillares 30, 33
— pectinati 26
Musculus papillaris magnus 30
— — subarteriosus 30
— — subatrialis 33
— — subauricularis 33
Myeloblasts 7
Myelocytes 7
Myocardium 19

Nervus, nervi
— cardiaci 37
— genitofemoralis D. 492; R. 493; O. 519
— iliohypogastricus O. 519
— ilioinguinalis O. 519
— intercostales D. 492; C. 493
— pudendus O. 519
Network, venous, at the dorsum of the penis 259
—, —, subcutaneous H. 557
Nodi haemales 280
Nodi lymphatici, nodus lymphaticus 378, 307
— abomasiales dorsales 325; O. 395; S. 414; G. 414
— — ventrales 325; O. 396; S. 414; G. 414
— anorectales 331; P. 377; O. 400; S. 416; G. 416; H. 435
— atriales 325; O. 393; S. 413; G. 413
— axillares accessorii 316; D. 342; C. 357; S. 410; H. 424
— — primae costae 316; C. 357; P. 370; O. 389; S. 409; G. 409; H. 424
— — proprii 314; D. 342; C. 356; O. 388; S. 408; G. 408; H. 424
— bifurcationis dextri 321; D. 345; C. 359; P. 372; O. 391; G. 412; H. 428

Nodi, *Continued*
— — medii 321; D. 345; C. 359; P. 372; O. 392
— — sinistri 321; D. 345; C. 359; P. 372; O. 391; S. 411; G. 411; H. 428
— caecales 329; C. 362; O. 398; S. 415; H. 433
— cervicales profundi caudales 313; D. 342; C. 356; P. 370; O. 387; S. 408; G. 408; H. 424
— — craniales 313; D. 342; P. 369; O. 387; S. 407; G. 407; H. 423
— — medii 313; D. 342; C. 356; P. 370; O. 387; S. 407; G. 407; H. 424
— — superficiales 312; D. 341; O. 386; S. 407; G. 407; H. 422
— — — accessorii 312; O. 386; S. 407
— — — dorsales 312; C. 355; P. 368
— — — medii 312; P. 369
— — — ventrales 312; C. 355, 369
— coeliaci 325; P. 374; H. 430
— — et mesenterici craniales 325; O. 393; S. 412; G. 412
— colici 329; D. 349; C. 362; P. 376; O. 398; S. 415; G. 415; H. 433
— costocervicalis 314; O. 388; S. 408; G. 408
— coxalis 334; O. 401; S. 417; H. 437
— — accessorius 334; O. 401
— cubitales 316; S. 410; H. 424
— epigastricus 333; O. 400
— — caudalis 333; C. 363
— — cranialis 319; C. 358
— femorales 333; D. 351; C. 363
— fossae paralumbalis 334; O. 402
— gastrici 325; D. 347; C. 360; P. 374; H. 430
— glutaeus 335; P. 380; O. 403
— hepatici 325; D. 347; C. 360; P. 375; O. 396; S. 414; G. 414; H. 431
— — accessorii 325; O. 396
— hyoideus caudalis 310; O. 385
— — rostralis 310; O. 385
— iliaci laterales 331; P. 377; O. 399; S. 416; G. 416; H. 435
— — mediales 331; D. 350; C. 362; P. 377; O. 399; S. 415; G. 415; H. 435
— iliocolici 329; P. 376; G. 415
— — iliofemorales 333; D. 350; C. 363; P. 379; O. 400; S. 417
— infraspinatus 316; O. 389
— inguinalis profundi 333; G. 417; H. 436
— — superficialis 333; D. 351; C. 363; P. 380; O. 401; S. 417; G. 417; H. 436
— intercostales 319; D. 344; C. 358; O. 389; S. 410; G. 410; H. 425
— ischiadici 335; C. 363; P. 380; O. 402; S. 417; G. 417; H. 437
—jejunales 329; D. 348; C. 361; P. 376; O. 397; S. 415; G. 415; H. 432

Nodi, *Continued*
— lienales 325; D. 346; C. 360; P. 374; H. 430
— — seu atriales 325; O. 393; S. 413; G. 413
— — seu atriales 325; O. 393; S. 413; G. 413
— lumbales aortici 324; D. 346; C. 360; P. 373; O. 393; S. 412; G. 412; H. 429
— — proprii 324; O. 393
— mammarii 333; D. 351; C. 363; P. 380; O. 401; S. 417; G. 417; H. 436
— mandibulares 309; D. 337; C. 354; P. 365; O. 383; S. 405; G. 405; H. 420
— — accessorii 309; C. 354; P. 366
— mediastinales caudales 320; P. 372; O. 391; S. 411; G. 411; H. 428
— — craniales 320; D. 344; C. 359; P. 372; O. 390; S. 410; G. 410; H. 427
— — medii 320; O. 391; S. 411; G. 411; H. 428
— mesenterici caudales 330; D. 358; C. 362; P. 377; O. 398; S. 415; G. 415; H. 433
— — craniales 328; P. 375; H. 432
— nuchalis 320; H. 428
— obturatorius 333; H. 436
— omasiales 325; O. 395; S. 414; G. 414
— omentales 325; H. 431
— ovarici 324; H. 429
— pancreaticoduodenales 325; D. 347; C. 360; P. 375; O. 397; S. 414; G. 414; H. 431
— parotidei 308; D. 337; C. 354; P. 364; O. 383; S. 405; G. 405; H 420
— phrenicoabdominalis 324; P. 373
— phrenicus 320; C. 359; O. 391
— poplitei profundi 335; P. 381; O. 403; S. 419; G. 419; H. 438
— — superficiales 335; D. 352; C. 364; P. 391
— portales 325; D. 347; C. 360; P. 375; O. 396; S. 414; G. 414; H.431
— pterygoideus 309; O. 383
— pulmonales 321; D. 346; C. 359; O. 392; G. 412; H. 428
— renales 324; P. 373; O. 393; S. 412; G. 412; H. 429
— reticulares 325; O. 395; S. 414; G. 414
— reticuloabomasiales 325; O. 395; S. 414; G. 414
— retropharyngei laterales 310; D. 341; C. 355; P. 368; O. 384; S. 406; H. 422
— — mediales 310; D. 340; C. 355; P. 366; O. 384; S. 406; G. 406; H. 422
— ruminales craniales 325
— — dextri 325; O. 394; S. 413; G. 413

Nodi, *Continued*
— — sinistri 325; O. 394; S. 414; G. 414
— ruminoabomasiales 325; O. 395; S. 414
— sacrales 331; D. 350; C. 362; P. 377; O. 399; S. 416; G. 416; H. 435
— scrotales 333; D. 351; C. 363; P. 380; O. 401; S. 417;. G. 417; H. 436
— sternales caudales 319; C. 358; O. 390; S. 410; H. 426
— — craniales 319; D. 344; C. 358; P. 372; O. 390; S. 410; G. 410; H. 426
— subiliaci 334; C. 363; P. 380; O. 401; S. 417; G. 417; H. 436
— subrhomboideus 314; O. 388
— testicularis 324; P. 373
— thoracici aortici 319; C. 357; P. 370; O. 389; S. 410; G. 410; H 425
— tracheobronchales craniales 321; P. 373; O. 392; S. 412; G. 412
— — dextri 321; D. 345; C. 359; P. 372; O. 391; G. 412; H. 428
— — medii 321; D. 345; C. 359; P. 372; O. 392
— — sinistri 321; D. 345; C. 359; P. 372; O. 391; S. 411; G. 411; H. 428
— tuberalis 335; O. 403; S. 418; G. 418
— uterini 333; P. 378; H. 435
— vesicalis 330; H. 434
Nodulus valvulae semilunaris 31
Nodus atrioventricularis 34, 35
— sinuatrialis 34
Normoblasts 7
Nail 482
Nail fold 482
— plate 482
Nail, sole of 482
Nasolabial plate O. 461
Nasolabiogram 450
Nutrition of the blood vessel wall 13

Oestrogens 474
Organs of blood formation 6
— of circulation 1
Organs of touch 460
Organum carpale P. 464
— caudae 466
— digitale 478; Cn. 493
— mentale P. 464
— metatarsale 465
— tactus 460
Os cordis 21
— unguiculare Cn. 493
Ostia papillaria 470; D. 491; C. 493; P. 499; O. 510; G. 520; H. 539
Ostium aortae 33
— atrioventriculare dextrum 27, 30
— — sinistrum 23, 32
— trunci pulmonalis 71
— venae cavae caudalis 25
— — — cranialis 25
— venarum pulmonarum 26
Outer hair 452; H. 537

Pads 476, 477; C. 495
Palear 461
Panniculus adiposus 445; P. 496
Papillae coriales H. 543
Papilla mammae 470; P. 499; O. 506
— pili 451
Papillary muscles 30
Paries corneus Cn. 481; H. 546
— ungulae H. 541
Pars membranacea septi interventricularis 21
— transversa / r. sinister / v. portae 261
— umbilicalis / r. sinister / v. portae 261
Penna pilorum 456
Pericardium 15
—, cavum 15
—, fibrosum 16
—, lamina parietalis 16
—, — visceralis 16
—, liquor 16
—, pleura 16
—, serosum 16
—, sinus obliquus 16
—, — transversus 16
—, vaginae serosae arteriorum et venarum 16
Pericytes 12
Perioplic corium P. 500; O. 525; R. 533; H. 543
— cushion O. 525; H. 542
— epidermis P. 502; O. 529
— horn O. 529; R. 533; H. 542; 546
— segment 481; P. 502; O. 524
Perioral glands C. 463
Peyer's patches 277
Pheromones 462
Pili lanei 452
— tactiles 454
Pilus 444
Planum nasale 461
— nasolabiale O. 461
— rostrale P. 461
Plasma cells 7, 274
Plate bed Cn. 481
Plate, nasolabial 461
Pleura pericardiaca 16
Plexus pampiniformis 266
— venae profundae faciei O. 225
— (venosus) ophthalmicus Cn. 229; 232
— (—) palatinus 224, 229
— (—) pharyngeus 224
— (—) pterygoideus 227
— (—) vertebralis externus dorsalis 187
— (—) — — ventralis 187
— (—) — internus vertralis 187
Plicae cutis 461
Plica vena cavae 233
Polymastia 473
Polythelia 473
Portal vein 260
Pregnancy grooves R. 485
Preorbital gland S. 463
Prepucial diverticulum P. 468
— glands 468
Primary follicle 275
— lymph 307
— stage 307

Processus cornualis 483
Proerythroblasts 6
Progesterone 474
Prolactin 474
Promyelocytes 7
Protective layer H. 546
Pulvinus 477
Purkinje fibres 36

Radix pili 451
Ramus rami
— acetabularis / a. circumflexa femoris medialis 139
— — / v. circumflexa femoris medialis 139
— acromialis P. 77; O. 80; 80, 198; Cn., P. 216
— ad rete mirabile epidurale rostrale / a. meningea media P. 112
— — — — / a. meningea rostralis P. 115
— anastomoticus / aa. metacarpeae dorsales H. 99
— — / v. temporalis superficialis Cn. 232
— cum a. carotide interna / a. meningea media Cn. 112
— — — — — / a ophthalmica externa D. 113
— — cum a. meningea media / a. ophthalmica externa D. 113
— — cum a. occipitali / a. vertebralis 74
— — cum a. ophthalmica interna / a. ophthalmica externa 113
— — cum plexu ophthalmico / vv. temporales profundae H. 229
— — — — / v. temporalis superficialis Cn. 232
— — cum v. ophthalmica externa dorsali / v. angularis oculi 225
— — — — — ventralis / v. profunda faciei Cn. 225
— — cum v. saphena mediali / r. caudalis / v. saphena lateralis 248
— — — — — — / r. cranialis / v. saphena lateralis 248
— — cum v. temporali superficiali / v. profunda faciei Cn. 225
— angularis oculi / a. malaris O. 115
— ascendens / a. cervicalis superficialis 77
— — / a. circumflexa femoris lateralis 142
— — / a. circumflexa femoris medialis 139
— — / v. circumflexa femoris lateralis 238, 241
— — / a. iliacofemoralis 157
— — / v. cervicalis superficialis 215
— — / v. circumflexa femoris medialis 241
— articularis temporomandibularis / a. maxillaris Cn. 111
— — — / aa. temporales profundae S., G. 111
— — — / a. temporalis superficialis 109

Ramus, *Continued*
— — — / a. transversa faciei P., O. 109
— auricularis / v. cervicalis superficialis P. 216, 231
— — intermedius / a. auricularis caudalis 109
— — — lateralis / a. auricularis caudalis O. 109
— — — medialis / a. auricularis caudalis O. 109
— — lateralis / a. auricularis caudalis 108
— — medialis / a. auricularis caudalis 109
— — — / a. auricularis rostralis O. 110
— bronchalis / a. broncho-oesophagea 72, 123, 126
— canalis vertebralis / aa. intercostales dorsales 121
— carpeus dorsalis / a. collateralis ulnaris 84
— — — / a. interossea cranialis 90
— — — / a. radialis 92
— — — / a. ulnaris 91
— — — / v. interossea cranialis 206
— — — / v. radialis 209
— — — / v. radialis proximalis H. 209
— carpei dorsales / v. ulnaris 207
— carpeus palmaris / a. collateralis ulnaris 84
— — — / a. interossea caudalis 90
— — — / a. radialis 92
— — — / a. ulnaris 91
— — — / v. interossea caudalis 206
— — — / v. radialis 209
— — — / v. radialis proximalis H. 209
— caudales / v. caudalis mediana 260
— — s. coccygei 159
— caudalis / a. circumflexa ilium profunda 131
— — / a. saphena 142
— — / v. circumflexa ilium profunda 236
— — / v. saphena lateralis 248
— — / v. saphena medialis (magna) 244
— — ad rete mirabile epidurale rostrale R. 113
— colici 179; R. 170
— collaterales / aa. intercostales dorsales 121
— collateralis / a. mesenterica cranialis 169
— — / v. mesenterica cranialis O. 261
— — / v. ruminalis dextra 261
— cranialis / a. circumflexa ilium profunda 131
— — / a. saphena Cn., H. 142
— — / v. saphena lateralis 248
— — / v. saphena medialis (magna) 243
— cricothyreoideus / a. thyreoidea cranialis 100

Ramus, *Continued*
— cutaneri laterales / aa. intercostales dorsales 121
— cutaneus medialis / r. dorsalis / aa. intercostales dorsales 121
— deltoideus / a. axillaris 78
— — / a. cervicalis superficialis 77
— dentales / a. alveolaris mandibularis 111
— — / a. infraorbitalis 115
— — / v. infraorbitalis 225
— descendens / a. circumflexa femoris lateralis 142
— — / a. vertebralis 74
— — / v. circumflexa femoris lateralis 249
— dexter / a. hepatica 162
— — / v. portae 261
— lateralis / a. hepatica 162
— medialis / a. hepatica 162
— dorsales / a. vertebralis 74
— linguae 103
— dorsalis / aa. intercostales dorsales 121
— — / aa. lumbales 127
— — / a. ulnaris 91
— — / r. carpeus dorsalis / a. collateralis ulnaris R., H. 84
— — / v. collateralis ulnaris 203
— — / v. costoabdominalis dorsalis 187
— — / vv. intercostales dorsales 187
— — / vv. lumbales 236
— — / v. ulnaris C. 207
— phalangis distalis 94; H. 99, 156
— — — mediae 94; H. 99, 156
— — — proximalis 94; H. 99, 156; P. 151
— ductus deferentis 177
— — / a. testicularis 176
— — / v. testicularis 266
— — / a. umbilicalis 176
— — / v. prostatica H. 266
— duodenales / a. pancreaticoduodenalis cranialis 166
— (venosus) dorsalis phalangis distalis 94; H. 215, 256
— (—) — — mediae 94; H. 215, 256
— (—) — — proximalis 94; H. 215, 256; R. 255
— epididymales / a. testicularis 176
— — / v. testicularis 266
— epiploici / a. gastroepiploica dextra 166
— — / a. gastroepiploica sinistra 167
— — / a. lienalis 161
— epiploicus / a. ruminalis dextra 168
— — / v. lienalis R. 261
— frontalis / a. malaris P. 115
— gastrici / a. gastrica dextra R. 165
— gastrolienalis / a. lienalis P. 161
— glandulares R. 103
— zygomatici Cn. 112
— glandularis 103; D. 108
— ilei antimesenterialis 170, 173

Ramus, *Continued*
— — mesenterialis 170
— interarcuales / plexus vertebralis internus ventralis D. 187
— intercostales ventrales / a. musculophrenica 76
— intercostalis ventralis / a. thoracica interna 76
— interosseus / a. interossea caudalis 90
— — / a. interossea cranialis 90
— — / v. interossea caudalis Cn., P. 206
— — / v. interossea cranialis R. 206
— — s. perforans C., P., O. 148
— interspinosus / r. dorsalis / a. intercostalis dorsalis 121
— labialis dorsalis / a. perinealis ventralis 158
— — — et mammarius / a. perinealis ventralis R. 158
— — ventralis / a. pudenda externa 137
— lacrimalis / a. temporalis superficialis S., O. 109
— laryngeus / a. laryngea cranialis 101
— — / v. thyreoidea cranialis 218
— — caudalis / a. thyreoidea cranialis 100
— lienales / a. lienalis 161
— lingualis / v. lingualis impar C. 222
— malleolares laterales / a. interossea cruris P., O. 148
— — mediales / a. interossea cruris P., O. 148
— — — / a. saphena 143
— — — / a. tibialis caudalis O. 145
— mammarii / a. epigastrica caudalis superficialis Cn., P. 137
— — / a. epigastrica cranialis superficialis 77
— — / aa. intercostales dorsales 121
— — / a. thoracica interna 76
— — laterales / a. thoracica lateralis Cn., P. 79
— — / v. epigastrica caudalis superficialis 240
— — / v. epigastrica cranialis superficialis 195
— — / vv. intercostales ventrales 195
— — / vv. perforantes Cn., P. 195
— massetericus / a. carotis externa O., H. 102
— — / a. transversa faciei 109
— mediastinales / aorta thoracica 126
— — / a. thoracica interna 76
— meningeus / a. auricularis caudalis S., G. 108
— — / a. auricularis rostralis O. 110
— mentales / a. alveolaris mandibularis Cn., P. 111
— musculares / a. ophthalmica externa 114
— muscularis / v. auricularis caudalis Cn., P. 230

Ramus, *Continued*
— mylohyoideus / a. alveolaris mandibularis 111
— obturatorius / a. circumflexa femoris medialis 139
— — / v. circumflexa femoris medialis 240
— occipitalis / a. auricularis caudalis 109
— — / a. occipitalis 102
— oesophagei / aorta thoracica 126
— oesophageus / a. broncho-oesophagea 72, 123
— — / a. gastrica dextra 165
— — / a. gastrica sinistra 161, 162
— — / a. reticularis 168
— palatini / a. pharyngea ascendens S., G. 101
— palmaris 90, 91
— — profundus / a. radialis 92
— — — / v. radialis 209
— — superficialis / a. radialis 92
— — — / v. radialis 209
— — phalangis distalis 94
— — — mediae 94
— — — proximalis 94
— pancreatici 166; R. 161, 169; H. 161, 162
— pancreaticus P. 161; C. 165
— parietalis / a. gastrica sinistra H. 162
— parotidei P. 102; R., H. 108
— perforantes / a. thoracica interna 76
— — / vv. metacarpeae palmares 95; Cn. 209; P. 211; R. 214
— — / vv. metatarseae plantares 93; Cn. 251; P. 254; R. 255
— — distales / aa. metacarpeae 93; Cn. 94; P. 95; R. 98; H. 99
— — — / aa. metatarseae 93; Cn. 150; P. 150; R. 151; H. 154
— — proximales / aa. metacarpeae 93; Cn. 94; C., P., 95; R. 98; H. 99
— — — / aa. metatarseae 93; Cn. 150; P. 150; R. 151; H. 154
— pericardiaci / aorta thoracica 126
— perihyoidei / a. lingualis 103
— pharyngei / a. pharyngea ascendens 101
— pharyngeus / a. laryngea cranialis 101
— — / a. thyreoidea cranialis 100
— phrenici / aa. lumbales P., R. 128
— — / aa. intercostales dorsales 121
— — / a. musculophrenica 76
— — / a. reticularis 168
— plantaris phalangis distalis 94
— — — mediae 94
— — — proximalis 94; Cn. 150; P. 150
— praeputiales / v. epigastrica caudalis superficialis 240
— praescapularis / a. cervicalis superficialis 77
— — / v. cervicalis superficialis 216
— profundus / a. circumflexa femoris medialis 139
— — / a. plantaris lateralis 144
— — / a. plantaris medialis 144

Ramus, *Continued*
— — / r. palmaris 90, 91
— — / v. circumflexa femoris medialis 240
— — / v. plantaris lateralis 244
— — / v. plantaris medialis 244
— prostaticus / a. prostatica 177
— pterygoidei / a. maxillaris 111
— retis / rete mirabile a. maxillaris C. 111
— rostrales ad rete mirabile epidurale rostrale R. 112
— sacrales H. 157; 159
— scrotalis dorsalis / a. perinealis ventralis 158
— — ventralis / a. pudenda externa 137
— sinister / a. hepatica Cn. 162
— — / v. portae 261
— spinales / a. vertebralis 74
— — / plexus (venosus) vertebralis internus ventralis 187
— — / rr. sacrales 159
— spinalis / aa. intercostales dorsales 121
— — / aa. lumbales 127
— sternales / rr. perforantes / a. thoracica interna 76
— — / vv. perforantes 195
— sternocleidomastoidei / a. carotis communis R. 100
— sternocleidomastoideus / a. auricularis caudalis D., P., G. 108
— — / a. thyreoidea cranialis 100
— sublingualis / plexus (venosus) pterygoideus 229
— — / sinus (venosus) pterygoideus 229
— submentalis / arcus (venosus) hyoideus 222
— superficialis / a. circumflexa ilium profunda 131
— — / a. plantaris lateralis 144
— — / a. plantaris medialis 144
— — / a. tibialis cranialis 148
— — / r. caudalis / v. circumflexa ilium profunda 236
— — / r. palmaris 91, 206
— — / v. plantaris lateralis 244
— — / v. plantaris medialis 244
— suprarenales 175
— — / aa. lumbales D., R. 128
— — caudales / a. coeliaca 159
— — — / a. renalis 175, 176
— — craniales 175
— — — / a. phrenica caudalis 130
— — — / v. phrenica caudalis Cn. 235
— suprascapularis / a. cervicalis superficialis O. 77
— — / a. suprascapularis O. 80
— — / v. cervicalis superficialis R. 189, 216
— — / v. subscapularis P. 200
— — / v. suprascapularis 189
— thymici / a. thoracica interna 76
— tonsillares / a. pharyngea ascendens O. 101
— tori digitalis 94

Ramus, *Continued*
— transversus / a. circumflexa femoris lateralis 142
— — / v. circumflexa femoris lateralis 242
— — (r. descendens) / a. circumflexa femoris medialis 138
— — (—) / v. circumflexa femoris medialis 241
— tubarius / a. ovarica 176
— — v. ovarica 266
— uretericus / a. renalis 176
— — / a. umbilicalis 176
— — / a. vesicalis caudalis 177
— urethralis / a. prostatica 183
— — / a. vesicalis caudalis 183
— uterinus / a. ovarica 178
— — / a. umbilicalis S. 178
— — / a. vaginalis 183
— — / v. ovarica 266
— — / v. vaginalis 268
— (venosi) colici R. 265
— (—) pancreatici H. 261
— (—) parotidei 230
— (—) sacrales 260
— (venosus) colicus 265
— (—) ilei antimesenterialis 265
— (—) — mesenterialis 265
— (—) infraorbitalis 225
— (—) interosseus s. perforans C., P., O. 251
— (—) palmaris 93, 206
— (—) — phalangis distalis 94
— (—) — — mediae 94
— (—) — — proximalis 94
— (—) plantaris phalangis distalis 94
— (—) — — mediae 94
— (—) — — proximalis 94; Cn. 251
— (—) profundus / r. palmaris 206
— (—) suprarenalis caudalis R., H. 266
— (—) tori digitalis 94
— (—) — metatarsei C. 251
— ventrales / a. vertebralis 74
— vestibularis H. 183
— visceralis / a. gastrica sinistra H. 162
Receptors, sensory 460
Recognition glands 462
Reflex, neurohormonal 474
Regional lymph nodes 307
Rete articulare cubiti 82, 85, 90
— — genus 145
— calcanei / a. saphena 143
— carpi dorsale 89, 92, 93; Cn. 95; P., R., 98; H. 99
— mirabile a. maxillaris C. 111
— — ophthalmicum R. 113
— patellae 145
— (venosum) articulare cubiti 202
— (—) carpi dorsale 93; Cn. 211; P. 212; R. 214; H. 215
Reticulating zone 277
Reticulocytes 3
Reticulo-endothelial system 6, 12, 273
Reticulo-histiocytic system 273
Reticulum cells 6, 272

Rootlets 446
Root sheath, epithelial 444, 451
Rough hair D. 488

Saccus lymphaticus 294
— (—) caudalis 294
— (—) inguinalis 294
— (—) jugularis 293
— (—) retroperitonealis 294
Scales 443
Scapus pili 450
Scent glands 458, 461; O. 504
Secondary follicles 276
— lymph 307
— stage 307
Sebum 458
Septum interatriale 23
— interventriculare 27, 32
— ventriculoconale aortale 21
Setae 454
Sheath cuticle 444, 451
Shield P. 496
Shock absorbing action 477
Short hair D. 488
Sinus aortae 34, 71
— coronarius 16, 40
— durae matris 229
— hairs 454, C. 490
— infraorbitalis S. 463
— inguinalis S. 468
— interdigitalis S. 465
— lactiferus O. 510
— obliquus pericardii 16
— petrosus ventralis 101
— transversus pericardii 16
— trunci pulmonalis 32, 71
— venae buccalis H. 237
— — profundae faciei H. 255
— — transversae faciei H. 232
— venarum cavarum 17, 25
— venosus, right atrium 184, 233
— — cavernosus 232
— (—) ophthalmicus P. 232
— (—) pterygoideus P. 227
Sinusoids 11
Size, weight and measurements of the heart 43
Skein glands 458
Skin 441; D. 487; C. 489; P. 496; O. 503; G. 505; S. 505; H. 537
—, blood supply 459
—, bursa 445
—, cleavage line 446
—, folds 461
—, glands, apocrine 445, 458; O. 513
— —, eccrine 458
— —, holocrine 458
— —, monotychial 458
— —, polyptychial 458
—, hairless organs 476
—, lamellar bodies 460
—, Langer's lines 446
—, modifications of 461
—, nerve supply 460
—, ontogenesis 443, 476
—, phylogenesis 443
—, pigments 442
—, scent glands 461

Skin, *Continued*
—, sebaceous glands 441, 445, 458; D. 489; C. 491; P. 497; O. 504; G. 505; S. 506; H. 538
—, sensory organs 441
—, specific hairless organs 476
—, sweat glands 441, 458; D. 489; C. 491; P. 497; O. 504; S. 506; H. 538
Slough 443
Smooth hair D. 488
Solea cornea Cn. 481; O. 530
— ungulae H. 541
Sole (solar) bed Cn. 481
— (—) corium P. 501; O. 527; R. 533; H. 545
— (—) epidermis O. 530
— (—) horn P. 501; O. 530; H. 542, 546
— (—) pad 477; D. 494; C. 496
— (—) segment 481; O. 524
— (—) subcutis H. 542
Solitary follicle 276
Spatium mediastini 15
Species characteristics, heart 41, 68
Spirals 455
Spleen 281
—, ontogenesis 282
Spina cunei H. 549
Sterile matrix P. 501; O. 530
Stratum adiposum C. 490
— basale 448; C. 489
— corneum 448; C. 489; P. 469
— externum parietis cornei H. 548
— fibrosum C. 490
— germinativum 448
— granulosum 448; C. 489
— internum parietis cornei II. 548
— lucidum 448; C. 489; G. 505; H. 537
— medium parietis cornei H. 548
— papillare 446; D. 487; C. 489
— reticulare 446; D. 487; C. 489
— spinosum 448; C. 489
Structural fat 477
Subcaudal gland G. 467
Subcutaneous venous networks H. 557
Subcutis 445, 480; D. 487; C. 489; P. 496; H. 542
Sulci cunei H. 549
Sulcus coronarius 16
— intermammarius 470; D. 511; P. 519; O. 530; H. 564
— interventricularis paraconalis 16
— — subsinuosus 17
— terminalis 25
— venae cavae hepatis 233
Sweat 458
Systema lymphaticum 269

Tactile hairs 444, 454; D. 489; C. 490; P. 497; O. 504; G. 505; S. 506; H. 538
Tail gland C. 466
Tail hair 454
Tassel 461; P. 497; G. 505
T-cells 275
Teat 470; P. 499; O. 506

Teat, *Continued*
— canal 470; D. 491; C. 493; P. 499; O. 510; G. 520
— — opening 470; H. 539
— cistern C. 493; P. 499; O. 510; G. 520; S. 522; H. 539
Teats, accessory 473; P. 499; O. 513; G. 521; H. 539
—, supernumerary 473; P. 499; O. 513; G. 521; H. 539
Tela subcutanea 445, 479; D. 487; C. 489; P. 496
— — coronae O. 525; H. 542
— — cunei P. 542
— — limbi P. 542
— — parietis P. 542;
— — soleae P. 542
— — tori O. 525; H. 542
— — ungulae O. 524; H. 542
Terminal circulation 7, 11
Terminal layers P. 502; R. 532
Thermoregulation 450
Thoracic duct 294, 295, 306; D. 352; C. 364; P. 382; O. 403; S. 419; G. 419; H. 438
Thrombin 2
Thrombocytes 5, 7
Throttle artery 9
— vein 10
Thymocytes 283
Thymus 283; Cn. 286; C. 286; P. 287; R. 288, 290; H. 292
—, accessory 290
—, blood supply O. 290
—, fine structure 283
—, function 283
—, involution 284
—, isthmus craniocervicalis 286
—, — cervicothoracalis 286
—, lobus dexter 286
—, — sinister 286
—, ontogenesis 283
—, pars cervicalis 286
—, — cranialis 286
—, — thoracalis 286
—, superficialis 287
T-lymphocytes 275, 285
Toe pads 477; Cn. 481; D. 494; C. 496
Tonsillar crypts 278
Tonsillectomy 278
Tonsils 277
—, ontogenesis 277
Tori digitales 477; Cn. 481; D. 494; H. 541
Torus 477
— carpeus 477; H. 550
— metacarpeus 477; D. 494
— metatarseus 477; D. 494
— tarseus 477; H. 550
— ungulae H. 541
Touch corpuscles 460
— disks 460
—, organs of 460
Trabeculae carneae 27, 32
Trabecula septomarginalis 30, 33
Tragi 454
Transport vessels 295, 302
Tunica elastica int. 7
— externa 7

Tunica, *Continued*
— intima 7
— media 7
Truncus bicaroticus 73
— brachiocephalicus 72
— costocervicalis 74
— fasciculi atrioventricularis 34; 36
— linguofacialis 103
— pudendoepigastricus 135
— pulmonalis 16, 27, 71
— thyreocervicalis P. 74, 77, 100
— (lymphaticus) coeliacus 325; H. 438
— (—) colicus 330
— (—) gastricus 325
— (—) hepaticus 325
— (—) intestinalis 325; H. 438
— (—) jejunalis 330
— (—) jugularis 314; D. 354; P. 382; O. 404; S. 419; G. 419; H. 439
— (—) — dexter 295, 306, 314
— (—) — sinister 295, 306, 314
— (—) lumbales 325; D. 353; P. 382; O. 404; S. 419; G. 419; H. 439
— (—) trachealis 314
— (—) visceralis 325; D. 353; P. 382; O. 404; S. 419
Tuberculum intervenosum 26
Tubular glands 445
Tubular horn H. 542
Tubuli epidermales H. 548

Unguicula 479; Cn. 493
Unguis 482
Ungula 479; P. 500; O. 524; H. 541
Ungulates 478
Underwool 452

Vaginae serosae arteriorum et venarum 16
Vallum Cn. 481; O. 525
Valva aortae 36
— atrioventricularis dext. 30
— — sin. 32, 33
— bicuspidalis s. mitralis 33
— tricuspidalis 30
— trunci pulmonalis 31
Valvulae semilunares 33, 71
Valvula foraminis ovalis 26
— sinus coronarii 26, 40
— venae cavae caudalis 25
Valve sinus 10
Vasa afferentia 301, 307
— efferentia 301, 307
— lymphatica, see lymph vessels 292
Vasoconstrictors 14
Vasodilators 14
Vasopotent hormones 14
Veins, adventitia 10
—, endothelium 10
—, forefoot 98; Cn. 202; P. 211; R. 214; H. 214
—, —, dorsal 99; Cn. 211; P. 212; R. 214; H. 215
—, —, palmar 98; Cn. 209; P. 211; R. 214; H. 214
—, head 223
—, heart Cn. 48; P. 53; O. 62; H. 65

Veins, *Continued*
—, hind foot 98; Cn. 251; P. 254; R. 255; H. 256
—, —, dorsal 99; Cn. 251; P. 254; R. 255; H. 256
—, —, plantar 98; Cn. 251; P. 254; R. 255; H. 256
—, intimal swellings 10
—, neck 115
—, networks R. 535; H. 555
—, pectoral limb 197
—, pelvic limb 240
—, pelvis 256
—, postcapillary 7
—, pulmonary circulation 184
—, structure of 10
—, tail 256
—, tunica externa 7, 10
—, —, intima 7, 10
—, —, media 7, 10
—, valves 10
—, valvular sinus 10
Velvet antler 487
Vena, venae 7, 10
— abdominalis caudalis Cn., R. 238
— — cranialis Cn., P. 233, 255
— alveolaris mandibularis 229
— angularis oculi 224
— — oris 224
— articulares temporomandibulares 229
— auricularis caudalis 229
— — intermedia 230
— — lateralis C. 230, 232
— — medialis H. 231, 232
— — profunda 232
— — rostralis 232
— axillaris 197
— axillobrachialis Cn. 216
— azygos dextra 69, 70, 185
— — sinistra 69, 70, 185, 187
— basivertebrales 187
— bicipitalis 202
— brachialis 202
— — superficialis Cn. 204, 216
— brachiocephalica Cn., P. 184, 196
— bronchales 184, 186
— broncho-oesophagea C. 184, 186
— buccalis 229
— bulbi penis 259
— — vestibuli 260
— caecalis 265
— — lateralis H. 265
— — medialis H. 265
— caudales femoris 244
— caudalis dorsalis C. 258
— — dorsolateralis 260
— — femoris distalis 244
— — — media 244
— — — proximalis 244
— — lateralis superficialis Cn. 258
— — mediana 260
— — ventrolateralis 260
— cava caudalis 16, 233
— — —, its visceral veins 260
— — —, its terminal subdivision 234
— — cranialis 16, 184
— cephalica 216
— — accessoria 217

Index

Vena, *Continued*
— cervicalis profunda 193
— — superficialis 215
— ciliares 233
— circumflexa femoris lateralis 241
— — — medialis 240
— — humeri caudalis 200
— — — cranialis 201
— — ilium profunda 233, 236
— — — superficialis Cn. 241
— — scapulae 200
— clitoridis 260
— — media H. 258
— colica dextra 265
— — media 265
— — sinistra 265
— colicae dextrae R. 265
— collateralis media 203
— — radialis 202
— — ulnaris 202
— comitans a. carotidis externae 221
— — a. lingualis 221
— — n. tibialis H. 246
— conjunctivales 233
— cordis magna 40
— — media 40
— cornualis R. 232
— coronalis 94
— — profunda R. 536; H. 555
— — superficialis R. 535
— costoabdominalis dorsalis 186, 187
— —, vessel of origin of 193
— costocervicalis 184, 192, 194
— cremasterica R. 240
— cricothyreoidea 218
— cysticae 261
— digitales dorsales communes 93; Cn. 211, 254; P. 213, 255; R. 215, 255; H. 256
— — — propriae 93; Cn. 211, 254; P. 213, 255; R. 214, 255
— — palmares communes 93; Cn. 211; P. 211; R. 212; H. 214
— — — propriae 93; Cn. 211; P. 211; R. 214; H. 215
— — palmaris I abaxialis 93; Cn. 211
— — — V abaxialis 93; Cn. 211; P. 213
— — — lateralis H. 215
— — — medialis H. 215
— — plantaris V. abaxialis 93; C. 251; P. 254
— — — lateralis H. 256
— — — medialis H. 256
— — plantares communes 93; Cn. 251; P. 254; R. 255; H. 256
— — — propriae 93; Cn. 251; P. 254; R. 255; H. 256
— — propriae 93
— digitalis dorsalis I abaxialis 93
— — — V abaxialis 93; Cn. 211; P. 213
— — — prop. axialis R. 535
— diploicae frontalis Cn. 233
— diploicae parietales 229
— — temporales 229
— diverticuli P. 261
— dorsales linguae 222

Vena, *Continued*
— dorsalis clitoridis 260
— — nasi 224
— — pedis 250
— — penis 259
— — phalangis mediae H. 555
— ductus deferentis 268
— emissariae 229
— emissaria canalis carotici 229
— — fissurae orbitalis Cn., H. 232
— — foraminis jugularis 217, 219
— — — laceri 229
— — — orbitorotundi P., R. 232
— — — ovalis 229
— — — retroarticularis 229; R. 232
— — — rotundi 229
— — occipitalis 219
— epigastrica caudalis 238
— — superficialis 240; C. 492
— — cranialis 195
— — — superficialis 195, 240; C. 493; D. 492; O. 519; H. 540
— ethmoidalis externa 233
— facialis 224
— femoralis 241
— frontalis (V. supratrochlearis) 224
— gastricae breves 261
— gastrica dextra 261
— — sinistra 261
— — parietalis H. 261
— — — visceralis H. 261
— gastroduodenalis 261
— gastroepiploica dextra 261
— — sinistra 261
— genus descendens 244
— — distalis lateralis 248
— — — medialis 248
— — media 248
— — proximalis lateralis 248
— — — medialis 248
— glandulares 222; R. 230
— glandularis D. 222; Cn. 228
— glutaea caudalis 258
— — cranialis 258
— hemiazygos dextra P., R. 186
— — sinistra Cn., H. 186
— hepaticae 233; 260
— ilei 261
— ileocolica 261
— iliaca communis 233, 236
— — externa 236
— — interna 252
— — —, visceral veins 266
— iliacofemoralis H. 238
— iliolumbalis 257
— infraorbitalis 225; C. 229
— intercostales dorsales 186, 187; D., P. 194
— — —, vessels of origin of 193
— — ventrales 195
— intercostalis suprema 194
— interdigitales 94, Cn. 211, 251; P. 212, 254; R. 214, 255
— interossea caudalis 205
— — communis 204
— — cranialis 205
— — cruris P., O. 250
— interspinosi 187
— intervertebralis 187
— jejunales 261

Vena, *Continued*
— jugularis communis 215, 217
— — externa 184, 215
— — interna 217
— labialis dorsalis 259
— — — et mammaria R. 259; O. 519; H. 540
— — mandibularis 224
— — maxillaris 224
— — ventralis 240; R. 523
— lacrimalis 233
— laryngea cranialis 224
— — impar Cn. 222
— lateralis nasi 224
— lienalis 261
— lingualis 222
— — impar C. 222
— linguofacialis 222
— lumbales 187, 233, 235
— —, vessels of origin of 235
— malaris D. 233
— malleolaris caudalis lateralis H. 250
— mammaria caudalis R., H. 240; O. 518
— — cranialis H. 240; O. 518; R. 524
— — media R. 524
— marginis solearis R. 535; H. 556
— masseterica 229
— — ventralis R., H. 228
— maxillaris 226
— mediana 206
— — cubiti 216
— mediastinales 195
— mentalis, mentales 229
— mesenterica caudalis 265
— — cranialis 261
— metacarpeae dorsales 93; Cn. 211; P. 212; R. 214
— — palmares 92; Cn. 209; P. 211; R. 214; H. 214
— metatarsea dorsales 93; Cn. 251; P. 254; R. 255; H. 256
— — plantares 93; Cn. 251; P. 254; R. 255; H. 256
— musculophrenica 195
— nervomedullares 187
— obliqua atrii sinistri 186
— obturatoria 258
— occipitalis 217
— oesophageae 186
— oesophagea caudalis 261
— omobrachialis D. 215
— ophthalmica externa dorsalis R. 232
— ovarica 233, 266
— palatinae 229
— palatina ascendens Cn. 224
— — descendens 225; P. 229
— — major, minor 225
— palmaris phalangis mediae H. 556
— palpebrae tertiae P., R. 233
— palpebralis inferior Cn. 224
— — — lateralis P., R. 232
— — — medialis P., O. 224; C., H. 225
— — superior lateralis P., R. 232
— — — medialis 225
— pancreaticae 261

Vena, *Continued*
— pancreaticoduodenalis caudalis 261
— — cranialis 261
— papillaris O. 518; R. 524
— penis 259
— — cranialis, media H. 240, 258
— perforantes 195
— — / v. profunda femoris 238
— pericardiacophrenica 195
— perinealis dorsalis Cn., P. 259; R. 268
— — ventralis 259
— phalangis distalis R. 536
— pharyngea Cn., P. 219
— — ascendens 223
— pharyngeae R., H. 229
— phrenica caudalis 233, 235
— phrenicae craniales 233
— plantaris lateralis 244
— — medialis 244
— poplitea 248
— portae 260
— profunda antebrachii 206
— — brachii 202
— — clitoridis 260
— — faciei 225
— — femoris 238
— — lingualis 222
— — penis 259
— prostatica 266
— pterygoideae 229
— pudenda externa 240; D. 592; O. 519; R. 523; H. 540
— — interna 259; O. 519; H. 540
— — —, visceral veins of 266
— pudendoepigastrica 238; O. 519
— pulmonales 16, 26, 184
— radiales superficiales Cn. 204
— radialis 209
— — proximalis H. 209
— radiculares dorsales 187
— — ventrales 187
— rectalis caudalis P. 259; Cn., S., O., H. 259; G., O. 265
— — cranialis 265
— — media 265

Vena, *Continued*
— recurrens interossea 206
— — ulnaris Cn. 207; R. 205
— renalis 233, 265
— reticularis 261
— ruminalis dextra, sinistra 261
— sacralis mediana 233, 260
— saphena lateralis 248
— — medialis (magna) 243
— scapularis dorsalis 194
— scrotalis dorsalis 259
— — ventralis 240
— sigmoideae 265
— sphenopalatina 226
— spinales 187
— sternocleidomastoidea 227
— stylomastoidea P., H. 219; D., R. 230
— subclavia 184, 197
— subcutanea abdominis 195; O. 519; H. 540
— sublingualis 222
— submentalis 223
— subscapularis 198
— superficialis ventralis linguae D. 223
— supraorbitalis 233
— suprarenales O., H. 233; 266
— suprascapularis 197
— supratrochlearis 224
— surales 248
— tarsea lateralis 250
— — medialis D. 244, 250
— — perforans distalis 93, 250
— — — proximalis 93; P., O. 250
— temporales profundae 229
— temporalis superficialis 231
— testicularis 233, 266
— thoracica externa 198
— — interna 184, 195; O. 519
— — lateralis Cn., P. 198; C. 593
— — superficialis O., H. 198; 202
— thoracodorsalis 202
— thymicae 195
— thyreoidea caudalis s. v. thyreoidea ima 197
— — cranialis 218

Vena, *Continued*
— — media 217
— tibialis caudalis 248
— — cranialis 250
— tori digitalis H. 555
— transversa cubiti 204
— — faciei 232
— ulnaris 206
— urethralis Cn., O. 268
— uterina 266
— vaginalis 268
— — accessoria O. 268
— vertebralis 184, 194
— — thoracia 186, 187, 194
— vesicalis caudalis 268
— — cranialis R. 266; P. 268
— — media C. 240
— vestibularis O. 268
— vorticosae 233
Venous angle 306
Venous ring of Fürstenberg O. 511, 518
Ventriculi cordis 27
Ventriculus cordis dexter 27
— — sinister 32
Venules 7
Vibrissae 454
Vitreous membrane 451
Vortex cordis 22
Vortices pilorum 455

Wall (parietal) corium P. 501; O. 527; R. 532; H. 544
—, epidermis P. 502; O. 527
—, horn O. 527; H. 542, 546
—, segment 481; O. 524
—, subcutis H. 542
Wavy hair D. 488
Weight and measurements of the heart D. 43; C. 45; P. 49; O. 57; H. 63
Whirring of uterine artery 177
White line O. 530; R. 532; H. 545, 548
Wire hair D. 488
Wool hairs 452

Zona alba R. 532; H. 545, 548

Atlas of Topographical Surgical Anatomy of the Dog
Atlas zur chirurgisch-topographischen Anatomie des Hundes

By Prof. Dr. Dr. h. c. Karl Ammann, Zurich, Prof. Dr. Dr. h. c. Eugen Seiferle, Zurich, Gertrud Pelloni, Zurich. 1978. 77 pages with 95 coloured illustrations. In five languages: English, German, French, Italian, Spanish. Cloth DM 180,–

Four-coloured drawings of parts of the body of particular surgical interest are based on preparations made from the Alsatian breed (German Shepherd Dog). They present the anatomical and topographical structure from the surface into deeper layers and regions. From the surgical point of view they enable the student and the practitioner to find the operational way and, used in anatomical teaching, they clearly illustrate the topographical relations.

Atlas of Radiographic Anatomy of the Dog and Cat
Atlas der Röntgenanatomie von Hund und Katze

By Prof. Dr. Horst Schebitz, Munich, and Prof. Dr. Helmut Wilkens, Hanover. 3rd revised edition. 1977. 197 pages, 103 radiographs, 103 radiographic-sketches and 68 positioning-drawings. Bilingual: English and German. Cloth DM 180,–

Atlas of Radiographic Anatomy of the Horse
Atlas der Röntgenanatomie des Pferdes

By Prof. Dr. Horst Schebitz, Munich, and Prof. Dr. Helmut Wilkens, Hanover. 3rd revised edition. 1978. 100 pages. 45 radiographs, 45 radiographic sketches and 38 positioning-drawings. Bilingual: English and German. Cloth DM 116,–

The large-sized atlases are directed towards the needs of both student and practitioner, illustrating the normal radiographic anatomy by means of x-ray pictures taken of live animals. Produced in negative print, they facilitate comparison with x-ray photographs viewed in the normal way in transmitted light. Each one is aided by a fully described sketch, so that the anatomical details can easily be recognized and retained. Technical data such as diaphragm, film, screen and setting are given and advice on taking radiographs as well as immobilization sketches also included.

Clinical Examination of Cattle

Edited by Prof. Dr. Dr. h. c. mult. Gustav Rosenberger, Hanover, in collaboration with Prof. Dr. Gerrit Dirksen, Munich, Prof. Dr. Hans-D. Gründer, Gießen, Prof. Dr. Eberhard Grunert, Hanover, Prof. Dr. Dietrich Krause, Hannover, and Prof. Dr. Mathaeus Stöber, Hanover. Translated from the German by Roy Mack, Woking, Surrey. This book is an authorized translation of Rosenberger, Klinische Untersuchung des Rindes, 2nd edition 1977. 1979. 469 pages with 478 illustrations in the text and on 17 colour plates, 52 tables. Cloth DM 148,–

Krankheiten des Rindes

Herausgegeben von Prof. Dr. Dr. h. c. mult. Gustav Rosenberger, Hannover, unter Mitarbeit von Prof. Dr. Gerrit Dirksen, München, Prof. Dr. Hans-D. Gründer, Gießen, und Prof. Dr. Mathaeus Stöber, Hannover. 2., unveränderte Auflage mit Neufassung des Therapeutischen Index. 1978. 1430 Seiten mit 747 Abbildungen im Text und auf 28 Farbtafeln. Ganzleinen DM 390,–

Published by   Spitalerstraße 12, D-2000 Hamburg 1, West Germany
VERLAG PAUL PAREY · BERLIN AND HAMBURG · GERMANY

Journal of Veterinary Medicine, Series C
Anatomia, Histologia, Embryologia
Journal of the World Association of Veterinary Anatomists

Edited by: Prof. Dr. Robert Barone (Lyon, France), Prof. Julian J. Baumel, Ph. D. (Omaha, Nebraska, USA), Prof. Dr. James Breazile (Stillwater, Oklahoma, USA), Prof. Dr. Horst Dieter Dellmann (Ames, Iowa, USA), Prof. Carl Gans (Ann Arbor, Michigan, USA), Prof. Dr. Ekkehard Kleiss (Mérida, Venezuela), Prof. Dr. Bernd Vollmerhaus (Munich, Germany)
Editors-in-Chief: Prof. Dr. James Breazile (Stillwater, Oklahoma, USA), Prof. Dr. Bernd Vollmerhaus (Munich, Germany)
Scientific Advisory Board: Prof. Dr. H. A. Bern (Berkeley, California, USA), Prof. Dr. Nils H. Björkman (Copenhagen, Denmark), Prof. Dr. Gunnar D. Bloom (Umeå, Sweden), Univ.-Prof. Dr. György Fehér (Budapest, Hungary), Prof. Dr. Giovanni Godina (Torino, Italy), Prof. Dr. H. Kobayashi (Misaki, Kanagawa-Ken, Japan), Prof. Dr. Willy Mosimann (Bern, Switzerland), Prof. Narciso L. Murillo-Ferrol (Zaragoza, Spain), Prof. R. O'Rahilly (Davis, California, USA), Prof. Dr. Fritz Preuß (Berlin, Germany), M.A., Oh.D.B.V.Sc., M.R.C.V.S. Janis Priedkalns (Adelaide, Australia), Prof. Dr. Dr. Oskar Schaller (Vienna, Austria), Dr. Brian Weatherhead (Birmingham, Great Britain), Dr. Mikio Yasuda (Nagoya, Japan)
Mode of Publication: Four issues per volume. Each issue consists of about 100 pages and appears quarterly
Publication languages: German, English, French or Spanish. Summaries in German, English, French and Spanish

Journal of Veterinary Medicine

Edited by: Prof. Dr. Dr. Max Berchtold (Zurich, Switzerland), Prof. Dr. Dr. h. c. Martin Lerche†(Berlin, Germany), Prof. Dr. Dr. h. c. Anton Mayr (Munich, Germany), Prof. Dr. Dr. h. c. Heinrich Spörri (Zurich, Switzerland), Prof. Dr. E. G. White (Merseyside, Great Britain). In collaboration with a great number of leading and international authorities
Mode of publication: Ten issues per volume. Each issue consists of about 90 pages
Publication languages: German, English, French or Spanish. Summaries in German, English, French and Spanish

Series A

Physiology, Endocrinology, Biochemistry, Pharmacology, Internal Medicine, Surgery, Genetics, Animal Breeding, Obstetrics, Gynaecology, Andrology, Animal Nutrition and Feeding, General and Special Pathology (except Infectious and Parasitic Diseases)

Series B

Infectious and Parasitic Diseases, Microbiology (Bacteriology, Virology, Mycology), Immunology, Parasitology, Animal Hygiene, Food Hygiene, Pathology of Infectious and Parasitic Diseases

A supplement series "Fortschritte der Veterinärmedizin – Advances in Veterinary Medicine" is being published in irregular sequence

Published by Spitalerstraße 12, D-2000 Hamburg 1, West Germany

Prices to be inquired from the publisher

VERLAG PAUL PAREY · BERLIN AND HAMBURG · GERMANY